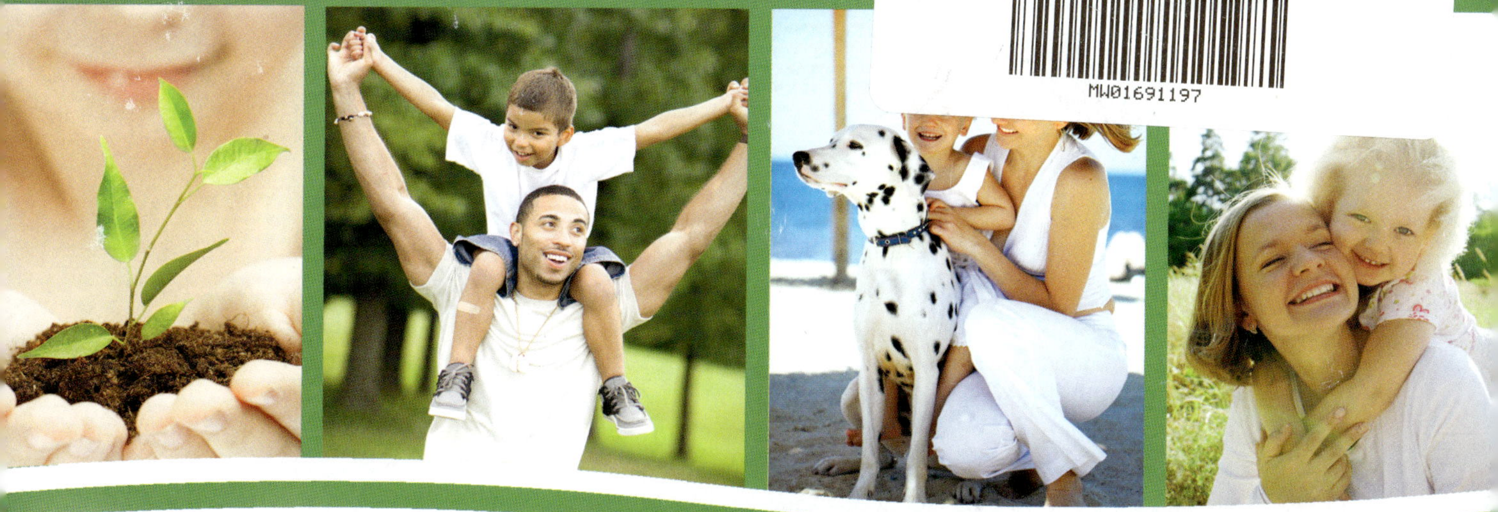

Reference Guide for Essential Oils

By Connie and Alan Higley

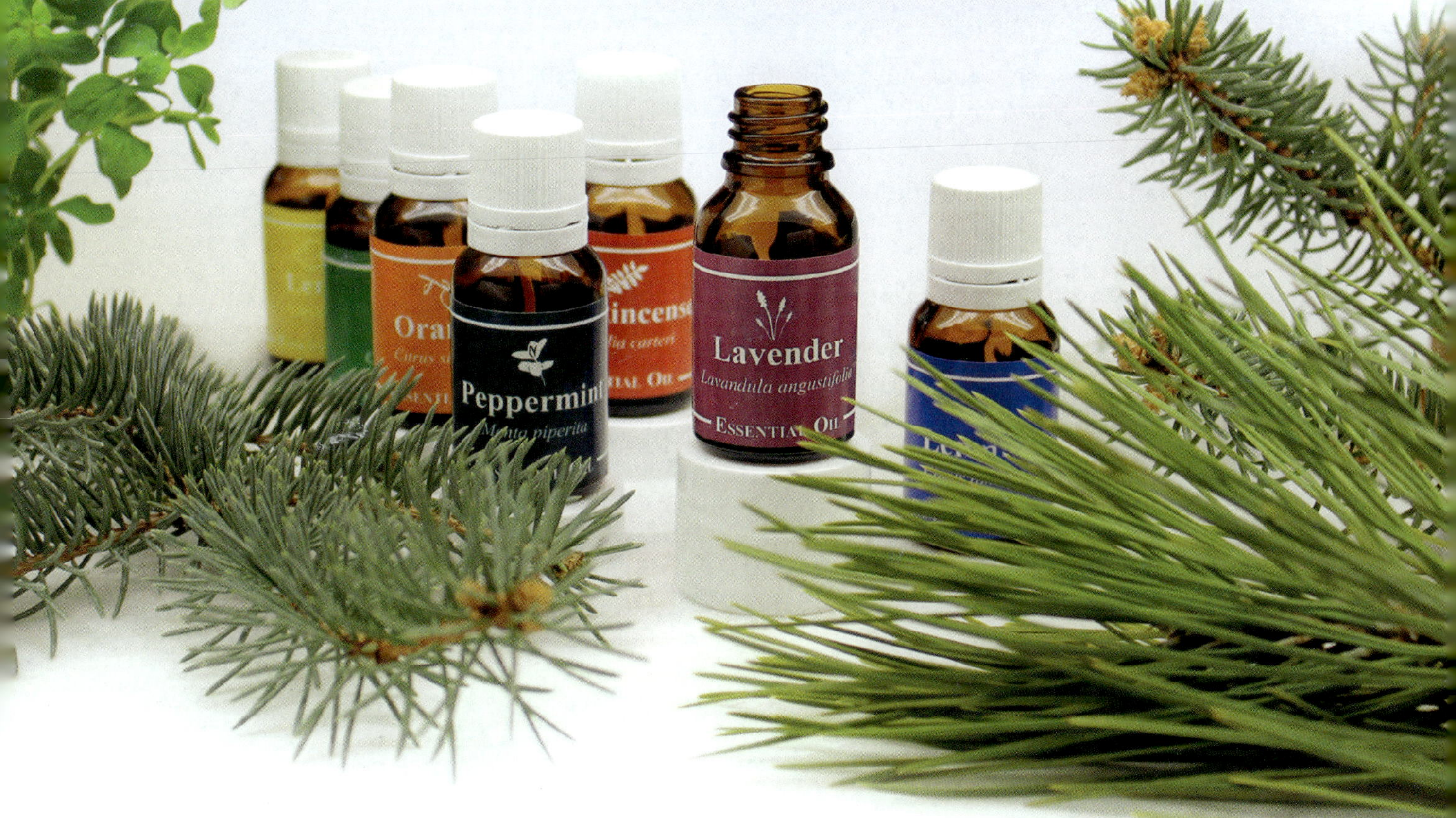

2013 Edition

This book has been designed to provide information to help educate the reader in regard to the subject matter covered. It is sold with the understanding that the publisher and the authors are not liable for the misconception or misuse of the information provided. It is not provided in order to diagnose, prescribe, or treat any disease, illness, or injured condition of the body. The authors and publisher shall have neither liability nor responsibility to any person or entity with respect to any loss, damage, or injury caused or alleged to be caused directly or indirectly by the information contained in this book. The information presented herein is in no way intended as a substitute for medical counseling. Anyone suffering from any disease, illness, or injury should consult a qualified health care professional.

Library of Congress Cataloging-in-Publication Data.

Higley, Connie.
Reference guide for essential oils / Connie and Alan Higley
p. ill. cm.
Includes bibliographical references.
1. Essences and essential oils–Therapeutic use–Handbooks, manuals, etc.
2. Aromatherapy–Handbooks, manuals, etc. 00-500404

Published and distributed by:

Abundant Health
222 W. 3560 N.
Spanish Fork, UT 84660

Phone: 1-888-718-3068 (toll-free) / 801-798-0642 (local)
Fax: 1-877-568-1988 (toll-free) / 801-798-0644 (local)

Internet: www.AbundantHealth4u.com
E-Mail: orders@abundanthealth4u.com

Printed and bound in the United States of America.

International Standard Book Number: 978-1-937702-07-6 (soft-cover, coil-bound)
978-1-937702-11-3 (hard-cover, coil-bound)

Dedication

We, the authors (compilers) of this information, were introduced to Young Living Essential Oils in 1995. At that time, there was no compiled information on the use of these valuable oils, so together with Pat Leatham, we set out to find what we could. We gathered notes from lectures and seminars by D. Gary Young and product information from Young Living Essential Oils. Extensive research into the works of other aromatherapy experts has shown us that Gary Young, through his own research and clinical study, not only supports but expands their solid foundation of knowledge and expertise. When this book was first made available in 1996, we made a conscious decision to keep the names of D. Gary Young and Young Living Essential Oils out of this book so as to remove all possibility of recrimination or harm to Gary Young or his company. However, all past, present, and future readers of this work need to understand that all of us, author and reader alike, are deeply indebted to Gary Young for his brilliant insight, extensive research, and incredible vision of the healing power of essential oils.

We, therefore, dedicate this book to D. Gary Young as a tribute to his vision of health for all who will embrace the oils and use them to their fullest potential. Gary Young is one of the foremost experts on the organic cultivation, distillation, and clinical use of essential oils in North America. His unwavering passion for maintaining the highest quality in his products has produced some astounding healing results. We applaud his heroic and often solitary effort to continue proving by clinical study the efficacy of essential oils as indispensable tools for combating disease.

Acknowledgments

To our 6 children who demonstrate much patience and responsibility with the freedom they are given during the on-going compilation and updating of this book.

To the late Pat Leatham who provided the initial impetus for its creation. Her many hours of research and meticulous note-taking will forever be appreciated.

And to all of you who are discovering, or re-discovering, for yourselves the healing powers of essential oils. May this book provide quick access to the information you need to help yourself and those you love progress on the road to better health.

A special thanks goes to our families and to all of our "Essential Oil" friends! Without your love, friendship, suggestions, support, patience, and prodding, we would have crumbled under the strain of compiling a book such as this while trying to raise a family and have a life.

Table of Contents

The section tabs shown on the right correspond to the individual sections listed below. By holding the spine of the book in the left hand and bending the right side back with the right hand, section markings become visible along the right edge. This should allow you quick and easy reference to any applicable section. ***NOTICE: The PERSONAL GUIDE tab is at the top of the tabs list to the right, even though the section itself is positioned after the middle of the book. This is to give it top priority on the edge of the book, as it is referred to most often.***

The sections on Personal Care Products and Supplements list commercially-available products that include pure essential oils either for additional therapeutic benefits or to enhance the bio-availability of the other ingredients.

Science and Application 7

Single Oils 47

Oil Blends 149

Personal Care Products 209

Supplements 245

Notes & New Products 287

(This section is for notes and information on newly-introduced products)

Personal Guide **(over 600 health-related topics)** 295

(NOTICE: It is the TOP TAB to the right and on the edge of the book!)

Appendix

- Body System Chart 543
- Single Oil Property Chart 549
- Single Oil Summary Information 552
- Oil Blend Summary Information 563
- Taxonomical Information 568
- Research References 573
- Bibliography 582

Index 583

Personal Guide | Science and Application | Single Oils | Oil Blends | Personal Care Products | Supplements | Notes & New Products | Appendix | Index

Science & Application

Basic Facts About Essential Oils

How long have essential oils been around?

Essential oils were mankind's first medicine. From Egyptian hieroglyphics and Chinese manuscripts, we know that priests and physicians have been using essential oils for thousands of years. In Egypt, essential oils were used in the embalming process, and well-preserved oils were found in alabaster jars in King Tut's tomb. Egyptian temples were dedicated to the production and blending of the oils, and recipes were recorded on the walls in hieroglyphics. There is even a sacred room in the temple of Isis on the island of Philae where a ritual called "Cleansing the Flesh and Blood of Evil Deities" was practiced. This form of emotional clearing required 3 days of cleansing using particular essential oils and oil baths.

There are 188 references to essential oils in the Bible. Oils such as frankincense, myrrh, rosemary, hyssop, and spikenard were used for anointing and healing the sick. In Exodus, the Lord gave the following recipe to Moses for "an holy anointing oil":

Myrrh ("five hundred shekels"— approximately 1 gallon)
Sweet Cinnamon ("two hundred and fifty shekels"— approximately ½ gallon)
Sweet Calamus ("two hundred and fifty shekels")
Cassia ("five hundred shekels")
Olive Oil ("an hin"— approximately 1 ⅓ gallons)

The 3 wise men presented the Christ child with essential oils of frankincense and myrrh. There are also accounts in the New Testament of the Bible where Jesus was anointed with spikenard oil: "And being in Bethany in the house of Simon the leper, as he sat at meat, there came a woman having an alabaster box of ointment of spikenard very precious; and she brake the box, and poured [it] on his head" (Mark 14:3). "Then took Mary a pound of ointment of spikenard, very costly, and anointed the feet of Jesus, and wiped his feet with her hair: and the house was filled with the odour of the ointment" (John 12:3). Some have even said that essential oils carry the consciousness of Christ.

What are *PURE, THERAPEUTIC-GRADE* essential oils?

Essential oils are the volatile liquids that are distilled from plants (including their respective parts such as seeds, bark, leaves, stems, roots, flowers, fruit, etc.). One of the factors that determines the purity and therapeutic value of an oil is its chemical constituents. These constituents can be affected by a vast number of variables including: the part(s) of the plant from which the oil was produced, soil condition, fertilizer (organic or chemical), geographical region, climate, altitude, harvest season and methods, and distillation process. For example, common thyme, or thyme vulgaris, produces several different chemotypes (biochemical specifics or simple species) depending on the conditions of its growth, climate, and altitude. High levels of thymol production depend on the time of year in which it is distilled. If distilled during mid-summer or late fall, there can be higher levels of carvacrol that can cause the oil to be more caustic or irritating to the skin. Low pressure and low temperature are also keys to maintaining the purity, the ultimate fragrance, and the therapeutic value of the oil.

As we begin to understand the power of essential oils in the realm of personal, holistic health care, we comprehend the absolute necessity for obtaining the purest therapeutic-grade essential oils possible. No matter how costly pure therapeutic-grade essential oils may be, there can be no substitutes. Chemists can replicate some of the known individual constituents, but they have yet to successfully recreate complete essential oils in the laboratory.

The information in this book is based upon the use of pure, therapeutic-grade essential oils. Those who are beginning their journey into the realm of aromatherapy and essential oils must actively seek for the purest quality and highest therapeutic-grade oils available. Anything less than pure, therapeutic-grade essential oil may not produce the desired results and can, in some cases, be extremely toxic.

Why is it so difficult to find *PURE, THERAPEUTIC-GRADE* essential oils?

Producing the purest of oils can be very costly because it may require several hundred pounds, or even several thousand pounds, of plant material to extract 1 pound of pure essential oil. For example, 1 pound of pure melissa oil sells for $9,000–$15,000. Although this sounds quite expensive, one must realize that 3 tons of plant material are required to produce that single pound of oil. Because the vast majority of all the oils produced in the world today are used by the perfume industry, the oils are being purchased for their aromatic qualities only. High pressure, high temperatures, rapid processing, and the use of chemical solvents are often employed during the distillation process so that a greater *quantity* of oil can be produced at a faster rate. These oils may smell just as good and cost much less, but they will lack most, if not all, of the chemical constituents necessary to produce the expected therapeutic results.

What benefits do *PURE, THERAPEUTIC-GRADE* essential oils provide?

1. Essential oils embody the regenerating, oxygenating, and immune-strengthening properties of plants.
2. Essential oils are so small in molecular size that they can quickly penetrate the skin.
3. Essential oils are lipid-soluble and are capable of penetrating cell walls, even if they have hardened because of an oxygen deficiency. In fact, essential oils can affect every cell of the body within 20 minutes and then be metabolized like other nutrients.
4. Essential oils contain oxygen molecules that help to transport nutrients to the starving human cells. Because a nutritional deficiency is an oxygen deficiency, disease begins when the cells lack the oxygen for proper nutrient assimilation. By providing the needed oxygen, essential oils also work to stimulate the immune system.
5. Essential oils are very powerful antioxidants. Antioxidants create an unfriendly environment for free radicals. Antioxidants prevent all mutations, work as free radical scavengers, prevent fungus, and prevent oxidation in the cells.
6. Essential oils are antibacterial, anticancerous, antifungal, anti-infectious, antimicrobial, antitumor, antiparasitic, antiviral, and antiseptic. Essential oils have been shown to destroy all tested bacteria and viruses, while simultaneously restoring balance to the body.

7. Essential oils may detoxify the cells and blood in the body.
8. Essential oils containing sesquiterpenes have the ability to pass the blood-brain barrier, enabling them to be effective in the treatment of Alzheimer's disease, Lou Gehrig's disease, Parkinson's disease, and multiple sclerosis.
9. Essential oils are aromatic. When diffused, they provide **air purification** by:
   A. Removing metallic particles and toxins from the air;
   B. Increasing atmospheric oxygen;
   C. Increasing ozone and negative ions in the area, which inhibits bacterial growth;
   D. Destroying odors from mold, cigarettes, and animals; and
   E. Filling the air with a fresh, aromatic scent.
10. Essential oils help promote emotional, physical, and spiritual healing.
11. Essential oils have a bioelectrical frequency that is several times greater than the frequency of herbs, food, and even the human body. Clinical research has shown that essential oils can quickly raise the frequency of the human body, restoring it to its normal, healthy level.

What is frequency and how does it pertain to essential oils?

Frequency is a measurable rate of electrical energy that is constant between any 2 points. Everything has an electrical frequency. Bruce Tainio of Tainio Technology in Cheny, Washington, developed new equipment to measure the biofrequency of humans and foods. Bruce Tainio and D. Gary Young, a North American expert on essential oils, used this biofrequency monitor to determine the relationship between frequency and disease. Some of the results of their studies are show in the following table.

Human Brain	72–90 MHz	Processed/canned food	0 MHz
Human Body (day)	62–68 MHz	Fresh Produce	up to 15 MHz
Cold Symptoms	58 MHz	Dry Herbs	12–22 MHz
Flu Symptoms	57 MHz	Fresh Herbs	20–27 MHz
Candida	55 MHz	Essential Oils	52–320 MHz
Epstein-Barr	52 MHz		
Cancer	42 MHz		
Death Begins	25 MHz		

Note: Due to the sensitivity of the instruments, these results are not easily duplicable. What is important is the relativity of the numbers and the fact that the higher frequency of the essential oils can help raise the frequency of the human body to a more normal level.

Another part of this same study measured the frequency fluctuations within the human body as different substances were introduced. The chart shown below illustrates the frequency reaction of the human body to the introduction of coffee. The subsequent time necessary for the frequency to return to its original measurement was shown to be substantially reduced with the use of essential oils.

Frequency Reaction to Substance

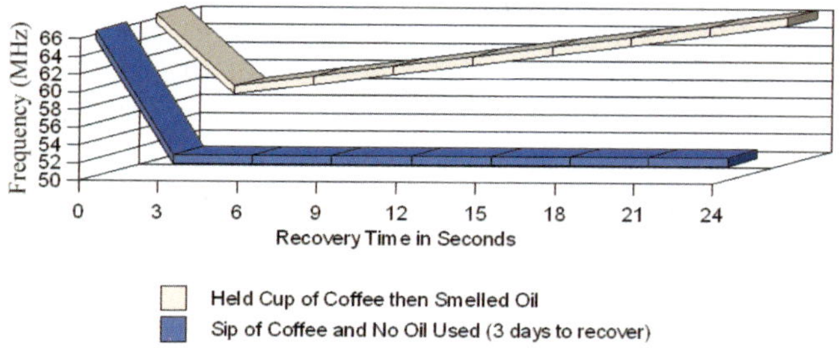

Initially, the frequency of each of 2 different individuals—the first a 26-year-old male and the second a 24-year-old male—was measured at 66 MHz for both. The first individual held a cup of coffee (without drinking any), and his frequency dropped to 58 MHz in 3 seconds. He then removed the coffee and inhaled an aroma of essential oils. Within 21 seconds, his frequency had returned to 66 MHz. The second individual took a sip of coffee, and his frequency dropped to 52 MHz in the same 3 seconds. However, no essential oils were used during the recovery time, and it took 3 days for his frequency to return to the initial 66 MHz.

Another very interesting result of this study was the influence that thoughts have on our frequency as well. Negative thoughts lowered the measured frequency by 12 MHz, and positive thoughts raised the measured frequency by 10 MHz. It was also found that prayer and meditation increased the measured frequency levels by 15 MHz.

How do *PURE, THERAPEUTIC-GRADE* essential oils affect the brain?

The blood-brain barrier is the barrier membrane between the circulating blood and the brain that prevents certain damaging substances from reaching brain tissue and cerebrospinal fluid. The American Medical Association (AMA) determined that if they could find an agent that would pass the blood-brain barrier, they would be able to cure Alzheimer's disease, Lou Gehrig's disease, multiple sclerosis, and Parkinson's disease. In June of 1994, it was documented by the Medical University of Berlin, Germany, and Vienna, Austria, that sesquiterpenes have the ability to go beyond the blood-brain barrier.

High levels of sesquiterpenes, found in the essential oils of frankincense and sandalwood, help increase the amount of oxygen in the limbic system of the brain, particularly around the pineal and pituitary glands. This leads to an increase in secretions of antibodies, endorphins, and neurotransmitters.

Also present in the limbic system of the brain is a gland called the amygdala. In 1989, it was discovered that the amygdala plays a major role in the storing and releasing of emotional trauma. The only way to stimulate this gland is with fragrance or the sense of smell. Therefore, with aromatherapy and essential oils, we are now able to release emotional trauma.

What enables *PURE, THERAPEUTIC-GRADE* essential oils to provide such incredible benefits?

Essential oils are chemically very heterogeneous—meaning they are very diverse in their effects and can perform several different functions. Synthetic chemicals are completely opposite in that they have basically one action. This heterogeneity gives essential oils a paradoxical nature that can be difficult to understand. However, essential oils can be compared to another paradoxical group—human beings. For example, a man can play many roles: father, husband, friend, coworker, accountant, school teacher, church volunteer, scout master, minister, etc. And so it is with essential oils: lavender can be used for burns, insect bites, headaches, PMS, insomnia, stress, and so forth.

The heterogeneous benefits of an oil depend greatly on its chemical constituents—and not only on the existence of specific constituents but also on the constituent amounts in proportion to the other constituents that are present in the same oil. Some individual oils may have anywhere from 200 to 800 different chemical constituents. However, of the possible 800 different constituents, only about 200 of those have so far been identified. Although not everything is known about all of the different constituents, most of them can be grouped into a few distinct families, each with some dominant characteristics. The following section provides greater insights into these constituent families.

Essential Oil Constituents

As was mentioned previously, the chemical constituents of an oil are affected by a vast number of variables. However, most of these variables are controlled by the oil producers. One thing that the student of aromatherapy can do is ask questions about the company from which they are purchasing the oils. Some of the most important questions should be, "Does the company utilize gas chromatography (GC) in their quality control process?" "Does their GC equipment utilize a column of at least 50 to 60 meters in length in order to properly identify the hundreds of natural constituents found in an essential oil?" A gas chromatogram shows a pattern of the separated constituents of an oil and helps a trained technician determine its purity and therapeutic quality. The following information can help us understand the functions of some of the main chemical constituents.

In general, *pure* essential oil constituents can be subdivided into 2 distinct groups: the **hydrocarbons,** which are made up almost exclusively of *terpenes* (monoterpenes, sesquiterpenes, and diterpenes), and the **oxygenated compounds,** which are mainly *esters, aldehydes, ketones, alcohols, phenols,* and *oxides.*

Terpenes

Terpenes are the largest family of natural products and are found throughout nature. High concentrations of terpenes are found directly after flowering[1]. The basic molecular structure of a terpene is an isoprene unit (which has a C5H8 molecular formula).

Classes of terpenes are named according to how many isoprene units are present.

- Monoterpenes (C10) = two isoprene units
- Sesquiterpenes (C15) = three isoprene units
- Triterpenes (C30) = six isoprene units
- Tetraterpenes (C40) = eight isoprene units

Terpenes may also have oxygen-containing functional groups. Terpenes with these oxygen-containing functional groups are referred to as terpenoids[2].

ISOPRENE UNIT (C_5H_8)

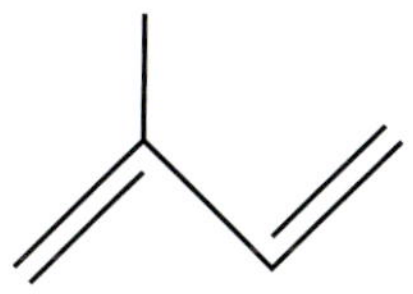

ISOPRENE UNIT (C_5H_8)

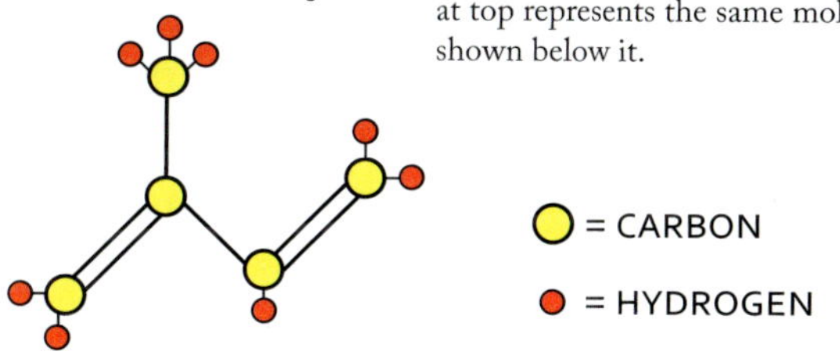

Figures such as the one shown at left represent the bonds between carbon (C) atoms in a molecule. Single lines represent a single bond, while double lines represent a double bond. Each intersecting point and the end of each line represents a carbon molecule along with any hydrogen molecules it is bonded to. Since each carbon molecule can have up to four bonds with other atoms, the number of hydrogen atoms can be determined by subtracting the number of bonds (lines) coming to each carbon atom from four. Thus, the shorthand figure at top represents the same molecule shown below it.

Monoterpenes—occur in practically all essential oils and have many different activities. Most tend to inhibit the accumulation of toxins and help discharge existing toxins from the liver and kidneys. Some are antiseptic, antibacterial, stimulating, analgesic (weak), and expectorant; while other specific terpenes have antifungal, antiviral, antihistaminic, antirheumatic, antitumor (antiblastic, anticarcinogenic), hypotensive, insecticidal, purgative, and pheromonal properties. Monoterpenes, in general, have a stimulating effect and can be very soothing to irritated tissues as well. Most citrus oils (not bergamot) and conifer oils contain a high proportion of terpenes.

Found as a Significant Constituent in ALL Essential Oils *Except*: Anise, basil, birch, calamus,

1 Paduch et al., 2007.

2 McGarvey et al., 1995.

cassia, cedarwood, German chamomile, cinnamon bark, clary sage, clove, blue cypress, davana, geranium, jasmine, melissa, lemon myrtle, onycha, palmarosa, patchouli, rosewood, sandalwood, vetiver, western red cedar, wintergreen, ylang ylang.

Pinenes (α- & β-) α- and β- pinene are isomers (meaning they have the same chemical formula but differing structures). They get their name because they are major constituents in pine resin or pine oil. They give off a resiny, piney smell. Pinenes have strong antiseptic, antibacterial, antifungal, and expectorant properties.

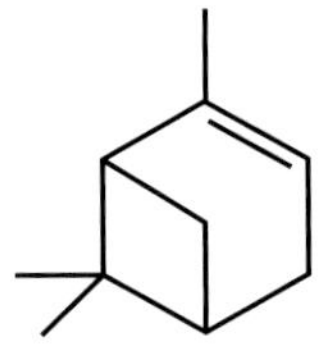

α- PINENE

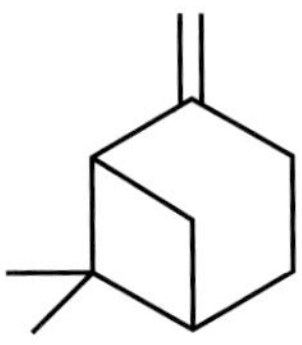

β- PINENE

Bone Resorption Inhibition: α- and β-pinene (found in pine oil) were found in animal studies to inhibit bone resorption. Bone resorption is the process by which osteoclasts—macrophage cells that reside in the bones—break down bone and release the minerals, which can lead to the loss of bone, such as in osteoporosis. Further studies have indicated that while α- and β-pinene may not directly influence osteoclast activity and bone resorption rates, a metabolite (a product created by the body from the original molecule when taken internally) of the pinenes, cis-verbenol, did directly inhibit bone resorption and the formation of osteoclasts[3,4].

Mosquito Larvicide: α-pinenes found in *Alpinia speciosa* and *Rosmarinus officinalis* (ginger and rosemary) demonstrated effective larvicidal activity against the mosquito *Aedes aegypti L.* The *A. aegypti* is a carrier of the dengue virus that causes dengue fever in tropical areas of the world[5].

Antibacterial: It has been observed that the larvae of the Douglas fir tussock moth have digestive systems that are relatively clear of bacterial flora. These larvae feed on terpenes found in the bark of Douglas fir trees, of which α-pinene is a major constituent. α-pinene inhibits the growth of *Bacillus* species (gram-positive bacteria). The concentration needed for maximum inhibition is well below the concentrations of α-pinene found in Douglas fir pine trees. Bacterial inhibition occurs because α-pinene disrupts the cytoplasmic membranes of the bacterial species. α-pinene seems to perform more effectively against gram-positive bacteria than gram-negative bacteria due to the extra outer membrane found in the cell walls of gram-negative bacteria[6,7].

Anti-inflammatory: $NF_{K}B$ is an important transcription factor in the body that regulates proinflammatory responses (signals proteins, specifically cytokines, to cause inflammation). When $NF_{K}B$ is activated, it goes to the nucleus of the cells, binds to DNA, and activates transcription needed to produce cytokines, chemokines, and cell adhesion molecules. These molecules all help in producing inflammation in the body.

α-pinene has been shown to inhibit/block $NF_{K}B$ from going to the nucleus. LPS (lipopolysaccharide, an endotoxin produced by gram-negative bacteria that causes inflammation in the body) was introduced to the cell culture of THP-1 cells to induce the activation of $NF_{K}B$. However, when α-pinene was present, activation was markedly reduced.

α-pinene inhibits $NF_{K}B$ by blocking the degradation of $I_{K}B\alpha$. $I_{K}B\alpha$ is a protein that binds to $NF_{K}B$ to prevent it from constantly transcribing proinflammatory genes. If LPS, a virus, or some stimulant of the immune system is recognized, $I_{K}B\alpha$ will degrade and release/activate $NF_{K}B$. $NF_{K}B$ will then transcribe genes to make proteins that cause

3 Eriksson et al., 1996.

4 Muhlbauer et al., 2003.

5 Freitas et al., 2010.

6 Andrews et al., 1980.

7 Uribe et al., 1985.

inflammation at the site of "invasion," such as a cut, scrape, or burn.

Even in the presence of an immune system stimulant (LPS), α-pinene blocks $I_K B\alpha$. During experimentation, it was also noted that the THP-1 cells received no cytotoxicity from the addition of α-pinene[8,9].

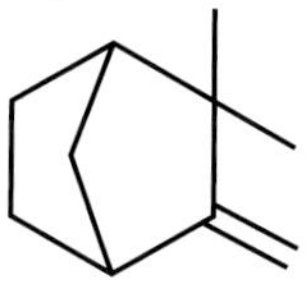

CAMPHENE

Camphene Camphene is found in many oils, such as cypress, citronella, neroli, ginger, and others. It is an insect repellent. According to the *Phytochemical Dictionary*, it is "used to reduce cholesterol saturation index in the treatment of gallstones."

β-Myrcene β-Myrcene is found in oils such as lemongrass, verbena, and bay. It has cancer–preventative properties.

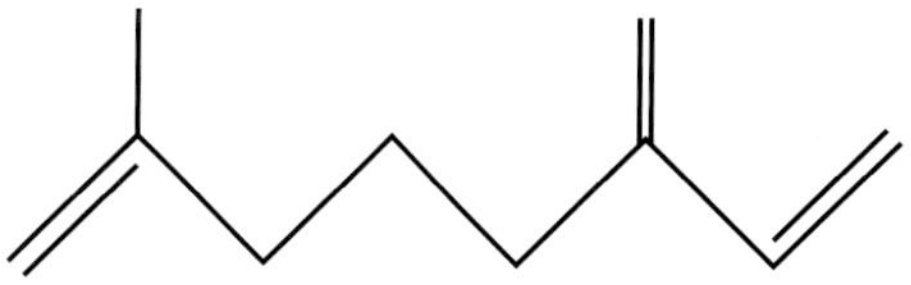

β-MYRCENE

Antioxidant: Studies have elucidated that β-myrcene can reverse and prevent the damaging effects of TCDD (2,3,7,8-Tetrachloro-p-dibenzodioxin) to the liver of rats by increasing GSH (glutathione), SOD (superoxide dismutase), and catalase activation[10,11].

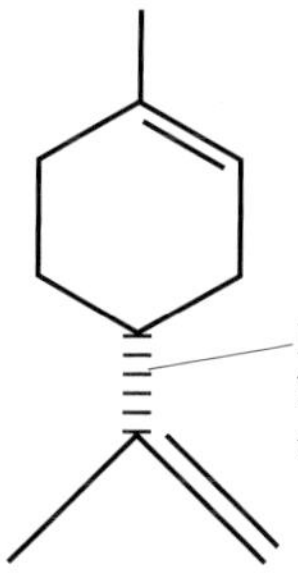

d-LIMONENE

d-Limonene d-Limonene is found in 90% of the citrus peel oils and in caraway seeds and dill. It is anticancer, antibacterial, antifungal, antiseptic (5x phenol), and highly antiviral.

Cancer Cell Inhibition: d-Limonene has been found to be cancer-preventive in vitro and in human mammary cells. It acts as a selective isoprenylation inhibitor. d-Limonene specifically inhibits small g-proteins known as Ras p21 (or p21ras). p21ras is a critical protein for oncogenesis (formation of cancer cells) in the body. In order for oncogenesis to commence, the p21ras protein must be transferred within the cell to the plasma membrane. Once p21ras is able to interact with the plasma membrane of the cell, it causes abnormal cell growth, intracellular localization, and transformations.

d-Limonene inhibits the transferral of p21ras within the cell, blocking its access to the plasma membrane.

Researchers also found that d-Limonene is selectively inhibitive. It targets only the transferral of Ras proteins and leaves all other ordinary cell functions alone. This makes d-Limonene a potentially effective chemopreventive agent because it targets areas of high oncogenic susceptibility and has no harmful side effects against critical cell components (low toxicity)[12,13,14].

Researchers have also observed that a continuous dose of limonene in the diets of rats with chemical-induced cancer helps inhibit the formation of secondary tumors and reduces the size of primary tumors. However, when limonene was removed from the rat's daily diet, tumors were more likely to return. This gives evidence that limonene works as a cytostatic agent (an agent that stops the tumor cells from creating new

8 Zhou et al., 2004.

9 Weaver, 2008.

10 Ciftci et al., 2011.

11 Gaetani et al., 1996.

12 Kato et al., 1992.

13 Crowell et al., 1991.

14 Morse et al., 1993.

tumor cells) rather than a cytotoxic agent (an agent that kills the tumor cells). These researchers also observed that little toxicity occurred to the rats from the high doses of d-Limonene[15].

Cholesterol Suppression: Researchers have discovered that when d-Limonene is included in the daily diet of rats treated with a chemical (7,12-dimetylbenzantracene) that induced high cholesterol, there was a 45% decrease in hepatic HMG-CoA reductase activity. HMG-CoA reductase is an enzyme that converts HMG-CoA (93-hydroxy-3-methylglutaryl coenzyme A) to mevalonic acid, which acts as a precursor to the production of cholesterol. Inhibiting HMG-CoA reductase halts this process and, in effect, lowers cholesterol rates[16,17].

Sesquiterpenes Sesquiterpenes are found in great abundance in essential oils. They are antibacterial, strongly anti-inflammatory, slightly antiseptic and hypotensive, and sedative. Some have analgesic properties, while others are highly antispasmodic. They are soothing to irritated skin and tissue and are calming. They also work as liver and gland stimulants. Research from the universities of Berlin and Vienna shows that sesquiterpenes increase oxygenation around the pineal and pituitary glands. Further research has shown that sesquiterpenes have the ability to surpass the blood-brain barrier and enter the brain tissue. They are larger molecules than monoterpenes and have a strong aroma.

Found as a Major Constituent In: Cedarwood, German chamomile, ginger, goldenrod, melissa, myrrh, patchouli, pepper, sandalwood, spikenard, vetiver, yarrow, ylang ylang.

Found as a Minor (but significant) Constituent In: Bergamot, carrot, cedar leaf, celery seed, Roman chamomile, cinnamon bark, clary sage, clove, cumin, cypress, blue cypress, elemi, *Eucalyptus citriadora* (lemon eucalyptus), *Eucalyptus globulus*, silver fir, white fir, frankincense, galbanum, geranium, helichrysum, hyssop, lavandin, lavender, ledum, lemongrass, *Melaleuca alternifolia* (tea tree), *Melaleuca ericifolia* (rosalina), *Melaleuca leucadendron* (cajeput), *Melaleuca quinquenervia* (niaouli), peppermint, pine, rosewood, sage, blue tansy, tsuga, valerian.

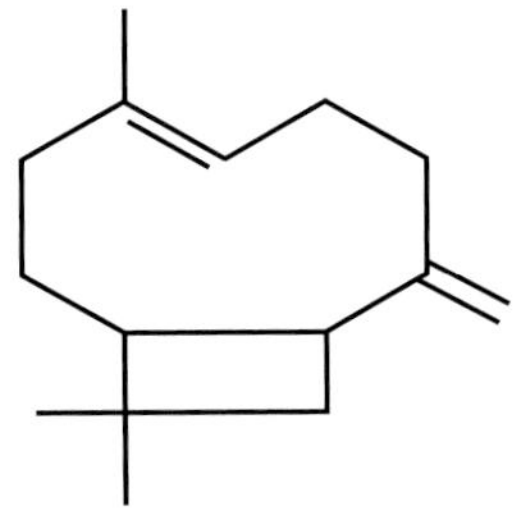

β-CARYOPHYLLENE

β-Caryophyllene β-caryophyllene is found in clove and cinnamon essential oils and is found in high proportions in plants from the Labiatae family. It is antiedema, anti-inflammatory, antispasmodic, and an insect and termite repellent.

Anesthetic: β-caryophyllene has been shown to act as a local anesthetic in vitro and in vivo. In an in vitro experiment, β-caryophyllene reduced the number of contractions electrically invoked in rat phrenic nerve-hemidiaphragms. Phrenic nerves are found in the spine, specifically at the 3rd, 4th, and 5th cervical vertebrae. These nerves provide sole motor control to the diaphragm. In this experiment, electrical impulses through the phrenic nerves induced diaphragm contractions, but the addition of β-caryophyllene reduced the number of contractions[18].

In an in vivo (real life) experiment, researchers performed a conjunctival reflex test on rabbits in which the conjunctival sac, found in the eye, was stimulated with a cat whisker to promote palpebral closure (or blinking). β-caryophyllene acted as a local anesthetic: when it was applied to the eye, more stimulation with the cat whisker was required in order to promote blinking in the rabbit[19].

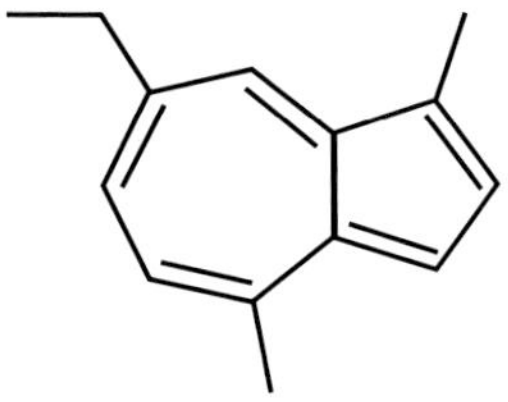

CHAMAZULENE

15 Haag et al., 1992.

16 Sorentino et al., 2005.

17 Qureshi et al., 1988.

18 Bulbring, 1946.

19 Ghelardini et al., 2001.

Chamazulene Chamazulene is found in chamomile oil and is very high in anti-inflammatory and antibacterial activity.

Farnesene Farnesene refers to several isomers with the chemical formula $C_{15}H_{24}$. Farnesene is found in ylang ylang, valerian, and German chamomile oil and is antiviral in action.

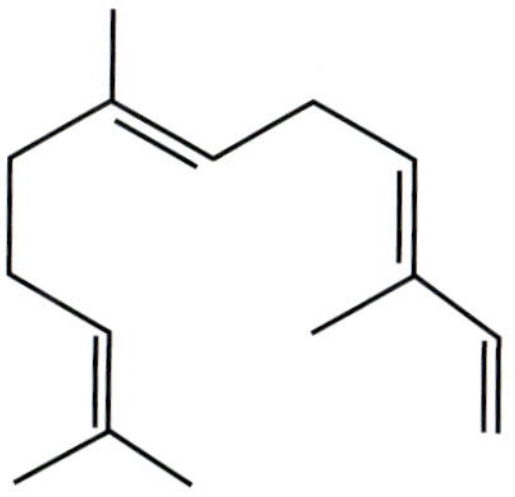

α-FARNESENE

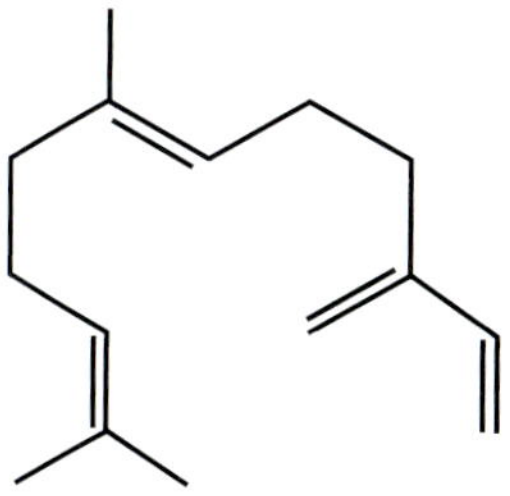

β-FARNESENE

Alcohols

Alcohols are any organic molecule with a carbon atom bound to a hydroxyl group. A hydroxyl group is an oxygen and hydrogen molecule (-OH). Alcohols are commonly recognized for their antibacterial, anti-infectious, and antiviral activities. They are somewhat stimulating and help to increase blood circulation. Because of their high resistance to oxidation and their low toxicity levels, they have been shown in animal studies to revert cells to normal function and activity. They create an uplifting quality and are regarded as safe and effective for young and old alike.

METHANOL (CH_3OH)

—OH

Shorthand model of methanol, the simplest alcohol, and the molecular model it represents, below.

METHANOL (CH_3OH)

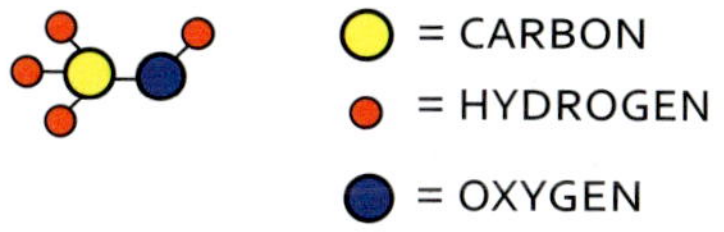

Monoterpene Alcohols (or Monoterpenols) Like monoterpenes, monoterpene alcohols are comprised of two isoprene units but have a hydroxyl group bound to one of the carbons instead of a hydrogen. Monoterpene alcohols are known for their ability to stimulate the immune system and to work as a diuretic and a general tonic. They are antibacterial and mildly antiseptic as well.

Linalool Linalool is found in rosewood, bergamot, coriander, rose, jasmine, and lavender essential oils. It has a flowery aroma and is used to scent soaps, shampoos, and perfumes. Linalool can help relieve discomfort. It has antibacterial, antifungal, antiseptic (5x phenol), antispasmodic, antiviral, and sedative properties.

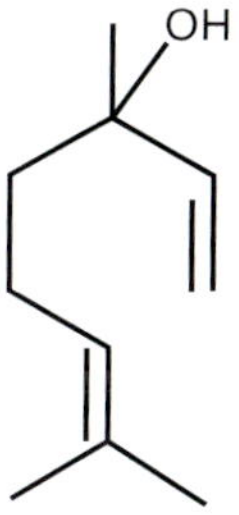

LINALOOL

Anti-inflammatory: Linalool has been used to reduce paw swelling induced by carrageenan in mice. The effects of linalool work against swelling in a dose-dependent manner[20,21]. Linalool also mediates pain caused by inflammation. In a particular study, acetic acid was administered to mice via intraperitoneal

20 Peana et al., 2002.

21 Skold et al., 2002.

(gut) injections. Mice that received a dose of linalool following administration of acetic acid exhibited less writhing (due to pain) than mice that acted as controls[22].

Antifungal: *Candida albicans* is the primary fungus responsible for yeast infections. Yeast infections are commonly exhibited as vulvovaginal candidiasis and thrush (oropharyngeal candidiasis, in the mouth). Thrush is commonly expressed in newborns and AIDS patients.

Candida albicans is also becoming a concern due to its emergence as a nosocomial infection (an infection contracted in a hospital) and its increasing resistance to fluconazole—an antifungal drug. *C. albicans* can form biofilms (aggregated colonies) on medical devices such as catheters and dentures[23,24].

Topical application of linalool to colonies of the polymorphic fungus *Candida albicans* results in growth inhibition and fungal death. Linalool affects growth by blocking passage beyond the G1 (cell growth) phase of the cell cycle[25].

Sedative: Linalool is a common sedative used in Brazilian folk medicine. According to studies using mice, inhaled linalool induces sleep or sedation[26,27].

Antiepileptic/Anticonvulsant: Epilepsy is characterized by seemingly spontaneous spasms of electrical activity in the brain. These spasms can cause seizures and convulsions. One hypothesis for the cause of epilepsy is excessive glutamate levels in neurons (nerve cells)[28,29,30,31]. Glutamates are a common form of neurotransmitter that are stored in special vesicles (storage containers) near nerve synapses (locations where nerve cells come close to each other in order to pass along electrical impulses and signals). Impulses along the nerve cause one nerve cell to release glutamate across the synapse where it is received by receptors on the second nerve cell, opening channels in that cell to allow it to pass ions through the cell membrane, changing the electrical potential of that cell[32].

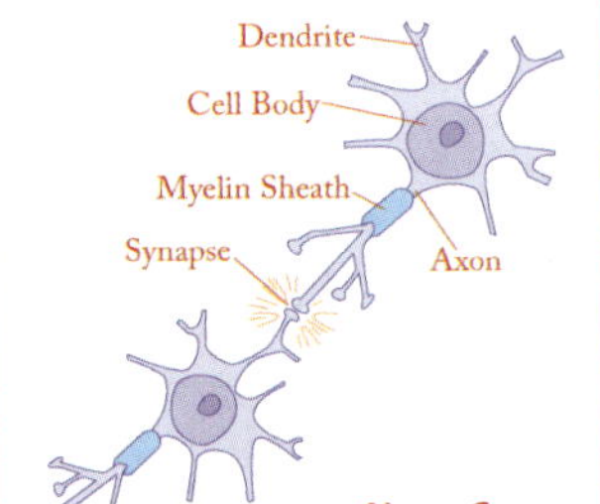

Nerve Cells

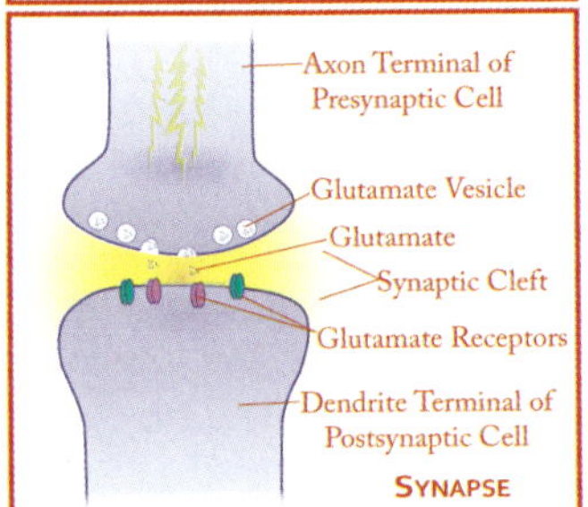

Synapse

Studies have shown that the release of large concentrations of glutamate will lead to too many open channels, which will cause high, intense depolarization sequences of the action potential. Disproportionate depolarizations are the basis for seizures and convulsions in epilepsy[33,34,35].

Using mouse models, researchers have found that applications of linalool on cortical synaptosomes (isolated nerve terminals, or synapses) significantly inhibited glutamate uptake. Inhibition of glutamate is a method to reduce occurrences

22 Peana et al., 2003.
23 Mukherjee et al., 2003.
24 Microbiology. 9th ed, 2007.
25 Zore et al., 2011.
26 Linck et al., 2009.
27 de Almeida et al., 2009.
28 Chapman et al., 2000.
29 Meldrum et al., 1999.
30 Meldrum, 1994.
31 Chapman, 1998.
32 Medical Physiology. 10th ed, 2000.
33 Chapman et al., 2000.
34 Meldrum et al., 1994.
35 Paolette et al., 2007.

of epileptic seizures. These observations provide significant evidence for linalool acting as a possible antiepileptic agent[36,37].

Citronellol Citronellol is found in citronella, rose, melissa, and eucalyptus essential oils. It has antibacterial, antifungal, antiseptic (3.8x phenol), and sedative properties.

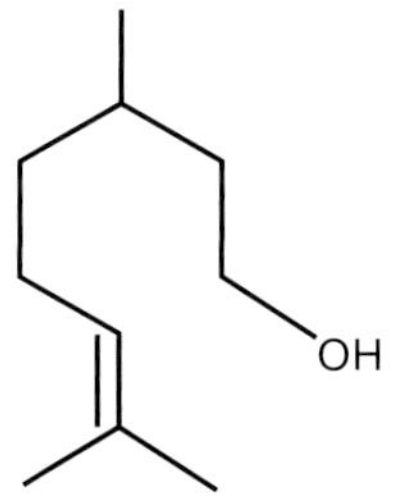

CITRONELLOL

Anticonvulsant Activity: Administered doses of citronellol given via the intraperitoneal cavity (gut) to rodents have been observed to reduce the convulsive effects in induced epileptic attacks. Epilepsy is studied in animal models by inducing convulsions with compounds such as pentylenetetrazol (PTZ) and picrotoxin. Citronellol, over time, reduces the amplitude of the compound action potential (CAP) in neurons. This decreases the effect and intensity of convulsions[38].

Blood Pressure: Injections of citronellol into the blood were found by researchers to reduce blood pressure in animal models. Citronellol is theorized to decrease the flux of Ca^{2+} ions into smooth vascular muscle cells by deactivating VOCCs (voltage-operated calcium channels).Calcium is the principle regulator of tension in vascular smooth muscle (blood vessels). When the transport of Ca^{2+} into the cell is blocked, smooth muscle relaxation occurs. This leads to increased vasodilation (an increase in the diameter of the blood vessels, allowing a higher volume of blood flow) and, thus, lowered blood pressure[39,40,41].

Geraniol Geraniol is found in rose, citronella, and lemon essential oils. It has antifungal, antiseptic (7x phenol), cancer preventative, and sedative properties.

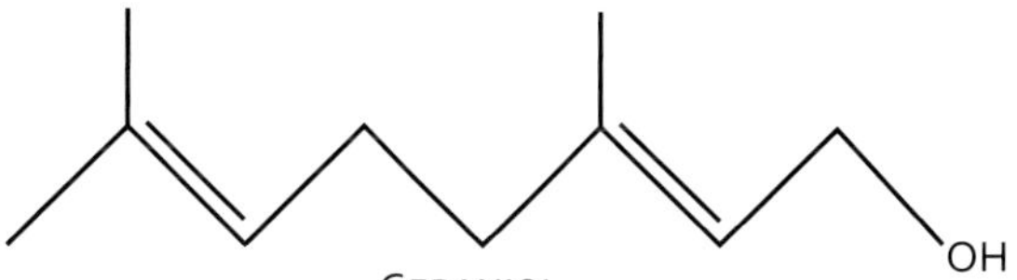

GERANIOL

Other Monoterpene Alcohols Other monoterpene alcohols include borneol, menthol, nerol, terpineol (which Dr. Gattefosse considered to be a decongestant), vetiverol, and cedrol.

Sesquiterpene Alcohols (Sesquiterpenols) are antiallergenic, antibacterial, anti-inflammatory, ulcer-protective (preventative), and a liver and glandular stimulant.

Farnesol Farnesol is found in rose, neroli, ylang ylang, and Roman chamomile essential oils. It is known to be good for the mucous membranes and to help prevent bacterial growth from perspiration.

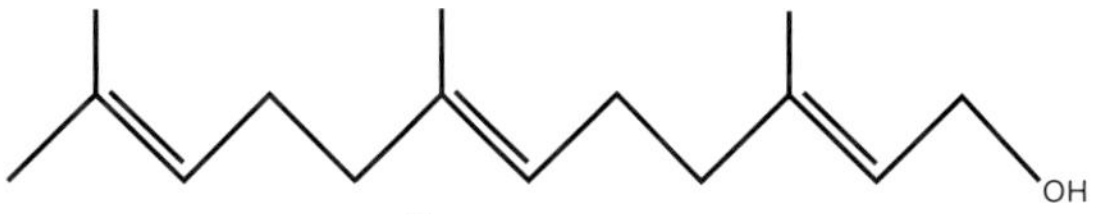

FARNESOL

Bisabolol Bisabolol is found in German chamomile essential oil. It is one of the strongest sesquiterpene alcohols.

Other Sesquiterpene Alcohols Others include nerolidol and zingiberol.

Found as a Significant Constituent in ALL Essential Oils *Except*: Anise, birch, calamus, cassia, celery seed, clove, cumin, davana, dill, *Eucalyptus*

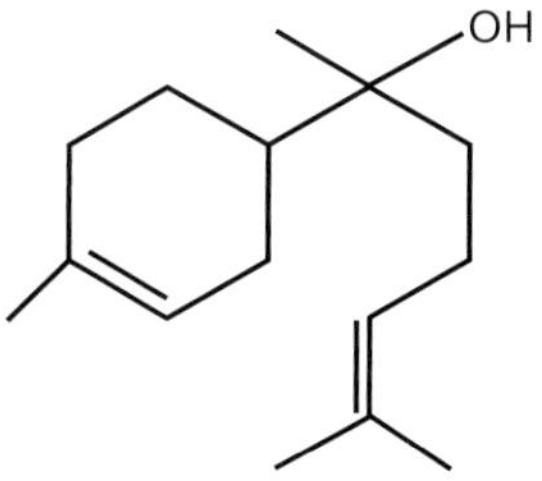

BISABOLOL

36 Silva Brum et al., 2001a.

37 Silva Brum et al., 2001b.

38 de Sousa et al., 2006.

39 Bastos et al., 2009.

40 Gurney, 1994.

41 Munzel et al., 2003.

polybractea, balsam fir, silver fir, white fir, galbanum, goldenrod, grapefruit, hyssop, juniper, melissa, mugwort, lemon myrtle, myrrh, onycha, oregano, pepper, pine, rosemary (CT verbenon), spruce, blue tansy, Idaho tansy, tarragon, tsuga, western red cedar, wintergreen, yarrow.

Esters

METHYL ACETATE (CH_3OOCH_3)

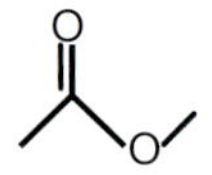

Methyl acetate (shown here) is a simple organic ester molecule.

METHYL ACETATE (CH_3OOCH_3)

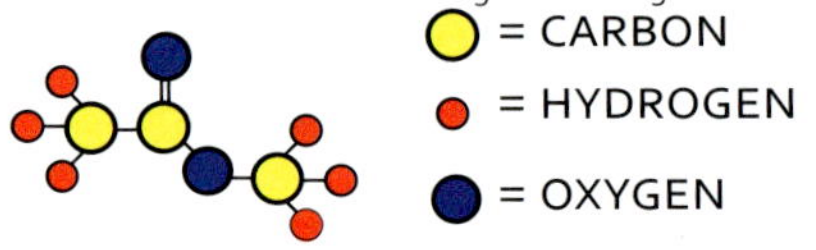

Esters are the compounds resulting from the reaction of an alcohol with an acid (known as esterification). Esters consist of a carboxyl group (a carbon atom double bonded to an oxygen atom) bound to a hydrocarbon group on one side and bound to an oxygen and a hydrocarbon group on the opposite side. Esters are very common and are found in the mildest essential oils. Mostly free of toxicity and irritants, they tend to be the most calming, relaxing, and balancing of all the essential oil constituents. They are also antifungal and antispasmodic. They have a balancing or regulatory effect, especially on the nervous system. Some examples are linalyl acetate, geranyl acetate (with strong antifungal properties), and bornyl acetate (effective on bronchial candida). Other esters include eugenyl acetate, lavendulyl acetate, and methyl salicylate.

Found as a Major Constituent In: Birch, bergamot, cardamom, Roman chamomile (85%), clary sage, geranium, helichrysum, jasmine, lavandin, lavender, onycha, petitgrain, spruce, tsuga, valerian, wintergreen, ylang ylang.

Found as a Minor (but significant) Constituent In: Angelica, carrot, cassia, cedar leaf, celery seed, cistus, clove, coriander, cypress, dill, *Eucalyptus citriadora* (lemon eucalyptus), balsam fir, Douglas fir, silver fir, white fir, fleabane, juniper, *Laurus nobilis*, lemon, lemongrass, mandarin, marjoram, melissa, myrtle, neroli, orange, palmarosa, rosemary (CT verbenon), sage lavender.

Aldehydes

ACETALDEHYDE (CH_3CHO)

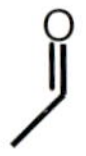

Acetaldehyde (shown here) is a simple organic aldehyde molecule.

ACETALDEHYDE (CH_3CHO)

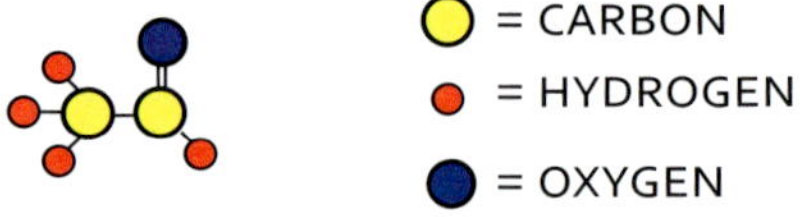

Aldehydes are often responsible for the fragrance of an oil. They exert powerful aromas and are often calming to the emotions. They are highly reactive and are characterized by a carboxyl group (a carbon atom double bonded to an oxygen atom) with a hydrogen atom on one side and a hydrocarbon group on the opposite side. In general, aldehydes are anti-infectious, anti-inflammatory, calming to the central nervous system, fever-reducing, hypotensive, and tonic. Some are antiseptic, antimicrobial, and antifungal, while others act as vasodilators. They can be quite irritating when applied topically (citrals being an example). However, it has been shown that adding an essential oil with an equal amount of d-Limonene can negate the irritant properties of a high citral oil.

Found as a Major Constituent In: Cassia, cinnamon bark, cumin, *Eucalyptus citriadora* (lemon eucalyptus), lemongrass, lemon myrtle, lemon verbena.

Found as a Minor (but significant) Constituent In: Calamus, cistus, citronella, *Eucalyptus radiata*, grapefruit, lemon, lime, mandarin, myrrh, orange, tangerine.

Citrals Citrals (like neral, geranial, and citronellal) are very common and have a distinct antiseptic action. They also show antiviral properties (as is the case with melissa oil) when applied topically on herpes simplex.

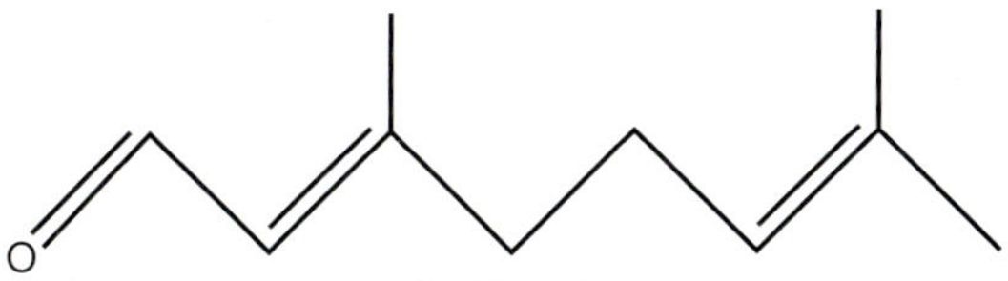

GERANIAL

Other Aldehydes include benzaldehyde, cinnamic aldehyde, cuminic aldehyde, and perillaldehyde.

Ketones

Ketones are organic compounds characterized by a carboxyl group (a carbon atom double bonded to an oxygen atom) with a hydrocarbon on both sides. Ketones are sometimes mucolytic and neurotoxic when isolated from other constituents. However, all recorded toxic effects come from laboratory testing on guinea pigs and rats. No documented cases exist where oils with a high concentration of ketones (such as mugwort, tansy, sage, and wormwood) have ever caused a toxic effect on a human being. Also, large amounts of these oils would have to be consumed for them to result in a toxic neurological effect. Ketones stimulate cell regeneration, promote the formation of tissue, and liquefy mucous. They are helpful with conditions such as dry asthma, colds, flu, and dry cough and are largely found in oils used for the upper respiratory system, such as hyssop, rosemary, and sage.

ACETONE (CH_3COCH_3)

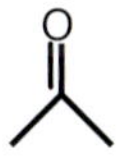

Acetone (shown here) is a simple ketone molecule.

ACETONE (CH_3COCH_3)

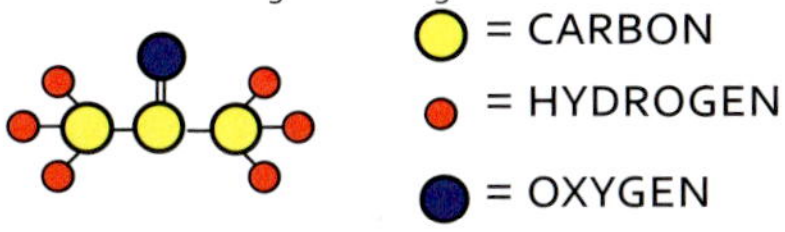

Found as a Major Constituent In: Calamus, cedar leaf, davana, dill, *Eucalyptus dives*, hyssop, rosemary (CT cineol), rosemary (CT verbenon), sage, sage lavender, spearmint, Idaho tansy, Western red cedar.

Found as a Minor (but significant) Constituent In: Cedarwood, Roman chamomile, cistus, coriander, *Eucalyptus polybractea*, fennel, geranium, helichrysum, juniper, lavandin, lemongrass, melissa, mugwort, myrrh, peppermint, spikenard, blue tansy, vetiver, yarrow.

Thujone Thujone is one of the most toxic members of the ketone family. It can be an irritant and upsetting to the central nervous system and may be neurotoxic when taken internally, such as in the banned drink absinthe. Although oils containing thujone may be inhaled to relieve respiratory distress and may stimulate the immune system, they should usually be used in dilution (1–2%) and/or for only short periods of time.

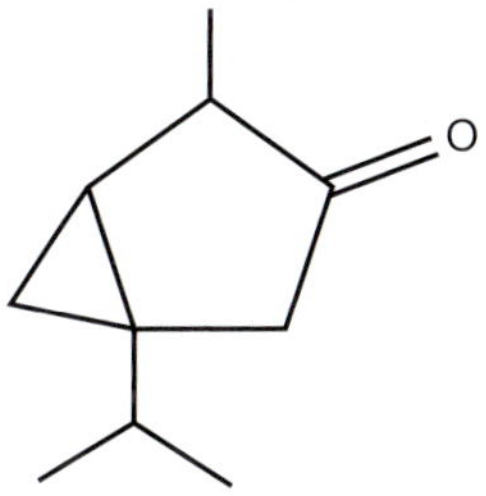

α-THUJONE

Jasmone is found in jasmine essential oil and is nontoxic.

Fenchone Fenchone is found in fennel essential oil and is nontoxic.

Other Ketones include camphor, carvone, menthone, methyl nonyl ketone, and pinocamphone.

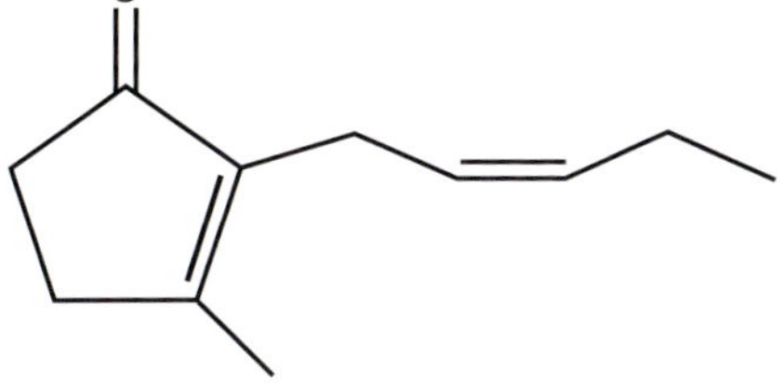

JASMONE

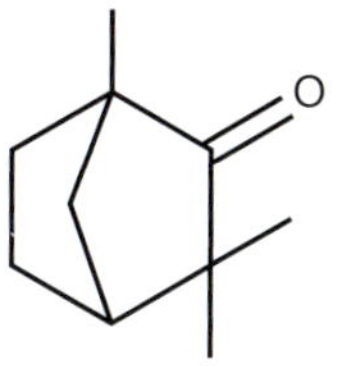

FENCHONE

Phenols

Phenols are a diverse group of compounds derived from a phenol group, which is comprised of a benzene ring (six carbon atoms bound in a circle) and a hydroxyl group (oxygen and hydrogen).

PHENOL (C_6H_6OH)

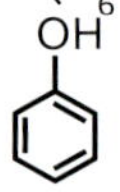

Phenol (shown here) is a simple phenol molecule.

PHENOL (C_6H_6OH)

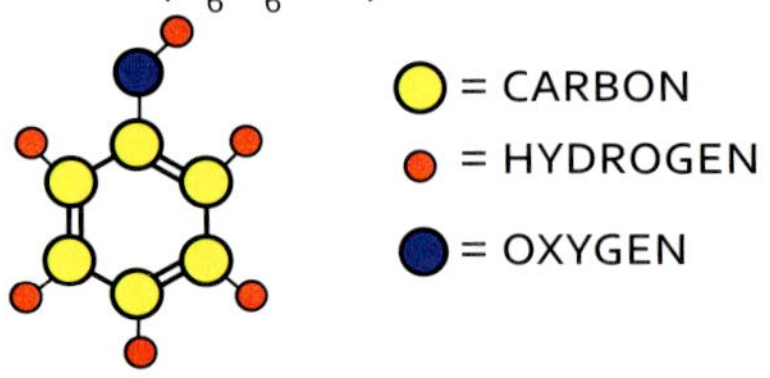

Phenols comprise some of the most powerful antibacterial, anti-infectious, and antiseptic constituents in the plant world. They are also very stimulating to both the nervous and immune systems. They contain high levels of oxygenating molecules and have antioxidant properties. However, they can be quite caustic to the skin, and they present some concerns regarding liver toxicity. Essential oils that contain a high proportion of phenols should be diluted and/or used only for short periods of time.

Found as a Major Constituent In: Anise, basil, birch, cinnamon bark, clove, fennel, *Melaleuca alternifolia* (tea tree), mountain savory, oregano, peppermint, tarragon, thyme, wintergreen.

Found as a Minor (but significant) Constituent In: Cassia, citronella, cumin, *Eucalyptus citriadora* (lemon eucalyptus), *Laurus nobilis*, marjoram, nutmeg, ylang ylang.

Eugenol Eugenol is found in clove, nutmeg, cinnamon, bay, and basil essential oils. It has analgesic, anesthetic (in dentistry), anticonvulsant, antifungal, anti-inflammatory, antioxidant, antiseptic, cancer-preventative, and sedative properties.

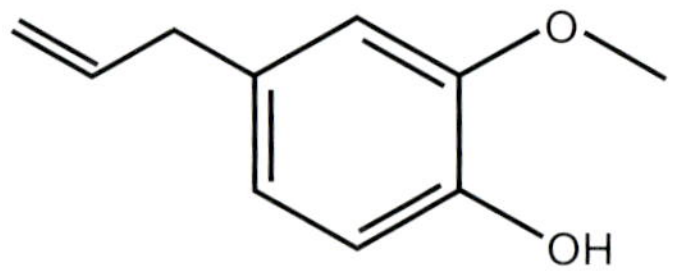

EUGENOL

Vasodilator: Eugenol was found to increase vasodilation (increase the diameter of the opening through the blood vessels) in animal models. When blood vessels expand, the result is larger amounts of blood flow and, thus, a decrease in heart rate. In these particular studies, it was observed that heart rate decreased in conjunction with increased vasodilation, as compared to controls[42,43].

Eugenol is thought to increase vasodilation by inhibiting the action of calcium (Ca^{2+}) in voltage-operated calcium channels (VOCCs). Ca^{2+} is the main regulator of vascular smooth muscle (blood vessel) tension. When Ca^{2+} is blocked, blood vessels relax and widen, allowing for an increase in blood flow[44,45].

Thymol Thymol is found in thyme and oregano essential oils. It may not be as caustic as other phenols. It has antibacterial, antifungal, anti-inflammatory, antioxidant, antiplaque, antirheumatic, antiseptic (20x phenol), antispasmodic, deodorizing, and expectorant properties.

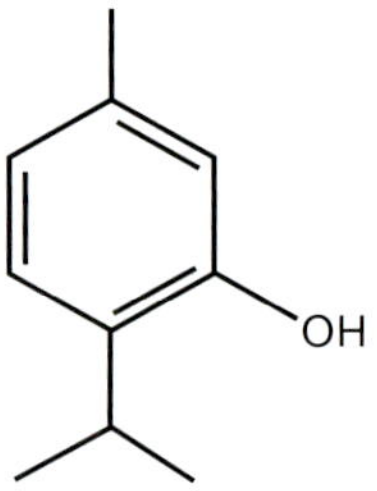

THYMOL

Antibacterial: Thymol has been shown to inhibit the growth of microorganisms such as *Escherichia coli*, *Campylobacter jejuni*, *Porphyromonas gingivalis*, *Staphylococcus aureus*, and *Pseudomonas aeruginosa*. Thymol is thought to disrupt (or impair) the cytoplasmic membranes of microbes, causing cell

42 Lahlou et al., 2004.

43 Damiani et al., 2003.

44 Gurney, 1994.

45 Munzel et al., 2003.

leakage. Without the protective barrier of the cytoplasmic membrane, viability of these microorganisms significantly decreases[46,47,48,49].

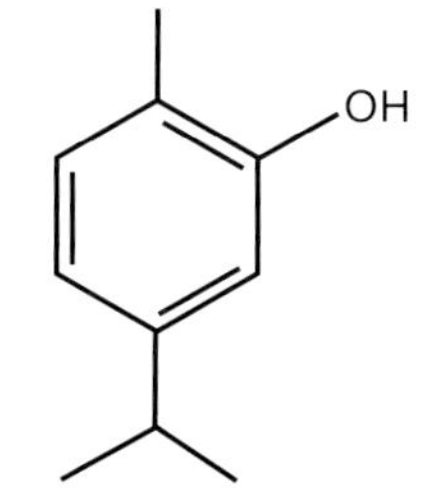

CARVACROL

Carvacrol Carvacrol is a product of auto-oxidation of d-Limonene. It is antibacterial, antifungal, anti-inflammatory, antiseptic (1.5x phenol), antispasmodic, and expectorant. Researchers believe it may possibly have some anticancer properties as well.

Other Phenols Others in the phenol family include methyl eugenol, methyl chavicol, anethole, and safrole.

Oxides—An organic oxide typically refers to an organic molecule (one that contains carbon and hydrogen) that has been oxidized, meaning an oxygen atom has become bound between two carbon atoms. According to the *American Heritage® Dictionary of the English Language*, an oxide is "a binary compound of an element or a radical with oxygen." Oxides often act as expectorants and are mildly stimulating.

Found as a Major Constituent In: Cardamom, German chamomile, *Eucalyptus globulus*, *Eucalyptus polybractea*, *Eucalyptus radiata*, *Laurus nobilis*, *Melaleuca leucadendron* (Cajeput), *Melaleuca quinquenervia* (Niaouli), myrtle, ravensara, rosemary (CT cineol).

Found as a Minor (but significant) Constituent In: Basil, carrot, *Eucalyptus citriadora* (lemon eucalyptus), lavandin, lemongrass, lime, *Melaleuca alternifolia* (tea tree), *Melaleuca ericifolia* (rosalina), melissa, mugwort, pepper, rosemary (CT verbenon), rosewood, sage, sage lavender, thyme, ylang ylang.

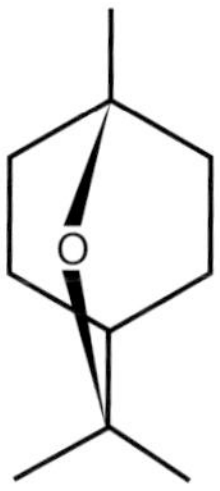

1,8-CINEOL
(EUCALYPTOL)

1,8-Cineol (Eucalyptol) 1,8-cineol is, by far, the most prevalent member of the oxide family and virtually exists in a class of its own. It is anesthetic, antiseptic, and works as a strong mucolytic as it thins mucus in respiratory tract infections.

Anti-Inflammatory: Researchers found in an animal experiment that rats that were given oral doses of 1,8-cineole before injection with lambda carrageenan (a sweetener that causes inflammation) had markedly decreased swelling when compared to rats that were given the injection without a dosage of 1,8-cineole.

It has been suggested by scientists that 1,8-cineole inhibits cytokine production. Inhibiting cytokine production would decrease inflammation despite having a stimulant present (such a carrageenan)[50,51].

Asthma: Asthma is a chronic inflammatory disease that restricts air flow to the lungs (specifically in the bronchial tubes). A double-blind, placebo-controlled study was performed to test the ability of 1,8-cineole to alleviate asthmatic symptoms. All subjects in the study suffered from bronchial asthma and required daily administration of oral glucocorticosteroids in order to maintain stable conditions.

At the conclusion of the study, which lasted over a course of 12 weeks, patients who received daily doses of 1,8-cineole were able to maintain stable conditions despite significantly reduced oral doses of glucocorticosteroids, as compared to the placebo group. Proper lung function was also maintained four times longer in the test group than in the placebo group[52,53].

46 Shapiro et al., 1995.
47 Xu et al., 2008.
48 Lambert et al., 2001.
49 Evans et al., 2000.
50 Santos et al., 2000.
51 Juergens et al., 2003.
52 Juergens et al., 2003.
53 Goodwin et al., 1986.

Pain: In one study, mice were injected in the hind paw with a dose of 1% formalin (a common substance used to model pain in experimental studies)/99% saline solution. A portion of mice were given 1,8-cineole. It was observed that these mice who received 1,8-cineole licked their paw substantially less (meaning they did not feel as much pain) than mice that did not receive the 1,8-cineole treatment. In this study, researchers found that 1,8-cineole treatment produced antinociceptive (pain-blocking) effects comparable to those observed for morphine[54,55].

Other Oxides Linalool oxide, ascaridol, bisabolol oxide, 1,4-cineol, and bisabolone oxide.

All pure essential oils have some antibacterial properties. They increase the production of white blood cells, which help fight infectious illnesses. It is because of these properties that aromatic herbs have been esteemed so highly throughout the ages and so widely used during the onsets of malaria, typhoid, and, of course, the epidemic plagues during the 16th century. Research has found that people who consistently use pure essential oils have a higher level of resistance to illnesses, colds, flues, and diseases than does the average person. Further indications show that such individuals after contracting a cold, flu, or other illness will recover 60–75 percent faster than those who do not use essential oils.

The Art Of Blending

Blending essential oils is an art and usually requires a little bit of training and experimentation. If you choose to create your own blends, it is important to understand that the order in which the oils are blended is key to maintaining the desired therapeutic properties in a synergistic blend. An alteration in the sequence of adding selected oils to a blend may change the chemical properties, the fragrance, and the desired results. The "Blend Classification," and "Blends With" listings under each oil in the Single Oils section of this book should assist one in the blending process. In general, oils that are from the same botanical family usually blend well together. In addition, oils with similar constituents also mix well.

Another method utilizes 4 blending classifications. The following information explains the characteristics of each classification, the order in which they should be added to the blend (i.e. Personifiers first, Enhancers second, Equalizers third, and Modifiers fourth), and the amount of each type of oil as a percentage of the blend.

1st—The **Personifier** (1–5% of blend) oils have very sharp, strong, and long-lasting fragrances. They also have dominant properties with strong therapeutic action.

Oils in this classification may include: Angelica, birch, cardamom, cinnamon bark, cistus, clary sage, clove, coriander, German chamomile, ginger, helichrysum, mandarin, neroli, nutmeg, orange, patchouli, peppermint, petitgrain, rose, spearmint, tangerine, tarragon, wintergreen, and ylang ylang.

2nd—The **Enhancer** (50–80% of blend) oil should be the predominant oil, as it serves to enhance the properties of the other oils in the blend. Its fragrance is not as sharp as the personifiers and is usually of a shorter duration.

Oils in this classification may include: Basil, bergamot, birch, cajeput, cedarwood, cumin, dill, eucalyptus, frankincense, galbanum, geranium, grapefruit, hyssop, jasmine, lavender, lemon, lemongrass, lime, marjoram, *Melaleuca alternifolia* (tea tree), melissa, myrtle, orange, oregano, palmarosa, patchouli, petitgrain, ravensara, Roman chamomile, rose, rosemary, sage, spruce, thyme, and wintergreen.

54 Santos et al., 2000.

55 Shibata et al., 1989.

3rd—The **Equalizer** (10–15% of blend) oils create balance and synergy among the oils contained in the blend. Their fragrance is also not as sharp as the personifier's and is of a shorter duration.

Oils in this classification may include: Basil, bergamot, cedarwood, cypress, fennel, fir, frankincense, geranium, ginger, hyssop, jasmine, juniper, lavender, lemongrass, lime, marjoram, *Melaleuca alternifolia* (tea tree), melissa, myrrh, myrtle, neroli, oregano, pine, Roman chamomile, rose, rosewood, sandalwood, spruce, tarragon, and thyme.

4th—The **Modifier** (5–8% of blend) oils have a mild and short fragrance. These oils add harmony to the blend.

Oils in this classification may include: Angelica, bergamot, cardamom, coriander, eucalyptus, fennel, grapefruit, hyssop, jasmine, lavender, lemon, mandarin, melissa, myrrh, neroli, petitgrain, rose, rosewood, sandalwood, tangerine, and ylang ylang.

Depending upon the topical application of your blend, you will want to add some carrier/base oil. When creating a **therapeutic essential oil blend**, you may want to use about **28 drops of essential oil to ½ oz. of V-6 Oil**. When creating a **body massage blend**, you will want to use a total of about **50 drops of essential oils to 4 oz. of V-6 Oil**. Remember to store your fragrant creation in dark-colored glass bottles.

As essential oils can vary in thickness, the following are approximate measurements:

25–30 drops	= 1/4 teaspoon	= 1–2 milliliters	= 5/8 dram
45–50 drops	= 1/2 teaspoon	= 2–3 milliliters	= 1 dram
75–80 drops	= 3/4 teaspoon	= 3–4 milliliters	= 1/8 oz.
100–120 drops	= 1 teaspoon	= 5 milliliters	= 1/6 oz.
160 drops	= 1½ teaspoons	= 6–8 milliliters	= 1/4 oz.
320–400 drops	= 3 teaspoons	= 13–15 milliliters	= 1/2 oz.
600–650 drops	= 6 teaspoons	= 25–30 milliliters	= 1 oz.

Learn to trust your nose, as it can help you decide which classification an oil should be in. More detailed information about these methods of blending is beyond the scope of this revision of the book. For additional information on using these classifications in your blending, we highly recommend Marcel Lavabre's *Aromatherapy Workbook*. Another very simple book about blending, with recipes and easy-to-follow guidelines, is Mindy Green's *Natural Perfumes*, which uses perfume notes (top, middle, base), odor, and odor intensity to help guide you in making your own fragrant blend creations (refer to the chart on the following page).

Essential Oils Odor Chart

(The following chart was compiled from the book *Natural Perfumes*, by Mindy Green, and from various other sources. It lists essential oils by note types in order of odor intensity, 1-lightest to 5-strongest.)

Essential Oil	Scent	Intensity
Top Notes	(5–20% of the blend)	
orange	Fresh, citrusy, fruity, sweet, light	1
bergamot	Sweet, lively, citrus, fruity	2
grapefruit	Clean, fresh, bitter, citrusy	2
citronella	Citrusy, slightly fruity, fresh, sweet	3
lemon	Sweet, sharp, clear, citrusy	3
lime	Sweet, tart, intense, lively	3
mandarin	Very sweet, citrusy, fruity	3
petitgrain	Fresh, floral, citrusy, slightly woody	3
ravensara	Slightly medicinal, eucalyptus-like	3
spearmint	Minty, slightly fruity	3
tangerine	Fresh, sweet, citrusy	3
euc. polybrac.	Fresh, woody, earthy	4
lemongrass	Grassy, lemony, pungent, earthy	4
euc. globulus	Fresh, medicinal, woody, earthy	5
galbanum	Warm, earthy, green, woody, spicy	5
lemon myrtle	Extremely lemony and crisp	5
Top to Middle Notes	(20–80% of the blend)	
anise	Licorice-like, rich, sweet	3
laurel	Sweet, fresh, spicy, medicinal	3
lavandin	Fresh, sweet, floral, herbaceous	3
myrtle	Sweet, slightly camphorous, floral hint	3
palmarosa	Lemony, fresh, green, hints of rose	3
angelica	Earthy, peppery, green, spicy	4
basil	Spicy, anise-like, camphorous, lively	4
fennel	Sweet, somewhat spicy, licorice-like	4
Middle Notes	(50–80% of the blend)	
carrot seed	Sweet, fruity, warm, earthy	2
dill	Fresh, sweet, herbaceous, slight earthy	2
fir, balsam	Fresh, clean, green, balsamic, sweet	2
lavender	Floral, sweet, balsamic, slightly woody	2
melissa	Delicate, lemony	2
cajeput	Fresh, camphorous, with fruity note	3
coriander	Woody, spicy, sweet	3
cypress	Fresh, herbaceous, slightly woody	3
elemi	Balsamic, fresh, citrusy, peppery, spicy	3
euc. citriodora	Sweet, lemony, fresh, slightly woody	3
euc. radiata	Slightly camphorous, sweet, fruity	3
fir	Fresh, woody, earthy, sweet	3
geranium	Sweet, green, citrus-rosy, fresh	3

Essential Oil	Scent	Intensity
Middle Notes (continued)	(50–80% of the blend)	
helichrysum	Rich, sweet, fruity, slightly honey-like	3
hyssop	Fresh, earthy, woody, fruity	3
juniper	Sweet, musky, tenacious	3
marjoram	Herbaceous, green, spicy	3
melaleuca	Medicinal, fresh, woody, earthy	3
neroli	Floral, citrusy, semi-sweet, delicate	3
niaouli	Earthy, musty, harsh	3
black pepper	Spicy, peppery, musky, warm	3
rosemary cin.	Strong, camphorous, slightly woody	3
rosewood	Sweet, woody, fruity, floral	3
spruce	Fresh, woody, earthy, sweet	3
cardamom	Sweet, spicy, balsamic, slightly floral	4
G. chamomile	Deep, rich, tenacious, cocoa-like	4
R. chamomile	Fresh, sweet, fruity, apple-like	4
ginger	Sweet, spicy-woody, warm, fresh, sharp	4
nutmeg	Sweet, musky, spicy	4
pine, scotch	Fresh, woody, earthy, balsamic	4
thyme	Fresh, medicinal, herbaceous	4
yarrow	Sharp, woody, herbaceous, slight floral	4
oregano	Herbaceous, sharp	5
peppermint	Minty, sharp, intense	5
Middle to Base Notes	(20–80% of the blend)	
clary sage	Spicy, hay-like, sharp, fixative	3
rose	Floral, spicy, rich, deep, sensual, green	3
clove bud	Spicy, warming, slightly bitter, woody	5
ylang ylang	Sweet, heavy, narcotic, tropical floral	5
Base Notes	(5–20% of the blend)	
onycha	Rich, warm, slightly woody, creamy	1
cedarwood	Warm, soft, woody	3
cypress, blue	Long-lasting, warm, woody, earthy	3
frankincense	Rich, deep, warm, balsamic, sweet	3
sandalwood	Soft, woody, sweet, earthy, balsamic	3
jasmine	Powerful, sweet, tenacious, floral	4
myrrh	Warm, earthy, woody, balsamic	4
patchouli	Earthy, sweet-balsamic, rich, wood-like	4
vanilla	Sweet, balsamic, heavy, warm	4
spikenard	Heavy, earthy, animal-like	5
vetiver	Heavy, earthy, balsamic, smoky	5

Methods Of Application

Topical Application

1. **Direct Application.** Apply the oils directly on the area of concern using 1 to 6 drops of oil. More oil is not necessarily better, since a large amount of oil can trigger a detoxification of the surrounding tissue and blood. Such a quick detoxification can be somewhat uncomfortable. To achieve the desired results, 1 to 3 drops of oil is usually adequate. A few guidelines for direct application of the oils are as follows:

   ✓ The feet are the second fastest area of the body to absorb oils because of the large pores. Other quick-absorbing areas include behind the ears and on the wrists.

   ✓ To experience a feeling of peace, relaxation, or energy, 3 to 6 drops per foot are adequate.

   ✓ When massaging a large area of the body, always dilute the oils by 15% to 30% with the V-6 Oil.

   ✓ When applying oils to infants and small children, dilute with V-6 Oil. Use 1 to 3 drops of an essential oil to 1 tablespoon (Tbs.) of V-6 Oil for infants and 1 to 3 drops of an essential oil to 1 teaspoon (tsp.) V-6 Oil for children from 2- to 5-years-old.

   ✓ Do not mix oil blends. Commercially available blends have been specially formulated by someone who understands the chemical constituents of each oil and which oils blend well. The chemical properties of the oils can be altered when mixed improperly, resulting in some undesirable reactions.

   ✓ Layering individual oils is preferred over mixing your own blends. Layering refers to the process of applying one oil, rubbing it in, and then applying another oil. There is no need to wait more than a couple of seconds between each oil, as absorption occurs quite rapidly. If dilution is necessary, the V-6 Oil may be applied on top. The layering technique is not only useful in physical healing but also when doing emotional clearing.

   ✓ The FDA has approved some essential oils for internal use and given them the designation of GRAS (Generally Regarded As Safe for internal consumption). *This designation is listed in the Single Oil Summary Information chart in the Appendix of this book under Safety Data.* **Oils without this designation should never be used internally.**

2. **Vita Flex Therapy.** A simple method of applying oils to contact points (or nerve endings) in the feet or hands; then a series of hand rotation movements at those control points create a vibrational healing energy that carries the oils along the neuroelectrical pathways. The oils help increase the frequency of this healing energy and serve to either help remove any blockage along the pathways or to travel the length of the pathway to benefit the particular organ. Refer to the following pages on Vita Flex therapy for more details.

3. **Raindrop Technique.** A simple application of dropping certain oils like little drops of rain from about 6 inches above the body along the entire length of the spine. It is also a tremendous boost to the immune system, as it releases toxins and kills viruses and bacteria that have accumulated along the spine. See the pages on Raindrop Technique in this section of the *Reference Guide* for more details.

4. **Auricular Therapy.** A method of applying the oils to the rim of the ears. This technique works extremely well for emotional clearing. Some physical benefits can also be obtained from this technique. See the pages on Auricular Therapy in this section of the *Reference Guide* for more details.

5. **Perfume or Cologne.** Wearing the oils as a perfume or cologne can provide wonderful emotional and physical support—not just a beautiful fragrance. (For some simple, yet exquisite, perfume/cologne blends, refer to the book *Natural Perfumes*, by Mindy Green.)

Compresses

1. **Basin.** Fill a wash basin with 2 quarts of hot or cold water, and add the desired essential oils. Stir the water vigorously, and then lay a towel on top of the water. Since the oils will float to the top, the towel will absorb the oils with the water. After the towel is completely saturated, wring out the excess water (leaving much of the oils in the towel), and place the towel over the area needing the compress. For a **hot** compress, cover with a dry towel and a hot water bottle. For a **cold** compress, cover with a piece of plastic or plastic wrap. Finally, put another towel on top and leave for as long as possible (1 to 2 hours is best).
2. **Massage.** Apply a hot wet towel and a dry towel on top of an already massaged area. The moist heat will force the oils deeper into the tissues of the body.

Inhalations

1. **Diffuser.** The easiest and simplest way of putting the oils into the air for inhalation is to use an aromatic diffuser. Diffusers that use a heat source (such as a light bulb ring) will alter the chemical makeup of the oil and its therapeutic qualities. A cold air diffuser uses room-temperature air to blow the oil up against some kind of a nebulizer. This breaks the oils up into a micro-fine mist that is then dispersed into the air, covering hundreds of square feet in seconds. The oils, with their oxygenating molecules, will then remain suspended for several hours to freshen and improve the quality of the air. The antiviral, antibacterial, and antiseptic properties of the oils kill bacteria and help to reduce fungus and mold. Essential oils, when diffused, have been found to reduce the amount of airborne chemicals and metallics as well as help to create greater spiritual, physical, and emotional harmony. The greatest therapeutic benefit is received by diffusing oils for only 15 minutes out of an hour so that the olfactory system has time to recover before receiving more oils. The easiest way to do this is by using a timer that can be set in 15 minute increments over a 24 hour period. Abundant Health offers a variety of cold-air diffusers and timers for your convenience.
2. **Cloth or Tissue.** Put 1 to 3 drops of an essential oil on a paper towel, tissue, cotton ball, handkerchief, towel, or pillow case. Hold it close to your face, and inhale.
3. **Hot Water.** Put 1 to 3 drops of an essential oil into hot water (or a hot mug or glass), and inhale. Again, heat reduces some of the benefits.
4. **Vaporizer or Humidifier.** Put oil in a vaporizer or a humidifier. The cold air types are best since heat reduces some of the benefits.
5. **Fan or Vent.** Put oil on a cotton ball, and attach it to a ceiling fan or to an air vent. This can also work well in a vehicle, as the area is so small.

Baths

1. **Bathwater.** Begin by adding 3 to 6 drops of oil to the bathwater while the tub is filling. Because the individual oils will separate as the water calms down, the skin will quickly draw the oils from the top of the water. People have commented that they were unable to endure more than 6 drops of oil. Such individuals may benefit from adding the oils to a bath and shower gel base first. Soak for 15 minutes.
2. **Bath and Shower Gel.** Begin by adding 3 to 6 drops of oil to ½ oz. of a bath and shower gel base. Add the mixture to the water while the tub is filling. The number of drops can be increased as described above under *Bathwater*. Adding the oils to a bath and shower gel base first allows one to obtain the greatest benefit from the oils, as they are more evenly dispersed throughout the water and not allowed to immediately separate.

3. **Washcloth.** When showering, add 3–6 drops of oil to a bath and shower gel base. Place on a washcloth, and wash the entire body.
4. **Body Sprays.** Fill a small spray bottle with distilled water, and add 10–15 drops of your favorite oil blend or single oils. Shake well, and spray onto the entire body just after taking a bath or shower.

Dishwater, Clothes Washers, And Dryers

The antibacterial properties of essential oils can effectively promote greater hygiene. Add a couple drops of melrose or lemon to dishwater for clean dishes and a great smelling kitchen. Use lemon or another citrus oil to take gum out of clothes. A few drops of Purification in the wash water will kill bacteria and germs in clothes. Put Purification, Joy, or other oil on a wet rag, and place in dryer or mist from a spray bottle directly into the dryer.

Cooking

Essential oils can easily be incorporated into your cooking, as long as you remember that they are very concentrated. Usually only 1 drop is necessary, and sometimes even less. Use a toothpick to help control the addition of smaller amounts of oil by dipping the toothpick into the oil (more oil on the toothpick = stronger flavor, etc.) and then stirring it into the food. Here are a couple examples of recipes where people have used the essential oils for flavoring.

Lemon Tarragon Dressing

1 tablespoon fresh tarragon diced, or 1 teaspoon dried tarragon
1 tablespoon fresh or 1 teaspoon dried basil leaves
1 cup organic extra-virgin, cold-pressed olive oil
dash of pepper
dash of red pepper
6 drops lemon essential oil

Mix well, and drizzle on salad or fish or anything! Keep unused portion in the fridge.
-Submitted by Jill Burk, Saginaw, Michigan (July 2004)

Cream Cheese Icing

8 oz. package of cream cheese
1½ cups of powdered sugar
1 stick of butter
3 drops of tangerine essential oil

Thoroughly cream together the cream cheese, powdered sugar, and butter with an electric beater. Stir in the tangerine oil. Enjoy!
-Submitted by Ellie Ayers (July 2004)

Cleaning and Disinfecting

Put a few drops of **lemon, spruce, or fir** oil on a dust cloth or 10 drops in water in a spray bottle to polish furniture and to clean and disinfect bathrooms and kitchens.

Painting

To effectively remove paint fumes and after smell, add one 15 ml bottle of oil to any 5 gallon bucket of paint. The Abundance blend and citrus oils have been favorites. Either a paint sprayer or brush and roller may be used to apply the paint after mixing the oils into the paint by stirring vigorously. Oils may eventually rise to the top if using a water-based paint. Occasional stirring may be necessary to keep the oils mixed.

Vita Flex Therapy

Vita Flex therapy is based on a small part of a complete system that was developed by Stanley Burroughs during a period of more than fifty years of research and application. Vita Flex uses the reflex system of internal body controls to release tensions, congestions, and maladjustments. When properly applied through specific application of hand rotation movements and control points, a vibrational healing energy is released along the neuroelectrical pathways to an exact point. This healing energy is created by the contact between the fingertips and the reflex (contact) points. The resulting spark of energy follows the neuro pathways of the nervous system to where there is a break in the electrical circuit. Upon reaching the break, any necessary changes are made automatically. This technique is believed to have originated in Tibet many thousands of years ago, long before acupuncture was ever discovered.

The Vita Flex Technique is a superior form of reflexology. Reflexology, as used today, has a tendency to ground out the electrical charge from constant compression and rotation, which causes cell separation, loss of oxygen to subdermal tissues, and further injury. With the Vita Flex technique, people experience less discomfort. Using the thumb and all 4 fingers, the application is much more efficient. There are more than 5,000 Vita Flex points throughout the body (in the complete system as developed by Stanley Burroughs), in comparison to the 365 acupuncture points used in reflexology. With Vita Flex, the weakened or injured areas are corrected on reflected points, thereby preventing further injury.

Combining the electrical frequency of the oils and the frequency of the person receiving the application creates rapid and phenomenal results. "Vita Flex" is derived from the term "vitality through the reflexes" and is a complete, workable system that, when combined with the healing properties of essential oils, can release an unlimited healing power.

Stanley Burroughs' book *Healing for the Age of Enlightenment* explains in detail the system that he designed over many years. For step-by-step instruction of the full Vita Flex treatment, refer to the video, *Vita Flex Instruction* with Tom Woloshyn. This video teaches the proper Vita Flex technique as developed by Stanley Burroughs, including the Atlas Adjustment (a nonchiropractic technique used to quickly and efficiently realign the spine or any other misalignment in the body). Stanley Burroughs also designed the **Vita Flex roller**, or "Relax-a-Roller" to assist one in doing Vita Flex on themselves. This device is a special type of roller with staggered, fine-pointed pegs, placed close enough together so as not to dig in too deeply with heavy pressure. Yet, they are far enough apart to reach all Vita Flex points as one rolls both feet back and forth. With just a few minutes of use, tensions, drowsiness, weariness, and discomfort disappear. Also, by adding the desired oils to the feet and rolling them back and forth on the roller, one can easily achieve the benefits of Vita Flex therapy. These rollers are produced in Canada and are available from Abundant Health.

Key Principles

1. **To reduce any discomfort, fingernails should be cut and filed short.**
2. Remove all jewelry and watches to prevent an interference of energy.
3. Always **DROP** the oils into the palm of your non-dominant hand, and use the dominant hand to stir the oils clockwise 3 times before application. This method will increase the electrical frequency of the oils and significantly improve the results. **To prevent contamination of the oils, do not touch the top of the bottle with any part of your body.**
4. Put a drop of White Angelica on each of your shoulders to protect yourself against any negative energies from the person you are working on.
5. Always start on the bottoms of the feet. Put 3 to 6 drops of Valor on the bottom of each foot. Some may be applied to the area above the brain stem if desired. Hold the bottoms of the feet with your hands: right hand to right foot and left hand to left foot. Continue holding the feet until you feel the body's energy balance. This usually feels like an energy pulse beating in both feet. Another way to balance, which may be preferable to some, is to put 1 drop of Valor on the wrists and hold the wrists crossed together for a few minutes, until you feel a pulse in the tips of the thumb and index finger.
6. Use the Vita Flex charts (*shown on the next couple of pages*) to determine where the oils should be placed during the therapy. One to three drops of oil may be applied to the specific Vita Flex points of the foot. Vita Flex points on the hand can be used as an alternative to extremely sensitive or sore feet. Apply the oil(s).
7. Apply the Vita Flex technique as follows: Starting with the fingers on their pads, curl the fingers up and over onto the nails (see photo examples on the next page). Increasing pressure is applied until the fingers are curled almost completely over on the nails. Pressure is then immediately released to create the spark of energy and send it on its way. The curling should be one continuous motion, not jerky, with medium to heavy pressure being placed on the contact point. Never press and hold while performing this technique. This may be done several times on the same spot to obtain the desired results. Some leverage can be achieved by placing the thumb of the same hand around to the other side of the foot or hand on which the Vita Flex is being performed. This allows the hand to operate in a fashion similar to a pipe wrench, which increases pressure on the pipe as it is twisted.

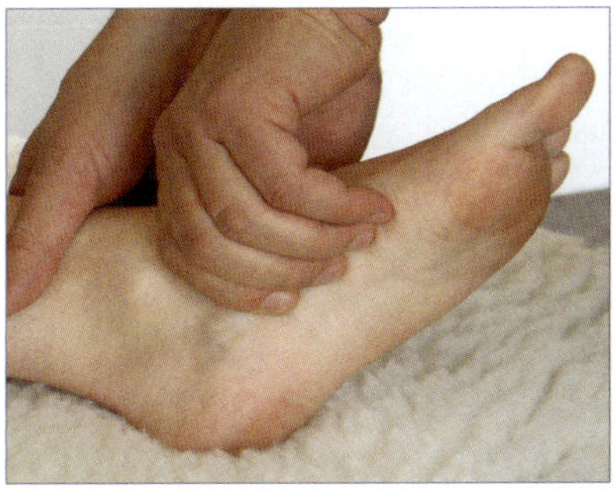

Vita Flex Start Position

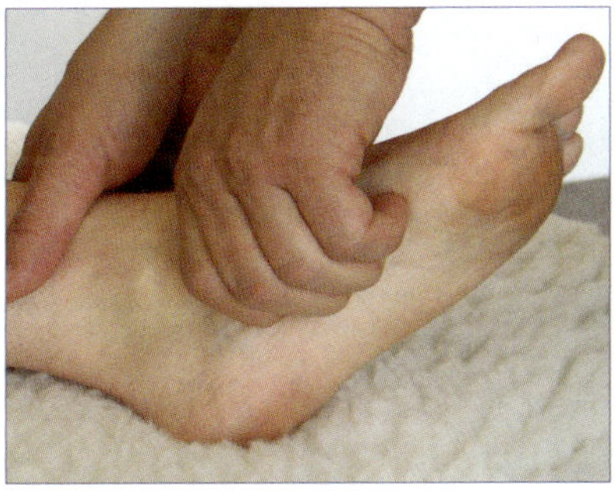

Vita Flex Middle Position

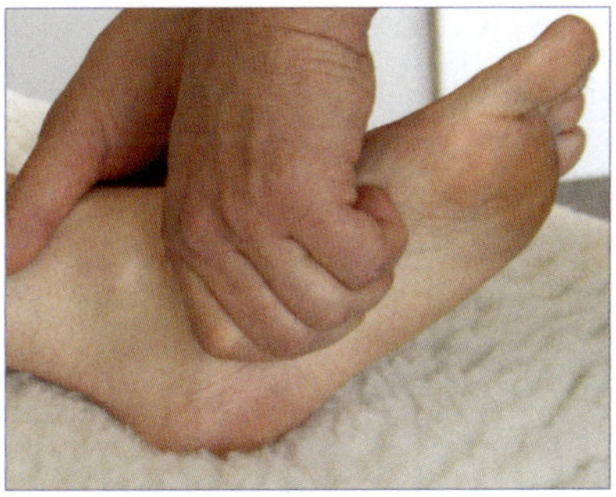

Vita Flex End Position

VITA FLEX HAND CHART

Vita Flex points in this hand chart correspond to those on the feet. Occasionally the feet can be too sensitive for typical Vita Flex therapy. Working with the hands will not only affect the specific body points but may also help to provide some pain relief to the corresponding points on the feet. (Refer to Stanley Burroughs' book *Healing for the Age of Enlightenment*, p. 78, for a more detailed explanation.)

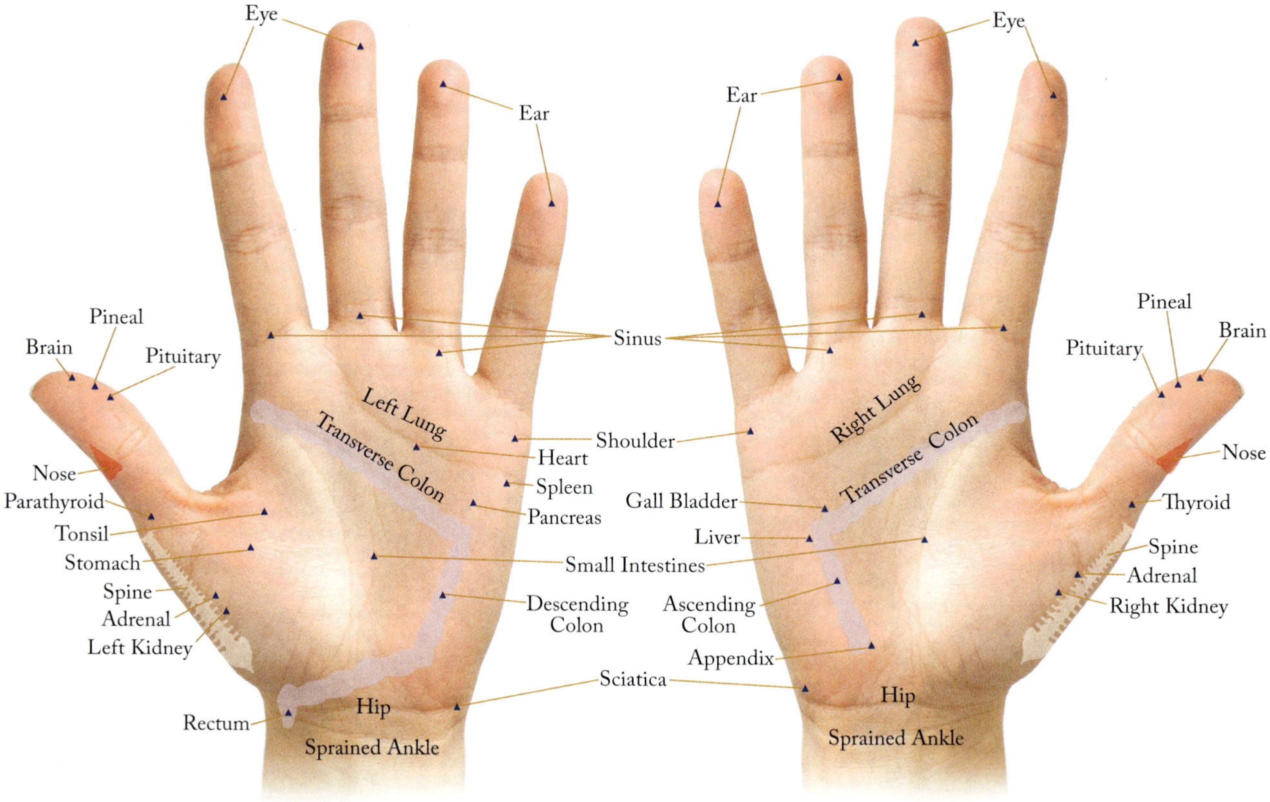

Vita Flex Feet Chart

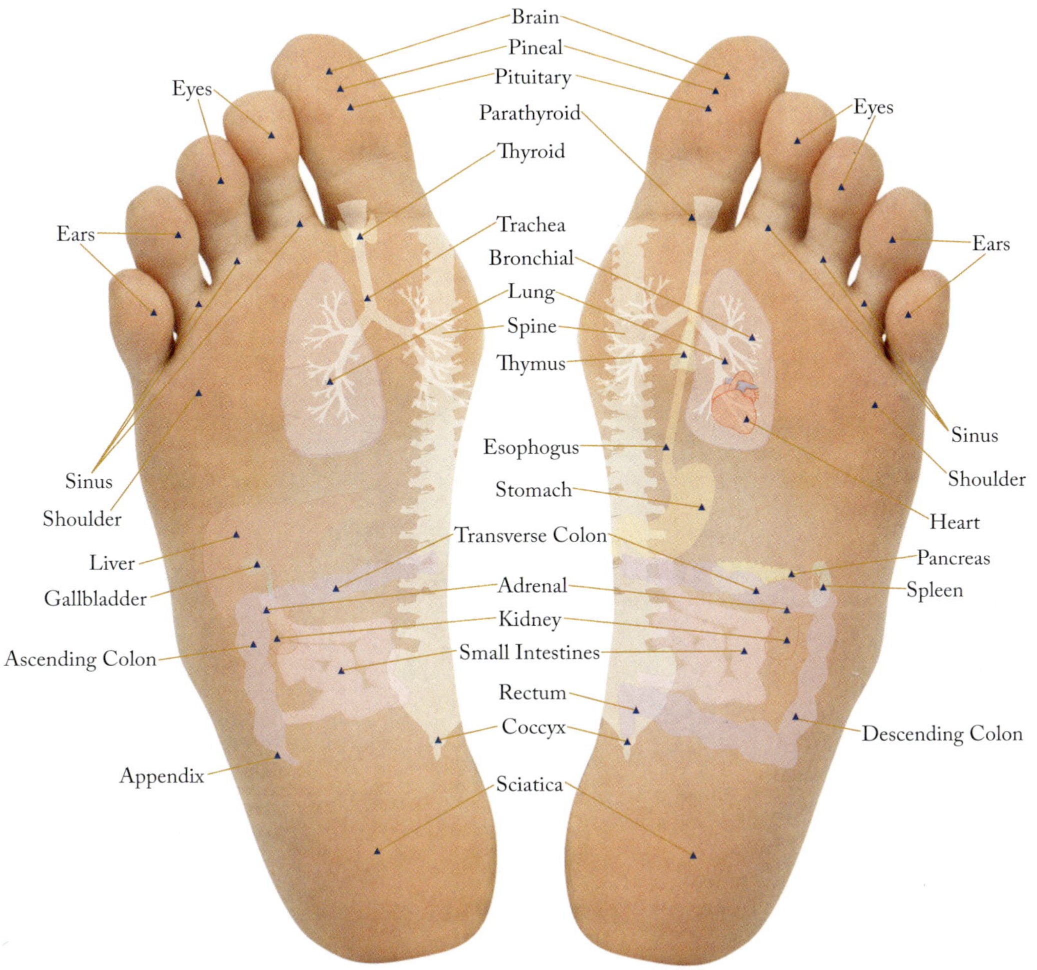

Right Foot **Left Foot**

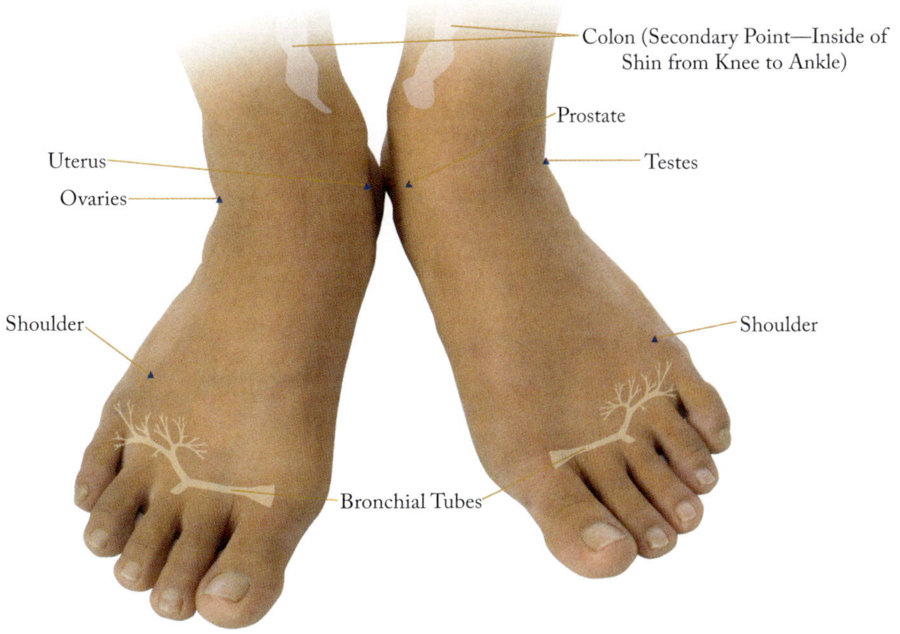

Note: This chart combines the work of Stanley Burroughs (Vita Flex Charting) and D. Gary Young (Electrical Frequency Tracing). Refer to their respective books, listed in the bibliography, for more detailed information.

Auricular Internal Body Points

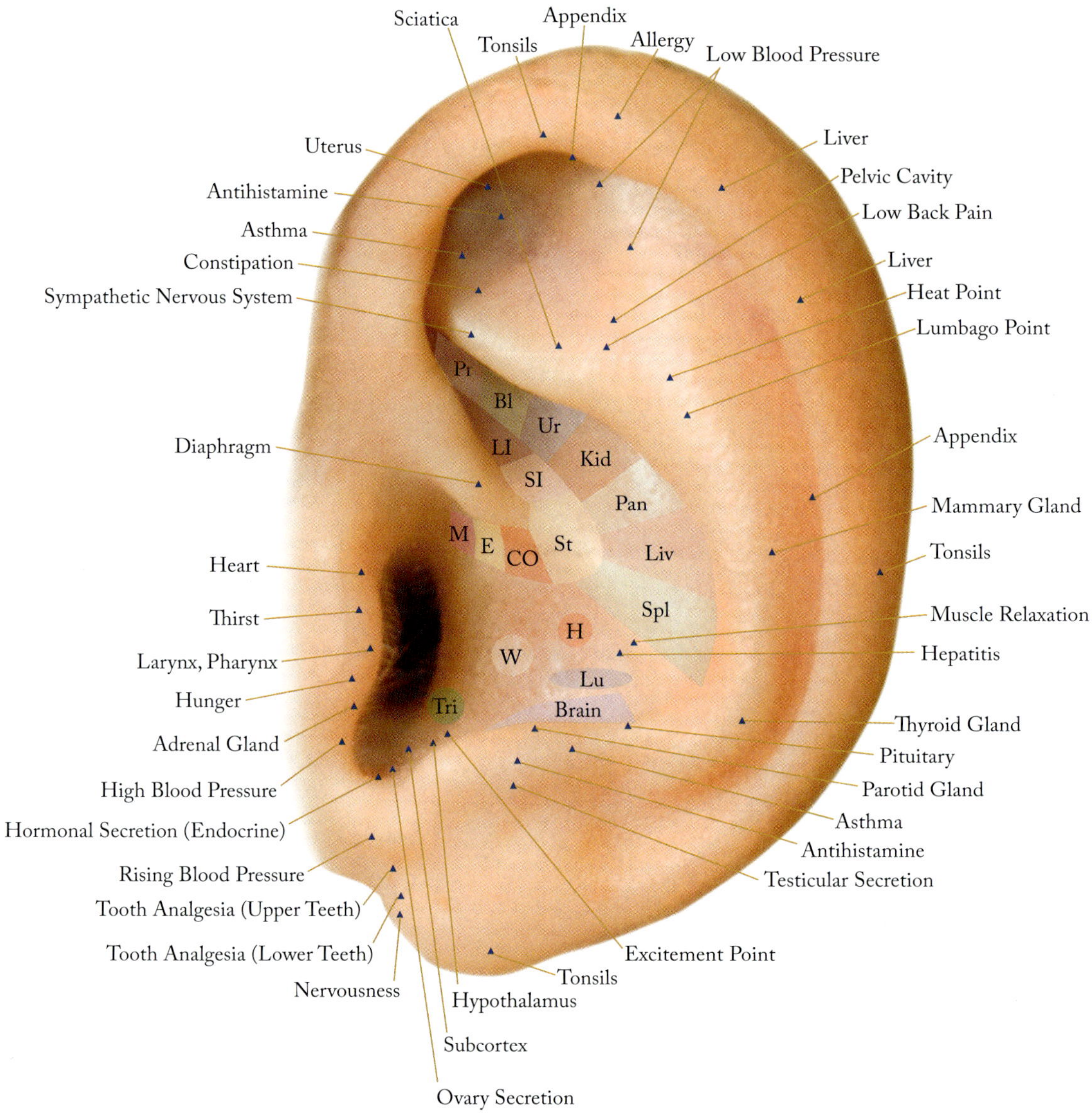

Bl: Bladder
CO: Cardiac Orifice
E: Esophogus
H: Heart
Kid: Kidney
LI: Large Intestine
Liv: Liver
Lu: Lungs
M: Mouth
Pan: Pancreas
Pr: Prostate
SI: Small Intestine
Spl: Spleen
ST: Stomach
Tri: Triple Warmer
Ur: Ureter
W: Windpipe/Trachea

Raindrop Technique

This application technique was developed by D. Gary Young, aromatologist and one of North America's leading experts on the art and science of aromatherapy. This technique involves dropping the oils directly onto the spine from about six inches above the body. The oils are then worked into the spine using light strokes with the fingers, which stimulate energy impulses and disperse the oils along the nervous system throughout the entire body. In this way, the body can be brought into balance and the energy centers can be cleared and realigned. This method also helps to reduce spinal inflammations and to kill viruses that hibernate along the spinal column, as well as to help straighten any spinal curvatures. Although a session only lasts from about 45 minutes to an hour, the oils will continue to work in the body for a week or more following the treatment. The Raindrop Technique that is explained below is an abbreviated form. The video entitled *Raindrop Technique* by D. Gary Young (*available from Abundant Health*) provides step-by-step instructions for this technique.

Oils Used in the Raindrop Technique

Valor—is the first and most important oil used in this technique because it helps balance the electrical energies within the body. It also helps create an environment where structural alignment can occur.

Thyme—is used for its ability to support the immune system by attacking any bacteria, fungus, infection, or virus that may be present. It may also help one overcome fatigue and physical weakness after an illness.

Oregano—works in conjunction with thyme to strengthen the immune system and to attack bacteria and viruses. It may also act as an antiseptic for the respiratory system, help balance metabolism, and help strengthen the vital centers of the body.

Cypress—is used for its antibacterial, anti-infectious, antimicrobial, and diuretic properties. In addition, it may function as a decongestant for the circulatory and lymphatic systems.

Birch/Wintergreen—is great for removing discomfort associated with the inflammation of bones, muscles, and joints. It may also help cleanse the lymphatic system.

Basil—is relaxing to spastic muscles and is stimulating to the nerves and to the adrenal glands.

Peppermint—is used to calm and strengthen the nerves, reduce inflammation, and is highly effective when dealing with conditions related to the respiratory system. It also has a synergistic and enhancing effect on all other oils.

Marjoram—is used to relax spastic muscles, soothe the nerves, relieve cramps, aches, and pains and to help calm the respiratory system.

Aroma Siez—may help to relax, calm, and relieve the tension of spastic muscles resulting from sports injury, fatigue, or stress.

Ortho Ease—is the crowning oil to this application. It is used to help relax all the muscles of the back and legs and to help reduce any stress, arthritic pain, or tension that may exist.

V-6 Oil—is used to help dilute any of the oils that may be somewhat caustic to the skin. It should always be used with oregano and thyme and can be used with any of the other oils based upon the person's skin sensitivity.

Note: The oils listed above have many more benefits. *For more specific information, please refer to the sections in this book on Singles and Blends.*

Raindrop Technique

1. Remove all jewelry or metal to allow the energy to flow freely. Put a drop of **White Angelica** on each of your shoulders to protect yourself against any negative energies coming from the person receiving the treatment.
2. Have the person lie face up on a table with their body as straight as possible on the table. The person receiving the treatment should be as comfortable as possible, so the arms can be resting along side the body or resting on the top of their hips, whichever they prefer (don't let their hands touch each other, as this will tend to short circuit the flow of energy through their body). Cover the person with a sheet to protect their privacy and to keep them warm as you roll them over and alternate between working on their back and working on their legs and feet.
3. Apply **3** drops of **Valor** on each shoulder as well as 6 drops on each foot. Hold right foot/shoulder with right hand and left foot/shoulder with left hand (crossing hands if necessary—see the photo illustration entitled, "Valor Balance on Feet") for 5 to 10 minutes or until you can feel an energy pulse in the person's feet. For this part of the application, it works best if there is another person assisting in the treatment. If you are working by yourself, do the feet only. **Valor** is used to balance, and it works well on the energy alignment of the body. **This is the most important oil that is used in this application.**

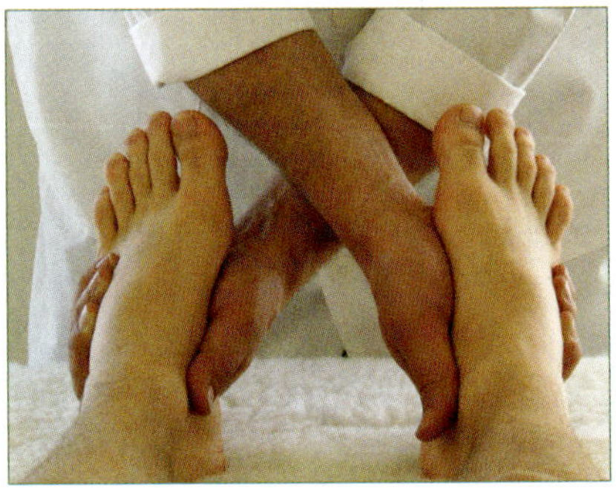

Valor Balance on Feet

4. First apply 2 drops of **thyme** to the Vita Flex spine points along the inside edge of each foot, working it in 3 times with the Vita Flex technique (*refer to Vita Flex Technique in this same section, Key Principle #7 and photo illustrations for an explanation of this technique*). Repeat this procedure with each of the following oils, one at a time: **oregano**, **cypress**, **birch/wintergreen**, **basil**, and **peppermint**. Then, have the person roll over onto their stomach, and perform steps 5 through 14 on their spine.
5. Hold the bottle of **thyme** about 6 inches from the spine, and evenly space **4 to 5** drops from the sacrum (tailbone) to the neck. Work it in evenly along the curvature of the spine with gentle upward strokes. Apply **5** drops of **oregano,** and work it in the same way. Then, apply **10 to 15** drops of **V-6 Oil** to prevent any discomfort, since both these oils can be quite caustic.
6. Using the very tips of the fingers, alternate between left hand and right hand as you very lightly work up the spine from the sacrum to the base of the neck with short, brush-like strokes. Follow the curvature of the spine, and repeat 2 more times.

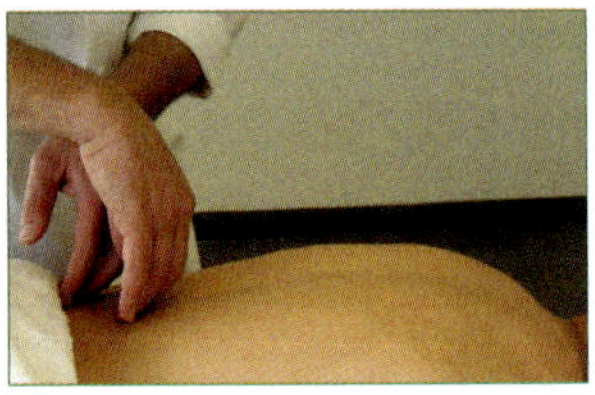
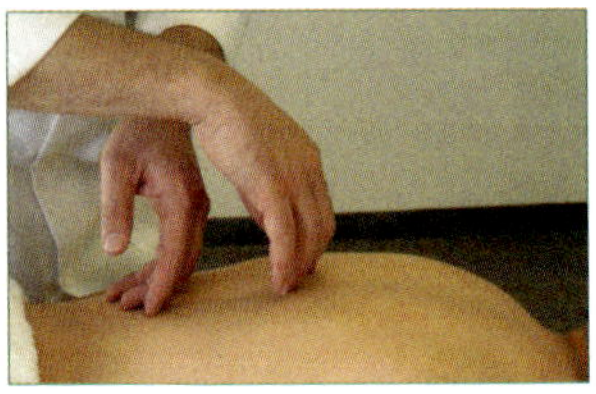
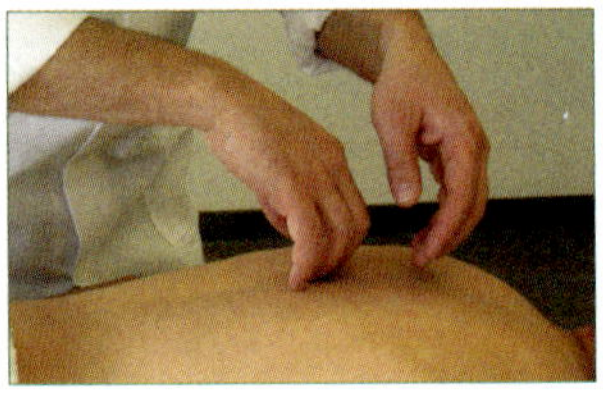

7. Using your finger tips again, softly brush up a few inches from the sacrum and then out to either side of the body; right hand to the right and left hand to the left.

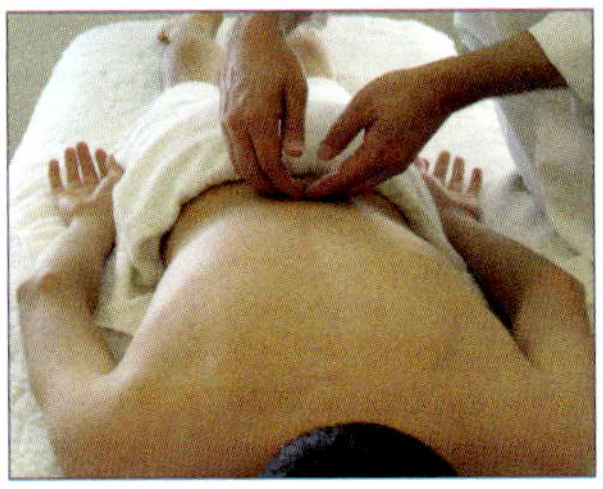
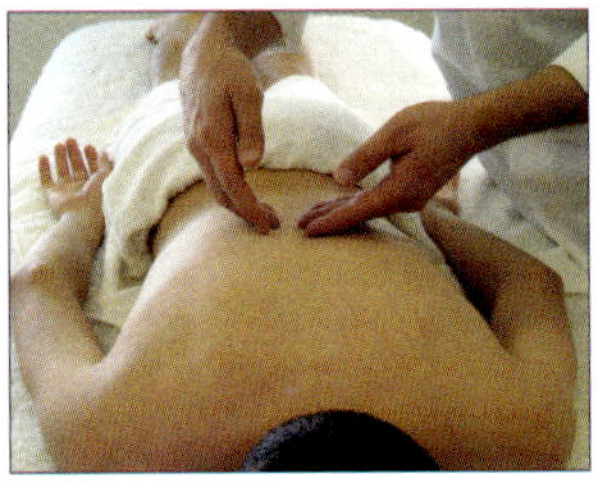
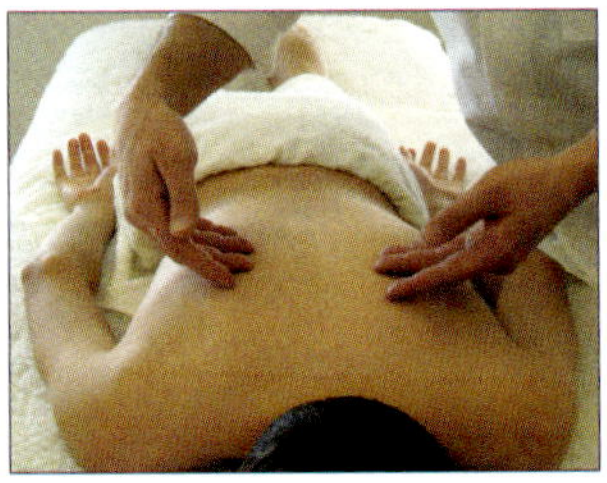
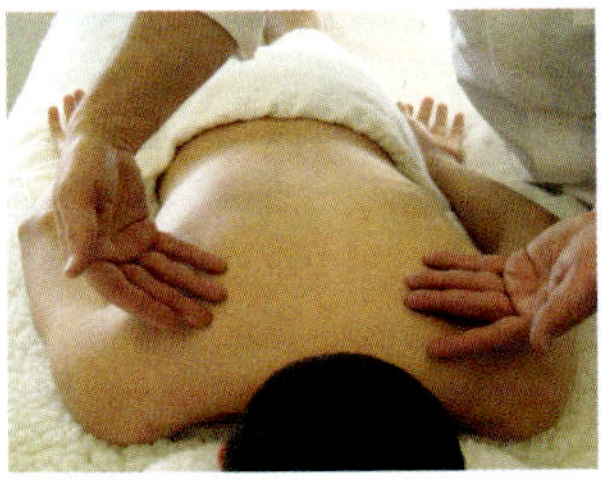

Repeat this step from the sacrum, but go a few more inches up the spine and then out to the sides. Then again from the sacrum, go up a few more inches and then out. Then do it again, each time going further up the spine until you reach the base of the neck and flare out along the shoulders. This entire step should then be repeated 2 more times.

8. Using your finger tips again, start at the sacrum and, in full-length strokes, lightly brush all the way up the spine to the base of the neck and then out over the shoulders. Repeat 2 more times.
9. Evenly space **4 to 5** drops of **cypress** from the sacrum to the neck. Work it in evenly along the curvature of the spine with gentle upward strokes. Then apply the oils of **birch/wintergreen, basil, and peppermint** in the same manner.
10. Place both hands side by side (parallel to the spine) and, using the tips of the fingers, massage in a circular, clockwise motion, just off to one side of the spine, from the sacrum up to the neck. **Remember to never work directly on the spine**. Apply moderate pressure, and move a finger's width at a time. This will help to loosen the muscles and allow the spine to straighten itself. After doing one side of the spine, move around the person, and work the other side of the spine from the sacrum to the neck in the same manner. Repeat 2 more times on either side.

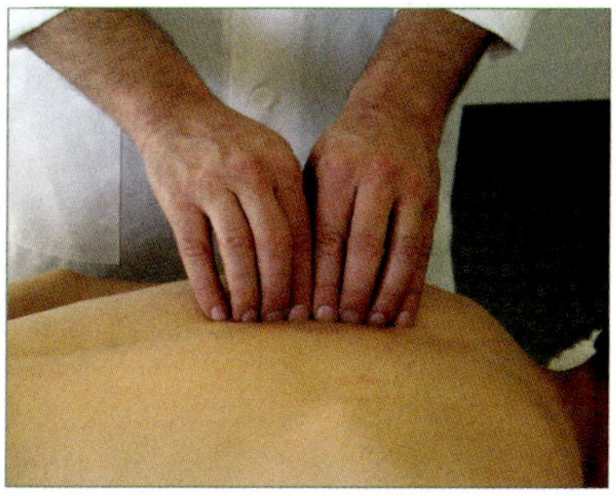

11. Using whichever hand is most comfortable to you, place the index and middle finger on either side of the spine at the sacrum. Place the other hand on top of the first, partway down the 2 fingers. Apply moderate pressure and, with a quick, forward and back continued sawing motion of the hand on top, slide the fingers a little at a time up the spine to the skull. Move the fingers upward slowly during the sawing motion. Once the skull is reached, apply gentle but firm pressure to push the skull forward, stretching the spine. Return to the sacrum, and repeat 2 more times.

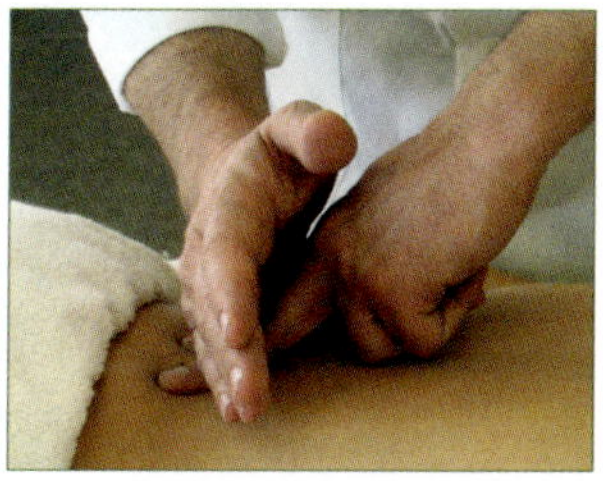

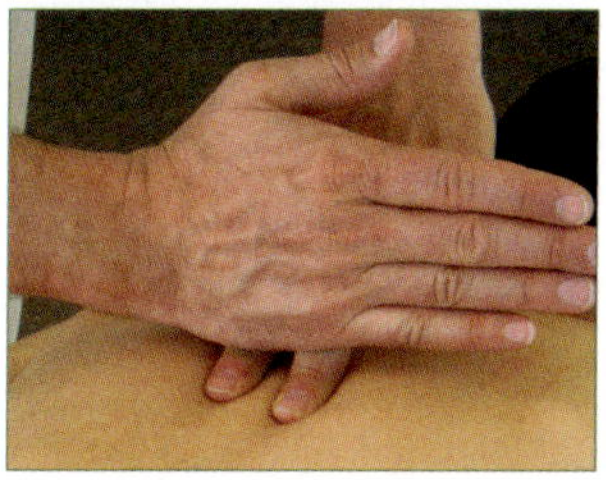

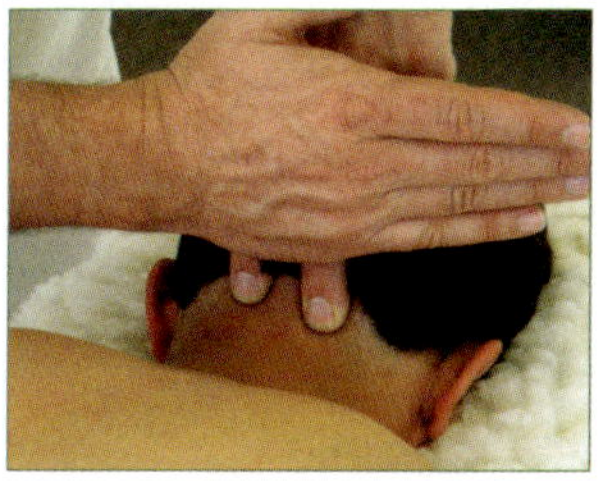

12. Place the thumbs of each hand on either side of the spine at the sacrum, and point them towards each other. Next, using the Vita Flex technique, roll the thumbs up and over onto the thumbnails, applying some pressure straight down during the roll. Then release and slide the thumbs up an inch or so, and repeat the roll with pressure. Continue up to the base of the neck, and then return to the sacrum and repeat 2 more times. This will become easier with practice.

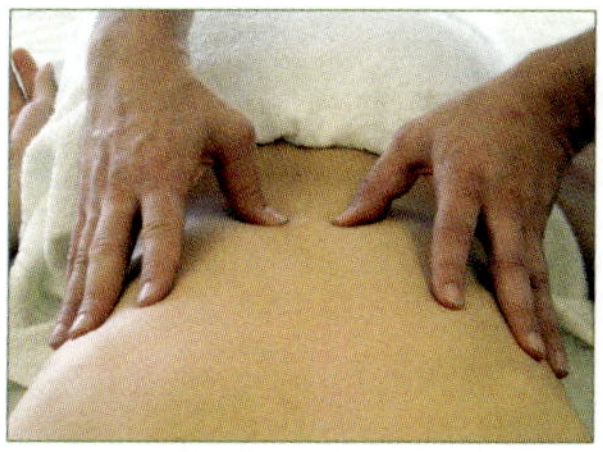

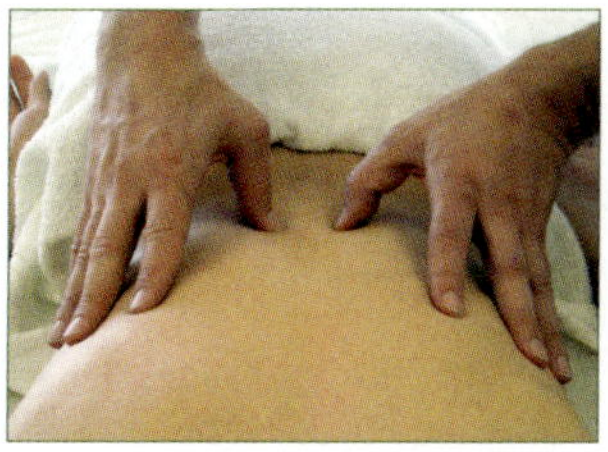

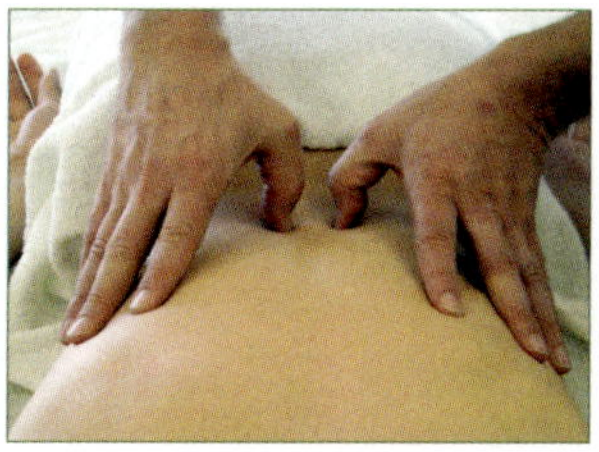

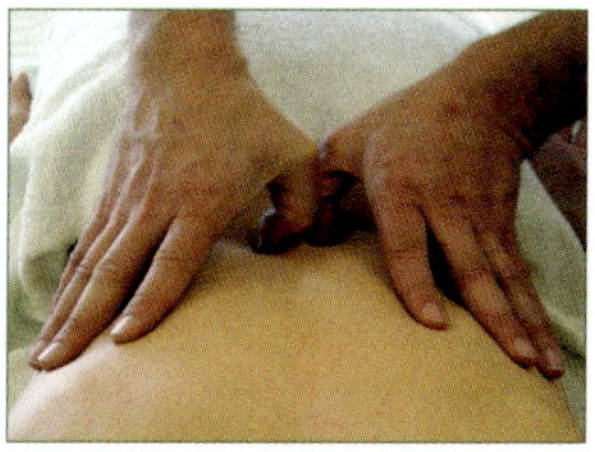

13. Apply 5 to 6 drops of **marjoram** up the spine, and work it in. Then apply 5 to 6 drops of **Aroma Siez** to each side and away from the spine. Gently massage these oils into the muscle tissue all over the back to soothe and relax the patient. After the oils have been massaged in well, you may cover the person with the sheet and rest for approximately 5 minutes. Apply **Ortho Ease** over the entire area of the back, and gently massage it in. Then cover the person to keep them warm, and massage **Ortho Ease** into the legs. This will help to relax the muscles that may be pulling on the spine.

14. Fold a hand towel, soak it in hot water, wring it out, and lay it along the entire length of the spine. Take a dry bath towel, fold it in half lengthwise, and place it over the hot wet towel. Be extremely sensitive to the feelings of the person, as the heat may build along the spine. The heat will gradually build for 5 to 8 minutes and then cool right down to normal. If the heat becomes too uncomfortable, remove the towels and apply V-6 Oil. Then replace the towels and continue until the wet towel becomes cold. If the person's back is still hot, cover with a dry towel and allow the back to cool down slowly.

15. After the person's back begins to cool down, gently stretch the spine by crossing hands and straddling the spine with your hands—one pointing towards the top of the spine and the other towards the bottom as shown in the adjacent photo. Starting in the middle, gently press the hands downwards and apart towards opposite ends of the spine. Then move the hands apart more, and repeat the stretch. Continue until the ends of the spine are reached.

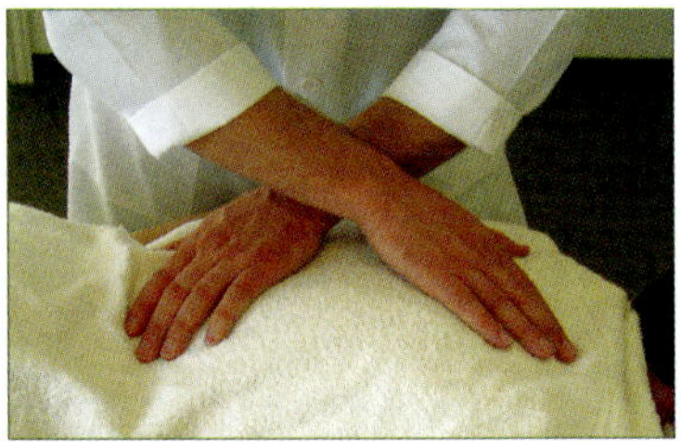

16. Remove the wet towels and have the person roll over onto their back. Apply 2 to 3 drops of **birch/ wintergreen** along the inside of each leg from the knee to the heel and up the inside of the foot to the big toe. Layer it in, and apply the oils of **cypress, basil, and peppermint** in the same fashion. Then work the same area using the Vita Flex technique. The inside of the shin corresponds to the colon. By working this area, you are opening the colon and allowing it to expel any toxins released during the Raindrop Technique.

17. The final step is to perform another gentle stretching of the spine. If you are working alone, put your right hand behind the base of the head and your left hand under the chin. Very gently pull to create a slight tension and release. Do this 3 times, and then move to the feet. Hold above the ankles, and gently pull and release 3 times. If you have an assistant, one person can hold the head and the other hold the feet. Then together, apply a gentle tension and hold for a few minutes. This is then completed by the person at the head doing a very slight pull and release 3 times.

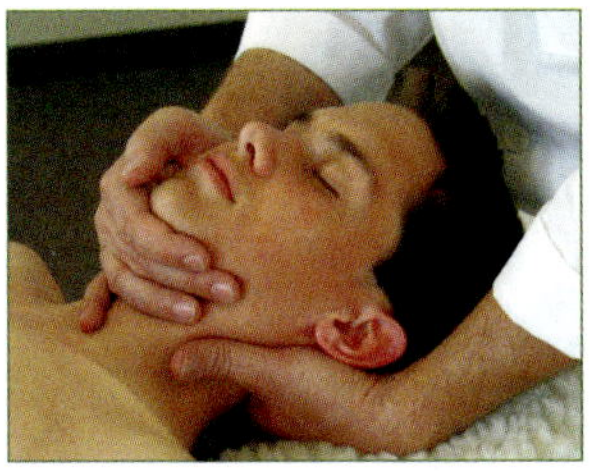

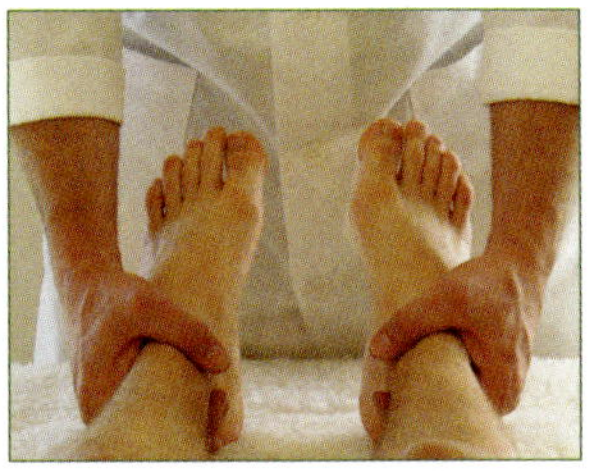

18. If certain systems of the body need work, have the person roll back over onto their stomach, and use the applicable blends and/or singles with the Vita Flex technique on the spine. Refer to the chart of the autonomic nervous system to help with placement of the oils along the spine.

By stimulating the Central Nervous System, you have just given someone a total treatment, affecting every system in the body, including emotional release and support. Even though the oils continue to work in the body for a week or more, one application may last months, or it may be necessary to repeat the application every week until the body begins to respond. The object is to develop a new memory in the tissues of the body and to train them to hold themselves in place. **(For a list of videos that effectively demonstrate this valuable application technique, refer to *Video Listing* in the Bibliography section of this book.)**

Another aspect of the Raindrop Technique is the ability to **customize it** to the needs of the receiver. Each Raindrop Technique session should begin with the **Valor** essential oil blend and the single oils of **oregano** (*Origanum compactum* CT carvacrol) and **thyme** (*Thymus vulgaris* CT thymol). However, after that, the remaining oils can be replaced with others more specific to the condition or body system needing to be affected. To assist with this customization, the following chart is a partial list of single oils and oil blends under the particular body system that they affect. This chart is a condensed excerpt from the Body System Chart shown in the Appendix of this book *(Refer to the full chart in the Appendix for other products that can assist in strengthening a particular body system)*.

Cardiovascular System	Digestive System	Emotional Balance*	Hormonal System	Immune System	Nervous System	Respiratory System
anise	anise	angelica	anise	Abundance	angelica	anise
Aroma Life	cardamon	Australian Blue	clary sage	cistus	Brain Power	Aroma Siez
basil	celery seed	chamomile (both)	coriander	Citrus Fresh	carrot	cajeput
cajeput	clove	fir, white	davana	clove	cedarwood	clove
carrot	coriander	frankincense	Dragon Time	cumin	celery seed	eucalyptus (all)
Christmas Spirit	cumin	Gathering	EndoFlex	cypress, blue	chamomile (both)	fir (all)
clove	cypress, blue	geranium	fennel	Exodus II	En-R-Gee	hyssop
copal	Di-Gize	jasmine	fleabane	frankincense	balsam fir	laurel
cypress	fennel	juniper	goldenrod	galbanum	frankincense	lavandin
fleabane	ginger	Lady Sclareol	jasmine	ImmuPower	hyssop	lemon
goldenrod	juniper	lavender	Mister	laurel	juniper	melaleuca (all)
grapefruit	JuvaFlex	onycha	myrrh	ledum	lavender	Melrose
helichrysum	Juva Cleanse	orange	myrtle	lemon	myrrh	myrtle
hyssop	laurel	palmarosa	nutmeg	lemongrass	nutmeg	peppermint
lavandin	lemon	petitgrain	sage	lime	PanAway	pine
lavender	mandarin	pine	sage lavender	melaleuca	Peace & Calming	Raven
Longevity	myrtle	sage lavender	SclarEssence	Mountain savory	pepper, black	ravensara
marjoram	orange	sandalwood	Sensation	myrrh	peppermint	RC
onycha	peppermint	spikenard	vetiver	nutmeg	sage lavender	rosemary ver-
palmarosa	Purification	spruce	yarrow	orange	sandalwood	banon
rosemary	rosemary	Tranquil	ylang ylang	ravensara	spruce	sage lavender
tsuga	SclarEssence	Valor		sage	tansy, blue	spruce
ylang ylang	spearmint	vetiver		Thieves	valerian	thyme linalol
	tarragon	ylang ylang		yarrow	vetiver	tsuga

**The majority of the essential oil blends in this book deal with emotional balance and are, therefore, too numerous to list here. Refer to the Body Systems Chart in the Appendix for more possible blends.*

The booklet entitled *A Statistical Validation of Raindrop Technique*, by David Stewart, PhD, RA (available from Abundant Health), is the result of research conducted by the distribution of over 3,000 surveys to individuals that have either received a Raindrop Technique session, administered Raindrop Technique sessions to others, or both. The results of the survey were tabulated, and the following are excerpts from these results, showing overwhelming evidence that "Raindrop is thought by the vast majority of its participants to benefit people in ways both objective and subjective, physical and emotional, social and spiritual."

	Perceived Results of Raindrop as Expressed by 416 clients receiving 3,584 Raindrops			**Perceived Results of Raindrop as Expressed by Clients to the 265 Facilitators Responding to this Survey for 11,256 Raindrop Procedures Administered**		
a.	Positive 97.0%	Neutral 2.5%	Negative 0.5%	Positive 96.3%	Neutral 3.5%	Negative 0.2%
b.	Pleasant 97.9%	Neutral 1.4%	Unpleasant 0.4%	Pleasant 96.4%	Neutral 3.0%	Unpleasant 0.6%
c.	Resulted in Healing 15.9%	No Perceptible Results 83.9%	Resulted in Harm or Injury 0.2%	Resulted in Healing 87.7%	No Perceptible Results 12.0%	Resulted in Harm or Injury 0.3%
d.	Felt Better Afterwards 97.7%	No Change in Feeling 1.4%	Felt Worse Afterwards 0.9%	Felt Better Afterwards 96.0%	No Change in Feeling 3.4%	Felt Worse Afterwards 0.6%
e.	Health Improved 89.1%	No Change in Health 10.9%	Health Got Worse 0.0%	Health Improved 90.8%	No Change in Health 9.2%	Health Got Worse 0.03%
f.	Emotional State Improved 86.2%	No Change in Emotions 13.4%	Emotional State Worsened 0.4%	Emotional State Improved 91.0%	No Change in Emotions 8.5%	Emotional State Worsened 0.5%
g.	Would Receive it Again 99.9%	Maybe So, Maybe Not 0.1%	Would Never Receive it Again 0.0%	Would Receive it Again 96.7%	Maybe So, Maybe Not 3.2%	Would Never Receive it Again 0.1%

–This information is included here with permission from the author, David Stewart.

Autonomic Nervous System

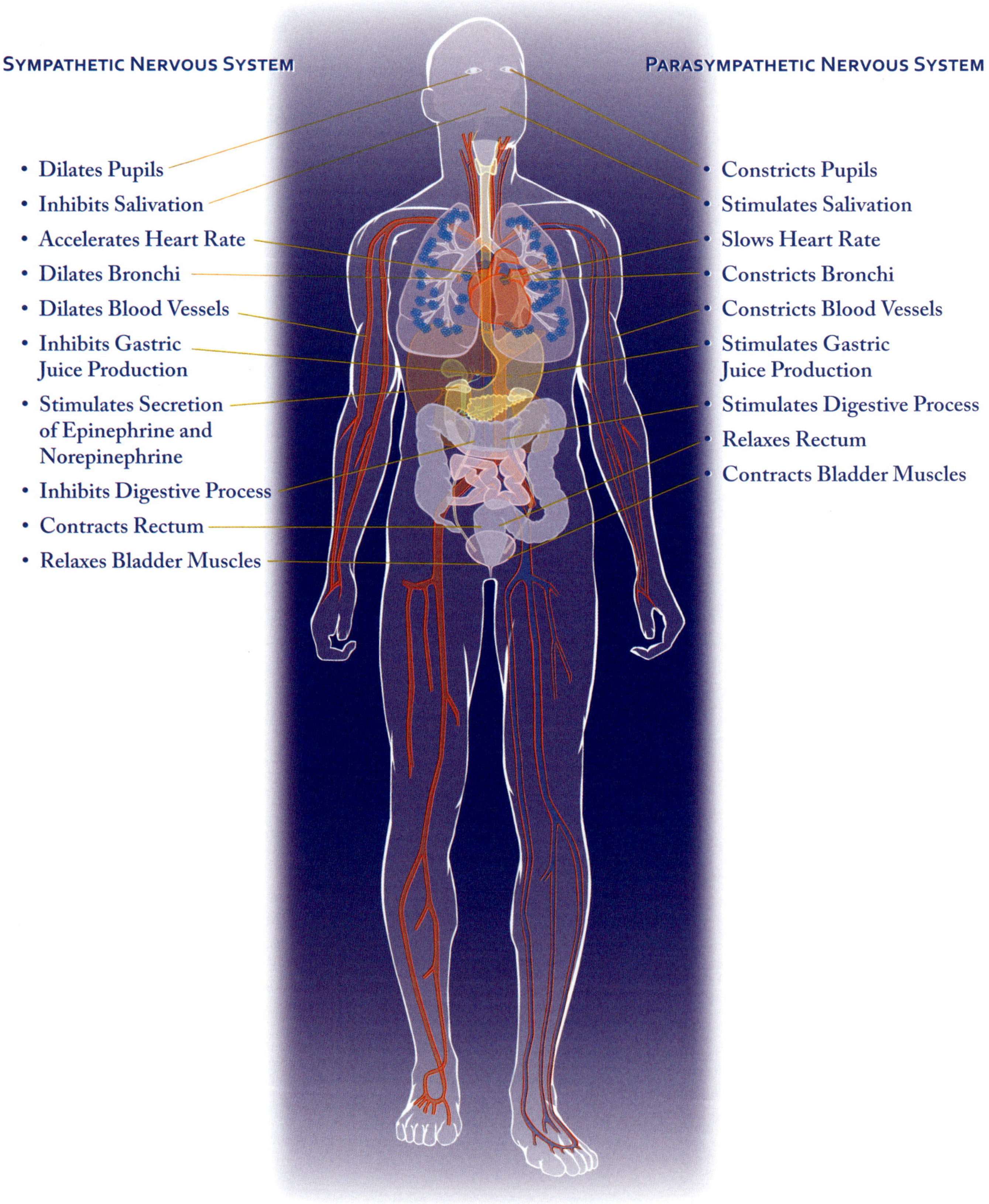

Digestive Tract

"The gastrointestinal (GI) tract is a tube, 25–32 feet in length, which begins at the mouth and ends at the anus. It comprises the mouth, pharynx, esophagus, stomach, small intestine (duodenum, jejunum, and ileum), large intestine (cecum, ascending colon, transverse colon, and descending colon), rectum, and anus. Accessory organs—the liver, pancreas, and gallbladder—all play an important role in digestion.

"Digestion begins when food mixes with enzymes in saliva. The process is then carried on in the stomach by hydrochloric acid (HCI) and pepsin. Food is liquefied in the stomach and passes into the small intestine, where it is further broken down by digestive enzymes from the pancreas (protease digests proteins, amylase digests carbohydrates, and lipase digests fats.) . . . The gallbladder secretes bile to aid absorption of fats and fat-soluble vitamins. . . .

"Most food absorption takes place in the small intestine, while water, electrolytes, and some of the final products of digestion are absorbed in the large intestine" (*Alternative Medicine—The Definitive Guide*, p. 715).

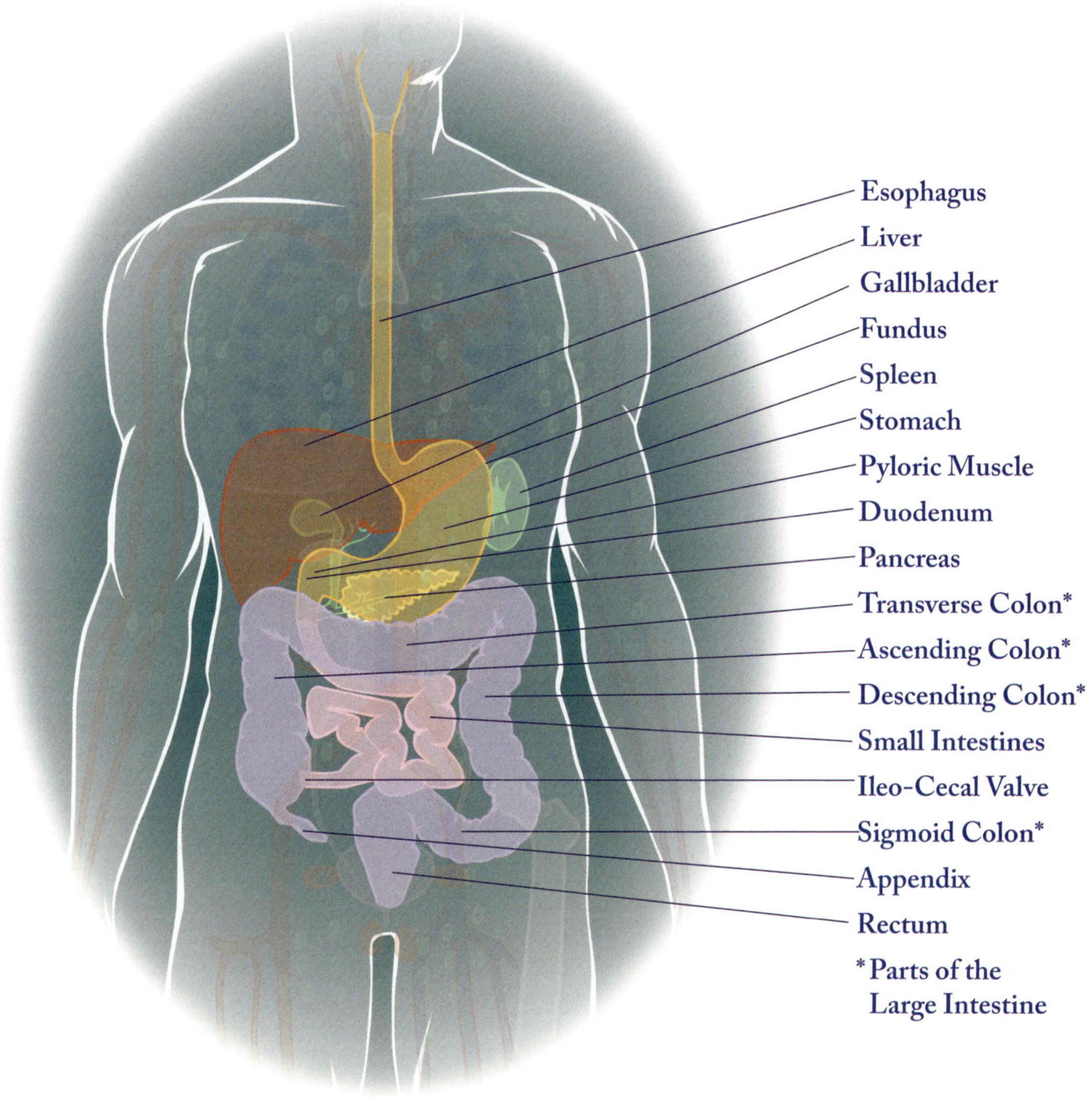

Nose And Olfactory System

When an odor molecule is inhaled into the nasal cavity, it is first sensed by the olfactory cells that are part of the olfactory epithelium. The olfactory epithelium is comprised of 2 small patches of olfactory nerves (each about 1 cm square) that lie on the roof of the nasal cavity. The olfactory cells within the olfactory epithelium are specialized nerve cells that extend cilia (small hair-like structures) from their dendrites into the nasal cavity. Each of these cilia has a receptor that binds it to a specific type of odor molecule. When an odor molecule binds to a receptor on the cilia of an olfactory cell, the olfactory cell passes the signal through the cribriform plate (the bone at the roof of the nasal cavity) to the olfactory bulb. The olfactory bulb, in turn, sends those impulses along the lateral olfactory tract to 5 different structures in the brain, including the amygdala (which is responsible for storing and releasing emotional trauma), the anterior olfactory nucleus (which helps process smells), the olfactory tubercle, the piriform cortex (which passes the signal on to other structures that create a conscious perception of the odor), and the entorhinal cortex (which processes stimuli before sending them on to the hippocampus, the long-term memory center of the brain). Anatomically, the olfactory system is closely connected to the limbic system of the brain. The limbic system includes structures such as the hippocampus (long-term memory), the amygdala (emotions), the hypothalamus (autonomic nervous system and hormones), and the cingulate gyrus (regulates blood pressure, heart rate, and attention). It is due to the fact that the olfactory system is so closely connected to the limbic system that essential oils have such profound physiological and psychological effects

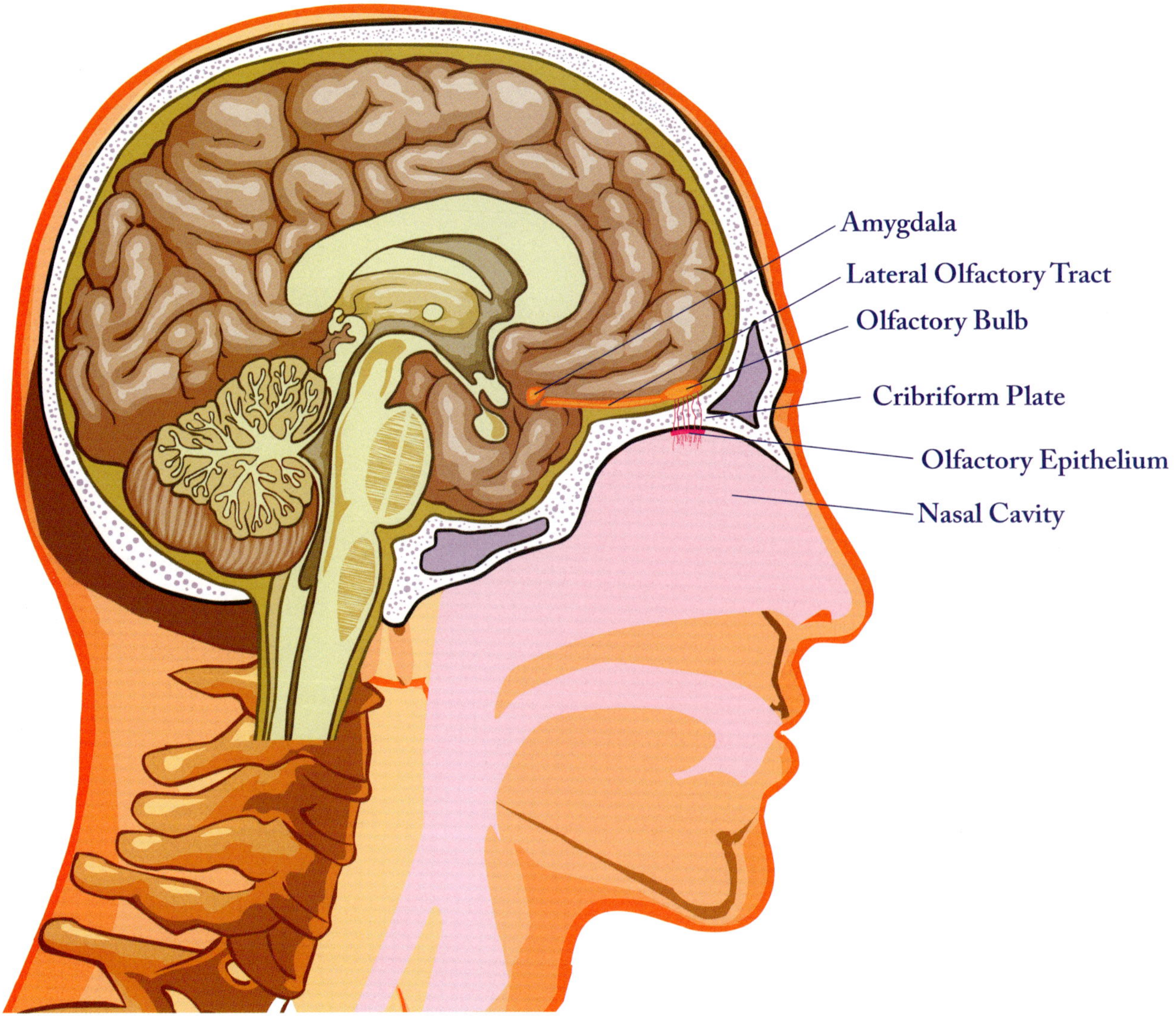

Auricular Emotional Therapy

**If more than one oil/blend is indicated, layer them on one at a time.*

***When working on the ear, apply Harmony and Forgiveness to the entire ear, and apply Valor on the feet.*

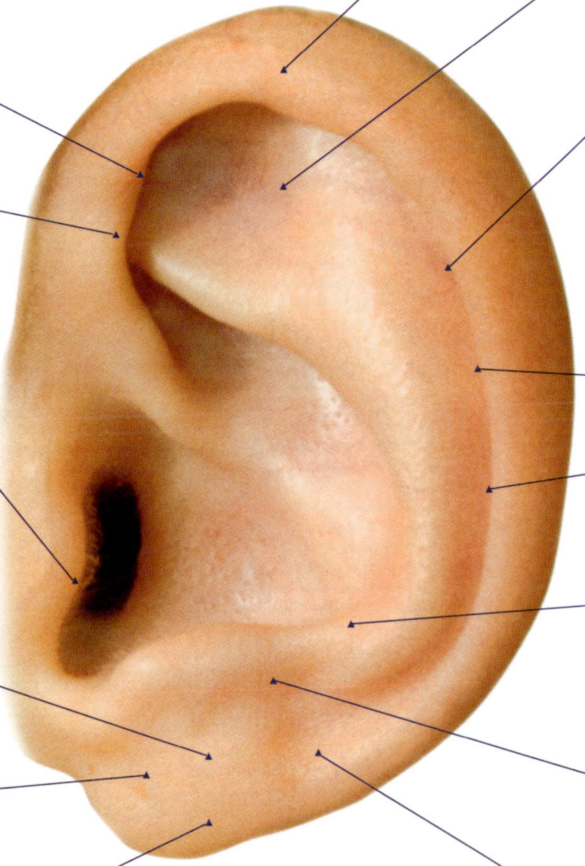

SYMPATHY & GUILT
Use Joy and Inspiration.

SELF PITY
Use Acceptance.

REJECTION
Use Forgiveness and Acceptance. Work the rejection points on both ears. For rejection from mother, use geranium. For rejection from father, use lavender. While applying the oils say, "I choose to accept my Mother/Father for what they have done or not done. It is their life and not mine."

EYES & VISION
To Improve Eyesight, use 10 drops lemongrass, 5 cypress, and 3 eucalyptus in ½ oz. (1 Tbsp) of V-6 Mixing Oil.

HEART
Use Joy to stimulate the pituitary.
Use Valor and Release to release the anger.

OPEN THE MIND
Use Valor and Motivation. Take deep breaths to express oneself.

MOTHER: Geranium
Sexual Abuse: Geranium, ylang ylang.
Abandonment: Geranium, Forgiveness, Acceptance.

FATHER: Lavender
Sexual Abuse: Lavender, ylang ylang.
Male Abuse: Helichrysum, lavender.

DEPRESSION
Any of the following: Valor, Joy, Hope, White Angelica, Peace & Calming, Citrus Fresh, Christmas Spirit, Gentle Baby.
Use whichever blend(s) works for you.

OVERWHELMED
Use Hope and Acceptance.

BEARING BURDENS OF THE WORLD
Use Release and Valor.

ANGER & HATE
Use Joy to stimulate the pituitary.
Use Valor and Release to release the anger.

SELF EXPRESSION
Use Valor and Motivation. Take deep breaths to express oneself.

FEAR
Apply Valor, Release, Joy.

Emotional Release

Apply each of the following oils in the order suggested. Smell each oil before applying. If you find an oil repulsive, you may choose to not use it in this procedure.

1. Apply 3 to 6 drops of Valor to the bottoms of the feet, and balance by holding the right foot in the right hand and the left foot in the left hand. Continue to hold the feet until an energy pulse can be felt in both feet. Valor helps balance electrical energies within the body, helps one overcome fear and opposition, and may give courage, confidence, and increased self-esteem. Known as the "Chiropractor in a Bottle," it works best on the bottoms of the feet or on the spine (top and bottom, or entire length—Raindrop style).
2. Apply 1 drop of Harmony either directly on the energy centers (chakras) or along the side of the body. Harmony brings about a harmonic balance to the chakras (energy centers), allowing the energy to flow more efficiently through the body. It may reduce stress and create a general overall feeling of well-being.
3. Apply 1 drop of 3 Wise Men on the crown of the head in a clockwise motion. 3 Wise Men opens crown chakra and stimulates the pineal gland to release emotions and deep-seated trauma. It brings a sense of grounding and uplifting through memory recall. It also helps to keep negative energy and negative emotions from reattaching to the body.
4. Apply 1 drop of Present Time on the thymus in a circular motion; then close eyes and tap the thymus 3 times with the energy fingers (pointer and middle). Present Time helps bring one into the moment. We must forget about the past and stop worrying about the future. We must live in the moment in order to heal.
5. Apply 1 drop of Inner Child around the navel and nose. Inner Child may stimulate memory response and help one reconnect with their inner-self or their own identity. This is one of the first steps to achieving emotional balance.
6. Apply 1 drop of Release over the liver. Release helps to enhance the release of memory trauma from the cells of the liver, where anger and hate emotions are stored. It may also help one let go of negative emotions so that progress is more effective and efficient.
7. Apply 1 drop of Grounding to the brain stem, back of neck, and sternum. Grounding may help one deal with the reality of their emotions in a peaceful way.
8. Apply 1 drop of Forgiveness on the navel in a clockwise motion. Forgiveness may help one move past the barriers in life. It also helps to bring a person into a higher spiritual awareness of their needs and helps raise their frequency to the point where they feel almost compelled to **forgive**, **forget**, **let go**, and go on with their lives.
9. Apply 1 drop of Hope on the outer edge of the ears. Hope helps support the body both physically and mentally. It may help one overcome suicidal depression and restore hope for tomorrow. By filling a person with a feeling of strength and grounding, it empowers them to go forward with hope and achievement.
10. Apply 1 drop of Joy over the heart in a clockwise motion. Joy gives one a glorious feeling of self-love, confidence, and creates a frequency around oneself of the energy of love: the true source of all healing.
11. Apply 1 drop of SARA over the energy centers (chakras), navel, and chest. SARA may enable one to relax and to release the memories of traumatic experiences.
12. Apply 1 drop of White Angelica to the energy centers on the crown and shoulders. White Angelica strengthens and fortifies one's aura, generating a feeling of protection and an awareness of one's potential. As the final oil in this emotional clearing process, it supports all that has taken place and prepares one to search inward for the strength to proceed with life and to search upward for the true source of love and light.

13. Meditate for 20 minutes.

Comments: This procedure has been used successfully by many practitioners.

Note: Energy centers are commonly known as chakras. For a complete listing of the appropriate oils for each chakra, refer to the Personal Guide section of this book under Chakras.

Energy Centers

Associated Glands:

- **Pineal:** Controls cerebrum, right brain hemisphere, central nervous system, right eye.
- **Pituitary:** Controls endocrine system, left brain hemisphere, left eye, nose, ears, sinuses, and parts of nervous system.
- **Thyroid:** Controls jaw, neck, throat, voice, airways, upper lungs, nape of neck, arms.
- **Thymus:** Controls heart, blood circulation, immune system, lower lungs, rib cage, skin, upper back, hands.
- **Pancreas:** Controls liver, digestive system, stomach, spleen, gall bladder, autonomic nervous system, lower back, muscles.
- **Reproductive Organs:** Controls pelvic area, sex organs, fluid functions, kidneys, bladder.
- **Adrenal:** Controls all solid parts—spinal column, bones, teeth, nails. Anus, rectum, colon prostate gland, blood, and building of cells.

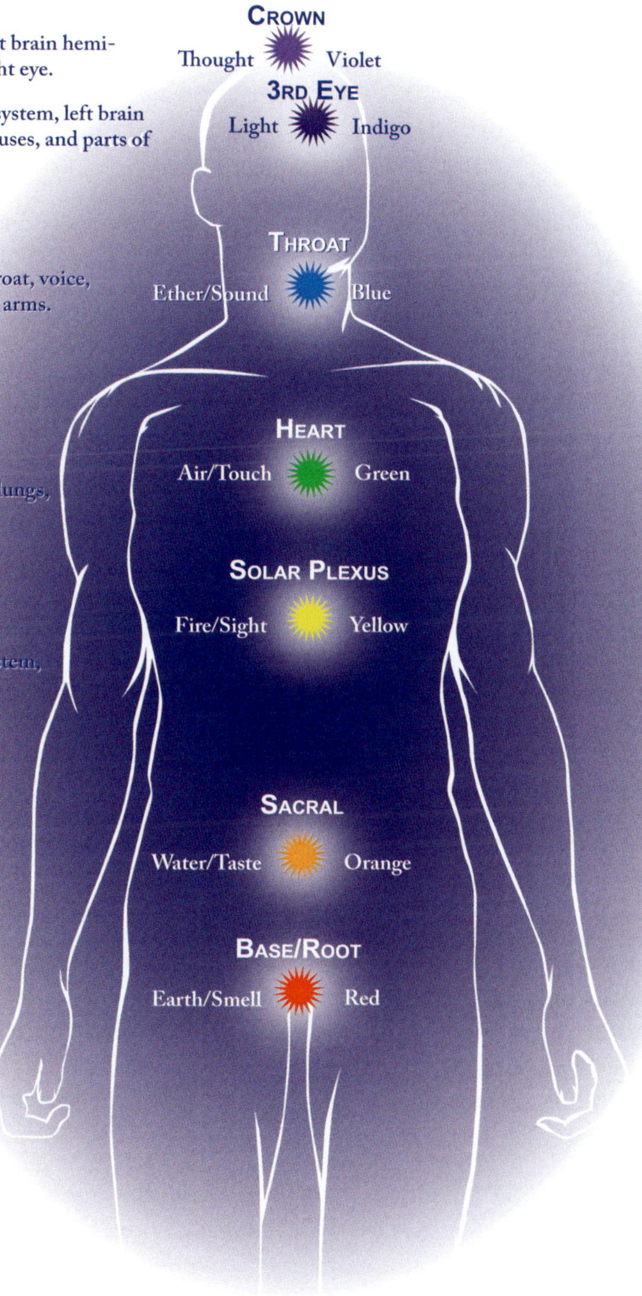

Applicable Oils:

- Lotus, rose, spruce
- Jasmine, peppermint, spearmint
- Eucalyptus, frankincense, sage
- Marjoram, rose, yarrow
- Bergamot, lavender, rosemary
- Sandalwood, ylang ylang
- Cedarwood, clove, pepper, vetiver

Music and Aromatherapy

Duets for Peaceful Emotional Healing
by Karyn Grant, Licensed Massage Therapist, Singer, Songwriter

Walking through life is like taking a journey. There are hidden treasures of knowledge along the path. There are precious traveling companions that enlighten our journey and make the way to healing more peaceful, more gentle, and more beautiful. Music has become that traveling companion for me. It has never left my side.

I didn't realize it then, but I am aware now that it was as a youth that I learned that music was healing to the soul. I didn't know why I sang, I just sang. I found that through singing my spirit was lifted and my mood was brightened. I began writing music by putting scriptures to simple guitar chords (I only knew three). Eventually, my own little handwritten verses became songs too. Just as the poetry of my heart turned into the lyrics of song, the simple everyday sorrows of a teenage girl turned into peaceful happy feelings. I was very happy as a youth. I took voice lessons, wrote songs, and sang about everything from a stubbed toe to a broken heart. I didn't know exactly how it worked, but I learned that I was the happiest when my heart was making music. Music became, for me, the peaceful way to handle any of life's problems.

I didn't understand then what was happening on a metaphysical level. I did not comprehend that music is a form of "light" and has healing vibrations of its own. I did not yet know what I now know—that music performs a massage on an atomic level in one's body and creates a way for less desirable energies to be transformed into more desirable ones. All I really knew was that when I sang, I got happy. When I wrote out my feelings and expressed them instead of holding them in, I got happy. And when I sang the heartfelt words I wrote, I got twice as happy. I had a quote on my wall at age sixteen that read, "I once wrote a poem that no one read, I once sang a song that no one heard, I once drew a picture that no one saw... and I was happy."

At nineteen, I was having my preschool class draw pictures as they listened to music blindfolded. I watched amused as they colored slower or scribbled faster to the tempos, rhythms, and beats of the songs that I selected for them. I wondered how music could have such a powerful effect over someone so little. Their feelings and demeanors changed so quickly! Even then, I began learning by exploring my own emotions and feelings and the mysterious power of music and the effect it had on myself and others.

As I reached my mid-twenties, the songs began coming again in the middle of the night. I learned that the combination of words and music could have a very softening effect on mind, heart, body and spirit. As my marriage grew more and more troubled, I realized that the gift of song was assuaging deep feelings of emotional isolation, spiritual bereavement, and loneliness that I could not bear alone. I would arise at 3:00 a.m. every morning to nurse my baby girl back to sleep. Those became my own "feedings" too. That's when I began journeying with song again.

As the isolation grew in my marital relationship, so did the spiritual gift of singing. Singing the praises and sorrows of my heart literally took the ache from my heart and transformed grief into comfort, serenity, and peace. I was able to focus on spiritual solutions for my less than desirable circumstance. The ability to express the innermost desires and feelings of my heart became easier. Not having developed the talent for writing the melodies, I sung them onto cassettes and hid them away in a drawer never imagining that these treasures would ever serve to bless other souls who were journeying through life carrying hidden wounds that could not be seen, diagnosed, or solaced.

Not until years later, following my divorce, when I became a massage therapist, did I begin to understand the healing effect of music as therapy. I would work with clients during the day and would help them as best I could. Then, later in the night, I would be awakened with songs of comfort, courage, and peace to sing to them at their next appointment. This I would do, and many wept tears of gratitude, saying that they never had anyone take the time to sing to them. N'Shama Sterling writes:

When a woman in a certain African tribe knows she is pregnant, she goes out into the wilderness with a few friends and together they pray and meditate until they hear the song of the child. They recognize that every soul has its own vibration that expresses its unique flavor and purpose. When the women attune to the song, they sing it out loud. They then return to the tribe and teach the song of the child to the village.

When the child is born, the community gathers and sings the child's song to him or her. Later, when the child enters education, the village gathers and chants the child's song. When the child passes through the initiation to adulthood, the people would again come together and sing. At the time of marriage, the person hears his or her song. Finally, when the soul is about to pass from this world, the family and friends gather at the person's bed, just as they did at their birth, and they sing the person to the next life.

In this African tribe there is one other occasion upon which the villagers sing to the child. If at any time during his or her life, the person commits a crime or aberrant social act, the individual is called to the center of the village and the people in the community form a circle around them. They sing their song to them. The tribe recognized that the correction for antisocial behavior is not punishment; it is love and the remembrance of your true identity. When you recognize your own song, you have no desire or need to do anything that would hurt another.

A friend is someone who knows your song and sings it to you when you have forgotten it. Those who love you are not fooled by mistakes you have made or by dark images you hold about yourself. They remember your beauty when you feel ugly; your wholeness when you are broken; your innocence when you feel guilty; and your purpose when you are confused. You may not have grown up in an African tribe that sings your song to you at crucial life transitions, but life is always reminding you when you are in tune with yourself and when you are not. When you feel good, what you are doing matches your song; and when you feel awful, it doesn't. In the end, we shall all recognize our song and sing it well. You may feel your voice is a bit "warbly" at the moment, but so have all the great singers at one time or another. Just keep singing.

I began learning that music was a vibrational soothing balm that could enter into places that the physical ointment could not reach. Combining aromatherapy with the music anchored in the affirmations and imageries of the songs with scent. I instinctively knew that to reach those hidden wounds that are infected with the energies of loneliness, resentment, anger, despair, sadness, fear, doubt, and other such emotions that are locked into the cellular memory of the glands, organs, tissues, and systems of the body, it would take the healing vibrations of touch, smell, visualization, and soothing sounds to transform those energies into positive and more joyful emotions.

From *The Book of Sound Therapy*, we read, "The human being is therefore likened to a very complex, unique, and finely-tuned musical instrument. Every atom, molecule, cell, tissue and organ of the body continually broadcasts the frequencies of physical, emotional, mental and spiritual life. The human voice is an indicator of its body's health on all these levels of existence. It establishes a relationship between the individual and the wondrous network of vibrations that is the cosmos."

In the ancient societies of Egypt, India, Greece, and China, to name a few, music played a vital role in just about everything—from health, to architecture, to politics. They believed that music was the bridge linking all things. Physical forms were considered manifestations of music, and it was held that life and health depended upon harmonic balance of rations and relationships. In ancient Greece, for instance, one could not become a physician until he had first become a musician, and prescriptions often included rhythmic singing and chanting from selected sacred melodic sequences.

If we could put a heart, broken and scarred, under a microscope and see the emotional aches manifesting themselves as rips and cuts and then pour the healing balm and vibrations of song and scent into those open and festering sores, I believe that we would watch in amazement as the rips began to mend and the cuts began to close in perfect alignment. For that is what I see in my mind's eye. I see song as living water. I see the vibrations of aromatherapy as more than just a scent, but as a healing balm for the soul. I see the wounds being cleansed and mended in perfect closure, having finally been acknowledged, addressed, and administered to.

An anonymous quote reads, "Man of himself is an instrument of music; and when the chords of which he is composed are touched as sound salutes the ear, the sound appeals to his spirit and the sentiment to his understanding. If the strains are harmonious, he endorses and enjoys them with supreme delight. Whether the tones are from a human voice or from an instrument, they arrest his attention and absorb his whole being."

I have stood at the side of my massage table and beheld as countenances have changed from tearful torment into peaceful, blissful expressions of tranquil gratitude. For the hidden wounds of the heart and the spirit, there are no scalpels, no knives, no needles, no thread, no numbing medications. There is only beauty all around—where there are flowers, where there are songs, where there are scents, where there is compassion, where there is pure touch, where there is hope, and, most of all, where there is love. We only give the gifts that do the real healing.

Single Oils

This section provides concise information about many of the pure essential oils that are available for use by the general public. The listings of possible uses are meant for external application unless otherwise directed. The included safety data is also based on the external use of the oils and may differ from other published information that is based on oral application.

Other seeming discrepancies between sources of published safety data arise when one does not take into consideration the certain constituents of the oil being reviewed. One glaring example of this is thyme. A linalol type of oil does not have the same caustic/irritant effects that a thymol type would, but the particular application may require the added strength of the thymol type of oil. In this book, care has been taken to differentiate between the different types of essential oil for each application. Since pure essential oils are powerful healing agents, please remember to check the safety data before using an oil. Because there are several different oils that can help the same health condition, it should not be difficult to find one that will work for any particular situation. Also, for a listing of products that contain these individual oils, please refer to the Single Oil Summary section in the Appendix.

Amazonian Ylang Ylang

(See Ylang Ylang, Amazonian)

Angelica

(Angelica archangelica)

Botanical Family: Apiaceae, Umbelliferae (parsley)

Extraction Method/Origin: Steam distillation of roots—France, Belgium

Chemical Constituents: Monoterpenes (up to 95%): d- and l-limonenes (up to 40%), α- and β-pinenes, α- and β-phellandrenes; Esters: bornyl acetate, verbenyl acetate; Terpene Alkaloids: bergaptene; Coumarins: umbelliferone.

Properties: **Anticoagulant**, **anti-inflammatory** (intestinal wall), **calming**, **expectorant**, **sedative** (nervous system), **stomachic**, and **tonic**.

Common Primary Uses: [T]**Cooling.**

Folklore: One possible source for this oil's unique name comes from an old legend which states that during a terrible plague an angel revealed this plant to a monk. History also records the use of the plant during the plague of 1660. The stems were chewed to prevent infection, and the seeds and roots were burned to help purify the air. The German people refer to the essence as the "oil of angels."

Other Possible Uses: Angelica may help with **anorexia**, **appetite** (loss of), **bruises**, **colds**, **colic**, **coughs**, **flatulence**, **indigestion**, **menopause**, **premenstrual tension**, **respiratory infections**, and **rheumatic conditions**.

Body System(s) Affected: **Emotional Balance**, **Nervous System**.

Aromatic Influence: It may help one release and let go of negative feelings by bringing one's memory back to a point of origin before **trauma** or **anger** was experienced.

Application: Apply to **shoulders, vita flex points**, bottoms of **feet**, and/or directly on **area** of concern; diffuse.

Oral Use As Dietary Supplement: Generally regarded as safe (GRAS) for human consumption by the FDA. ***Dilute** one drop oil in 1 tsp. honey or in 4 oz. of beverage (i.e. soy/rice milk). **Not for children under 6 years old; use with caution and in greater dilution for children 6 years old and over.***

Safety Data: ***Avoid if diabetic. Use with caution during pregnancy. Avoid direct sunlight for 12 hours after use.***

Blend Classification: Personifier, Modifier.

Blends With: Clary sage, patchouli, vetiver, florals, woods, and most citrus oils.

Odor: Type: *Top to Middle Notes (20–80% of the blend)*; Scent: *Herbaceous, earthy, peppery, green, spicy*; Intensity: *4.*

Frequency: Physical and Emotional; approximately 85 MHz.

Anise

(Pimpinella anisum)

Botanical Family: Umbelliferae (dainty, white-flowered annual)

Extraction Method/Origin: Steam distillation from seeds (fruit)—Turkey

Chemical Constituents: Phenolic Ethers: anethol (up to 95%) and estragole (1–4%); Alcohols: anisol, linalol, α-terpineol; Phenols: p-anol; Aldehydes: anisicaldehyde.

Properties: **Antifungal**[1] **antiseptic, antispasmodic, estrogen-like, diuretic, stimulant** (heart), and **tonic** (heart).

Historical Uses: This oil has been used for dry irritable **coughs, bronchitis, whooping cough**.

Other Possible Uses: **Alkalosis, blood oxygenation, bronchitis, colitis, constipation, digestion** (accelerates), **diverticulitis, estrogen** (increases), **fertility, flatulence, hormonal imbalance, irritable bowel syndrome, menopause, parasites, PMS, prostate cancer** (blend with frankincense), and **respiratory system** (strengthens).

Body System(s) Affected: **Cardiovascular, Digestive, Hormonal**, and **Respiratory Systems**.

Application: Apply to **Vita Flex Points** and directly on **area** of concern; diffuse.

Oral Use As Dietary Supplement: Generally regarded as safe (GRAS) for human consumption by the FDA. ***Dilute** one drop oil in 1 tsp. honey or in 4 oz. of beverage (i.e. soy/rice milk). **Not for children under 6 years old; use with caution and in greater dilution for children 6 years old and over.***

Safety Data: ***Can irritate sensitive skin and has been known to cause dermatitis in some individuals. Best if used in moderation.***

Blend Classification: Difficult to use in blending. Use only in very small amounts.

Blends With: Bergamot, blue tansy, fennel, ginger, juniper, lemongrass, patchouli, black pepper, peppermint, tangerine, tarragon, and ylang ylang.

Odor: Type: *Top to Middle Notes (20–80% of the blend).*

Balsam Fir

(See Fir, Balsam)

Basil

(Ocimum basilicum CT methyl chavicol)

Botanical Family: Lamiaceae or Labiatae (mint)

Extraction Method/Origin: Steam distillation of leaves, stems, and flowers—Egypt, India, Utah, France

Chemical Constituents: Phenolic Ethers: methyl chavicol (or estragole—up to 89%), methyl eugenol; Alcohols (up to 20%): linalool (up to 19%), citronellol, α-fenchol, α-terpineol; Oxides (up to 9%): 1,8 cineol, ocimene oxide; Esters (<5%); Monoterpenes (<4%); Ketones (<2%).

Properties: **Antibacterial**[2], **anti-infectious**, **anti-inflammatory**, **antioxidant**[3], **antiseptic** (stomach/intestinal), **antispasmodic** (powerful), **antiviral**, **decongestant** (veins, arteries of the lungs, prostate), **stimulant** (nerves, adrenal cortex), and **uplifting**. Basil may also be **anticatarrhal**, **antidepressant**, **energizing**, and **restorative**.

Common Primary Uses: ^T^**Autism**, ^T^**carpal tunnel**, ^T^**chronic fatigue**, ^IT^**cramps (abdominal)**, ^T^**infection (skin)**, ^AT^**mental fatigue**, ^T^**migraine**, ^T^**muscle spasms**, ^T^**muscular dystrophy**, ^T^**snake bites**, ^T^**spider bites**, ^A^**whooping cough**, ^T^**wounds**.

Folklore: Considered by the ancient Greeks as the "king of plants," basil was used to anoint kings. Hindus placed sprigs of basil on the chests of deceased loved ones to protect them from evil and to provide safe passage into the next life. Due to its supposed aphrodisiac qualities, Italian women displayed basil to attract possible suitors, and the men would present the women with basil sprigs.

Historical Uses: Basil was used anciently for respiratory problems, digestive and kidney ailments, epilepsy, poisonous insect or snake bites, fevers, epidemics, and malaria.

French Medicinal Uses: **Migraines** (especially from liver and gallbladder problems), **mental fatigue**, **menstrual periods** (scanty).

Other Possible Uses: This oil may be used for **aches/pains**, **anxiety**, **bronchitis**[4], **chronic colds**, **concentration**, nervous **depression**, **digestion**, **earache**, **fainting**, **fatigue** (mental), **fever**, **gout**, **headaches**, **hemorrhoids**, **hiccups**, **insect bites** (soothing), **repelling insects**[5], **insomnia** (from nervous tension), **intestinal problems**, poor **memory**, chronic **mucus**, **muscle spasms**, **ovarian cysts**, **prostate problems**, **rhinitis** (inflammation of nasal mucus membranes), loss of **smell**, **snake bites**, **vomiting**, **wasp stings**, and **whooping cough**.

Body System(s) Affected: **Cardiovascular System**, **Muscles** and **Bones**.

Aromatic Influence: Helps one maintain an **open mind** and increases **clarity** of thought. **Application:** Apply to **temples**, tip of **nose**, **Vita Flex Points**, and/or directly on **area** of concern; diffuse. May also be added to food or water as a dietary supplement.

Oral Use As Dietary Supplement: Generally regarded as safe (GRAS) for human consumption by the FDA. ***Dilute** one drop oil in 1 tsp. honey or in 4 oz. of beverage (i.e. soy/rice milk).* ***Not for children under 6 years old; use with caution and in greater dilution for children 6 years old and over.***

Safety Data: ***Avoid during pregnancy. Not for use by people with epilepsy. It may also irritate sensitive skin (test a small area first).***

Blend Classification: Enhancer and Equalizer.

Blends With: Bergamot, cypress, fir, geranium, helichrysum, lavender, lemongrass, marjoram, peppermint, spruce, wintergreen.

Odor: Type: *Top to Middle Notes (20–80% of the blend)*; Scent: *Herbaceous, spicy, anise-like, camphorous, lively*; Intensity: *4*.

Frequency: Low (Physical); approximately 52 MHz.

Bergamot
(Citrus bergamia)

Botanical Family: Rutaceae (citrus)

Extraction Method/Origin: Solvent extraction or vacuum distillation; pressed from rind or peel; rectified and void of terpenes—Italy, Ivory Coast

Chemical Constituents: Monoterpenes: d-limonene (>30%), γ-terpinene, α & β-pinenes; Esters: linalyl acetate (usually around 20%); Alcohols: linalool (10%), geraniol, nerol, α-terpineol; Sesquiterpenes: β-caryophyllene, β-bisabolene; Furanocoumarins; Aldehydes.

Properties: **Analgesic, antibacterial** (strep and staph infection), **anti-infectious, anti-inflammatory, antiparasitic, antiseptic, antispasmodic, digestive, sedative**[6], and **uplifting**.

Common Primary Uses: **ᵀAutism, ᵀcold sores, ᴬᵀdepression, ᴬgrief/sorrow, ᵀhoarse (voice), ᴬinsomnia, ᵀoily skin, ᴬᵀphysical stress**.

Folklore: Christopher Columbus is credited with bringing bergamot to Italy from the Canary Islands.

Historical Uses: Bergamot was used by the Italians to cool and relieve fevers, protect against malaria, and expel intestinal worms.

French Medicinal Uses: **Agitation, appetite** (loss of), **colic, depression, indigestion, infection, inflammation, insect repellent, insomnia, intestinal parasites, rheumatism, stress**, and **vaginal candida**.

Other Possible Uses: This oil may help **acne, anxiety**, regulate **appetite, boils, bronchitis, carbuncles, cold sores**, oily **complexion, coughs, cystitis, digestion, eczema, emotions, endocrine system functioning, fever, gallstones, gonorrhea, infectious disease, insect bites**, soothe **lungs, psoriasis, respiratory infection, scabies, sore throat**, nervous **tension, thrush**, acute **tonsillitis, ulcers, urinary tract infection**, spot **varicose veins**, and **wounds**.

Body System(s) Affected: **Digestive System, Emotional Balance, Skin**.

Aromatic Influence: It may help to **relieve anxiety, depression, stress**, and **tension**. It is **uplifting** and **refreshing**. It helps to expand and open the **heart chakra** and to radiate **love energy**.

Application: Apply to **forehead, temples, Vita Flex Points**, and/or directly on **area** of concern; diffuse. May also be applied as a **deodorant** or added to food or water as a dietary supplement.

Oral Use As Dietary Supplement: Generally regarded as safe (GRAS) for human consumption by the FDA. ***Dilute** one drop oil in 1 tsp. honey or in 4 oz. of beverage (i.e. soy/rice milk). **Not for children under 6 years old; use with caution and in greater dilution for children 6 years old and over.***

Safety Data: ***Repeated use can result in extreme contact sensitization. Avoid direct sunlight or ultraviolet light for 72 hours after use.***

Blend Classification: Equalizer, Modifier, and Enhancer.

Blends With: Chamomile, cypress, eucalyptus, geranium, jasmine, juniper, lavender, lemon, palmarosa, patchouli, and ylang ylang.

Odor: Type: *Top Note (5–20% of the blend)*; Scent: *Sweet, lively, citrusy, fruity*; Intensity: *2*.

Biblical Sweet Myrrh
(See Myrrh, Biblical Sweet)

Black Pepper
(See Pepper, Black)

Blue Cypress

(See Cypress, Blue)

Blue Spruce

(See Spruce, Idaho Blue)

Cajeput

(Melaleuca leucadendra)

Botanical Family: Myrtaceae (myrtle shrubs and trees)

Chemical Constituents: Oxides: 1,8 cineol (<50%); Alcohols: α-terpineol (>8%), viridiflorol, nerolidol; Monoterpenes: α- & β-pinenes, l-limonene; Sesquiterpenes: β-caryophyllene; Aldehydes: benzoicaldehyde; Esters: α-terpinyl acetate.

Properties: **Analgesic** (mild), **anticatarrhal, anti-infectious, anti-inflammatory, antimicrobial, antineuralgic, antiseptic** (pulmonary, urinary, intestinal), **antispasmodic, expectorant, insecticidal,** and **tonic.**

Common Primary Uses: **TOily skin, TAviral infection.**

Historical Uses: In Malaysia and other Indonesian islands, cajeput was considered valuable for cholera, colds, flu, headaches, rheumatism, throat infections, toothache, various skin conditions, and sore muscles.

Other Possible Uses: Cajeput may help with **acne, arthritis, asthma, bronchitis, bursitis, catarrh, colds, coughs, cystitis, dysentery, enteritis, flu, hay fever, headaches, infections** of the **urethra, insect bites, intestinal problems,** stiff **joints, laryngitis, pneumonia, psoriasis, respiratory infections, rheumatism, sinusitis, skin** (oily and spots), **sore throat, toothache, urinary complaints, viral infections.**

Body System(s) Affected: **Cardiovascular** and **Respiratory Systems.**

Application: Apply to **Vita Flex Points** and/or directly on **area** of concern. **Diffuse** for **respiratory infections.**

Oral Use As Dietary Supplement: Approved by the FDA for use as a Food Additive (FA) or Flavoring Agent (FL). ***Dilute** one drop oil in 1 tsp. honey or in 4 oz. of beverage (i.e. soy/rice milk).* ***Not for children under 6 years old; use with caution and in greater dilution for children 6 years old and over.***

Safety Data: ***If not absolutely pure, cajeput could cause further blistering and skin eruptions! Even when pure, it can irritate sensitive skin. Use with caution.***

Blend Classification: Enhancer.

Blends With: Eucalyptus, juniper, peppermint, and wintergreen.

Odor: Type: *Top Note (5–20% of the blend).*

Caraway

(Carum carvi)

Botanical Family: Umbelliferae (dainty, white-flowered annual)

Extraction Method/Origin: Steam distillation from seeds (fruit)—Netherlands

Chemical Constituents: Ketones: carvone (up to 60%); Monoterpenes: limonene (>45%), phellandrene, pinene, carvene; Monoterpene Alcohols (>6%): cis-carveol (<5%), furfurol, carvacrol, hydrocarveols; Coumarins: herniarine; Aldehydes: acetaldehyde, cuminic aldehyde.

Properties: **Antiparasitic, antihistamine, antimicrobial, antispasmodic, antitumoral**[7], **expectorant, diuretic, stimulant** (circulatory, urinary), and **tonic**[8] (digestive).

Common Primary Uses: ¹**Irritable bowel syndrome (IBS)**.

Historical Uses: Caraway is a very old, well-known spice and has been used as far back as the Stone Age. Egyptians used it as food flavoring, the Romans used it in bread-making, and in the Middle Ages the Germans and Austrians used it in their cooking. Traditionally this herb is associated with sharp eyesight and sweet breath.

Other Possible Uses: **Acne, appetite** (aids poor), **asthma** (bronchial), **boils, bowels** (general complaints), **breath** (sweetens), **bronchitis** (acute catarrhal), **bruises, colic, colitis, cough, diarrhea, dizziness, dyspepsia, gas, indigestion, intestines** (calms muscle fibers), **laryngitis, liver** and **gallbladder** (promotes bile), **lymph** (stimulates flow), **menstrual period** (eases pains), **nursing** (increases milk), itchy **scalp, scabies, skin** (oily, stimulates pale skin), **toxins**[9] (flushes), **urine** (increases), **vertigo, wounds**.

Body System(s) Affected: **Digestive System**.

Aromatic Influence: Caraway is **warming** to the **emotions**. It helps to ease **mental strain** and **fatigue** and helps one replenish lost **energy**.

Application: Apply to **Vita Flex Points** and directly on **area** of concern; **diffuse**.

Oral Use As Dietary Supplement: Generally regarded as safe (GRAS) for human consumption by the FDA. ***Dilute** one drop oil in 1 tsp. honey or in 4 oz. of beverage (i.e. soy/rice milk).* ***Not for children under 6 years old; use with caution and in greater dilution for children 6 years old and over.***

Safety Data: ***Avoid during pregnancy. Can irritate sensitive skin and has produced contact sensitivity. Best if used in moderation.***

Blend Classification: Difficult to use in blending. Use only in very small amounts.

Blends With: Basil, chamomile, coriander, frankincense, ginger, lavender, and orange.

Odor: Type: *Top Note (20–80% of the blend)*

Cardamom

(Elettaria cardamomum)

Botanical Family: Zingiberaceae (ginger)

Chemical Constituents: Esters (>40%): α-terpenyl acetate (30–45%), linalyl acetate (3%); Oxides: 1,8 cineol (up to 35%); Alcohols (7%): linalol, terpinen-4-ol, α-terpineol; Monoterpenes (6%): sabinene, myrcene, l-limonene; Aldehyde: geranial.

Properties: **Antibacterial, anti-infectious, anti-inflammatory**[10], **antiseptic, antispasmodic**[11], **aphrodisiac, digestive**[12], **diuretic, stomachic**, and **tonic**.

Historical Uses: Anciently, cardamom was used for epilepsy, spasms, paralysis, rheumatism, cardiac disorders, all intestinal illnesses, pulmonary disease, fever, and digestive and urinary complaints. It is said to be able to neutralize the lingering odor of garlic.

Other Possible Uses: Cardamom may help with **appetite** (loss of), **colic, coughs, debility, dyspepsia, flatulence, halitosis, headaches, mental fatigue, nausea, pyrosis** (or **heartburn**), **sciatica**, and **vomiting**. It may also help with **menstrual periods, menopause**, and nervous **indigestion**. *Note: Cardamom has the same properties as ginger but is less of an irritant.*

Body System(s) Affected: **Digestive System**.

Aromatic Influence: Cardamom is **uplifting, refreshing**, and **invigorating**. It may be beneficial for **clearing confusion**.

Application: Apply to **Vita Flex Points** and/or directly on **area** of concern. Dilute with base oil, and **massage** over the stomach, solar plexus, and thighs. Excellent as a **bath** oil.

Oral Use As Dietary Supplement: Generally regarded as safe (GRAS) for human consumption by the FDA. ***Dilute*** *one drop oil in 1 tsp. honey or in 4 oz. of beverage (i.e. soy/rice milk).* ***Not for children under 6 years old; use with caution and in greater dilution for children 6 years old and over.***

Blend Classification: Personifier and Modifier.

Blends With: Bergamot, cedarwood, cinnamon bark, cistus, clove, neroli, orange, rose, and ylang ylang.

Odor: Type: *Middle Note (50–80% of the blend)*; Scent: *Sweet, spicy, balsamic, with floral undertones*; Intensity: *4.*

Carrot

(Daucus carota)

Botanical Family: Umbelliferae (parsley)

Chemical Constituents: Alcohols: carotol (up to 50%), daucol (up to 5%), linalol; Monoterpenes: α- & β-pinenes, sabinene; Sesquiterpenes: β-bisabolene (10%), β-caryophyllene (4%), daucene; Oxides: epoxy β-caryophyllene; Esters: geranyl acetate; Phenols: β-asarone.

Properties: **Antifungal**[13], **carminative, hepatic** (cleanses the liver), **stomachic**.

Common Primary Uses: [T]**Wrinkles**.

Historical Uses: Carrots have been used as a blood cleanser, for liver and skin problems, pulmonary conditions, allergies, inflammation of the intestines, as a tonic for the nervous system, and for eyesight. Carrots were used during the Second World War to help pilots with their night vision.

Other Possible Uses: Carrot oil may help with **anemia, colic** (with fennel), **constipation, diarrhea, eye problems, gallbladder problems, liver problems, rheumatism**, and **skin problems** (**aging skin, wrinkles, sunburn**, and **dryness**).

Body System(s) Affected: **Cardiovascular** and **Nervous Systems, Skin**.

Application: Apply to **Vita Flex Points** and/or directly on **area** of concern. To promote a healthy **suntan**, apply carrot oil (dilute with hazelnut oil) for a few days before exposure to the sun.

Oral Use As Dietary Supplement: Generally regarded as safe (GRAS) for human consumption by the FDA. ***Dilute*** *one drop oil in 1 tsp. honey or in 4 oz. of beverage (i.e. soy/rice milk).* ***Not for children under 6 years old; use with caution and in greater dilution for children 6 years old and over.***

Blend Classification: Considered as more of an active carrier oil (same as Vitamin E Oil and Wheatgerm Oil).

Blends With: Citrus oils, fennel, frankincense, geranium, spice oils.

Odor: Type: *Middle Note (50–80% of the blend)*; Scent: *Sweet, fruity, warm, earthy*; Intensity: *2.*

Cassia

(Cinnamomum cassia)

Botanical Family: Lauraceae (laurel)

Extraction Method/Origin: Steam distillation from bark—China

Chemical Constituents: Aldehydes: trans-cinnamaldehyde (up to 85%), benzaldehyde; Phenols (>7%): eugenol, chavicol, phenol, 2-vinyl-phenol; Esters: cinnamyl acetate, benzyl acetate.

Properties: **Antibacterial, antifungal, antiviral**.

Historical Uses: Cassia has been used extensively as a domestic spice. Medicinally, it has been used for colds, colic, flatulent dyspepsia, diarrhea, nausea, rheumatism, and kidney and reproductive complaints.

Other Possible Uses: This oil is best not used individually in aromatherapy as it can be extremely sensitizing to the dermal tissues. Can provide some powerful support to blends when used in very small quantities.

Application: None.

Oral Use As Dietary Supplement: Generally regarded as safe (GRAS) for human consumption by the FDA. **Dilute** *one drop oil in 2 tsp. honey or in 8 oz. of beverage (i.e. soy/rice milk). May need to increase dilution even more due to this oil's potential for irritating mucus membranes.* ***Not for children under 6 years old; use with caution and in greater dilution for children 6 years old and over.***

Safety Data: ***Repeated use can result in extreme contact sensitization. Avoid during pregnancy. Can cause extreme skin irritation. Diffuse with caution; it will irritate the nasal membranes if it is inhaled directly from the diffuser.***

Blend Classification: Personifier/Enhancer.

Odor: Type: *Middle Note (50–80% of the blend)*; Scent: *Spicy, warm, sweet*; Intensity: *5.*

Cedar, Western Red

(Thuja plicata)

Botanical Family: Cupressaceae (conifer: cypress)

Extraction Method/Origin: Steam distillation from leaves and twigs—USA

Chemical Constituents: Ketones: α- & β-thujones (>60%), fenchone (<7%), camphor (<3%); Monoterpenes (<7%): sabinene, α- & β-pinenes; Esters: methyl thujate; Sesquiterpene Alcohols: muurolol.

Properties: **Antibacterial** and **antiseptic**.

Historical Uses: The western red cedar has been referred to as the "Tree of Life." It has been used by ancient civilizations to enhance their potential for spiritual communication during rituals and other ceremonies. It has also been used for coughs, fevers, intestinal parasites, cystitis, and venereal diseases.

Other Possible Uses: This oil may help with **hair loss, skin** (nourishing), **rheumatism, warts**, and **psoriasis**. It has powerful effects on the **subconscious** and **unconscious mind**.

Body System(s) Affected: **Skin**.

Aromatic Influence: It is **calming** and may help enhance **spiritual awareness** or **meditation**.

Application: Apply to **Vita Flex Points** and/or directly on **area** of concern. **Diffuse**.

Oral Use As Dietary Supplement: None.

Safety Data: ***For Topical Use Only. Due to high Thujone content, use sparingly and dilute well with V-6 Oil.***

Cedar Leaf (Thuja)

(Thuja occidentalis)

Botanical Family: Cupressaceae (conifer: cypress)

Extraction Method/Origin: Steam distillation from leaves, twigs, and bark—Canada, USA

Chemical Constituents: Ketones: α- & β-thujones (>60%), fenchone (up to 14%), camphor (<3%), piperitone; Monoterpenes: sabinene (<35%), l-limonene; Esters: bornyl acetate (up to 12%); Sesquiterpene Alcohols: occidentalol, occidol, α-, β-, & γ-eudesmols; Phenolic Alcohols: terpinen-4-ol (<6%).

Properties: **Antirheumatic, astringent, expectorant, insect repellent, and stimulant** (nerves, immune system, uterus and heart muscles).

Historical Uses: Has been used by ancient civilizations to enhance their potential for spiritual communication during rituals and other ceremonies. It has also been used for coughs, fevers, intestinal parasites, cystitis, and venereal diseases.

Other Possible Uses: May help with **rheumatism, warts**, and **psoriasis**.

Aromatic Influence: May help enhance **spiritual awareness** or **meditation**.

Application: Apply to **Vita Flex Points** and directly on **area** of concern. **Diffuse**.

Oral Use As Dietary Supplement: *Has been approved by the FDA for use as a Food Additive (FA) or Flavoring Agent (FL) as long as the finished food is thujone-free (see 21CFR172.510). It is **best not to use this oil as a dietary supplement.***

Safety Data: ***For Topical Use Only**. Due to high Thujone content, use **sparingly** and **dilute well** with V-6 Oil.*

Cedarwood

(Cedrus atlantica)

Botanical Family: Pinaceae (conifer)

Extraction Method/Origin: Steam distillation from bark—Morocco, USA

Chemical Constituents: Sesquiterpenes (up to 90%): α-, β-, & γ-himachalenes (>55%), cadinene; Sesquiterpene Alcohols (up to 40%): alantol (<20%), α-caryophyllenol (<10%), β-cubenol (<10%), cedrol, cedrenol; Sesquiterpene Ketones (20%): α- & β-alantones.

Properties: **Antifungal, anti-infectious, antiseptic** (urinary and pulmonary), **astringent, diuretic, insect repellent**, and **sedative**.

Common Primary Uses: **ATCalming**, **Tcellulite**, **Thair loss**, **ATtension**, **ATtuberculosis**, **Turinary infection**, **Ayoga**.

Folklore: *Cedrus atlantica* is supposed to be the species most closely related to the biblical Cedars of Lebanon.

Historical Uses: Cedarwood was used traditionally by the North American Indians to enhance their spiritual communication. It creates the symbolic effect of the umbrella protecting the earth and bringing energy in from the universe. At night the animals in the wild lie down under the tree for the protection, recharging, and rejuvenation the trees bring them.

French Medicinal Uses: **Anger** (calming effect), **arteriosclerosis, bronchitis, calming, cellulite, diuretic, hair loss, nervous tension, tuberculosis, urinary infections**.

Other Possible Uses: This oil is recognized for its **purifying** properties. It may also help **acne, anxiety, arthritis, congestion, coughs, cystitis, dandruff, psoriasis, purification, sinusitis, skin diseases**, and **water retention**. It may help **open** the **pineal gland**. It also helps to reduce **oily secretions**.

Body System(s) Affected: **Nervous** and **Respiratory Systems**.

Application: Apply to **Vita Flex Points** and/or directly on **area** of concern.

Oral Use As Dietary Supplement: None.

Safety Data: *Use with caution during **pregnancy**.*

Blend Classification: Enhancer and Equalizer.

Blends With: Bergamot, clary sage, cypress, eucalyptus, floral oils, juniper, resinous oils, rosemary.

Odor: Type: *Base Note (5–20% of the blend)*; Scent: *Warm, soft, woody*; Intensity: *3*.

Biblical References: Lev. 14:4, 6, 49, 51, 52.

Celery Seed

(Apium graveolens)

Botanical Family: Umbeliferae

Extraction Method/Origin: Steam distilled from seed—France

Chemical Constituents: Monoterpenes (up to 85%): d-limonene (>60%), ocimene (<11%), α & γ-terpinenes; Esters (<23%): carvyl acetate, geranyl acetate; Lactones (approx. 15%): 3-n-butylphthalide (up to 7%), sedanenolides (>1%), 4-dihydro-phthalide (1%), dihydro-ligustilide (3%); Sesquiterpenes (up to 12%): α- & β-selinenes; Ketones: d-carvone (<10%); Carboxylic Acids: sedanolic acid; Alcohols: α-terpineol.

Properties: **Antioxidant**, **antirheumatic**, **antiseptic** (urinary), **antispasmodic**, **antitumoral**[14], **hepatic** (stimulates drainage), **stimulant** (uterine), **tonic** (neuromuscular).

Possible Uses: Celery seed may help with **arthritis**, **bloating**, **bronchitis**, **congestion** (respiratory), **cystitis**, **flatulence**, **glands** (swollen), **gout** (reduces uric acid), **hemorrhoids**, **indigestion**, **jaundice**, **kidney** detoxification (after illness), **lactation** (increases flow of breast milk), **liver** congestion (after infection), **lymphatic** drainage, **menstruation** (induces), **Nervous** disorders, **neuralgia**, **rheumatism**, **sciatica**, **sexual** problems (minimizes), **skin** (puffiness, redness, spots, water-logged), and **urine** flow (increases). It may help to balance the **endocrine system** to help with glandular problems. It is also a sedative and a tonic for the **central nervous system** and may help provide more **restful sleep**.

Body Systems Affected: **Digestive System**, **Muscles** and **Bones**, **Nervous System**.

Aromatic Influence: Celery seed has a spicy, warm, sweet, tenacious odor. It is fairly strong and long-lasting. The aroma is **calming** and **relaxing** to the mind and the body.

Application: Apply to **Vita Flex Points** on the feet and directly on **area** of concern.

Oral Use As Dietary Supplement: Generally regarded as safe (GRAS) for human consumption by the FDA. ***Dilute** one drop oil in 1 tsp. honey or in 4 oz. of beverage (i.e. soy/rice milk).* ***Not for children under 6 years old; use with caution and in greater dilution for children 6 years old and over.***

Safety Data: ***Repeated use can possibly result in contact sensitization or skin irritation. Avoid during pregnancy.***

Blend Classification: Personifier.

Odor: Type: *Middle Note (50–80% of the blend)*; Scent: *Spicy, warm, sweet, tenacious*; Intensity: *3*.

Chamomile, German (Blue)

(Matricaria recutita)

Botanical Family: Compositae (daisy)

Extraction Method/Origin: Steam distillation from flowers—Egypt, Hungary, Utah

Chemical Constituents: Sesquiterpenes (up to 60%): α- & β-farnesenes (>20%), chamazulene (<20%), dihydrochamazulene I & II, cadinene, bisabolenes; Oxides: bisabolol oxide-A (>24%), bisabolone oxide (<20%), bisabolol oxide-B (<10%), 1,8 cineol (<5%); Sesquiterpene Alcohols: α-bisabolol (<8%), fanesol, spathulenol; Ethers; Monoterpenes.

Properties: **Analgesic**, **anti-infectious**, **anti-inflammatory**, **antioxidant**, **antispasmodic**, **decongestant**, **digestive tonic**[15], and **hormone-like**.

Common Primary Uses: **ᵀAcne**, **ᵀchapped lips**, **ᵀcolic**, **ᵀdermatitis/eczema**, **ᴬᵀmeasles**, **ᵀsensitive skin**, **ᵀteething pain**, **ᴵulcer**.

Historical Uses: Native to Europe, it is no longer grown in Germany. It has a long history of use for all symptoms related to or resulting from tension.

French Medicinal Uses: Acne, cystitis, decongestant, digestive tonic, eczema, gallbladder, hormone-like, liver, ulcers.

Other Possible Uses: Chamomile neutralizes allergies[16] and increases the ability of the skin to regenerate. It is a cleanser of the blood and also helps open the liver, increase liver function and secretion, and support the pancreas. This oil may be used for abscesses, acne, boils, burns, cuts, cystitis, dermatitis, eczema, gallbladder, chronic gastritis, hair care, inflamed joints, ingrown nails (infected), insomnia, liver problems, menopausal problems, migraine headaches, open leg sores, rashes, skin disorders, stress-related complaints, teething pains, toothaches, ulcers, and wounds.

Body System(s) Affected: Emotional Balance, Nervous System, Skin.

Aromatic Influence: It can dispel anger, stabilize the emotions, and help release emotions linked to the past. It may also be used to soothe and clear the mind, creating an atmosphere of peace and patience.

Application: Apply to Vita Flex Points and directly on area of concern; diffuse.

Oral Use As Dietary Supplement: Generally regarded as safe (GRAS) for human consumption by the FDA. *Dilute one drop oil in 1 tsp. honey or in 4 oz. of beverage (i.e. soy/rice milk).* ***Not for children under 6 years old; use with caution and in greater dilution for children 6 years old and over.***

Safety Data: ***Use with caution during pregnancy. Can irritate sensitive skin.***

Blend Classification: Personifier.

Blends With: Fir, geranium, helichrysum, hyssop, lavender, lemongrass, marjoram, sandalwood, spearmint, spruce, melaleuca (tea tree), and wintergreen.

Odor: Type: *Middle Note (50–80% of the blend)*; Scent: *Deep, rich, tenacious, cocoa-like, herbaceous*; Intensity: *4*.

Frequency: Emotional; approximately 105.

Chamomile, Roman

(Chamaemelum nobile or Anthemis nobilis)

Botanical Family: Compositae (daisy)

Extraction Method/Origin: Steam distillation from flowers—Egypt, Utah

Chemical Constituents: Esters (up to 75%): isobutyl angelate (up to 25%), isoamyl methacylate (up to 25%), amyl butyrate (<15%), other angelate, butyrate, acetate, and tiglate esters; Monoterpenes (<35%): α- & β-pinenes (<20%), terpinenes, sabinene, camphene, d-limonene, p-cymene, myrcene; Ketones: pinocarvone (14%); Sesquiterpenes (up to 12%): β-caryophyllene, chamazulene; Alcohols (>7%): trans-pinocarveol, farnesol, nerolidol.

Properties: Anti-infectious, anti-inflammatory[17], antiparasitic, antispasmodic, calming, and relaxing.

Common Primary Uses: ^AT^Allergies (airborne), ^AT^anxiety, ^T^bee stings, ^A^crying, ^T^diaper rash, ^T^dry skin, ^T^dysentery, ^T^muscle spasms, ^T^neuralgia, ^T^neuritis, ^T^shock, ^T^spina bifida, ^TI^tooth abscess, ^T^wounds.

Historical Uses: It was traditionally used by the ancient Romans to give them a clear mind and to empower them with courage for their battles. According to Roberta Wilson, "Chamomile was nicknamed the 'plant's physician' because it supposedly cured any ailing plant placed near it."

French Medicinal Uses: Intestinal parasites, neuritis, neuralgia, shock (nervous).

Other Possible Uses: Chamomile neutralizes allergies and increases the ability of the skin to regenerate. It is a cleanser of the blood and also helps the liver to reject poisons and to discharge them. This oil may help with allergies, bruises, cuts, depression, insomnia, muscle tension, nerves (calming and promoting nerve health), restless legs, and skin conditions like acne, boils, dermatitis,

eczema, rashes, and **sensitive skin**. Chamomile is mild enough to use on **infants** and **children**. For centuries, mothers have used chamomile to **calm crying children**, ease **earaches**, fight **fevers**, soothe **stomachaches** and **colic**, and relieve **toothaches** and **teething pain**. It can safely and effectively reduce **irritability** and minimize **nervousness** in children, especially **hyperactive children**.

Body System(s) Affected: **Emotional Balance, Nervous System, Skin**.

Aromatic Influence: Because it is calming and relaxing, chamomile can combat **depression, insomnia**, and **stress**. It eliminates some of the emotional charge of **anxiety, irritability**, and **nervousness**. It can dispel **anger**, stabilize the **emotions**, and help to release emotions that are linked to the past. It may also be used to **soothe** and **clear** the **mind**, creating an atmosphere of **peace** and **patience**.

Application: Apply to **Vita Flex Points** and/or directly on **area** of concern; diffuse. Applied over the **throat**, it can help a person express his or her true feelings.

Oral Use As Dietary Supplement: Generally regarded as safe (GRAS) for human consumption by the FDA. ***Dilute*** *one drop oil in 1 tsp. honey or in 4 oz. of beverage (i.e. soy/rice milk).* ***Not for children under 6 years old; use with caution and in greater dilution for children 6 years old and over.***

Safety Data: ***Can irritate sensitive skin.***

Blend Classification: Personifier.

Blends With: Lavender, rose, geranium, or clary sage.

Odor: Type: *Middle Note (50–80% of the blend)*; Scent: *Fresh, sweet, fruity-herbaceous, apple-like, no tenacity*; Intensity: *4*.

Cinnamon Bark

(Cinnamomum verum or C. zeylanicum)

Botanical Family: Lauraceae (laurel)

Extraction Method/Origin: Steam distillation from bark—India, Madagascar, Sri Lanka

Chemical Constituents: Aldehydes: trans-cinnamaldehyde (<50%), hydroxycinnamaldehyde, benzaldehyde, cuminal; Phenols (up to 30%): eugenol (<30%), phenol, 2-vinyl-phenol; Alcohols: linalol, cinnamic alcohol, benzyl alcohol, α-terpineol, borneol; Sesquiterpenes: β-caryophyllene; Carboxylic Acids: cinnamic acid.

Properties: **Antibacterial**[18], **antidepressant, antifungal**[19], **anti-infectious** (intestinal, urinary), **anti-inflammatory, antimicrobial, antioxidant, antiparasitic, antiseptic, antispasmodic** (light), **antiviral, astringent, immune-stimulant, purifier, sexual stimulant**, and **warming**. It also **enhances** the action and activity of other oils.

Common Primary Uses: [TA]**Antibacterial**, [TA]**antifungal**, [IT]**diabetes**, [T]**diverticulitis**, [A]**pneumonia**, [TI]**staph/MRSA**, [T]**vaginal infections**, [T]**warming oils**, [A]**whooping cough**.

Historical Uses: This most ancient of spices was included in just about every prescription issued in ancient China. It was regarded as a tranquilizer, tonic, and stomachic and as being good for depression and a weak heart.

French Medicinal Uses: **Sexual stimulant, tropical infection, typhoid, vaginitis**.

Other Possible Uses: This oil may be beneficial for **circulation, colds, coughs, digestion, exhaustion, flu, infections, rheumatism**, and **warts**. This oil fights **viral** and **infectious diseases**, and testing has yet to find a **virus, bacteria**, or **fungus** that can survive in its presence.

Body System(s) Affected: **Immune System**.

Application: Apply to **Vita Flex Points** and directly on **area** of concern. Best if diluted with V-6 Oil, as the high amount of phenols can irritate the skin.

Oral Use As Dietary Supplement: Generally regarded as safe (GRAS) for human consumption by the FDA. **Dilute** *one drop oil in 2 tsp. honey or in 8 oz. of beverage (i.e. soy/rice milk). May need to increase dilution even more due to this oil's potential for irritating mucus membranes.* ***Not for children under 6 years old; use with caution and in greater dilution for children 6 years old and over.***

Safety Data: ***Repeated use can result in extreme contact sensitization. Avoid during pregnancy. Can cause extreme skin irritation. Diffuse with caution; it will irritate the nasal membranes if it is inhaled directly from the diffuser. Use extreme caution when diffusing cinnamon bark because it may burn the nostrils if you put your nose directly next to the nebulizer of the diffuser.***

Blend Classification: Personifier.

Blends With: All citrus oils, cypress, frankincense, geranium, juniper, lavender, rosemary, and all spice oils.

Odor: Type: *Base Note (5–60% of the blend)*; Scent: *Spicy, warm, sweet*; Intensity: *5*.

Frequency: Traditionally thought to have a frequency that attracted wealth.

Bible: Exod. 30:23, Prov. 7:17, Song. 4:14, Rev. 18:13.

Cistus (Labdanum)

(Cistus ladanifer)

Botanical Family: Cistaceae

Extraction Method/Origin: Steam distillation from branches—France, Spain

Chemical Constituents: Monoterpenes (up to 65%): α-pinene (50%), camphene (4%), sabinene, myrcene, phellandrene, limonene, cymene; Alcohols: α-terpineol (>5%), pinocarveol, borneol; Esters: linalyle acetate, bornyl & geranyl acetates (3%), methyl benzoate, phenyl propanoate; Ketones: 2,2,6-trimethylcyclohexanone (2%), fenchone (1%); Aldehydes: benzaldehyde (>3%), neral; Carboxylic Acids.

Properties: **Antimicrobial, antiseptic, astringent, diuretic, expectorant**, and **tonic**.

Common Primary Uses: [T]**Sciatica**.

Folklore: Anciently, cistus was among the first aromatic substances used.

Historical Uses: Used for catarrh, diarrhea, dysentery, and promoting menstruation.

Other Possible Uses: Cistus may help with **bleeding** (stop), **boils, bronchitis, colds, coughs, rhinitis, urinary infections, wounds**, and **wrinkles**.

Body System(s) Affected: **Immune System**. It may also assist the **auto-immune system**.

Aromatic Influence: **Stimulating** to the **senses** of touch, feeling, sight, and sound. It affects the upper part of the **brain**. It may also help quiet the **nerves**, calm the **insomniac**, and elevate the emotions in **meditation**.

Application: Apply to **Vita Flex Points** and/or directly on **area** of concern; diffuse.

Oral Use As Dietary Supplement: Approved by the FDA for use as a Food Additive (FA) or Flavoring Agent (FL). **Dilute** *one drop oil in 1 tsp. honey or in 4 oz. of beverage (i.e. soy/rice milk).* ***Not for children under 6 years old; use with caution and in greater dilution for children 6 years old and over.***

Safety Data: ***Use with caution during pregnancy.***

Blend Classification: Personifier.

Blends With: Bergamot, calamus, chamomile, clary sage, cypress, juniper, lavender, lavandin, patchouli, pine, sandalwood, and vetiver.

Citronella

(Cymbopogon nardus)

Botanical Family: Gramineae (grasses)

Extraction Method/Origin: Steam distillation from grass—Egypt, Philippines, Sri lanka

Chemical Constituents: Alcohols (>35%): geraniol (>16%), citronnellol (8%), borneol (6%); Phenols: methyl ether (<10%), methyl isoeugenol (<10%), isoeugenol (7%); Monoterpenes: d-limonene (<10%); Aldehydes: citronnellal (<7%).

Properties: **Antibacterial, antifungal, anti-inflammatory, antiseptic, antispasmodic, deodorizing**, and **insecticidal**[20].

Common Primary Uses: AT**Bug repellent**, AT**insect repellent**.

Historical Uses: This oil belongs to the same family of aromatic, oil-rich tropical grasses as lemongrass and palmarosa. It has been used as an insecticide and for rheumatic problems or other aches and pains. The leaves of citronella have been utilized by many diverse cultures for fever, intestinal parasites, digestive and menstrual problems, and as a stimulant. This oil is hardly used alone in therapy, but because of its highly antiseptic and deodorizing properties, it is used a great deal in commercial preparations and in some aromatherapy blends.

Other Possible Uses: Citronella may help with **colds, fatigue, flu, headaches**, minor **infections, migraines, neuralgia**, excessive **perspiration**, and **oily skin**. Can be used as an antiseptic to **sanitize** and **deodorize surfaces** where food has been prepared. Combined with cedarwood, it makes an excellent insect repellent.

Body System(s) Affected: **Muscles** and **Bones, Skin**.

Aromatic Influence: May increase the heart rate.

Application: Dilute, and apply directly on **area** of concern.

Oral Use As Dietary Supplement: Generally regarded as safe (GRAS) for human consumption by the FDA. ***Dilute** one drop oil in 1 tsp. honey or in 4 oz. of beverage (i.e. soy/rice milk).* ***Not for children under 6 years old; use with caution and in greater dilution for children 6 years old and over.***

Safety Data: ***Repeated use can result in extreme contact sensitization. Use with caution during pregnancy. Can irritate sensitive skin. Inhaling citronella can increase the heart rate.***

Blend Classification: Personifier.

Blends With: Bergamot, cedarwood, geranium, lemon, orange, and pine.

Odor: Type: *Top Note (5–20% of the blend)*; Scent: *Citrusy, slightly fruity, fresh, sweet*; Intensity: *3.*

Clary Sage

(Salvia sclarea)

Botanical Family: Labiatae (mint)

Extraction Method/Origin: Steam distillation from flowing plant—France, Utah

Chemical Constituents: Esters (up to 75%): linalyl acetate (20–75%); Alcohols (20%): linalol (10–22%), geraniol, α-terpineol; Sesquiterpenes (<14%): germacrene-D (up to 12%), β-caryophyllene; Diterpene alcohols: sclareol (normally 0.5–2.5%, but 5–7% from double distillation in Utah); Monoterpenes: myrcene, α- and β-pinenes, l-limonene, ocimene, terpinolene; Oxides: 1,8 cineol, linalol oxide, sclareol oxide; Ketones: α- and β-thujone; Sesquiterpene alcohols; Aldehydes; Coumarins. *(More than 250 constituents).*

Properties: **Anticonvulsive, antifungal, antiseptic, antispasmodic, astringent, nerve tonic, sedative, soothing**[21], **tonic**, and **warming**.

Common Primary Uses: [T]**Autism**, [T]**cholesterol**, [T]**cramps (abdominal)**, [T]**cramps (menstrual)**, [T]**epilepsy**, [T]**hair loss**, [T]**hemorrhoids**, [T]**hot flashes**, [T]**PMS**, [T]**seizure**.

Historical Uses: Nicknamed "clear eyes," it was famous during the Middle Ages for its ability to clear eye problems. During that same time, it was widely used for female complaints, kidney/digestive/skin disorders, inflammation, sore throats, and wounds.

French Medicinal Uses: **Bronchitis, cholesterol, frigidity, genitalia, hemorrhoids, hormonal imbalance, impotence, infections, intestinal cramps, menstrual cramps, PMS, premenopause, weak digestion.**

Other Possible Uses: This oil may be used for **amenorrhea, cell regulation, circulatory problems, depression, insect bites, insomnia, kidney disorders**, dry **skin**, **throat infection, ulcers**, and **whooping cough**.

Body System(s) Affected: **Hormonal System**.

Aromatic Influence: It may calm and enhance the **dream state**, helping to bring about a feeling of **euphoria**.

Application: Apply to **Vita Flex Points** and/or directly on **area** of concern; diffuse.

Oral Use As Dietary Supplement: Generally regarded as safe (GRAS) for human consumption by the FDA. **Dilute** *one drop oil in 1 tsp. honey or in 4 oz. of beverage (i.e. soy/rice milk).* ***Not for children under 6 years old; use with*** **caution** ***and in*** **greater dilution** ***for children 6 years old and over.***

Safety Data: ***Use with caution during*** **pregnancy*****. Not for babies. Avoid during and after consumption of*** **alcohol.**

Blend Classification: Personifier.

Blends With: Bergamot, cedarwood, citrus oils, cypress, geranium, juniper, and sandalwood.

Odor: Type: *Middle to Base Notes (5–60% of the blend)*; Scent: *Herbaceous, spicy, hay-like, sharp, fixative*; Intensity: *3*.

Clove

(Syzygium aromaticum)

Botanical Family: Myrtaceae (shrubs and trees)

Extraction Method/Origin: Steam distillation from bud and stem—Madagascar, Spice Islands

Chemical Constituents: Phenols: eugenol (up to 85%), chavicol, 4-allylphenol; Esters: eugenyl acetate (up to 15%), styralyl, benzyl, terpenyl, ethyl phenyl acetates, methyl salicylate (tr.); Sesquiterpenes (up to 14%): β-caryophyllene (<12%), humulene, α-amorphene, α-muurolene, calamenene; Oxides (<3%): caryophyllene oxide, humulene oxide; Carboxylic Acids; Ketones.

Properties: **Analgesic, antibacterial**[22]**, antifungal**[23]**, anti-infectious, anti-inflammatory**[24]**, antioxidant**[25]**, antiparasitic**, strong **antiseptic, antitumoral, antiviral**[26]**, disinfectant**, and **immune-stimulant**.

Common Primary Uses: [TA]**Antifungal**, [AI]**antioxidant**, [TA]**antiviral**, [IT]**blood clots**, [AT]**bug repellent**, [T]**candida**, [T]**cavities (pain)**, [T]**corns**, [IT]**fever**, [T]**herpes simplex**, [AT]**insect repellent**, [T]**lupus**, [T]**muscle aches**, [T]**pain**, [TI]**tooth abscess**, [T]**tumor**, [T]**wounds**.

Folklore: Some old tales say that walking near clove trees while wearing a hat would frighten the trees into no longer bearing fruit. While the trees may have been afraid of hats, they were not afraid of viruses. History has it that the people of Penang (among the "Spice Islands") were free from epidemics until the sixteenth century when Dutch conquerors destroyed the clove trees that flourished on those islands. Many of the islanders died from the epidemics that followed.

Historical Uses: Cloves were historically used for skin infections, digestive upsets, intestinal parasites, childbirth, and most notably for toothaches. The Chinese also used cloves for diarrhea, hernia, bad breath, and bronchitis.

French Medicinal Uses: **Impotence, intestinal parasites, memory deficiency, pain, plague, toothache, wounds** (infected).

Other Possible Uses: This oil may help **amebic dysentery, arthritis, bacterial colitis, blood clots**[27], **bones, bronchitis, cholera, cystitis, dental infection, diarrhea, infectious acne, fatigue, flatulence** (gas), **flu, halitosis** (bad breath), tension **headaches, hypertension, infection** (wounds and more), **insect bites and stings, elmiminating insects**[28], **lupus, nausea, neuritis, nettles** and **poison oak** (takes out sting), **rheumatism, sinusitis, skin cancer**, chronic **skin disease, smoking** (removes desire), **sores** (speeds healing of mouth and skin sores), **tuberculosis, thyroid dysfunction**, leg **ulcers, viral hepatitis, vomiting**, and **warts**. (*See WARTS in the Personal Guide section of this book.*)

Body System(s) Affected: **Cardiovascular, Digestive, Immune**, and **Respiratory Systems**.

Aromatic Influence: It may influence **healing**, improve **memory** (mental stimulant), and create a feeling of **protection** and **courage**. Septimas Piesse considered clove scent to **vibrate** in the **key** of **B** and in the color of **violet**. It can also cause a good sleep, generally culminating in stimulating dreams.

Application: Apply to **Vita Flex Points** and/or directly on **area** of concern. Rub directly on the **gums** surrounding an infected tooth. Place on **tongue** with finger to remove desire to smoke, or place on back of tongue to fight a tickling cough. **Diffuse**.

Oral Use As Dietary Supplement: Generally regarded as safe (GRAS) for human consumption by the FDA. ***Dilute*** *one drop oil in 1 tsp. honey or in 4 oz. of beverage (i.e. soy/rice milk).* ***Not for children under 6 years old; use with caution and in greater dilution for children 6 years old and over.***

Safety Data: ***Repeated use can result in extreme contact sensitization. Use with caution during pregnancy. Can irritate sensitive skin.***

Blend Classification: Personifier.

Blends With: Basil, bergamot, cinnamon bark, clary sage, grapefruit, lavender, lemon, nutmeg, orange, peppermint, rose, rosemary, and ylang ylang.

Odor: Type: *Middle to Base Notes (20–80% of the blend)*; Scent: *Spicy, warming, slightly bitter, woody, reminiscent of true clove buds, but richer*; Intensity: *5*.

Copaiba (Copal)

(Copaifera reticulata or Copaifera L. genus)

Botanical Family: Leguminosae (flowering plants)

Extraction Method/Origin: Steam distillation from oleoresin—Brazil, Ecuador

Chemical Constituents: Sesquiterpenes (up to 90%): β-caryophyllene (up to 52%), copaene (>15%), trans-α-bergamotene (>8%), α-cubebene, γ- & β-elemene, β-cubebene.

Properties: **Analgesic**[29], **powerful anti-inflammatory, antibacterial**[30], **antiseptic**, and **stimulant** (circulatory, pulmonary systems).

Common Primary Uses: **ATAnxiety, Tmuscle aches, Tpain**.

Historical Uses: The oleoresin has traditionally been used for **inflammation** (internal and external), **skin disorders**[31], **respiratory problems** including **bronchitis** and **sinusitis**, and **urinary tract problems** including **cystitis** and **bladder and kidney infections**. It has also been used for **bleeding, gonorrhea, hemorrhages, herpes, incontinence, insect bites, pain, pleurisy, sore throats, stomach ulcers, syphilis, tetanus, tonsillitis, tuberculosis**, and **tumors**[32]. All of these traditional uses have been verified by modern research.

Other Possible Uses: Copaiba may also help with **colds, constipation, diarrhea, dyspepsia, edema, flatulence, flu, bacterial infections** (internal and external), **hemorroids, muscular aches and pains, nervous exhaustion, piles, poor circulation, stiffness**, and **wounds**.

Body System(s) Affected: **Cardiovascular, Respiratory, and Nervous Systems, Muscles** and **Bones, Emotional Balance, and Skin.**

Aromatic Influence: Copaiba helps to **elevate** the mood and lift **depression**. It also helps to combat **nervous tension, stress problems**, and **anxiety**[33]. Copaiba is believed to amplify the effects of any other essential oil.

Application: Apply to **Vita Flex Points** and directly on **area** of concern.

Oral Use As Dietary Supplement: The oleoresin is generally regarded as safe (GRAS) for human consumption by the FDA when taken in small doses (less than 5 ml). It is also approved by the FDA for use as a Food Additive (FA) or Flavoring Agent (FL). **Dilute** *one drop oil in 1 tsp. honey or in 4 oz. of beverage (i.e. soy/rice milk).* ***Not for children under 6 years old; use with*** **caution** ***and in*** **greater dilution** ***for children 6 years old and over.***

Safety Data: ***Repeated use can possibly result in*** **contact sensitization**.

Odor: Type: *Base Note (5–20% of the blend)*; Scent: *Soft, sweet, balsamic*; Intensity: *3.*

Found In: Deep Relief.

Single Oils

Coriander

(Coriandrum sativum L.)

Botanical Family: Umbelliferae (parsley)

Extraction Method/Origin: Steam distillation from seeds—India, Russia

Chemical Constituents: Alcohols (up to 80%): linalol (up to 70%), coriandrol (<30%), geraniol, terpinen-4-ol, borneol; Monoterpenes (up to 24%): α-pinene, γ-terpinene, l-limonene, p-cymene, myrcene, camphene; Esters: geranyl acetate, linalyl acetate; Ketones: camphor, carvone; Aldehydes: decanal.

Properties: **Analgesic, antibacterial, antifungal, antioxidant, antirheumatic, antispasmodic**[34], and **stimulant** (cardiac, circulatory, and nervous systems). It also has **anti-inflammatory** and **sedative** properties.

Folklore: The seeds were found in the ancient Egyptian tomb of Rameses II.

Historical Uses: The Chinese have used coriander for dysentery, piles, measles, nausea, toothache, and painful hernias.

Other Possible Uses: Coriander may help with **anorexia, arthritis, colds, colic, diarrhea, digestive spasms, dyspepsia, flatulence, flu, gout, infections** (general), **measles, migraines, muscular aches and pains, nausea, nervous exhaustion, neuralgia, piles, poor circulation, rheumatism, skin** (oily skin, blackheads, and other impurities), and **stiffness**. Current research at Cairo University indicates that coriander lowers **glucose** levels by normalizing insulin levels and supporting **pancreas function**. Coriander may also help during **convalescence** and after a difficult childbirth. Because of its estrogen content, it may regulate and help control pain related to **menstruation**.

Body System(s) Affected: **Digestive** and **Hormonal Systems**.

Aromatic Influence: Coriander is a gentle stimulant for those with **low physical energy**. It also helps one relax during times of **stress, irritability, and nervousness**. It may provide a **calming** influence to those suffering from **shock** or **fear**.

Application: Apply to **Vita Flex Points** and directly on **area** of concern; **diffuse**.

Oral Use As Dietary Supplement: Generally regarded as safe (GRAS) for human consumption by the FDA. **Dilute** *one drop oil in 1 tsp. honey or in 4 oz. of beverage (i.e. soy/rice milk).* ***Not for children under 6 years old; use with*** **caution** ***and in*** **greater dilution** ***for children 6 years old and over.***

Safety Data: ***Use sparingly as coriander can be*** **stupifying** ***in large doses.***

Blend Classification: Personifier and Modifier.

Blends With: Bergamot, cinnamon bark, citronella, clary sage, cypress, ginger, jasmine, neroli, petitgrain, pine, sandalwood, and other spice oils.

Odor: Type: *Middle Note (50–80% of the blend)*; Scent: *Woody, spicy, sweet*; Intensity: *3.*

Cumin

(Cuminum cyminum)

Botanical Family: Umbelliferae (parsley)

Extraction Method/Origin: Steam distillation from seeds—Egypt

Chemical Constituents: Monoterpenes (up to 75%): α- and γ-terpinenes (<40%), β-pinene, p-cymene, camphene; Aldehydes (<60%): p-menthadienals (up to 35%), cuminal (up to 32%), dihydro-cuminal, p-mentha-3-en-7-ol; Phenols: p-cuminol; Sesquiterpenes: β-caryophyllene; Coumarins: scopoletin.

Properties: **Antibacterial, antifungal**[35], **antioxidant, antiparasitic, antiseptic, antispasmodic, antitoxic, antiviral, aphrodisiac, digestive, stimulant** (heart, immune and nervous systems), and **tonic**.

Common Primary Uses: **AT AIDS/HIV**, **IT diabetes**.

Folklore: Cumin seeds were found in Egyptian tombs. Cumin seeds were also used by the Romans as a food preservative.

Historical Uses: In biblical times, cumin was used by the Hebrews as an antiseptic during their ceremony of circumcision. Traditionally one of the main ingredients in curry, cumin was also used to help with flatulence, the digestive system, rheumatic conditions, the heart, and the nervous system.

Other Possible Uses: This oil may help with **cellulite**, poor **circulation, colic, deafness** following a bad viral **flu** infection, **digestive spasms, dyspepsia, epilepsy**[36], **flatulence, headaches, indigestion, lymphatic congestion, migraines, morphine withdrawal**[37], **nervous debility**, and **exhaustion**.

Body System(s) Affected: **Digestive** and **Immune Systems**.

Aromatic Influence: Used by one source to encourage **bowel movements** in a child. It has also been used at dinner parties to **stimulate appetite**.

Application: Apply to **Vita Flex Points** and directly on **area** of concern; **diffuse**.

Oral Use As Dietary Supplement: Generally regarded as safe (GRAS) for human consumption by the FDA. ***Dilute** one drop oil in 1 tsp. honey or in 4 oz. of beverage (i.e. soy/rice milk).* ***Not for children under 6 years old; use with caution and in greater dilution for children 6 years old and over.***

Safety Data: ***Use with caution during pregnancy. Avoid direct sunlight for up to 12 hours after use.***

Blend Classification: Enhancer.

Blends With: Cinnamon bark, jasmine, patchouli, rose, sandalwood, and ylang ylang.

Cypress

(Cupressus sempervirens)

Botanical Family: Cupressaceae (conifer: cypress)

Extraction Method/Origin: Steam distillation from branches—France, Spain

Chemical Constituents: Monoterpenes: α-pinene (>55%), δ-3-carene (<22%), l-limonene, terpinolene, sabinene, β-pinene; Sesquiterpene Alcohols: cedrol (up to 15%), cadinol; Alcohols: borneol (<9%), α-terpineol, terpinene-4-ol,linalol sabinol; Esters: α-terpinyl acetate (<5%), isovalerate, terpinen-4-yl acetate; Sesquiterpenes: δ-cadinene, α-cedrene; Diterpene Alcohols; labdanic alcohols, manool, sempervirol; Diterpene Acids; Oxides.

Properties: **Antibacterial, anti-infectious, antimicrobial, mucolytic, antiseptic, astringent, deodorant, diuretic, lymphatic** and **prostate decongestant, refreshing, relaxing**, and a **vasoconstrictor.**

Common Primary Uses: [A]**Aneurysm**, [T]**bunion**, [T]**bursitis**, [T]**carpal tunnel**, [T]**cataracts**, [TA]**concussion (brain)**, [T]**deodorant**, [T]**hemorrhoids**, [T]**herniated disc**, [T]**jock itch**, [TA]**Lou Gehrig's disease**, [T]**muscle fatigue**, [T]**nose bleed**, [T]**Raynaud's disease**, [T]**shingles**, [AT]**stroke**, [T]**toxemia**, [AT]**tuberculosis**, [T]**varicose veins.**

Folklore: According to Roberta Wilson, "The evergreen branches of the cypress tree were considered symbolic of life after death. In fact, *sempervirens* means 'ever-living.'"

Historical Uses: It was used anciently for its benefits to the urinary system and in other instances where there is excessive loss of fluids, such as perspiration, diarrhea, and menstrual flow. The Chinese valued cypress for its benefits to the liver and the respiratory system.

French Medicinal Uses: **Arthritis, bronchitis, circulation, cramps, hemorrhoids, insomnia, intestinal parasites, lymphatic decongestion, menopausal problems, menstrual pain, pancreas insufficiencies, pleurisy, prostate decongestion, pulmonary tuberculosis, rheumatism, spasms, throat problems, varicose veins, and water retention.**

Other Possible Uses: This oil may be beneficial for **asthma**, strengthening **blood capillary walls**, reducing **cellulite, circulatory system functioning, colds**, strengthening **connective tissue**, spasmodic **coughs, diarrhea, edema, energy, fever, gallbladder**, bleeding **gums, hemorrhaging, influenza, laryngitis, liver disorders, lung circulation, muscular cramps, nervous tension, nose bleeds, ovarian cysts**, increasing **perspiration, skin care, scar tissue, whooping cough**, and **wounds.**

Body System(s) Affected: **Cardiovascular System, Muscles** and **Bones.**

Aromatic Influence: It influences and strengthens, and it helps ease the feeling of **loss**. It creates a feeling of **security and grounding**, and it helps to heal **emotions.**

Application: Apply to **Vita Flex Points** and directly on **area** of concern; **diffuse.**

Oral Use As Dietary Supplement: None.

Safety Data: *Use with caution during* ***pregnancy.***

Blend Classification: Equalizer.

Blends With: Bergamot, clary sage, juniper, lavender, lemon, orange, and sandalwood.

Odor: Type: *Middle Note (50–80% of the blend)*; Scent: *Fresh, herbaceous, slightly woody with evergreen undertones*; Intensity: *3.*

Cypress, Blue

(Callitris intratropica)

Botanical Family: Cupressaceae

Extraction Method/Origin: Steam distillation from the heartwood, which makes up 70% of the tree trunk—Australia

Chemical Constituents: Sesquiterpene Alcohols (up to 70%): guaiol (<26%), α- and β-eudesmols (<25%), bulnesol (<15%); Sesquiterpenes (<22%): β-elemene (<10%), β-selinene (<10%), δ-guaiazulene (<2%); Lactones.

Properties: **Anti-inflammatory, antiviral, insect repellent**, and **stimulant** (to amygdalla, pineal gland, pituitary gland, and hypothalamus).

Common Primary Uses: [T]**Shingles.**

Historical Uses: Blue cypress has been used historically for incense, perfume, and embalming. The resin was used for sores, cuts, and upset stomachs. The aboriginal Tiwi people of Australia would throw the wood onto the fire to drive away the mosquitoes and midges. The guaiazulene gives blue cypress oil its azure blue color.

Other Possible Uses: Blue cypress may help with **abdominal cramps, aches** and **pain** (minor), **brain** function (improves circulation and oxygenates), **cold sores, herpes simplex, herpes zoster**, and the **human papilloma virus (HPV)**.

Body System(s) Affected: **Digestive** and **Immune Systems**.

Application: Apply to **Vita Flex Points** and directly on **area** of concern; diffuse.

Safety Data: ***None available.***

Blends With: Cedarwood, frankincense, helichrysum, lavender, melissa, and sandalwood.

Odor: Type: *Base Note (5–20% of the blend)*; Scent: *Long-lasting, warm, woody, earthy*; Intensity: *3*.

Found In: Brain Power, Australian Blue, AromaGuard Mountain Mint Deodorant.

Davana

(Artemisia pallens)

Botanical Family: Compositae (daisy)

Extraction Method/Origin: Steam distillation of the stems and leaves—India

Chemical Constituents: Ketones: davanone (47–52%), nordavanone (<3%), artemone (<3%); Alcohols: nerol (10%), geraniol (5%), nerolidol (<3%), borneol, davanol, farnesol, linalol; Ethers: davana ether (<6%); Furanoids: davana furan (<4%); Terpenes: cadinene, para-cymene, camphene, sabinene; Carboxylic Acids: davanic acid (<3%); Esters: cinnamyl cinnamate (2%), ethyl davanate; Oxides: linalol oxide; Aldehydes: lilac aldehyde.

Properties: **Antibacterial, antifungal, anti-infectious, nervine.**

Historical Uses: Davana has been widely used in Iraqi and Indian folk medicine for the treatment of diabetes mellitus. According to one research study, "Oral administration of an aqueous/methanolic extract from the aerial parts of the plants led to significant blood glucose lowering effect in glucose-fed hyperglycemic and alloxan-induced diabetic rabbits and rats" (Twaij HA and Al-Badr AA, 1988 and Subramoniam A et al. 1996).

Possible Uses: This oil may help stimulate the **endocrine system**, improve **hormonal balance**, and soothe **rough, dry,** and **chapped skin**. It may also help with **coughing attacks,** with **thick mucus** and **spasmodic coughs,** and may also help ease **anxious feelings** and **nervousness**.

Body System(s) Affected: **Hormonal System**.

Oral Use As Dietary Supplement: Approved by the FDA for use as a Food Additive (FA) or Flavoring Agent (FL). ***Dilute*** *one drop oil in 1 tsp. honey or in 4 oz. of beverage (i.e. soy/rice milk).* ***Not for children under 6 years old; use with caution and in greater dilution for children 6 years old and over.***

Safety Data: ***Use with caution during pregnancy.***

Dill

(Anethum graveolens)

Botanical Family: Umbelliferae (parsley)

Extraction Method/Origin: Steam distillation from whole plant—Austria, Hungary

Chemical Constituents: Monoterpenes (up to 65%): d-limonene (up to 25%), α- & β-pinenes (<30%), α- & β-phellandrenes, p-cymene; Ketones: d-carvone (<45%); Ethers (<11%).

Properties: **Antispasmodic, antibacterial, expectorant**, and **stimulant**.

Common Primary Uses: **ᵀCholesterol**.

Folklore: The dill plant is mentioned in the Papyrus of Ebers from Egypt (1550 B.C.). Roman Gladiators would rub it into their skin before a fight.

Possible Uses: This oil may help **bronchial catarrh, colic, constipation, dyspepsia, flatulence, headaches, indigestion, liver deficiencies, lower glucose levels, nervousness, normalize insulin levels, promote milk flow** in nursing mothers, **support pancreas functioning**, and clear **toxins**[38].

Body System(s) Affected: **Digestive System**.

Aromatic Influence: It calms the autonomic nervous system and, when diffused with Roman chamomile, may help fidgety children

Application: Apply to **Vita Flex Points** and/or directly on **area** of concern; diffuse. A drop or two on the **wrists** can help remove **addictions** to **sweets**.

Oral Use As Dietary Supplement: Generally regarded as safe (GRAS) for human consumption by the FDA. ***Dilute** one drop oil in 1 tsp. honey or in 4 oz. of beverage (i.e. soy/rice milk).* ***Not for children under 6 years old; use with caution and in greater dilution for children 6-years-old and over.***

Safety Data: ***Use with caution if susceptible to epilepsy.***

Blend Classification: Enhancer.

Blends With: Nutmeg and citrus oils.

Odor: Type: *Middle Note (50–80% of the blend)*; Scent: *Fresh, sweet, herbaceous, slightly earthy*; Intensity: *2*.

Dorado Azul

(Hyptis suaveolens)

Botanical Family: Labiatae (mint)

Extraction Method/Origin: Steam distillation from whole plant—Ecuador

Chemical Constituents: Oxides: 1,8 cineol (<40%); Monoterpenes (<30%): α- & β-pinenes, sabinene, limonene; Alcohols: α-fenchol (10–15%); Ketones: fenchone (7%).

Properties: **Anti-inflammatory**.

Possible Uses: This oil may also be used to help balance the **hormonal system** (balances estrogen), modulate **brain function**, and control **asthma** and **emphysema**.

Body System(s) Affected: **Hormonal**, **Nervous**, and **Respiratory Systems**.

Application: Apply to **Vita Flex Points** and/or directly on **area** of concern; diffuse.

Odor: Scent: *Fresh, herbaceous.*

Douglas Fir

(See Fir, Douglas)

Elemi

(Canarium luzonicum)

Botanical Family: Burseraceae

Extraction Method/Origin: Steam distillation from the gum of the tree—Philippines

Chemical Constituents: Monoterpenes (up to 90%): l-limonene (up to 70%), α- phellandrene (<24%), sabinene (<10%), β-phellandrene (5%), dipentene, terpinolene; Alcohols: elemol (up to 25%), α-terpineol; Ethers: elemicin; Sesquiterpenes: elemene; Ketones: d-carvone.

Properties: **Anticatarrhal, antidepressant, anti-infectious, antiseptic, expectorant**, and **sedative**.

Common Primary Uses: [T]**Chapped/cracked skin**, [T]**rashes**, [T]**tissue repair**.

Folklore: The name *elemi* comes from an Arabic phrase meaning "As above, so below." This helps us to understand its action on both the emotional and spiritual planes. Because of the similar properties and uses, it has come to be known as the "poor man's frankincense."

Historical Uses: Native to the Philippine islands and the Moluccas, it is used locally for skin conditions and respiratory problems. Anciently, the Egyptians used the oil that was distilled from the resin in part of the embalming process.

Other Possible Uses: This oil may help with **bronchitis** (chronic), **chest infections, childbirth, coughs** (unproductive), **cuts** (infected), **gangrene, inflammation** (breast and uterus), **pregnancy, rashes** (allergic), **rejuvenation, skin** (chapped), **thymus gland, tissue** (builds), **ulcers, wounds** (infected), and **wrinkles**. (See FRANKINSENSE and MYRRH for other possible uses.)

Body System(s) Affected: **Skin**.

Aromatic Influence: When diffused, this oil may help with **nervous exhaustion, stress, sinusitis**, and other **bronchial infections**. During **meditation**, it may help to **calm** and Chakras (Energy Centers) **center** the individual. It may also help to bring the **mind, body**, and **spirit** into alignment with each other. It is psychologically **balancing** and **strengthening** as well as **fortifying** to the **psychic centers**.

Application: Apply to **Vita Flex Points** and/or directly on **area** of concern. May be used as a **compress** for infected **wounds** and **abscesses**. May also be diluted for use during a **massage** or be added to a **bath**.

Oral Use As Dietary Supplement: Approved by the FDA for use as a Food Additive (FA) or Flavoring Agent (FL). ***Dilute** one drop oil in 1 tsp. honey or in 4 oz. of beverage (i.e. soy/rice milk).* ***Not for children under 6 years old; use with caution and in greater dilution for children 6 years old and over.***

Blend Classification: Enhancer; the hint of lemon gives it more of a middle note.

Blends With: Cinnamon bark & other spices, frankincense, lavender, myrrh, rosemary, sage.

Odor: Type: *Middle Note (50–80% of the blend)*; Scent: *Balsamic, fresh, citrusy, peppery, spicy*; Intensity: *3*.

Eucalyptus

(Eucalyptus globulus)

Botanical Family: Myrtaceae (Myrtle shrubs and trees)

Extraction Method/Origin: Steam distillation from leaves—Australia, Brazil

Chemical Constituents: Oxides: 1,8 cineol (up to 78%); Monoterpenes (>20%): α- & β-pinenes, l-limonene, ρ-cymene, α-phellandrene; Sesquiterpene Alcohols: globulol (>7%), trans-pinocarveol (<5%), ledol (>2%), linalol, terpinen-4-ol, eudesmol; Sesquiterpenes: aromadendrene (>7%), allo-aromadendrene (>2%), δ-guaiazulene, humulene; Ketones: pinocarvone, d-carvone, fenchone; Aldehydes: butyricaldehyde, caproicaldehyde, geranial, myrtenal, valericaldehyde; Phenols: myrtenol, p-cuminol; Alcohols: α-fenchol, α-terpineol; Esters: α-terpenyl acetate.

Properties: **Analgesic**[39], **antibacterial**[40], **anticatarrhal, anti-infectious, anti-inflammatory**[41], **antiseptic, antiviral**[42], **diuretic, expectorant, insect repellent**[43], and **stimulant**.

Common Primary Uses: [AT]**Asthma**, [AT]**bronchitis**, [T]**carpal tunnel**, [T]**cataracts**, [TA]**congestion**, [T]**cooling**, [AT]**coughs**, [T]**deodorant**, [T]**dysentery**, [A]**emphysema**, [T]**fever**, [AT]**high blood pressure**,

Thypoglycemia, Tinflammation, Tjet lag, Tkidney stones, ATmeasles, Tmigraine, Tneuralgia, Tneuritis, Tpain, Tshingles, ATsinusitis, Tsore throat, Tspina bifida, ATstimulating, Tstrep throat, Ttennis elbow, ATtuberculosis.

Historical Uses: Australian aborigines used the eucalyptus leaves to bind up serious wounds. This would not only prevent infection but also expedite healing.

French Medicinal Uses: **Asthma, candida, coughs, diabetes, fever, hypoglycemia, lungs, measles, migraines, respiratory stimulant, sinusitis, tuberculosis, urinary stimulant.**

Other Possible Uses: This oil may be used for **aches/pains, acne, allergies, bronchitis**[44], **burns, colds, cystitis, diarrhea, endometriosis**, increasing **energy, flu, gallstones, gonorrhea, hay fever, herpes, high blood pressure**[45], **inflammation** of the **ear, inflammation** of the **iris, inflammation** of the **nasal mucous membrane, malaria, nasopharynx, rheumatism, skin infection/sores, sore throat, ulcers, vaginitis, viruses**, and **wounds.**

Body System(s) Affected: **Muscles** and **Bones, Respiratory System.**

Aromatic Influence: It promotes **health, well-being, purification**, and **healing.**

Application: Apply to **Vita Flex Points** and/or directly on **area** of concern; diffuse. *Apply under the nose and on each side of the nose for quick* ***sinus relief.***

Oral Use As Dietary Supplement: Approved by the FDA for use as a Food Additive (FA) or Flavoring Agent (FL). **Dilute** *one drop oil in 1 tsp. honey or in 4 oz. of beverage (i.e. soy/rice milk).* ***Not for children under 6 years old; use with caution and in greater dilution for children 6 years old and over.***

Blend Classification: Enhancer.

Blends With: Geranium, lavender, lemon, sandalwood, juniper, lemongrass, melissa, pine, thyme.

Odor: Type: *Top Note (5–20% of the blend)*; Scent: *Fresh, medicinal, woody, earthy*; Intensity: *5.*

Eucalyptus Blue

(Eucalyptol natriol azul)

Botanical Family: Myrtaceae (Myrtle shrubs and trees)

Extraction Method/Origin: Steam distillation from leaves —Ecuador

Chemical Constituents: Oxides (<85%): 1,8 cineol (<68%), α-pinene (<26%); Monoterpenes: limonene (6%); Alcohols: α-terpineol (<2%); Esters: α-terpinyl acetate (<2%); Sesquiterpenes: aromadendrene (<2%).

Properties: **Anti-inflammatory, antiviral.**

Other Possible Uses: This oil may also be used for **respiratory infections** and to help increase **metabolism.**

Body System(s) Affected: **Respiratory System, Immune System.**

Aromatic Influence: It is stimulating to the hypothalmus, bringing a sense of peace and balance. It is also invigorating.

Application: Apply to **Vita Flex Points** and/or directly on **area** of concern; diffuse. *Apply under the nose and on each side of the nose.*

Odor: Type: *Top Note (5–20% of the blend)*; Scent: *Fresh, medicinal, sweet, refreshing*; Intensity: *5.*

Eucalyptus Citriodora (or Lemon Eucalyptus)

(Eucalyptus citriodora)

Botanical Family: Myrtaceae (Myrtle shrubs and trees)

Extraction Method/Origin: Steam distillation from leaves—China

Chemical Constituents: Aldehydes: citronellal (<80%); Alcohols: citronellol (<20%), geraniol, trans-pinocarveol, cis- & trans-p-menthane-3,8-diols; Phenols (<21%): isopulegol, eugenol, p-cuminol; Oxides (<18%): 1,8 cineol, linalool oxide, rose oxide; Esters (<12%): citronellyl acetate (<8%), citronellyl butyrate, citronellyl citronellate.

Properties: **Antibacterial, antifungal, anti-infectious, anti-inflammatory**[46]**, antirheumatic, antiseptic, antiviral, deodorant, expectorant**, and **insecticidal**.

Historical Uses: *Eucalyptus citriodora* has been used to perfume the linen closet and to repel insects, especially cockroaches and silverfish.

Other Possible Uses: *Eucalyptus citriodora* may help with **asthma, athlete's foot** and other **fungal infections, colds, cuts, dandruff, fevers, herpes, infectious skin conditions** such as **chickenpox, infectious diseases, insect repellent, laryngitis, scabs, sore throat, sores, wounds**.

Body System(s) Affected: **Respiratory System**.

Application: Apply to **Vita Flex Points** and/or directly on **area** of concern.

Oral Use As Dietary Supplement: None.

Safety Data: ***Repeated use can possibly result in* contact sensitization**.

Odor: Type: *Middle Note (50–80% of the blend)*; Scent: *Sweet, lemony, fresh, with a woody hint;* Intensity: *3.*

Eucalyptus Dives

(Eucalyptus dives var. piperitone)

Botanical Family: Myrtaceae (Myrtle shrubs and trees)

Extraction Method/Origin: Steam distillation from leaves—Australia, Brazil

Chemical Constituents: Ketones: piperitone (up to 50%); Monoterpenes (<47%): α- & β-phellandrenes (<30%), p-cymene (<10%), α-thujene (<6%); Phenolic Alcohols: terpinen-4-ol (<6%); Sesquiterpenes (<4%): α-cubebene, β-caryophyllene, δ-cadinene, γ-elemene, longifolene; Alcohols (<3%): α-terpineol, linalol, piperitol; Oxides (<1%): α-pinene oxide, 1,8 cineol oxide.

Properties: **Antibacterial** (*more specific than other varieties of eucalyptus oil*).

Possible Uses: See other varieties of eucalyptus for possible uses.

Body System(s) Affected: **Respiratory System**.

Application: **Diffuse**; apply to **Vita Flex Points** and directly on **area** of concern.

Oral Use As Dietary Supplement: None.

Eucalyptus Polybractea

(Eucalyptus polybractea)

Botanical Family: Myrtaceae (Myrtle shrubs and trees)

Extraction Method/Origin: Steam distillation from leaves—Australia, Brazil

Chemical Constituents: Oxides: 1,8 cineol (up to 95%); Monoterpenes (<6%): l-limonene, α-pinene, p-cymene; Ketones: cryptone; Aldehydes: cuminal; Phenols: p-cuminol.

Properties: **Antibacterial, anti-infectious, anti-inflammatory**[47]**, antiviral, expectorant, mucolytic**, and **insecticidal**.

Possible Uses: **Acne, cystitis**. See other varieties of eucalyptus for possible uses.

Body System(s) Affected: **Respiratory System**.

Application: **Diffuse**; apply to **Vita Flex Points** and directly on **area** of concern.

Oral Use As Dietary Supplement: None.

Odor: Type: *Top Note (5–20% of the blend)*; Scent: *Fresh, woody, earthy*; Intensity: *4*.

Eucalyptus Radiata

(Eucalyptus radiata)

Botanical Family: Myrtaceae (myrtle shrubs and trees)

Extraction Method/Origin: Steam distillation from leaves—Australia

Chemical Constituents: Oxides: 1,8 cineol (62–72%), caryophyllene oxide; Monoterpenes (up to 24%): α- & β-pinenes (<12%), l-limonene (<8%), myrcene, p-cymene; Alcohols (<19%): α-terpinol (14%), geraniol, borneol, linalol; Aldehydes (8%): myrtenal, citronellal, geranial, neral.

Properties: **Antibacterial, anticatarrhal, anti-infectious, anti-inflammatory**[47]**, antiviral**, and **expectorant**.

Common Primary Uses: **TACongestion, Aemphysema, ATflu (influenza), Tpink eye, ATtuberculosis.**

Other Possible Uses: This oil, when combined with bergamot, has been used effectively on **herpes simplex**. It may also help with **acne, bronchitis, ear inflammation, endometriosis, flu, hay fever, iris inflammation, nasal mucous membrane inflammation, sinusitis**, and **vaginitis**.

Body System(s) Affected: **Respiratory System, Skin.**

Application: Apply to **Vita Flex Points** and/or directly on **area** of concern; diffuse.

Odor: Type: *Middle Note (50–80% of the blend)*; Scent: *Slightly camphorous, sweet, fruity*; Intensity: *3*.

Eucalyptus Staigeriana

(Eucalyptus staigeriana)

Botanical Family: Myrtaceae (myrtle shrubs and trees)

Extraction Method/Origin: Steam distillation from leaves—Brazil

Chemical Constituents: Aldehydes: citral (up to 40%), geranial (12%), neral; Monoterpenes: limonene (up to 25%), p-cymene (2%), many others; Alcohols: geraniol (6%), nerol; Oxides: 1,8 cineol (5%); Ester: geranyl acetate (4%), methyl geraniate.

Properties: **Analgesic, antifungal, anti-infectious, anti-inflammatory, antiviral, antiseptic** (pulmonary, urinary), powerful **antispasmodic, purifying**, and **sedative** (CNS, heart).

Possible Uses: This oil may help with **bronchitis, colds, congestion, cystitis, dermatitis, fevers, infections, hypertension** (lowers blood pressure), **inflammation** (joint and muscle), **leucorrhea** (increases urine flow), **neck aches, solar plexus** (relaxes), **stress-related disorders**, and **vaginitis**. It is also very soothing and calming.

Body System(s) Affected: **Muscles** and **Bones, Respiratory System, Skin.**

Application: Apply to **Vita Flex Points** and/or directly on **area** of concern; diffuse.

Fennel

(Foeniculum vulgare)

Botanical Family: Umbelliferae (parsley)

Extraction Method/Origin: Steam distillation from the crushed seeds—Australia, Spain

Single Oils

Chemical Constituents: Phenolic Ethers (up to 80%): trans-anethole (70%), methyl chavicol (or estragole) (>3%); Monoterpenes (up to 50%): trans-ocimene (<12%), l-limonene (<12%), γ-terpinene (<11%), α- & β-pinenes (<10%), p-cymene, α- & β-phellandrenes, terpiolene, myrcene, sabinene; Alcohols (up to 16%): linalol (<12%), α-fenchol (<4%); Ketones (<15%): fenchone (12%), camphor; Oxides; Phenols.

Properties: **Antiparasitic, antiseptic, antispasmodic**[48]**, antitoxic, diuretic**, and **expectorant**.

Common Primary Uses: **A Alcoholism**, **IT blood clots**, **T bruises**, **T colic**, **IT gas/flatulence**, **IT gastritis**, **T gout**, **IT obesity**, **IT parasites**, **T PMS**, **IA vomiting**, **T wrinkles**.

Folklore: During Medieval times, fennel was believed to ward off evil spirits and to block spells cast by witches.

Historical Uses: The ancient Egyptians and Romans awarded garlands of fennel as praise to victorious warriors because fennel was believed to bestow strength, courage, and longevity. It has been used for thousands of years for snakebite, to stave off hunger pains, to tone the female reproductive system, for earaches, eye problems, insect bites, kidney complaints, lung infections, and to expel worms.

French Medicinal Uses: **Cystitis**, sluggish **digestion, flatulence, gout, intestinal parasites, intestinal spasms**, increase **lactation, menopause problems, premenopause, urinary stones, vomiting**.

Other Possible Uses: Fennel oil may be used for **colic**, stimulating the **cardiovascular system, constipation, digestion** (supports the liver), balancing **hormones, kidney stones, nausea, obesity**, supporting **pancreatic function**, and **PMS**. It may break up **fluids** and **toxins**, and **cleanse** the **tissues**.

Body System(s) Affected: **Digestive** and **Hormonal Systems**.

Aromatic Influence: It influences and increases **longevity, courage,** and **purification**. It **stimulates** sympathetic nervous system activity[49].

Application: Apply to **Vita Flex Points** and directly on **area** of concern; diffuse.

Oral Use As Dietary Supplement: Generally regarded as safe (GRAS) for human consumption by the FDA. ***Dilute** one drop oil in 1 tsp. honey or in 4 oz. of beverage (i.e. soy/rice milk).* ***Not for children under 6 years old; use with caution and in greater dilution for children 6 years old and over.***

Safety Data: ***Repeated use can possibly result in contact sensitization. Use with caution if susceptible to epilepsy. Use with caution during pregnancy.***

Blend Classification: Equalizer and Modifier.

Blends With: Basil, geranium, lavender, lemon, rosemary, and sandalwood.

Odor: Type: *Top to Middle Notes (20–80% of the blend)*; Scent: *Sweet, somewhat spicy, licorice-like*; Intensity: *4*.

Fir (Silver Fir or Fir Needle)

(Abies alba)

Botanical Family: Pinaceae (conifer)

Extraction Method/Origin: Steam distillation from needles—Balkans

Chemical Constituents: Monoterpenes (75–95%): l-limonene (34%), α-pinene (24%), camphene (21%), santene, δ-3-carene; Esters: bornyle acetate (up to 10%).

Properties: **Analgesic, antiarthritic, anticatarrhal, antiseptic** (pulmonary), **expectorant**, and **stimulant**.

Common Primary Uses: **A Antioxidant**, **T bathroom/kitchen cleaning**, **AT bronchitis**, **AT energizing**, **T furniture polish**, **T muscle aches**, **T muscle fatigue**.

Historical Uses: The fir tree is the classic Christmas tree (short with the perfect pyramidal shape and silvery white bark). Though highly regarded for its fragrant scent, the fir tree has been prized through the ages for its medicinal virtues in regards to respiratory complaints, fever, and muscular and rheumatic pain.

French Medicinal Uses: **Bronchitis**[50], **respiratory congestion, energy**.

Other Possible Uses: Fir creates the symbolic effect of the umbrella protecting the earth and bringing energy in from the universe. At night the animals in the wild lie down under the trees for the protection, recharging, and rejuvenation the trees bring them. This oil may be beneficial for reducing **aches/pains** from **colds** and the **flu**, fighting **airborne germs/bacteria, arthritis, asthma**, supporting the **blood, bronchial** obstructions, **coughs, fevers, oxygenating** the cells, **rheumatism, sinusitis**, and **urinary tract infections**.

Body System(s) Affected: **Respiratory System**.

Aromatic Influence: It creates a feeling of **grounding, anchoring**, and **empowerment**. It can **stimulate** the **mind** while allowing the body to relax.

Application: Apply to **Vita Flex Points** and/or directly on **area** of concern; diffuse.

Oral Use As Dietary Supplement: Approved by the FDA for use as a Food Additive (FA) and Flavoring Agent (FL). ***Dilute** one drop oil in 1 tsp. honey or in 4 oz. of beverage (i.e. soy/rice milk).* ***Not for children under 6 years old; use with caution and in greater dilution for children 6 years old and over.***

Safety Data: ***Can irritate sensitive skin***.

Blend Classification: Equalizer.

Blends With: German chamomile, cedarwood, frankincense, lavender, myrtle, and rosewood.

Odor: Type: *Middle Notes (50–80% of the blend)*; Scent: *Fresh, woody, earthy, sweet*; Intensity: *3*.

Fir, Balsam (Canadian Balsam)

(Abies balsamea)

Botanical Family: Pinaceae (conifer)

Extraction Method/Origin: Steam distillation from branches—Canada, USA

Chemical Constituents: Monoterpenes (up to 90%): α- & β-pinenes (<73%), δ-3-carene (<35%), camphene (<20%), l-limonene (<20%), β-phellandrene, bisabolene, dipentene; Esters (<23%): bornyl acetate (<23%), terpinyl acetate.

Properties: **Antiseptic**[51] (genito-urinary, pulmonary), **astringent, diuretic, expectorant, anti-inflammatory, sedative** (nerves), and **tonic**.

Common Primary Uses: **ᵀMuscle fatigue**.

Historical Uses: This fir tree is tall and graceful with a perfect conical shape. Though highly regarded for its fragrant scent, the fir tree has been prized through the ages for its medicinal virtues in regards to respiratory complaints, fever, and muscular and rheumatic pain. The oleoresin from the balsam fir tree has been used extensively for ritual purposes and for the external treatment of burns, sores, cuts, heart and chest pains, and coughs.

Other Possible Uses: This oil may be beneficial for **asthma, bronchitis, burns, catarrh, chronic coughs, cuts, cystitis, depression, hemorrhoids, stress-related conditions, sore throat, tension** (nervous), **tumors**[52], **urinary infections**, and **wounds**. This oil may help with **anxiety, colds, flu, infections**, and **pain** (reduces). It may help enhance the production of hGH (human growth hormone) and reduce the levels of cortisol. It has been found to be very effective for soothing **overworked** or **tired muscles, ligaments, tendons**, and **joints**. It may also help with back pain.

Body System(s) Affected: **Emotional Balance, Muscles and Bones, Nervous** and **Respiratory Systems**.

Aromatic Influence: It creates a feeling of **grounding, anchoring**, and **empowerment**. It can **stimulate** the **mind** while allowing the **body** to **relax**. It has been described as **appeasing, elevating**, and **opening**. It is also very **emotionally balancing**.

Application: **Diffuse**; apply to **Vita Flex Points** and directly on **area** of concern.

Oral Use As Dietary Supplement: Approved by the FDA for use as a Food Additive (FA) and Flavoring Agent (FL). ***Dilute** one drop oil in 1 tsp. honey or in 4 oz. of beverage (i.e. soy/rice milk).* ***Not for children under 6 years old; use with caution and in greater dilution for children 6 years old and over.***

Safety Data: ***Can irritate sensitive skin. Avoid direct sunlight for 3 to 6 hours after use.***

Blend Classification: Equalizer.

Blends With: German chamomile, cedarwood, cypress, frankincense, juniper, lavender, lemon, myrtle, pine, sandalwood, and rosewood.

Odor: Type: *Middle Note (50–80% of the blend)*; Scent: *Fresh, clean, green, balsamic, coniferous, sweet*; Intensity: *2.*

Fir, Douglas

(Pseudotsuga menziesii)

Botanical Family: Pinaceae (conifer)

Extraction Method/Origin: Steam distillation of leaves and twigs—Canada, USA

Chemical Constituents: Monoterpenes (up to 80%): α- & β-pinenes (<65%), l-limonene (<18%), δ-3-carene, camphene, terpinolene; Esters (up to 15%): bornyl acetate (<15%), geranyl acetate (<4%), bornyl & geranyl coproates; Alcohols (up to 10%): borneol (<6%), geraniol (<6%); Aldehydes: benzoicaldehyde, citrals; Ketones: camphor; Oxides: 1,8 cineol.

Properties: **Antiseptic, astringent, diuretic, expectorant, sedative** (joints, muscles, nerves), and **tonic**.

Historical Uses: Though highly regarded for its fragrant scent, the fir tree has been prized through the ages for its medicinal virtues in regards to respiratory complaints, fever, and muscular and rheumatic pain.

Other Possible Uses: This oil may help with **anxiety, asthma, bronchitis, catarrh, colds, coughs, flu, infections, respiratory weakness, rheumatism, tension** (nervous), and **wounds**. It is very soothing for **sore muscles** and has been found to be very effective for calming **overworked** or **tired muscles** and **joints**.

Body System(s) Affected: **Respiratory System, Muscles and Bones**.

Aromatic Influence: It creates a feeling of **grounding, anchoring**, and **empowerment**. It can **stimulate** the **mind** while allowing the **body** to **relax**.

Application: **Diffuse**; apply to **Vita Flex Points** and directly on **area** of concern.

Oral Use As Dietary Supplement: None.

Safety Data: ***Can irritate sensitive skin.***

Blend Classification: Equalizer.

Blends With: German chamomile, cedarwood, cypress, frankincense, juniper, lavender, lemon, myrtle, pine, sandalwood, and rosewood.

Fir, Idaho Balsam

(See Fir, Balsam)

Fir, White (or Giant Fir)

(Abies grandis or Abies concolor)

Botanical Family: Pinaceae (conifer)

Extraction Method/Origin: Steam distillation of leaves/twigs—Canada, France, USA

Chemical Constituents: Monoterpenes (up to 75%): α- & β-pinenes (<42%), β-phellandrene (<16%), camphene (<15%); Sesquiterpenes: δ-cadinene (<7%); Esters: bornyl acetate (<14%); Alcohols: borneol (<2%).

Properties: **Analgesic, antiseptic, astringent, diuretic, expectorant, sedative** (joints, muscles, nerves), and **tonic**.

Common Primary Uses: [T]**Muscle aches**.

Historical Uses: Though highly regarded for its fragrant scent, the fir tree has been prized through the ages for its medicinal virtues in regards to respiratory complaints, fever, muscular and rheumatic pain.

Other Possible Uses: This oil may help with **anxiety, asthma, bronchitis, catarrh, colds, coughs, flu, infections, respiratory weakness, rheumatism, tension** (nervous), and **wounds**. It has been found to be very effective for calming **overworked** or **tired muscles** and **joints** and for relieving **pain** resulting **from inflammation**.

Body System(s) Affected: **Emotional Balance, Muscles and Bones, Respiratory System**.

Aromatic Influence: It creates a feeling of **grounding, anchoring**, and **empowerment**. It can **stimulate** the **mind** while allowing the **body** to **relax**.

Application: **Diffuse**; apply to **Vita Flex Points** and/or directly on **area** of concern.

Oral Use As Dietary Supplement: None.

Safety Data: ***Can irritate sensitive skin.***

Blend Classification: Equalizer.

Blends With: German chamomile, cedarwood, cypress, frankincense, juniper, lavender, lemon, myrtle, pine, sandalwood, and rosewood.

Fleabane

(Conyza canadensis)

Botanical Family: Compositae (daisy)

Extraction Method/Origin: Steam distillation from stems, leaves, and flowers—Canada

Chemical Constituents: Monoterpenes (up to 83%): l-limonene (up to 75%), β-ocimene (<7%), β-pinene, myrcene; Furanocoumarins: α-bergamotene (<11%); Esters: methyl esters (<6%), methyl acetate; Alcohols: α-terpineol (<6%); Sesquiterpene Alcohols: nerolidol (<4%); Lactones; lachnophyllum lactone (<2%); Sesquiterpenes: β-farnesene.

Properties: **Antirheumatic, antispasmodic, cardiovascular dilator, hormone-like**.

French Medicinal Uses: Used by Daniel Pénoël, M.D., to treat children with **retarded puberty.**

Other Possible Uses: May help stimulate the **liver** and **pancreas**. It is a **mood enhancer** and a promoter of hGH.

Body System(s) Affected: **Cardiovascular** and **Hormonal Systems**.

Application: Apply to **Vita Flex Points** and directly on **area** of concern; diffuse.

Oral Use As Dietary Supplement: None.

Safety Data: ***This oil is still under study. Best to dilute with V-6 Oil.***

Frankincense (Olibanum)

(Boswellia carterii)

Botanical Family: Burseraceae (resinous trees and shrubs)

Extraction Method/Origin: Steam distillation from gum/resin—Somalia, Oman, Yemen

Chemical Constituents: Monoterpenes (up to 90%): α- & β-pinenes (35–45%), α-thujene (7–8%), d-limonene (11–14%), myrcene (<12%), sabinene (<7%), p-cymene (<5%), α-terpinene, camphene, α-phellandrene (2.5–3.5%); Sesquiterpenes (<10%): β-caryophyllene (<8%), α-gurjunene, α-guaiene; Alcohols (<5%): incensol, borneol, olibanol, trans-pinocarveol, farnesol.

Properties: **Anticatarrhal, anticancer**[53]**, antidepressant**[54]**, anti-infectious, anti-inflammatory**[55]**, antiseptic, antitumoral**[53]**, expectorant, immune-stimulant**[56], and **sedative**.

Common Primary Uses: **TArthritis, ATasthma, ATbrain injury, Tcoma, TAconcussion (brain), Aconfusion, ATcoughs, ATdepression, Tinfection (skin), Tinflammation, Alaryngitis, TALou Gehrig's disease, ATmental fatigue, Tmoles (skin), Tmultiple sclerosis, TParkinson's disease, Tscarring, Ttumor, Iulcer, Twarts, Twrinkles.**

Folklore: There are over 52 references to frankincense in the Bible (considering that "incense" is translated from the Hebrew/Greek "frankincense" and either refers to the same oil or to a mixture of which frankincense was one of the ingredients).

Historical Uses: Frankincense is a **holy oil** in the Middle East. As an ingredient in the holy incense, it was used anciently during sacrificial ceremonies to help improve communication with the **Creator**.

French Medicinal Uses: **Asthma, depression, ulcers.**

Other Possible Uses: This oil may help with **aging, allergies, bites** (insect and snake), **bronchitis, cancer, carbuncles, catarrh, colds, coughs, diarrhea, diphtheria, gonorrhea, headaches, healing, hemorrhaging, herpes, high blood pressure, inflammation, jaundice, laryngitis, meningitis, nervous** conditions, **prostate** problems, **pneumonia, respiratory problems**, preventing **scarring, sciatic pain, sores, spiritual awareness, staph, strep, stress, syphilis, T.B., tension, tonsillitis, typhoid, wounds**, and **warts**. It contains sesquiterpenes, enabling it to go beyond the blood-brain barrier. It may also help **oxygenate** the **pineal** and **pituitary glands**. It increases the activity of **leukocytes** in defense of the body against infection. Frankincense may also help one have a better attitude, which may help to strengthen the **immune system**.

Body System(s) Affected: **Emotional Balance, Immune** and **Nervous Systems, Skin.**

Aromatic Influence: It increases **spiritual awareness** and **meditation**.

Application: Apply to **Vita Flex Points** and/or directly on **area** of concern; **diffuse**.

Oral Use As Dietary Supplement: Approved by the FDA for use as a Food Additive (FA) and Flavoring Agent (FL). ***Dilute** one drop oil in 1 tsp. honey or in 4 oz. of beverage (i.e. soy/rice milk).* ***Not for children under 6 years old; use with caution and in greater dilution for children 6 years old and over.***

Blend Classification: Enhancer and Equalizer.

Blends With: All oils.

Odor: Type: *Base Note (5–20% of the blend)*; Scent: *Rich, deep, warm, balsamic, sweet, with incense-like overtones*; Intensity: *3*.

Frequency: High (Spiritual).

Bible: Exod. 30:34, Lev. 2:1, 2, 15, 16; 5:11; 6:15; 24:7, Num. 5:15, Matt 2:11, Rev. 18:13.

Frankincense, Sacred

(Boswellia sacra)

Botanical Family: Burseraceae (resinous trees and shrubs)

Extraction Method/Origin: Steam distillation from gum/resin—Oman

Chemical Constituents: Monoterpenes (up to 93%): α-pinene (<85%), l-limonene (<5%), camphene, myrcene, sabinene, p-cymene, β-pinene, α- & β-thujene, α- & β-phellandrene, δ-3-carene; Alcohols (<5%): incensol, trans-pinocarveol, trans-verbenol; Sesquiterpenes (<2%): β-elemene, β-selinene; Ketones: verbenone; Esters: Bornyl Acetate.

Properties: **Anticatarrhal, anticancer**[53]**, antidepressant**[54]**, anti-infectious, anti-inflammatory**[55]**, antiseptic, antitumoral**[53]**, anxiolytic**[54]**, expectorant, immune-stimulant**[56], and **sedative**.

Common Primary Uses: **ATBrain injury**, **ATmental fatigue**.

Folklore: The Omani frankincense resin this oil is distilled from is often regarded as the most highly-prized form of frankincense and is thought by many to be the type of frankincense referred to in the Bible and one of the gifts given to Christ at His birth. There are over 52 references to frankincense in the Bible (considering that "incense" is translated from the Hebrew/Greek "frankincense" and either refers to the same oil or to a mixture of which frankincense was one of the ingredients).

Historical Uses: Frankincense is a **holy oil** in the Middle East. As an ingredient in the holy incense, it was used anciently during sacrificial ceremonies to help improve communication with the **Creator**.

French Medicinal Uses: **Asthma, depression, ulcers**.

Other Possible Uses: This type of frankincense oil may help deepen **spiritual awareness** beyond the ability of typical frankincense oil. It has also shown an ability to help reduce brain "noise," while enhancing **calmness**, allowing the brain to better use its own innate abilities for **learning** and **decision making**. This oil may also help with **aging, allergies, bites** (insect and snake), **bronchitis, cancer, carbuncles, catarrh, colds, coughs, diarrhea, diphtheria, gonorrhea, headaches, healing, hemorrhaging, herpes, high blood pressure, inflammation, jaundice, laryngitis, meningitis, nervous** conditions, **prostate** problems, **pneumonia, respiratory problems**, preventing **scarring, sciatic pain, sores, spiritual awareness, staph, strep, stress, syphilis, T.B., tension, tonsillitis, typhoid, wounds**, and **warts**. It contains sesquiterpenes, enabling it to go beyond the blood-brain barrier. It may also help **oxygenate** the **pineal** and **pituitary glands**. It increases the activity of **leukocytes** in defense of the body against infection. Frankincense may also help one have a better attitude, which may help to strengthen the **immune system**.

Body System(s) Affected: **Emotional Balance, Immune** and **Nervous Systems, Skin**.

Aromatic Influence: It increases **meditation** and **spiritual awareness**.

Application: Apply to **Vita Flex Points** and/or directly on **area** of concern; **diffuse**.

Oral Use As Dietary Supplement: Approved by the FDA for use as a Food Additive (FA) and Flavoring Agent (FL). ***Dilute** one drop oil in 1 tsp. honey or in 4 oz. of beverage (i.e. soy/rice milk).* ***Not for children under 6 years old; use with caution and in greater dilution for children 6 years old and over.***

Blend Classification: Enhancer and Equalizer.

Blends With: All oils.

Odor: Type: *Base Note (5–20% of the blend)*; Scent: *Rich, deep, warm, balsamic, sweet, with incense-like overtones*; Intensity: *3*.

Frequency: High (Spiritual).

Bible: Exod. 30:34, Lev. 2:1, 2, 15, 16; 5:11; 6:15; 24:7, Num. 5:15, Matt 2:11, Rev. 18:13.

Galbanum

(Ferula gummosa or F. galbaniflua)

Botanical Family: Umbelliferae (parsley)

Extraction Method/Origin: Steam distillation from resin derived from stems and branches—Iran, Turkey, Afghanistan, Lebanon

Chemical Constituents: Monoterpernes (up to 95%): α- & β-pinenes (<90%), δ-3-carene (<16%), myrcene, sabinene, camphene, tricyclene, limonene, terpinolene, β-phellandrene; Sesquiterpene Alcohols: α-, β-, & γ-eudesmols (=galbanol), guaiol, bulnesol, 10-γ-epijunenol, α-cadinol; Esters: fenchyl acetate, linalyl acetate, terpenyl acetate; Coumarins.

Properties: **Analgesic, anti-infectious, anti-inflammatory, antimicrobial, antiseptic, antispasmodic**[57], **antiviral, diuretic, expectorant, restorative**, and **tonic**.

Historical Uses: Galbanum was used anciently as an incense and for embalming. It was also combined with frankincense as a holy incense (Exodus 30:34-38) and was only used in the tabernacle during sacrifices. It has been used for treating wounds, inflammation, and skin disorders.

Other Possible Uses: Galbanum is similar to hyssop, oregano, and frankincense and is recognized for its **antiviral, body-strengthening**, and **supporting** properties. It may also help with **abscesses, acne, asthma, boils, bronchitis, catarrh, chronic coughs, cramps, cuts, flatulence, indigestion, inflammation, muscular aches** and **pains, nervous tension**, the **pineal gland, poor circulation, rheumatism, scar tissue, skin** (tones), **stress-related complaints, swollen glands, wrinkles**, and **wounds**. Some very interesting research is being done with galbanum. It has a low frequency, but when combined with other oils such as frankincense or sandalwood, the frequency changes drastically. This oil is more than just a medicinal oil.

Body System(s) Affected: **Immune System**.

Aromatic Influence: It may help increase **meditation** and **spiritual awareness** and may have a **harmonizing** and **balancing** effect on the psyche.

Application: Apply to **Vita Flex Points** and directly on **area** of concern; **diffuse**.

Oral Use As Dietary Supplement: Approved by the FDA for use as a Food Additive (FA) and Flavoring Agent (FL). ***Dilute*** *one drop oil in 1 tsp. honey or in 4 oz. of beverage (i.e. soy/rice milk).* ***Not for children under 6 years old; use with caution and in greater dilution for children 6 years old and over.***

Blend Classification: Enhancer and Equalizer.

Blends With: All oils.

Odor: Type: *Top Note (5–20% of the blend)*; Scent: *Warm, earthy, green, woody, spicy*; Intensity: *5*.

Frequency: Low (Physical); approximately 56.

Bible: Exodus 30:34.

Geranium

(Pelargonium graveolens)

Botanical Family: Geraniaceae

Extraction Method/Origin: Steam distillation from leaves—Egypt, India

Chemical Constituents: Alcohols (up to 70%): citronellol (>32%), geraniol (<23%), linalol (<14%), nerol, γ-eudesmol, α-terpineol, menthol; Esters (up to 30%): citronellyl formate (14%), geranyl formate & acetate (<12%), other propionates, butyrates, & tiglates; Ketones: isomenthone (<8%), menthone, piperitone; Sesquiterpenes: 4-guaiadiene-6,9, αcopaene, δ- & γ-cadinenes, δ-guaiazulene, β-farnesene;

Aldehydes: geranial (<6%), neral, citronellal; Monoterpenes (<5%): α- & β-pinenes, l-limonene, myrcene, ocimene; Sesquiterpene Alcohols: farnesol (<3%).

Common Primary Uses: ^A^**Air purification**, ^T^**autism**, ^T^**bleeding**, ^T^**bruises**, ^T^**chapped lips**, ^T^**cradle cap**, ^IT^**diarrhea**, ^T^**dry skin**, ^T^**jaundice**, ^T^**paralysis**, ^AT^**physical stress**, ^T^**sensitive skin**, ^TI^**staph/MRSA**.

Properties: **Antibacterial**[58], **Antidepressant, antiseptic, astringent, diuretic, insect repellent, refreshing, relaxing, sedative**, and **tonic**.

Folklore: During the 1600's, European gardeners would plant geraniums around their houses to keep the evil spirits out. However, this oil is not produced from the same geranium as the house plants.

Historical Uses: Geranium oil has been used for dysentery, hemorrhoids, inflammations, heavy menstrual flow, and possibly even cancer (if the folktale is correct). It has also been said to be a remedy for bone fractures, tumors, and wounds.

French Medicinal Uses: **Diabetes, diarrhea, gallbladder, gastric ulcer, jaundice, liver, sterility, urinary stones.**

Other Possible Uses: This oil may be used for **acne, bleeding** (increases to eliminate toxins, then stops), **burns, circulatory problems** (improves blood flow), **convulsions**[59], **depression, digestion, eczema, hormonal imbalance, inflammation**[60], **insomnia, kidney stones**, dilating biliary ducts for **liver detoxification, menstrual problems, neuralgia** (severe pain along the nerve), regenerating **tissue** and **nerves, pancreas** (balances), **ringworm, shingles, skin** (may balance the sebum, which is the fatty secretion in the sebaceous glands of the skin that keeps the skin supple. This is good for expectant mothers as a cleanser for oily skin and for livening up pale skin), **sores, sore throats**, and **wounds**. Geranium opens the **liver chakra** and discharges the toxins from the liver that prevent balance.

Body System(s) Affected: **Emotional Balance, Skin**.

Aromatic Influence: It may help to release **negative memories** and take us back to **peaceful, joyful moments**. It may also help **ease nervous tension** and **stress, balance** the **emotions, lift** the **spirit**, and foster **peace, well-being**, and **hope**. It may also help lower defenses that prevent individuals from being **open** and **receptive to new ideas**.

Application: Apply to **Vita Flex Points** and directly on **area** of concern; **diffuse**.

Oral Use As Dietary Supplement: Generally regarded as safe (GRAS) for human consumption by the FDA. ***Dilute** one drop oil in 1 tsp. honey or in 4 oz. of beverage (i.e. soy/rice milk).* ***Not for children under 6 years old; use with caution and in greater dilution for children 6 years old and over.***

Safety Data: ***Repeated use can possibly result in some contact sensitization.***

Blend Classification: Enhancer and Equalizer.

Blends With: All oils.

Odor: Type: *Middle Note (50–80% of the blend)*; Scent: *Sweet, green, citrus-rosy, fresh*; Intensity: *3*.

German Chamomile

(See Chamomile, German)

Ginger

(Zingiber officinale)

Botanical Family: Zingiberaceae (ginger)

Extraction Method/Origin: Steam distillation from rhizomes—China, West Indies, and many others

Chemical Constituents: Sesquiterpenes (up to 90%): zingiberene (up to 50%), α- & β-curcumene (<33%), β-farnesene (<20%), β-sesquiphellandrene (<9%), β- & γ-bisabolene (<7%), β-ylangene, β-elemene, α-selinene, germacrene-D; Monoterpenes: camphene (8%), β-phellandrene, l-limonene, p-cymene, α and β-pinenes, myrcene; Alcohols: nonanol (<8%), citronellol (<6%), linalol (<5%), borneol, butanol, heptanol; Sesquiterpene Alcohols: nerolidol (<9%), zingeberol, elemol; Ketones (<6%): heptanone, acetone, 2 hexanone; Aldehydes: butanal, citronellal, geranial; Sesquiterpene Ketones: gingerone.

Properties: **Antiseptic, laxative, stimulant, tonic**, and **warming**.

Common Primary Uses: **TAAngina, ITdiarrhea, ITgas/flatulence, Tindigestion, IAmorning sickness, Amotion sickness, IAnausea, Trheumatic fever, Tscurvy, Tteething pain, Itonsillitis, Tvertigo, IAvomiting**.

Historical Uses: Anciently esteemed as a spice and recognized for its affinity for the digestive system, ginger has been used in gingerbread (up to 4,000 years ago in Greece), in Egyptian cuisine to ward off epidemics, in Roman wine (for its aphrodisiac powers), in Indian tea (to soothe upset stomachs), and in Chinese tonics (to strengthen the heart and relieve head congestion). It has been used by the Hawaiians to scent clothing, cook with, and cure indigestion. The Hawaiians have also added it to their shampoos and massage oils.

French Medicinal Uses: **Angina**, prevention of **contagious diseases, cooking, diarrhea, flatulence, impotence, rheumatic pain, scurvy**, and **tonsillitis**.

Other Possible Uses: Ginger may be used for **alcoholism**, loss of **appetite, arthritis**[61], **broken bones, catarrh** (mucus), **chills, colds, colic, congestion, coughs, cramps, digestive** disorders, **fevers, flu, impotence, indigestion, infectious diseases, memory, motion sickness, muscular aches/pains, nausea**[62], **rheumatism, sinusitis, sore throats**, and **sprains**. Ginger is also used in **cooking**.

Body System(s) Affected: **Digestive** and **Nervous Systems**.

Aromatic Influence: The aroma may help influence physical energy, sex, love, money, and courage.

Application: Apply to **Vita Flex Points** and directly on **area** of concern; **diffuse**.

Oral Use As Dietary Supplement: Generally regarded as safe (GRAS) for human consumption by the FDA. ***Dilute** one drop oil in 1 tsp. honey or in 4 oz. of beverage (i.e. soy/rice milk). **Not for children under 6 years old; use with caution and in greater dilution for children 6 years old and over.***

Safety Data: ***Repeated use can possibly result in contact sensitization. Avoid direct sunlight for 3 to 6 hours after use.***

Blend Classification: Personifier and Equalizer.

Blends With: All spice oils, all citrus oils, eucalyptus, frankincense, geranium, myrtle, rosemary, and spearmint.

Odor: Type: *Middle Note (50–80% of the blend)*; Scent: *Sweet, spicy-woody, warm, tenacious, fresh, sharp*; Intensity: *4*.

Goldenrod

(Solidago canadensis)

Botanical Family: Asteraceae or Compositae (daisy)

Extraction Method/Origin: Steam distillation from stems, leaves, and flowers—Eastern Canada

Chemical Constituents: Monoterpenes (up to 55%): α-pinene (<18%), myrcene (<15%), l-limonene (<12%), sabinene (<11%), α-phellandrene (<2%); Sesquiterpenes (up to 35%): germacrene-D (<35%), isolongifolene; Alcohols: borneol; Esters: bornyl acetate, bornyl benzoate.

Properties: **Relaxing** and **calming**.

Traditional Uses: **Diphtheria, dyspepsia, hypertension, influenza, nervousness, respiratory mucus, tonsillitis** and **pharyngitis** (these uses have not been substantiated by modern clinical research).

Other Possible Uses: According to Franchomme (1990) and as mentioned in the Swiss Pharmacopia, *faltrank*, goldenrod supports the **circulatory system** including **cardiovascular problems** (like tachycardia and arrhythmia), the **urinary tract**, and **liver function**. According to the University of Montreal in Canada, goldenrod shows great potential for help with **impotence**.

Body System(s) Affected: **Cardiovascular System, Hormonal System**.

Application: Apply to **Vita Flex Points** and/or directly on **area** of concern; **diffuse**. According to literature from Young Living Essential Oils, goldenrod may also be used as a dietary supplement by diluting one drop oil in 4 oz. of liquid (i.e. soy/rice milk or honey).

Oral Use As Dietary Supplement: None. *Although Young Living Essential Oils recommends the use of this oil as a dietary supplement, the FDA has* ***not yet*** *approved it for use as a food additive (FA) or flavoring agent (FL) (see 21CFR172.510 and 21CFR182.20).*

Grapefruit

(Citrus x paradisi)

Botanical Family: Rutaceae (hybrid between *Citrus maxima* and *Citrus sinensis*)

Extraction Method/Origin: Cold pressed from rind—California

Chemical Constituents: Monoterpenes (up to 95%): d-limonene (<92%), myrcene, α-pinene, sabinene, β-phellandrene; Tetraterpenes: β-carotene, lycopene; Aldehydes (>2%): nonanal, decanal, citral, citronellal; Furanocoumarins: aesculetine, auraptene, bergaptole; Sesquiterpene Ketones (<2%): nootketone (used to determine harvest time); Alcohols: octanol.

Properties: **Antidepressant, antiseptic, disinfectant, diuretic, stimulant**, and **tonic**.

Common Primary Uses: [A]**Anorexia**, [A]**appetite suppressant**, [A]**bulimia**, [TI]**cellulite**, [TA]**hangover**, [T]**indigestion**, [IT]**obesity**, [IT]**overeating**, [AT]**postpartum depression**, [IA]**weight loss**.

French Medicinal Uses: **Cellulite, digestion, dyspepsia, lymphatic decongestant, water retention**.

Other Possible Uses: Grapefruit oil may help with **depression, drug withdrawal, eating** disorders, **fatigue, gallstones, jet lag, liver** disorders, **migraine headaches, obesity, premenstrual tension**, and **stress**. It may also have a cleansing effect on the **kidneys**, the **lymphatic system**, and the **vascular system**.

Body System(s) Affected: **Cardiovascular System**.

Aromatic Influence: It may help prevent one from drowning in his or her own negativity. It is **balancing** and **uplifting** to the mind and may help **relieve anxiety**.

Application: Apply to **Vita Flex Points** and/or directly on **area** of concern; **diffuse**. *Because grapefruit oil has many of the same uses as other citrus oils, it can be used in their place when immediate exposure to the sun is unavoidable. This is because grapefruit oil does not have the photosensitivity that the other citrus oils have.*

Oral Use As Dietary Supplement: Generally regarded as safe (GRAS) for human consumption by the FDA. **Dilute** *one drop oil in 1 tsp. honey or in 4 oz. of beverage (i.e. soy/rice milk).* ***Not for children under 6 years old; use with caution and in greater dilution for children 6 years old and over.***

Blend Classification: Modifier and Enhancer.

Blends With: Basil, bergamot, cedarwood, chamomile, cypress, frankincense, geranium, juniper, lavender, peppermint, rosemary, rosewood, and ylang ylang.

Odor: Type: *Top Note (5–20% of the blend)*; Scent: *Clean, fresh, bitter, citrusy*; Intensity: *2*.

Helichrysum

(Helichrysum angustifolia var. italicum)

Botanical Family: Compositae

Extraction Method/Origin: Steam distilled from flowers—Yugoslavia, France, Italy *(Note: Since the supply of pure, therapeutic-grade helichrysum can be somewhat erratic at times, similar therapeutic results have been achieved by using a blend of 3 oils as follows: 5 drops elemi, 5 drops Idaho tansy, 1 drop wintergreen)*

Chemical Constituents: Esters (up to 60%): neryl acetate (up to 50%), neryl propionate & butyrate (<10%); Ketones: italidione (<20%), β-diketone; Sesquiterpenes: γ-curcumene (<20%), β-caryophyllene (<5%); Monoterpenes: l-limonene (<13%), α-pinene; Alcohols: nerol (<5%), linalol (<4%), geraniol; Oxides: 1,8 cineol; Phenols: eugenol.

Properties: **Antibacterial**[63], **anticatarrhal**, **anticoagulant**, **antioxidant**[64], **antispasmodic**, **antiviral**[65], **expectorant**, and **mucolytic**.

Common Primary Uses: [AT]**AIDS/HIV**, [A]**aneurysm**, [AI]**antioxidant**, [TA]**antiviral**, [T]**bleeding**, [T]**blood clots**, [T]**bone bruises**, [T]**bruises**, [T]**burns**, [T]**cholesterol**, [T]**colitis**, [T]**dermatitis/eczema**, [T]**herpes simplex**, [T]**nose bleed**, [T]**psoriasis**, [T]**scarring**, [T]**sciatica**, [T]**shock**, [AT]**stroke**, [T]**sunscreen**, [T]**tennis elbow**, [T]**tinnitus**, [T]**tissue repair**, [TI]**tooth abscess**.

Folklore: Helichrysum as an ornamental dried flower retains its fragrance, color, and shape almost forever. Hence came the other names "Everlasting" or "Immortelle" by which it is commonly known.

Historical Uses: Helichrysum has been used for asthma, bronchitis, whooping cough, headaches, liver ailments, and skin disorders.

French Medicinal Uses: **Blood cleansing**, **chelating agent** for **metallics**, **chemicals**, and **toxins**, viral **colitis**, **detoxification**, **gallbladder infection**, **hematoma**, **hypocholesterol**, **liver cell function stimulant**, **lymph drainage**, **pain reducer**, **pancreas stimulant**, **phlebitis**, **sciatica**, **sinus infection**, **skin conditions** (eczema, dermatitis, psoriasis), **stomach cramps**, **sun screen**.

Other Possible Uses: This oil may help **anger**, stop **bleeding**, **circulatory** functions, **gallbladder infection**, improve **hearing**, **hematoma** (swelling or tumor full of diffused blood), detoxify the liver and stimulate **liver** cell function, **lymph drainage**, **pain** (acute), relieve **respiratory** conditions, reduce **scarring**, **scar tissue**, reduce **tissue pain**, regenerate **tissue**, and **varicose veins**.

Body System(s) Affected: **Cardiovascular System**, **Muscles and Bones**.

Aromatic Influence: It is **uplifting** to the subconscious and may possess the ability to cut through **barriers** of anger, allowing one to forgive trespasses and move forward in life.

Application: Apply to **Vita Flex Points** and directly on **area** of concern; **diffuse**.

Oral Use As Dietary Supplement: Generally regarded as safe (GRAS) for human consumption by the FDA. ***Dilute*** *one drop oil in 1 tsp. honey or in 4 oz. of beverage (i.e. soy/rice milk).* ***Not for children under 6 years old; use with caution and in greater dilution for children 6 years old and over.***

Blend Classification: Personifier,

Blends With: Geranium, clary sage, rose, lavender, spice oils, and citrus oils.

Odor: Type: *Middle Note (50–80% of the blend)*; Scent: *Rich, sweet, fruity, with tea and honey undertones*; Intensity: *3*.

Frequency: High (Spiritual); approximately 181 MHz.

Hinoki (Japanese Cypress)

(Chamaecyparis obtusa)

Botanical Family: Cupressaceae (conifer: cypress)

Extraction Method/Origin: Steam distilled from leaves and bark—Japan

Chemical Constituents: Monoterpenes (up to 50%): sabinene (<15%), limonene (<7%), α-pinene (<7%), myrcene (<7%), terpinene-4-ol (<6%) γ-terpinene (<5%) β-pinene (<1%); Esters: α-terpinyl acetate (<15%), bornyl acetate (<12%); Alcohols: elemol (<7%).

Properties: **Anti-infectious, antiseptic, antiviral, disinfectant,** and **insecticidal**.

Common Primary Uses: [T]**Bathroom/kitchen cleaning**, [A]**calming**, [A]**colds**, [T]**cuts/scrapes**, [T]**rashes**.

Historical Uses: Hinoki wood has long been used in Japan for building royal palaces and sacred baths because of its beautiful look, wonderful smell, and its natural properties that allow it to resist insects, bacteria, and fungi—allowing the wood to last for hundreds of years.

Other Possible Uses: Hinoki may be beneficial for respiratory conditions such as **colds**, **coughs**, and **bronchitis**. It is also often used as an **antiseptic** to help clean and aid in tissue healing for **abrasions**, **cuts**, **scrapes**, and **rashes**. It may also be an effective insect repellent

Body System(s) Affected: **Emotional Balance, Immune** and **Respiratory Systems, Skin**.

Aromatic Influence: Hinoki oil is believed to impart a **calming** influence, helping to alleviate **stress** and **anxiety**. It also **uplifts** the mind and increases **spiritual awareness**.

Application: Diffuse into the air. Apply to **Vita Flex Points** and/or directly on **area** of concern.

Oral Use As Dietary Supplement: None.

Safety Data: ***Avoid during* pregnancy. *Keep out of reach of children.***

Blend Classification: Enhancer.

Blends With: Sacred frankincense, ravensara.

Odor: Type: *Top Note (5–20% of the blend)*; Scent: *Clean, woody, citrusy, spicy.*

Hong Kuai (Formosan Cypress)

(Chamaecyparis formosensis)

Botanical Family: Cupressaceae (conifer: cypress)

Extraction Method/Origin: Steam distilled from wood—Taiwan

Chemical Constituents: Sesquiterpenes (up to 50%); Sesquiterpene alcohols (up to 30%); Monoterpenes (up to 5%); Ketones.

Properties: **Antiseptic**.

Common Primary Uses: [A]**Air purification**, [A]**calming**, [AT]**relaxing**, [A]**mental support**.

Historical Uses: Hong kuai trees are ancient cypress trees that grow high in the mountains of Taiwan, where they can grow to enormous sizes and live for up to two millennia. Hong kuai wood has long been used in the building of temples, royal palaces, and baths because of its beautiful look, wonderful smell, and its natural properties that allow it to resist insects, bacteria, and fungi—allowing the wood to last for hundreds of years.

Other Possible Uses: Hong kuai may be beneficial for respiratory conditions such as **colds**, **coughs**, and **bronchitis**.

Body System(s) Affected: **Emotional Balance, Immune** and **Respiratory Systems**.

Aromatic Influence: Hong kuai oil is believed to impart a **calming** influence, helping to alleviate **stress** and **anxiety**. It may also help enhance mental clarity and focus.

Application: Diffuse into the air. Use in bathwater for a relaxing bath. Apply to **Vita Flex Points** and/or directly on **area** of concern.

Oral Use As Dietary Supplement: None.

Safety Data: ***Keep out of reach of children.***

Blend Classification: Enhancer.

Blends With: Micromeria.

Odor: Type: *Base Note (5–10% of the blend)*; Scent: *Clean, woody, earthy, long-lasting.*

Hyssop

(Hyssopus officinalis)

Botanical Family: Labiatae (mint)

Extraction Method/Origin: Steam distilled from stems/leaves—France, Hungary

Chemical Constituents: Ketones (>58%): isopinocamphone (>40%), pinocamphone (>12%), α and β-thujones, camphor; Monoterpenes (>25%); α- & β-pinenes (15–22%), l-limonene, ocimene, sabinene camphene, myrcene, p-cymene; Sesquiterpenes (<7%): germacrene-D, β-caryophyllene, aromadendrene, phellandrene; Phenols (4%): myrtenal methyl-ether, myrtenol, eugenol (methyl chavicol); Alcohols: borneol, linalol, nerolidol, geraniol; Esters: methyl myrtenate, bornyl acetate; Oxides: linalol oxide, 1,8 cineol.

Properties: **Antiasthmatic, anticatarrhal, anti-infectious, anti-inflammatory, antioxidant, antiparasitic, antiseptic, antispasmodic, antiviral, astringent, decongestant, diuretic, mucolytic**, and **sedative**.

Common Primary Uses: [IT]**Kidney stones.**

Historical Uses: Hyssop is mentioned in Exodus Chapter 12 as the oil in lamb's blood. It was used to prevent the plague, which may have been similar to AIDS today.

Other Possible Uses: This oil may be beneficial for **anxiety**, restoring **appetite, arthritis, asthma, bruises, cleansing** and purifying, **colds, concentration** (stimulating alertness and clearing the mind), **coughs, cuts, dermatitis, digestion, fatigue** (strengthens and enlivens the body), **fever**, expelling **gas** from intestines, **gout, grief**, regulating **lipid metabolism**, raising **low blood pressure**, clearing **lungs**, promoting and regulating **menstrual flow**, discharging **mucus, nervous tension, parasites** (expelling worms), increasing **perspiration, rheumatism**, preventing **scarring, scar tissue, sore throats, stress**-related conditions, **tonsillitis**, discharging **toxins, viral infections**, and **wounds**.

Body System(s) Affected: **Cardiovascular, Nervous**, and **Respiratory Systems**.

Aromatic Influence: It may help stimulate **creativity** and **meditation** and promote **centering**.

Application: Apply to **Vita Flex Points** and directly on **area** of concern; **diffuse**.

Oral Use As Dietary Supplement: Generally regarded as safe (GRAS) for human consumption by the FDA. **Dilute** *one drop oil in 1 tsp. honey or in 4 oz. of beverage (i.e. soy/rice milk). However, due to high ketone content, extreme caution should be taken.* ***Best avoided by children of any age.***

Safety Data: ***According to some sources, the pinocamphone can cause toxic effects. Avoid during pregnancy. Avoid if dealing with high blood pressure. Not for use by people with epilepsy. Use extreme caution and dilute well when unsure!***

Blend Classification: Enhancer, Equalizer, and Modifier.

Odor: Type: *Middle Note (50–80% of the blend)*; Scent: *Fresh, earthy, woody, fruity, slightly sweet*; Intensity: *3.*

Bible: According to the Bible, hyssop ***purges*** and ***cleanses***. See the following: Exodus 12:22; Lev. 14:4, 6, 49,51,52; Num. 19:6,18; 1 Kings 4:33; Psalms 51:7.

Idaho Balsam Fir
(See Fir, Balsam)

Idaho Blue Spruce
(See Spruce, Idaho Blue)

Idaho Tansy
(See Tansy, Idaho)

Jasmine
(Jasminum officinale)

Botanical Family: Oleaceae (olive)

Extraction Method/Origin: Absolute extraction from flowers (jasmine is actually an "essence" not an essential oil. The flowers must be picked at night to maximize the fragrance)—India

Chemical Constituents: Esters (up to 50%): benzyl acetate (<28%), benzyl benzoate (<21%), methyl anthranilate, methyl jasmonate; Diterpene Alcohols: phytol (<12%), isophytol (<7%); Alcohols: linalool (<8%), benzyl alcohol, farnesol; Triterpenes: squalene (<7%); Pyrroles: indole, scatole; Ketone: cis-jasmone.

Properties: **Anticatarrhal, antidepressant**, and **antispasmodic**[66].

Common Primary Uses: ^T^**Hoarse (voice)**, ^T^**pink eye**, ^T^**sensitive skin**.

Historical Uses: Known in India as the "queen of the night" and "moonlight of the grove," women have treasured it for centuries for its beautiful, aphrodisiac-like fragrance. According to Roberta Wilson, "In many religious traditions, the jasmine flower symbolizes hope, happiness, and love." Jasmine has been used for hepatitis, cirrhosis of the liver, dysentery, depression, nervousness, coughs, respiratory congestion, reproductive problems, and "to stimulate uterine contractions in pregnant women as childbirth approached." It was also used in teas, perfumes, and incense.

Other Possible Uses: This oil may help with **catarrh** (mucus), **conjunctivitis, coughs, dysentery, eczema** (when caused by emotions), **frigidity, hepatitis** (cirrhosis of the liver), **hoarseness, labor pains, laryngitis, lethargy** (abnormal drowsiness), **menstrual pain** and **problems, muscle spasms, nervous exhaustion** and **tension, pain relief, respiratory** conditions, **sex, skin care** (dry, greasy, irritated, and sensitive), **sprains**, and **uterine** disorders. Jasmine is an oil that affects the **emotions**; it penetrates the deepest layers of the soul, opening doors to our emotions. It produces a feeling of **confidence, energy, euphoria**, and **optimism**. It helps to reduce **anxiety, apathy, depression, indifference, listlessness, and relationship dilemmas**. As cologne, it increases feelings of **attractiveness**.

Body System(s) Affected: **Emotional Balance, Hormonal System**[67].

Aromatic Influence: It is very **uplifting** to the **emotions** and may help increase **intuitive** powers and **wisdom**. It may also help to promote powerful, inspirational **relationships**.

Application: Apply to **Vita Flex Points** and directly on **area** of concern; **diffuse**.

Oral Use As Dietary Supplement: Generally regarded as safe (GRAS) for human consumption by the FDA. ***Dilute*** *one drop oil in 1 tsp. honey or in 4 oz. of beverage (i.e. soy/rice milk).* ***Not for children under 6 years old; use with caution and in greater dilution for children 6 years old and over.***

Blend Classification: Equalizer, Modifier, and Enhancer.

Blends With: Bergamot, frankincense, geranium, helichrysum, lemongrass, mandarin, melissa, orange, palmarosa, rose, rosewood, sandalwood, spearmint.

Odor: Type: *Base Note (5–20% of the blend)*; Scent: *Powerful, sweet, tenacious, floral with fruity-herbaceous undertones*; Intensity: *4*.

Note: *One pound of jasmine oil requires about 1,000 pounds of jasmine or 3.6 million fresh picked blossoms. The blossoms must be collected before sunrise, or much of the fragrance will have evaporated. The quality of the blossoms can also be compromised if they are squashed. A single 1 lb. can of pure jasmine oil can cost from $1,200 to $4,500. In contrast, synthetic jasmine oils can be obtained for $3.50 per pound, but these synthetic oils obviously do not possess the same therapeutic qualities as pure jasmine oil. The above mentioned properties and possible uses are based on pure jasmine oil, not synthetic oil.*

Juniper (or Rocky Mountain Juniper)

(Juniperus osteosperma and/or J. scopulorum)

Botanical Family: Cupressaceae (conifer: cypress)

Extraction Method/Origin: Steam distilled from berries and twigs—Utah

Chemical Constituents: Monoterpenes (>50%): α-pinene (up to 40%), sabinene (<18%), myrcene (<8%), l-limonene (<6%); Esters: bornyl acetate (up to 20%); Ketones (up to 19%): camphor (<18%), junionone, pinocamphone; Sesquiterpenes: muurolene (<3%).

Properties: **Antiseptic, antispasmodic, astringent, cleanser, detoxifier, diuretic, stimulant**, and **tonic**.

Common Primary Uses: [T]**Acne**, [A]**alcoholism**, [T]**dermatitis/eczema**, [T]**kidney stones**, [T]**tinnitus**.

Folklore: According to Roberta Wilson, "During biblical times, juniper was often used to banish evil spirits." Also, during Medieval times, "Bundles of juniper berries were hung over doors to ward off witches, and burning juniper wood supposedly deterred demons."

Historical Uses: Over the centuries, juniper has been used for physical and spiritual purification, for cleansing infections and healing wounds, for liver complaints, for embalming, for relieving arthritis and urinary tract infections, for warding off plagues, epidemics, and contagious diseases, and for headaches, kidney and bladder problems, pulmonary infections, and fevers.

French Medicinal Uses: **Acne, dermatitis, eczema.**

Other Possible Uses: This oil may work as a **detoxifier** and a **cleanser**, which may reduce **acne, dermatitis**, and **eczema**. It may also help **coughs, depression, energy, infection**, increase circulation through **kidneys, kidney stones, liver problems**, aching **muscles, nerve function** and **regeneration, obesity, rheumatism** (promotes excretion of uric acid and toxins), **ulcers, urinary infections, water retention**, and **wounds**.

Body System(s) Affected: **Digestive System, Emotional Balance** (aromatic), **Nervous System, Skin**.

Aromatic Influence: Juniper evokes feelings of **health, love**, and **peace** and may help to **elevate** one's **spiritual awareness**.

Application: Apply to **Vita Flex Points** and/or directly on **area** of concern; **diffuse**. Juniper may also be applied to the **forehead** to enhance feelings of **optimism** or on the **cheeks** for **confidence** and **euphoria**.

Oral Use As Dietary Supplement: *As of the printing of this book, the FDA has NOT given this variety of juniper the designation of GRAS (Generally Regarded As Safe for human consumption) (see 21CFR182.20). However, the more common variety of Juniper berry (Juniperus communis L.) has been designated GRAS by the FDA. Since chemical constituents are very similar,* ***use with caution and dilute well when unsure!***

Blend Classification: Equalizer.

Blends With: Bergamot, all citrus oils, cypress, geranium, lavender, melaleuca (tea tree), Melrose, and rosemary.

Odor: Type: *Middle Note (50–80% of the blend)*; Scent: *Sweet, musky, tenacious*; Intensity: *3*.

Frequency: Emotional; approximately 98 MHz.

Bible: Job 30:4.

Laurel (Bay or Sweet Bay)

(Laurus nobilis)

Botanical Family: Lauraceae

Extraction Method/Origin: Steam distilled from leaves—France

Chemical Constituents: Oxides: 1,8 cineol (up to 50%); Alcohols: linalol (>15%), α-terpineol (<10%), borneol, geraniol, cis-thujanol-4; Monoterpenes (up to 28%): α and β-pinenes (<18%), sabinene (>10%), limonene; Esters: α-terpinyl acetate (up to 10%), bornyl, geranyl & linalyl acetates (<10%); Phenols: eugenol (<9%), terpinen-4-ol (<3%); Lactones: costunolide (<2%), artemorine, laurensolide; Sesquiterpenes: β-caryophyllene, humulene, β-elemene, phellandrene.

Properties: **Antiseptic, digestive, diuretic, antifungal, anti-inflammatory**[68].

Folklore: Ancient Greek and Roman generals would wear crowns of laurel leaves when victorious in battle. Both the Greeks and the Romans believed that the laurel tree had great powers of divination and prophecy and that all one had to do to avoid thunder and lightning or evil spirits was to run under a laurel tree.

Historical Uses: Both the leaves and the black berries were also used to alleviate colic, indigestion, and loss of appetite. During the Middle Ages, laurel was used for angina pectoris, asthma, fever, gout, migraine, palpitations, and liver and spleen complaints. Laurel has also been used as a fragrance component in cosmetics and perfumes.

Other Possible Uses: Laurel oil is primarily produced in the country formerly known as Yugoslavia. Laurel may help with loss of **appetite, asthmatic conditions, chronic bronchitis, dyspepsia, flatulence, flu, hair loss** (after an infection), **pediculosis, scabies, and viral infections**.

Body System(s) Affected: **Digestive, Immune**, and **Respiratory Systems**.

Application: Apply to **Vita Flex Points** and/or directly on **area** of concern.

Oral Use As Dietary Supplement: Generally regarded as safe (GRAS) for human consumption by the FDA. **Dilute** *one drop oil in 1 tsp. honey or in 4 oz. of beverage (i.e. soy/rice milk).* ***Not for children under 6 years old; use with caution and in greater dilution for children 6 years old and over.***

Safety Data: ***Repeated use can possibly result in contact sensitization. Moderate use is recommended. Avoid during pregnancy.***

Odor: Type: *Top to Middle Notes (20–80% of the blend)*; Scent: *Sweet, fresh, spicy, camphorous, medicinal*; Intensity: *3*.

Lavandin
(Lavandula x hybrida)

Botanical Family: Labiatae

Chemical Constituents: Alcohols (up to 60%): linalol (> 40%), α-terpineol (<5%), borneol, geraniol, lavendulol, nerol; Esters (<55%): linalyl acetate (<50%), lavandulyl acetate, geranyl acetate, bornyl acetate, neryl acetate; Monoterpenes (up to 24%): β-ocimene (<16%), d-limonene (<7%), myrcene, camphene; Ketones: camphor (>5%); Oxides: 1,8 cineol (<10%), caryophyllene oxide, linalol oxide; Phenols: terpinen-4-ol (<6%); Coumarins.

Properties: **Antibacterial, antifungal**, and strong **antiseptic**. *(See* LAVENDER *for additional properties.)*

Historical Uses: Also known as *Lavandula x intermedia*, lavandin is a hybrid plant developed by crossing true lavender with spike lavender or aspic (*Lavandula Latifolia*). It has been used to sterilize the animal cages in veterinary clinics and hospitals throughout Europe. There is not a long history of the therapeutic use of lavandin as it was most often used to adulterate true lavender oils.

Other Possible Uses: Lavandin can be used in the same way as true lavender (*see* LAVENDER) ***except NOT for burns***. It is more penetrating and has a much sharper scent than lavender. Some have even had success with using it to help reduce the itching and swelling associated with **insect bites** and **stings**.

Body System(s) Affected: **Cardiovascular System, Muscles and Bones, Respiratory System**.

Aromatic Influence: It has the same calming effects as lavender.

Application: Apply to **Vita Flex Points** and/or directly on **area** of concern; diffuse.

Oral Use As Dietary Supplement: Generally regarded as safe (GRAS) for human consumption by the FDA. ***Dilute** one drop oil in 1 tsp. honey or in 4 oz. of beverage (i.e. soy/rice milk). **Not for children under 6 years old; use with** **caution** **and in** **greater dilution** **for children 6 years old and over.***

Safety Data: ***Use with caution if susceptible to* epilepsy. *Avoid during* pregnancy. Do not use for burns!**

Blends With: Bergamot, cinnamon bark, citronella, clove, cypress, clary sage, geranium, lime, patchouli, pine, rosemary, and thyme.

Odor: Type: *Top to Middle Notes (20–80% of the blend)*; Scent: *Fresh, sweet, floral, more herbaceous than lavender*; Intensity: *3*.

Lavender
(Lavandula angustifolia)

Botanical Family: Labiatae (mint)

Extraction Method/Origin: Steam distilled from flowering top—France, Idaho, Utah

Chemical Constituents: Alcohols (up to 58%): linalool (23–41%), α-terpineol, borneol, lavendulol, geraniol, nerol; Esters (approx. 50%): linalyl acetate (up to 40%), lavendulyl & geranyl acetates, α-terpenyl acetate; Monoterpenes (up to 24%): β-ocimene (<16%), d-limonene (<5%), α- & β-pinenes, camphene, δ-3-carene; Sesquiterpenes: β-caryophyllene (<7%), χ-farnesene; Phenols: terpinen-4-ol (<9%); Aldehydes: benzaldehyde, cuminal, geranial, hexanal, myrtenal, neral; Oxides: 1,8 cineol, caryophyllene oxide, linalol oxide; Coumarins (<4%); Ketones: octanone (<3%), camphor; Lactones.

Properties: **Analgesic**[69], **anticoagulant, anticonvulsive**[70], **antidepressant, antifungal**[71], **antihistamine, anti-infectious, anti-inflammatory**[72], **antimicrobial**[73], **antimutagenic**[74], **antiseptic, antispasmodic, antitoxic, antitumor**[75], **cardiotonic, regenerative**, and **sedative**[76].

Common Primary Uses: **TAcne, AADD/ADHD, AIalertness, ATallergies (airborne), Tallergies (skin), ATanxiety, ATatherosclerosis, Tblister, ATbug repellent, Tburns, ATcalming, Tcandida, Tcarpal tunnel, Tchapped lips, Tchicken pox, Tcholesterol, Aconcentration (poor), Tcooling,**

[A]crying, [T]dandruff, [AT]depression, [T]diaper rash, [T]dry skin, [IT]gas/flatulence, [T]hair loss, [T]heatstroke, [T]herpes simplex, [AT]high blood pressure, [T]hives, [T]impetigo, [T]indigestion, [T]inflammation, [AT]insect repellent, [A]insomnia, [T]itching, [T]jock itch, [A]laryngitis, [T]mastitis, [AT]measles, [T]mosquito bites, [T]mumps, [IA]nausea, [T]neuritis, [T]pain, [T]Parkinson's disease, [AT]physical stress, [T]poison ivy, [AT]postpartum depression, [AT]relaxing, [T]rubella, [T]scabies, [T]scarring, [AT]sedative, [T]seizure, [T]sensitive skin, [AT]sleep, [T]spina bifida, [AT]stress, [T]stretch marks, [T]sunburn, [A]teeth grinding, [T]teething pain, [AT]tension, [T]thrush, [T]wounds, [T]wrinkles.

Historical Uses: During Medieval times, people were obviously divided on the properties of lavender regarding love. Some would claim that it could keep the wearer chaste, while others claimed just the opposite—touting its aphrodisiac qualities. The list of uses is long.

French Medicinal Uses: **Acne, allergies**[77], **burns** (cell renewal), **cramps** (leg), **dandruff, diaper rash, flatulence, hair loss, herpes, indigestion, insomnia**[78], **lowering blood pressure**[79], **lymphatic system drainage, menopausal conditions, mouth abscess, nausea, phlebitis, premenstrual conditions, scarring** (minimizes), **stretch marks, tachycardia, thrush, water retention.**

Other Possible Uses: Lavender is a universal oil that has traditionally been known to balance the body and to work wherever there is a need. If in doubt, use lavender. It may help **anxiety**[80], **arthritis, asthma, body systems balance, boils, bronchitis**[81], **bruises, carbuncles, cold sores, convulsions, depression, earaches, fainting, gallstones, hay fever,** relieve **headaches, heart** irregularities, reduce **high blood pressure, hives** (urticaria), **hysteria, insect bites** and **bee stings, infection, influenza, injuries, repel insects**[82], **laryngitis, mental clarity**[83], **migraine headaches, mouth abscess,** reduce **mucus, nervous tension, pineal gland** (activates), **respiratory function, rheumatism, skin conditions** (eczema, psoriasis, rashes), **sprains, stress**[84], **sunburns** (including lips), **sunstroke, tension, throat infections, tuberculosis, typhoid fever, whooping cough,** and **wounds.** One of our readers suggested putting a drop of lavender in the mascara bottle to thin it out and get more shine from eyelashes.

Body System(s) Affected: **Cardiovascular System, Emotional Balance, Nervous System, Skin.**

Aromatic Influence: It promotes **consciousness, health, love, peace** and a general sense of **well-being.**

Application: Apply to **Vita Flex Points** and directly on **area** of concern; **diffuse.**

Oral Use As Dietary Supplement: *As of the printing of this book, the FDA has NOT given this variety of lavender the designation of GRAS (Generally Regarded As Safe for human consumption) (see 21CFR182.20). However, Lavandula officinalis Chaix. has been designated GRAS by the FDA. Since chemical constituents are very similar,* ***use with caution and dilute well when unsure!***

Blend Classification: Enhancer, Modifier, and Equalizer.

Blends With: Most oils, especially citrus oils, chamomile, clary sage, and geranium.

Odor: Type: *Middle Note (50–80% of the blend)*; Scent: *Floral, sweet, herbaceous, balsamic, woody undertones*; Intensity: *2.*

Frequency: Emotional and Spiritual; approximately 118.

Ledum (or Labrador Tea)

(Ledum groenlandicum)

Botanical Family: Ericaceae (heather)

Extraction Method/Origin: Steam distilled from leaves—Canada

Chemical Constituents: Monoterpenes (up to 50%): l-limonene (up to 35%), p-menthatriene (<15%), α- and β-pinenes, sabinene, γ-terpinenes; Sesquiterpene Alcohols: p-menthadiene-8-ol (<17%), ledol

(<3%); Alcohols: α-terpineol; Aldehydes: myrtenal; Esters: bornyl acetate & butyrate; Sesquiterpene Ketones: germacrone; Sesquiterpenes: α-selinene, selinadiene; Phenols: terpinen-4-ol.

Properties: **Anticancerous, antimutagenic**[85]**, antitumoral, antiviral, nerve-stimulant**, and **tonic**.

Common Primary Uses: ^{T}**Tumor.**

Historical Uses: Ledum tea has been used for all types of skin problems, kidney-related problems, coughs, and hoarseness. Some sources say it was used by the Eskimos of the arctic region to fight cancer. Other natives of North America have used ledum tea to fight scurvy for thousands of years. According to Laurie Lacey, "The Cree named this plant **muskeko-pukwan**, and used it to treat fevers, colds, and other conditions."

Other Possible Uses: This oil may be beneficial for **ADD, allergies, bronchitis, colds, edema, fever, hepatitis** (viral), **influenza, laryngitis, lymph nodes** (inflamed), **skin problems** (all kinds), and **thyroid regulation**. It may also be a wonderful support to the **urinary tract, respiratory system**, and **immune system** as well as a powerful **liver** support and detoxifier (best when combined with JuvaTone). Research has indicated that this oil may contain more anticancerous and antitumoral properties than frankincense.

Body System(s) Affected: **Digestive** and **Immune Systems, Skin**.

Application: **Diffuse**, or apply to **Vita Flex Points** and/or directly on **area** of concern. Best **diluted** in one teaspoon of V-6 Oil for topical application. According to literature from Young Living Essential Oils, may also be used as a dietary supplement by diluting one drop of oil in 4 oz. of liquid (i.e. soy/rice milk or honey).

Oral Use As Dietary Supplement: None. *Although Young Living Essential Oils recommends the use of this oil as a dietary supplement, the FDA has* ***not yet*** *approved it for use as a food additive (FA) or flavoring agent (FL) (see 21CFR172.510 and 21CFR182.20).*

Lemon

(Citrus limon)

Botanical Family: Rutaceae (citrus)

Extraction Method/Origin: Cold pressed from rind (requires 3,000 lemons to produce a kilo of oil)—California, Italy

Chemical Constituents: Monoterpenes (up to 90%): d-limonene (up to 72%), α- & β-pinenes (<30%), α- & γ-terpinenes (7–14%), sabinene, p-cymene, terpinolene, α- & β-phellandrenes; Aldehydes (up to 12%): citral, citronellal, neral, geranial, heptanal, hexanal, nonanal, octanal, undecanal; Alcohols: hexanol, octanol, nonanol, decanol, linalol, αterpineol; Esters (<5%): geranyl acetate, neryl acetate, methyl anthranilate; Sesquiterpenes (<5%): β-bisabolene, β-caryophyllene; Tetraterpenes (<4%): β-carotene, lycopene; Phenols: terpinen-4-ol; Coumarins and Furocoumarins (<3%): umberlliferone, bergaptene, α-bergamotene, limettine, psoralen, bergamottin, bergaptole, citroptene scopoletin.

Properties: **Anticancer**[86]**, antidepressant**[87]**, antiseptic, antifungal**[88]**, antioxidant**[89]**, antiviral, astringent, invigorating, refreshing**, and **tonic**.

Common Primary Uses: ^{A}**Air purification**, ^{AI}**antioxidant**, ^{TA}**antiviral**, ^{AT}**anxiety**, ^{IT}**atherosclerosis**, ^{T}**autism**, ^{T}**bathroom/kitchen cleaning**, ^{AT}**brain injury**, ^{T}**carpets**, ^{AIT}**colds (common)**, ^{A}**concentration (poor)**, ^{T}**constipation**, ^{T}**Cushing's syndrome**, ^{AT}**depression**, ^{T}**dishes (sanitizing)**, ^{T}**disinfecting**, ^{T}**dysentery**, ^{IT}**fever**, ^{T}**furniture polish**, ^{IT}**gout**, ^{A}**grief/sorrow**, ^{T}**gum/grease removal**, ^{TA}**hangover**, ^{T}**heartburn**, ^{IT}**kidney stones**, ^{T}**laundry**, ^{I}**malaria**, ^{T}**mumps**, ^{IT}**overeating**, ^{AT}**postpartum depression**, ^{AT}**relaxing**, ^{AT}**stress**, ^{A}**uplifting**, ^{T}**varicose veins**, ^{IT}**water purification**.

Historical Uses: Lemon has been used to fight food poisoning, malaria and typhoid epidemics, and scurvy (in fact, sources say that Christopher Columbus carried lemon seeds to America—probably just the leftovers from the fruit that was eaten during the trip). Lemon has also been used to lower blood pressure and to help with liver problems, arthritis, and muscular aches and pains.

French Medicinal Uses: **Air disinfectant, anemia, asthma, cold, fever** (reduces), **germicide, gout, heartburn, intestinal parasites, red blood cell formation, rheumatism, throat infection, ureter infections, varicose veins, water purification, white blood cell formation.**

Other Possible Uses: This oil may be beneficial for **anxiety**[90], **blood pressure**, soothing broken **capillaries**, dissolving **cellulite, improving clarity** of thought, **debility, digestive problems**[91], **energy, gallstones, hair** (cleansing), promoting **leukocyte formation, liver** deficiencies in children, **lymphatic system cleansing, memory improvement, nails** (strengthening and hardening), **nerves**[92], **nervous conditions, respiratory problems**, cleaning dirty kids' **skin**, eliminating **sore throats, reducing stress**[93], and promoting a sense of **well-being**. It works extremely well in **removing gum, wood stain, oil**, and **grease spots**. It may also brighten a pale, dull **complexion** by removing dead skin cells.

Body System(s) Affected: **Digestive, Immune**, and **Respiratory Systems**.

Aromatic Influence: It promotes **health, healing, physical energy**, and **purification**. Its fragrance is **invigorating, enhancing**, and **warming**.

Application: Apply to **Vita Flex Points** and directly on **area** of concern; **diffuse**.

Oral Use As Dietary Supplement: Generally regarded as safe (GRAS) for human consumption by the FDA. ***Dilute** one drop oil in 1 tsp. honey or in 4 oz. of beverage (i.e. soy/rice milk).* ***Not for children under 6 years old; use with caution and in greater dilution for children 6 years old and over.***

Safety Data: ***Avoid direct sunlight for 12 hours after use. Can cause extreme skin irritation.***

Blend Classification: Modifier and Enhancer.

Blends With: Chamomile, eucalyptus, fennel, frankincense, geranium, juniper, peppermint, sandalwood, and ylang ylang.

Odor: Type: *Top Note (5–20% of the blend)*; Scent: *Sweet, sharp, clear, citrusy*; Intensity: *3*.

Lemongrass

(Cymbopogon flexuosus)

Botanical Family: Gramineae (grasses)

Extraction Method/Origin: Steam distilled from leaves—India, Guatemala

Chemical Constituents: Aldehydes (up to 80%): geranial (<42%), neral (<38%), farnesal (<3%), decanal; Alcohols (<15%): geraniol (<10%), α-terpineol (<3%), borneol (<2%), nerol, linalol, citronellol; Sesquiterpene Alcohols: farnesol (<13%); Esters (<11%): geranyl & linalyl acetates; Monoterpenes (<9%): myrcene (<5%), d-limonene (<3%), β-ocimene; Sesquiterpenes: β-caryophyllene (<6%); Oxides: caryophyllene oxide (<4%); Ketones: methyl heptanone (<3%).

Properties: **Analgesic, antibacterial**[94], **anticancer**[95], **anti-inflammatory, antiseptic, insect repellent, revitalizer, sedative, tonic**, and **vasodilator**.

Common Primary Uses: **[A]Air purification, [TA]antibacterial, [T]carpal tunnel, [T]cataracts, [IT]cholesterol, [IT]gastritis, [T]Grave's disease, [TA]Hashimoto's disease, [T]hyperthyroidism, [T]muscular dystrophy, [T]paralysis, [T]tissue repair, [T]varicose veins, [T]whiplash.**

Historical Uses: Lemongrass has been used for infectious illnesses and fever, as an insecticide, and as a sedative to the central nervous system.

French Medicinal Uses: Bladder infection (cystitis), connective tissue (regenerates), digestive system, edema, fluid retention, kidney disorders, lymphatic drainage, parasympathetic nervous system (regulates), varicose veins, vascular walls (strengthens).

Other Possible Uses: This oil may help cholesterol[96], improve circulation, improve digestion, improve eyesight, fevers, flatulence, headaches, clear infections, repair ligaments, wake up the lymphatic system, get the oxygen flowing, purification, respiratory problems[97], sore throats, tissue regeneration, and water retention.

Body System(s) Affected: Immune System, Muscles and Bones.

Aromatic Influence: It promotes psychic awareness and purification.

Application: Apply to Vita Flex Points or directly on area of concern; diffuse.

Oral Use As Dietary Supplement: Generally regarded as safe (GRAS) for human consumption by the FDA. *Dilute one drop oil in 1 tsp. honey or in 4 oz. of beverage (i.e. soy/rice milk).* ***Not for children under 6 years old;*** *use with* **caution** *and in* **greater dilution** ***for children 6 years old and over.***

Safety Data: *Can cause extreme* **skin irritation.**

Blend Classification: Enhancer and Equalizer.

Blends With: Basil, cedarwood, clary sage, eucalyptus, geranium, jasmine, lavender, melaleuca (tea tree), and rosemary.

Odor: Type: *Top Note (5–20% of the blend)*; Scent: *Grassy, lemony, pungent, earthy, slightly bitter*; Intensity: *4*.

Lemongrass, Red

(See Xiang Mao)

Lime

(Citrus aurantifolia)

Botanical Family: Rutaceae (citrus)

Extraction Method/Origin: Cold expressed from peel—India, Guatemala

Chemical Constituents: Monoterpenes (up to 80%): d-limonene (<65%), α- & β-pinenes (<17%), camphene, sabinene, p-cymene, myrcene, bisabolene, dipentene, phellandrene, cadinene; Oxides (<22%): 1,8 cineol (<20%), 1,4 cineol; Aldehydes (<20%): geranial (<8%), neral (<5%), citral, citronellal, octanal, nonanal, decanal, lauric aldehyde; Alcohols (4%): α-terpineol (<2%), borneol, α-fenchol, linalol; Coumarins: limettine; Furanoids: furfural, garanoxycoumarin.

Properties: Antibacterial, antiseptic, antiviral, restorative, and tonic.

Common Primary Uses: [IT]Fever.

Historical Uses: For some time, lime was used as a remedy for dyspepsia with glycerin of pepsin. It was often used in place of lemon for fevers, infections, sore throats, colds, etc.

Other Possible Uses: This oil may be beneficial for anxiety, blood pressure, soothing broken capillaries, dissolving cellulite, clarity of thought, debility, energy, fevers, gallstones, hair (cleansing), promoting leukocyte formation, liver deficiencies in children, lymphatic system cleansing, memory improvement, nails (strengthening), nervous conditions, cleaning dirty kids' skin, sore throats, water and air purification, and promoting a sense of well-being. It works extremely well in removing gum, wood stain, oil, and grease spots. It may also help brighten a pale, dull complexion by removing the dead skin cells. Lime oil is capable of tightening skin and connective tissue.

Body System(s) Affected: Digestive, Immune, and Respiratory Systems.

Aromatic Influence: Lime oil has a fresh, lively fragrance that is **stimulating** and **refreshing**. It helps one overcome **exhaustion, depression**, and **listlessness**. Although unverifiable, some sources claim that inhaling the oil may stimulate the muscles around the eyes.

Application: Apply to **Vita Flex Points** and/or directly on **area** of concern; **diffuse**. Excellent addition to **bath** and **shower gels, body lotions**, and **deodorants**.

Oral Use As Dietary Supplement: Generally regarded as safe (GRAS) for human consumption by the FDA. ***Dilute*** *one drop oil in 1 tsp. honey or in 4 oz. of beverage (i.e. soy/rice milk).* ***Not for children under 6 years old; use with caution and in greater dilution for children 6 years old and over.***

Safety Data: ***Avoid direct sunlight for up to 12 hours after use.***

Blend Classification: Enhancer and Equalizer.

Blends With: Citronella, clary sage, lavandin, lavender, neroli, rosemary, other citrus oils.

Odor: Type: *Top Note (5–20% of the blend)*; Scent: *Sweet, tart, intense, lively*; Intensity: 3.

Limette (or Combava)

(Citrus hystrix)

Botanical Family: Rutaceae (citrus)

Extraction Method/Origin: Cold pressed from peel—Madagascar

Chemical Constituents: Aldehydes: citronellal (66%); Oxides: citronellol (up to 10%), nerol; Monoterpenes: limonene.

Properties: **Anti-infectious, antiseptic, decongestant** (liver), **stimulant** (gallbladder), **tonic** (nerves)

Common Primary Uses: **AT Bug repellent, AT insect repellent.**

Historical Uses: Limette has been used to repel flies and other household pests.

Other Possible Uses: This oil may be beneficial for **anxiety, clarity** of thought, **debility, energy, insect repellent**[98]**, memory improvement, nervous conditions, air purification, trauma**, and promoting a sense of **well-being**.

Body System(s) Affected: **Nervous System**.

Aromatic Influence: Limette oil has a crisp, tart fragrance that is dominating and penetrating at first, but after a little getting used to, it becomes uniquely **refreshing** and **uplifting**. It helps one overcome **exhaustion, depression**, and **listlessness**.

Application: **Diffuse**.

Safety Data: ***Avoid direct sunlight for 12 hours after use.***

Blends With: Orange, angelica, lemon, and jasmine.

Mandarin

(Citrus reticulata)

Botanical Family: Rutaceae (citrus)

Extraction Method/Origin: Cold pressed from peel—China, Italy, Madagascar

Chemical Constituents: Monoterpenes (up to 95%): d-limonene (up to 75%), γ-terpinene (<22%), α- & β-pinenes (<5%), p-cymene (<4%), myrcene, α-phellandrene, terpinolene; Alcohols (<10%): linalol (<6%), octanol, α-terpineol, citronellol, nonanol, geraniol; Tetraterpenes (<8%): β-carotene (<6%), lycopene; Aldehydes (<4%): α-sinensal, decanal, perillaldehyde, octanal, citronellal; Esters: benzyl acetate, methyl anthranilate (>1%).

Properties: **Antifungal, antiseptic, antispasmodic, digestive, sedative** (nervous system), **stimulant** (digestive, lymphatic), **tonic.**

Folklore: The name of the fruit is said to have originated from a group of Imperial Chinese officials called the Mandarins. The fruit was a traditional gift given to these officials.

Historical Uses: Mandarin has been used in children's remedies for indigestion, hiccups, etc. Also for the elderly to strengthen the digestive function and the liver.

Other Possible Uses: This oil may help with **acne, digestive problems, dyspepsia, fluid retention, hepatic duct function, hiccups, insomnia, intestinal problems, skin problems** (congested and oily skin, **scars, spots,** tones the skin), **stretch marks** (when combined with either jasmine, lavender, sandalwood, and/or frankincense), **nervous tension, obesity, restlessness.** Mandarin is recommended for **children** and **pregnant women** because it is very gentle.

Body System(s) Affected: **Digestive System, Skin.**

Aromatic Influence: It is **appeasing, gentle,** and promotes **happiness.** It is also **refreshing, uplifting,** and **revitalizing.** Because of its sedative and slightly hypnotic properties, it is very good for **stress** and **irritability.**

Application: Apply to **Vita Flex Points** and/or directly on **area** of concern; **diffuse.** During pregnancy, combine with olive oil or wheat germ oil, and **massage** on the **abdomen.**

Oral Use As Dietary Supplement: Generally regarded as safe (GRAS) for human consumption by the FDA. ***Dilute*** *one drop oil in 1 tsp. honey or in 4 oz. of beverage (i.e. soy/rice milk).* ***Not for children under 6 years old; use with caution and in greater dilution for children 6 years old and over.***

Safety Data: ***Avoid direct sunlight for 3 to 6 hours after use.***

Blend Classification: Personifier and Modifier.

Blends With: Lavender, neroli (and other citrus oils), cinnamon bark, clove, nutmeg, and other spice oils.

Odor: Type: *Top Note (5–20% of the blend)*; Scent: *Very sweet, citrusy, fruity*; Intensity: *3.*

Manuka

(Leptospermum scoparium)

Botanical Family: Myrtaceae (Myrtle: shrubs and trees)

Extraction Method/Origin: Steam distilled from the leaves and branches—New Zealand

Chemical Constituents: Monoterpenes: pinenes; Sesquiterpenes: caryophyllene, humulene; Alcohols: linalol, geraniol; Cyclic Triketones (20–30%): leptospermone, iso-leptospermone, flavesone.

Properties: **Analgesic, antiallergic, antibacterial**[99]**, antifungal, anti-infectious, antiviral, antihistamine, antiseptic, decongestant, insecticidal,** and highly **bactericidal**[99] **(antimicrobial)** across a wide spectrum.

Historical Uses: This oil has a long history of use by the Maori people for bronchitis, rheumatism and similar conditions. Also, manuka oil has been used to treat a range of skin problems including chronic sores, ringworm, eczema, fungal infections (athlete foot and fungal nail infections), scalp itch, and dandruff. A decoction of leaves was used for urinary complaints and to reduce fever. The leaves were boiled in water and inhaled for head colds, blocked sinuses, hay fever, and even bronchitis and asthma. Leaves and bark were boiled together, and the warm liquid was rubbed on stiff backs and rheumatic joints. The leaves and young branches were put into vapor baths. The crushed leaves were applied as a poultice for many skin diseases and were directly applied to wounds and deep gashes to enhance healing and to reduce the risk of infection. The young shoots were chewed and swallowed for dysentery. The bark, the sap, and the seed capsules of the manuka were also used extensively for treating various ailments.

Other Possible Uses: This oil may help with **abrasions**, **acne**, **bronchitis**, **catarrh**, **chafing**, **colds**, **cuts**, **dandruff**, **fungal infections** (athletes foot, skin, and nails), **infections** (staph and strep), **insect bites** and **stings**, **muscle** and **joint pains**, **odor** (foot and body), **rashes**, **scratches**, oily **skin**, **skin irritation**, **sinusitis**, mild **sunburn**, and **ulcers** (Active Manuka Honey, a unique honey produced from the blossoms of the manuka tree, has been shown to naturally kill *Helicobacter pylori*).

Body System(s) Affected: **Muscles and Bones, Respiratory System, Skin.**

Aromatic Influence: Manuka helps to **calm oversensitive nerves** and **strengthen the psyche**, producing an almost sensual feeling of well-being. It's **stabilizing** and **calming** aroma makes it very good for combating **stress** and **irritability**.

Application: Apply to **Vita Flex Points** and/or directly on **area** of concern; **diffuse**. Can also be used in the **bath** or as a **gargle**.

Blend Classification: Enhancer and Equalizer.

Blends With: All citrus oils, cypress, eucalyptus, lavender, rosemary, and thyme.

Single Oils

Marjoram

(Origanum majorana)

Botanical Family: Labiatae (mint)

Extraction Method/Origin: Steam distilled from leaves—France

Chemical Constituents: Monoterpenes (up to 60%): α- & γ-terpinenes (<30%), sabinene (<8%), myrcene (<7%), terpinolene, ocimene, δ-3-carene, p-cymene, α- and β-pinenes, δ-cadinene, α- & β-phellandrenes, l-limonene; Alcohols (<30%): α-terpineol (<15%), cis- & trans-thujanol-4 (<12%), linalol (<8%); Phenols: terpinen-4-ol (>21%), terpinen-1-ol-3; Esters: geranyl acetate (<7%), linalyl acetate, α-terpenyl acetate; Aldehydes: citral (<6%); Sesquiterpenes (<5%): β-caryophyllene, humulene; Phenolic Ethers: trans-anethole.

Properties: **Antibacterial, anti-infectious, antiseptic, antisexual, antispasmodic, arterial vasodilator, digestive stimulant, diuretic, expectorant, sedative**, and **tonic**.

Common Primary Uses: **ᵀArthritis, ᵀCarpal tunnel, ᵀcolic, ᵀconstipation, ᵀcramps (muscle), ᴬcroup, ᴬᵀhigh blood pressure, ᵀmuscle fatigue, ᵀmuscle spasms, ᵀmuscular dystrophy, ᵀneuralgia, ᵀParkinson's disease, ᴬᵀphysical stress, ᵀwhiplash.**

Folklore: Known as the "herb of happiness" to the Romans and "joy of the mountains" to the Greeks, marjoram was used to decorate at both weddings and funerals. Not only would it warm both the body and the emotions, but many believed it would increase longevity. It was grown on grave sites to comfort the departed soul.

Historical Uses: Marjoram was used for poisoning (as an antidote), fluid retention, muscle spasms, rheumatism, sprains, stiff joints, bruises, obstructions of the liver and spleen, and respiratory congestions. According to Roberta Wilson, "Those curious about their futures anointed themselves with marjoram at bedtime so that they might dream of their future mates."

French Medicinal Uses: **Aches, arthritis**[100]**, asthma, bronchitis, colic, constipation, cramps, insomnia, intestinal peristalsis, migraine headache, muscles, neuralgia, pains, parasympathetic nervous system** (tones), **blood pressure** (regulates), **rheumatism, sprains.**

Other Possible Uses: It may be **relaxing** and **calming** to the **muscles** that constrict and sometimes contribute to **headaches**. It may help **anxiety, boils, bruises, burns, carbuncles, celibacy** (vow not to marry), **colds, cold sores, cuts, fungus** and **viral infections, hysteria, menstrual problems**, calm the **respiratory system, ringworm, shingles, shock, sores**, relieve **spasms, sunburns, tension**, and **water retention**.

Body System(s) Affected: **Cardiovascular System, Muscles and Bones**.

Aromatic Influence: It promotes **peace** and **sleep**.

Application: Apply to **Vita Flex Points** and directly on **area** of concern; **diffuse**.

Oral Use As Dietary Supplement: Generally regarded as safe (GRAS) for human consumption by the FDA. ***Dilute** one drop oil in 1 tsp. honey or in 4 oz. of beverage (i.e. soy/rice milk).* ***Not for children under 6 years old; use with caution and in greater dilution for children 6 years old and over.***

Safety Data: ***Use with caution during pregnancy.***

Blend Classification: Enhancer and Equalizer.

Blends With: Bergamot, cedarwood, chamomile, cypress, lavender, orange, nutmeg, rosemary, rosewood, ylang ylang.

Odor: Type: *Middle Note (50–80% of the blend)*; Scent: *Herbaceous, green, spicy*; Intensity: *3*.

Melaleuca (Tea Tree)

(Melaleuca alternifolia)

Botanical Family: Myrtaceae (Myrtle: shrubs and trees)

Extraction Method/Origin: Steam distilled from leaves—Australia

Chemical Constituents: Monoterpenes (up to 70%): α- & γ-terpinenes (<40%), p-cymene (<12%), α- and β-pinenes (<8%), terpinolene, l-limonene, sabinene, myrcene, α-thujene; Phenols: terpinen-4-ol (<40%); Sesquiterpenes (up to 20%): α- & δ-cadinenes (<8%), aromadendrene (<7%), viridiflorene (<5%), β-caryophyllene, α-phellandrene; Oxides: 1,8 cineol (<14%), 1,4 cineol (<3%), caryophyllene oxide; Alcohols: α- & β-terpineols (<8%); Sesquiterpene Alcohols (<5%): globulol, viridiflorol.

Properties: **Analgesic, antibacterial**[101]**, antifungal**[102]**, anti-infectious, anti-inflammatory**[103]**, antioxidant, antiparasitic**, a strong **antiseptic, antiviral**[104]**, decongestant, digestive, expectorant, immune-stimulant, insecticidal, neurotonic, stimulant**, and **tissue regenerative**.

Common Primary Uses: [T]**Acne**, [T]**allergies (skin)**, [TA]**antibacterial**, [TA]**antifungal**, [AI]**antioxidant**, [TA]**antiviral**, [T]**athlete's foot**, [T]**boils**, [T]**candida**, [T]**cavities**, [T]**chicken pox**, [T]**cold sores**, [AIT]**colds (common)**, [T]**cooling**, [AT]**coughs**, [T]**dandruff**, [T]**deodorant**, [T]**ear infection/earache**, [AT]**flu (influenza)**, [T]**gum disease**, [T]**herpes simplex**, [T]**hives**, [T]**infection (skin)**, [T]**inflammation**, [T]**jock itch**, [AT]**measles**, [T]**mumps**, [T]**rashes**, [T]**ringworm**, [T]**rubella**, [T]**scabies**, [T]**shingles**, [I]**sore throat**, [TI]**staph/MRSA**, [I]**strep throat**, [T]**sunburn**, [T]**thrush**, [I]**tonsillitis**, [T]**vaginal infections**, [TA]**viral infection**, [T]**wounds**.

Historical Uses: The leaves of the melaleuca tree (or tea tree) have been used for centuries by the aborigines to heal cuts, wounds, and skin infections. With twelve times the antiseptic power of phenol, it has some strong immune-building properties.

French Medicinal Uses: **Athlete's foot, bronchitis, colds, coughs, diarrhea, flu, periodontal (gum) disease, rash, skin healing, sore throat, sunburn, tonsillitis, vaginal thrush**.

Other Possible Uses: This oil may help **acne**[105]**, boils**[106]**, burns, candida, cold sores, digestion, fungal infections, hysteria, infectious diseases, inflammation, mites**[107]**, shock, ticks**[108]**, viral infections, tinea pedis, warts**, and **wounds** (promotes healing).

Body System(s) Affected: **Immune** and **Respiratory Systems, Muscles and Bones, Skin**.

Aromatic Influence: It promotes **cleansing** and **purity**.

Application: Apply to **Vita Flex Points** and/or directly on **area** of concern; **diffuse**.

Oral Use As Dietary Supplement: Approved by the FDA for use as a Food Additive (FA) or Flavoring Agent (FL). **Dilute** *one drop oil in 1 tsp. honey or in 4 oz. of beverage (i.e. soy/rice milk).* ***Not for children under 6 years old; use with* caution *and in* greater dilution *for children 6 years old and over.***

Safety Data: ***Repeated use can possibly result in* contact sensitization.**

Blend Classification: Enhancer and Equalizer.

Blends With: All citrus oils, cypress, eucalyptus, lavender, rosemary, and thyme.

Odor: Type: *Middle Note (50–80% of the blend)*; Scent: *Medicinal, fresh, woody, earthy, herbaceous*; Intensity: *3*.

Melaleuca Ericifolia (or Rosalina)

(Melaleuca ericifolia)

Botanical Family: Myrtaceae (Myrtle: shrubs and trees)

Origin: Australia

Chemical Constituents: Alcohols (up to 52%): linalol (<46%), α-terpineol (<5%); Monoterpenes (up to 30%): β-phellandrene (up to 12%), α-pinene (<10%), p-cymene (<6%), l-limonene (<2%), γ-terpinene (<2%); Oxides (up to 20%): 1,8 cineol (<19%), 1,4 cineol; Sesquiterpenes (up to 8%): aromandrene (<6%), viridiflorene (<2%); Phenols: terpinen-4-ol.

Properties: **Antibacterial, antifungal, anti-infectious**, powerful **antimicrobial, calming**, and **sedative**.

Other Possible Uses: Because this variety of melaleuca oil is **very gentle** and **nonirritating** to the skin, it is well suited for **youth** and others who may be more sensitive to the oils. Research by Dr. Daniel Pénoël, M.D. has shown this oil to help with **bronchitis, dermatitis, ear infections, eczema, influenza, insomnia, nervous tension, pneumonia**, and **sinusitis**.

Body System(s) Affected: **Respiratory System, Skin**.

Application: Apply to **Vita Flex Points** and/or directly on **area** of concern. May also be applied to the **chest, face, temples, throat**, or **wrists**. For a **full-body massage**, dilute 4–8 drops of *Melaleuca ericifolia* oil in 30 ml. of a pure vegetable oil. May also be diffused or added to bathwater. *Caution: Heating or burning this oil can cause it to lose all therapeutic value.*

Oral Use As Dietary Supplement: Approved by the FDA for use as a Food Additive (FA) or Flavoring Agent (FL). **Dilute** *one drop oil in 1 tsp. honey or in 4 oz. of beverage (i.e. soy/rice milk).* ***Not for children under 6 years old; use with* caution *and in* greater dilution *for children 6 years old and over.***

Blend Classification: Personifier, Enhancer, Equalizer, and Modifier.

Melaleuca Leucadendron

(See Cajeput)

Melaleuca Quinquenervia (or Niaouli)

(Melaleuca quinquenervia)

Botanical Family: Myrtaceae (Myrtle: shrubs and trees)

Extraction Method/Origin: Steam distilled from leaves and limbs—Australia

Chemical Constituents: Oxides: 1,8 cineol (>60%), 1,4 cineol; Monoterpenes (<29%): α- & β-pinenes (<21%), l-limonene (<8%), β-phellandrene, α- & γ-terpinenes; Sesquiterpene Alcohols (<22%): viridiflorol (>14%), nerolidol (<6%), globulol; Alcohols (<15%): α-terpineol (<12%), linalol; Sesquiterpenes (<4%): β- caryophyllene, aromadendrene, viridiflorene, δ-cadinene; Phenols: terpinen-4-ol (2%); Aldehydes: isovaleraldehyde, benzaldehyde.

Properties: **Antibacterial, antifungal** (very strong and powerful), **anti-inflammatory, antiseptic, antiviral, digestive tonic, protector against radiation,** and a strong **tissue regenerator**.

Other Possible Uses: This oil may help with **respiratory allergies, infections, hemorrhoids,** and other conditions as listed under MELALEUCA.

Body System(s) Affected: **Muscles and Bones, Respiratory System.**

Aromatic Influence: Some people may prefer this oil to melaleuca (*M. alternifolia*) because of its sweet, delicate scent. It aids in **concentration**, is **reviving**, and helps **clear** the **head**.

Application: Apply to **Vita Flex Points** and/or directly on **area** of concern; **diffuse**, especially for respiratory problems.

Oral Use As Dietary Supplement: Approved by the FDA for use as a Food Additive (FA) or Flavoring Agent (FL). ***Dilute** one drop oil in 1 tsp. honey or in 4 oz. of beverage (i.e. soy/rice milk).* ***Not for children under 6 years old; use with caution and in greater dilution for children 6 years old and over.***

Safety Data: ***Repeated use can possibly result in contact sensitization.*** Odor: Type: *Middle Note (50–80% of the blend)*; Scent: *Earthy, musty, harsh*; Intensity: *3.*

Melissa (Lemon Balm)

(Melissa officinalis)

Botanical Family: Labiatae (mint)

Extraction Method/Origin: Steam distilled from leaves and flowers—France, Idaho, Utah

Chemical Constituents: Aldehydes (up to 65%): geranial (<35%), neral (<28%), citronellal (<3%), α-cyclocitral; Sesquiterpenes (<35%): β-caryophyllene (<19%), α-copaene (<5%), germacrene-D (<4%), β-bourbonene, δ- & γ-cadinenes, humulene, β-elemene; Oxides (<11%): caryophyllene oxide (<7%), 1,8 cineol (<4%); Alcohols (<7%): linalol, octen-3ol, nerol, geraniol, citronnellol, isopulegol, caryophyllenol, farnesol; Esters (<7%): methyl citronellate (<5%), citronellyl, geranyl, neryl, & linalyl acetates; Ketones (<7%): methyl heptanone (<5%), farnesylacetone, octanone; Monoterpenes (<3%): cis- & trans-ocimenes, l-limonene; Sesquiterpene Alcohols: elemol, α-cadinol; Furanocoumarins: aesculetine.

Properties: **Antibacterial, antidepressant, antihistamine, antimicrobial, antispasmodic, antiviral**[109], **hypertensive, nervine, sedative**[110], **tonic**, and **uterine**.

Common Primary Uses: **TAAntiviral, ATanxiety, ATcalming, Tcold sores, Tcolic, Therpes simplex, ATtuberculosis, TAviral infection.**

Folklore: Melissa, the "Elixir of Life," is one of the earliest known medicinal herbs.

Historical Uses: Anciently, melissa was used for nervous disorders and for many different ailments dealing with the heart or the emotions. It was also used to promote fertility. Melissa was the main ingredient in Carmelite water, distilled in France since 1611 by the Carmelite monks.

Other Possible Uses: **Allergies, anxiety, asthma, bronchitis, chronic coughs, colds, cold-sore blisters** (apply directly three times per day), **colic, depression, dysentery, eczema, erysipelas, fevers, heart conditions** (where there is overstimulation or heat), **hypertension, indigestion, insect bites, insomnia, menstrual problems, migraine, nausea, nervous tension, palpitations, shock, sterility** (in women), **throat infections, vertigo,** and **vomiting**. Dr. Dietrich Wabner, a professor at the Technical University of Munich, reported that a onetime application of true melissa oil led to complete remission of **herpes simplex lesions**. According to Robert Tisserand, "Melissa is the nearest one can find to a rejuvenator—not something which will make us young again, but which helps to cushion the effect of our mind and the world outside on our body."

Body System(s) Affected: Emotional Balance, Skin.

Aromatic Influence: Melissa has a delicate, delightful, lemony scent that is unique among essential oils, providing a wonderful support to both body and mind. It has been known to bring out gentle characteristics within people. It is calming and uplifting and may help to balance the emotions. It may also help to remove emotional blocks and instill a positive outlook on life.

Application: Apply to Vita Flex Points and/or directly on area of concern.

Oral Use As Dietary Supplement: Generally regarded as safe (GRAS) for human consumption by the FDA. *Dilute one drop oil in 1 tsp. honey or in 4 oz. of beverage (i.e. soy/rice milk).* ***Not for children under 6 years old; use with caution and in greater dilution for children 6 years old and over.***

Blend Classification: Enhancer, Equalizer, and Modifier

Blends With: Geranium, lavender, and other floral and citrus oils.

Odor: Type: *Middle Note (50–80% of the blend)*; Scent: *Delicate, lemony*; Intensity: 2.

Frequency: Emotional and Spiritual; approximately 102 MHz.

Single Oils

Micromeria (White Savory)

(Micromeria fruticosa)

Botanical Family: Labiatae (mint)

Extraction Method/Origin: Steam distilled from leaf, stem, and flowers—Israel

Chemical Constituents: Ketones (up to 80%): piperitenone, pulegone, isomenthone, piperitone; Monoterpenes: α-thujene, α-pinene, β-pinene, limonene; Oxides: 1,8-cineole; Sesquiterpenes: germacrene-D; Alcohols: spathulenol.

Properties: Antibacterial, antifungal, cardiotonic, immune-stimulant.

Common Primary Uses: [TA]Antibacterial, [T]candida, [AT]insect repellent, [T]herbicide.

Historical Uses: Micromeria was traditionally used as a natural herbicide and insect repellent. It was also used as a tea and used by the Bedouins to support digestion and cardiovascular functions.

Other Possible Uses: May also be useful to help support respiratory health and digestion.

Body System(s) Affected: Immune System.

Aromatic Influence: It may help energize the spirit and refresh the mind.

Application: Apply diluted to Vita Flex points and on area of concern; diffuse.

Oral Use As Dietary Supplement: Traditionally used as a tea and in cooking. *Dilute one drop of oil in 2 tsp. of honey or in 8 oz. of beverage (i.e. soy/rice milk).* ***Not for children under 6 years old; use with caution and in greater dilution for children 6 years old and over.***

Safety Data: ***Do not use if pregnant or trying to conceive, due to the high levels of pulegone in this oil.***

Mountain Savory (or Winter Savory)

(Satureja montana)

Botanical Family: Labiatae (mint)

Extraction Method/Origin: Steam distilled from flowering plant—France

Chemical Constituents: Phenols (up to 58%): carvacrol (<35%), thymol (<24%), carvacrol methyl-ether (<9%), eugenol; Monoterpenes (<32%): p-cymene (<20%), α- & γ-terpinenes (20%); Alcohols (<25%): linalol (<11%), α-terpineol (<9%), cis- & trans-thujanol-4 (<4%), geraniol, borneol, myrtenol; Sesquiterpenes (<7%): β-caryophyllene (<7%); Oxides: 1,8 cineol (<1%), caryophyllene oxide; Ketones: camphor, damasceneone.

Properties: **Antibacterial, antifungal**, strong **anti-infectious** (genito-urinary & gastrointestinal—superior to thyme, rosemary, and lavender), **antiparasitic, antiviral, immune-stimulant**, and a general **tonic** for the body.

Common Primary Uses: TA**Antibacterial**, T**candida**.

Historical Uses: This oil has been used as a digestive remedy for colic and diarrhea.

Other Possible Uses: Due to its high phenol content, mountain savory is a very strong antiseptic and has been used to hasten the **formation** of **scar tissue** and to help with **abscesses, burns**, and **cuts**. It is also known to stimulate the **adrenal gland**.

Body System(s) Affected: **Immune System**.

Aromatic Influence: It may produce **strong psychological effects** and can help revitalize and stimulate the nervous system. It is a powerful **energizer** and **motivator**.

Application: Apply diluted to **Vita Flex Points** and on **area** of concern; **diffuse**.

Oral Use As Dietary Supplement: Generally regarded as safe (GRAS) for human consumption by the FDA. ***Dilute** one drop oil in 2 tsp. honey or in 8 oz. of beverage (i.e. soy/rice milk). May need to increase dilution even more due to this oil's potential for irritating mucus membranes.* ***Not for children under 6 years old; use with caution and in greater dilution for children 6 years old and over.***

Safety Data: ***Robert Tisserand has classified mountain savory as a dermal toxin, dermal irritant, and mucous membrane irritant. He recommends it never be used on the skin. However, other sources recommend its use but emphasize that it must always be used in dilution. Can cause extreme skin irritation.*** *Avoid during* ***pregnancy*** *and use with* ***extreme caution.*** *Also, it is best if used only for short durations, as it may be toxic to the liver during long-term use.*

Mugwort

(Artemisia vulgaris)

Botanical Family: Asteraceae or Compositae (daisy)

Extraction Method/Origin: Steam distillation from the leaves and root—Europe

Chemical Constituents: Monoterpenes (up to 45%): myrcene (up to 25%), sabinene (<14%), l-limonene (<3%), β-phellandrene (<3%), α- & β-pinenes, camphene, p-cymene, γ-cadinene; Ketones (<18%): α- & β-thujones (up to 12%), camphor (<2%); Oxide: 1,8 cineol; Lactones: vulgarin, pilostachyn.

Properties: **Antiseptic, antispasmodic**[111], **calming, diuretic, expectorant**[111].

Historical Uses: Having been associated with superstition and witchcraft, mugwort was seen as a protective charm against danger and evil. It has been used for painful or delayed menstruation, amenorrhea and dysmenorrhea, for hysteria and epilepsy, to expel worms, and to control fever. According to some sources, mugwort was used by the Jews as one of the bitter herbs eaten during Passover.

Other Possible Uses: **Antioxidant**[112], **mucus** (expels), **nerves** (calms), **parasites** (blend with thyme).

Body System(s) Affected: **Hormonal** and **Nervous Systems**.

Aromatic Influence: This strongly aromatic oil was anciently believed to increase psychic powers.

Application: Apply to **Vita Flex Points** and/or directly on **area** of concern.

Oral Use As Dietary Supplement: *Has been approved by the FDA for use as a Food Additive (FA) or Flavoring Agent (FL) as long as the finished food is thujone-free. (See 21CFR172.510)* ***Best not to use this oil as a dietary supplement.***

Safety Data: ***For topical use only.** Due to high thujone content, use **sparingly** and **dilute well** with V-6 Oil. Avoid during **pregnancy**, as it may contribute to a miscarriage.*

Blends With: Anise, German chamomile, ginger, peppermint, rosemary, tangerine, and tarragon.

Found In: ComforTone.

Myrrh

(Commiphora myrrha)

Botanical Family: Burseraceae (resinous trees and shrubs)

Extraction Method/Origin: Steam distilled from gum/resin—Somalia

Chemical Constituents: Sesquiterpenes (up to 75%): lindestrene (up to 30%), β-, γ-, & δ-elemenes (<40%), α-copaene (<12%), β-bourbonene (<5%), muurolene, δ-cadinene, humulene, curzerene; Furanoids (<27%): methoxyfurogermacrene (<9%), furoendesmadiene (<8%), α-bergamotene (<5%), methylisopropenylfurone (<5%), furfural (<3%), furanodione (<2%), rosefuran; Ketones: (<20%): curzenone (<11%), methylisobutyl ketone (<6%), germacrone (<4%); Triterpenes (<7%): α-amyrin (<4%), α-amyrenone (<3%); Monoterpenes (<6%): ocimene, p-cymene, α-thujene, l-limonene, myrcene; Aldehydes: methylbutynal (<3%), cinnamaldehyde, cuminal; Arenes: xylene; Carboxylic Acids: acetic acid, formic acid, palmitic acid; Phenols: eugenol, cresol.

Properties: **Anti-infectious, anti-inflammatory**[113], **antiseptic, antitumor**[114], **astringent**, and **tonic**.

Common Primary Uses: **[T]Allergies (skin), [T]chapped/cracked skin, [T]dysentery, [TA]Hashimoto's disease, [T]hyperthyroidism, [T]impetigo, [T]inflammation, [T]stretch marks, [I]ulcer.**

Folklore: Well over 2,000 years before the baby Jesus received myrrh as a gift, it was one of the most desired and most expensive items in the world. According to Roberta Wilson, "In Greek mythology, Aphrodite forced the goddess Myrrha into an incestuous relationship with her father, Cinyras. Cinyras avenged the act by turning his daughter into a myrrh tree. When the tree sprouted its blooms, their child Adonis was born. The resinous drops that exude from cuts in the tree's bark were said to be Myrrha's tears."

Historical Uses: Myrrh was used as incense in religious rituals, in embalming, and as a cure for cancer, leprosy, and syphilis. Myrrh, mixed with coriander and honey, was used to treat herpes.

French Medicinal Uses: **Bronchitis, diarrhea, dysentery, hyperthyroidism, stretch marks, thrush, ulcers, vaginal thrush, viral hepatitis.**

Other Possible Uses: This oil may help **appetite (increase), asthma, athlete's foot, candida, catarrh** (mucus), **coughs, eczema, digestion, dyspepsia** (impaired digestion), **flatulence** (gas), **fungal infection, gingivitis, gum infection, hemorrhoids, mouth ulcers**, decongest **prostate gland, ringworm, sore throats, skin conditions** (chapped, cracked, and inflammation), **wounds**, and **wrinkles**.

Body System(s) Affected: **Hormonal, Immune**, and **Nervous Systems; Skin**.

Aromatic Influence: It promotes **spiritual awareness** and is **uplifting**.

Application: Apply to **Vita Flex Points** and/or directly on **area** of concern.

Oral Use As Dietary Supplement: Approved by the FDA for use as a Food Additive (FA) and Flavoring Agent (FL). ***Dilute** one drop oil in 1 tsp. honey or in 4 oz. of beverage (i.e. soy/rice milk). **Not for children under 6 years old; use with caution and in greater dilution for children 6 years old and over.***

Safety Data: *Use with caution during **pregnancy**.*

Blend Classification: Modifier and Equalizer.

Blends With: Frankincense, lavender, patchouli, sandalwood, and all spice oils.

Odor: Type: *Base Note (5–20% of the blend)*; Scent: *Warm, earthy, woody, balsamic*; Intensity: *4*.

Frequency: Emotional and Spiritual; approximately 105 MHz.

Comments: Myrrh is a true gift. When we open our **hearts** and **minds** to receive the gifts, they will be given.

Myrrh, Biblical Sweet™

(Commiphora erythraea)

Botanical Family: Burseraceae (resinous trees and shrubs)

Extraction Method/Origin: Steam distilled from gum/resin—Socotra Island, Yemen

Chemical Constituents: Furanosesquiterpenoids (40-45%): 4-furanodien-6-one (20-30%), 1,10(15)-furanogermacra-dien-6-one (10-15%), dihydropyrocurzerenone, rel-3R-methoxy-4S-furanogermacra-1E,10(15)-dien-6-one, rel-2R-methoxy-4R-furanogermacra-1(10)E-en-6-one; Sesquiterpenes (up to 40%): δ-elemene (<2%), α-copaene (<5%), β-elemene (5-8%), α-gurjunene (<5%), β-caryophyllene (<2%), aromadendrene (<5%), α-humulene, alloaromadendrene, germacrene-D, β-selinene, α-selinene, γ-cadinene, δ-cadinene, germacrone; Monoterpenes (up to 6%): α-pinene (<6%); Sesquiterpene alcohols (up to 6%): alismol, eudesmol; Ketones: curzerenone.

Properties: **Anti-infectious, anti-inflammatory, antiseptic.**

Common Primary Uses: ᵀ**Bruises** ᵀ**chapped/cracked skin**, ᵀ**inflammation**, ᵀ**stretch marks**, ᵀ**wounds**.

Historical Uses: This type of myrrh was traditionally used to help promote healthy, elastic skin and to support the immune system.

Other Possible Uses: This oil may have **neuro-protective** properties and may also help **gingivitis, gum infection, hemorrhoids, mouth ulcers, skin conditions** (chapped, cracked, and inflammation), **wounds**, and **wrinkles**.

Body System(s) Affected: **Immune** and **Nervous Systems, Skin**.

Aromatic Influence: It promotes **spiritual awareness** and is **uplifting**.

Application: Apply directly on **area** of concern.

Oral Use As Dietary Supplement: Approved by the FDA for use as a Food Additive (FA) and Flavoring Agent (FL). ***Dilute** one drop of oil in 1 tsp. of honey or in 4 oz. of beverage (i.e. soy/rice milk).* ***Not for children under 6 years old; use with caution and in greater dilution for children 6 years old and over.***

Safety Data: ***Use with caution during pregnancy.***

Blend Classification: Modifier and Equalizer.

Blends With: Frankincense, ylang ylang, and blue spruce.

Odor: Type: *Middle Note (15–20% of the blend)*; Scent: *Warm, earthy, woody, mild, balsamic*; Intensity: *4*.

Myrtle

(Myrtus communis ssp. red)

Botanical Family: Myrtaceae (Myrtle: shrubs and trees)

Extraction Method/Origin: Steam distilled from leaves—Morocco, Tunisia

Chemical Constituents: Oxides (up to 48%): 1,8 cineol (<45%), caryophyllene oxide; Monoterpenes (up to 45%): α-pinene (>24%), l-limonene (<11%), β-pinene (<5%), camphene; Esters (<22%): myrtenyl acetate (<10%), geranyl acetate (<5%), terpenyl acetate (<3%), methyl myrtenate (<3%), also linalyl, neryl, bornyl, & trans-carvyl acetates; Alcohols (<18%): α-terpineol (<8%), linalol (<5%), myrtenol (<4%), nerol, geraniol; Aldehydes: myrtenal, decanal, hexanal, methylbutynal; Phenols: myrtenol, terpinen-4-ol; Furanoids: methylfuran, furfural; Lactones: myrtecommulone.

Properties: **Antibacterial, anti-inflammatory, antiparasitic, antiseptic, astringent, expectorant, decongestant**, and **deodorizer**.

Common Primary Uses: **[AT]Coughs, [A]deodorizing, [AT]flu (influenza), [T]hypothyroidism.**

Folklore: According to Susanne Fischer-Rizzi, "Myrtle, considered the sacred plant of the goddess Aphrodite, was worshiped as a plant of mystery. Aphrodite, goddess of beauty and love, and born as a beautiful adult woman from sea foam, sought refuge in her newborn nakedness in a myrtle bush. That's why myrtle also stands for chaste beauty. Many brides today still wear myrtle as a symbol for innocence."

Historical Uses: Myrtle was used for diarrhea, dysentery, catarrhal conditions (asthma, bronchitis, chronic coughs, tuberculosis), lung and bladder infections, sinus infections, and skin care.

French Medicinal Uses: **Bronchitis, coughs, flu, hypothyroidism, insomnia, ovaries** (hormone-like effects), **prostate decongestant, sinus infection, tuberculosis, ureter infections**.

Other Possible Uses: This oil may help **anger, asthma, catarrh, children** (see comment), **colds, cystitis, diarrhea, dysentery, dyspepsia** (impaired digestion), **flatulence** (gas), **hemorrhoids**, support **immune system, infections, infectious diseases, pulmonary disorders, skin conditions** (acne, blemishes, bruises, oily skin, psoriasis, etc.), and **sinusitis**. Useful on **children** for **chest** complaints and **coughs**.

Body System(s) Affected: **Digestive, Hormonal**, and **Respiratory Systems, Muscles and Bones**.

Aromatic Influence: It is **elevating** and **euphoric**. It also soothes **anger**.

Application: Apply to **Vita Flex Points** or directly on **area** of concern; **diffuse**.

Oral Use As Dietary Supplement: Approved by the FDA for use as a Food Additive (FA) and Flavoring Agent (FL). ***Dilute** one drop oil in 1 tsp. honey or in 4 oz. of beverage (i.e. soy/rice milk). **Not for children under 6 years old; use with caution and in greater dilution for children 6 years old and over.***

Blend Classification: Equalizer and Enhancer.

Blends With: Bergamot, lavender, lemon, lemongrass, rosewood, rosemary, spearmint, thyme, and melaleuca (Tea Tree).

Odor: Type: *Top to Middle Notes (20–80% of the blend)*; Scent: *Sweet, slightly camphorous, with a floral hint*; Intensity: *3*.

Myrtle, Lemon

(Backhousia citriodora)

Botanical Family: Myrtaceae (Myrtle: shrubs and trees)

Extraction Method/Origin: Steam distilled from leaves—Australia

Chemical Constituents: Aldehydes (>90%): geranial (57%), neral (37%), citronellal; Alcohols (<4%): cis- & trans-verbenol (<3%), linalol, nerol. Other trace elements include linalyl acetate, myrcene, methylheptenone, and geranic acid.

Properties: **Antibacterial, antifungal, antimicrobial, antiseptic, antiviral**[115], **calming, corrective**, and **sedative**.

Common Primary Uses: **[TA]Antibacterial, [TA]antifungal, [T]candida, [TI]staph/MRSA**.

Historical Uses: The leaves from the lemon myrtle trees have been dried and used as food flavoring for poultry and seafood as well as for air fresheners in wardrobes, shoe cabinets, and vehicles. Lemon myrtle is said to smell more "lemony than lemon." Research is showing that lemon myrtle oil has very good antibacterial activity and excellent antifungal activity, maybe even more so than *Melaleuca alternifolia*. Other tests have shown lemon myrtle to possess strong germicidal powers, twice that of *Eucalyptus citriodora* and even 19.5 times that of citral alone.

Other Possible Uses: This oil may help with **viral, bacterial**, and **fungal infections**. It has also been reported to help with sprained or torn **ligaments** and **tendons**. Due to its antibacterial, antifungal, and antimicrobial actions, it would work well as an additive to any natural cleaning product. And what a better way to clean than with the strong lemon scent from the oil.

Body System(s) Affected: **Immune and Respiratory Systems, Muscles and Bones**.

Aromatic Influence: It is **elevating** and **refreshing**.

Application: Apply to **Vita Flex Points** or directly on **area** of concern; **diffuse**.

Odor: Type: *Top Note (5–20% of the blend)*; Scent: *Extremely lemony and crisp, more "lemony" than true lemon oil*; Intensity: *5*.

Neroli (or Orange Blossom)

(Citrus aurantium bigaradia)

Botanical Family: Rutaceae (citrus)

Extraction Method/Origin: Absolute extraction from flowers of the orange tree—Morocco, Tunisia

Chemical Constituents: Alcohols (up to 53%): linalol (<44%), α-terpineol (<6%), geraniol (<3%), nerol; Sesquiterpene Alcohols (<7%): trans-nerolidol (<5%), farnesol (<2%); Monoterpenes (up to 40%); d-limonene (<18%), β-pinene (<17%), ocimene (<8%), myrcene (<4%) α-pinene, neptadecene, sabinene, camphene; Esters (>25%): linalyl acetate (<15%), methyl anthranilate (<10%), neryl & geranyl acetates; Aldehydes: decanal, benzaldehyde, vinylhexanal; Phenols: phenylethanol, benzyl alcohol; Pyrroles: indole, scatole.

Properties: **Antibacterial, antidepressant, anti-infectious, antiparasitic, antiseptic, antispasmodic, antiviral, aphrodisiac, deodorant, sedative**, and **tonic**.

Common Primary Uses: **ᵀSensitive skin**.

Folklore: The name of this oil is said to originate from a beloved princess of Nerola, Italy, who lavished it on everything. Brides adorned themselves and their bouquets with orange blossoms to signify their purity and beauty.

Historical Uses: Neroli has been regarded traditionally by the Egyptian people for its great attributes for healing the **mind, body**, and **spirit**. It brings everything into the focus of one and at the moment.

Other Possible Uses: It may support the **digestive system** and fight **bacteria, infections, parasites**, and **viruses**. It may also help with **anxiety, chronic diarrhea, colic, depression, digestive spasms, fear, flatulence, headaches, heart** (regulates rhythm), **hysteria, insomnia, mature** and **sensitive skin, nervous dyspepsia, nervous tension, palpitations, PMS, poor circulation, scars, shock, stress-related conditions, stretch marks, tachycardia, thread veins**, and **wrinkles**. In support of the skin, it works at the cell level to help shed the old skin cells and **stimulate new cell growth**.

Body System(s) Affected: **Digestive System, Skin**.

Aromatic Influence: As a **natural tranquilizer**, neroli has some **powerful psychological effects**. It has been used successfully to treat **depression, anxiety**, and **shock**. It is **calming** and **relaxing** to the body and spirit. It may also help to **strengthen** and **stabilize** the emotions and **bring relief** to seemingly hopeless situations. It encourages **confidence, courage, joy, peace**, and **sensuality**. Neroli is said to vibrate in the 2nd and 4th chakra. In the words of one author, "Neroli offers the gift of strength and courage that helps us see life's beauty."

Application: Apply to **Vita Flex Points** and directly on **area** of concern; **diffuse**.

Oral Use As Dietary Supplement: Generally regarded as safe (GRAS) for human consumption by the FDA. ***Dilute*** *one drop oil in 1 tsp. honey or in 4 oz. of beverage (i.e. soy/rice milk).* ***Not for children under 6 years old; use with caution and in greater dilution for children 6 years old and over.***

Blend Classification: Equalizer, Modifier, and Personifier.

Blends With: Rose, lavender, sandalwood, jasmine, cedarwood, geranium, lemon.

Odor: Type: *Middle Note (50–80% of the blend)*; Scent: *Floral, citrusy, sweet, delicate, slightly bitter*; Intensity: *3*.

Niaouli

(See Melaleuca Quinquenervia)

Nutmeg

(Myristica fragrans)

Botanical Family: Myristicaceae

Extraction Method/Origin: Steam distilled from fruits and seeds—Indonesia, Tunisia

Chemical Constituents: Monoterpenes (up to 80%): α- & β-pinenes (<46%), sabinene (25%), myrcene (<12%), d-limonene (<7%), α- & γ-terpinenes (<11%), p-cymene, δ-3-carene, terpinolene, camphene, α- & β-phellandrenes; Phenolic Ethers (<16%): myristicin (<12%), elemicin (<3%), safrole (<2%), eugenol; Phenols: terpinen-4-ol (<8%); Oxides: 1,8-cineol (<4%); Alcohols: α-terpineol (<2%); Sesquiterpenes: β-caryophyllene.

Properties: **Anti-inflammatory**[116], **antiparasitic, antiseptic, stimulant** (cerebral, circulatory), **laxative**, and **tonic**.

Common Primary Uses: ^T^**Addison's disease**, ^I^**bad breath (halitosis)**.

Historical Uses: Nutmeg has been used for centuries for digestive and kidney problems.

French Medicinal Uses: **Appetite** (loss of), **chronic diarrhea, debility, digestion** (helps with starchy foods and fats), **gallstones, halitosis** (bad breath), **rheumatism**.

Other Possible Uses: This oil has adrenal cortex-like activity that helps support the **adrenal glands** for **increased energy**. Nutmeg may also help **arthritis, bacterial infection, circulation**, revive **fainting, flatulence** (gas), **frigidity, gout, impotence, immune function** (support), **joints, menstruation** (regulates scanty periods and soothes pains), **muscles** (also muscle aches and pains), **nausea, nervous fatigue, neuralgia** (severe pain along nerve), support the **nervous system**, and **vomiting**.

Body System(s) Affected: **Hormonal, Immune**, and **Nervous Systems**.

Application: Apply to **Vita Flex Points** and/or directly on **area** of concern.

Oral Use As Dietary Supplement: Generally regarded as safe (GRAS) for human consumption by the FDA. ***Dilute*** *one drop oil in 1 tsp. honey or in 4 oz. of beverage (i.e. soy/rice milk).* ***Not for children under 6 years old; use with caution and in greater dilution for children 6 years old and over.***

Safety Data: ***Not for use by people with epilepsy. Use with caution during pregnancy. If over-used (several undiluted drops at once), it may cause mental discomfort or delirium and convulsions and could overstimulate the heart. Dilute well or use a single undiluted drop; then wait for a period of time.***

Blend Classification: Personifier.

Blends With: Cinnamon bark, clove, cypress, frankincense, lemon, orange, patchouli, rosemary, melaleuca, melissa.

Odor: Type: *Middle Note (50–80% of the blend)*; Scent: *Sweet, musky, spicy*; Intensity: *4*.

Ocotea

(Ocotea quixos)

Botanical Family: Lauraceae

Extraction Method/Origin: Steam distilled from stem and leaves—Ecuador.

Chemical Constituents: Sesquiterpenes (<50%): β-caryophyllene, α-humulene, β-selinene, α-copaene, α-selinene, δ-cadinene; Esters (<21%): methyl cinnamate, cinnamyl acetate; Monoterpenes (<5%): α-pinene, β-pinene; Oxides: eucalyptol; Aldehydes: trans-cinnamaldehyde.

Properties: **Anesthetic, antibacterial, antidiarrheal, antifungal** (yeast), **anti-inflammatory**[117], **disinfectant,** and **eupeptic** (promotes good digestion).

Historical Uses: Ocotea was traditionally used as a disinfectant and for digestive support.

Other Possible Uses: This oil may help with **blood clots**[118] and **digestion**. It may also help to reduce **swelling** and—in conjunction with proper exercise and healthy eating—may help enhance **weight loss** by helping to balance the pituitary and endocrine systems.

Body System(s) Affected: **Cardiovascular System, Emotional Balance, Skin.**

Application: Dilute with V-6 Oil and apply to **Vita Flex Points** and/or directly on **area** of concern; **diffuse**.

Oral Use As Dietary Supplement: *Although Young Living Essential Oils recommends the use of this oil as a dietary supplement, the FDA has* ***not yet*** *approved it for use as a food additive (FA) or flavoring agent (FL) (see 21CFR172.510 and 21CFR182.20).* ***Dilute*** *1–4 drops oil in V-6 Oil or olive oil and place in capsule and swallow up to once daily.* ***Not for children under 6 years old; use with caution and in greater dilution for children 6 years old and over.***

Blends With: Copaiba.

Onycha (Benzoin)

(Styrax benzoin)

Botanical Family: Styracaceae

Extraction Method/Origin: Absolute extraction from the resin (Onycha is actually an "essence" not an essential oil)—India, China, Laos, Thailand, or Vietnam.

Chemical Constituents: **Non-Volatile Fraction:** Esters (<70%): coniferyl benzoate; **Volatile Fraction:** Carboxylic Acids: benzoic acid (up to 20%), cinnamic acid (<10%), hydroxyoleanic acid; Esters (<9%): cinnamyl benzoate & cinnamoate (<7%), propyl cinnamoate, benzyl cinnamate (tr.); Aldehydes: vanillin aldehyde; Alcohols: benzoresinol, siaresinotannol.

Properties: **Anti-inflammatory, antiseptic, antioxidant, astringent, deodorant, diuretic, expectorant,** and **sedative.**

Common Primary Uses: **[T]Warming.**

Historical Uses: Onycha (or benzoin), as either a resin or an absolute, has been used for thousands of years in the East for rituals and ceremonies as either incense or for anointings. It is mentioned in the Bible as one of the ingredients for a "Holy Anointing Oil" (Exodus 30:34). The Chinese used it for its heating and drying qualities, and in the West it was used for respiratory complaints.

Other Possible Uses: This oil may help **arthritis, asthma, bleeding** (slow or stop), **bronchitis, chills, circulation** (poor), **colic, cuts, flatulence** (gas), **flu, gout, laryngitis, mucus** (helps remove), **nervous tension, rheumatism, skin** (lesions; chapped, inflamed, and irritated conditions), **stomach** (gripping pains), **stress**-related conditions, **urinary tract infection**, and **wounds**. It is very **warming**, which makes it good for **colds, coughs**, and **sore throats**.

Body System(s) Affected: **Cardiovascular System, Emotional Balance, Skin**.

Aromatic Influence: Onycha is **warming** and **soothing** to the **heart**. According to Marguerite Maury, "This essence creates a kind of euphoria; it interposes a padded zone between us and events." It may also help one overcome **sadness, loneliness, depression**, and **anxiety**. When combined with rose, it can be very **comforting** and **uplifting**.

Application: Apply to **Vita Flex Points** and/or directly on **area** of concern; **massage** (combine with rose and add to V-6 Oil). Because of its thick, resinous nature, thin heavily with lavender or peppermint oils for diffusion.

Oral Use As Dietary Supplement: Approved by the FDA for use as a Food Additive (FA) and Flavoring Agent (FL). ***Dilute*** *one drop oil in 1 tsp. honey or in 4 oz. of beverage (i.e. soy/rice milk).* ***Not for children under 6 years old; use with caution and in greater dilution for children 6 years old and over.***

Blend Classification: Enhancer and Equalizer.

Blends With: Coriander, cypress, frankincense, jasmine, juniper, lemon, myrrh, rose, sandalwood, and other spice oils.

Odor: Type: *Base Note (5–20% of the blend)*; Scent: *Rich, warm, slightly woody, creamy, vanilla-like*; Intensity: *1*.

Orange

(Citrus sinensis)

Botanical Family: Rutaceae (citrus)

Extraction Method/Origin: Cold pressed from rind.—USA, South Africa, Italy, China

Chemical Constituents: Monoterpenes (up to 95%): d-limonene (<90%), terpinolene, myrcene, α-pinene; Tetraterpenes (<8%): β-carotene (<6%), lycopene; Aldehydes (<8%): citral, decanal, citronellal, dodecanal, nonanal, octanal, α-sinensal; Alcohols (<6%): linalol, cis & trans-carveol, α-terpineol, geraniol; Ketones (<4%): l- & d-carvone (<3%), α-ionone; Esters (<3%): citronellyl acetate, geranyl acetate, linalyl acetate, methyl anthranilate; Furanoids: auraptene, bergaptole, imperatarine; Sesquiterpene Ketones: nootkatone.

Properties: **Anticancer**[119] **antidepressant, antiseptic, antispasmodic, digestive, sedative**[120], and **tonic**.

Common Primary Uses: ^{AT}**Anxiety**, ^{AT}**calming**, ^{TI}**constipation**, ^{T}**indigestion**, ^{IT}**obesity**, ^{T}**oily skin**, ^{A}**uplifting**, ^{IT}**water purification**.

Folklore: According to Roberta Wilson, "From early times, oranges have been associated with generosity and gratitude. Once called 'golden apples,' oranges symbolized innocence and fertility."

Historical Uses: Oranges, particularly the bitter orange, have been used for palpitation, scurvy, jaundice, bleeding, heartburn, relaxed throat, prolapse of the uterus and the anus, diarrhea, and blood in the feces.

French Medicinal Uses: **Angina** (false), **cardiac spasm, constipation, diarrhea** (chronic), **dyspepsia** (nervous), **insomnia, menopause, palpitation**.

Other Possible Uses: This oil may help **appetite, bones** (rickety), **bronchitis, colds, colic** (dilute for infants; helps them sleep), **complexion** (dull and oily), **dermatitis, digestive system, fever, flu**, lower **high cholesterol, mouth ulcers, muscle soreness, obesity, sedation, tissue repair**[121], **water retention**, and **wrinkles**.

Body System(s) Affected: Digestive and Immune Systems, Emotional Balance, Skin.

Aromatic Influence: Orange brings peace and happiness to the mind and body and joy to the heart, which provide emotional support to help one overcome depression.

Application: Apply to Vita Flex Points and directly on area of concern; diffuse.

Oral Use As Dietary Supplement: Generally regarded as safe (GRAS) for human consumption by the FDA. *Dilute one drop oil in 1 tsp. honey or in 4 oz. of beverage (i.e. soy/rice milk). **Not for children under 6 years old; use with caution and in greater dilution for children 6 years old and over.***

Safety Data: *Avoid direct* ***sunlight*** *for up to 12 hours after use.*

Blend Classification: Enhancer and Personifier.

Blends With: Cinnamon bark, frankincense, geranium, juniper, lavender, nutmeg, rosewood.

Odor: Type: *Top Note (5–20% of the blend)*; Scent: *Fresh, citrusy, fruity, sweet*; Intensity: 1.

Oregano

(Origanum compactum, CT Carvacrol)

Botanical Family: Labiatae

Extraction Method/Origin: Steam distilled from leaves—Morocco, France

Chemical Constituents: Phenols (up to 80%): carvacrol (<75%), thymol (<5%), terpinen-4-ol; Monoterpenes (<25%): p-cymene (<10%), γ-terpinene (<9%), myrcene (<3%), α- and β-pinenes, camphene, l-limonene, α-terpinene; Sesquiterpenes (<6%): β-caryophyllene (<5%), β-bisabolene; Carboxylic Acids: rosmaric acid (<5%); Esters: linalyl acetate (<4%); Ketones: camphor, d-carvone; Alcohols: borneol, linalol, α-terpineol.

Properties: Antibacterial[122], antifungal[123], antiparasitic[124], antiseptic (to the respiratory system), antiviral, antispasmodic, and immune-stimulant[125].

Common Primary Uses: [TA]Antibacterial, [TA]antifungal, [T]calluses, [TI]candida, [T]carpal tunnel, [IT]parasites (intestinal), [A]pneumonia, [I]sore throat, [TI]staph/MRSA, [I]strep throat, [TA]viral infection, [T]warming oils, [T]warts, [A]whooping cough.

French Medicinal Uses: Asthma, bronchitis (chronic), mental disease, pulmonary tuberculosis, rheumatism (chronic), whooping cough.

Other Possible Uses: This oil may help colds, digestion problems, metabolism balance, viral and bacterial pneumonia, and vital centers strengthening.

Body System(s) Affected: Immune and Respiratory Systems, Muscles and Bones.

Aromatic Influence: Strengthens one's feeling of security.

Application: Apply to Vita Flex Points and directly on area of concern; diffuse.

Oral Use As Dietary Supplement: Generally regarded as safe (GRAS) for human consumption by the FDA. *Dilute one drop oil in 1 tsp. honey or in 4 oz. of beverage (i.e. soy/rice milk). **Not for children under 6 years old; use with caution and in greater dilution for children 6 years old and over.***

Safety Data: ***Can cause extreme skin irritation.***

Blend Classification: Enhancer and Equalizer.

Blends With: Basil, fennel, geranium, lemongrass, myrtle, pine, thyme, rosemary.

Odor: Type: *Middle Note (50–80% of the blend)*; Scent: *Herbaceous, sharp*; Intensity: 5.

Oregano, Plectranthus

(Plectranthus amboinicus)

Botanical Family: Lamiaceae

Extraction Method/Origin: Steam distilled from leaves and stem—Ecuador

Chemical Constituents: Monoterpenes (up to 40%): γ-terpinene (17.9%), para-cymene (12.2%), limonene, myrcene, α-terpinene, α-thujene, α-pinene; Phenols (up to 35%): carvacrol (<33%), terpinen-4-ol; Sesquiterpenes (up to 15%): trans-β-caryophyllene (<12%), trans-β-farnesene, α-humulene, β-bisabolene, δ-cadinene; Furanoids: trans-α-bergamotene (<7%); Oxides: caryophyllene oxide, eucalyptol; Alcohols: α-terpineol, geraniol; Aldehydes: neral; Ketones: pulegone.

Properties: **Antibacterial, insecticidal**.

Common Primary Uses: TA**Antibacterial**, TA**insect repellent**.

Other Possible Uses: This oil may help relieve **tired** and **sore joints** and **muscles**.

Body System(s) Affected: **Immune System, Muscles and Bones**.

Aromatic Influence: Promotes feelings of **relaxation**.

Application: Dilute and apply to **Vita Flex Points** and directly on **area** of concern; **diffuse**.

Oral Use As Dietary Supplement: Traditionally used in cooking and as a tea. ***Dilute*** *one drop oil in 1 tsp. honey or in 4 oz. of beverage (i.e. soy/rice milk).* ***Not for children under 6 years old; use with caution and in greater dilution for children 6 years old and over.***

Safety Data: ***Can cause extreme skin irritation***.

Odor: Scent: *Herbaceous, sharp*; Intensity: 5.

Palmarosa

(Cymbopogon martinii)

Botanical Family: Graminaceae

Extraction Method/Origin: Steam distilled from leaves—India, Conoros

Chemical Constituents: Alcohols (up to 90%): geraniol (<85%), linalol, nerol, citronellol (tr.), farnesol (tr.); Esters (<30%): geranyl formate, acetate, & isovalerate (<27%); Monoterpenes: d-limonene; Oxides: geranyl epoxide; Sesquiterpene Alcohols: elemol.

Properties: **Antibacterial, antifungal, antimicrobial, antiseptic, antiviral, hydrating, stimulant** (digestive and circulatory), and **tonic**.

Folklore: Once known as Turkish geranium oil or Indian geranium oil, palmarosa was used for centuries by the Turks to adulterate the more costly Turkish rose oil.

Historical Uses: Used to prevent infections and fight fever, palmarosa was also added to many culinary dishes to kill bacteria and aid digestion.

Other Possible Uses: This oil may be beneficial for **candida, circulation, digestion, fever, infection, nervous system**, and **rashes**. It is valuable for all types of **skin** problems because it stimulates new cell growth, regulates oil production, moisturizes, and speeds healing.

Body System(s) Affected: **Cardiovascular System, Emotional Balance, Skin**.

Aromatic Influence: Strengthens one's feeling of **security**. It also helps to reduce **stress** and **tension** and promotes recovery from **nervous exhaustion**. If uplifts the **emotions**, refreshes the **mind**, and clarifies **thoughts**. Inhaling palmarosa may also have a normalizing effect on the **thyroid gland**.

Application: Apply to **Vita Flex Points** and directly on **area** of concern; **diffuse**.

Oral Use As Dietary Supplement: Generally regarded as safe (GRAS) for human consumption by the FDA. ***Dilute** one drop oil in 1 tsp. honey or in 4 oz. of beverage (i.e. soy/rice milk). **Not for children under 6 years old; use with caution and in greater dilution for children 6 years old and over.***

Blend Classification: Enhancer and Equalizer.

Blends With: Basil, fennel, geranium, lemongrass, myrtle, pine, thyme, rosemary.

Odor: Type: *Top to Middle Notes (20–80% of the blend)*; Scent: *Lemony, fresh, green, with hints of rose and geranium*; Intensity: *3*.

Palo Santo ("Holy Wood")

(Bursera graveolens)

Botanical Family: Burseraceae (resinous trees and shrubs)

Extraction Method/Origin: Steam distilled from wood chips of dead heartwood—Ecuador.
Note: The wood must be dead for at least 2 years before the oil is pulled into the heartwood. The wood must be cut into sawdust to get at the oil (9 kg of sawdust to produce 500 ml of oil). Also, this oil is distilled from the red wood, which produces a much better quality oil.

Chemical Constituents: Monoterpenes: d-limonene (75–76%), α-pinene; Alcohols: α-terpineol; Sesquiterpenes: eudesmene; Ketones: carvone (<4%); Furanoids: menthofuran, agarofuran; Phenols: carvacrol, terpinen-4-ol; Sesquiterpene Alcohols: eudesmol.

Properties: **Anti-infectious, antiseptic, antitumoral, immune-stimulant**, and **sedative**.

Common Primary Uses: [TA]**Antiviral**.

Historical Uses: Palo Santo (also known as Holy Wood) is a natural wood aromatic incense. It has been used for centuries by the indigenous peoples of the Amazon in rituals and ceremonies for the purifying and cleansing of evil spirits, misfortune, and calamity.

Other Possible Uses: This oil may help with **cancer, healing, muscle pain, nervous** conditions, acute **rheumatism**, and **spiritual awareness**.

Body System(s) Affected: **Emotional Balance, Immune** and **Nervous Systems**.

Aromatic Influence: It has a wonderfully **calming, soothing** aroma with a **powerful energy**. It may help to increase **spiritual awareness** and focus **meditation** while **clearing** the space of **negative energy**.

Application: Apply to **Vita Flex Points** and/or directly on **area** of concern; **diffuse**. Some say that because it is a shamanic oil, the user must have a firm intention in mind before applying this oil to the **forehead** (3rd eye chakra) so that the oil can change the energy both inside and outside the person to assist in the fulfillment of that intention.

Blend Classification: Enhancer and Equalizer.

Blends With: Benzoin, frankincense, myrrh, and sandalwood.

Odor: Type: *Base Note (5–20% of the blend)*; Scent: *Rich, citrusy, balsamic, sweet, with incense-like overtones*; Intensity: *4*.

Frequency: High (Spiritual).

Patchouli (or Patchouly)

(Pogostemon cablin)

Botanical Family: Labiatae (mint)

Extraction Method/Origin: Steam distilled from leaves and flowers—Sumatra, Java, Malaysia, China, Brazil, Indonesia

Chemical Constituents: Sesquiterpenes (up to 63%): α-bulnesene (<20%), β-bulnesene (<16%), aromadendrene (<15%), α-gaiene (>12%), seychellene (6%), α-, β- & γ-patchoulenes (<12%), β-caryophyllene (<4%), δ-cadinene (<3%), β-gaiene, β-elemene, humulene; Sesquiterpene Alcohols (<38%): patchoulol (up to 35%), pogostol, bulnesol, guaiol, patchoulenol; Oxides (<5%): bulnesene oxide, caryophyllene oxide, guaiene oxide; Ketones: patchoulenone (<3%); Monoterpenes: α- & β-pinenes, l-limonene.

Properties: **Anti-infectious, anti-inflammatory, antifungal, antiseptic, antitoxic, astringent, decongestant, deodorant, diuretic, insecticidal**[126], **stimulant** (digestive), and **tonic**.

Common Primary Uses: ^T^**Allergies (skin)**, ^AT^**bug repellent**, ^T^**dermatitis/eczema**, ^T^**hemorrhoids**, ^AT^**insect repellent**, ^T^**jock itch**, ^T^**snake bites**, ^T^**wrinkles**.

Historical Uses: For centuries, the Asian people used patchouli to fight infection, cool fevers, tone the skin (and entire body), and as an antidote for insect and snake bites. It was also used to treat colds, headaches, nausea, vomiting, diarrhea, abdominal pain, and halitosis (bad breath).

French Medicinal Uses: **Allergies, dermatitis, eczema, hemorrhoids, tissue regeneration**.

Other Possible Uses: This oil is a **digester** of **toxic material** in the body. It may also help **acne, appetite** (curbs), **bites** (**insect** and **snake**), **cellulite, congestion, dandruff, depression, the digestive system**, relieve itching from **hives, skin conditions** (chapped; tightens loose skin), **UV radiation** (protects against), **water retention, weeping wounds, weight reduction**, and prevent **wrinkles**.

Body System(s) Affected: **Skin**.

Aromatic Influence: It is **sedating, calming**[127], and **relaxing**, allowing it to reduce **anxiety**. It may have some particular influence on **sex, physical energy**, and **money**.

Application: Apply to **Vita Flex Points** and directly on **area** of concern; **diffuse**.

Oral Use As Dietary Supplement: Approved by the FDA for use as a Food Additive (FA) and Flavoring Agent (FL). ***Dilute** one drop oil in 1 tsp. honey or in 4 oz. of beverage (i.e. soy/rice milk).* ***Not for children under 6 years old; use with caution and in greater dilution for children 6 years old and over.***

Blend Classification: Enhancer.

Blends With: Bergamot, clary sage, frankincense, geranium, ginger, lavender, lemongrass, myrrh, pine, rosewood, sandalwood.

Odor: Type: *Base Note (5–20% of the blend)*; Scent: *Earthy, herbaceous, sweet-balsamic, rich, with woody undertones*; Intensity: *4*.

Pepper, Black

(Piper nigrum)

Botanical Family: Piperaceae

Extraction Method/Origin: Steam distilled from berries—Egypt, India, Madagascar

Chemical Constituents: Monoterpenes (up to 70%): l-limonene (<15%), δ-3-carene (<15%), β-pinene (<14%), sabinene (<10%), α-phellandrene (<9%), α-pinene (<9%), α-thujene (<4%), γ- & α-terpinene (<7%), p-cymene (<3%), myrcene (<3%), terpinolene (<2%); Sesquiterpenes (up to 60%): β-caryophyllene (up to 35%), β-selinene (<8%), β-bisabolene (<5%), α-, β-, & δ-elemenes, β-farnesene, humulene, α-copaene, α-guaiene, α- & β-cubebenes; Oxides: caryophyllene oxide (<8%); Ketones (<2%): acetophenone, hydrocarvone, piperitone; Aldehydes: piperonal; Carboxylic Acids: piperonylic acid; Furanocoumarin: α-bergamotene.

Properties: **Analgesic, anticatarrhal, anti-inflammatory, antiseptic, antispasmodic, antitoxic, aphrodisiac, expectorant, laxative, rubefacient**, and **stimulant**[128] (nervous, circulatory, digestive).

Common Primary Uses: ^A**Fainting**.

Folklore: Pepper was used by the Egyptians in mummification as evidenced by the discovery of black pepper in the nostrils and abdomen of Ramses II. Indian monks ate several black pepper corns a day to maintain their incredible stamina and energy.

Historical Uses: Pepper has been used for thousands of years for malaria, cholera, and several digestive problems.

Other Possible Uses: This oil may increase **cellular oxygenation**[128], support **digestive glands**, stimulate the **endocrine system**, increase **energy**, and help **rheumatoid arthritis**. It may also help with **addiction**[129], loss of **appetite, catarrh, chills, cholera, colds, colic, constipation, coughs, diarrhea, dysentery, dyspepsia, dysuria, flatulence** (combine with fennel), **flu, heartburn, influenza, nausea, neuralgia, poor circulation, poor muscle tone, quinsy, sprains, toothache, vertigo, viruses**, and **vomiting**.

Body System(s) Affected: **Digestive** and **Nervous Systems**.

Aromatic Influence: Pepper is considered to be good for the **1st chakra**. It is **comforting** and **stimulating**.

Application: Apply to **Vita Flex Points** and/or directly on **area** of concern; **diffuse**. Mix very sparingly with juniper and lavender in a **bath** to help with **chills** or to warm one up in the winter.

Oral Use As Dietary Supplement: Generally regarded as safe (GRAS) for human consumption by the FDA. ***Dilute** one drop oil in 1 tsp. honey or in 4 oz. of beverage (i.e. soy/rice milk).* ***Not for children under 6 years old; use with caution and in greater dilution for children 6 years old and over.***

Safety Data: ***Can cause extreme skin irritation.***

Blends With: Cumin, fennel, frankincense, lavender, marjoram, rosemary, sandalwood, and other spice oils.

Odor: Type: *Middle Note (50–80% of the blend)*; Scent: *Spicy, peppery, musky, warm, with herbaceous undertones*; Intensity: *3*.

Pepper, Pink (or Brazilian Peppertree)

(Schinus molle)

Botanical Family: Anacardiaceae

Extraction Method/Origin: Steam distilled from leaves—South America

Chemical Constituents: Monoterpenes: α- & β-pinenes, camphene, phellandrene; Sesquiterpenes: caryophyllene, and others; Phenols: carvacrol.

Properties: **Antibacterial, antifungal** (especially candida), **anti-inflammatory, antitumoral, antiviral, antimicrobial, antispasmodic, astringent, diuretic, stimulant** (digestive), **tonic**, and **wound healer**.

Common Primary Uses: ^TA**Antifungal**.

Historical Uses: According to Leslie Taylor, ND, "Virtually all parts of this tropical tree, including its leaves, bark, fruit, seeds, resin, and oleoresin (or balsam) have been used medicinally by indigenous peoples throughout the tropics."

Other Possible Uses: This oil may help with **bronchitis, gingivitis, gonorrhea, gout, heart problems** (hypertension and irregular heart beat), **inflammation** (general), **menstrual disorders** (excessive bleeding), **pain relief, rheumatism, sores, swellings, tuberculosis, tumors, ulcers, urethritis, urogenital disorders, venereal diseases, warts**, and **wounds**. According to Leslie Taylor, ND, "More recently, in 2002, researchers in Argentina documented that it was toxic in vitro against a human liver cancer cell line."

Body System(s) Affected: **Immune** and **Respiratory Systems, Skin**.

Application: Apply to **Vita Flex Points** and/or directly on **area** of concern.

Oral Use As Dietary Supplement: Generally regarded as safe (GRAS) for human consumption by the FDA. ***Dilute** one drop oil in 1 tsp. honey or in 4 oz. of beverage (i.e. soy/rice milk).* ***Not for children under 6 years old; use with caution and in greater dilution for children 6 years old and over.***

Safety Data: ***Avoid during pregnancy.***

Peppermint

(Mentha piperita)

Botanical Family: Labiatae (mint)

Extraction Method/Origin: Steam distilled from leaves, stems, flower buds—North America

Chemical Constituents: Phenolic Alcohols (up to 55%): menthol (<52%), piperitols; Ketones (<25%): menthone (17–32% and up to 65% if distilled in September when flowering), pulegone (<5%), piperitone (<2%), carvone, jasmone; Monoterpenes (< 15%): α and β-pinenes (<6%), l-limonene (<6%), ocimene, myrcene, p-cymene, β-phellandrene, sabinene, α-terpinene, terpinolene, camphene; Sesquiterpenes (<10%): germacrene-D (<5%), β-bourbonene, ζ-bulgarene, γ-cadinene, β-caryophyllene, β-elemene, β-farnesene, muurolene; Esters (<9%): menthyl acetate (<9%), also menthyl butyrate & isovalerate; Oxides (<9%): 1,8 cineol (<5%), piperitone oxide, caryophyllene oxide; Furanoids: menthofuran (<8%); Phenols: terpinen-4-ol (<3%); Alcohols (<3%): α-terpineol, linalol; Sesquiterpene Alcohols: viridiflorol; Furanocoumarins: aesculetine; Sulphides: mint sulfide, di-menthyl sulfide.

Properties: **Analgesic, antibacterial**[130], **anticarcinogenic, anti-inflammatory**[131] (prostate and nerves), **antiseptic, antispasmodic**[132], **antiviral**[133], and **invigorating**.

Common Primary Uses: [AI]**Alertness**, [AT]**allergies (airborne)**, [T]**allergies (skin)**, [TA]**antibacterial**, [AI]**antioxidant**, [AT]**asthma**, [T]**autism**, [I]**bad breath (halitosis)**, [AT]**brain injury**, [TI]**candida**, [T]**carpal tunnel**, [T]**chronic fatigue**, [T]**cold sores**, [A]**concentration (poor)**, [T]**constipation**, [T]**cooling**, [IT]**cramps (abdominal)**, [IT]**Crohn's disease**, [IT]**diarrhea**, [AT]**energizing**, [A]**fainting**, [IT]**fever**, [AT]**flu (influenza)**, [IT]**gas/flatulence**, [IT]**gastritis**, [TA]**headache**, [T]**heartburn**, [T]**heatstroke**, [T]**hemorrhoids**, [T]**herpes simplex**, [T]**hives**, [T]**hot flashes**, [T]**indigestion**, [I]**irritable bowel syndrome (IBS)**, [T]**itching**, [T]**jet lag**, [A]**memory**, [T]**migraine**, [IA]**morning sickness**, [A]**motion sickness**, [T]**multiple sclerosis**, [T]**muscle fatigue**, [IA]**nausea**, [T]**paralysis**, [IA]**polyps (colon)**, [I]**radiation (gamma)**, [T]**ringworm**, [T]**scabies**, [T]**sciatica**, [T]**shock**, [AT]**stimulating**, [T]**tennis elbow**, [T]**varicose veins**, [IA]**vomiting**.

Folklore: According to Roberta Wilson, "In Roman mythology, when Pluto professed his love for the nymph Mentha, his wife Persephone, afire with jealousy, crushed Mentha into dust on the ground. Pluto, unable to change her back, transformed her into a peppermint plant and gave her a fresh fragrance so she would smell sweet whenever stepped upon."

Historical Uses: For centuries, peppermint has been used to soothe digestive difficulties, freshen breath, and relieve colic, gas, headaches, heartburn, and indigestion.

French Medicinal Uses: **Asthma, bronchitis, candida, diarrhea, digestive aid**[134], **fever** (reduces), **flu, halitosis, heartburn, hemorrhoids, hot flashes, indigestion**[135], **menstrual irregularity, migraine headache, motion sickness, nausea, respiratory function** (aids), **shock, skin** (itchy), **throat infection, varicose veins, vomiting.**

Other Possible Uses: This oil may help **anger, arthritis, colic, depression, fatigue, food poisoning, headaches**[136], **hives, hysteria, inflammation, irritable bowel syndrome (IBS)**[137], **liver problems, memory**[138], **morning sickness, nerves** (regenerate and support)[139], **radiation exposure**[140], **rheumatism**, elevate and open **sensory system**, soothe and cool **skin** (may help keep body cooler on hot days), **toothaches, tuberculosis**, and add flavor to **water**.

Body System(s) Affected: **Digestive, Nervous,** and **Respiratory Systems, Muscles and Bones, Skin.**

Aromatic Influence: It is **purifying** and **stimulating** to the **conscious mind**. Reduces **fevers**. Dr. Dembar of the University of Cincinnati discovered in a research study that inhaling peppermint oil **increased** the **mental accuracy** of the students by up to 28%.

Application: Apply to **Vita Flex Points** and/or directly on **area** of concern.

Oral Use As Dietary Supplement: Generally regarded as safe (GRAS) for human consumption by the FDA. ***Dilute** one drop oil in 1 tsp. honey or in 4 oz. of beverage (i.e. soy/rice milk).* ***Not for children under 6 years old; use with caution and in greater dilution for children 6 years old and over.***

Safety Data: ***Repeated use can possibly result in contact sensitization. Use with caution if dealing with high blood pressure. Use with caution during pregnancy.***

Blend Classification: Personifier.

Odor: Type: *Middle Note (50–80% of the blend)*; Scent: *Minty, sharp, intense*; Intensity: *5*.

Frequency: Physical; approximately 78.

Petitgrain

(Citrus aurantium)

Botanical Family: Rutaceae (citrus)

Extraction Method/Origin: Steam distilled from bitter orange tree leaves—Italy

Chemical Constituents: Esters (up to 65%): linalyl acetate (<55%), geranyl acetate (<5%), neryl & α-terpenyl acetates, methyl anthranilate; Alcohols (40%): linalol (<28%), α-terpineol (<8%), geraniol (<5%), nerol, citronellol; Monoterpenes (<28%): myrcene (<6%), β-cymene (<5%), cis- & trans-ocimenes (<5%), p-cymene (<3%), β-pinene, γ-terpinene, d-limonene, phellandrene, sabinene, terpinolene; Aldehydes: decanal, geranial, neral; Phenols: thymol, terpinen-4-ol; Furanocoumarins: bergaptene, citroptene.

Properties: **Antibacterial, anti-infectious, anti-inflammatory, antiseptic, antispasmodic, deodorant, nervine**, and **stimulant** (digestive, nervous).

Common Primary Uses: **[T]Greasy/oily hair.**

Folklore: Petitgrain derives its name from the extraction of the oil, which at one time was from the green unripe oranges when they were still about the size of a cherry.

Historical Uses: Because of its very pleasing scent, petitgrain has been used extensively in high-quality perfumes and cosmetics.

Other Possible Uses: This oil may help re-establish **nerve equilibrium**. It may also help with **acne, dyspepsia, fatigue, flatulence, greasy hair, insomnia**, and excessive **perspiration**.

Body System(s) Affected: **Emotional Balance.**

Aromatic Influence: It is **uplifting** and **refreshing** and helps to refresh the **senses**, clear **confusion**, reduce **mental fatigue**, and reduce **depression**. It may also stimulate the **mind**, support **memory**, and gladden the **heart**.

Application: Apply to **Vita Flex Points** and directly on **area** of concern; **diffuse**.

Oral Use As Dietary Supplement: Generally regarded as safe (GRAS) for human consumption by the FDA. ***Dilute** one drop oil in 1 tsp. honey or in 4 oz. of beverage (i.e. soy/rice milk).* ***Not for children under 6 years old; use with caution and in greater dilution for children 6 years old and over.***

Blend Classification: Enhancer, Modifier, and Personifier.

Blends With: Bergamot, cistus, clary sage, clove, geranium, jasmine, lavender, neroli, orange, palmarosa, and rosemary.

Odor: Type: *Top Note (5–20% of the blend)*; Scent: *Fresh, floral, citrusy, lighter in fragrance than neroli and slightly woody*; Intensity: *3.*

Pine (or Scotch Pine)

(Pinus sylvestris)

Botanical Family: Pinaceae (conifer)

Extraction Method/Origin: Steam distilled from needles—Austria, Canada, Russia

Chemical Constituents: Monoterpenes (up to 80%): α-pinene (>41%), δ-3-carene (<17%), l-limonene (<16%), β-pinene (<15%), camphene, β-phellandrene, terpinolene, ocimene, p-cymene, γ-terpinene, sabinene; Sesquiterpenes (<12%): β-caryophyllene (<6%), γ-cadinene (<5%), α-copaene, β-guaiene, longifolene, muurolene; Alcohols: borneol (2%); Esters: bornyl acetate (<3%); Sesquiterpene Alcohols: α-cadinol, muurolol; Diterpenes: cembrene; Aldehydes: citronellal; Phenols: terpinen-4-ol.

Properties: **Antibacterial, antimicrobial, antineuralgic, antiseptic** (pulmonary, urinary, hepatic), **antiviral, expectorant,** and **stimulant** (adrenal cortex, circulatory, nervous).

Common Primary Uses: [T]**Gout,** [AT]**sinusitis.**

Folklore: In some cultures, pine branches were placed on coffins to signify immortality.

Historical Uses: Pine was used by the American Indians to prevent scurvy. They also stuffed mattresses with pine to repel lice and fleas. Pine was used to treat pneumonia and lung infections and was even added to baths to revitalize people suffering from mental or emotional fatigue and nervous exhaustion.

French Medicinal Uses: **Asthma, bronchitis, diabetes, infections** (severe), **rheumatoid arthritis, sinusitis.**

Other Possible Uses: This oil may help dilate and open the **respiratory system**, particularly the **bronchial tract**. It may also help with **colds, coughs, cuts, cystitis, fatigue, feet** (excessive sweating), **flu, gout, lice, nervous exhaustion, scabies, skin parasites, sores, stress,** and **urinary infection.** Pine oil may also help increase **blood pressure** and **stimulate** the **adrenal glands** and the **circulatory system**. Pine is a good recommendation for any first aid kit.

Body System(s) Affected: **Emotional Balance, Respiratory System.**

Aromatic Influence: It helps soothe **mental stress**, relieve **anxiety, freshen** and **deodorize** a room, and **revitalize** the entire body.

Application: Apply to **Vita Flex Points** and/or directly on **area** of concern; **diffuse**. Pine is an excellent tonic when added to water and sprinkled on hot rocks in the **sauna**.

Oral Use As Dietary Supplement: Approved by the FDA for use as a Food Additive (FA) and Flavoring Agent (FL). **Dilute** *one drop oil in 1 tsp. honey or in 4 oz. of beverage (i.e. soy/rice milk).* ***Not for children under 6 years old; use with* caution *and in* greater dilution *for children 6 years old and over.***

Safety Data: ***Repeated use can possibly result in* skin irritation.**

Blends With: Cedarwood, eucalyptus, juniper, lemon, marjoram, melaleuca, and rosemary.

Odor: Type: *Middle Note (50–80% of the blend)*; Scent: *Fresh, woody, earthly, balsamic*; Intensity: *4.*

Plectranthus Oregano

(See Oregano, Plectranthus)

Ravensara

(Ravensara aromatica)

Botanical Family: Lauraceae

Extraction Method/Origin: Steam distilled from leaves and branches—Madagascar

Chemical Constituents: Oxides: 1,8-cineol (up to 61%); Monoterpenes (<32%): sabinene (<15%), α- and β-pinenes (<14%), l-limonene (<4%); Alcohols: α-terpineol (<7%); Phenols: terpinen-4-ol; Esters: α-terpenyl acetate; Sesquiterpenes: β-caryophyllene.

Properties: **Antibacterial, antifungal, anti-infectious, antiseptic**, powerful **antiviral**, and **expectorant**.

Common Primary Uses: ^{T}**Burns**, ^{T}**cholera**, ^{AT}**colds (common)**, ^{T}**shingles**, ^{TA}**viral infection**.

French Medicinal Uses: **Bronchitis, cholera, herpes, infectious mononucleosis, insomnia, muscle fatigue, rhino pharyngitis, shingles, sinusitis, viral hepatitis.**

Other Possible Uses: Ravensara is part of the laurel family (akin to *Laurus nobilis*) and is another universal oil like lavender. It may help **asthma, bladder, bunions, burns** (healing), **cancer, colds, cuts, ears, flu, liver, lungs**, support the **nerves, pneumonia, scrapes, viral infections**, and **wounds**. As a cross between clove and nutmeg, it may be very supportive to the **adrenal glands**. It has also demonstrated **antimutagenic**[141] properties.

Body System(s) Affected: **Immune** and **Respiratory Systems**.

Application: Apply to **Vita Flex Points** and/or directly on **area** of concern; **diffuse**.

Blend Classification: Enhancer.

Odor: Type: *Top Note (5–20% of the blend)*; Scent: *Slightly medicinal, eucalyptus-like, slightly sweet with a fruity hint*; Intensity: *3*.

Frequency: High (Spiritual); approximately 134 MHz.

Roman Chamomile

(See Chamomile, Roman)

Rosalina

(See Melaleuca Ericifolia)

Rose (or Bulgarian Rose)

(Rosa damascena)

Botanical Family: Rosaceae

Extraction Method/Origin: Steam distilled from flowers (a two-part process)—Bulgaria, Turkey

Chemical Constituents: Alcohols (up to 70%): citronellol (up to 45%), geraniol (up to 28%), nerol (<9%), linalol, borneol, α-terpineol; Monoterpenes (<25%): stearoptene (<22%), α & β-pinenes, camphene, α-terpinene, l-limonene, myrcene, p-cymene, ocimene; Alkanes (<19%): nonadecane (<15%), octadecane, eicosane, and others; Esters (<5%): geranyl, neryl, & citronellyl acetates; Phenols (<4%): eugenol, phenylethanol; Sesquiterpene Alcohols: farnesol (<2%); Oxides: rose oxide; Ketones: α- & β-damascenone, β-ionone; Furanoids: rosefuran; Many other trace elements.

Properties: **Antibacteral**[142], **antihemorrhaging, anti-infectious, aphrodisiac**, and **sedative**[142].

Common Primary Uses: ^{AT}**Calming**, ^{T}**poison ivy**, ^{AT}**relaxing**, ^{T}**scarring**.

Historical Uses: The healing properties of the rose have been utilized in medicine throughout the ages and still play an important role in the East. Rose has been used for digestive and menstrual problems, headaches and nervous tension, liver congestion, poor circulation, fever (plague), eye infections, and skin complaints.

Other Possible Uses: This oil may help **asthma**, chronic **bronchitis**, **frigidity**, **gingivitis**, **hemorrhaging**, **herpes simplex**, **impotence**, **infections**, prevent **scarring**, **sexual debilities**, **skin disease**, **sprains**, **thrush**, **tuberculosis**, **ulcers**, **wounds**, and **wrinkles**.

Body System(s) Affected: **Emotional Balance**, **Skin**.

Aromatic Influence: It is **stimulating** and **elevating** to the **mind**, creating a sense of **well-being**. Its beautiful fragrance is almost intoxicating and **aphrodisiac-like**.

Application: Apply to **Vita Flex Points** and/or directly on **area** of concern; **diffuse**.

Oral Use As Dietary Supplement: Generally regarded as safe (GRAS) for human consumption by the FDA. **Dilute** *one drop oil in 1 tsp. honey or in 4 oz. of beverage (i.e. soy/rice milk).* ***Not for children under 6 years old; use with caution and in greater dilution for children 6 years old and over.***

Safety Data: ***Use with caution during pregnancy.***

Blend Classification: Personifier, Enhancer, Equalizer, and Modifier.

Odor: Type: *Middle to Base Notes (20–80% of the blend)*; Scent: *Floral, spicy, rich, deep, sensual, green, honey-like*; Intensity: *3*.

Frequency: Highest of all the oils (Spiritual); approximately 320 MHz. It enhances the frequency of every cell, bringing balance and harmony to the body.

Rosehip

(Rosa canina or R. rubiginosa)

Botanical Family: Rosaceae

Properties: **Regenerative.**

Possible Uses: Rosehip oil has been used effectively in the treatment of **skin conditions**. It promotes **tissue regeneration** and may help heal **burns**, reduce **scarring**, retard **premature aging**, and soften **scar tissue**.

Application: Apply directly on **area** of concern.

Oral Use As Dietary Supplement: Generally regarded as safe (GRAS) for human consumption by the FDA. **Dilute** *one drop oil in 1 tsp. honey or in 4 oz. of beverage (i.e. soy/rice milk).* ***Not for children under 6 years old; use with caution and in greater dilution for children 6 years old and over.***

Rosemary Cineol

(Rosmarinus officinalis, CT 1,8 Cineol)

Botanical Family: Labiatae (mint)

Extraction Method/Origin: Steam distilled from flowering plant—France, Tunisia, USA

Chemical Constituents: Oxides: 1,8 cineol (up to 55%), caryophyllene oxide, humulene oxide; Monoterpenes: α-pinene (<14%), β-pinene (<9%), camphene (<8%), l-limonene, myrcene, p-cymene, α- & β-phellandrenes, α- & γ-terpinenes; Ketones (<32%): camphor (<30%), β-thujone, verbenone, d-carvone, hexanone, heptanone; Alcohols (<20%): borneol (<12%), α-terpineol (<5%), linalol, verbenol; Sesquiterpenes (<3%): β-caryophyllene, humulene; Phenols: terpinen-4-ol; Esters: bornyl & fenchyl acetates; Acids: rosemaric acid.

Properties: **Analgesic**[144] **antibacterial**[145], **anticancer**[146], **anticatarrhal**, **antifungal**[147], **anti-infectious**, **anti-inflammatory**[148], **antioxidant**[149], and **expectorant**.

Common Primary Uses: **^A^Alcoholism**, **^AI^antioxidant**, **^T^arthritis**, **^T^autism**, **^T^cellulite**, **^T^cholera**, **^AT^colds (common)**, **^T^constipation**, **^T^cramps (muscle)**, **^T^dandruff**, **^IT^diabetes**, **^A^fainting**, **^AT^flu (influenza)**, **^T^hair loss**, **^TA^headache**, **^A^low blood pressure**, **^A^memory**, **^AT^mental fatigue**, **^T^muscular dystrophy**, **^AT^sinusitis**, **^AT^stimulating**, **^T^vaginal infections**.

Historical Uses: The rosemary plant was regarded as sacred by many civilizations. It was used as a fumigant to help drive away evil spirits, and to protect against plague and infectious illness.

French Medicinal Uses: **Arthritis**[150], **blood pressure** (low), **bronchitis**[151], **cellulite**, **cholera**, **colds**, **dandruff**, **depression** (nervous), **diabetes**, **fatigue** (nervous/mental), **flu**, **fluid retention**, **hair loss**[152], **headache**, **hepatitis** (viral), **menstrual periods** (irregular), **sinusitis**, **tachycardia**, **vaginitis**.

Other Possible Uses: This oil may help **arteriosclerosis**, **bronchitis**, **chills**, **colds**, **colitis**, **cystitis**, **dyspepsia**, nervous **exhaustion**, **flu**, oily **hair**, **the immune system** (stimulate), **otitis**, **palpitations**, prevent **respiratory infections**, **sinusitis**, sour **stomach**, **stress-related illness**. *Note: This chemotype is said to be best used for* ***pulmonary congestion***[153], *slow* ***elimination***, ***candida***, *chronic* ***fatigue***, *and* ***infections*** *(especially staph and strep).*

Body System(s) Affected: **Immune**, **Respiratory**, and **Nervous Systems**.

Aromatic Influence: Stimulates **memory**[154] and opens the **conscious mind**.

Application: Apply to **Vita Flex Points** and/or directly on **area** of concern; **diffuse**.

Oral Use As Dietary Supplement: Generally regarded as safe (GRAS) for human consumption by the FDA. ***Dilute*** *one drop oil in 1 tsp. honey or in 4 oz. of beverage (i.e. soy/rice milk).* ***Not for children under 6 years old; use with caution and in greater dilution for children 6 years old and over.***

Safety Data: ***Avoid during pregnancy. Not for use by people with epilepsy. Avoid if dealing with high blood pressure.***

Blend Classification: Enhancer.

Blends With: Basil, cedarwood, frankincense, lavender, peppermint, rosewood, eucalyptus, marjoram, pine.

Odor: Type: *Middle Note (50–80% of the blend)*; Scent: *Herbaceous, strong, camphorous, with woody-balsamic and evergreen undertones*; Intensity: *3*.

Rosemary Verbenon

(Rosmarinus officinalis, CT Verbenon)

Botanical Family: Labiatae (mint)

Extraction Method/Origin: Steam distilled from flowering plant—Corsica

Chemical Constituents: Ketones (up to 50%): verbenon (<37%), camphor (<15%); Monoterpenes (<45%): α-pinene (<34%), camphene (<10%), l-limonene (<4%), β-pinene, myrcene, α-terpinene, terpinolene; Oxides: 1,8 cineol (<15%); Esters: bornyl acetate (<11%); Alcohols: borneol (<7%); Sesquiterpenes: β-caryophyllene, humulene.

Properties: **Antibacterial**, **anticatarrhal**, **anti-infectious**, **antispasmodic**, **cardiac** regulator, **endocrine** regulator (pituitary: regulates ovaries and testicles), **expectorant**, **mucolytic**, and **nervous** regulator.

Historical Uses: (See Rosemary Cineol)

French Medicinal Uses: (See Rosemary Cineol)

Other Possible Uses: This oil may help **asthma**, **baldness**, **candida**, **cholesterol**, **circulation**, **gout**, balance **heart function**, support the **immune system**, **injuries**, decongest the **liver**, **muscular aches/pains**, stimulate **nerves**, **obesity**, regulate **ovary** function, **respiratory functions**, **rheumatism**, **skin**

conditions, energize **solar plexus, the spine, sprains**, regulate **testicular** function, **viruses**, and **wounds**. *Note: This chemotype is said to be best used for* ***liver*** *and* ***gallbladder*** *support, rejuvenation of* ***skin*** *(especially chronic* ***dry skin****), middle* ***ear infections****, and* ***endocrine*** *problems (regulates hypothalamic / pituitary / sexual glands).*

Body System(s) Affected: **Digestive** and **Hormonal Systems, Skin and Hair**.

Aromatic Influence: Stimulates **memory** and opens the **conscious mind**.

Application: Apply to **Vita Flex Points** and directly on **area** of concern; **diffuse**.

Oral Use As Dietary Supplement: Generally regarded as safe (GRAS) for human consumption by the FDA. **Dilute** *one drop oil in 1 tsp. honey or in 4 oz. of beverage (i.e. soy/rice milk). Not for children under 6 years old; use with* ***caution*** *and in* ***greater dilution*** *for children 6 years old and over.*

Safety Data: *Avoid during* ***pregnancy****. Not for use by people with* ***epilepsy****. Avoid if dealing with* ***high blood pressure****.*

Blend Classification: Enhancer.

Blends With: Basil, eucalyptus, lavender, marjoram, peppermint, pine.

Rosewood

(Aniba rosaeodora)

Botanical Family: Lauraceae

Extraction Method/Origin: Steam distilled from wood—Brazil

Chemical Constituents: Alcohols (up to 95%): linalol (<90%), α-terpineol (<7%), geraniol; Oxides (<6%): 1,8 cineol, linalol oxide; Sesquiterpenes: α-copaene; Ketones: heptanone.

Properties: **Antibacterial, antifungal, anti-infectious, antiparasitic**, and **antiviral**.

Common Primary Uses: **[T]Acne**, **[T]dermatitis/eczema**, **[T]dry skin**, **[T]vaginal infections**, **[T]wrinkles**.

Historical Uses: According to Roberta Wilson, "The original site of production of *bois de rose*, as the French called rosewood, was French Guiana, on the northern coast of South America. So great was the demand among the French for rosewood oil, . . . that they depleted the colony's rosewood forests." Even now, this tropical evergreen tree is one of the trees that is being extensively felled in the clearing of the South American rainforests.

French Medicinal Uses: **Acne, candida, depression, eczema, oral infections, skin** (dry), **vaginitis**.

Other Possible Uses: This oil may create **skin elasticity** and is **soothing** to the **skin**. It is recognized for its ability to get rid of **candida** of the **skin** and to slow the **aging** process. It may also be beneficial for **cuts, nausea, tissue regeneration**, and **wounds**. It helps to create a synergism with all other oils.

Body System(s) Affected: **Skin**.

Aromatic Influence: It is **appeasing** to the **mind, relaxing** to the **body**, and creates a feeling of **peace** and **gentleness**.

Application: Apply to **Vita Flex Points** and/or directly on **area** of concern; **diffuse**.

Oral Use As Dietary Supplement: Generally regarded as safe (GRAS) for human consumption by the FDA. **Dilute** *one drop oil in 1 tsp. honey or in 4 oz. of beverage (i.e. soy/rice milk). Not for children under 6 years old; use with* ***caution*** *and in* ***greater dilution*** *for children 6 years old and over.*

Blend Classification: Modifier and Equalizer.

Odor: Type: *Middle Note (50–80% of the blend)*; Scent: *Sweet, woody, floral aroma*; Intensity: *3*.

Sacred Frankincense

(See Frankincense, Sacred)

Sage

(Salvia officinalis)

Botanical Family: Labiatae (mint)

Extraction Method/Origin: Steam distilled from leaves and flowers—Croatia, France, Spain

Chemical Constituents: Ketones (approx. 60%): α-thujone (<33%), camphor (<24%), β-thujone (<14%); Monoterpenes (<30%): camphene (<12%), α- & β-pinenes (<8%), l-limonene (<4%), p-cymene (<2%), myrcene, salvene, α- & β-phellandrene, sabinene, α- & γ-terpinenes, α-thujene; Alcohols (<28%): borneol (<14%), linalol (<11%), α-terpineol (<9%); Oxides: 1,8 cineol (<13%); Sesquiterpenes (<12%): β-caryophyllene (<7%), humulene (<5%), aromadendrene, α- & β-cadinenes, β-copaene, ledene, α-maalene; Sesquiterpene Alcohols: viridiflorol (<10%); Esters (<5%): bornyl, linalyl, & sabinyl acetates; Phenols: terpinen-4-ol (<4%), estragole, thymol; Diterpene Alcohols: sclareol.

Properties: **Antibacterial**[155], **anticancerous, antimutagenic**[156], **antiseptic, antispasmodic, decongestant, diuretic**, and **disinfectant**. It contains estriol and has **estrogen-like properties**.

Common Primary Uses: **^IT^Diabetes**, **^T^gum disease**, **^AT^stimulating**.

Folklore: Sage is recognized by the Lakota Indians as a purifier and as the master healer. It was called *herba sacra* or "sacred herb" by the Romans.

Historical Uses: Sage has been used for respiratory infections, menstrual difficulties, digestive complaints, inflammations of the mouth, tongue, and throat, and to strengthen the senses.

French Medicinal Uses: **Asthma, bronchitis** (chronic), **digestion** (sluggish), **gingivitis, glandular disorders, lymphatic system, menopause, menstrual irregularity, night sweats**.

Other Possible Uses: This oil may help improve **estrogen** and **progesterone-testosterone balance**. It is believed to contain elements that contribute to the **secretion** of **progesterone-testosterone**. It activates the **nervous system** and **adrenal cortex** and may help with illness that is related to **digestion** and **liver problems**. It may also be beneficial for **acne, Alzheimer's**[157], **arthritis, bacterial infections, catarrh** (mucus), **dandruff, depression, eczema, fibrositis, hair loss, low blood pressure, mental fatigue, metabolism, respiratory problems, rheumatism, skin conditions, sores, sprains, tissue** (firms), and strengthening the **vital centers** of the body. It may also **balance** the **pelvic chakra** where negative emotions from denial and sexual abuse are stored.

Body System(s) Affected: **Hormonal** and **Immune Systems**.

Aromatic Influence: Helps to relieve **depression, mental fatigue**, and **strain**.

Application: Apply to **Vita Flex Points** and/or directly on **area** of concern; **diffuse**.

Oral Use As Dietary Supplement: Generally regarded as safe (GRAS) for human consumption by the FDA. ***Dilute*** *one drop oil in 2 tsp. honey or in 8 oz. of beverage (i.e. soy/rice milk). However, due to thujone content, more dilution may be necessary.* ***Best avoided by children of all ages.***

Safety Data: ***Classified by Robert Tisserand as an oral toxin due to thujone content. However, other sources indicate that for thujone to be toxic, undiluted oil in excess of 30 ml must be ingested in a short period of time. Therefore, use with caution. Best kept away from children. Avoid during pregnancy. Not for use by people with epilepsy. Avoid if dealing with high blood pressure.***

Blend Classification: Enhancer.

Blends With: Bergamot, lemon, lavender, peppermint, rosemary, lemongrass, pine.

Sage Lavender (or Spanish Sage)

(Salvia lavandulafolia)

Botanical Family: Labiatae

Extraction Method/Origin: Steam distilled from flowering plant—Spain

Chemical Constituents: Monoterpenes (up to 43%): α- & β-pinenes (up to 34%), camphene (<10%), sabinene (<8%), limonene (<5%), myrcene (<5%), p-cymene (3%), α- & γ terpinenes (<3%), α-phellandrene, cis- & trans-ocimene, tricyclene, α-thujene; Ketones (<30%): camphor (<30%), α-thujone; Oxides (<26%): 1,8 cineol (<25%), caryophyllene oxide; Esters (<11%): α-terpenyl, linalyl, & bornyl acetates; Alcohols (<14%): α-terpineol (<6%), borneol (<5%), linalol (<3%), geraniol; Sesquiterpenes (<6%): β-caryophyllene, humulene, δ-cadinene, aromadendrene, bicyclogermacrene; Sesquiterpene Alcohols: viridiflorol, caryophyllenol; Phenols: terpinen-4-ol.

Properties: **Anticatarrhal, antidepressant, anti-inflammatory, antimicrobial, antiseptic, anti-infectious, antispasmodic, astringent, analgesic, regulator** (seborrhea), **stimulant** (liver, adrenal, and circulatory), **tonic**.

Common Primary Uses: [AI]**Alertness**, [A]**memory**.

Possible Uses: Sage lavender may be beneficial for Alzheimer's disease. It has been shown to inhibit cholinesterase activity and mimic **hormones** (increasing both estradiol and testosterone levels). It may also be beneficial for **aches/pains** (muscle), **acne, arthritis, asthenia, asthma, bronchitis, chills, circulation** (poor), **colds, coughs, cuts, dandruff, debility, dermatitis, eczema, exhaustion** (nervous), **fever, flu, gum** infections, **hair** loss, **headaches, jaundice, laryngitis, liver** congestion, **menstruation** (induces), **neuralgia, periods** (painful and difficult), **rheumatism, rhinitis, sinusitis, sterility, sweating** (excessive).

Body System(s) Affected: **Emotional Balance, Hormonal System, Muscles and Bones, Nervous System, Respiratory System, Skin.**

Aromatic Influence: Sage lavender helps improve **mood** and **memory**[158]. It may also help **harmonize** and **balance** the **emotions** and reduce **stress-related** conditions.

Application: Apply to **Vita Flex Points** on feet and/or directly on **area** of concern; **diffuse**.

Oral Use As Dietary Supplement: Generally regarded as safe (GRAS) for human consumption by the FDA. ***Dilute** one drop oil in 1 tsp. honey or in 4 oz. of beverage (i.e. soy/rice milk).* ***Not for children under 6 years old; use with caution and in greater dilution for children 6 years old and over.***

Blend Classification: Personifier and Equalizer.

Blends With: Clary sage, fennel, frankincense, geranium, sandalwood, ylang ylang.

Sandalwood

(Santalum album)

Botanical Family: Santalaceae (sandalwood)

Extraction Method/Origin: Steam distilled from wood—India, Indonesia

Chemical Constituents: Sesquiterpene Alcohols: α- & β-santalols (<80%); Sesquiterpenes : α- & β-santalenes (<11%); Sesquiterpene Aldehydes: teresantalal (<3%); Carboxylic Acids : nor-tricyclo-eka-santalic acid (<2%).

Properties: **Antidepressant, antiseptic, antitumor**[159]**, aphrodisiac, astringent, calming, sedative,** and **tonic.**

Common Primary Uses: [T]**Back pain**, [T]**coma**, [A]**confusion**, [T]**hemorrhoids**, [AT]**hiccups**, [A]**laryngitis**, [TA]**Lou Gehrig's disease**, [T]**multiple sclerosis**, [T]**radiation (UV)**, [T]**wrinkles**, [A]**yoga**.

Folklore: Sandalwood purportedly awakens the latent life force energy during meditation, and frees the souls of the deceased at funerals. Many cultures still consider sandalwood to be sacred.

Historical Uses: Sandalwood was traditionally used as an incense during ritual work for enhancing meditation. The Egyptians also used sandalwood for embalming.

French Medicinal Uses: **Bronchitis** (chronic), **diarrhea** (obstinate), **hemorrhoids, impotence**.

Other Possible Uses: Sandalwood is very similar to frankincense in action. It may support the **cardiovascular system**, remove **negative programming** from **cells**, and relieve symptoms associated with **lumbago** and the **sciatic nerves.** It may also be beneficial for **acne**, regenerating **bone cartilage, catarrh, circulation** (similar in action to frankincense), **coughs, cystitis, depression, hiccups, lymphatic system, meditation, menstrual problems, nerves** (similar in action to frankincense), **nervous tension**, increasing **oxygen** around the **pineal** and **pituitary glands, skin infection** and **regeneration, tuberculosis**, and **yoga**.

Body System(s) Affected: **Emotional Balance, Muscle and Bone, Nervous System, Skin**.

Aromatic Influence: Slowly and powerfully **calms, harmonizes**, and **balances** the **emotions**. It helps one accept others with an open heart while diminishing one's own egocentricity. It may help **enhance meditation** by opening the third eye. It can also be stimulating as well as grounding, as it is said to vibrate between the 7th and 1st chakra.

Application: Apply to **Vita Flex Points** of the feet and/or directly on **area** of concern; **diffuse**.

Oral Use As Dietary Supplement: Approved by the FDA for use as a Food Additive (FA) and Flavoring Agent (FL). ***Dilute** one drop oil in 1 tsp. honey or in 4 oz. of beverage (i.e. soy/rice milk).* ***Not for children under 6 years old; use with caution and in greater dilution for children 6 years old and over.***

Blend Classification: Modifier and Equalizer.

Blends With: Cypress, frankincense, lemon, myrrh, ylang ylang, patchouli, spruce.

Odor: Type: *Base Note (5–20% of the blend)*; Scent: *Soft, woody, sweet, earthy, balsamic, tenacious*; Intensity: *3*.

Frequency: Physical and Emotional; approximately 96 MHz.

Spearmint

(Mentha spicata, CT Carvone)

Botanical Family: Labiatae (mint)

Extraction Method/Origin: Steam distilled from leaves—Utah, USA

Chemical Constituents: Ketones (up to 70%): l-carvone (<58%), dihydrocarvone (<10%), menthone (<2%), pulegone; Monoterpenes (<30%): l-limonene (<25%), myrcene (<3%), camphene, α- & β-pinenes, α-phellandrene; Alcohols (<10%): carveol (<3%), linalol, trans-thujanol-4, octanol, borneol; Sesquiterpenes (<5%): β-caryophyllene, β-bourbonene, α-elemene, β-farnesene; Esters: carvyl acetates (<4%); Oxides: 1,8 cineol (<3%); Sesquiterpene Alcohols: α-cadinol, farnesol, elemol; Phenolic Alcohols: menthol.

Properties: **Antibacterial**[160]**, anticatarrhal, antifungal, anti-inflammatory, antiseptic, antispasmodic, hormone-like, insecticidal**, and **stimulant**.

Historical Uses: Spearmint has been used to relieve hiccough, colic, nausea, indigestion, flatulence, headaches, sores, and scabs.

French Medicinal Uses: **Bronchitis, candida, cystitis, hypertension**.

Other Possible Uses: This oil may balance and increase **metabolism**, which may help **burn up fats** and **toxins** in the body. It may aid the **glandular, nervous**, and **respiratory systems**. It may also help with **acne, appetite** (stimulates), **bad breath, balance, childbirth** (promotes easier labor), **constipation,**

depression, diarrhea, digestion, dry skin, eczema, fevers, headaches, intestines (soothes), **kidney stones, menstruation** (slow, heavy periods), **migraines, nausea, sore gums, stomach** (relaxes muscles), **urine retention, vaginitis, weight** (reduces), and bring about a feeling of **well-being**.

Body System(s) Affected: **Digestive System, Emotional Balance**.

Aromatic Influence: Its **hormone-like** activity may help open and release emotional blocks to bring about a feeling of balance. It acts as an antidepressant by relieving mental strain and fatigue, and by lifting one's spirits.

Application: Apply to **Vita Flex Points** and directly on **area** of concern; **diffuse**.

Oral Use As Dietary Supplement: Generally regarded as safe (GRAS) for human consumption by the FDA. ***Dilute*** *one drop oil in 1 tsp. honey or in 4 oz. of beverage (i.e. soy/rice milk).* ***Not for children under 6 years old; use with caution and in greater dilution for children 6 years old and over.***

Safety Data: ***Use with caution during pregnancy. Not for use on babies.***

Blend Classification: Personifier.

Blends With: Basil, lavender, peppermint, rosemary.

Odor: Type: *Top Note (5–20% of the blend)*; Scent: *Minty, slightly fruity, less bright than peppermint*; Intensity: *3*.

Spikenard

(Nardostachys jatamansi)

Botanical Family: Valerianaceae

Extraction Method/Origin: Steam distilled from roots—India

Chemical Constituents: Sesquiterpenes (up to 50%): β-gurjunene (<30%), β-maalene (<9%), aristoladiene (<7%), aristolene (5%), seychellene, dihydroazulene, β-patchoulene; Monoterpenes (up to 45%): calarene (<35%), β-ionene (<8%), α- & β-pinenes, limonene, aristolene; Sesquiterpene Alcohols (<11%): patchoulol (<7%), nardol, calarenol, maaliol, valerianol; Ketones (<10%): aristolenone (<7%), β-ionone, nardostachone, valerianone (=jatamansone); Phenolic Aldehydes: valerianal; Coumarins; Oxides: 1,8 cineol; Carboxylic Acids: jatamanshinic acid.

Properties: **Antibacterial, antifungal, anti-inflammatory, deodorant, relaxing**, and **skin tonic**.

Folklore: Spikenard has also been known as "nard" and "'false' Indian valerian root" oil. Prized in early Egypt, it was used in a preparation called *kyphi* with other oils like saffron, juniper, myrrh, cassia, and cinnamon. According to Roberta Wilson, "The Egyptians believed that in addition to appeasing the gods, Kyphi incense quelled fear and anxiety, improved meditation, and induced restful sleep with pleasant dreams."

Historical Uses: In India, spikenard was notably regarded as a perfume, medicinal herb, and as a skin tonic. Highly prized in the Middle East during the time of Christ, there are several passages in the Bible referring to spikenard. Spikenard was also used in the preparation of *nardinum*, a scented oil of great renown during ancient times.

Other Possible Uses: The oil is known for helping in the treatment of **allergic skin reactions**, and according to Victoria Edwards, "The oil redresses the skin's physiological balance and causes permanent regeneration." Spikenard may also help with **allergies, candida, flatulent indigestion, insomnia, menstrual difficulties, migraine, nausea, rashes, staph infections, stress, tachycardia, tension**, and **wounds** that will not heal.

Body System(s) Affected: **Emotional Balance, Skin**.

Aromatic Influence: Spikenard has a peaty, earthy, animal-like fragrance, reminiscent of goats. It is **balancing, soothing**, and **harmonizing**.

Application: Apply to **Vita Flex Points** and/or directly on **area** of concern.

Oral Use As Dietary Supplement: None.

Blends With: Cistus, lavender, patchouli, pine, and vetiver.

Odor: Type: *Base Note (5–20% of the blend)*; Scent: *Heavy, earthy, animal-like, similar to valerian*; Intensity: *5*.

Bible: Song of Solomon 1:12, 4:13-14; Mark 14:3; John 12:3.

Spruce (or Black Spruce)

(Picea mariana)

Botanical Family: Pinaceae (conifer) **Extraction Method/Origin:** Steam distilled from needles—Canada

Chemical Constituents: Monoterpenes (up to 55%): camphene (<25%), α-pinene (<19%), δ-3carene (<10%), β-pinene (<8%), l-limonene (<7%), santene, tricyclene; Esters: bornyl acetate (>35%); Alcohols: borneol, longiborneol; Sesquiterpenes: longifolene, longicyclene.

Properties: **Anti-infectious, anti-inflammatory, antispasmodic, cortisone-like, disinfectant**, and **tonic**.

Common Primary Uses: **[T]Bathroom/kitchen cleaning**, **[T]cooling**, **[T]furniture polish**, **[T]hyperthyroidism**, **[A]yoga**.

Historical Uses: It was used by the Lakota Indians to enhance their communication with the Great Spirit.

French Medicinal Uses: **Arthritis, candida, hyperthyroidism, immune-depression, prostatitis, rheumatism, solar plexus.**

Other Possible Uses: Spruce oil creates the symbolic effect of an umbrella that protects the earth and brings energy in from the universe. At night the animals in the wild lie down under the trees for the protection, recharging, and rejuvenation the trees bring them. Spruce may be beneficial for **bone pain, glandular system**, aching **joints**, opening the **pineal gland, sciatica pain**, and stimulating the **thymus** and **adrenal** glands.

Body System(s) Affected: **Emotional Balance, Nervous** and **Respiratory Systems.**

Aromatic Influence: Spruce oil **grounds** the body, creating the feeling of **balance** necessary to receive and to give. Helps release **emotional blocks.**

Application: Apply to **Vita Flex Points** and/or directly on **area** of concern.

Oral Use As Dietary Supplement: Approved by the FDA for use as a Food Additive (FA) and Flavoring Agent (FL). ***Dilute** one drop oil in 1 tsp. honey or in 4 oz. of beverage (i.e. soy/rice milk).* ***Not for children under 6 years old; use with caution and in greater dilution for children 6 years old and over.***

Blend Classification: Equalizer and Enhancer.

Blends With: Eucalyptus, frankincense, helichrysum, ravensara, wintergreen.

Odor: Type: *Middle Note (50–80% of the blend)*; Scent: *Fresh, woody, earthy, sweet, with a hint of a fruity note*; Intensity: *3*.

Spruce, Idaho Blue

(Picea pungens)

Botanical Family: Pinaceae (conifer)

Extraction Method/Origin: Steam distilled from wood, bark, and needles—Idaho

Chemical Constituents: Monoterpenes: camphene, α-pinene, limonene, δ-3carene, β-pinene, santene, tricyclene; Esters: bornyl acetate; Alcohols: borneol, longiborneol; Sesquiterpenes: longifolene, longicyclene: Ketones: camphor.

Properties: **Anti-infectious, anti-inflammatory, antispasmodic, cortisone-like, disinfectant**, and **tonic**.

Common Primary Uses: [A]**aphrodisiac**, [T]**Bathroom/kitchen cleaning**, [T]**cooling**, [T]**furniture polish**, [T]**hyperthyroidism**, [A]**yoga**.

Historical Uses: Spruce was used by the Lakota Indians to enhance their communication with the Great Spirit.

French Medicinal Uses: **Arthritis, candida, hyperthyroidism, immune-depression, prostatitis, rheumatism, solar plexus.**

Other Possible Uses: Spruce oil creates the symbolic effect of an umbrella that protects the earth and brings energy in from the universe. At night the animals in the wild lie down under the trees for the protection, recharging, and rejuvenation the trees bring them. Spruce may be beneficial for **bone pain, glandular system**, aching **joints**, opening the **pineal gland, sciatica pain**, and stimulating the **thymus** and **adrenal** glands.

Body System(s) Affected: **Emotional Balance, Nervous** and **Respiratory Systems**.

Aromatic Influence: Spruce oil **grounds** the body, creating the feeling of **balance** necessary to receive and to give. Helps release **emotional blocks**.

Application: Apply to **Vita Flex Points** and/or directly on **area** of concern.

Oral Use As Dietary Supplement: Approved by the FDA for use as a Food Additive (FA) and Flavoring Agent (FL). ***Dilute** one drop oil in 1 tsp. honey or in 4 oz. of beverage (i.e. soy/rice milk).* ***Not for children under 6 years old; use with caution and in greater dilution for children 6 years old and over.***

Blend Classification: Equalizer and Enhancer.

Blends With: Eucalyptus, frankincense, helichrysum, ravensara, wintergreen.

Odor: Type: *Middle Note (50–80% of the blend)*; Scent: *Fresh, woody, earthy, sweet, with a hint of a fruity note*; Intensity: *3*.

Sweet Myrrh

(See Myrrh, Biblical Sweet)

Tamanu

(Calophyllum inophyllum)

NOTE: This is a vegetal oil, not an essential oil. It is listed here because of its value as a fixed oil in formulations. Available through Creer Labs 801-418-8870.

Botanical Family: Gutiferae or Hypericaceae

Extraction Method/Origin: Cold pressed from the nut of the Polynesian tamanu tree—Tahiti

Chemical Constituents: Terpenic essences, benzoic & oxibenzoic acids, vitamin F, lipids, glycerides, saturated fatty acids, calophyllolide (3,4-dihydro-5-methoxyl-22-dimethyl-6), calophyllic acid, coumarin derivatives, and phospho-amino acids.

Properties: **Antibacterial, anti-infectious, anti-inflammatory, antirheumatic**.

Common Primary Uses: [T]**Burns**, [T]**sunscreen**.

Historical Uses: The natives of Tahiti believe that tamanu oil is a "sacred" gift of nature. The women use the oil as a natural moisturizing cosmetic on their faces and bodies. It was also used for protection against sunburns.

Other Possible Uses: **Burns** and **wounds** (when mixed with helichrysum), **hair** (creates healthy), and **natural sun screen**[161].

Body System(s) Affected: **Skin**

Aromatic Influence: **Grounding** and **soothing**. It has an earthy, musky, slightly nutty odor.

Application: Apply directly on area of concern.

Oral Use As Dietary Supplement: None.

Safety Data: ***Avoid if allergic to any kind of nuts.***

Blends With: Helichrysum (burns and wounds), rosemary camphor (hair growth).

Tangerine

(Citrus nobilis or Citrus reticulata var. tangerine)

Botanical Family: Rutaceae (citrus)

Extraction Method/Origin: Cold pressed from rind—USA, Mexico, Brazil, South Africa

Chemical Constituents: Monoterpenes (up to 95%): d-limonene (<80%), γ-terpinene (<20%), myrcene (<4%), p-cymene, α- & β-phellandrenes, β-ocimene, α- & β-pinenes, terpinolene, cadinene; Tetraterpenes (<10%): β-carotene (<6%), lycopene (<4%); Alcohols: linalol, citronellol; Aldehydes: citral, neral.

Properties: **Anticoagulant, anti-inflammatory, laxative**, and **sedative**.

Possible Uses: It may help **cellulite** (dissolve), **circulation, constipation, diarrhea, digestive system disorders, fat digestion, dizziness, fear, flatulence, gallbladder, insomnia, intestinal spasms, irritability, limbs** (tired and aching), **liver problems**, decongest the **lymphatic system** (helps to stimulate draining), **obesity, parasites, sadness, the stomach** (tonic), **stretch marks** (smooths when blended with lavender), **stress, swelling**, and alleviate **water retention (edema).**

Body System(s) Affected: **Emotional Balance, Immune System, Skin.**

Aromatic Influence: Tangerine oil contains esters and aldehydes, which are **sedating** and **calming** to the **nervous system**. When diffused together with marjoram, tangerine can soothe emotions such as grief, anger, and shock.

Application: Apply to **Vita Flex Points** and directly on **area** of concern; **diffuse**.

Oral Use As Dietary Supplement: Generally regarded as safe (GRAS) for human consumption by the FDA. ***Dilute** one drop oil in 1 tsp. honey or in 4 oz. of beverage (i.e. soy/rice milk).* ***Not for children under 6 years old; use with caution and in greater dilution for children 6 years old and over.***

Blend Classification: Modifier and Personifier.

Blends With: Basil, bergamot, chamomile, clary sage, frankincense, geranium, grapefruit, lavender, lemon, orange.

Odor: Type: *Top Note (5–20% of the blend)*; Scent: *Fresh, sweet, citrusy*; Intensity: *3.*

Tansy, Blue

(Tanacetum annum)

Botanical Family: Compositae (daisy)

Extraction Method/Origin: Steam distilled from leaves and flowers—France, Morocco

Chemical Constituents: Monoterpenes (up to 65%): sabinene (<17%), myrcene (<13%), d-limonene (<11%), β-pinene (<10%), α-phellandrene (<10%), p-cymene (<8%); Ketones: camphor (<17%); Sesquiterpenes: chamazulene (<12%).

Properties: **Analgesic, antibacterial, anti-inflammatory, antihistamine, hypotensive, hormone-like**, and **nervine**.

Possible Uses: May help with **low blood pressure**, relieve **itching**, reduce **pain**, and sedate the **nerves**.

Body System(s) Affected: **Nervous System**.

Application: Apply to **Vita Flex Points** and/or directly on **area** of concern.

Safety Data: ***This oil should only be used externally and with caution.***

Tansy, Idaho

(Tanacetum vulgare)

Botanical Family: Compositae (daisy)

Extraction Method/Origin: Steam distilled from leaves—Idaho, Washington

Chemical Constituents: Ketones: β-thujone (approx. 65%, can be as high as 81%), camphor (<8%), α-thujone (<5%), piperitone, artemisia ketone, davanone, isothujone, umbellulone, isopinocamphone; Monoterpenes (<10%): sabinene (<4%), α-pinene (<3%), camphene, α-terpinene; Sesquiterpenes: germacrene-D (<7%); Alcohols: borneol, α-terpineol, lyratol, chrysanthenol, vulgerol, thujyl alcohol; Sesquiterpene Lactones: artemarin, chrysanthemine, crispolid, parthenolide, santamarin, tatridin; Esters: bornyl, α-terpinyl, lyratyl, and chrysanthenyl acetates; Oxides: 1,8-cineol; Coumarins: scopoletin.

Properties: **Antibacterial**, **antifungal**, **anti-infectious**, **anti-inflammatory**, **antispasmodic**, **antiviral**, **nervine**, and **stimulant**.

Common Primary Uses: **[T]Mosquito bites**.

Carrier Oils: Some commercial companies will dilute this oil with almond oil.

Historical Uses: Wild tansy (similar in chemical makeup to Idaho tansy) was used historically among the gypsies as a sort of "cure all." It has been used for worms, colds, fever, miscarriage, dyspepsia, cramping pains, scabies, bruises, sprains, nervous disorders, and to keep flies and vermin away.

Other Possible Uses: Idaho tansy may be supportive to the **immune system** in helping to **fight colds**, **flu**, and **infections**. It may also be beneficial for **stomach** conditions, **arthritis** symptoms, and possibly **tumors**. It has been shown to soothe the **bowels** and to tone the entire system. The properties of this oil suggest that it may help with **aneurysms**, **bruises**, **diarrhea**, **dyspepsia**, **freckles**, **gout**, **heart disorders**, **inflamed eyes**, **irritable bowel syndrome**, **jaundice**, **kidneys**, **liver spots**, **menstruation** (promotes), **palpitations**, **respiratory infections**, **rheumatism**, **sciatica**, **sprains**, **sunburn**, **toothaches**, **tuberculosis**, and **vomiting**.

Body System(s) Affected: **Immune System**.

Aromatic Influence: It encourages an **uplifting feeling**, a **positive attitude**, and a general feeling of **well-being**.

Application: Apply to **Vita Flex Points** and/or directly on **area** of concern.

Oral Use As Dietary Supplement: None.

Safety Data: *Because Idaho tansy contains a high concentration of thujone, this oil has been classified (along with wild tansy) as an* ***oral toxin*** *by Robert Tisserand. However, other sources indicate that for thujone to be toxic, undiluted oil in excess of 30 ml must be ingested in a short period of time. Best for this oil to only be used* ***externally*** *and with* ***caution****. Avoid during* ***pregnancy****. Not for use by people with* ***epilepsy****.*

Blends With: Most oils; perfumers in France have found that wild tansy (similar in chemical makeup to Idaho tansy) has a greater fixative capability than any other oil.

Frequency: Emotional; approximately 105 MHz.

Tarragon

(Artemisia dracunculus)

Botanical Family: Compositae

Extraction Method/Origin: Steam distilled from leaves—France, Slovenia

Chemical Constituents: Phenolic Ethers (up to 85%): methyl chavicol/estragole (<75%), anethole (<10%); Monoterpenes (<30%): cis- & trans-β-ocimenes (<24%), l-limonene (<6%), α- & β-pinenes, camphene; Coumarins: herniarin, scopoletin, scoparone, artemidin, esculetin; Also: nerol, thujone, cineol, and linalyl acetate in trace amounts.

Properties: **Antibacterial, anticancerous, anti-infectious, anti-inflammatory, antiseptic, antispasmodic[162], antiparasitic, antiviral, diuretic, laxative, neuromuscular**, and **stimulant**.

Common Primary Uses: [A]**Anorexia**, [T]**colitis**, [IT]**gas/flatulence**, [AT]**hiccups**, [T]**PMS**, [T]**rheumatic fever**, [T]**sciatica**.

Folklore: The name *tarragon* is said to come from its ancient use as a remedy for bites from venomous creatures.

Historical Uses: Tarragon was used to induce appetite, for digestive and menstrual irregularities, and as a remedy for toothache.

French Medicinal Uses: **Colitis, hiccups, intestinal spasms, parasites, rheumatic pain, sciatica**.

Other Possible Uses: It may be beneficial for **abdominal discomfort** and **spasms, arthritis, dyspepsia** (impaired digestion), preventing **fermentation, genital urinary tract infection, kidneys, nausea, nervous** and **sluggish digestion, premenstrual** discomfort, and **weeping wounds**.

Body System(s) Affected: **Digestive System**. It may also help balance the **Autonomic Nervous System**.

Application: Apply to **Vita Flex Points** and/or directly on **area** of concern. Best to **dilute** with V-6 Oil.

Oral Use As Dietary Supplement: Generally regarded as safe (GRAS) for human consumption by the FDA. ***Dilute** one drop oil in 1 tsp. honey or in 4 oz. of beverage (i.e. soy/rice milk).* ***Not for children under 6 years old; use with caution and in greater dilution for children 6 years old and over.***

Safety Data: ***Avoid during pregnancy. Not for use by people with epilepsy.***

Blend Classification: Equalizer.

Blends With: Chamomile, clary sage, fir, juniper, lavender, pine, rosewood, orange, and tangerine.

Thyme

(Thymus vulgaris, CT Thymol)

Botanical Family: Labiatae (mint)

Extraction Method/Origin: Steam distilled from leaves, stems, and flowers—Utah, Idaho, France

Chemical Constituents: Phenols (up to 60%): thymol (<55%), carvacrol (<10%); Monoterpenes (<54%): p-cymene (<28%), γ-terpinene (<11%), terpinolene (<6%), α-pinene (<6%), myrcene (<3%); Oxides: 1,8 cineol (<15%); Alcohols (<14%): linalol (<8%), borneol (<7%), thujanol, geraniol; Sesquiterpenes: β-caryophyllene (<8%); Carboxylic Acids: rosmaric acid (<2%), triterpenic acids (tr.); Ethers: methyl thymol (tr.), methyl carvacrol (tr.); Ketone: camphor (tr.); Also trace elements of menthone.

Properties: Highly **antibacterial[163], antifungal[164], antioxidant[165] antiviral, antiseptic**.

Common Primary Uses: [T]**Aging**, [TA]**antibacterial**, [TA]**antifungal**, [AI]**antioxidant**, [AT]**bronchitis**, [AT]**colds (common)**, [T]**colitis**, [A]**croup**, [T]**dermatitis/eczema**, [T]**hair loss**, [T]**indigestion**, [A]**laryngitis**, [IT]**parasites (intestinal)**, [A]**pneumonia**, [T]**psoriasis**, [T]**ringworm**, [T]**sciatica**, [T]**spider bites**, [T]**thrush**, [TA]**viral infection**, [T]**warming oils**.

Historical Uses: It was used by the Egyptians for embalming and by the ancient Greeks as protection against infectious illnesses. It has also been used for respiratory problems, digestive complaints, the prevention and treatment of infection, dyspepsia, chronic gastritis, bronchitis, pertussis, asthma, laryngitis, tonsillitis, and enuresis in children.

French Medicinal Uses: **Anthrax, asthma, bronchitis, colitis** (infectious), **cystitis, dermatitis, dyspepsia, fatigue** (general), **pleurisy, psoriasis, sciatica, tuberculosis, vaginal candida**.

Other Possible Uses: This oil is a general **tonic** for the **nerves** and **stomach**. It may also help with **bacterial infections, colds, circulation, depression, digestion, physical weakness** after **illness, flu, headaches, immunological** functions, **insomnia, rheumatism, urinary infections, viruses** along the **spine**, and **wounds**.

Body System(s) Affected: **Immune System, Muscles and Bones**.

Aromatic Influence: It helps **supply energy** in times of **physical weakness** and **stress**. It has also been thought to increase **intelligence** and aid **concentration**. It is **uplifting** and helps to relieve **depression**.

Application: Apply to **Vita Flex Points** and/or directly on **area** of concern.

Oral Use As Dietary Supplement: Generally regarded as safe (GRAS) for human consumption by the FDA. ***Dilute** one drop oil in 2 tsp. honey or in 8 oz. of beverage (i.e. soy/rice milk). However, more dilution may be necessary due to this oil's potential for irritating mucus membranes.* ***Not for children under 6 years old; use with caution and in greater dilution for children 6 years old and over.***

Safety Data: ***This type of thyme oil may be somewhat irritating to the mucous membranes and dermal tissues (skin). This type of thyme should be avoided during pregnancy. Use this type with caution when dealing with high blood pressure.***

Blend Classification: Equalizer and Enhancer.

Blends With: Bergamot, cedarwood, juniper, melaleuca, oregano, and rosemary.

Odor: Type: *Middle Note (50–80% of the blend)*; Scent: *Fresh, medicinal, herbaceous*; Intensity: *4*.

Thyme Linalol

(Thymus vulgaris, CT Linalol)

Botanical Family: Labiatae (mint)

Extraction Method/Origin: Steam distilled from leaves, stems, and flowers—France

Chemical Constituents: Alcohols (up to 85%): linalol (<78%), thujanol (<4%), geraniol (<3%), α-terpineol; Monoterpenes (<21%): myrcene (<8%), p-cymene (<7%), γ-terpinene (<%); Phenols: terpinen-4-ol (<12%), thymol, carvacrol; Esters: linalyl acetate (<5%), geranyl acetate; Sesquiterpenes (tr.): β-caryophyllene, humulene; Also (tr.): 1,8 cineol, camphor.

Properties: **Antibacterial, antifungal, anti-infectious, anti-inflammatory, antimicrobial, antiparasitic, antiseptic, antiviral, cardiotonic, neurotonic**, and **uterotonic**.

Historical Uses: It was used by the Egyptians for embalming and by the ancient Greeks to protect against infectious illnesses. It has also been used for respiratory problems, digestive complaints, the prevention and treatment of infection, dyspepsia, chronic gastritis, bronchitis, pertussis, asthma, laryngitis, tonsillitis, and enuresis in children.

French Medicinal Uses: **Anthrax, asthma, bronchitis, colitis** (infectious), **cystitis, dermatitis, dyspepsia, fatigue** (general), **pleurisy, psoriasis, sciatica, tuberculosis, vaginal candida**.

Other Possible Uses: This oil is a general **tonic** for the **nerves** and **stomach**. It may also help with **bacterial infections, colds, circulation, depression, digestion, physical weakness** after **illness, flu, headaches, immunological** functions, **insomnia, rheumatism, urinary infections, viruses** along the **spine**, and **wounds**. *Note: This chemotype is said to be the best suited to kill* ***bacteria****, relieve discomfort in stomach or gut (****candida, parasites****), and combat nervous* ***fatigue****. It is nonirritating, especially for children, elderly, and the infirm.*

Body System(s) Affected: **Respiratory System, Skin.**

Aromatic Influence: It helps **supply energy** in times of **physical weakness** and **stress**. It has also been thought to increase **intelligence** and aid **concentration**. It is **uplifting** and helps to relieve **depression**.

Application: Apply to **Vita Flex Points** and/or directly on **area** of concern.

Oral Use As Dietary Supplement: Generally regarded as safe (GRAS) for human consumption by the FDA. **Dilute** *one drop oil in 1 tsp. honey or in 4 oz. of beverage (i.e. soy/rice milk). Not for children under 6 years old; use with* ***caution*** *and in* ***greater dilution*** *for children 6 years old and over.*

Safety Data: *Because this type of thyme oil is a "linalol type," it is safe for use on the skin and with children. Other varieties of thyme oil can contain large amounts of thymol and carvacrol, making them somewhat toxic, irritating to the mucous membranes, and dermal (skin) irritants. While this type of thyme may be used during pregnancy, the other types should be avoided! Use this type with caution when dealing with* ***high blood pressure****.*

Blend Classification: Equalizer and Enhancer.

Blends With: Bergamot, citrus oil, cedarwood, juniper, melaleuca, oregano, and rosemary.

Tsuga (or Hemlock Spruce)

(Tsuga canadensis)

Botanical Family: Pinaceae (pine)

Extraction Method/Origin: Steam distilled from leaves and twigs—Idaho, Canada *This oil is not to be confused with hemlock (Conium maculatum), which contains toxic alkaloids and is not a source of essential oil.*

Chemical Constituents: Monoterpenes (up to 50%): α- & β-pinenes (<25%), camphene (<18%), l-limonene (<5%), tricyclene (<8%), α- & β-phellandrenes (<5%), myrcene (<3%); Esters: bornyl acetate (<38%); Sesquiterpenes (<14%): tricyclene (<8%), dipentene (<4%), δ-cadinene (<3%); Ketones: α-thujone (<3%).

Properties: **Antimicrobial, antiseptic, astringent, diuretic, expectorant, nervine, tonic.**

Common Primary Uses: [A]**Yoga**.

Historical Uses: It has been used for diarrhea, cystitis, mucous colitis, leucorrhea, uterine prolapse, pharyngitis, stomatitis, gingivitis, wounds, sores, digestive disorders, diseases of the mouth and throat, and scurvy.

Other Possible Uses: This oil may help with **anxiety, asthma, bronchitis**, poor **circulation, colds, coughs, flu, infections, muscular aches** and **pains, periodontal (gum) disease, respiratory weakness** (opens and dilates for better oxygen exchange), **rheumatism, stress-related conditions**, and **wounds**. It can also be used in **veterinary liniments**.

Body System(s) Affected: **Cardiovascular** and **Respiratory Systems**.

Aromatic Influence: It is **uplifting** to the **emotions** as it **opens** and **elevates** while **grounding** at the same time. Some have found it excellent for **yoga** and **meditation**.

Application: **Diffuse**. Apply to **Vita Flex Points** and/or directly on **area** of concern. For topical use, **dilute** in one teaspoon V-6 Oil.

Oral Use As Dietary Supplement: Approved by the FDA for use as a Food Additive (FA) or Flavoring Agent (FL) (see 21CFR172.510). **Dilute** *one drop oil in 1 tsp. honey or in 4 oz. of beverage (i.e. soy/rice milk).* ***Not for children under 6 years old; use with* caution *and in* greater dilution *for children 6 years old and over.***

Safety Data: ***Repeated use can possibly result in* skin irritation.**

Companion Products: Di-Gize, Essentialzyme, Thieves Fresh Essence Plus Mouthwash, K&B Tincture, Rose Ointment.

Blends With: Pine, cedarwood, galbanum, lavender, lavandin, and rosemary.

Valerian

(Valeriana officinalis)

Botanical Family: Valerianaceae

Extraction Method/Origin: Steam distilled from roots—Belgium, Croatia, France

Chemical Constituents: Esters (up to 50%): bornyl acetate (<44%), myrtenyl acetate (<5%), bornyl formate, butyrate, & isovalerate (responsible for odor & therapeutic effects), eugenyl isovalerate; Monoterpenes (<41%): camphene (<21%), α-fenchene (<13%), α-pinene (<8%), β-pinene (<6%); Alcohols (<6%): borneol, α-terpineol, geraniol, patchouli alcohol, valerianol; Sesquiterpenes (5%): vitivene, δ-cadinene, α-farnescene, valerazulene, β-caryophyllene; Sesquiterpene Aldehydes: valerianal; Sesquiterpene Ketones: valerianone, ionone; Carboxylic Acids: valerinic acid, isovaleric acid, chlorogenic acid, malic acid; Sesquiterpene Lactones: actinidine, valerianine.

Properties: **Antianxiety**[166], **antibacterial, anti-dandruff, antispasmodic, depressant** (central nervous system), **diuretic, hypnotic, regulator, sedative.**

Common Primary Uses: **TAAngina**, **ATanxiety**, **Ainsomnia**, **ATsleep**.

Folklore: Once called "all heal," valerian has been treasured since medieval times.

Historical Uses: Down through the centuries, valerian has been used for insomnia, migraine, dysmenorrhea, intestinal colic, rheumatism, cholera, epilepsy, skin complaints, backache, colds, menstrual problems, and sores. During the last few decades, it has been studied for its tranquilizing properties.

Other Possible Uses: Because of its effect on the nervous system, it may help with **insomnia, nervous indigestion, migraine, restlessness, sleep disturbances**, and **tension**. Valerian has also been shown to naturally inhibit the re-uptake of 5HT (serotonin). It also helps with the free-flow of blood platelets and may help relieve symptoms of heart pain due to restricted blood flow[167].

Body System(s) Affected: **Nervous System**.

Aromatic Influence: It may be useful in meditation, as it helps cut through the tension and stress of our everyday lives to help us focus on our inner self, where true peace and calm can be found. It is profoundly **calming, relaxing, grounding**, and **balancing**.

Application: Apply to **Vita Flex Points** and/or directly on **area** of concern. May also be applied to the **wrists** or bottoms of the **feet**. Is actually more effective when taken internally as a dietary supplement.

Oral Use As Dietary Supplement: Approved by the FDA for use as a Food Additive (FA) and Flavoring Agent (FL). **Dilute** *one drop oil in 1 tsp. honey or in 4 oz. of beverage (i.e. soy/rice milk).* ***Not for children under 6 years old; use with* caution *and in* greater dilution *for children 6 years old and over.***

Safety Data: ***Repeated use can possibly result in* contact sensitization**.

Blends With: Cedarwood, lavender, mandarin, patchouli, petitgrain, pine, and rosemary.

Vetiver

(Vetiveria zizanoides)

Botanical Family: Gramineae (grasses)

Extraction Method/Origin: Steam distilled from roots—India, Haiti (best)

Chemical Constituents: Sesquiterpene Alcohols (up to 42%): isovalencenol (<15%), bicyclovetiverol (<13%), khusenol (<11%), tricyclovetiverol (<4%), vetiverol, zizanol, furfurol; Sesquiterpene Ketones (<22%): α- & β-vetivones (<12%), khusimone (<6%), nootkatone (<5%); Sesquiterpenes (<4%): vitivene, tricyclovetivene, vetivazulene, β- & δ-cadinenes; Sesquiterpene Esters: vetiveryl acetate; Carboxylic Acids: benzoic, palmitic, and vetivenic acids.

Properties: **Antiseptic, antispasmodic, calming, grounding, immune-stimulant, rubefacient** (locally warming), **sedative** (nervous system), **stimulant** (circulatory, production of red corpuscles).

Folklore: Known in India as "oil of tranquility," vetiver is distilled from the root of a scented grass native to India that is botanically related to citronella and lemongrass

Historical Uses: The distillation of vetiver is a painstaking, labor-intensive activity. The roots and rootlets of vetiver have been used in India as a perfume since antiquity.

Other Possible Uses: Vetiver may help **acne, anorexia, anxiety, arthritis, breasts** (enlarge), **cuts, depression** (including postpartum), **insomnia, muscular rheumatism, nervousness** (extreme), **skin care** (oily, aging, tired, irritated), **sprains**, and **stress**. It may also be effective at **repelling** termites.

Body System(s) Affected: **Emotional Balance, Hormonal** and **Nervous Systems, Skin**.

Aromatic Influence: Vetiver has a heavy, smokey, earthy fragrance reminiscent of patchouli with lemon-like undertones. Because of its **psychologically grounding, calming**, and **stabilizing** properties, vetiver has also been valuable for relieving **stress** and helping people recover from **emotional traumas** and **shock**. As a natural tranquilizer, it may help induce a **restful sleep**. It is known to affect the **parathyroid gland**. According to Susanne Fischer-Rizzi, "Sexual energies become more peaceful and grounded."

Application: Apply to **Vita Flex Points** and/or directly on **area** of concern; **diffuse**. Also excellent in **baths** or in **massage** blends. A very small amount of vetiver oil is all that is needed in most applications. Mix with geranium and ylang ylang to help with breast enlargement.

Oral Use As Dietary Supplement: Approved by the FDA for use as a Food Additive (FA) and Flavoring Agent (FL). ***Dilute*** *one drop oil in 1 tsp. honey or in 4 oz. of beverage (i.e. soy/rice milk).* ***Not for children under 6 years old; use with caution and in greater dilution for children 6 years old and over.***

Safety Data: ***Use with caution during pregnancy.***

Blends With: Clary sage, jasmine, lavender, patchouli, rose, sandalwood, ylang ylang.

Odor: Type: *Base Note (5–20% of the blend)*; Scent: *Heavy, earthy, balsamic, smoky, sweet undertones*; Intensity: *5*.

Vitex

(Vitex negundo)

Botanical Family: Labiatae (mint)

Extraction Method/Origin: Steam distilled from the inner bark, small branches, and leaves of the Chaste tree (this essential oil is different from the extract of the chaste berry, which is used for PMS symptoms and hormone balance)—Turkey

Chemical Constituents: Sesquiterpenes (up to 65%): β-caryophyllene (<40%), germacrene-B (<10%), β-farnesene (<7%), logifolene (<6%), α-gurjunene (5%); Monoterpenes (<20%): sabinene (<15%), α-pinene (<6%), l-limonene (<3%); Oxides (<18%): caryophyllene oxide (<10%), 1,8 cineol (<8%); Esters: α-terpinyl acetate.

Historical Uses: Vitex has been historically used in Europe and Asia for its benefits relating to **rheumatism, hernias, deafness**, and **mental unrest**.

Other Possible Uses: Research is being conducted on the use of vitex oil for reversing the symptoms of Parkinson's Disease.

Oral Use As Dietary Supplement: None.

Safety Data: ***Use with caution during pregnancy.***

Western Red Cedar

(See Cedar, Western Red)

White Fir

(See Fir, White)

White Lotus

(Nymphaea lotus)

Botanical Family: Nymphaeaceae

Extraction Method/Origin: Steam distilled from flower—Egypt

(NOTE: This oil is only available periodically in very small amounts.)

Properties: **Anticancerous**.

Historical Uses: White lotus was traditionally used by the Egyptians for **spiritual, emotional**, and **physical** application; every recipe contained white lotus. Research in China found that white lotus contains **anticancerous** and strong **immune-supporting** properties.

Other Possible Uses: **Eyes** (inflamed), **jaundice, kidneys, liver spots, menstruation** (promotes), **palpitations, rheumatism, sciatica, sprains, sunburn, toothaches, tuberculosis, vomiting**.

Body System(s) Affected: **Immune System**.

Aromatic Influence: White lotus has a euphoric fragrance that **lifts** and **stabilizes** the **emotions**, creating a powerful sense of **emotional, physical**, and **spiritual well-being**.

Blends With: Most oils.

Wintergreen

(Gaultheria procumbens)

Botanical Family: Ericaceae (heather)

Extraction Method/Origin: Steam distillation from leaves—Canada

Chemical Constituents: Phenolic Esters: methyl salicylate (>90%); Carboxylic Acids: salicylic acid.

Properties: **Analgesic, anti-inflammatory**[169], **antirheumatic, antiseptic, antispasmodic, disinfectant**[170], **diuretic, stimulant** (bone), and **warming**.

Common Primary Uses: ᵀ**Dandruff**, ᵀ**gout**, ᵀ**muscle aches**.

Historical Uses: Wintergreen oil has a strong, penetrating aroma. The American Indians and early European settlers enjoyed a tea that was flavored with birch bark or wintergreen. According to Julia Lawless, "This has been translated into a preference for 'root beer' flavourings [sic]." A synthetic methyl salicylate is now widely used as a flavoring agent, especially in root beer,'chewing gum, toothpaste, etc. *In fact, the true essential oil is produced in such small quantities (compared to the very extensive uses of the synthetic methyl salicylate) that those desiring to use wintergreen essential oil for therapeutic uses should **verify the source** of their oil to make sure they have a true oil, not a synthetic one.*

French Medicinal Uses: **Rheumatism, muscular pain, cramps, arthritis, tendonitis, hypertension, inflammation**.

Other Possible Uses: This oil may be beneficial for **acne, bladder infection, cystitis, dropsy, eczema, edema**, reducing **fever, gallstones, gout, infection**, reducing discomfort in **joints, kidney stones**, draining and cleansing the **lymphatic system, obesity, osteoporosis, skin diseases, ulcers**, and **urinary tract disorders**. It is known for its ability to alleviate **bone pain**. It has a cortisone-like action due to the high content of methyl salicylate. For nerve or tissue pain, use Relieve It.

Body System(s) Affected: **Muscles and Bones**.

Aromatic Influence: It influences, elevates, opens, and increases **awareness** in the **sensory system**.

Application: Apply to **Vita Flex Points** and/or directly on **area** of concern; **diffuse**. Apply topically on location, and use only small amounts (dilute with V-6 Oil for application on larger areas).

Safety Data: *Avoid during* **pregnancy**. *Not for use by people with* **epilepsy**. *Some people are very allergic to methyl salicylate.* **Test a small area of skin first for allergies!**

Blend Classification: Personifier and Enhancer.

Blends With: Basil, bergamot, chamomile, cypress, geranium, juniper, lavender, lemongrass, marjoram, peppermint, and rosewood.

Yarrow

(Achillea millefolium)

Botanical Family: Compositae (daisy)

Extraction Method/Origin: Steam distilled from flowering top—Utah

Chemical Constituents: Monoterpenes (up to 65%): sabinene (<40%), α- & β-pinenes (<16%), camphene (<6%), γ-terpinene; Sesquiterpenes (<55%): chamazulene (<30%), germacrene-D (<13%), trans-β-caryophyllene (<8%), humulene (<7%), dihydroazulenes; Ketones (<30%): camphor (<18%), isoartemisia ketone (<10%), thujone; Alcohols (<10%): borneol (<9%), terpineol; Oxides (<12%): 1,8 cineol (<10%), caryophyllene oxide; Phenols: terpinen-4-ol (<5%); Esters: bornyl acetate; Lactones: achillin; Sesquiterpene Alcohols: α-cadinol.

Properties: **Anti-inflammatory, antiseptic**[171], **astringent**, and **styptic**.

Folklore: The Greek Achilles, hero of the Trojan Wars, was said to have used yarrow to help cure the injury to his Achilles tendon. Yarrow was considered sacred by the Chinese, who recognized the harmony of the Yin and Yang energies within it. It has been said that the fragrance of yarrow makes possible the meeting of heaven and earth.

Historical Uses: Yarrow was used by Germanic tribes to treat battle wounds.

Other Possible Uses: It is a powerful decongestant of the **prostate** and helps to balance **hormones**. It may also help with **acne, amenorrhea, appetite** (lack of), **bladder** or **kidney weakness, cellulite, colds, catarrh, digestion** (poor), **dysmenorrhea, eczema, fevers, flatulence, gallbladder inflam-**

mation, gastritis, gout, hair (promotes hair growth), **headaches, hemorrhoids, hypertension, injuries, kidney stones, liver, menopause problems, neuritis, neuralgia, open leg sores, pelvic infections, prostatitis, rheumatism, scarring** (reduces or prevents), **sprains, stomach flu, sunburn, thrombosis, ulcers, urinary infections, vaginitis, varicose veins**, and **wounds** (promotes healing).

Body System(s) Affected: **Hormonal** and **Immune Systems, Skin**.

Aromatic Influence: Balancing highs and lows, both external and internal, yarrow may allow us to have our heads in the clouds while our feet remain firm on the ground. Its **balancing** properties may also make it useful during **meditation**. It is **supportive** to **intuitive energies** and helps reduce **confusion** and **ambivalence**. One source suggests that it may help open our awareness to **cosmic energies**.

Application: Apply to **Vita Flex Points** and/or directly on **area** of concern; **diffuse**. Also excellent for **baths** or **massage** blends.

Safety Data: ***Repeated use can possibly result in contact sensitization. Use with caution during pregnancy.***

Blends With: Clary sage, hyssop, myrtle, pine, valerian, and vetiver.

Odor: Type: *Middle Note (50–80% of the blend)*; Scent: *Sharp, woody, herbaceous, with a slight floral undertone*; Intensity: *4*.

Xiang Mao (Red Lemongrass)

(Cymbopogon citratus)

Botanical Family: Gramineae (grasses)

Extraction Method/Origin: Steam distilled from grass and stem—Taiwan

Chemical Constituents: Aldehydes (up to 87%): geranial, neral, citronellal, isovaleric aldehyde, furfural, n-decyclic aldehyde; Monoterpenes (10–20%): myrcene, limonene, dipentene; Alcohols: citronellol, nerol, geraniol, linalool, terpineol, isopulegol; Esters: valeric, caprylic, capric.

Properties: **Analgesic, antibacterial, antifungal, anti-inflammatory, antiseptic, diuretic, sedative**, and **tonic**.

Common Primary Uses: ^A^**Air purification**, ^TA^**antibacterial**, ^A^**calming**, ^T^**moisturizing**.

Historical Uses: Xiang mao has been used traditionally to help purify the air and to help enhance mental clarity and relaxation.

Other Possible Uses: This oil may help with **digestion**, lowering **cholesterol**, **fevers, flatulence, headaches**, clearing **infections, purification, respiratory problems, sore throats**, and **water retention**.

Body System(s) Affected: **Immune System, Digestive System, Muscles and Bones**.

Aromatic Influence: It may help promote **purification** and help **clear the mind**.

Application: Massage on the feet to support the immune system; **diffuse**.

Oral Use As Dietary Supplement: Generally regarded as safe (GRAS) for human consumption by the FDA. ***Dilute*** *one drop of oil in 1 tsp. honey or in 4 oz. of beverage (i.e. soy/rice milk).* ***Not for children under 6 years old; use with caution and in greater dilution for children 6 years old and over.***

Safety Data: ***Can cause skin irritation.***

Blend Classification: Enhancer and Equalizer.

Blends With: Basil, cedarwood, clary sage, eucalyptus, geranium, jasmine, lavender, melaleuca (tea tree), and rosemary.

Odor: Type: *Top Note (5–20% of the blend)*; Scent: *Grassy, lemony, pungent, earthy, slightly bitter*; Intensity: *4*.

Ylang Ylang
(Cananga odorata)

Botanical Family: Annonaceae (tropical trees and shrubs: custard-apple)

Extraction Method/Origin: Steam distilled from flowers—Commores, Madagascar, Indonesia, Philippines *(Flowers are picked early in the morning to maximize oil yield. The highest quality oil is drawn from the first hour of distillation.)*

Chemical Constituents: Sesquiterpenes (up to 55%): β-caryophyllene (<22%), germacrene-D (<25%), α-farnesene (<12%), humulene (<5%); Esters (<50%): benzyl acetate & benzoate (<25%), methyl salicylate & benzoate (<17%), farnesyl acetate (<7%), geranyl acetate (<4%), linalyl acetate; Alcohols (<45%): linalool (13%), geraniol; Ethers: paracresyl methyl ether (<15%); Phenols (<10%): methyl p-cresol (<9%), methyl chavicol (estragole), eugenol, isoeugenol; Oxides: caryophyllene oxide (<7%); Sesquiterpene Alcohols: farnesol.

Properties: **Antidepressant, antiseptic, antispasmodic, sedative**[172], and **tonic**.

Common Primary Uses: ATCalming, Acrying, Thair loss, AThigh blood pressure, Ahyperpnea, ATmental fatigue, ATrelaxing, ATstress, ATtension.

Historical Uses: Interestingly enough, the original wild flowers had no fragrance. Through selection and cloning, we have this unique fragrance today. Ylang ylang has been used to cover the beds of newlywed couples on their wedding night, for skin treatments, to soothe insect bites, and in hair preparations to promote thick, shiny, lustrous hair (it is also reported to help control split ends). It has also been used to treat colic, constipation, indigestion, stomachaches, and to regulate the heartbeat and respiration.

French Medicinal Uses: **Anxiety, arterial hypertension, depression, diabetes, fatigue** (mental), **frigidity, hair loss, hyperpnea** (reduces), **insomnia, palpitations, tachycardia**.

Other Possible Uses: Ylang ylang may help balance **male-female energies** so one can move closer towards being in spiritual attunement and focus his or her thoughts together, filtering out the ever-present garbage. It may help with lowering **blood pressure**[173], rapid **breathing**, balancing **equilibrium, frustration**, balancing **heart function, impotence, infection, intestinal problems, sex drive problems, shock**, and **skin problems**.

Body System(s) Affected: **Emotional Balance, Cardiovascular** and **Hormonal Systems**.

Aromatic Influence: It influences **sexual energy** and enhances **relationships**. It may help stimulate the adrenal glands. It is **calming** and **relaxing** and may also help with **anger** and possibly **rage** and **low self-esteem**. It brings back feelings of **self-love, confidence, joy,** and **peace**.

Application: Apply to **Vita Flex Points** and/or directly on **area** of concern; **diffuse**. It may be beneficial when applied over the **thymus** (to help stimulate the immune system).

Oral Use As Dietary Supplement: Generally regarded as safe (GRAS) for human consumption by the FDA. ***Dilute** one drop oil in 1 tsp. honey or in 4 oz. of beverage (i.e. soy/rice milk).* ***Not for children under 6 years old; use with caution and in greater dilution for children 6 years old and over.***

Safety Data: ***Repeated use can possibly result in contact sensitization.***

Blend Classification: Personifier and Modifier.

Blends With: Anise, bergamot, cardamom, chamomile, cumin, geranium, grapefruit, lemon, marjoram, sandalwood, vetiver.

Odor: Type: *Middle to Base Notes (20–80% of the blend)*; Scent: *Sweet, heavy, narcotic, cloying, tropical floral, with spicy-balsamic undertones*; Intensity: *5*.

Ylang Ylang, Amazonian

(Cananga odorata equitoriana)

Botanical Family: Annonaceae (tropical trees and shrubs: custard-apple)

Extraction Method/Origin: Steam distilled from flowers—Ecuador *(Flowers are picked early in the morning to maximize oil yield. The highest quality oil is drawn from the first hour of distillation.)*

Chemical Constituents: Sesquiterpenes (up to 55%): β-caryophyllene (<5%), germacrene-D (<18%), α-farnesene (<8%), α-humulene (<5%), δ-cadinene, α-copaene; Esters (<50%): benzyl acetate & benzoate (<30%), methyl salicylate & benzoate (<15%), farnesyl acetate (<3%), geranyl acetate (<3%), linalyl acetate; Alcohols (<45%): linalool (<20%), para-methyl anisol (<7%), geraniol; Sesquiterpene Alcohols: τ-cadinol, farnesol, τ-muurolol.

Properties: **Antidepressant, antiseptic, antispasmodic, aphrodisiac, sedative**[172].

Common Primary Uses: ^AT^**Calming**, ^A^**crying**, ^T^**hair loss**, ^AT^**high blood pressure**, ^A^**hyperpnea**, ^AT^**mental fatigue**, ^AT^**relaxing**, ^AT^**stress**, ^AT^**tension**.

Historical Uses: Traditionally grown in Madagascar, Indonesia, and the Philippines, Amazonian ylang ylang is a new variety of oil distilled from trees grown in the lush farmland of Ecuador.

Other Possible Uses: Amazonian ylang ylang may help harmonize and balance **male-female energies**. It may help with lowering **blood pressure**[173], rapid **breathing**, balancing **equilibrium**, **frustration**, balancing **heart function**, **impotence**, **infection**, **intestinal problems**, **sex drive problems**, **shock**, and **skin problems**.

Body System(s) Affected: **Emotional Balance**, **Cardiovascular** and **Hormonal Systems**.

Aromatic Influence: It influences **sexual energy** and enhances **relationships**. It may help stimulate the adrenal glands. It is **calming** and **relaxing** but can help enhance alertness and attentiveness.

Application: Apply to **Vita Flex Points** and/or directly on **area** of concern; **diffuse**. It may be beneficial when applied over the **thymus** (to help stimulate the immune system).

Oral Use As Dietary Supplement: Generally regarded as safe (GRAS) for human consumption by the FDA. ***Dilute** one drop oil in 1 tsp. of honey or in 4 oz. of beverage (i.e. soy/rice milk).* ***Not for children under 6 years old; use with caution and in greater dilution for children 6 years old and over.***

Safety Data: ***Repeated use can possibly result in contact sensitization.***

Blend Classification: Personifier and Modifier.

Blends With: Anise, bergamot, cardamom, chamomile, cumin, geranium, grapefruit, lemon, marjoram, sandalwood, vetiver.

Odor: Type: *Middle to Base Notes (20–80% of the blend)*; Scent: *Sweet, heavy, narcotic, cloying, tropical floral, with spicy-balsamic undertones*; Intensity: *5.*

Yuzu

(Citrus junos)

Botanical Family: Rutaceae (citrus)

Extraction Method/Origin: Hydro-distilled from peel—Shikoku Island, Japan

Chemical Constituents: Monoterpenes (up to 95%): limonene (<80%), α- & γ-terpinenes (<10%), α- & β-pinenes (<5%), camphene, sabinene, β-myrcene, β-phellandrene; Alcohols (<4%): terpineol, linalool; Coumarins: limettine; Sesquiterpenes (<1%): β-farnesene.

Properties: **Antibacterial, calming**, and **warming**.

Common Primary Uses: ^AT^**Calming**, ^T^**warming.**

Historical Uses: Yuzu fruit has been used traditionally in Japan since the eighteenth century in a bath taken at winter solstice to help warm the body, improve circulation, promote healthy looking skin, and prevent illness.

Other Possible Uses: This oil may be beneficial for **acne**, **arthritic pain**, **circulation**, **clarity**, **concentration**, **focus**, **moisturizing skin**, **neuralgia**, **skin tone**, **sore throat**, and **sore muscles**.

Body System(s) Affected: **Digestive** and **Immune Systems** , **Skin and Hair**.

Aromatic Influence: Yuzu oil has a refreshing, citrusy aroma that is often used to help improve **focus** and **concentration** and that may be beneficial for helping **purify** the air.

Application: Apply directly on **area** of concern; **diffuse**. Yuzu is an excellent addition to **bath** and **shower gels**, **body lotions**, or directly in **baths**.

Oral Use As Dietary Supplement: ***Dilute*** *1–2 drops of oil in 1 tsp. honey or in 4 oz. of beverage (i.e. soy/rice milk).* ***Not for children under 6 years old; use with caution and in greater dilution for children 6 years old and over.***

Safety Data: ***May irritate very young or sensitive skin.***

Blend Classification: Enhancer and Equalizer.

Blends With: Citronella, clary sage, lavandin, lavender, neroli, rosemary, other citrus oils.

Odor: Type: *Top Note (5–20% of the blend)*; Scent: *Sweet, citrusy*; Intensity: 3.

> ***I am so grateful to have these oils!***
>
> ***My daughter, Haley, at age 18 was ill one Sunday, and later in the evening was feeling quite worse. When we checked, she had a fever of 105 degrees. I filled a gel capsule with 10 drops of clove oil and had her take it with some water. In 1/2 hour I checked her temperature, and it was down to 102. I gave her 5 more drops in another capsule, and in another 1/2 hour her fever was totally gone!***
>
> ***-Submitted by Sally Donahue, Wilsonville, Oregon***

Endnotes

Note: *This list contains summaries of research articles referenced in this section. For the full article references, please see Research References in the appendix of this book. Please note that much of this research is still preliminary and is meant as an educational reference to guide further research and study. It should not be used to attempt to diagnose or prescribe any medical condition. Consult with a certified medical professional with regard to any medical condition.*

1. Anethol from star anise was found to inhibit three Aspergillus strains at concentrations of 2 mg/ml (Hitokoto et al., 1980).

   Essential oil of anise was found to be highly antifungal against several Candida species at low concentrations and was found to have stronger antifungal properties than a fluid extract from anise (Kosalec et al., 2005).
2. Basil oil was found to strongly inhibit several multidrug-resistant bacteria (Opalchenova et al., 2003).
3. In patients with chronic bronchitis, rosemary, basil, fir, and eucalyptus oils were found to demonstrate an antioxidant effect. Lavender was found to promote normalization of lipid levels (Siurin, 1997).

   Basil and its component, linalool, were found to reduce spontaneous mutagenesis in bacteria cells (Berić et al., 2008).
4. In patients with chronic bronchitis, rosemary, basil, fir, and eucalyptus oils were found to demonstrate an antioxidant effect (Siurin, 1997).
5. Two basil oils (*Ocimum basilicum* and *O. gratissimum*) were found to be insecticidal against the cowpea weevil (an agricultural pest) beetle and eggs in both a diffused and an aromatized powder form (Kéita et al., 2001).
6. Study participants listening to soft music and inhaling bergamot oil were found to be more relaxed with enhanced parasympathetic activity compared to the control group (Peng et al., 2009).
7. Supplementation with caraway was found to inhibit development of aberrant crypt foci (precursors to polyps) in the colorectal area of rats induced to develop aberrant crypt foci (Deeptha et al., 2006).

   Perillyl alcohol (found in caraway) was found to inhibit hyperproliferation of mammary epithelial cells prior to tumorigenisis (Katdare et al., 1997).
8. A combination of peppermint and caraway oil was found to reduce visceral hyperalgesia (pain hypersensitivity in the gastrointestinal tract) after induced inflammation in rats (Adam et al., 2006).

   In patients with dyspepsia (indigestion), treatments with capsules containing peppermint and caraway oil were found to decrease pain and pain frequency (Freise et al., 1999).

   An enteric-coated capsule with peppermint and caraway oil was found to reduce pain and symptoms in patients with non-ulcer dyspepsia (indigestion) compared to a control (May et al., 1996).
9. Carvone, found in dill and caraway oil, was found to induce the glutathione S-transferase enzyme (which helps to remove toxins from the body) in several target mouse tissues (Zheng et al., 1992).
10. Linalool and linalyl acetate (found in caraway oil) were found to exhibit anti-inflammatory activity in rats subjected to carrageenin-induced edema (inflammation) (Peana et al., 2002).

    Oil from cardamom seeds was found to have anti-inflammatory, analgesic, and antispasmodic effects on rats, mice, and a rabbit intestine preparation (respectively) (al-Zuhair et al., 1996).
11. Oil from cardamom seeds was found to have anti-inflammatory, analgesic, and antispasmodic effects on rats, mice, and a rabbit intestine preparation (respectively) (al-Zuhair et al., 1996).
12. Various extract of cardamom (including the essential oil) were found to significantly reduce gastric lesions induced by ethanol and aspirin (Jamal et al., 2006).
13. Carrot essential oil was found to demonstrate antifungal activity against yeasts and *Aspergillus* fungi at concentrations that were not cytotoxic to mouse skin dendritic cells (Tavares et al., 2008).
14. Treatment with 3-n-butyl phthalide and sedanolide, two chemicals extracted from celery seed oil, was found to reduce benzo[a]pyrene-induced tumors from 68% to 30% and 11% (respectively) in adult and juvenile female mice (Zheng et al., 1993).
15. Oral administration of German chamomile and melissa extracts was found to delay upper gastrointestinal transit in mice (Capasso et al., 2007).

    Colicky infants treated with a blend extracted from melissa, German chamomile, and fennel were found to have less crying time than infants treated with a placebo (Savino et al., 2005).
16. Oral administration of German chamomile oil (dissolved in 10% ethanol, 10% Tween, and 80% saline) was found to significantly reduce itching caused by compound 48/80 injection (Kobayashi et al., 2005).
17. Chamazulene, a chemical in chamomile oil, was found to block formation of leukotriene (a signaling chemical involved in the inflammation process) in neutrophilic (immune system) granulocytes (white blood cells containing granules). It also demonstrated an antioxidant effect (Safayhi et al., 1994).
18. Cinnamon, thyme, and clove essential oils demonstrated an antibacterial effect on several respiratory tract pathogens (Fabio et al., 2007).

    Cinnamon oil exhibited a strong antimicrobial activity against two detrimental oral bacteria (Filoche et al., 2005).

    Cinnamon bark, lemongrass, and thyme oils were found to have the highest level of activity against common respiratory pathogens among 14 essential oils tested (Inouye et al., May 2001).

    Oils with aldehyde or phenol as major component demonstrated a high level of antibacterial activity (Inouye et al., Dec. 2001).

    Bay, cinnamon, and clove oils reduced production of alpha-toxin and enterotoxin A by *Staphylococcus aureus* bacteria (Smith-Palmer et al., 2004).

Single Oils

19. In a test of nine oils, clove, followed by cinnamon, oregano, and mace oils, was found to be inhibitory to two toxin-producing fungi. It was also shown that whole and ground cloves stored with grain reduced the amount of aflatoxin contamination (Juglal et al., 2002).

    Vapor of cinnamon bark oil and cinnamic aldehyde was found to be effective against fungi involved in respiratory tract mycosis (fungal infections) (Singh et al., 1995).

    Cinnamon, thyme, oregano, and cumin oils inhibited the production of aflatoxin by aspergillus fungus (Tantaoui-Elaraki et al., 1994).

20. Clove, citronella, and patchouli oils were found to effectively repel 3 species of mosquitoes, with clove giving the highest level of 100% repellency for 2–4 hours) (Trongtokit et al., 2005).

    Citronella oil was found to effectively repel nymphs of *Amblyomma cajennense* (a type of tick known to carry Rocky Mountain spotted fever) at high concentrations for up to 35 hours (Soares et al., 2009).

    A slow-release citronella formula was found to significantly reduce infection with head lice in elementary school children compared to a control (Mumcuoglu et al., 2004).

21. Nurses working in an ICU setting demonstrated decreased perception of stress when receiving a topical application of *Lavandula angustifolia* and *Salvia sclarea* essential oils (Pemberton et al., 2008).

22. Cinnamon, thyme, and clove essential oils demonstrated an antibacterial effect on several respiratory tract pathogens (Fabio et al., 2007).

    Bay, cinnamon, and clove oils reduced production of alpha-toxin and enterotoxin A by *Staphylococcus aureus* bacteria (Smith-Palmer et al., 2004).

23. Eugenol from clove and thymol from thyme were found to inhibit the growth of *Aspergillus flavus* and *Aspergillus versicolor* at concentrations of .4 mg/ml or less (Hitokoto et al., 1980).

    Clove oil was also found to display an antifungal effect against tested candida strains (Chaieb et al., 2007).

24. Eugenol (found in clove EO) was found to increase the anti-inflammatory activity of cod liver oil (lowered inflammation by 30%) (Reddy et al., 1994).

25. Clove oil was found to have very strong radical scavenging activity (antioxidant) (Chaieb et al., 2007).

    Various essential oils demonstrated an antioxidant effect toward skin lipid squalene oxidized by UV irradiation, with a blend of thyme and clove oil demonstrating the highest inhibitory effect (Wei et al., 2007).

26. Eugenol was found to be virucidal to *Herpes Simplex* and to delay the development of herpes-induced keratitis (inflammation of the cornea) in mice (Benencia et al., 2000).

27. Clove oil demonstrated an ability to prevent the aggregation of platelets that can lead to blood clots and thrombosis both in vivo and in vitro (Saeed et al., 1994).

28. A blend of eugenol, alpha-terpineol, and cinnamic alcohol was found to be insecticidal against American cockroaches, carpenter ants, and German cockroaches (Enan, 2001).

    Vetiver oil was found to repel termites and prevent tunnelling with long-lasting effects, while clove oil was found to be highly termiticidal (Zhu et al., 2001).

29. Oral administration of copaiba oil was found to have antinociceptive (blocks transmission of pain-causing stimuli) activity in rodents (Gomes et al., 2007).

30. Copaiba oil demonstrated inhibitory activities on several species of bacteria (Santos et al., May 2008).

31. Copaiba oil was found to inhibit the parasite *Leishmania amazonensis* (a protozoa that causes skin lesions) (Santos et al., Nov. 2008).

32. Beta-caryophyllene (found in copaiba oil) was found to increase the anticancer activities of paclitaxel (a chemotherapy drug derived from the yew tree) (Legault et al., 2007).

33. In the elevated plus-maze, copaiba oil was found to demonstrate anxiolitic effects on rats comparable to the antianxiety drug diazepam (Curio et al., 2009).

34. Linalool, found in several essential oils, inhibited induced convulsions in rats by directly interacting with the NMDA receptor complex (Brum et al., 2001).

35. Cinnamon, thyme, oregano, and cumin oils inhibited the production of aflatoxin by aspergillus fungus (Tantaoui-Elaraki et al., 1994).

36. Cumin oil demonstrated an ability to reduce the frequency of epileptic activity induced by pentylenetetrazol in Helix aspersa (garden snails) (Janahmadi et al., 2006).

37. Rats with morphine-induced conditioned place preference who received injections of cumin essential oil demonstrated decreased morphine-induced conditioning, while those receiving a control substance (Tween-80) did not (Khatibie et al., 2008).

38. Three compounds derived from dill and caraway oil—anethofuran, carvone, and limonene—were found to induce the enzyme glutathione S-transferase (involved in transforming or binding to toxins in tissues) in several mice tissues (Zheng et al., 1992).

39. 1,8 cineole (eucalyptol) was found to have antinociceptive (pain-reducing) properties similar to morphine. Beta-pinene was found to reverse the effects of morphine in a degree similar to naloxone (a drug used to counter the effects of morphine overdose) (Liapi et al., 2007).

    1,8 cineole (eucalyptol) was found to display an anti-inflammatory effect on rats in several tests and was found to exhibit antinociceptive (pain-reducing) effects in mice, possibly by depressing the central nervous system (Santos et al., 2000).

40. Subjects using a mouthwash containing thymol, menthol, methyl salicylate, and eucalyptol for 6 months were found to not have developed oral bacteria that were resistant to the oils (Charles et al., 2000).

    Eucalyptus globulus oil was found to inhibit several bacteria types (Cermelli et al., 2008).

41. Eucalyptus oil was shown to ameliorate inflammatory processes by interacting with oxygen radicals and interfering with leukocyte activation (Grassmann et al., 2000).

Therapy with 1,8 cineole (eucalyptol) in both healthy and bronchitis-afflicted humans was shown to reduce production of LTB4 and PGE2, both metabolites of arachidonic acid, a known chemical messenger involved in inflammation, in white blood cells (Juergens et al., 1998).

Eucalyptus oil was found to have an anti-inflammatory and mucin-inhibitory effect on rats with lipopolysaccharide-induced bronchitis (Lu et al., 2004).

1,8 cineole (eucalyptol) displayed an anti-inflammatory effect on rats in several tests and was found to exhibit antinociceptive (pain-reducing) effects in mice, possibly by depressing the central nervous system (Santos et al., 2000).

Oils of three eucalyptus species (*citriodora*, *tereticornis*, and *globulus*) demonstrated analgesic (pain-relieving) and anti-inflammatory properties in rats (Silva et al., 2003).

42. Tea tree and eucalyptus oil demonstrated ability to inhibit *Herpes simplex* virus (Schnitzler et al., 2001).

43. A blend of eugenol, alpha-terpineol, and cinnamic alcohol was found to be insecticidal against American cockroaches, carpenter ants, and German cockroaches (Enan, 2001).

A eucalyptus-based repellent containing p-menthane-3,8-diol as the active ingredient was found to be as effective as DEET in repelling the mosquito commonly known to carry a deadly malaria disease (complete protection for 6–7.75 hours) (Trigg, 1996).

44. Therapy with 1.8 cineole (eucalyptol) in both healthy and bronchitis-afflicted humans was shown to reduce production of LTB4 and PGE2, both metabolites of arachidonic acid, a known chemical messenger involved in inflammation, in white blood cells (Juergens et al., 1998).

In patients with chronic bronchitis, rosemary, basil, fir, and eucalyptus oils were found to demonstrate an antioxidant effect. Lavender was found to promote normalization of lipid levels (Siurin, 1997).

45. Treatment of rats with 1,8-cineole (or eucalyptol, found in eucalyptus and rosemary) demonstrated an ability to lower mean aortic pressure (blood pressure), without decreasing heart rate, through vascular wall relaxation (Lahlou et al., 2002).

46. Oils of three eucalyptus species (*citriodora*, *tereticornis*, and *globulus*) demonstrated analgesic (pain-relieving) and anti-inflammatory properties in rats (Silva et al., 2003).

47. Therapy with 1.8 cineole (eucalyptol) in both healthy and bronchitis-afflicted humans was shown to reduce production of LTB4 and PGE2, both metabolites of arachidonic acid, a known chemical messenger involved in inflammation, in white blood cells (Juergens et al., 1998).

1,8 cineole (eucalyptol) displayed an anti-inflammatory effect on rats in several tests, and exhibited antinociceptive (pain-reducing) effects in mice, possibly by depressing the central nervous system (Santos et al., 2000).

48. Fennel oil was found to reduce contraction frequency and intensity in rat uterus induced to contract (Ostad et al., 2001).

49. Inhalation of essential oils such as pepper, estragon, fennel, and grapefruit was found to have a stimulating effect on sympathetic activity in healthy adults, while inhalation of essential oils of rose or patchouli caused a decrease in sympathetic activity (Haze et al., 2002).

50. In patients with chronic bronchitis, rosemary, basil, fir, and eucalyptus oils demonstrated an antioxidant effect. Lavender was found to promote normalization of lipid levels (Siurin, 1997).

51. Balsam fir oil and three of its constituents (alpha-pinene, beta-caryophyllene, and alpha humulene) were found to inhibit *Staphylococcus aureus* (Staph) bacteria (Pichette et al., 2006).

52. Balsam fir oil and its constituent, alpha-humulene, were found to be active against several solid tumor cell lines (Legault et al., 2003).

53. An extract from frankincense was found to produce apoptosis in human leukemia cells (Ghushan et al., 2007).

Boswellic acid reduced induced inflammation and tumors in mice and was found to inhibit DNA synthesis in human leukemia cells in culture (Huang et al., 2000).

Boswellic acid was found to cause differentiation in premyelocytic leukemia cells, while inhibiting growth of these cells in mice (Jing et al., 1992).

Boswellic acids demonstrated an antiproliferative and apoptotic effect on liver cancer cells (Liu et al., Oct. 2002).

Boswellic acids demonstrated antiproliferative and apoptotic effects on human colon cancer cells (Liu et al., Dec. 2002).

Boswellic acid induced apoptosis in prostate cancer cells (Lue et al., 2008).

Boswellic acids from frankincense were found to induce apoptosis (cell death) in human leukemia cell lines (Xia et al., 2005).

Boswellic acid was found to prevent and inhibit invasion and metastasis of melanoma (skin pigment) and fibrosarcoma (connective tissue cancer) cells (Zhao et al., 2003).

54. Incensole acetate (found in frankincense) was found to open TRPV3 ion channels in mice brain neurons, while also demonstrating anxiolytic (anti-anxiety) and antidepressive effects in mice (Moussaieff et al., 2008).

55. Triterpene acids isolated from frankincense exhibited a marked anti-inflammatory activity on TPA-induced inflammation in mice (Banno et al., 2006).

Boswellic acid reduced induced inflammation and tumors in mice and was found to inhibit DNA synthesis in human leukemia cells in culture (Huang et al., 2000).

Incensole acetate, isolated from frankincense resin demonstrated an anti-inflammatory and neuroprotective effect on mice with closed head injuries (Moussaieff et al., 2008).

Boswellic acid from frankincense was found in vitro to prevent expression and activity of several proteins involved in the inflammatory response. In vivo, boswellic acid was found to protect against experimental arthritis (Roy et al., Mar. 2006).

Boswellic extract effected genes related to the inflammatory response in human microvascular cells. Additionally, boswellic extract was found to reduce inflammation in carrageenan induced rat paw inflammation (Roy et al, Apr. 2006).

56. Boswellic acids from frankincense inhibited TH1 cytokines while potentiating TH2 cytokines when delivered with sesame seed oil, demonstrating their ability to modulate the immune response (Chevrier et al., 2005).

57. In isolated rat Ileum tissue, galbanum oil demonstrated an antispasmodic effect against contractions induced by KCl (potassium chloride) (Sadraei et al., 2001).

58. A combination of citricidal and geranium oil demonstrated strong antibacterial effects on MRSA. Geranium and tea tree demonstrated strong antibacterial effects on *Staphylococcus aureus* (Edwards-Jones et al., 2004).

    A formulation of lemongrass and geranium oil was found to reduce airborne bacteria by 89% in an office environment after diffusion for 15 hours (Doran et al., 2009).

59. Linalool, found in several essential oils, inhibited induced convulsions in rats by directly interacting with the NMDA receptor complex (Brum et al., 2001).

60. Topical application of geranium oil was found to reduce the inflammatory response of neutrophil (white blood cell) accumulation in mice (Maruyama et al., 2005).

61. Powdered ginger supplementation was found to lower pain and swelling in arthritic patients and to relieve pain from muscle discomfort (Srivastava et al., 1992).

    Eugenol and ginger oil taken orally were found to reduce paw and joint swelling in rats with induced severe arthritis (Sharma et al., 1994).

    Elderly persons with knee pain were found to have less pain and more knee function when receiving a massage with ginger and orange oil compared to a group receiving massage without the oils, or a group not receiving the massage (Yip et al., 2008).

62. In a trial of women receiving gynaecological surgery, women receiving ginger root had less incidences of nausea compared to a placebo. Ginger root demonstrated results similar to the antiemetic drug (a drug effective against vomiting and nausea) metoclopramide (Bone et al., 1990).

    Ginger root given one hour before major gynecological surgery resulted in lower nausea and fewer incidences of vomiting compared to control (Nanthakomon et al., 2006).

    Ginger root given orally to pregnant women was found to decrease the severity of nausea and frequency of vomiting compared to control (Vutyavanich et al., 2001).

63. Helichrysum oil exhibited definite antibacterial activity against six test Gram (+/-) bacteria (Chinou et al., 1996).

    Helichrysum was found to inhibit both the growth and the formation of some enzymes of *Staphylococcus aureus* (staph) bacteria (Nostro et al., 2001).

64. Arzanol (extracted from helichrysum) at non-cytotoxic concentrations showed a strong inhibition of TBH-induced oxidative stress in VERO cells (Rosa et al., 2007).

    In fruit flies, essential oils of helichrysum, ledum, and ravensara demonstrated antimutagenic properties against urethane-induced genetic mutations (Idaomar et al., 2002).

65. Helichrysum showed significant antiviral activity against the herpes virus at non-cytotoxic concentrations (Nostro et al., 2003).

66. While inhaled jasmine has been shown to stimulate in vivo, jasmine applied to guinea pig and rat tissue was shown to be spasmolytic (antispasm) (Lis-Balchin et al., 2002).

67. Jasmine flowers applied to the breast were found to be as effective as the anti-lactation drug bromocriptine at reducing breast engorgement, milk production, and analgesic (pain-relieving drug) intake in women after giving birth (Shrivastav et al., 1988).

68. The essential oil of laurel (*Laurus nobilis*) was found to reduce pain and inflammation in rats in a manner similar to morphine and piroxicam (an anti-inflammatory drug) in mice and rats (Sayyah et al., 2003).

69. Lavender oil was found to work as an anaesthetic (reducing pain) in rabbit reflex test (Ghelardini et al., 1999).

    Oil from Lavandula angustifolia was found to reduce writhing in induced writhing in rats, and to reduce edema (swelling) in carrageenan-induced paw edema, indicating an anti-inflammatory effect (Hajhashemi et al., 2003).

70. Linalool, found in several essential oils, inhibited induced convulsions in rats by directly interacting with the NMDA receptor complex (Brum et al., 2001).

71. Lavender oil demonstrated both fungistatic (stopped growth) and fungicidal (killed) activity against *Candida albicans* (D'Auria et al., 2005).

72. Oil from *Lavandula angustifolia* was found to reduce writhing in induced writhing in rats, and to reduce edema (swelling) in carrageenan-induced paw edema, indicating an anti-inflammatory effect (Hajhashemie et al., 2003).

    Linalool and linalyl acetate (from lavender, and other essential oils) exhibited anti-inflammatory activity in rats subjected to carrageenin-induced edema (inflammation) (Peana et al., 2002).

73. Essential oil from *Lavandula angustifolia* demonstrated an ability to eliminate protozoal pathogens *Giardia duodenalis*, *Thrichomonas vaginalis*, and *Hexamita inflata* at concentrations of 1% or less (Moon et al., 2006).

74. In tests for mutagenicity, both tea tree and lavender oils were found to not be mutagenic. In fact, lavender oil was found to have strong antimutagenic activity, reducing mutations of cells exposed to a known mutagen (Evandri et al., 2005).

75. Mice treated with perillyl alcohol (found in lavender and mint plants) had a 22% reduction in tumor incidence and a 58% reduction in tumor multiplicity during a mouse lung tumor bioassay (Lantry et al., 1997).

    Rats with liver tumors that were treated with perillyl alcohol had smaller tumor sizes than untreated rats due to apoptosis in cancer cells in treated rats.

    Rats fed diets containing perillyl alcohol (derived from lavender plants) were found to have less incidence of colon tumors and less multiplicity of tumors in the colon compared to control. Colon tumors of animals fed perillyl alcohol were found to exhibit increased apoptosis of cells compared to control (Reddy et al., 1997).

76. Exposure to lavender odor was found to decrease anxiety in gerbils in the elevated plus maze, with a further decrease in anxiety in females after prolonged (2 week) exposure (Bradley et al., 2007).

    Exposure to lavender oil and to its constituents, linalool and linalyl acetate, was found to decrease normal movement in mice as well as to return mice to normal movement rates after caffeine-induced hyperactivity (Buchbauer et al., 2001).

    In patients admitted to an intensive care unit, those receiving lavender aromatherapy reported a greater improvement in mood and perceived levels of anxiety compared to those receiving massage or a period of rest (Dunn et al., 1995).

    Swiss mice fed lavender oil diluted in olive oil were found to be more sedate in several common tests (Guillemain et al., 1989).

    Female patients being treated with chronic hemodialysis demonstrated less anxiety when exposed to lavender aroma (Itai et al., 2000).

    Inhaling lavender oil was found to lower agitation in older adults suffering from dementia (Lin et al., 2007).

    Lavender oil was found to inhibit sympathetic nerve activity in rats while exciting parasympathetic nerve activity. Linalool, a component of lavender, was shown to have similar effects (Shen et al., 2005).

    Lavender oil was found to demonstrate anticonflict effects in mice similar to the anxiolytic (antianxiety) drug diazepam (Umezu, 2000).
77. Lavender oil was found to inhibit immediate-type allergic reactions in mice and rats by inhibiting mast cell degranulation (Kim et al., 1999).
78. Female students suffering from insomnia were found to sleep better and to have a lower level of depression during weeks they used a lavender fragrance when compared to weeks they did not use a lavender fragrance (Lee et al., 2006).
79. Lavender oil scent was found to lower sympathetic nerve activity and blood pressure in rats while elevating parasympathetic nerve activity. It was further found that applying an anosmia-inducing agent (something that causes a loss of smell) eliminated the effects of the lavender oil scent (Tanida et al., 2006).
80. Patients waiting for dental treatment were found to be less anxious and to have a better mood when exposed to the odor of lavender or orange oil compared to a control (Lehrner et al., 2005).

    Oral supplementation of lavender oil was found to decrease anxiety in females in conditions of low anxiety (Bradley et al., 2009).

    An office environment featuring a soothing DVD video presentation and diffused lavender oil was found to reduce anxiety in patients awaiting a gastroscopy procedure, compared to a regular office environment (Hoya et al., 2008).
81. In patients with chronic bronchitis, lavender was found to promote normalization of lipid levels (Siurin, 1997).
82. Lavender oil was found to be comparable to DEET in its ability to repel ticks (*Hyalomma marginatum*) (Mkolo et al., 2007).

    An infestation of the red bud borer pest was reduced by more than 95% in the grafted buds of apple trees by application of the essential oil of *Lavandula angustifolia* (van Tol et al., 2007).
83. Subjects exposed to 3 minutes of lavender aroma were more relaxed and were able to perform math computations faster and more accurately (Diego et al., 1998).

    Subjects who smelled a cleansing gel with lavender aroma were more relaxed and wereable to complete math computations faster (Field et al., 2005).
84. Lavender odor was found to reduce mental stress while increasing arousal (Motomura et al., 2001).

    Nurses working in an ICU setting demonstrated decreased perception of stress when receiving a topical application of *Lavandula angustifolia* and *Salvia sclarea* essential oils (Pemberton et al., 2008).
85. In fruit-flies, essential oils of helichrysum, ledum, and ravensara demonstrated antimutagenic properties against urethane-induced genetic mutations (Idaomar et al., 2002).
86. In a study of older individuals, it was found that there was a dose-dependent relationship between citrus peel (which are high in d-limonene) consumption and a lower degree of squamous cell carcinoma (SCC) of the skin (Hakim et al., 2000).

    In clinical trials, d-Limonene (found in most citrus oils and in dill, caraway, citronella, and nutmeg) was found to elicit a response (kept patients stable) in some patients in advanced stages of cancer (1 breast and 3 colorectal carcinoma of 32 total patients). A secondary trial with just breast-cancer patients did not elicit any responses (Vigushin et al., 1998).
87. Lemon oil and its component, citral, were found to decrease depressed behavior in a similar manner to antidepressant drugs in rats involved in several stress tests (Komori et al., 1995).
88. Lemon oil was found to be an effective antifungal agent against two bread-mold species (Caccioni et al., 1998).
89. Lemon oil and one of its components, gamma-terpinene, was found to inhibit oxidation of low-density lipoprotein (LDL). Oxidation of LDL has been found to increase the risk of atherosclerosis and cardiac disease (Grassmann et al., 2001).
90. Rats exposed long-term to lemon essential oil were found to demonstrate different anxiety and pain threshold levels than untreated rats. It was also found that exposure to lemon oil induced chemical changes in the neuronal circuits involved in anxiety and pain (Ceccarelli et al., 2004).
91. The use of rosemary, lemon, and peppermint oils in massage demonstrated an ability to reduce constipation and to increase bowel movements in elderly subjects, compared to massage without the oils (Kim et al., 2005).
92. Pretreatment of human and rat astrocyte cells (cells found in the nerve and brain that support the blood-brain barrier and help repair the brain and spinal cord following injuries) with lemon oil was found to inhibit heat-shock induced apoptosis of these cells (Koo et al., 2002).

    Several constituents of lemon oil and their metabolites (chemicals made by these chemicals in the body) were found to increase the release of monoamines (various chemicals responsible for neurotrasmission and neuromodulation) in rat brain tissue, indicating a possible effect on brain nerve cell behavior (Fukumoto et al., 2006).
93. Lemon oil vapor was found to have strong antistress and antidepressant effects on mice subjected to several common stress tests (Komiya et al., 2006).

    Lemon odor was found to enhance the positive mood of volunteers exposed to a stressor (Kiecolt-Glaser et al., 2008).

94. A formulation of lemongrass and geranium oil was found to reduce airborne bacteria by 89% in an office environment after diffusion for 15 hours (Doran et al., 2009).

    Lemongrass and lemon verbena oil were found to be bactericidal to *Helicobacter pylori* at very low concentrations. Additionally, it was found that this bacteria did not develop a resistance to lemongrass oil after 10 passages, while this bacteria did develop resistance to clarithromycin (an antibiotic) under the same conditions (Ohno et al., 2003).

    Two components of lemongrass demonstrated antibacterial properties, while the addition of a third component, myrcene enhanced the antibacterial activities (Onawunmi et al., 1984).

95. Geraniol, found in lemongrass oil (among others), was found to inhibit colon cancer cell growth while inhibiting DNA synthesis in these cells (Carnesecchi et al., 2001).

    Lemongrass oil and its constituent, isointermedeol, were found to induce apoptosis in human leukemia cells (Kumar et al., 2008).

    An extract from lemon \grass was found to inhibit hepatocarcinogenesis (liver cancer genesis) in rats (Puatanachokchai et al., 2002).

    Lemongrass oil was found to inhibit multiple cancer cell lines, both in vitro and in vivo, in mice (Sharma et al., 2009).

96. Internal use of lemongrass capsules was found to reduce cholesterol in some subjects (Elson et al., 1989).

97. Cinnamon bark, lemongrass, and thyme oils were found to have the highest level of activity against common respiratory pathogens among 14 essential oils tested (Inouye et al., 2001).

98. *Citrus hystrix* essential oil was found to be an effective repellent against three types of cockroaches, exhibiting 100% repellency against two and 87% repellency against the third (Thavara et al., 2007).

99. Among several oils tested, tea tree (melaleuca), manuka, and eucalyptus demonstrated strong antibacterial activity against detrimental oral bacteria (Takarada et al., 2004).

    Cinnamon oil exhibited a strong antimicrobial activity against two detrimental oral bacteria. Manuka, tea tree, and the component thymol also exhibited antimicrobial potency (Filoche et al., 2005).

100. In patients suffering from arthritis, it was found that a blend of lavender, marjoram, eucalyptus, rosemary, peppermint, and carrier oils reduced perceived pain and depression compared to a control (Kim et al., 2005).

101. MRSA (methicillin-resistant staph) and MSSA (methicillin-sensitive staph) in biofilms (plaque/microcolonies) were eradicated by a 5% solution of tea tree oil, as were 5 of 9 CoNS (coagulase-negative staph) (Brady et al., 2006).

    66 isolates of *Staphylococcus aureus* (Staph), including 64 methicillin-resistant (MRSA) and 33 mupirocin-resistant strains, were inhibited by tea tree essential oil (Carson et al., 1995).

    Tea tree oil was found to disrupt the cellular membrane and inhibited respiration in *Candida albicans*, Gram-negative *E. coli*, and Gram-positive *Staphylococcus aureus* (Staph) (Cox et al., 2000).

    Tea tree oil and its component terpinen-4-ol demonstrated an effective antibacterial activity against *Staphylococcus aureus* (Staph) bacteria, superior to the activities of several antibiotic drugs, even against antibiotic-resistant strains (Ferrini et al., 2006).

    Geranium and tea tree demonstrated strong antibacterial effects on *Staphylococcus aureus* (Edwards-Jones et al., 2004).

    Tea tree oil was found to kill transient skin flora at lower concentrations than it killed resident skin flora (Hammer et al., 1996).

    Gram-positive strains of *Staphylococcus aureus* and *Enterococcus faecalis* were shown to have very low frequencies of resistance to tea tree oil (Hammer et al., 2008).

    Tea tree oil demonstrated ability to kill *Staphylococcus aureus* (Staph) bacteria both within biofilms and in the stationary growth phase at concentrations below 1% (Kwieciński et al., 2009).

102. Tea tree oil was found to inhibit 301 different types of yeasts isolated from the mouths of cancer patients suffering from advanced cancer, including 41 strains that are known to be resistant to antifungal drugs (Bagg et al., 2006).

    Eleven types of Candida were found to be highly inhibited by tea tree oil (Banes-Marshall et al., 2001).

    Topical application of 100% tea tree oil was found to have results similar to topical application of 1% clotrimazole (antifungal drug) solution on onychomycosis (also known as tinea, or fungal nail infection) (Buck et al., 1994).

    Tea Tree oil was found to alter the membrane properties and functions of *Candida albicans* cells, leading to cell inhibition or death (Hammer et al., 2004).

    Terpinen-4-ol, a constituent of tea tree oil, and tea tree oil were found to be effective against several forms of vaginal candida infections in rats, including azole-resistant forms (Mondello et al., 2006).

    Patients with tinea pedis (athlete's foot) were found to have a higher rate of cure and a higher clinical response when treated topically with 25 or 50% tea tree oil solution compared to control (Satchell et al., 2002).

103. Tea tree oil was found to reduce swelling during a contact hypersensitivity response in the skin of mice sensitized to the chemical hapten (Brand et al., 2002).

    Melaleuca alternifolia oil was found to reduce reactive oxygen species (ROS) production in neutrophils (a type of white blood cell), indicating an antioxidant effect and decreased Interleukin 2 (a chemical messenger that helps trigger an inflammatory response) secretion, while increasing the secretion of Interleukin 4 (a chemical messenger involved in turning off the inflammatory response) (Caldefie-Chézet et al., 2006).

    Melaleuca alternifolia oil was found to mediate the Reactive Oxygen Species (ROS) production of leukocytes (white blood cells), indicating a possible anti-inflammatory activity (Caldefie-Chézet et al., 2004).

    Inhaled tea tree oil was found to have anti-inflammatory influences on male rats with induced peritoneal inflammation (Golab et al., 2007).

    The water-soluble terpinen-4-ol component of tea tree was found to supress the production of pro-inflammatory mediators in human monocytes (a type of white blood cell that is part of the human immune system) (Hart et al., 2000).

    Tea tree oil applied to histamine-induced weal and flare in human volunteers was found to decrease the mean weal volume when compared to a control (Koh et al., 2002).

104. Tea tree and eucalyptus oil demonstrated ability to inhibit *Herpes simplex* virus (Schnitzler et al., 2001).

105. A gel with 5% tea tree oil was found to be as effective as a 5% benzoyl peroxide (a common chemical used to treat acne) lotion, with fewer side effects (Bassett et al., 1990).

A topical gel containing 5% tea tree oil was found to be more effective than a placebo at preventing acne vulgaris lesions and severity in patients suffering from acne vulgaris (Enshaieh et al., 2007).

Tea tree oil and several of its main components were found to be active against *Propionibacterium acnes*, a bacteria involved in the formation of acne. This oil was also found to be active against two types of staphylococcus bacteria (Raman et al., 1995).

106. In a human trial, most patients receiving treatment with *Melaleuca alternifolia* oil placed topically on boils experienced healing or reduction of symptoms, while of those receiving no treatment (control), half required surgical intervention, and all still demonstrated signs of the infection (Feinblatt, 1960).

107. Tea tree oil scrub and shampoo were found to reduce demodex mite infestation on the eyelids of patients suffering from ocular irritation and inflammation who used this treatment daily for six weeks. There was also a dramatic decrease in ocular irritation and inflammation (Kheirkhah et al., 2007).

Tea tree oil was found to be effective against both lice an dust mites in a mite chamber assay (Williamson et al., 2007).

108. Essential oil of *Melaleuca alternifolia* was found to be lethal for more than 80% of *Ixodes ricinus* tick nymphs (a carrier or Lyme disease) when ticks inhaled a 10 microl dose of the oil for 90 minutes or more (Iori et al., 2005).

109. Melissa oil demonstrated inhibition of *Herpes simplex* type 1 and 2 viruses (Schnitzler et al., 2008).

110. Results of a clinical trial indicate that a combination of melissa and valerian oils may have anxiety reducing properties at some doses (Kennedy et al., 2006).

Melissa (lemon balm) oil applied topically in a lotion was found to reduce agitation and improve quality of life factors in patients suffering severe dementia, compared to those receiving a placebo lotion (Ballard et al., 2002).

111. An extract from *Artemisia vulgaris* (mugwort) was found to have antispasmodic and bronchodilating activities in several different animal and animal tissue tests (Khan et al., 2009).

112. The volatile oil of *Artemisia vulgaris* demonstrated strong antioxidative activity in two laboratory tests (Xiufen et al., 2004).

113. At subtoxic levels, myrrh oil was found to reduce interleukin (chemical signals believed to play a role in the inflammation response) by fibroblast cells in the gums (Tipton et al., 2003).

114. Treatment with elemene (found in myrrh oil) was found to increase survival time and to reduce tumor size in patients with malignant brain tumor versus chemotherapy (Tan et al., 2000).

115. In children with *Molloscum contagiosum* (a viral infection causing skin lesions), application of a 10% solution of lemon myrtle oil was found to reduce lesions by more than 90% in 56% of patients; while in children receiving application of a control (olive oil), none had a reduction of lesions greater than 90% (Burke et al., 2004).

116. A chloroform extract of nutmeg was found to exhibit anti-inflammatory, analgesic (pain-reducing), and antithrombotic (blood clot–reducing) effects in rodents (Olajide et al., 1999).

117. Ocotea oil was found to demonstrate anti-inflammatory effects in rats without damaging gastric mucosa (Ballabeni et al., 2009).

118. Oral administration of ocotea oil in mice was found to prevent collagen-epinephrine induced thrombosis (blood clots) (Ballabeni et al., 2007).

119. In a study of older individuals, it was found that there was a dose-dependent relationship between citrus peel (which are high in d-limonene) consumption and a lower degree of squamous cell carcinoma (SCC) of the skin (Hakim et al., 2000).

In clinical trials, D-Limonene (found in most citrus oils and in dill, caraway, citronella, and nutmeg) was found to elicit a response (kept patients stable) in some patients in advanced stages of cancer (1 breast and 3 colorectal carcinoma of 32 total patients). A secondary trial with just breast-cancer patients did not elicit any responses (Vigushin et al., 1998).

120. Female patients waiting for dental treatment were found to be less anxious, more positive, and more calm when exposed to orange oil odor than patients who were not exposed to the orange oil odor (Lehrner et al., 2000).

Patients waiting for dental treatment were found to be less anxious and to have a better mood when exposed to the odor of lavender or orange oil compared to control (Lehrner et al., 2005).

121. Elderly persons with knee pain were found to have less pain and more knee function when receiving a massage with ginger and orange oil compared to a group receiving massage without the oils or a group not receiving the massage (Yip et al., 2008).

122. Oregano oil was found to inhibit MRSA (Nostro et al., 2004).

Oregano oil was found to kill antibiotic-resistant strains of Staph, *E. coli*, *Klebsiella pneumoniae*, *Helicobacter pylori*, and *Mycobacterium terrae* (Preuss et al., 2005).

123. The vapor of oregano oil was found to be fungicidal against the *Trichophyton mentagrophytes* fungi (a fungi that causes a skin infection known as Malabar itch) (Inouye et al., 2006).

In a test of nine oils, clove, followed by cinnamon, oregano, and mace oils, was found to be inhibitory to two toxin-producing fungi (Juglal et al., 2002).

Cinnamon, thyme, oregano, and cumin oils inhibited the production of aflatoxin by aspergillus fungus (Tantaoui-Elaraki et al., 1994).

Mice infected with *Candida albicans* who were fed origanum oil or carvacrol diluted in olive oil had an 80% survival rate after 30 days, while infected mice fed olive oil alone all died after 10 days (Manohar et al., 2001).

124. Oregano oil administered orally was found to improve gastrointestinal symptoms in 7 of 11 patients who had tested positive for the parasite *Blastocystis hominis* and to cause disappearance of this parasite in 8 cases (Force et al., 2000).

125. Growth-retarded pigs receiving a supplementation of oregano leaves and flowers enriched with cold-pressed oregano oil were found to have increased growth, decreased mortality, and higher numbers of immune-system cells and compounds when compared to control pigs who did not receive supplementation (Walter et al., 2004).

126. In a test of 34 different essential oils, patchouli (*Pogostemon cablin*) oil proved to be the most effective insecticide against the common house fly (Pavela, 2008).

    Both patchouli oil and its constituent, patchouli alcohol (patchoulol), were found to be repellent and insecticidal to Formosan termites when applied topically (Zhu et al., 2003).

    Clove, citronella, and patchouli oils were found to effectively repel 3 species of mosquitoes (Trongtokit et al., 2005).

127. Inhalation of essential oils such as pepper, estragon, fennel, and grapefruit was found to have a stimulating effect on sympathetic activity, while inhalation of essential oils of rose or patchouli caused a decrease in sympathetic activity in healthy adults (Haze et al., 2002).

128. Inhalation of black pepper oil was found to increase cerebral blood flow and improve the swallowing reflex in elderly patients who had suffered a stroke (Ebihara et al., 2006).

129. Inhaled vapor of black pepper oil was found to reduce craving for cigarettes and symptoms of anxiety in smokers deprived from smoking compared to a control (Rose et al., 1994).

130. Subjects using a mouthwash containing thymol, menthol, methyl salicylate, and eucalyptol for 6 months were found to not have developed oral bacteria that were resistant to the oils (Charles et al., 2000).

    Peppermint and spearmint oil inhibited resistant strains of Staphylococcus, *E. Coli*, Salmonella, and *Helicobacter pylori* (Imai et al., 2001).

    Peppermint and rosemary oils were each found to be more effective at preventing dental biofilm (plaque) formation than chlorhexidine (an antiseptic) (Rasooli et al., 2008).

131. A combination of peppermint and caraway oil was found to reduce visceral hyperalgesia (pain hypersensitivity in the gastrointestinal tract) after induced inflammation in rats (Adam et al., 2006).

    L-menthol was found to inhibit production of inflammation mediators in human monocytes (a type of white blood cell involved in the immune response) (Juergens et al., 1998).

132. Peppermint oil was found to be as effective as Buscopan (an antispasmodic drug) at preventing spasms during a barium enema (a type of enema used to place barium in the colon for X-ray imaging purposes) (Asao et al., 2003).

133. Peppermint oil demonstrated a direct virucidal activity against Herpes type 1 and type 2 viruses (Schuhmacher et al., 2003).

134. The use of rosemary, lemon, and peppermint oils in massage demonstrated an ability to reduce constipation and to increase bowel movements in elderly subjects, compared to massage without the oils (Kim et al., 2005).

135. In patients with dyspepsia (indigestion), treatments with capsules containing peppermint and caraway oil were found to decrease pain and pain frequency (Freise et al., 1999).

    An enteric coated capsule with peppermint and caraway oil was found to reduce pain and symptoms in patients with nonulcer dyspepsia (indigestion) compared to a control (Mimica-Dukić et al., 2003).

136. A combination of peppermint oil and ethanol was found to have a significant analgesic effect with a reduction in sensitivity to headache, while a combination of peppermint, eucalyptus, and ethanol was found to relax muscles and increase cognitive performance in humans (Göbel et al., 1994).

137. In irritable bowel syndrome patients without bacterial overgrowth, lactose intolerance, or celiac disease, peppermint oil was found over 8 weeks to reduce IBS symptoms significantly more than a placebo (Cappello et al., 2007).

    Children suffering from irritable bowel syndrome (IBS) who received peppermint oil in enteric-coated capsules (encapsulated so the capsules wouldn't open until they reached the intestines) reported a reduced severity of pain associated with IBS (Kline et al., 2001).

    Patients with IBS symptoms who took a peppermint-oil formulation in an enteric-coated capsule were found to have a significantly higher reduction of symptoms than did patients taking a placebo (Liu et al., 1997).

    Peppermint oil in enteric-coated capsules was found to relieve symptoms of irritable bowel syndrome better than a placebo in patients suffering from IBS (Rees et al., 1979).

138. In human trials, the aroma of peppermint was found to enhance memory and increase alertness, while ylang ylang aroma was found to increase calmness (Moss et al., 2008).

139. Pretreatment of human and rat astrocyte cells (cells found in the nerve and brain that support the blood-brain barrier and help repair the brain and spinal cord following injuries) with peppermint oil was found to inhibit heat-shock induced apoptosis of these cells (Koo et al., 2001).

140. Mice pretreated with peppermint leaf extract demonstrated less bone marrow cell loss than mice not pretreated with peppermint when exposed to gamma radiation (Samarth et al., 2007).

    In mice exposed to whole-body gamma irradiation, only 17% of mice who had been fed peppermint oil died, while 100% of mice who did not receive peppermint oil died. It was also found that mice pre-fed peppermint oil were able to return blood cell levels to normal after 30 days, while control mice were not, suggesting a protective or stimulating effect of the oil on blood stem cells (Samarth et al., 2004).

    Peppermint extract fed orally to mice demonstrated the ability to protect the testis from gamma radiation damage (Samarth et al., 2009).

141. In fruit flies, essential oils of helichrysum, ledum, and ravensara demonstrated antimutagenic properties against urethane-induced genetic mutations (Idaomar et al., 2002).

142. Rose essential oil demonstrated strong antibacterial activity against several pathogenic bacteria (Ulusoy et al., 2009).

143. In human volunteers wearing breathing masks to prevent aroma inhalation, rose oil applied to the skin was found to significantly decrease breathing rate, blood oxygen saturation, and systolic blood pressure compared to a placebo, and volunteers receiving rose oil rated themselves more calm and relaxed than subjects receiving the placebo (Hongratanaworakit et al., 2009).

Rose oil was found to have similar effects as the antianxiety drug diazepam (Valium) in mice, but through a different cellular mechanism (Umezu, 1999).

Geraniol and eugenol, two components of rose oil (among others), were found to demonstrate antianxiety effects on mice in several tests (Umezu et al., 2002).

Inhalation of essential oils such as pepper, estragon, fennel, and grapefruit was found to have a stimulating effect on sympathetic activity in healthy adults, while inhalation of essential oils of rose or patchouli caused a decrease in sympathetic activity (Haze et al., 2002).

144. An ethanol extract of rosemary was found to demonstrate antinociceptive (pain-blocking) and anti-inflammatory activity in mice and rats (González-Trujano et al., 2007).

145. Peppermint and rosemary oils were each found to be more effective at preventing dental biofilm (plaque) formation than chlorhexidine (an antiseptic) (Rasooli et al., 2008).

146. An ethanol extract of rosemary was found to have an antiproliferative effect on human leukemia and breast carcinoma cells as well as an antioxidant effect (Cheung et al., 2007).

Rosemary extract injected in rats was found to decrease mammary adenocarcinomas in rats (Singletary et al., 1997).

Carnosic acid (derived from rosemary) was found to inhibit the proliferation of human leukemia cells in vitro (Steiner et al., 2001).

147. Rosemary oil was found to inhibit aflatoxin production by aspergillus fungi (a highly toxic and carcinogenic substance produced by these fungi (Rasooli et al., 2008).

148. Rosemary oil was found to have anti-inflammatory and peripheral antinociceptive (pain sensitivity–blocking) properties in mice (Takaki et al., 2008).

149. Extracts from rosemary were found to have high antioxidant properties. Rosmarinic acid and carnosic acid from rosemary were found to have the highest antioxidant activities of studied components of rosemary (Almela et al., 2006).

Extracts from rosemary were found to have high antioxidant levels. Additionally, a methanol extract with 30% carnosic acid, 16% carnosol, and 5% rosmarinic acid was found to be effective against Gram-positive and negative bacteria and against yeast (Moreno et al., 2006).

An ethanol extract of rosemary demonstrated a protective effect against the oxidative damage to DNA in cells exposed to H2O2 and light-excited Methylene Blue (Slamenova et al., 2002).

150. In patients suffering from arthritis, it was found that a blend of lavender, marjoram, eucalyptus, rosemary, peppermint, and carrier oils reduced perceived pain and depression compared to control (Kim et al., 2005).

151. In patients with chronic bronchitis, rosemary, basil, fir, and eucalyptus oils were found to demonstrate an antioxidant effect (Siurin, 1997).

152. Patients with alopecia areata (hair loss) that massaged carrier oils containing a blend of thyme, rosemary, lavender, and cedarwood oils into their scalps were more likely to show improvement when compared to a control group that massaged carrier oils alone into their scalps (Hay et al., 1998).

153. Rosemary oil demonstrated a relaxant effect on smooth muscle from the trachea of rabbit and guinea pig (Aqel et al., 1991).

154. Subjects exposed to rosemary aroma were more alert, and completed math computations faster (but not more accurately) (Diego et al., 1998).

Volunteers completing a battery of tests were found to be more content when exposed to lavender and rosemary aromas. Rosemary aroma also was found to enhance quality of memory compared to control (Moss et al., 2003).

155. Tea tree, peppermint, and sage oils were found to inhibit oral bacteria, with thymol and eugenol being the most active components of these oils (Shapiro et al., 1994).

156. The terpenoid fractions of sage were found to inhibit mutation of cells by the mutagen (mutation-causing agent) mitomycin C in mice (Vujosević et al., 2004).

Sage and several of its monoterpene constituents (thujone, 1,8-cineole, camphor, and limonene) were found to have antimutagenic effects on cells exposed to UV radiation (Vuković-Gacić et al., 2006).

157. Oils of *Salvia fruticosa* and *Salvia officinalis* were found to inhibit butyrylcholinesterase, an enzyme that has been studied for its potential role in increasing the chances of developing Alzheimer's disease (Savelev et al., 2004).

158. In a small human trial, oral administration of sage lavender oil was found to improve speed of memory as well as alertness and calmness in healthy volunteers compared to a placebo (Tildesley et al., 2005).

159. Alpha-santalol, derived from sandalwood EO, was found to delay and decrease the incidence and multiplicity of skin tumor (papilloma) development in mice (Dwivedi et al., 2003).

Various concentrations of alpha-santalol (from sandalwood) were tested against skin cancer in mice. All concentrations were found to inhibit skin cancer development (Dwivedi et al., 2005).

Alpha-santalol was found to induce apoptosis in human skin cancer cells (Kaur et al., 2005).

160. Peppermint and spearmint oil inhibited resistant strains of Staphylococcus, *E. Coli*, Salmonella, and *Helicobacter pylori* (Imai et al., 2001).

161. Calophyllum inophyllum (tamanu) oil was found to demonstrate UV filtering properties in the SPF 18–22 range at low concentrations, and was also found to not be cytotoxic to human eye cells at concentrations up to 1% (Said et al., 2007).

162. In animal testing, the essential oil of tarragon demonstrated anticonvulsant and sedative properties at low concentrations (Sayyah et al., 2004).

163. Subjects using a mouthwash containing thymol, menthol, methyl salicylate, and eucalyptol for 6 months were found to not have developed oral bacteria that were resistant to the oils (Charles et al., 2000).

Cinnamon, thyme, and clove essential oils demonstrated an antibacterial effect on several respiratory tract pathogens (Fabio et al., 2007).

Thyme oil demonstrated a strong antibacterial effect against Staph and E. Coli bacteria (Mohsenzadeh et al., 2007).

164. Thyme oil was found to inhibit Candida species by causing lesions in the cell membrane as well as inhibiting germ tube (an outgrowth that develops when the fungi is preparing to replicate) formation (Pina-Vaz et al., 2004).

Cinnamon, thyme, oregano, and cumin oils inhibited the production of aflatoxin by aspergillus fungus (Tantaoui-Elaraki et al., 1994).

165. Older rats whose diets were supplemented with thyme oil were found to have higher levels of the antioxidant enzymes superoxide dismutase and glutathione peroxidase in the heart, liver, and kidneys than did older rats without this supplementation (Youdim et al., 1999).

Aging rats fed thyme oil or the constituent thymol were found to have higher levels of the antioxidant enzymes superoxide dismutase and glutathione peroxidase in the brain than did aging rats not fed the oil or constituent (Youdim et al., 2000).

166. Results of a clinical trial indicate that a combination of melissa and valerian oils may have anxiety-reducing properties at some doses (Kennedy et al., 2006).

Two chemical components found in valerian were found to have sedative, sleep-enhancing, and anxiolytic (anxiety-lowering) properties (Marder et al., 2003).

Subjects suffering from insomnia who took an extract from valerian demonstrated results similar to subjects who took oxazepam (an antianxiety and insomnia drug) (Ziegler et al., 2002).

167. In a human trial in China, a preparation of volatile oil fractionated from valerian root was effective in remitting symptoms, decreasing attack frequency, and shortening duration of angina pectoris (heart pain due to restricted blood flow). It aslo demonstrated an ability to lower plasma lipids (Yang et al., 1994).

168. Vetiver oil was found to repel termites and prevent tunnelling with long-lasting effects (Zhu et al., 2001).

169. Methyl salicylate (found in wintergreen or birch oils) was found to inhibit leukotriene C4 (a chemical messenger involved in inflammatory response), while also demonstrating gastroprotective effects against ethanol-induced gastric injury in rats (Trautmann et al., 1991).

170. Subjects using a mouthwash containing thymol, menthol, methyl salicylate, and eucalyptol for 6 months were found to not have developed oral bacteria that were resistant to the oils (Charles et al., 2000).

171. The essential oil of yarrow demonstrated antioxidant and antimicrobial activity against several different pathogenic bacteria and fungi (Candan et al., 2003).

172. In human trials ylang ylang aroma was found to increase calmness (Moss et al., 2008).

173. Subjects who had ylang ylang oil applied to their skin had decreased blood pressure, increased skin temperature, and reported feeling more calm and relaxed compared to subjects in a control group (Hongratanaworakit et al., 2006).

Inhaled ylang ylang oil was found to decrease blood pressure and pulse rate and to enhance attentiveness and alertness in volunteers compared to an odorless control (Hongratanaworakit et al., 2004).

Goodbye to Fibroid Lumps

I had suffered for 32 years with massive fibrocystic breast lumps. They were so painful that I could not even hug my children when they were young. I took vitamin E during those years, which seemed to help. Then I heard about the research done on therapeutic-grade essential oils and breast cancer. I stopped using deodorants with aluminum. I also mixed 40 drops of frankincense essential oil with 4 oz. of pure apricot oil and applied this mixture under my arms during the day as often as I would think about it. Every night before I went to bed, I applied 4–5 drops each of frankincense and lavender to both breasts. A little over 4 weeks later, all fibroid lumps, pain and tenderness were completely gone and have not returned.

-Submitted by Ann Gaither, Corpus Christi, Texas

Special recognition is given to Dr. Ann Blake Tracy for her assistance with this essential oil regimen.

Oil Blends

This section contains proprietary blends and detailed information about each. Other commercial blends exist on the market, but the authors (and many others) find the blends mentioned in this section to be superior in synergy and potency. An approximate frequency is indicated for many of the blends. However, please keep in mind that there are many variables involved in an oil's frequency. Consequently, these numbers may be difficult to duplicate. These product names are all trademarks of Young Living Essential Oils, and although these product names appear throughout other sections of this book without the trademark symbol, they still refer to these same trademarked products.

Abundance™

This blend was specifically designed to enhance **magnetic energy** and to create the law of attraction through the magnetic field around us, to enhance one's thoughts by electrical stimulation of the somatides and the cells, and to put out a frequency charge of **prosperity** and **abundance**. It may **attract riches** to **oneself**. It also contains tremendous **antiviral** and **antifungal** properties, which may make it a very powerful **support** to the **immune system**, possibly giving one an abundance of **health** as well.

Single Oils Contained in This Blend:

- Orange—brings **peace** and **happiness** to the **mind** and **body** and **joy** to the **heart**, which feelings provide **emotional** support.
- Frankincense—contains sesquiterpenes, which may help **oxygenate** the **pineal** and **pituitary glands**. It may help **promote** a **positive attitude**.
- Patchouli—is **sedating, calming**, and **relaxing**—allowing it to reduce **anxiety**. It may have some particular influence on **sex, physical energy**, and **money**.
- Clove—may influence **healing**, improve **memory**, and create a feeling of **protection** and **courage**.
- Ginger—is **warming, uplifting**, and **empowering**. Emotionally, it may help influence **physical energy, love**, and **courage**. Because of its calming influence on the digestive system, it may help reduce feelings of **nausea** and **motion sickness**.
- Myrrh—is part of the formula the Lord gave Moses (Exodus 30:22-27). It is a **true gift**. When we **open** our **hearts** and **minds** to receive the gifts, they will be given.
- Cinnamon Bark—is part of the formula the Lord gave Moses (Exodus 30:22-27). It has very specific purposes: (1) it is a **powerful purifier**, (2) it is a powerful **oxygenator**, and (3) it **enhances** the action and the activity of **other oils**. It may have a **stimulating** and **toning** effect on the whole body and particularly on the circulatory system. It may also help bring about feelings of **joy**.
- Spruce—**grounds** the **body**, creating the **balance** and the **opening** necessary to **receive** and to **give**. It may help **dilate** the **bronchial tract** to **improve** the **oxygen exchange**. It also helps one release **emotional blocks**.

Body System(s) Affected: The oils in this blend may help it be effective for dealing with various problems related to the **Immune** and **Respiratory Systems** and to **Emotional Balance**.

Aromatic Influence: When diffused, this oil creates harmonic energy in the surrounding area.

Application: May be worn on the **wrists**, behind the **ears**, and on the **neck** and **face**. Individuals with sensitive skin may want to dilute the blend with V-6 Oil or Genesis Hand and Body Lotion. May be worn as a **perfume** or **cologne** or placed on your **checkbook, car dash, computer, phone, wallet**, or in your **purse**. Try **cooking** with it. To create more business, add ½ bottle of Abundance to 5 gallons of paint before painting the office.

Safety Data: *Repeated use can result in extreme* **contact sensitization**. *Can be irritating to sensitive* **skin**.

Companion Oils: Acceptance, Awaken, or Release may be used first to help release the emotions that stop us from receiving abundance. It may then be followed by Envision, Into the Future, Joy, Magnify Your Purpose, Motivation, or Live with Passion.

Frequency: Physical; approximately 78 MHz—same frequency as the brain.

Bible: "For as he thinketh in his heart, so [is] he . . ." (Proverbs 23:7). We can create the kind of abundance we want, even that of poverty by believing we can't receive.

Acceptance™

This blend was formulated to help stimulate the mind to open up and **accept new things** in **life**, enabling us to reach toward our higher potential. It may also be beneficial in helping one **overcome denial** or **procrastination** and to help create a feeling of **security**.

Single Oils Contained in This Blend:

Rosewood—is **soothing** to the **skin, appeasing** to the **mind, relaxing** to the **body**, and creates a feeling of **peace** and **gentleness**.

Geranium—may help with **hormonal balance, liver** and **kidney functions**, and the **discharge** of **toxins** from the **liver** that keep us from having balance. Geranium **opens** the **liver chakra** (solar plexus). Note: The liver is the place where fear and anger are stored.

Frankincense—contains sesquiterpenes, which may help **oxygenate** the **pineal** and **pituitary glands**. As one of the ingredients for the holy incense, frankincense was used anciently to help **enhance** one's **communication with the Creator**. It may help **promote** a **positive attitude**.

Blue Tansy—may help **cleanse** the **liver** and **calm** the **lymphatic system** to help rid oneself of **anger** and promote a feeling of **self-control**.

Sandalwood—like frankincense—is high in sesquiterpenes, which were discovered to **increase** the amount of **oxygen** around the **pineal** and **pituitary glands**, thus helping to **improve** one's **attitude**. It **alleviates depression** and assists in the removal of **negative programming** from the cells of the body. It helps one **accept others** with an open heart, while diminishing one's own egocentricity.

Neroli—has been regarded traditionally by the Egyptian people for its great ability to **heal** the **mind, body**, and **spirit**. It is **calming** and **relaxing** to the body and spirit. It may also help to **strengthen** and **stabilize** the emotions and **bring relief** to seemingly hopeless situations. It encourages **confidence, courage, joy, peace**, and **sensuality**.

Carrier Oil Contained in This Blend: Almond oil.

Body System(s) Affected: The oils in this blend may help it be effective for dealing with numerous problems related to the **Nervous System** and **Emotional Balance**. Even when dealing with a physical problem, emotional acceptance of the present situation, rather than denial, helps one move forward in the healing process.

Aromatic Influence: When inhaled or diffused, this blend may help **calm** a troubled mind and promote feelings of **confidence** and **courage**. By calming the raging storms of mental frustration, we are finally capable of viewing our true position in life. We can then accept where we are and move forward with confidence on our path to achieving loftier goals.

Application: Best when rubbed over the **liver** (when the liver is toxic, the mind and emotions are lethargic), behind the **ears**, and on the **chest, face, heart, neck, thymus**, and **wrists**. It may also be applied over the **sacral chakra** (base) and worn as a **perfume** or **cologne**. It can be **diffused** for some great results.

Frequency: Physical and Emotional; approximately 102 MHz.

Aroma Life™

This is a blend of oils that, through extensive research, were found to help **strengthen** and **improve** the **cardiovascular, lymphatic**, and **circulatory systems**. This blend may also help to lower **high blood pressure, reduce stress**, and **alleviate hemorrhoids**.

Oil Blends

Single Oils Contained in This Blend:

Cypress—is **anti-infectious, mucolytic, antiseptic, lymphatic decongestant, refreshing**, and **relaxing**. It may help improve **lung circulation** and relieve other **respiratory problems**.

Marjoram—is **relaxing, calming**, and **appeasing** to the **muscles** that constrict and sometimes contribute to **headaches**.

Helichrysum—may help **cleanse** the **blood** and improve **circulatory functions**. It is **anticatarrhal** in structure and nature. On a spiritual level, it may help one **let go of angry feelings** that prevent one from forgiving and moving forward in life.

Ylang Ylang—may help **balance** the **male-female energies** so one can move closer towards being in **spiritual attunement** and be able to focus their thoughts, filtering out the ever-present garbage.

Carrier Oil Contained in This Blend: Sesame seed oil.

Body System(s) Affected: The oils in this blend may help it be effective for dealing with various problems related to the **Cardiovascular System**.

Application: Best when massaged over the **heart** (left side of the chest). It can be diluted with V-6 Oil for a full-body massage. It can also be applied to the **Vita Flex Heart Points** including, under the **left ring finger** and the **left ring toe**, on the left arm just **above** the **elbow**, and on the **arteries** of the **neck**. It may also help to apply this blend along the spine from the 1st to the 4th thoracic vertebrae, which correspond to the cardiopulmonary nerves (*Refer to the Autonomic Nervous System chart in the Science and Application section of this book*).

Companion Oils: It may be beneficial to combine Joy with this blend when the heart is in stress or combine it with Valor to give the heart courage. Adding some grapefruit oil to this blend may help improve circulation and dissolve fat more quickly. May also add helichrysum, rosemary, or ylang ylang.

Frequency: Physical; approximately 84 MHz.

Comments: This blend may work as a natural hemostat and chelating agent. Red spots on the body may indicate a biotin deficiency. If so, using Super C may be beneficial.

Aroma Siez™

The oils in this blend were selected specifically for their ability to **relax, calm,** and **relieve** the **tension** of **spastic muscles** resulting from **sports injury, fatigue,** or **stress.** This blend may also help to relieve **headaches.**

Single Oils Contained in This Blend:

Basil—has **anti-inflammatory** and **antispasmodic** properties. It is relaxing to **spastic muscles,** including those that contribute to **headaches** and **migraines.**

Marjoram—is an **antispasmodic** and is **relaxing, calming,** and **appeasing** to the **muscles** that constrict and sometimes contribute to **headaches.** It has been useful for **muscle spasms, sprains, bruises, migraines,** and **sore muscles.**

Lavender—is an oil that has traditionally been known to **balance** the **body** and to work wherever there is a need. It has **antispasmodic** and **analgesic** properties. It may help with **sprains, sore muscles, headaches,** and general **healing.**

Peppermint—is an **anti-inflammatory** to the **nerves** and helps **reduce inflammation** in **damaged tissue.** It is **soothing, cooling,** and **dilating** to the **system.** It may help to **reduce fevers, candida, nausea, and vomiting** and help strengthen the **respiratory system.**

Cypress—is **anti-infectious, mucolytic, antiseptic, lymphatic decongestant, refreshing,** and **relaxing.** It may help improve **lung circulation** as well as help relieve other **respiratory problems.** It may also help relieve **muscle cramps** and improve overall **circulation.**

Body System(s) Affected: The oils in this blend may help it be effective for dealing with various problems related to the **Respiratory System** and to **Muscles and Bones.**

Application: Best if applied on location for all **muscles** and on back of **neck** for **stress headaches.** It may also be applied over the **heart** or diluted with V-6 Oil for a full-body **massage.** It is also beneficial when applied to **Vita Flex points** on **feet** or placed in **bathwater.**

Companion Oils: Basil, elemi, helichrysum, Idaho tansy, marjoram, spruce, wintergreen. Ortho Ease Massage Oil or Ortho Sport Massage Oil may also be used to enhance the effects of this blend.

Frequency: Low (Physical); approximately 64 MHz.

Australian Blue™

With a base of blue cypress oil, this blend has an exotic, tropical scent that is **grounding** and **stabilizing,** yet **uplifting** and **inspiring.** Topically, it may help relieve minor **aches** and **pains.** It may help calm **anger** and bring about **self-control** as it balances and stabilizes the **emotions.**

Single Oils Contained in This Blend:

Blue Cypress (*Callitris intratropica*)—is an abundant source of sesquiterpenes. It is the only oil obtained from wood that contains guaiol and guaiazulene, which give it a deep blue color. It is grounding and stabilizing, with a fragrance that uplifts and inspires.

Ylang Ylang—may help **balance** the **male-female energies** so one can move closer towards being in **spiritual attunement** and be able to focus their thoughts, filtering out the ever-present garbage.

Cedarwood—was used traditionally by the North American Indians to enhance their potential for **spiritual communication.** It may help **open** the **pineal gland.**

Blue Tansy—may help **cleanse** the **liver** and **calm** the **lymphatic system** to help rid oneself of **anger** and promote a feeling of **self-control.**

White Fir (*Abies concolor*)—creates a feeling of **grounding, anchoring**, and **empowerment**. It can **stimulate** the **mind** while allowing the **body** to **relax**. Topically, it helps relieve **pain** from **inflammation**.

Body System(s) Affected: **Emotional Balance**.

Aromatic Influence: When diffused, this special blend of oils can be **calming** and **balancing** to the emotions. It may aleviate **stress** and **anger**, relieve **anxiety** and **tension**, and help **relax** the entire body. Mentally, it can be **stimulating** and **inspiring**.

Application: **Diffuse**, wear as **perfume** or **cologne**, or apply topically to areas of concern.

Safety Data: ***Could possibly result in contact sensitization or skin irritation.***

Awaken™

This blend may help **awaken** one to the possibility of their **higher potential**, that they may make the necessary transitions in their lives to achieve greater things. This blend may also be beneficial for **spiritual** and/or **emotional enhancement**.

Oil Blends Contained In This Blend:

Joy—is a blend that may help to open the heart and promote feelings of **self-love** and **love for others** so that one can experience ultimate joy.

Present Time—is a blend of oils that was designed to bring one both mentally and emotionally into the **present time**. In order for us to **awaken** to **our higher potential**, we must be living in the moment "**now,**" not fretting about the past or daydreaming about the future.

Forgiveness—is a blend that was formulated to help move people into a mental state where they can forgive and forget. Inhaling this blend may stimulate one to **forgive themself** and **others** of **transgression**.

Dream Catcher—is an oil blend that was created to **open** the **mind** and to **enhance** one's **dreams**—to help one **visualize** their dreams and **hang onto** them until they become a **reality**.

Harmony—Without **harmony** none of the other states of mind would come to be. We must be in **harmony** with ourselves, with our Creator, and with the world and all those around us. When we have harmony in our lives, then many other things will come to balance and fruition.

Carrier Oil Contained in This Blend: Almond oil.

Body System(s) Affected: The oils in this blend may help it be effective for dealing with various problems related to **Emotional Balance**.

Aromatic Influence: We enjoy diffusing this blend while we are sleeping at night because it helps us wake up feeling **invigorated** and **refreshed**.

Application: Best when applied on the **chest, heart, forehead, neck, sternum** (clearing allergies), **temples**, and **wrists**. It may be used as an **aftershave**, a **cologne**, or a **perfume**. It may also be diluted with V-6 Oil for a **full-body massage** or added to the **bathwater**. En-R-Gee may be put on the feet and Awaken on the temples or cheeks for one to feel like they have had eight hours of sleep.

Companion Oils: Dream Catcher, En-R-Gee, Envision, Harmony, Into the Future, Joy, Motivation, Live with Passion, Valor, White Angelica

Frequency: Physical; approximately 89 MHz.

Believe™

This blend has been specifically formulated to calm and ground the spirit while stimulating the mind, allowing us to believe in our own limitless potential to create and improve in an atmospher of peace and awareness. It is **grounding** and **empowering**, helping to promote positive action toward the accomplishment of goals and fulfillment of dreams.

Single Oils Contained in This Blend:

Idaho Balsam Fir—creates a feeling of **grounding, anchoring**, and **empowerment**. It can **stimulate** the **mind** while allowing the **body** to **relax**. Topically, it helps relieve **overworked** and **tired muscles** and **joints**.

Coriander—is **balancing** to the emotions, and may help soothe **stress** and **anxiety**.

Bergamot—may help to **relieve anxiety, depression, stress**, and **tension**. It is **uplifting** and **refreshing**.

Frankincense—contains sesquiterpenes, which may help **oxygenate** the **pineal** and **pituitary glands**. As one of the ingredients for the holy incense, frankincense was used anciently to help **enhance** one's **communication with the Creator**. It may help **promote** a **positive attitude**.

Idaho Blue Spruce—may help **ground** the body, creating the feeling of **balance** necessary to receive and to give. Helps release **emotional blocks**.

Ylang Ylang (Amazonian)—may help **harmonize** and **balance** the mind and emotions. It is **peaceful**, and **calming**, and may help increase **attentiveness** and **alertness**.

Geranium—may also help **ease nervous tension** and **stress, balance** the **emotions, lift** the **spirit**, and foster **peace, well-being**, and **hope**. It may also help lower defenses that prevent individuals from being **open** and **receptive to new ideas**.

Body System(s) Affected: The oils in this blend may help it be effective for dealing with various problems related to the **Nervous** and **Immune Systems, Muscles and Bones**, and to **Emotional Balance**.

Aromatic Influence: This blend of oils has a **calming, stabilizing**, and **mentally-energizing** aroma. Diffusing this blend may help to **release** the unlimited **potential** to **create** and to **improve** our surroundings. The mentally uplifting and energizing aroma may help **promote belief** in ourselves and our capabilities.

Application: **Diffuse**, or apply 2–4 drops to the **forehead, temples**, and over the **heart**. May also be worn as a **perfume** or **cologne**.

Companion Oils: frankincense, sacred frankincense, palmarosa, orange, Abundance

Safety Data: ***Can be irritating to young or sensitive skin.***

Brain Power™

This blend has been specifically formulated to include those oils that are high in sesquiterpene compounds. Research has shown that sesquiterpenes play a role in **dissolving petrochemicals** along the receptor sites near the **pituitary, pineal**, and **hypothalamus**. This helps to increase normal receptivity along those sites and increase the amount of oxygen in those areas. **Increased oxygen** around the pineal, pituitary, and hypothalamus can lead to **increased mental capacity, mental clarity**, and **reduced symptoms** of what has come to be known as "**brain fog.**"

Single Oils Contained in This Blend:

Sandalwood—like frankincense—is high in sesquiterpenes, which were discovered to **increase** the amount of **oxygen** around the **pineal** and **pituitary glands**, thus helping to **improve** one's **at-**

titude. It alleviates depression and assists in the removal of negative programming from the cells of the body. It helps one accept others with an open heart, while diminishing one's own egocentricity.

Cedarwood—was used traditionally by the North American Indians to enhance their potential for spiritual communication. It may help open the pineal gland.

Melissa—is powerful as an antiviral agent, yet it is very gentle and very delicate because of the nature of the plant. It has the ability to work with and enhance the gentle aspects of the human body. It is calming and uplifting and may also help to balance the emotions. It may help to remove emotional blocks and instill a positive outlook on life.

Frankincense—contains sesquiterpenes, which may help oxygenate the pineal and pituitary glands. As one of the ingredients for the holy incense, frankincense was used anciently to help enhance one's communication with the Creator. It may help promote a positive attitude.

Blue Cypress (*Callitris intratropica*)—comes from Australia and has been shown to improve circulation and increase the flow of oxygen to the brain.

Lavender—is an oil that has traditionally been known to balance the body and to work wherever there is a need. It has antispasmodic and analgesic properties. It may help with sprains, sore muscles, headaches, and general healing.

Helichrysum—may help cleanse the blood and improve circulatory functions. It is anticatarrhal in structure and nature. On a spiritual level, it may help one let go of angry feelings that prevent one from forgiving and moving forward in life.

Body System(s) Affected: The oils in this blend may help it be effective for dealing with various problems related to the Nervous System and to Emotional Balance.

Aromatic Influence: This blend of oils has a powerfully-uplifting and mentally-energizing aroma. Diffusing this blend may help to provide deep concentration and focus during strenuous mental activity.

Application: May be applied to the neck, throat, under the nose, or to the roof of the mouth using the thumb, or it may be worn as a perfume or cologne. May also be applied inside the mouth with a finger, either under the tongue or on the inside of each cheek (*See* SMELL *in the Personal Guide section of this book*).

Companion Oils: Clarity, Envision, RC, Raven

Frequency: Physical; approximately 78 MHz–same frequency as the brain.

Breathe Again™

(Essential Oil Roll-On)

This blend was specially formulated to promote healthy respiration. With the blend's combination of four different eucalyptus oils, its main functions are to help support immune system function and to open the nasal passages to help clear up nasal congestion. Because this blend is offered as a roll-on, it provides a no-mess application in just about any situation. With the small, steel ball applicator, it delivers a precise amount of oil with no runs or drips and no need to rub it in with a finger.

Single Oils Contained in This Blend:

Eucalyptus staigeriana—is analgesic, antifungal, antiviral, anti-inflammatory, antiseptic, purifying, and antiseptic. It may help with bronchitis, colds, congestion, infections, and fevers.

Eucalyptus globulus—promotes health, well-being, purification, and healing. It also has strong antibacterial, anticatarrhal, and antiseptic properties.

Laurel—is **antiseptic, diuretic,** and **antifungal**. It may help with **asthmatic conditions** and with **chronic bronchitis**.

Rose hip—is **antiseptic, antioxidant,** and **astringent**. It promotes **tissue regeneration** and helps to retard **premature aging**.

Peppermint—is **antiseptic, antispasmodic**, and **anti-inflammatory**. It is **soothing, cooling**, and **dilating** to the **system** and may help with **asthma, bronchitis, flu,** and **respiratory function**.

Eucalyptus radiata—may have a profound **antiviral** effect upon the **respiratory system**. It may also help reduce **inflammation** of the **nasal mucous membrane**.

Copal (or Copaiba)—is extremely high in β-caryophyllene, which has been well documented for its **anti-inflammatory** actions. It may help with **colds, bacterial infections, sinusitis, sore throats,** and **respiratory problems**.

Myrtle—is a **decongestant** of the **respiratory system**. It may help **improve oxygenation** and work as an **expectorant** in **discharging mucus**. It is **antiseptic , antibacterial, euphoric,** and **elevating**.

Manuka—is **antiallergic, antiviral, antihistamine,** and **decongestant**. It may help with **colds, bronchitis, sinusitis, hay fever,** and **asthma**. Its **stabilizing** and **calming** aroma makes it very good for combating **stress** and **irritability**.

Eucalyptus blue—is **invigorating** and brings a sense of **peace** and **balance**. The high **cineol** content helps promote **proper respiratory function**.

Carrier Oils Contained In This Blend: Coconut oil

Body System(s) Affected: The oils in this blend may be helpful for dealing with problems relating to the **Respiratory** and **Immune Systems**.

Aromatic Influence: This blend helps to **revive** and **invigorate the senses**.

Application: May be applied every fifteen minutes to either the **chest** or under the **nose**. Limit use to four applications.

Safety Data: ***Can be irritating to sensitive skin. Use with caution during pregnancy. Do not use on or near eyes or mucus membranes. Keep out of reach of children.***

Christmas Spirit™

This blend is effective for enhancing the **feeling** and **memory** of the beautiful times of **Christmas** and for enhancing the desire to be in that happy and joyful moment that Christmas brings. It may be very beneficial for **protecting** against **airborne viruses** and **bacteria** because it contains several very powerful **antiviral** and **antiseptic** oils. It may also be quite **soothing** and **healing** to the **respiratory system**.

Single Oils Contained in This Blend:

Orange—spreads a little sunshine on gloomy thoughts and depression. It may help encourage a positive outlook on life, bringing **peace** and **happiness** to the mind and body. Orange is **antiseptic** and **antidepressant**.

Cinnamon Bark—is part of the formula the Lord gave Moses (Exodus 30:22-27). It has very specific purposes: (1) it is a **powerful purifier**, (2) it is a powerful **oxygenator**, and (3) it **enhances** the action and the activity of **other oils**. It may have a **stimulating** and **toning** effect on the whole body and particularly on the circulatory system. It may also help bring about feelings of **joy**. It is **antiseptic, antibacterial**, and **antiviral**.

Spruce—**grounds** the **body**, creating the balance and opening necessary to receive and to give. This oil is **warming, healing, uplifting**, and **soothing**. It may also help **relieve anxiety** and act as an **antiseptic**.

Body System(s) Affected: The oils in this blend may help it be effective for dealing with various problems related to the **Cardiovascular** and **Nervous Systems** and to **Emotional Balance**.

Aromatic Influence: This blend of oils has a delightful **fragrance** and is wonderful for creating the **feeling** of **security** that usually accompanies the **holiday season**. It is also nice for **air purification**.

Application: May be applied to the **crown** of the **head** or worn as a **perfume** or **cologne**. The beautiful fragrance of this blend can be further enhanced by placing it on pine boughs, pine cones, cedar chips, and on logs to burn in the fireplace. It makes an excellent addition to potpourri.

Safety Data: ***Repeated use on the skin can result in extreme contact sensitivity. Can cause extreme skin irritation.***

Companion Oils: Mandarin, clove, and nutmeg.

Frequency: Emotional and Spiritual; approximately 104 MHz.

Citrus Fresh™

Citrus Fresh is a blend that may help to enhance the **feeling** of **well-being** in **children**. Because many of the oils contained in this blend are strong **antiseptics**, it may work well for **killing airborne bacteria**. It may be useful for **relaxing, calming**, and for alleviating **insomnia**. It may also help to **balance** the **systems**. It is a fragrance that can be enjoyed by everyone. Flavoring drinking water with this oil blend may help **open** the **lymphatic system** and **stimulate** the **immune system**.

Single Oils Contained in This Blend:

Orange—brings **peace** and **happiness** to the **mind** and **body** and **joy** to the **heart**, which feelings provide **emotional** support to help one overcome depression.

Tangerine—contains esters and aldehydes, which are **sedating** and **calming** to the **nervous system**. It is also a **diuretic** and a **decongestant** of the **lymphatic system**.

Mandarin—is **appeasing, gentle**, and promotes **happiness**. It is also **refreshing, uplifting**, and **revitalizing**. Because of its sedative and slightly hypnotic properties, it is very good for **stress** and **irritability**.

Grapefruit—is an **antidepressant**, an **antiseptic**, and a **diuretic**. It is **balancing** and **uplifting** to the mind and may help to **relieve anxiety**.

Lemon—promotes **health, healing, physical energy**, and **purification**. Its fragrance is **invigorating, enhancing**, and **warming**.

Spearmint—is **antifungal** and **antiseptic**. It also acts as an **antidepressant** by **relieving mental strain and fatigue** and by **lifting** one's **spirits**.

Body System(s) Affected: The oils in this blend may help it be effective for dealing with various problems related to the **Immune System** and to **Emotional Balance**.

Aromatic Influence: This blend of oils may create an enjoyable aromatic fragrance in the **home** or **workplace**. Simple diffusion can be achieved by applying a few drops of this blend on a cotton ball and placing it on the desk at work or in an air vent.

Application: May be applied on the **ears, heart**, and **wrists** or worn as a **perfume** or **cologne**. It may be diluted with V-6 Oil for a **full-body massage**. It may also be added to water for a **relaxing bath**. This blend can also help **purify drinking water**. Children may like to add this blend to water and freeze it to make **popsicles**. It is excellent for children, though dilution with V-6 Oil is highly recommended.

Safety Data: ***Can cause extreme skin irritation. Avoid exposure to direct sunlight for up to 12 hours after use.***

Frequency: Physical and Emotional; approximately 90 MHz.

Comments: A university in Japan experimented with diffusing different oils in the office. When they diffused lemon there were 54% fewer errors made in the office, with jasmine there were 33% fewer errors, and with lavender there were 20% fewer errors. When oils are diffused while students are studying for a test and then the same oils are smelled during the test via a hanky, cotton ball, or plastic nasal inhaler, test scores may increase by as much as 50%. Different oils should be used for different tests, but the same oil should be used during the test as was used while studying for that particular test. The smell of the oil may help bring back the memory of what was studied.

Clarity™

This blend may help with **memory retention** and **mental alertness**; it may even help **oxygenate** the **brain**. One may want to **study** with this blend diffusing and then smell this same blend during the test to help recall what was studied earlier. It may also be a **stimulant** for **low energy** and may help keep one from going into **shock**.

Single Oils Contained in This Blend:

Basil—has been found beneficial for **alleviating mental fatigue**. It may help **sharpen** the **senses** and **encourage concentration**. It may also **stimulate** the **nerves** and the **adrenal cortex**.

Cardamom—is **uplifting**, **refreshing**, and **invigorating**. It may be beneficial for **clearing confusion**.

Rosemary verbenon—may help **balance heart function**, **energize** the **solar plexus**, and **reduce mental fatigue**. It also stimulates **memory** and opens the **conscious mind**.

Peppermint—is an **anti-inflammatory** to the **nerves** and helps **reduce inflammation** in **damaged tissue**. It is **soothing**, **cooling**, and **dilating** to the **system**. Dr. Dembar, of the University of Cincinnati, discovered in a research study that inhaling peppermint oil **increased** the **mental accuracy** of the students tested by up to 28%.

Rosewood—may help improve **skin elasticity**. It is **soothing** to the **skin**, **appeasing** to the **mind**, **relaxing** to the **body**, and creates a feeling of **peace** and **gentleness**.

Geranium—may help with **hormonal balance**, **liver** and **kidney functions**, and the **discharge** of **toxins** from the **liver** that keep us from having balance. Geranium **opens** the **liver chakra**.

Lemon—promotes **health**, **healing**, **physical energy**, and **purification**. Its fragrance is **invigorating**, **enhancing**, and **warming**.

Palmarosa—is valuable for all types of **skin** problems because it **stimulates** new **cell growth**, regulates oil production, **moisturizes**, and **speeds healing**.

Ylang Ylang—may help **balance** the **male-female energies** so one can move closer towards being in **spiritual attunement** and be able to focus their thoughts, filtering out the ever-present garbage and establishing a sense of relaxation. It brings back feelings of **self-love**, **confidence**, **joy**, and **peace**.

Bergamot—is **soothing** to the **endocrine system** and to the **hormones**. It may **uplift** and **calm** the **emotions** and help relieve **anxiety**, **stress**, and **tension**.

Roman Chamomile—neutralizes **allergies** and helps to cleanse the **blood** and **expel toxins** from the **liver**.

Jasmine—is very **uplifting** to the **emotions**; it may produce a feeling of **confidence, energy, euphoria**, and **optimism**. As an **antispasmodic**, it has been used effectively for **menstrual** discomfort, **muscle spasms**, and **uterine** disorders.

Body System(s) Affected: The oils in this blend may help it be effective for dealing with various problems related to the **Nervous System** and to **Emotional Balance**.

Aromatic Influence: The oils in this blend are known for their ability to help increase **mental alertness**. Simple diffusion can be achieved by applying a few drops of this blend on a cotton ball and placing it on the desk at work or in an air vent. *Plastic nasal inhalers are also available from Abundant Health for more discreet, direct, and long-lasting personal use.*

Application: Best when applied across the **brow**, on the back of the **neck**, on the **temples**, and on the **wrists**. This blend may be added to one's **bathwater** or worn as a **perfume** or **cologne**.

Safety Data: ***Can be irritating to sensitive* skin*. Use with caution during* pregnancy*. Avoid exposure to direct* sunlight *for up to 12 hours after use.***

Companion Oils: This blend and En-R-Gee together may help one stay awake while driving late at night. Others include Brain Power, lemon, and peppermint.

Frequency: Emotional; approximately 101 MHz.

Comments: Since this blend contains cardamom and high levels of transphenol, it may cause headaches when inhaled if there is petrochemical or heavy metal accumulation in the brain.

Oil Blends

Common Sense™

This blend has been specially formulated from essential oils that can help individuals remain **calm** and **relaxed**, helping to enhance **clarity of thought** and **rational decision making**.

Single Oils Contained in This Blend:

Frankincense—This oil has sedative and antidepressant properties that may help reduce stress in individuals.

Ylang Ylang—This oil has **calming** and **sedative** properties and may help to **relax** and to **reduce anger**.

Ocotea—This oil has **anti-inflammatory** properties to help enhance the optimal functioning of the body.

Goldenrod—is **relaxing** and **calming** and may help relieve **nervousness**.

Rue—is **relaxing** to the body and mind and can help **calm stressed nerves** and promote better **sleep**.

Dorado Azul—This oil may help **balance** the **hormonal system** and modulate **brain function**. It also has **anti-inflammatory** properties.

Lime—This oil has a **stimulating** and **uplifting** aroma that can help one overcome feelings of **exhaustion** and **depression**.

Body System(s) Affected: The oils in this blend may help it be effective for dealing with various problems related to the **Nervous System** and to **Emotional Balance**.

Aromatic Influence: The oils in this blend are known to be **calming** and **relaxing**, helping to balance irrational thinking and rash decisions. Simple diffusion can be achieved by applying a few drops of this blend on a cotton ball and placing it on the desk at work or in an air vent. *Plastic nasal inhalers are also available from Abundant Health for more discreet, direct, and long-lasting personal use.*

Application: **Diffuse** into the air or place on a cotton ball or ribbon and attach to an air vent. **Inhale** directly. Dilute heavily for topical use.

Safety Data: ***Keep out of the reach of children. Use with caution during* pregnancy*. Consult with healthcare professional before use if you are nursing, taking medication, or if you have a pre-existing medical condition exists.***

Companion Oils: This blend works well with Brain Power, Clarity, and peppermint.

Deep Relief™

(Essential Oil Roll-On)

This blend contains a powerful combination of essential oils that are highly regarded for their anti-inflammatory properties. These oils have been formulated in such a way as to provide deep and lasting relief for **sore muscles, joints,** and **ligaments, stressed nerves**, and **tension headaches**. This blend may also help with **sports injuries, sprains, muscle spasms, bumps**, and **bruises**. Because this blend is offered as a roll-on, it provides a no-mess application in just about any situation. With the small, steel ball applicator, it delivers a precise amount of oil with no runs or drips and no need to rub it in with a finger.

Single Oils Contained in This Blend:

Peppermint—is **anti-inflammatory** to the **nerves** and helps **reduce inflammation** in **damaged tissue**. It is **soothing, cooling**, and **dilating** to the **system**. It **enhances** the effects of other oils in a blend and helps the entire blend to quickly **penetrate** the tissues of the body.

Lemon—is an **astringent** and **tonic**. It promotes **health, healing, physical energy**, and **purification**. Its fragrance is **invigorating, enhancing**, and **warming**. It has historically been used for **arthritis** and **muscle soreness**.

Balsam Fir—creates a feeling of **grounding, anchoring**, and **empowerment**. It can **stimulate** the **mind** while allowing the **body** to **relax**. Topically, it helps relieve **overworked** and **tired muscles** and **joints**.

Copal (or Copaiba)—is extremely high in β-caryophyllene, which has been well documented for its **anti-inflammatory** actions. It has traditionally been used for **muscle aches and pains, stiffness**, and **nervous exhaustion**.

Clove—is **anti-infectious, anti-inflammatory, strongly antiseptic, disinfectant, immune-stimulant**, and **topically analgesic**. It is also good for **arthritis** and **rheumatism** where penetrating pain relief is needed.

Wintergreen—contains 99% methyl salicylate, which gives it cortisone-like properties. It may be beneficial for **arthritis, rheumatism, tendinitis**, and any other discomfort that is related to the inflammation of **bones, muscles**, and **joints**.

Helichrysum—may help **cleanse** the **blood** and improve **circulatory functions**. It is **anticatarrhal** in structure and nature. As a powerful **anti-inflammatory**, it may even help reduce inflammation in the meninges of the brain.

Vetiver—is **antispasmodic** and locally **warming**. Vetiver has also been valuable for relieving **stress** and helping people recover from **emotional traumas** and **shock**.

Palo Santo—promotes healing and helps to relieve **muscle pain, nervous conditions**, and acute **rheumatism**. Historically it was used to diffuse **negative energy**.

Carrier Oils Contained In This Blend: Fractionated coconut oil and virgin coconut oil.

Body System(s) Affected: The oils in this blend may help it be effective for dealing with various problems related to the **Nervous System** and to **Muscles and Bones**.

Application: Apply on location for **muscles, cramps, bruises**, or any place that hurts. For **tension headaches**, apply across the **brow**, on the back of the **neck**, and on the **temples**.

Companion Oils: Add helichrysum (to enhance) or wintergreen (for bone pain), or use with Ortho Ease or Ortho Sport Massage Oil.

Di-Gize™

This blend may be useful for **improving digestive function**. The oils in this blend have been found to be beneficial in **digesting toxic material** and for **alleviating indigestion, stomach cramps, upset stomach, belching, bloating**, and **heartburn**. Placing a little of this blend behind the ears may help alleviate **morning sickness**. It has been found to rid animals and people of **parasites** when applied to their feet. It has also been reported that this blend helps to alleviate discomfort from **parasites** by massage and compress application across the stomach.

Single Oils Contained in This Blend:

Tarragon—may help to reduce **anorexia, dyspepsia, flatulence, intestinal spasms, nervous** and **sluggish digestion**, and **genital or urinary tract infections**.

Ginger—is **warming, uplifting**, and **empowering**. Emotionally, it may help influence **physical energy, love**, and **courage**. Because of its calming influence on the digestive system, it may help reduce feelings of **nausea** and **motion sickness**.

Peppermint—is an **anti-inflammatory** to the **prostate** and **nerves**. It is **soothing, cooling** and **dilating** to the **system**. It may also be beneficial when dealing with **food poisoning, vomiting, diarrhea, constipation, flatulence, halitosis, colic, nausea**, and **motion sickness**.

Juniper—has **antiseptic, cleansing**, and **detoxifying** properties. It may help to **improve circulation** through the **kidneys**.

Fennel—may help **improve digestive function** by **supporting** the **liver**. It may also help **balance** the **hormones**.

Lemongrass—is **vasodilatory, antiseptic, antibacterial, anti-inflammatory**, and **sedative**. It may help improve **circulation**, wake up the **lymphatic system**, and increase the flow of **oxygen**. It may also help to **lift** the **spirit**.

Anise—may help **calm** and **strengthen** the **digestive system**.

Patchouli—is **sedating, calming**, and **relaxing**, allowing it to reduce **anxiety**. It is a digester of toxic material in the body.

Body System(s) Affected: The oils in this blend may help it be effective for dealing with various problems related to the **Digestive System**.

Application: May be applied to the **Vita Flex points** on the **feet** and **ankles**. It may also be applied topically over the **stomach**, as a **compress** on the **abdomen**, on other **Vita Flex points** on the **body**, and at the bottom of the **throat** (for gagging). As a **dietary supplement**, dilute one drop in 4 oz. of water or soy/rice milk and sip slowly. May also be used in a **retention enema** for ridding the **colon** of **parasites** and for combating **digestive candida**. Apply to **animal paws** for **parasites**.

Safety Data: *Use with caution during* ***pregnancy*** *(only a drop massaged on the outer ear for morning sickness). Not for use by people with* ***epilepsy****.*

Companion Oils: Peppermint and spearmint.

Companion Supplements: ComforTone, Essentialzyme, JuvaTone

Frequency: Emotional; approximately 102 MHz.

Dragon Time™

This is a blend of single oils that have historically been used to help **alleviate premenstrual** and **menstrual cramps** and discomfort. This blend may also help **men** with **prostate** problems.

Single Oils Contained in This Blend:

Clary Sage—is beneficial for **regulating cells** and **balancing** the **hormones**. It may help with **menstrual cramps, PMS**, and **premenopause** symptoms. It may also help with **circulatory problems**.

Fennel—may help **improve digestive function** by **supporting** the **liver**. It may also help **balance** the **hormones**.

Lavender—is an oil that has traditionally been known to **balance** the **body** and to work wherever there is a need. It may help with **PMS/menopausal problems, stress, stretch marks, tension**, and **water retention**.

Marjoram—is **relaxing, calming**, and **appeasing** to the **muscles** that constrict and sometimes contribute to **headaches**.

Yarrow—is a **powerful decongestant** of the **prostate** and a **hormone balancer**.

Jasmine—is very **uplifting** to the **emotions**; it may produce a feeling of **confidence, energy, euphoria**, and **optimism**. As an **antispasmodic**, it has been used for **menstrual** discomfort, **muscle spasms**, and **uterine** disorders.

Body System(s) Affected: The oils in this blend may help it be effective for dealing with various problems related to the **Hormonal System** and to **Emotional Balance**.

Aromatic Influence: This blend of oils may be beneficial in times of **hormonal stress**. It may be diffused in the home or office, or a few drops can be placed on a cotton ball and be put in the car vent.

Application: May be applied to the **Vita Flex points** on the **feet** and around the **ankles**, both inside and out. It may be diluted with V-6 Oil for application on the other **Vita Flex points** on the **body**. It may also be applied as a hot **compress** or rubbed over the **abdomen**, across the **lower back**, or anywhere it **hurts**.

Safety Data: *Use with caution during* ***pregnancy***.

Companion Oils: Combining this blend with <u>Mister</u> or <u>EndoFlex</u> may help **alleviate hot flashes (power surges)** in women.

Frequency: Physical; approximately 72 MHz.

Dream Catcher™

This blend may help to open the **mind**, to **enhance dreams**, and to help one **visualize** their **dreams** and **hang onto** them until they become **reality**. It may also serve to **protect** one from the **negative dreams** that tend to steal our **vision**. Children love the smell of this blend, and it may even help them to sleep more soundly. Our little girl asked for this blend every night for a while, until she felt comfortable with sleeping in her own bed. Later, if she was having a bad dream, she would come ask for some to be put on her forehead and would go right back to bed and sleep soundly for the rest of the night.

Single Oils Contained in This Blend:

Sandalwood—like frankincense—is high in sesquiterpenes, which were discovered to **increase** the amount of **oxygen** around the **pineal** and **pituitary glands**, thus helping to **improve** one's **attitude**. It **alleviates depression** and assists in the removal of **negative programming** from the cells of the body.

Tangerine—contains esters and aldehydes, which are **sedating** and **calming** to the **nervous system**. It is also a **diuretic** and a **decongestant** of the **lymphatic system**.

Ylang Ylang—may help **balance** the **male-female energies** so one can move closer towards being in **spiritual attunement** and be able to focus their thoughts, filtering out the ever-present garbage. It brings back feelings of **self-love, confidence, joy,** and **peace**.

Pepper, Black—may help **stimulate** the **endocrine system** and **increase energy**. It may also help **increase cellular oxygenation**.

Bergamot—is **soothing** to the **endocrine system** and to the **hormones**. It may **uplift** and **calm** the **emotions** and help relieve **anxiety, stress**, and **tension**.

Juniper—evokes feelings of **health, love**, and **peace** and may help to **elevate** one's **spiritual awareness**.

Anise—may help **calm** and **strengthen** the **digestive system**.

Blue Tansy—encourages an **uplifting feeling**, a **positive attitude**, and a general sense of **well-being**.

Body System(s) Affected: The oils in this blend may help it be effective for dealing with various problems related to **Emotional Balance**.

Aromatic Influence: This blend may be diffused during the day, but it seems to be most effective during sleep. This blend may also be useful during **meditation**.

Application: Best when applied to the **forehead** (3rd **eye** or **brow chakra**), **eye brows, temples**, behind the **ears**, and on the **throat chakra** (base of neck). It may be worn as a **perfume** or **cologne**. For a lasting aroma, place a drop under the **nose** or on the **pillow**. Add to **bathwater**.

Safety Data: *Avoid exposure to direct* **sunlight** *for 3 to 6 hours after use.*

Companion Oils: To enhance **dream awareness**, put a couple drops of this blend on a **pillow**, Awaken on the **temples**, and Motivation on the **chest**. Other choices include Envision, Gathering, Into the Future, and Live with Passion.

Frequency: Physical and Emotional; approximately 98 MHz.

Comments: Indian dream catchers have been used to help keep bad dreams away. This blend may accomplish the same purpose. However, if bad dreams do come, continued use of this oil may be necessary as something in the subconscious may need to be processed. Hold onto your dreams, and visualize them into reality by bringing them from the mind to the heart to make them come true.

Egyptian Gold™

This special blend was formulated with oils that were used for various purposes in ancient Egypt, including mummification. Blended specifically to combat the "super bugs," the oils in this blend are highly **antibacterial, antifungal**, and **antiviral**. This blend may help stimulate the **hypothalamus** and **pituitary glands**. Its intoxicating fragrance is reminiscent of the grandeur of ancient Egypt. **Note**: The commercial availability of this blend may be somewhat erratic due to the occasional unavailability of some of the oils (i.e. hyssop).

Single Oils Contained in This Blend:

Frankincense—contains sesquiterpenes, which may help **oxygenate** the **pineal** and **pituitary glands**. As one of the ingredients for the holy incense, frankincense was used anciently to help **enhance** one's **communication with the Creator**. It was considered a prize possession and was given to Christ at his birth. It may help **promote** a **positive attitude**.

Lavender—is an oil that has traditionally been known to **balance** the **body** and to work wherever there is a need. It may help with **stress and tension**.

Balsam Fir—creates a feeling of **grounding, anchoring**, and **empowerment**. It can **stimulate** the **mind** while allowing the **body** to **relax**. Topically, it helps relieve **overworked** and **tired muscles** and **joints**.

Myrrh—is part of the formula the Lord gave Moses (Exodus 30:22-27). It is a **true gift**. When we **open** our **hearts** and **minds** to receive the gifts, they will be given.

Spikenard—was highly prized in the Middle East during the time of Christ and is referred to several times in the Bible. It is **antifungal, anti-inflammatory, relaxing, regenerative**, and helpful for allergic skin reactions.

Hyssop—was used by Moses during the Lord's Passover in Egypt (Exodus 12). It has **anti-inflammatory** and **antiviral** properties. It may also have the ability to **open** up the **respiratory system** and **discharge toxins** and **mucus**.

Cedarwood—was used traditionally by the North American Indians to enhance their potential for **spiritual communication**. It may help **open** the **pineal gland**.

Rose—possesses the highest frequency of any oil. It may help **enhance** the **frequency** of every cell, which could help bring **balance** and **harmony** to the body. It is thought by some to produce a magnetic energy that attracts **love** and enhances the frequency of **self-love**, bringing **joy** to the heart.

Cinnamon Bark—is part of the formula the Lord gave Moses (Exodus 30:22-27). It has very specific purposes: (1) it is a **powerful purifier**, (2) it is a powerful **oxygenator**, and (3) it **enhances** the action and the activity of **other oils**. It may have a **stimulating** and **toning** effect on the whole body and particularly on the circulatory system. It is **antiseptic, antibacterial**, and **antiviral**.

Body System(s) Affected: The oils in this blend may help it be effective for dealing with various problems related to the **Immune System** and to **Emotional Balance**.

Aromatic Influence: This blend of oils may help **lift** and **balance** one's **emotions**. It is also **stabilizing** and **empowering**. Simple diffusion can be achieved by applying a few drops of this blend on a cotton ball and placing it in the air vent of a car or on the heat registers of the home or hotel room.

Application: Best when applied on the **wrists** and behind and on the **ears**. It may also be massaged across the **base** of the **neck** and **temples**. Dilute with V-6 Oil to wear as a **perfume** or **cologne**.

Safety Data: ***Could possibly result in contact sensitization. Use with caution if susceptible to epilepsy.***

Companion Oils: Sandalwood.

En-R-Gee™

En-R-Gee is a blend that may help **improve one's energy** in a natural way without overstimulating or creating problems that may be uncomfortable. It may also help with **mental alertness**.

Single Oils Contained in This Blend:

Rosemary cineol—may help **balance heart function, energize** the **solar plexus**, and **reduce mental fatigue**.

Juniper—has **antiseptic, cleansing**, and **detoxifying** properties. It may help to **improve circulation** through the **kidneys**.

Lemongrass—is **vasodilatory, antiseptic, antibacterial, anti-inflammatory**, and **sedative**. It may help improve **circulation**, wake up the **lymphatic system**, and increase the flow of **oxygen**. It may also help to **lift** the **spirit**.

Nutmeg—has adrenal cortex–like activity, which helps support the **adrenal glands** for **increased energy**.

Balsam Fir—creates a feeling of **grounding, anchoring**, and **empowerment**. Topically, it helps relieve **overworked** and **tired muscles** and **joints**.

Clove—may influence **healing**, improve **memory**, and create a feeling of **protection** and **courage**. It may also help one overcome **fatigue**.

Pepper, Black—may help **stimulate** the **endocrine system** and **increase energy**.

Body System(s) Affected: The oils in this blend may help it be effective for dealing with various problems related to the **Nervous System** and to **Emotional Balance**.

Aromatic Influence: This blend of oils may help boost one's **energy** when diffused. It is also **purifying**. Simple diffusion can be achieved by applying a few drops of this blend on a cotton ball and placing it in the air vent of a car or on the heat registers of the home or hotel room.

Application: Best when applied to the **wrists** and behind and on the **ears**. It may also be massaged across the **base** of the **neck** and on the **temples** and be rubbed on the **feet** in the morning. Dilute with V-6 Oil for **full-body massage**, or wear as a **perfume** or **cologne**.

Safety Data: ***Can cause extreme skin irritation. Use with caution if susceptible to epilepsy.***

Companion Oils: One may feel like they have had eight hours of sleep by rubbing this blend on the feet and Awaken on the **temples**. This blend and Clarity together may help one stay awake while driving late at night.

Frequency: Emotional; approximately 106 MHz.

Endoflex™

This is a beautiful blend that may help provide overall **balance** and **support** to the **endocrine system** and may work to **improve** the **vitality** of the body. It may **support** the **pineal** and **pituitary** glands, **parathyroid**, **thymus**, and **adrenal** glands. It may also help **alleviate hot flashes** and **stimulate weight loss** by **improving metabolic function**. It may support the **thyroid** for **metabolic** and **hormonal balance**.

Single Oils Contained in This Blend:

Spearmint—is an oil that may balance and increase **metabolism**, helping to **burn up fats** and **toxins** in the body.

Sage—may help improve **estrogen** and **progesterone-testosterone balance**. It is believed to contain elements that contribute to the **secretion** of **progesterone-testosterone**.

Geranium—may help with **hormonal balance**, **liver** and **kidney functions**, and the **discharge** of **toxins** from the **liver** that keep us from having balance. Geranium **opens** the **liver chakra**.

Myrtle—may help **regulate thyroid function**. For **hypo-thyroid**, it may **increase activity** and **improve balance**.

Nutmeg—has adrenal cortex–like activity, which helps support the **adrenal glands** for **increased energy**.

German Chamomile—has been found to help **open** the **liver**, **increase liver function** and **secretion**, and **support** the **pancreas**.

Carrier Oil Contained in This Blend: Sesame seed oil.

Body System(s) Affected: The oils in this blend may help it be effective for dealing with various problems related to the **Hormonal (Endocrine) System**.

Application: May be applied over the **thyroid**, **kidneys**, **liver** (front right, 2" down from bra line), **pancreas** (front left), and all **glands**. It may also work well when applied to the **Vita Flex points** on the **feet**, including under the **big toe** and on the **throat** or **endocrine gland locations**.

Safety Data: ***Can be irritating to sensitive skin. Use with caution if susceptible to epilepsy.***

Frequency: Emotional and Spiritual; approximately 138 MHz.

Envision™

This blend is comprised of essential oils that provide powerful **support** and **balance** to the **emotions.** This type of emotional support is necessary for us to move forward with renewed faith in the future toward **achieving** our **dreams** and **goals.**

Single Oils Contained in This Blend:

Spruce—**grounds** the **body**, creating the **balance** and the **opening** necessary to **receive** and to **give.** It may help **dilate** the **bronchial tract** to **improve** the **oxygen exchange.** It also helps one release **emotional blocks.**

Geranium—may help with **hormonal balance, liver** and **kidney functions,** and the **discharge** of **toxins** from the **liver** that keep us from having balance. Geranium **opens** the **liver chakra.**

Orange—brings **peace** and **happiness** to the **mind** and **body** and **joy** to the **heart**, which feelings provide **emotional** support to help one overcome depression.

Lavender—is an oil that has traditionally been known to **balance** the **body** and to work wherever there is a need. It may help with **PMS/menopausal problems, stress, stretch marks, tension**, and **water retention.**

Sage—may help improve **estrogen** and **progesterone-testosterone balance.** It is believed to contain elements that contribute to the **secretion** of **progesterone-testosterone.**

Rose—possesses the highest frequency of any oil. It may help **enhance** the **frequency** of every cell, which could help bring **balance** and **harmony** to the body. It is thought by some to produce a magnetic energy that attracts **love** and enhances the frequency of **self-love**, bringing **joy** to the heart.

Body System(s) Affected: The oils in this blend may help it be effective for dealing with various problems related to **Emotional Balance.**

Aromatic Influence: This blend was structured specifically to **expel negative emotions, elevate** the **mind, balance, empower**, and **propel** one forward to achieve their desired goals.

Application: Apply to **Vita Flex points** on **feet** and/or directly on **area** of concern. This blend may also be **diffused**, applied to the **wrists** or **temples**, or added to warm **bathwater** (best when first combined with a bath gel base). For an uplifting massage, dilute first with a pure carrier oil.

Safety Data: ***Because this blend contains sage, it should be used with caution by those individuals who are susceptible to high blood pressure, epileptic seizures, or who are pregnant.***

Companion Oils: Acceptance, Clarity, Into the Future, Magnify Your Purpose, Motivation, Valor.

Frequency: Physical and Emotional; approximately 90 MHz.

Evergreen Essence™

This blend is a combination of oils distilled from a variety of aromatic cedar, pine, and spruce trees. Now the **peace, serenity, grounding**, and even **sacred feelings** of the evergreen forests can be brought into the home or workplace. All of these oils are grounding to the body, creating the **balance** and **opening** necessary to receive and to give. This blend is **healing, uplifting**, and **soothing.** It may help **relieve anxiety** and facilitate the **release** of **emotional blocks** as well as promote feelings of **protection, strength**, and **security.** *More detailed information for many of these oils is not readily available. In those cases, only the common names and the Latin names are listed.*

Single Oils Contained in This Blend:

Colorado Blue Spruce (*Picea pungens*)

Ponderosa Pine (*Pinus ponderosa*)

Pine—may help **dilate** and **open** the **respiratory system**, particularly the **bronchial tract**. It may also help **improve circulation throughout** the **lungs**. It helps soothe **mental stress**, relieve **anxiety**, and **revitalize** the entire body.

Red Fir (*Abies magnifica*)

Western Red Cedar (*Thuja plicata*)—is **calming** and has powerful effects on the **subconscious** and **unconscious mind**.

White Fir (*Abies grandis*)—creates a feeling of **grounding, anchoring**, and **empowerment**. It can **stimulate** the **mind** while allowing the **body** to **relax**. Topically, it helps relieve **pain** from **inflammation**.

Black Pine (*Pinus nigra*)

Pinyon Pine (*Pinus edulis*)

Lodge Pole Pine (*Pinus contorta*)

Contains other conifers, which may include black spruce, fir, and cedarwood.

Body System(s) Affected: The oils in this blend may help it be effective for dealing with various problems related to **Emotional Balance**.

Aromatic Influence: When diffused, this blend of conifer oils, each with their own powerful antiseptic properties, helps to **freshen** and **deodorize** the air. It may help soothe **mental stress**, relieve **anxiety**, and **revitalize** the entire body. The individual oils in this blend have also been described as **appeasing, elevating**, and **opening**.

Application: **Diffuse!** Can also be sprinkled on logs in the fireplace or used to scent potpourri. Dilute well with V-6 Oil for any topical application.

Safety Data: *Could possibly result in* **contact sensitization** *or* **skin irritation.**

Oil Blends

Exodus II™

This blend is comprised of many powerful and precious essential oils that are mentioned numerous times in the Bible (see Exodus, chapter 30). The intent behind this particular blend of oils is to enhance the ability of the body to **expel disease** and **dead tissue**. It is also specifically designed to work with the Exodus food supplement to help build one's defenses.

Single Oils Contained in This Blend:

Cassia—is part of the formula the Lord gave Moses (Exodus 30:22-27). It is **antibacterial, anticoagulant, anti-infectious** and **antimicrobial**.

Myrrh—is part of the formula the Lord gave Moses (Exodus 30:22-27). It is a **true gift**. When we **open** our **hearts** and **minds** to receive the gifts, they will be given.

Cinnamon Bark—is part of the formula the Lord gave Moses (Exodus 30:22-27). It has very specific purposes: (1) it is a **powerful purifier**, (2) it is a powerful **oxygenator**, and (3) it **enhances** the action and the activity of **other oils**. It may have a **stimulating** and **toning** effect on the whole body and particularly on the circulatory system. It is **antiseptic, antibacterial**, and **antiviral**.

Calamus—is part of the formula the Lord gave Moses (Exodus 30:22-27). It is **antibacterial, antiseptic**, and **antispasmodic**. It was once highly regarded as an aromatic stimulant and as a tonic for the digestive system.

Hyssop—was used by Moses during the Lord's Passover in Egypt (Exodus 12). It has **anti-inflammatory** and **antiviral** properties. It may also have the ability to **open** up the **respiratory system** and **discharge toxins** and **mucus**.

Galbanum—combined with frankincense—was used biblically to make a holy incense that would **enhance** one's **communication** with the **Creator**. It is recognized for its **antiviral** properties and its overall **strengthening** and **supporting** properties. It contains a low frequency in itself, but when combined with any other oils, such as frankincense or sandalwood, the frequency changes drastically.

Frankincense—contains sesquiterpenes, which may help **oxygenate** the **pineal** and **pituitary glands**. As one of the ingredients for the holy incense, frankincense was used anciently to help **enhance** one's **communication with the Creator**. It was considered a prize possession and was given to Christ at his birth. It may help **promote** a **positive attitude**.

Spikenard—was highly prized in the Middle East during the time of Christ and is referred to several times in the Bible. It is **antifungal, anti-inflammatory, relaxing, regenerative**, and helpful for allergic skin reactions.

Carrier Oil Contained in This Blend: Olive oil.

Body System(s) Affected: The oils in this blend may help it be effective for dealing with various problems related to the **Immune System**.

Application: Apply to **Vita Flex points** on **feet** and/or directly on **area** of concern. This blend may also be applied along the spine using the Raindrop Technique. **Dilution of this blend may be necessary due to the presence of cinnamon bark.**

Safety Data: ***Repeated use on the skin can result in extreme contact sensitization. Can cause extreme skin irritation. Avoid during pregnancy.***

Companion Supplements: Exodus, ImmuneTune.

Frequency: High (Spiritual); approximately 180 MHz.

Bible: "Purge me with Hyssop and I shall be clean" (Psalms 51:7). Several of the oils in this blend come from Chapter 30 in the book of Exodus.

Forgiveness™

The oils in this blend all have powerful emotional effects that may help people move past the barriers in life by bringing them to a **higher spiritual awareness** of their needs. This awareness leaves an angelic feeling in their souls that raises their frequency to the point where they are almost compelled to **forgive, forget, let go**, and go on with their lives.

Single Oils Contained in This Blend:

Melissa—is powerful as an **antiviral** agent, yet it is very gentle and very delicate because of the nature of the plant. It has the ability to work with and enhance the gentle aspects of the human body. It is **calming** and **uplifting** and may also help to **balance** the **emotions**. It may also help to remove **emotional blocks** and **instill** a **positive outlook** on **life**.

Geranium—may help with **hormonal balance, liver** and **kidney functions**, and the **discharge** of **toxins** from the **liver** that keep us from having balance. Geranium **opens** the **liver chakra**.

Frankincense—contains sesquiterpenes, which may help **oxygenate** the **pineal** and **pituitary glands**. As one of the ingredients for the holy incense, frankincense was used anciently to help **enhance** one's **communication with the Creator**. It may help **promote** a **positive attitude**.

Rosewood—may help improve **skin elasticity**. It is **soothing** to the **skin, appeasing** to the **mind, relaxing** to the **body**, and creates a feeling of **peace** and **gentleness**.

Sandalwood—like frankincense—is high in sesquiterpenes, which were discovered to **increase** the amount of **oxygen** around the **pineal** and **pituitary glands**, thus helping to **improve** one's **attitude**. It **alleviates depression** and assists in the removal of **negative programming** from the cells of the body. It helps one **accept others** with an open heart, while diminishing one's own egocentricity.

Angelica—may help one **release** and **let go** of **negative feelings**.

Lavender—is an oil that has traditionally been known to **balance** the **body** and to work wherever there is a need. It may help promote **consciousness, health, love, peace**, and a general sense of **well-being**.

Lemon—promotes **health, healing, physical energy**, and **purification**. Its fragrance is **invigorating, enhancing**, and **warming**.

Jasmine—is very **uplifting** to the **emotions**; it may produce a feeling of **confidence, energy, euphoria**, and **optimism**. As an **antispasmodic**, it has been used effectively for **menstrual** discomfort, **muscle spasms**, and **uterine** disorders.

Roman Chamomile—neutralizes **allergies** and helps to cleanse the **blood** and **expel toxins** from the **liver**.

Bergamot—is **soothing** to the **endocrine system** and to the **hormones**. It may **uplift** and **calm** the **emotions** and help relieve **anxiety, stress**, and **tension**.

Ylang Ylang—may help **balance** the **male-female energies** so one can move closer towards being in **spiritual attunement** and be able to focus their thoughts, filtering out the ever-present garbage and establishing a sense of relaxation. It brings back feelings of **self-love, confidence, joy**, and **peace**.

Palmarosa—is valuable for all types of **skin** problems because it **stimulates** new **cell growth**, regulates oil production, **moisturizes**, and **speeds healing**.

Helichrysum—may help **cleanse** the **blood** and improve **circulatory functions**. It is **anticatarrhal** in structure and nature. On a spiritual level, it may help one **let go of angry feelings** that prevent one from forgiving and moving forward in life.

Rose—possesses the highest frequency of any oil. It may help **enhance** the **frequency** of every cell, which could help bring **balance** and **harmony** to the body.

Carrier Oil Contained in This Blend: Sesame seed oil.

Body System(s) Affected: The oils in this blend may help it be effective for dealing with various problems related to **Emotional Balance**.

Aromatic Influence: When diffused, this blend of oils may stimulate one to feel the need to **forgive** themselves and others of transgression.

Application: Best when massaged clockwise over the **navel** (key area, lasts longer) and the **heart** and also placed behind the **ears** and on the **wrists**. It may also be worn as a **perfume** or **cologne**.

Companion Oils: Valor on the **feet, cheeks**, and **face**; Joy on the **ears** and **chest**; Gathering on the **forehead**.

Frequency: High (Spiritual); approximately 192 MHz.

Bible: Matthew 6:14-15.

Gathering™

The oils in this blend may help **increase** the **oxygen** around the **pituitary** and **pineal glands**, bringing us more into a **harmonic frequency** to be a receptor of the communications that we desire to receive. As many of these single oils tend to move people in a profound way, this blend may help **bring people together** in **spiritual oneness** with **god**. This blend may also **help bring** not only the **physical** but also the **emotional** and **spiritual thoughts** and **feelings together** for **greater focus** and **clarity**. By helping to prevent the **fracturing** of **thought energy**, this blend may help one find a greater **peace** and **balance** in life. It may help to keep one **focused, grounded, connected**, and **clear**, and may even help **gather** one's **potential** for **self-improvement**. It may be a very powerful blend for **supporting** and **protecting** the **body** from **outside attacks**, especially when there has been a **lack** of **sleep**. Because it tends to act as an **amplifier**, refer to the comments below regarding its use.

Single Oils Contained in This Blend:

Lavender—is an oil that has traditionally been known to **balance** the **body** and to work wherever there is a need. It may help promote **consciousness, health, love, peace**, and a general sense of **well-being**.

Galbanum—combined with frankincense—was used biblically to make a holy incense that would **enhance** one's **communication** with the **Creator**. It is recognized for its **antiviral** properties and its overall **strengthening** and **supporting** properties. It contains a low frequency in itself, but when combined with any other oils, such as frankincense or sandalwood, the frequency changes drastically.

Frankincense—contains sesquiterpenes, which may help **oxygenate** the **pineal** and **pituitary glands**. As one of the ingredients for the holy incense, frankincense was used anciently to help **enhance** one's **communication with the Creator**. It was considered a prize possession and was given to Christ at his birth. It may help **promote** a **positive attitude**.

Geranium—may be **healing, calming**, and **balancing** to the **skin**. It may help **balance** the **sebum**, which is the fatty secretion in the sebaceous glands of the skin that **keeps** the **skin supple**. It helps **open** and **elevate** the **mind**.

Ylang Ylang—may help **balance** the **male-female energies** so one can move closer towards being in **spiritual attunement** and be able to focus their thoughts, filtering out the ever-present garbage. It brings back feelings of **self-love, confidence, joy**, and **peace**.

Spruce—**grounds** the **body**, creating the **balance** and the **opening** necessary to **receive** and to **give**. It may help **dilate** the **bronchial tract** to **improve** the **oxygen exchange**. It also helps one release **emotional blocks**.

Cinnamon Bark—is part of the formula the Lord gave Moses (Exodus 30:22-27). It has very specific purposes: (1) it is a **powerful purifier**, (2) it is a powerful **oxygenator**, and (3) it **enhances** the action and the activity of **other oils**. It may have a **stimulating** and **toning** effect on the whole body and particularly on the circulatory system. It is **antiseptic, antibacterial**, and **antiviral**.

Rose—possesses the highest frequency of any oil. It may help **enhance** the **frequency** of every cell, which could help bring **balance** and **harmony** to the body.

Sandalwood—like frankincense—is high in sesquiterpenes, which were discovered to **increase** the amount of **oxygen** around the **pineal** and **pituitary glands**, thus helping to **improve** one's **attitude**. It **alleviates depression** and assists in the removal of **negative programming** from the cells of the body. It helps one **accept others** with an open heart, while diminishing one's own egocentricity.

Body System(s) Affected: The oils in this blend may help it be effective for dealing with various problems related to **Emotional Balance**.

Aromatic Influence: When diffused, this blend of oils may help one **gather** their **thoughts** so they can become **focused**. It may also help the **heart** and **mind** to work harmoniously, allowing **goals** and **dreams** to be **manifest** in **physical forms**.

Application: Best when applied to the **forehead, heart, right temple** across to the **left temple**, bottom front of the **neck, thymus, face, chest**, and on each side of the upper chest **near** the **shoulders**. It can be applied anywhere on the body or be worn as a **perfume** or **cologne**.

Companion Oils: Forgiveness on the **navel**, Sacred Mountain on the **crown** (to bring a person with a negative attitude to a clear space). This blend also works well with Valor (on crown or feet), 3 Wise Men (crown), Clarity (temples), and Dream Catcher.

Frequency: Physical and Emotional; approximately 99 MHz.

Bible: Galbanum and frankincense are talked about in Exodus and were used by Moses as the holy incense. Cinnamon is part of the formula that the Lord gave Moses to help him "become single unto God."

Comments: Gathering has a specific purpose for each individual use. One must use this blend with the right intent, as it may amplify negative as well as positive attitudes. Wear with caution when feeling negative because it may amplify the negative feelings. It may be necessary to use Sacred Mountain first in order to bring oneself to a clear space before using Gathering.

Gentle Baby™

This is a wonderful blend, designed specifically for **expectant mothers** and **newborn babies**. It is **comforting, soothing**, and **relaxing**. It may help **relieve stress** during **pregnancy** and may even be **beneficial** during the **birthing process**. It helps to **enhance** the **youthful appearance** of the **skin** and may be beneficial for men to use on **chapped skin** and as an **aftershave**. It may also help with **skin elasticity** and **stretch marks**. Every oil in **Gentle Baby** is for **skin regeneration** and may help to **prevent** and **retard wrinkles**. This blend is so gentle and soothing to the skin that it could possibly be used for **diaper rashes** (dilute at least by ½).

Oil Blends

Single Oils Contained in This Blend:

Rosewood—may help improve **skin elasticity**. It is **soothing** to the **skin, appeasing** to the **mind, relaxing** to the **body**, and creates a feeling of **peace** and **gentleness**.

Geranium—may be **healing, calming**, and **balancing** to the **skin**. It may help **balance** the **sebum**, which is the fatty secretion in the sebaceous glands of the skin that **keeps** the **skin supple**. It helps **open** and **elevate** the **mind**.

Palmarosa—is valuable for all types of **skin** problems because it **stimulates** new **cell growth**, regulates oil production, **moisturizes**, and **speeds healing**.

Lavender—is an oil that has traditionally been known to **balance** the **body** and to work wherever there is a need. It may help prevent **scarring** and **stretch marks** and promote a general sense of **well-being**.

Roman Chamomile—neutralizes **allergies** and helps in **skin regeneration**. It may also help reduce **irritability** and minimize **nervousness** in children, especially **hyperactive children**.

Ylang Ylang—may help **balance** the **male-female energies** so one can move closer towards being in **spiritual attunement** and be able to focus their thoughts, filtering out the ever-present garbage. It brings back feelings of **self-love, confidence, joy**, and **peace**.

Lemon—promotes **health, healing, physical energy**, and **purification**. Its fragrance is **invigorating, enhancing**, and **warming**.

Jasmine—is very **uplifting** to the **emotions**; it may produce a feeling of **confidence, energy, euphoria**, and **optimism**.

Bergamot—is **soothing** to the **endocrine system** and to the **hormones**. It may **uplift** and **calm** the **emotions** and help relieve **anxiety, stress**, and **tension**.

Rose—has a **beautiful fragrance** and contains the highest frequency of any oil. It may help **enhance** the **frequency** of every cell, which could help bring **balance** and **harmony** to the body.

Body System(s) Affected: The oils in this blend may help it be effective for dealing with various problems related to **Emotional Balance** and to the **Skin**.

Aromatic Influence: The aroma of this blend of oils is very **relaxing** and **calming**. It may also help one **create** a **space** for **being** in one's **childhood** again.

Application: Best when applied to the **Vita Flex points** on the **inner ankles**, across the **lower back** and **abdomen** (to reduce cramping and stretch marks), and on the **feet, face** and **neck** areas. Dilute with V-6 Oil for **full-body massage**, or wear as a **perfume** or **cologne**. It may also be added to **bathwater**.

Baby—When using on a baby, dilute at least by ½. Dilute with V-6 Oil for **full-body massage**. It may also be applied to the **feet, abdomen, lower back, face**, and **neck** areas.

Delivery—Massage it on the **perineum** to help it **stretch** and possibly help **avoid** an **episiotomy**.

Frequency: High (Spiritual); approximately 152 MHz.

GLF™

This blend was formulated with specific oils to help encourage the proper functioning of the **gallbladder** and the **liver**. This blend makes a wonderful addition to other liver supporting supplements such as Juva Power and JuvaTone.

Single Oils Contained in This Blend:

Grapefruit—is an **antidepressant**, an **antiseptic**, and a **diuretic**. It is **balancing** and **uplifting** to the mind and may help to **relieve anxiety**.

Helichrysum—may help **cleanse** the **blood** and improve **circulatory functions**. It is **anticatarrhal** in structure and nature. In the last few years, research has documented its **antioxidant** and **liver protective** properties.

Celery Seed—is **antioxidative** and **antiseptic** to the **urinary tract**. It helps **decongest** the **liver** by stimulating drainage. It has also been shown to aid **lymphatic drainage** and may help **balance** the **endocrine system**.

Ledum—has a long history of use as a tea by the natives of North America, where it was used to fight **cancer, scurvy**, and **urinary problems**. It may be a wonderful support to the **urinary tract** and a powerful **liver** support and detoxifier.

Hyssop—was used by Moses during the Lord's Passover in Egypt (Exodus 12). It has **anti-inflammatory** and **antiviral** properties. It may also have the ability to **open** up the **respiratory system** and **discharge toxins** and **mucus**.

Spearmint—is **antifungal** and **antiseptic**. It is an oil that may balance and increase **metabolism**, helping to **burn up fats** and **toxins** in the body.

Body System(s) Affected: The oils in this blend may help it be effective for dealing with various problems related to the **Digestive System** (especially the **gallbladder** and the **liver**).

Application: For topical use, dilute 1 part GLF with 1 part vegetable oil (e.g., olive oil, V-6 Enhanced Vegetable Oil Complex). Apply 4–6 drops **over liver** or on **Vita Flex points** on the **feet**. Avoid contact with eyes.

Safety Data: *Could possibly result in* **skin irritation**. *Use with caution during* **pregnancy**. *Avoid exposure to* **direct sunlight** *for 3 to 6 hours after use.*

Companion Products: JuvaFlex, Juva Cleanse, Juva Power, JuvaTone.

Gratitude™

This blend was specifically formulated to **elevate, soothe**, and **appease** the **mind** while **bringing relief** and **relaxation** to the body. While the body is relaxing, the heart and mind can be opened to receive the gifts that are given each day.

Single Oils Contained in This Blend:

Balsam Fir—creates a feeling of **grounding, anchoring**, and **empowerment**. It can **stimulate** the **mind** while allowing the **body** to **relax**. Topically, it helps relieve **overworked** and **tired muscles** and **joints**.

Frankincense—contains sesquiterpenes, which may help **oxygenate** the **pineal** and **pituitary glands**. As one of the ingredients for the holy incense, frankincense was used anciently to help **enhance** one's **communication with the Creator**. It was considered a prize possession and was given to Christ at his birth. It may help **promote** a **positive attitude**.

Rosewood—is **soothing** to the **skin, appeasing** to the **mind, relaxing** to the **body**, and creates a feeling of **peace** and **gentleness**.

Myrrh—is part of the formula the Lord gave Moses (Exodus 30:22-27). It promotes **spiritual awareness** and is a **true gift**. When we **open** our **hearts** and **minds** to receive the gifts, they will be given.

Galbanum—combined with frankincense—was used biblically to make a holy incense that would **enhance** one's **communication** with the **Creator**. It is recognized for its **antiviral** properties and its overall **strengthening** and **supporting** properties. It contains a low frequency in itself, but when combined with any other oils, such as frankincense or sandalwood, the frequency changes drastically.

Ylang Ylang—may help **balance** the **male-female energies** so one can move closer towards being in **spiritual attunement** and be able to focus their thoughts, filtering out the ever-present garbage. It brings back feelings of **self-love, confidence, joy**, and **peace**.

Body System(s) Affected: The oils in this blend may help it be effective for dealing with various problems related to the **Nervous** and **Immune Systems, Muscles and Bones**, and to **Emotional Balance**.

Aromatic Influence: This blend of oils may help **soothe** and **appease** the **mind**. It is **relaxing** and **elevating**, promoting a sense of gratitude for blessings received.

Application: Rub over the **heart** and on **forehead** and **temples**. **Diffuse**, or wear as **perfume** or **cologne**.

Companion Oils: Acceptance, Believe, Forgiveness, Inner Child, Inspiration, Peace & Calming.

Grounding™

This blend may help to **stabilize** and **ground** us in order **to deal with reality** in a logical, peaceful manner. It can be easy for us to disconnect from reality. We are either excited about new ideas or want to escape into our own fantasy world. However, doing this allows us to make choices that can lead to some very unfortunate circumstances. This blend may **help us deal** with **reality**.

Single Oils Contained in This Blend:

White Fir (*Abies concolor*)—creates a feeling of **grounding, anchoring**, and **empowerment**. It can **stimulate** the **mind** while allowing the **body** to **relax**. Topically, it helps relieve **pain** from **inflammation**.

Spruce—**grounds** the **body**, creating the **balance** and the **opening** necessary to **receive** and to **give**. It may help **dilate** the **bronchial tract** to **improve** the **oxygen exchange**. It also helps one release **emotional blocks**.

Ylang Ylang—may help **balance** the **male-female energies** so one can move closer towards being in **spiritual attunement** and be able to focus their thoughts, filtering out the ever-present garbage. It brings back feelings of **self-love, confidence, joy,** and **peace**.

Pine—may help **dilate** and **open** the **respiratory system**, particularly the **bronchial tract**. It may also help **improve circulation throughout** the **lungs**. It helps soothe **mental stress**, relieve **anxiety**, and **revitalize** the entire body.

Cedarwood—was used traditionally by the North American Indians to enhance their potential for **spiritual communication**. It may help **open** the **pineal gland**.

Angelica—may help one **release** and **let go** of **negative feelings**.

Juniper—evokes feelings of **health, love**, and **peace** and may help to **elevate** one's **spiritual awareness**.

Body System(s) Affected: The oils in this blend may help it be effective for dealing with various problems related to **Emotional Balance**.

Aromatic Influence: The aroma of this blend may help **ground** and **balance** the **emotions**.

Application: Best when worn on the back of the **neck** and on the **temples**.

Safety Data: ***Could possibly result in skin irritation.***

Frequency: Emotional and Spiritual; approximately 140 MHz.

Harmony™

This blend may help to establish **spiritual** and **emotional harmony** within us. We must be in **harmony** with ourselves, our Creator, others, and the world around us before we can truly feel and **overcome** our **negative emotions**. When we have **harmony** in our lives, many other things will come to balance and fruition. It may promote **physical** and **emotional healing** by bringing about a **harmonic balance** to the **chakras (energy centers)** of the **body**, allowing us to **relax** and feel **safe** and **secure**. Balancing and unblocking the **chakras** may allow the energy to flow more efficiently through the body, helping to **reduce stress** and creating a general overall **feeling** of **well-being**.

Single Oils Contained in This Blend:

Lavender—is an oil that has traditionally been known to **balance** the **body** and to work wherever there is a need. It may help promote **consciousness, health, love, peace**, and a general sense of **well-being**.

Sandalwood—like frankincense—is high in sesquiterpenes, which were discovered to **increase** the amount of **oxygen** around the **pineal** and **pituitary glands**, thus helping to **improve** one's **attitude**. It **alleviates depression** and assists in the removal of **negative programming** from the cells of the body. It helps one **accept others** with an open heart, while diminishing one's own egocentricity.

Ylang Ylang—may help **balance** the **male-female energies** so one can move closer towards being in **spiritual attunement** and be able to focus their thoughts, filtering out the ever-present garbage. It brings back feelings of **self-love, confidence, joy,** and **peace**.

Frankincense—contains sesquiterpenes, which may help **oxygenate** the **pineal** and **pituitary glands**. As one of the ingredients for the holy incense, frankincense was used anciently to help **enhance** one's **communication with the Creator**. It was considered a prize possession and was given to Christ at his birth. It may help **promote** a **positive attitude**.

Orange—brings **peace** and **happiness** to the **mind** and **body** and **joy** to the **heart**, which feelings provide **emotional** support to help one overcome depression.

Angelica—may help one **release** and **let go** of **negative feelings**.

Geranium—may help with **hormonal balance, liver** and **kidney functions,** and the **discharge** of **toxins** from the **liver** that keep us from having balance. Geranium **opens** the **liver chakra** (solar plexus). Note: The liver is the place where fear and anger are stored.

Hyssop—was used by Moses during the Lord's Passover in Egypt (Exodus 12). It may help stimulate **meditation** and promote **centering**.

Spruce—**grounds** the **body**, creating the **balance** and the **opening** necessary to **receive** and to **give**. It also helps one release **emotional blocks**.

Sage Lavender—has been shown to increase both estradiol and testosterone levels. It may also help **harmonize** and **balance** the **emotions** and reduce **stress-related** conditions.

Rosewood—may help improve **skin elasticity**. It is **soothing** to the **skin, appeasing** to the **mind, relaxing** to the **body**, and creates a feeling of **peace** and **gentleness**.

Lemon—promotes **health, healing, physical energy**, and **purification**. Its fragrance is **invigorating, enhancing**, and **warming**.

Jasmine—is very **uplifting** to the **emotions**; it may produce a feeling of **confidence, energy, euphoria**, and **optimism**.

Roman Chamomile—neutralizes **allergies** and helps with **skin regeneration**. It may also help reduce **irritability** and minimize **nervousness** in children, especially **hyperactive children**.

Bergamot—is **soothing** to the **endocrine system** and to the **hormones**. It may **uplift** and **calm** the **emotions** and help relieve **anxiety, stress**, and **tension**.

Palmarosa—is valuable for all types of **skin** problems because it **stimulates** new **cell growth**, regulates oil production, **moisturizes,** and **speeds healing**.

Rose—has a **beautiful fragrance** and contains the highest frequency of the oils. It may help **enhance** the **frequency** of every cell, which could help bring **balance** and **harmony** to the body.

Body System(s) Affected: The oils in this blend may help it be effective for dealing with various problems related to **Emotional Balance**.

Aromatic Influence: The fragrance of this blend of oils may help one establish and maintain a **positive attitude**, which is essential for **physical** and **emotional healing**.

Application: Best when applied on **each chakra** (or rub this blend between the hands in a circular, clockwise motion and place over the chakras), on the **ears** and **feet**, over the **heart**, and over areas of poor **circulation**. One may want to start at the **feet** and go up the **energy centers** and then over the **crown**. Application of this blend to each chakra or "energy center" will help open them and balance the electrical fields surrounding the body. Wear it as **perfume** or **cologne**. If there is an **allergy** or irritation to the smell of an oil, do the following:

1. Rub this blend between both hands in a circular, clockwise motion.
2. Put one hand over the **navel** and the other hand over the **thymus** (above the heart). Hold for **20 seconds. Change hands** and **repeat**.

Safety Data: *Use with caution during* **pregnancy**. *Not for use by people with* **epilepsy**. *Use with caution if dealing with* **high blood pressure**. *Avoid exposure to* **direct sunlight** *for 3 to 6 hours after use.*

Frequency: Emotional; approximately 101 MHz.

Highest Potential™

This blend contains the biblical oils of frankincense, galbanum, cedarwood, and sandalwood to help you tap into the divine power within yourself, **empowering** and **enabling** you to achieve your full potential. In addition, ylang ylang and lavender help to balance physical and emotional energies so you can focus on the higher goal, while the emotionally uplifting scent of jasmine helps to promote confidence and energy to reach that goal. This unique blend of oils is **uplifting** and **inspiring**, while promoting feelings of **stability** and **peace**.

Blends and Single Oils Contained in This Blend:

Australian Blue—is emotionally uplifting and helps to empower the physical and spiritual bodies. It helps to build **courage**, **confidence**, and **self-esteem** while promoting **calmness**, **peace**, and **relaxation**.

Gathering—helps to keep one **focused**, **grounded**, **connected**, and **clear** and may even help **gather** one's **potential** for **self-improvement**.

Jasmine—is very **uplifting** to the **emotions**; it penetrates the deepest layers of the soul, opening doors to our emotions. It produces feelings of **confidence**, **energy**, and **optimism**.

Ylang Ylang—may help **balance** the **male-female energies** so one can move closer towards being in **spiritual attunement** and be able to focus their thoughts, filtering out the ever-present garbage. It brings back feelings of **self-love**, **confidence**, **joy**, and **peace**.

Body System(s) Affected: **Emotional Balance**.

Aromatic Influence: When diffused or worn as perfume, this special blend of oils helps to **balance** the emotions. It may help relieve **anxiety**, **revitalize** the entire body, and **empower** both mind and soul.

Application: Rub over the **heart**, and on **forehead**, and **temples**. **Diffuse** or wear as **perfume**.

Companion Oils: Magnify Your Purpose, Live with Passion

Hope™

The single oils in this blend have the ability to help **support the body physically and mentally** to give us **hope**. These oils when inhaled together may give us the feeling of **going forward** with **hope** and **achievement**. This blend reconnects us with a feeling of **strength** and **grounding**. It may also help **relieve depression** and **suicidal thoughts**.

Single Oils Contained in This Blend:

Melissa—is powerful as an **antiviral** agent, yet it is very gentle and very delicate because of the nature of the plant. It has the ability to work with and enhance the gentle aspects of the human body. It is **calming** and **uplifting** and may help to **balance** the **emotions**. It may also help to remove **emotional blocks** and **instill** a **positive outlook** on **life**.

Myrrh—is part of the formula the Lord gave Moses (Exodus 30:22-27). It is a **true gift**. When we **open** our **hearts** and **minds** to receive, the gifts will be given.

Juniper—evokes feelings of **health**, **love**, and **peace** and may help to **elevate** one's **spiritual awareness**.

Spruce—**grounds** the **body**, creating the **balance** and the **opening** necessary to **receive** and to **give**. It may help **dilate** the **bronchial tract** to **improve** the **oxygen exchange**. It also helps one release **emotional blocks**.

Carrier Oil Contained in This Blend: Almond oil.

Body System(s) Affected: The oils in this blend may help it be effective for dealing with various problems related to **Emotional Balance**.

Aromatic Influence: This blend of oils may be instrumental in giving one feelings of **peace**, **security**, **hope**, and **achievement**.

Application: Apply on **ears** (outer edge). It may also be placed on the **chest, heart, temples, solar plexus**, across the **nape** of the **neck** (in back), **feet, wrists**, or **any place** on the **body**. To eliminate **suicidal thoughts**, use on **ears** and **wrists**. Wear as **perfume** or **cologne**.

Frequency: Physical and Emotional; approximately 98 MHz.

Comments: The first time this blend was used was for a lady in Arkansas for whom they could not find a diagnosis. She was dying from a mysterious disease. She was given Hope, and her life was spared. At different times in our lives we may experience feelings of hopelessness that can cause us to lose the vision of our goals and desires. Hope helps us reconnect with a feeling of strength and grounding, which may restore hope for tomorrow and help us go forward in life.

Humility™

Having humility and forgiveness **helps us heal ourselves and our earth**. Humility is an integral ingredient in forgiveness and seeking a closer relationship with God. Through its frequency and fragrance, you may find that special place where your own healing can begin.

Single Oils Contained in This Blend:

Rosewood—is **soothing** to the **skin, appeasing** to the **mind, relaxing** to the **body**, and creates a feeling of **peace** and **gentleness**.

Ylang Ylang—may help **balance** the **male-female energies** so one can move closer towards being in **spiritual attunement** and be able to focus their thoughts, filtering out the ever-present garbage. It brings back feelings of **self-love, confidence, joy,** and **peace**.

Geranium—may help with **hormonal balance, liver** and **kidney functions,** and the **discharge** of **toxins** from the **liver** that keep us from having balance. Geranium **opens** the **liver chakra** (solar plexus). It may help **ease nervous tension** and **stress, balance** the **emotions, lift** the **spirit**, and foster **peace, well-being**, and **hope**.

Melissa—is powerful as an **antiviral** agent, yet it is very gentle and very delicate because of the nature of the plant. It has the ability to work with and enhance the gentle aspects of the human body. It is **calming** and **uplifting** and may help to **balance** the **emotions**. It may also help to remove **emotional blocks** and **instill** a **positive outlook** on **life**.

Frankincense—contains sesquiterpenes, which may help **oxygenate** the **pineal** and **pituitary glands**. As one of the ingredients for the holy incense, frankincense was used anciently to help **enhance** one's **communication with the Creator**. It was considered a prize possession and was given to Christ at his birth. It may help **promote** a **positive attitude**.

Spikenard—was highly prized in the Middle East during the time of Christ and is referred to several times in the Bible. It is **antifungal, anti-inflammatory, relaxing, regenerative**, and helpful for allergic skin reactions.

Myrrh—is part of the formula the Lord gave Moses (Exodus 30:22-27). It promotes **spiritual awareness** and is a **true gift**. When we **open** our **hearts** and **minds** to receive the gifts, they will be given.

Rose—possesses the highest frequency of any oil. It may help **enhance** the **frequency** of every cell, which could help bring **balance** and **harmony** to the body.

Neroli—has been regarded traditionally by the Egyptian people for its great ability to **heal** the **mind, body,** and **spirit**. It is **calming** and **relaxing** to the body and spirit. It may also help to **strengthen** and **stabilize** the emotions and **bring relief** to seemingly hopeless situations. It encourages **confidence, courage, joy, peace**, and **sensuality**. It brings everything into the **focus** of one and at the moment.

Carrier Oil Contained in This Blend: Sesame seed oil.

Body System(s) Affected: The oils in this blend may help it be effective for dealing with various problems related to **Emotional Balance**.

Aromatic Influence: It may help one find that special, peaceful place where healing can begin.

Application: Rub over the **heart**, on **neck**, on **temples**, etc.

Companion Oils: Acceptance, Envision, Forgiveness, Inner Child, Inspiration, Peace & Calming

Frequency: Physical and Emotional; approximately 88 MHz.

Immupower™

This is a powerful oil blend for **building, strengthening** and **protecting** the **body** and supporting its defense mechanism. This blend raises the frequency of the **immune system** which helps one overcome the **flu, colds, respiratory problems, infections**, etc. It should be worn and diffused in the home daily, especially during the seasons of cold and flu. It should be used to **protect** the **home environment**.

Single Oils Contained in This Blend:

Hyssop—was used by Moses during the Lord's Passover in Egypt (Exodus 12). It has **anti-inflammatory** and **antiviral** properties. It may also have the ability to **open** up the **respiratory system** and **discharge toxins** and **mucus**.

Mountain Savory—has **immune-stimulant, antiviral, antifungal, anti-infectious, antimicrobial**, and **antiparasitic** properties.

Cistus—has **antibacterial, anti-infectious**, and **antiviral** properties. Because it is high in oxygenating molecules, it may also assist the **auto-immune system**; it may help strengthen the **immune system.**

Ravensara—is a powerful **antiviral, antibacterial, antifungal**, and **anti-infectious** oil. It may help **dilate, open**, and **strengthen** the **respiratory system**. As a cross between clove and nutmeg, it may also help support the **adrenal glands**.

Frankincense—contains sesquiterpenes, which may help **oxygenate** the **pineal** and **pituitary glands**. As one of the ingredients for the holy incense, frankincense was used anciently to help **enhance** one's **communication with the Creator**. It may help **promote** a **positive attitude** and has **anti-infectious** and **antiseptic** properties.

Oregano—has **antibacterial, antifungal, antiseptic, antiviral**, and **immune-stimulant** properties. It strengthens one's feeling of **security**.

Clove—is **antiparasitic, antitumoral, antiviral,** and **immune-stimulant**.

Cumin—is an **antiseptic** and an **immune-stimulant**.

Idaho Tansy—is **antiviral** and may help support the **immune system**.

Body System(s) Affected: The oils in this blend may help it be effective for dealing with various problems related to the **Immune System**.

Aromatic Influence: This blend of oils should be worn and diffused every other day (alternate with Thieves), especially during **cold** and **flu** season.

Application: To protect oneself from our chemical environment and during the cold and flu season, diffuse ImmuPower in the morning and again in the evening and apply Thieves to the feet. The next day, alternate with Thieves. Diffuse Thieves and apply ImmuPower to the **throat, chest, spine**, and **feet** (best to **dilute** for topical application—see Safety Data below). Apply two to three drops on **thymus** in a clockwise motion. Stimulate by tapping the **thymus** with energy fingers (pointer and middle).

Also apply oil on **jugular veins** in **neck** and on **arm pits**. Apply ImmuPower by Raindrop Technique up the spine for a **fever, virus**, or to strengthen the **immune system**.

Safety Data: ***Can be irritating to sensitive skin; best to dilute with V-6 Oil for topical application. Use with caution during pregnancy. Use with caution if susceptible to epilepsy.***

Companion Oils: Thieves or Exodus II (good to alternate with ImmuPower). Single oils that may be added for extra strength include the following: cistus, clove, frankincense, melissa, mountain savory, oregano, rosewood.

Companion Supplements: ComforTone, Essentialzyme, Exodus, ImmuneTune, Super C / Super C Chewable.

Frequency: Physical and Emotional; approximately 89 MHz.

Inner Child™

This blend has a fragrance that may **stimulate memory response** and help one **reconnect with** their inner-self or **own identity**, which is one of the first steps to finding **emotional balance**. When children have been abused and misused, they become disconnected from their inner child, or identity, which causes confusion. This can contribute to multiple personalties. These problems may not manifest themselves until their early- to mid-adult years, often labeled as a mid-life crisis.

Single Oils Contained in This Blend:

Orange—is **uplifting** and **calming**. It brings **peace** and **happiness** to the **mind** and **body** and **joy** to the **heart**, which feelings provide **emotional** support to help one overcome depression.

Tangerine—contains esters and aldehydes, which are **sedating** and **calming** to the **nervous system**. It is also a **diuretic** and a **decongestant** of the **lymphatic system**.

Jasmine—is very **uplifting** to the **emotions**; it may produce a feeling of **confidence, energy, euphoria**, and **optimism**.

Ylang Ylang—may help **balance** the **male-female energies** so one can move closer towards being in **spiritual attunement** and be able to focus their thoughts, filtering out the ever-present garbage. It brings back feelings of **self-love, confidence, joy,** and **peace**.

Spruce—**grounds** the **body**, creating the **balance** and the **opening** necessary to **receive** and to **give**. It also helps one release **emotional blocks**.

Sandalwood—like frankincense—is high in sesquiterpenes, which were discovered to **increase** the amount of **oxygen** around the **pineal** and **pituitary glands**, thus helping to **improve** one's **attitude**. It **alleviates depression** and assists in the removal of **negative programming** from the cells of the body. It helps one **accept others** with an open heart, while diminishing one's own egocentricity.

Lemongrass—is **vasodilatory, antiseptic, antibacterial, anti-inflammatory**, and **sedative**. It may help improve **circulation**, wake up the **lymphatic system**, and increase the flow of **oxygen**. It may also help to **lift** the **spirit**.

Neroli—has been regarded traditionally by the Egyptian people for its great ability to **heal** the **mind, body,** and **spirit**. It is **calming** and **relaxing** to the body and spirit. It may also help to **strengthen** and **stabilize** the emotions and **bring relief** to seemingly hopeless situations. It encourages **confidence, courage, joy, peace**, and **sensuality**. It brings everything into **focus** and into the moment.

Body System(s) Affected: The oils in this blend may help it be effective for dealing with various problems related to **Emotional Balance**.

Aromatic Influence: The oils in this blend are very **calming** to the **nerves** and **emotions** when diffused.

Application: Apply around **navel** and on **chest, temples**, and **nose**.

Safety Data: *Avoid exposure to direct* ***sunlight*** *for up to 12 hours after use. Could possibly result in* ***skin irritation.***

Companion Oils: Acceptance, Awaken, Citrus Fresh, Envision, Forgiveness, Gentle Baby, Surrender.

Frequency: Physical and Emotional; approximately 98 MHz.

Inspiration™

This blend includes oils that have been combined to help those desirous of **communicating with** and getting closer to the **Creator** and enjoying the spiritual aspects of life. It **relieves negative thoughts** and **enhances spiritual awareness.** It creates a space for **prayer** and **inner awareness** during meditation and prayer.

Single Oils Contained in This Blend:

Cedarwood—was used traditionally by the North American Indians to enhance their potential for **spiritual communication.** It may help **open** the **pineal gland.**

Spruce—**grounds** the **body**, creating the **balance** and the **opening** necessary to **receive** and to **give.** It also helps one release **emotional blocks.** It was used by the Lakota Indians to enhance their communication with the Great Spirit. It may also **open** the **pineal gland.**

Rosewood—is **soothing** to the **skin, appeasing** to the **mind, relaxing** to the **body**, and creates a feeling of **peace** and **gentleness.**

Myrtle—is a **decongestant** of the **respiratory system.** It is **euphoric, elevating**, and may help to soother **anger.**

Sandalwood—like frankincense—is high in sesquiterpenes, which were discovered to **increase** the amount of **oxygen** around the **pineal** and **pituitary glands**, thus helping to **improve** one's **attitude.** It **alleviates depression** and assists in the removal of **negative programming** from the cells of the body. It helps one **accept others** with an open heart, while diminishing one's own egocentricity.

Frankincense—contains sesquiterpenes, which may help **oxygenate** the **pineal** and **pituitary glands.** As one of the ingredients for the holy incense, frankincense was used anciently to help **enhance** one's **communication with the Creator.**

Mugwort (*Artemisia vulgaris*)—was seen as a protective charm against danger and evil and anciently believed to **increase psychic powers.**

Body System(s) Affected: The oils in this blend may help it be effective for dealing with various problems related to **Emotional Balance.**

Aromatic Influence: When diffused, this blend of oils is wonderful for creating a spiritual environment in the home during times of **prayer, meditation**, or when seeking **inspiration** and direction. Put oil on a cotton ball near a vent in the car.

Application: Apply to **horns** (right and left sides of **forehead**), **crown, shoulders**, along **spine**, and on back of **neck.**

Companion Oils: Acceptance, Forgiveness, Humility, Surrender, 3 Wise Men.

Frequency: High (Spiritual); approximately 141 MHz.

Into The Future™

This blend may help one leave the past behind in order to go forward with vision and excitement. The single oils contained in this blend are all invigorating and uplifting. So many times we find ourselves settling for mediocrity and sacrificing our own potential and success because of the fear of the unknown and what the future may or may not hold. This blend was formulated to **support** the **emotions in** helping us create the feeling of **moving forward** and not being afraid to let determination and that pioneering spirit come through. Living on the edge with tenacity and integrity brings the excitement of the challenge and the joy of success.

Single Oils Contained in This Blend:

Clary Sage—may be beneficial for **regulating cells** and **balancing** the **hormones**. It may calm and enhance the **dream state**, helping to bring about a feeling of **euphoria**.

Ylang Ylang—may help **balance** the **male-female energies** so one can move closer towards being in **spiritual attunement** and be able to focus their thoughts, filtering out the ever-present garbage. It brings back feelings of **self-love, confidence, joy,** and **peace**.

White Fir (*Abies concolor*)—creates a feeling of **grounding, anchoring**, and **empowerment**. It can **stimulate** the **mind** while allowing the **body** to **relax**.

Idaho Tansy—is **antiviral** and may help support the **immune system**.

Juniper—may help to **improve circulation** through the **kidneys**. It has **antiseptic, antispasmodic, astringent, cleansing, detoxifying, diuretic, stimulant**, and **tonic** properties.

Jasmine—is very **uplifting** to the **emotions**; it may produce a feeling of **confidence, energy, euphoria**, and **optimism**.

Frankincense—contains sesquiterpenes, which may help **oxygenate** the **pineal** and **pituitary glands**. As one of the ingredients for the holy incense, frankincense was used anciently to **enhance communication** with the **Creator**.

Orange—is rich in compounds noted for their **stress-reducing** effects. It brings **peace** and **happiness** to the **mind** and **body** and **joy** to the **heart**.

Cedarwood—was used traditionally by the North American Indians to enhance their potential for **spiritual communication**. It may help **open** the **pineal gland**.

Carrier Oil Contained in This Blend: Almond oil.

Body System(s) Affected: The oils in this blend may help it be effective for dealing with various problems related to **Emotional Balance**.

Aromatic Influence: Diffusing this blend of oils may helps **lift** the **spirit** and **stabilize** the **emotions,** making it easier for one to recognize their own potential.

Application: **Diffuse**, put in **bathwater**, apply over the **heart**, on **wrists, neck**, as a **compress**, and dilute with V-6 Oil for **full-body massage**.

Companion Oils: Awaken, Clarity, Dream Catcher, Envision, Inspiration, Magnify Your Purpose, Live with Passion.

Frequency: Physical and Emotional; approximately 88 MHz.

Joy™

This blend is a beautiful complimentary blend of oils. When inhaled, it brings back **memories** of **being loved, being held, sharing loving times**, feeling and opening those blocks in our lives where perhaps we have shut down to love or receiving love or love of self. When there is grief, the adenoids and the adrenal glands shut down; Joy opens these glands.

Single Oils Contained in This Blend:

Bergamot—is **soothing** to the **endocrine system** and to the **hormones**. It may **uplift** and **calm** the **emotions** and help relieve **anxiety, stress**, and **tension**.

Ylang Ylang—may help **balance** the **male-female energies** so one can move closer towards being in **spiritual attunement** and be able to focus their thoughts, filtering out the ever-present garbage. It brings back feelings of **self-love, confidence, joy**, and **peace**.

Geranium—may help with **hormonal balance, liver** and **kidney functions**, and the **discharge** of **toxins** from the **liver** that keep us from having balance. Geranium **opens** the **liver chakra** (solar plexus). It may help **ease nervous tension** and **stress, balance** the **emotions, lift** the **spirit**, and foster **peace, well-being**, and **hope**.

Rosewood—may help improve **skin elasticity**. It is **soothing** to the **skin, appeasing** to the **mind, relaxing** to the **body**, and creates a feeling of **peace** and **gentleness**.

Lemon—promotes **health, healing, physical energy**, and **purification**. Its fragrance is **invigorating, enhancing**, and **warming**.

Mandarin—is **appeasing, gentle**, and promotes **happiness**. It is also **refreshing, uplifting**, and **revitalizing**. Because of its sedative and slightly hypnotic properties, it is very good for **stress** and **irritability**.

Jasmine—is very **uplifting** to the **emotions**; it may produce a feeling of **confidence, energy, euphoria**, and **optimism**.

Roman Chamomile—neutralizes **allergies** and helps with **skin regeneration**. It may also help reduce **irritability** and minimize **nervousness** in children, especially **hyperactive children**.

Palmarosa—is valuable for all types of **skin** problems because it **stimulates** new **cell growth**, regulates oil production, **moisturizes**, and **speeds healing**.

Rose—possesses the highest frequency of any oil. It may help **enhance** the **frequency** of every cell, which could help bring **balance** and **harmony** to the body. It is thought by some to produce a magnetic energy that attracts **love** and enhances the frequency of **self-love**, bringing **joy** to the heart.

Body System(s) Affected: The oils in this blend may help it be effective for dealing with various problems related to **Emotional Balance**.

Aromatic Influence: The fragrance of this blend of oils promotes feelings of **love, self-love**, and **confidence**. Emotional blockages to love may produce a dislike for the fragrance of this blend (see *HARMONY; Application* for method of correcting fragrance dislikes). Remember, the **energy** of **love** is the true source of all healing!

Application: Rub over **heart, ears, neck, thymus, heart chakras, temples, across brow**, and on **wrists**. Apply on **heart Vita Flex point**. Put four drops in KidScents Lotion for an aftershave. Put in **bathwater**. Use as **compress**; dilute with V-6 Oil for a full-**body massage**. Place on **areas** of **poor circulation**. Wear as **perfume** or **cologne** especially over the heart. Put two drops on a wet cloth and put in the dryer for **great smelling clothes**.

Safety Data: ***Avoid exposure to direct sunlight for up to 12 hours after use.***

Companion Oils: Hope, Magnify Your Purpose, Motivation, Live with Passion, Valor

Frequency: High (Spiritual); approximately 188 MHz.

Juva Cleanse™

In today's chemically polluted environment, there is a desperate need for natural, effective products that **cleanse** and **detoxify** the **liver**. This blend was created with three of the most powerful and effective liver-cleansing oils.

Single Oils Contained in This Blend:

Helichrysum—may help **cleanse** the **blood** and improve **circulatory functions.** It is **anticatarrhal** in structure and nature. In the last few years, research has documented its **antioxidant** and **liver-protective** properties.

Ledum—has a long history of use as a tea by the natives of North America, where it was used to fight **cancer, scurvy**, and **urinary problems**. It may be a wonderful support to the **urinary tract** and a powerful **liver** support and detoxifier.

Celery Seed—is **antioxidative** and **antiseptic** to the **urinary tract.** It helps **decongest** the **liver** by stimulating drainage. It has also been shown to aid **lymphatic drainage** and may help **balance** the **endocrine system**.

Body System(s) Affected: **Digestive System**.

Application: Apply to **Vita Flex points** on **feet** and especially over the **liver**.

Safety Data: *Can be irritating to sensitive* **skin** *(test first for sensitivity).*

JuvaFlex™

This blend contains oils that have been recognized medically and traditionally for aiding the body in **cleansing** the **liver** and **building** a **stronger system.** It may help **detoxify** the **lymphatic system** and provide **digestive support**. Anger and hate are stored in the liver, which creates extreme toxicity. Liver cancer is caused by solidified hate. JuvaFlex supports **getting off addictions**. The helichrysum contained in JuvaFlex is for chelating and may possess the ability to cut through **anger barriers**.

Single Oils Contained in This Blend:

Fennel—may help **improve digestive function** by **supporting** the **liver.** It is an **antiseptic** and a **tonic** for the **liver**. It may break up **fluids** and **toxins** and help **cleanse** the **tissues** in the body. It may also help **balance** the **hormones**.

Geranium—may help with **hormonal balance, liver** and **kidney functions,** and the **discharge** of **toxins** from the **liver** that keep us from having balance. Geranium **opens** the **liver chakra** (solar plexus). It may help **dilate** the **biliary ducts** for **liver detoxification**.

Rosemary cineol—may help **balance heart function, energize** the **solar plexus**, and **reduce mental fatigue.** It is an **antiseptic** and may help decongest the **liver**.

Roman Chamomile—**neutralizes allergies** and increases the ability of the **skin** to **regenerate.** It may help the **liver** to **reject** and **discharge poisons.** This oil is **soothing, relaxing, calming**, and may help **remove fears**.

Blue Tansy—may help **cleanse** the **liver** and **calm** the **lymphatic system**.

Helichrysum—may help **cleanse** the **blood** and improve **circulatory functions.** It is **anticatarrhal** in structure and nature. On a spiritual level, it may help one **let go of angry feelings** that prevent one from forgiving and moving forward in life.

Carrier Oil Contained in This Blend: Sesame seed oil.

Body System(s) Affected: The oils in this blend may help it be effective for dealing with various problems related to the **Digestive System** and to **Emotional Balance**.

Application: Apply to **Vita Flex points** on **feet, spine** (using the Raindrop Technique), and especially over the **liver.** Also apply over the **entire body** (dilute with V-6 Oil).

Oil Blends

Safety Data: ***Can be irritating to sensitive skin.***

Companion Oils: Enhance results by using this blend with Di-Gize.

Companion Supplements: Use JuvaTone and ComforTone together with this blend for maximum results. Best taken an hour apart. Also use Essentialzyme to help expel ingested toxins.

Frequency: Physical; approximately 82 MHz.

Lady Sclareol™

This blend was formulated to have a **seductive** and **alluring** scent with oils that are beneficial for the **skin** as well.

Single Oils Contained in This Blend:

Rosewood—is **soothing** to the **skin, appeasing** to the **mind, relaxing** to the **body**, and creates a feeling of **peace** and **gentleness**.

Vetiver—is **antispasmodic** and locally **warming**. Vetiver has also been valuable for relieving **stress** and helping people recover from **emotional traumas** and **shock**. According to Susanne Fischer-Rizzi, "Sexual energies become more peaceful and grounded."

Geranium—may help with **hormonal balance, liver** and **kidney functions,** and the **discharge** of **toxins** from the **liver**.

Orange—is rich in compounds noted for their **stress-reducing** effects. It brings **peace** and **happiness** to the **mind** and **body** and **joy** to the **heart**.

Clary Sage—is beneficial for **regulating cells** and **balancing** the **hormones**. It may help with **menstrual cramps, PMS**, and **premenopause** symptoms. It may also help with **circulatory problems**.

Ylang Ylang—may help **balance** the **male-female energies** so one can move closer towards being in **spiritual attunement** and be able to focus their thoughts, filtering out the ever-present garbage. It brings back feelings of **self-love, confidence, joy,** and **peace**.

Sandalwood—helps to **alleviate depression** and assists in the removal of **negative programming** from the cells of the body. It helps one **accept others** with an open heart, while diminishing one's own egocentricity.

Sage Lavender—has been shown to increase both estradiol and testosterone levels. It may also help **harmonize** and **balance** the **emotions** and reduce **stress-related** conditions.

Jasmine—is very **uplifting** to the **emotions**; it penetrates the deepest layers of the soul, opening doors to our emotions. It produces feelings of **confidence, energy**, and **optimism**.

Idaho Tansy—is **antiviral** and may help support the **immune system**. Its aroma is **uplifting** and promotes a general sense of **well-being**.

Body System(s) Affected: **Emotional Balance, Skin**.

Aromatic Influence: Because the aroma of this blend of oils is so **seductive** and **arousing**, it promotes feelings of **excitement** and **romance**.

Application: Apply on **location** (most effective when applied by the male partner), use for **massage**, and add to your Bath and Shower Gel Base. May also be used with a **compress** over the abdomen. **Diffuse,** or wear as a **perfume**.

Legacy

This is an incredible and comprehensive blend of 91 different essential oils. Its exquisite aroma **fine-tunes** and **energizes** the entire body. *Note: Since the blend includes oils that are only available on a seasonal basis, this blend may not always be available either.*

Body System(s) Affected: The oils in this blend may help it be effective for dealing with various problems related to **Emotional Balance**.

Aromatic Influence: Because of all the oils contained in this blend, it is **empowering** and **energizing**—not just for the emotions but for the entire body.

Application: Apply to **Vita Flex Points** on **feet** and/or directly on **area** of concern. May also **diffuse** this blend.

Safety Data: ***Because of the diversity of the oils that this blend contains, it should be used with caution by those individuals who are susceptible to epileptic seizures or who are pregnant. Repeated use could possibly result in contact sensitization or skin irritation. For topical use only.***

Companion Oils: **Any single oil may be used with this blend.**

Live with Passion™

The oils in this blend are all **emotionally balancing** and **uplifting**, helping to enhance our **passion** for life. By **strengthening** and **stabilizing** the emotions, not only may this blend help **bring relief** to seemingly hopeless situations, but it may also help to instill a **positive attitude** that can bring back the passion in our lives to help **propel** us toward **accomplishing our goals**.

Single Oils Contained in This Blend:

Clary Sage—is beneficial for **regulating cells** and **balancing** the **hormones**. It may help with **menstrual cramps, PMS**, and **premenopause** symptoms. It may also help with **circulatory problems**.

Ginger—is **warming, uplifting**, and **empowering**. Emotionally, it may help influence **physical energy, love**, and **courage**. Because of its calming influence on the digestive system, it may help reduce feelings of **nausea** and **motion sickness**.

Sandalwood—like frankincense—is high in sesquiterpenes, which were discovered to **increase** the amount of **oxygen** around the **pineal** and **pituitary glands**, thus helping to **improve** one's **attitude**. It **alleviates depression** and assists in the removal of **negative programming** from the cells of the body.

Jasmine—is very **uplifting** to the **emotions**; it may produce a feeling of **confidence, energy, euphoria**, and **optimism**.

Angelica—is referred to by the German people as the "oil of angels." It may help one **release** and **let go** of **negative feelings**.

Cedarwood—was used traditionally by the North American Indians to enhance their potential for **spiritual communication**. It may help **open** the **pineal gland**.

Helichrysum—may help **cleanse** the **blood** and improve **circulatory functions**. It is **anticatarrhal** in structure and nature. As a powerful **anti-inflammatory**, it may even help reduce inflammation in the meninges of the brain. On a spiritual level, it may help one **let go of angry feelings** that prevent one from forgiving and moving forward.

Patchouli—is **sedating, calming**, and **relaxing**, allowing it to reduce **anxiety**.

Neroli—has been regarded traditionally by the Egyptian people for its great ability to **heal** the **mind, body**, and **spirit**. It is **calming** and **relaxing** to the body and spirit. It may also help to **strength-**

en and **stabilize** the emotions and **bring relief** to seemingly hopeless situations. It encourages **confidence, courage, joy, peace**, and **sensuality**. It brings everything into the **focus** of one and at the moment.

Melissa—is powerful as an **antiviral** agent, yet it is very gentle and very delicate because of the nature of the plant. It has the ability to work with and enhance the gentle aspects of the human body. It is **calming** and **uplifting** and may help to **balance** the **emotions**. It may also help to remove **emotional blocks** and **instill** a **positive outlook** on **life**.

Body System(s) Affected: The oils in this blend may help it be effective for dealing with various problems related to the **Nervous System** and to **Emotional Balance**.

Aromatic Influence: This blend is **uplifting, empowering**, and **stabilizing** to the emotions. It may help to improve one's **attitude** by encouraging **confidence** and **courage**.

Application: Apply on the **wrists, temples, chest area**, and **forehead**. Add two to four drops to **bathwater**. May also be worn as **perfume** or **cologne**.

Companion Oils: Acceptance, Clarity, Gathering, Harmony, Inspiration, Magnify Your Purpose, Motivation, 3 Wise Men

Frequency: Physical and Emotional; approximately 89 MHz.

Longevity™

This blend contains oils that have powerful **antioxidant** properties. As measured on the ORAC (oxygen radical absorbent capacity) scale, this blend has scored near 150,000! When taken as a dietary supplement, it may help to **promote longevity** and **prevent premature aging**. *For easier supplement use, refer to Longevity Capsules in the Supplements section of this book.*

Single Oils Contained in This Blend:

Thyme (*CT Thymol*)—has been shown in studies to **dramatically boost glutathione levels** in the heart, liver, and brain. Because it can also help to **prevent** the **oxidation** of **fats** in the body, it may help to slow the aging process. It is also **antifungal** and **antiviral**.

Orange—is rich in compounds noted for their **stress-reducing** effects, lipid-soluble traits, and **antioxidant** properties that **enhance vitamin absorption**.

Clove—has one of the highest ORAC (oxygen radical absorbent capacity) scores. It is **antibacterial, antifungal, anti-infectious, antiparasitic**, a strong **antiseptic, antiviral**, and an **immune stimulant**; it helps preserve the integrity of fatty acids. Clove may also influence **healing** and help improve **memory**.

Frankincense—has powerful **antitumoral** and **anti-inflammatory** properties. It has been used in several clinical applications for fighting cancer. Frankincense also contains sesquiterpenes, which may help **oxygenate** the **pineal** and **pituitary glands**.

Body System(s) Affected: The oils in this blend may help it be effective for dealing with various problems related to the **Cardiovascular System**.

Application: Can be taken as a **dietary supplement** by diluting one drop in 4 oz. of liquid (i.e. soy/rice milk); **Diffuse**. This blend of oils has been put into gel capsules for easier consumption as a dietary supplement (*refer to Longevity Capsules in the Supplements section of this book*).

Safety Data: ***Repeated use can possibly result in* contact sensitization*. Can be irritating to sensitive* skin*. Avoid eye contact. Avoid exposure to direct* sunlight *for 3 to 6 hours after use.***

M-Grain™

This blend contains single oils that have traditionally been used to help **relieve migraine** and **stress headaches**. This blend may also help with **nausea** and **depression**.

Single Oils Contained in This Blend:

Basil—has **antidepressant, anti-inflammatory**, and **antispasmodic** properties. It is relaxing to **spastic muscles**, including those that contribute to **headaches** and **migraines**.

Marjoram—is **relaxing, calming**, and **appeasing** to the **muscles** that constrict and sometimes contribute to **headaches**.

Lavender—is an oil that has traditionally been known to **balance** the **body** and to work wherever there is a need. It has **antispasmodic** and **analgesic** properties. It may help with **sprains, sore muscles, headaches**, and general **healing**.

Peppermint—is **anti-inflammatory** to the **nerves**. It has a **soothing** and **cooling effect** on **headaches**. It is **purifying** and **stimulating** to the **conscious mind**.

Roman Chamomile—is **anti-inflammatory** and **antispasmodic**. It is **calming** and **relaxing** and helps to relieve **muscle tension** and **stress** that can lead to migraine headaches.

Helichrysum—may help **cleanse** the **blood** and improve **circulatory functions**. It is **anticatarrhal** in structure and nature. As a powerful **anti-inflammatory**, it may even help reduce inflammation in the meninges of the brain. On a spiritual level, it may help one **let go of angry feelings** that prevent one from forgiving and moving forward.

Body System(s) Affected: The oils in this blend may help it be effective for dealing with various problems related to the **Nervous System** and to **Muscles and Bones**.

Aromatic Influence: It is very effective for clearing **headaches** when inhaled.

Application: It is most effective when **inhaled**; for **migraines**, place two drops in **palms** of **hands** and then cup over nose and **inhale**. **Massage** along the **brain stem** or through the **thumbs**. Have someone cross their hands and rub your thumbs using their middle finger to push toward your hand. Also put on **forehead, crown, shoulders, back** of **neck, temples**, and **Vita Flex points** on the **feet**.

Companion Oils: Aroma Siez, Clarity, PanAway.

Frequency: Physical; approximately 72 MHz.

Magnify Your Purpose™

The emotionally-uplifting properties of the single oils in this blend make it excellent for helping us to **overcome negative emotions** and such self-defeating behaviors as procrastination and self-pity. By being able to deal with belittling feelings such as abandonment, rejection, and betrayal, we are able to more fully understand and **magnify** our life's purpose.

Single Oils Contained in This Blend:

Sandalwood—like frankincense—is high in sesquiterpenes, which were discovered to **increase** the amount of **oxygen** around the **pineal** and **pituitary glands**, thus helping to **improve** one's **attitude**. It **alleviates depression** and assists in the removal of **negative programming** from the cells of the body. It helps one **accept others** with an open heart, while diminishing one's own egocentricity.

Rosewood—is **soothing** to the **skin, appeasing** to the **mind, relaxing** to the **body**, and creates a feeling of **peace** and **gentleness**.

Sage—may help improve **estrogen** and **progesterone-testosterone balance.** It is believed to contain elements that contribute to the **secretion** of **progesterone-testosterone.**

Nutmeg—has adrenal cortex–like activity, which helps support the **adrenal glands** for **increased energy.**

Patchouli—is **sedating, calming,** and **relaxing,** allowing it to reduce **anxiety.**

Cinnamon Bark—is part of the formula the Lord gave Moses (Exodus 30:22-27). It has very specific purposes: (1) it is a **powerful purifier,** (2) it is a powerful **oxygenator,** and (3) it **enhances** the action and the activity of **other oils.** It may have a **stimulating** and **toning** effect on the whole body and particularly on the circulatory system. It is **antiseptic, antibacterial,** and **antiviral.**

Ginger—is **warming, uplifting,** and **empowering.** Emotionally, it may help influence **physical energy, love,** and **courage.** Because of its calming influence on the digestive system, it may help reduce feelings of **nausea** and **motion sickness.**

Body System(s) Affected: The oils in this blend may help it be effective for dealing with various problems related to the **Nervous System** and to **Emotional Balance.**

Aromatic Influence: Because of the oils contained in this blend, it is **empowering** and **uplifting,** helping us to rise above our negative emotions.

Application: Apply to **Vita Flex points** on **feet** and/or directly on **area** of concern. This blend may also be **diffused,** applied to the **wrists** or **temples,** or added to warm **bathwater** (best when first combined with a bath gel base). For an uplifting massage, dilute first with a pure carrier oil.

Safety Data: ***Because of the existing contraindications for nutmeg, cinnamon bark, and sage, this blend should be used with caution by those individuals who are susceptible to* epileptic seizures *or who are* pregnant. *Repeated use could possibly result in* contact sensitization *or* skin irritation.**

Companion Oils: Clarity, Harmony, Gathering, Into the Future, Live with Passion, Sensation.

Frequency: Physical and Emotional; approximately 99 MHz.

Melrose™

The strong antiseptic properties of the single oils in this blend make it excellent for cleansing and healing **cuts, bruises, scrapes, and insect bites**; but it's primary use is helping with **tissue regeneration** from damage or injury. It also helps with **skin abrasions, burns, rashes, earaches, gums, cold sores, canker sores,** and **candida.** It fights **infection** and kills **anaerobic bacteria** and **fungus.** It has been used to help horses (and other animals) with skin cuts. ***Avoid use on cats.***

Single Oils Contained in This Blend:

Melaleuca—has **antibacterial, antifungal, anti-infectious, antiviral, strong antiseptic,** and **tissue regenerating** properties.

Melaleuca quinquenervia—is a very strong, very powerful **antifungal, antiviral,** and **antibacterial** oil. It may help **protect** against **radiation** and is a **strong tissue regenerator.**

Rosemary cineol—may help **balance heart function, energize** the **solar plexus,** and **reduce mental fatigue.** It has **analgesic, antiseptic,** and **anti-infectious** properties.

Clove—is **antibacterial, anti-infectious, anti-inflammatory,** a **strong antiseptic, disinfectant, immune-stimulant,** and a **topical anesthetic.**

Body System(s) Affected: The oils in this blend may help it be effective for dealing with various problems related to the **Respiratory System** and to the **Skin.**

Aromatic Influence: Dispels **odors.**

Application: Rub across brow, thumb Vita Flex points, and liver. Apply topically on cuts, scrapes, burns, rashes, or any infection. Put one to two drops on a piece of cotton, and place in the ear for earaches.

Safety Data: *Repeated use can possibly result in* **contact sensitization**. *Can be irritating to sensitive* **skin**.

Companion Oils: *Melaleuca ericifolia*.

Companion Products: Rose Ointment (delays evaporation of oil and promotes healing).

Frequency: Very Low (Physical); approximately 48 MHz.

Mister™

This blend was initially formulated to help balance male energy and help regulate prostate function. However, it has also been used successfully in eliminating hot flashes for women. Generally, Mister is good for women age 30–45, while EndoFlex is for women age 45+, and Dragon Time is for women up to age 30.

Single Oils Contained in This Blend:

Sage—may help improve estrogen and progesterone-testosterone balance. It is believed to contain elements that contribute to the secretion of progesterone-testosterone.

Fennel—may help improve digestive function by supporting the liver. It may also help balance the hormones.

Lavender—is an oil that has traditionally been known to balance the body and to work wherever there is a need. It is anti-inflammatory and may help reduce inflammation of the prostate.

Myrtle—is a decongestant of the prostate and respiratory system.

Peppermint—is anti-inflammatory to the prostate.

Yarrow—is a powerful decongestant of the prostate and a hormone balancer.

Carrier Oil Contained in This Blend: Sesame seed oil.

Body System(s) Affected: The oils in this blend may help it be effective for dealing with various problems related to the Hormonal System.

Application: Apply to Vita Flex points on ankles, to lower pelvis as a compress, and to Vita Flex points on body. Use directly on area of concern. Use on prostate (may want to dilute).

Safety Data: *Avoid during* **pregnancy**. *Use with caution if susceptible to* **epilepsy**.

Companion Oils: Dragon Time is a good companion with Mister for ladies. Single oils may include sage and clary sage.

Companion Supplements: FemiGen (capsules), Estro (tincture).

Frequency: High (Spiritual); approximately 147 MHz.

Motivation™

The single oils in this blend were combined to help people overcome fear and procrastination and take action in their lives. The authors of this book have used this blend several times to help push us through the difficult tasks of reformatting and editing.

Single Oils Contained in This Blend:

Roman Chamomile—was used by the ancient Romans traditionally to empower them to go into battle. It was also to give them a clear mind. This oil is soothing, relaxing, calming, and may help remove fears.

Spruce—**grounds** the **body**, creating the **balance** and the **opening** necessary to **receive** and to **give**. This is **empowering, anchoring** and **encouraging**.

Ylang Ylang—may help **balance** the **male-female energies** so one can move closer towards being in **spiritual attunement** and be able to focus their thoughts, filtering out the ever-present garbage. It brings back feelings of **self-love, confidence, joy,** and **peace**.

Lavender—is an oil that has traditionally been known to **balance** the **body** and to work wherever there is a need. It may help promote **consciousness, health, love, peace**, and a general sense of **well-being**.

Body System(s) Affected: The oils in this blend may help it be effective for dealing with various problems related to the **Nervous System** and to **Emotional Balance**.

Aromatic Influence: This blend of oils is wonderful for helping one **overcome** the **fear** of **achieving goals** and **dreams** and for **motivating** the **body** and **mind** into action.

Application: Wear on the **chest** or on the **nape** of the **neck** to stimulate the mind to want to take action. Place on **solar plexus, sternum** (key area), **feet** (especially the **big toe**), **navel** area, **ears** (on and behind), **wrist, palms** of **hands**, and **under nose** (sniff). Wear as **perfume** or **cologne**.

Frequency: Emotional; approximately 103 MHz.

PanAway™

Due to the aspirin-like properties of wintergreen and the powerful anti-inflammatory properties of the other oils, this blend helps to **reduce pain**. It also **stimulates quicker healing** by the **induction** of **oxygen** into the **tissue site**. It has been used to **relieve pain during surgery** with no anesthetic (helichrysum and clove were also used). It alleviates the symptoms of **sciatica**, relieves **bone pain** and pain from **arthritis** and **rheumatism**, and promotes **healthy circulation**. It also helps with **sports injuries, sprains, muscle spasms, bumps**, and **bruises**.

Single Oils Contained in This Blend:

Wintergreen—contains 99% methyl salicylate, which gives it cortisone-like properties. It may be beneficial for **arthritis, rheumatism, tendinitis**, and any other discomfort that is related to the inflammation of **bones, muscles**, and **joints**.

Helichrysum—may help **cleanse** the **blood** and improve **circulatory functions**. It is **anticatarrhal** in structure and nature. As a powerful **anti-inflammatory**, it may even help reduce inflammation in the meninges of the brain. On a spiritual level, it may help one **let go of angry feelings** that prevent one from forgiving and moving forward.

Clove—is **anti-infectious, anti-inflammatory, strongly antiseptic, disinfectant, immune-stimulant**, and **topically anesthetic**. It is also good for **arthritis, infection**, and **rheumatism**.

Peppermint—is **anti-inflammatory** to the **prostate** and to **damaged tissues**. It has a **soothing** and **cooling** effect that may help with **arthritis** and **rheumatism**.

Body System(s) Affected: The oils in this blend may help it be effective for dealing with various problems related to the **Nervous System** and to **Muscles and Bones**.

Application: Apply as a **compress** on **spine**, and apply to **Vita Flex points** on **feet**. Apply on location for **muscles, cramps, bruises**, or any painful area.

Companion Oils: Add helichrysum (to enhance) or wintergreen (for bone pain), or use with Ortho Ease or Ortho Sport Massage Oil. For deep tissue pain, use Relieve It.

Frequency: Emotional; approximately 112 MHz.

Peace & Calming™

The oils in this blend have historically been used to help reduce **depression, anxiety, stress,** and **tension.** This blend may help **hyperactive children** get off **Ritalin.** It may also help children with **hypertension.** It may be useful at the end of a stressful day to promote **relaxation** and **peace** or to relieve **insomnia.**

Single Oils Contained in This Blend:

Tangerine—contains esters and aldehydes, which are **sedating** and **calming** to the **nervous system.** It is also a **diuretic** and a **decongestant** of the **lymphatic system.**

Orange—brings **peace** and **happiness** to the **mind** and **body** and **joy** to the **heart,** which feelings provide **emotional** support to help one overcome depression.

Ylang Ylang—may help **balance** the **male-female energies** so one can move closer towards being in **spiritual attunement** and be able to focus their thoughts, filtering out the ever-present garbage. It brings back feelings of **self-love, confidence, joy,** and **peace.**

Patchouli—is **sedating, calming,** and **relaxing,** allowing it to reduce **anxiety.**

Blue Tansy—may help **cleanse** the **liver** and **calm** the **lymphatic system.**

Body System(s) Affected: The oils in this blend may help it be effective for dealing with various problems related to the **Nervous System** and to **Emotional Balance.**

Aromatic Influence: This blend of oils is perfect for **calming** the **nerves** or **emotions** at the end of a long day or in times of stress. It may help one **relax** before going to bed. By helping the body relax, more blood is able to circulate to the brain, allowing **goals** and **dreams** to be visualized more vividly and accurately.

Application: Apply **under nose,** on back of **neck,** on **back** (dilute with V-6 Oil), and on **feet.** Put in **bathwater.** Apply to **navel, feet,** or **back** of **neck** for **insomnia.** Wear as **perfume** or **cologne.**

Safety Data: *Avoid exposure to direct* ***sunlight*** *for 3 to 6 hours after use.*

Companion Oils: Lavender (for **insomnia**), chamomile (for **calming**).

Frequency: Emotional; approximately 105 MHz.

Present Time™

This blend was specifically created to helped **bring people** into the **moment.** We must live in the moment in order to heal. We cannot live yesterday; we cannot live tomorrow; we have to live **today.**

Single Oils Contained in This Blend:

Neroli—has been regarded traditionally by the Egyptian people for its great ability to **heal** the **mind, body,** and **spirit.** It is **calming** and **relaxing** to the body and spirit. It may also help to **strengthen** and **stabilize** the emotions and **bring relief** to seemingly hopeless situations. It encourages **confidence, courage, joy, peace,** and **sensuality.** It brings everything into the **focus** of one and at the moment.

Spruce—**grounds** the **body,** creating the **balance** and the **opening** necessary to **receive** and to **give.** It also helps one release **emotional blocks.** It was used by the Lakota Indians to enhance their communication with the Great Spirit.

Ylang Ylang—may help **balance** the **male-female energies** so one can move closer towards being in **spiritual attunement** and be able to focus their thoughts, filtering out the ever-present garbage. It brings back feelings of **self-love, confidence, joy,** and **peace.**

Carrier Oil Contained in This Blend: Almond oil.

Body System(s) Affected: The oils in this blend may help it be effective for dealing with various problems related to **Emotional Balance**.

Application: It is most effective when rubbed clockwise over the **thymus** (down the sternum—middle front of ribs) in a circular motion; close eyes and tap three times with energy fingers (pointer and middle). Also apply to **neck** and **forehead**.

Companion Oils: Harmony, Hope.

Frequency: Physical and Emotional; approximately 98 MHz.

Purification™

The individual oils in this blend have some powerful antiseptic, antibacterial, antifungal, and sanitizing properties. This blend is therefore useful for **killing odors** and their **bacteria, molds,** and **fungus**. It **kills anaerobic bacteria**. It **purifies** and **cleanses bacteria** in the **air** and neutralizes **mildew, cigarette smoke**, and other noxious **odors**. It **repels bugs, insects**, and **mice** that like to live in homes, offices, and other confined areas. It has also been beneficial in **neutralizing poison from insect bites**, such as those from **spiders, bees, hornets**, and **wasps**. It is good for first-aid in sterilizing **wounds** and **cuts**.

Single Oils Contained in This Blend:

- **Citronella**—has **antiseptic, antibacterial, antispasmodic, anti-inflammatory, deodorizing, insecticidal, purifying**, and **sanitizing** properties.
- **Lemongrass**—is **vasodilatory, antiseptic, antibacterial, anti-inflammatory**, and **sedative**. It may help improve **circulation**, wake up the **lymphatic system**, and increase the flow of **oxygen**. It may also help to **lift** the **spirit**.
- **Rosemary cineol**—may help **balance heart function, energize** the **solar plexus**, and **reduce mental fatigue**. It may **improve circulation** and help **stimulate** the **nerves**. It is **antiseptic** and **anti-infectious**.
- **Melaleuca**—may help **balance heart function** and act as a **cleanser** and **detoxifier** of the **blood**. It has **antibacterial, antifungal, anti-infectious, antiseptic, antiviral**, and **immune-stimulant** properties.
- **Lavandin**—is an **antifungal**, an **antibacterial**, a **strong antiseptic**, and a **tissue regenerator**.
- **Myrtle**—is a **decongestant** of the **respiratory system**. It may help **improve oxygenation** and work as an **expectorant** in **discharging mucus**. It is **antiseptic, antibacterial, euphoric**, and **elevating**.

Body System(s) Affected: The oils in this blend may help it be effective for dealing with various problems related to the **Digestive System**, to **Emotional Balance**, and to the **Skin**.

Aromatic Influence: This blend is great for **air purification** when diffused. When illness is in the **home**, diffuse for one hour and then wait for two. Repeat this pattern as desired. **Diffuse** in the **office, barn, or garbage areas**; or put oil on a cotton ball and place in an air vent to freshen the **car**.

Application: **Apply** to **Vita Flex points** of the **body, ears, feet**, and **temples**. Apply topically for infections and cleansing. Put on cotton balls and place in air vents for an **insect repellent** at home or at work. Can also be added to **paint** to help **reduce fumes**.

Safety Data: *Repeated use can possibly result in* **contact sensitization**. *Can be irritating to sensitive* **skin**.

Companion Oils: Citrus Fresh, Melrose, Thieves

Frequency: Very Low (Physical); approximately 46 MHz.

Raven™

The properties of the individual oils in this blend make it well suited to help alleviate the symptoms of **tuberculosis** and **pneumonia**. It goes beyond RC for **upper respiratory problems** and is especially useful for **viral infections**. It has been very beneficial for alleviating the symptoms of **asthma**.

Single Oils Contained in This Blend:

Ravensara—is a powerful **antiviral, antibacterial, antifungal**, and **anti-infectious** oil. It may help **dilate, open**, and **strengthen** the **respiratory system**. As a cross between clove and nutmeg, it may also help support the **adrenal glands**.

Lemon—promotes **health, healing, physical energy**, and **purification**. Its fragrance is **invigorating, enhancing**, and **warming**. It is an **antiseptic** and is great for the **respiratory system**.

Wintergreen—contains 99% methyl salicylate, which gives it cortisone-like properties. It may be beneficial for **arthritis, rheumatism, tendinitis**, and any other discomfort that is related to the inflammation of **bones, muscles**, and **joints**. It is also a **lymphatic cleanser**.

Peppermint—is **antiseptic, antispasmodic**, and **anti-inflammatory**. It is **soothing, cooling**, and **dilating** to the **system**.

Eucalyptus radiata—may have a profound **antiviral** effect upon the **respiratory system**. It may also help reduce **inflammation** of the **nasal mucous membrane**.

Body System(s) Affected: The oils in this blend may help it be effective for dealing with various problems related to the **Respiratory System** and to the **Skin**.

Aromatic Influence: This blend of oils is excellent for opening the **respiratory system** when diffused or inhaled.

Application: Apply to **Vita Flex points** of the **body**. Apply topically to **lungs** and **throat**. Put on pillow at night. It was traditionally used in **suppository** or **enema** application with V-6 Oil and retained throughout the night. This method of application can directly benefit the **lungs** within seconds.

Safety Data: ***Can be irritating to sensitive skin.***

Companion Oils: Melrose, RC, Thieves.

Frequency: Physical; approximately 70 MHz.

RC™

Although not as powerful against viral infections as Raven, the properties of the oils in this blend make it extremely effective against **allergies, colds, bronchitis, respiratory congestion, flu, cold sores, pneumonia, sinusitis, sore throat, mucus**, and **bone spurs**.

Single Oils Contained in This Blend:

Eucalyptus (*E. globulus*)—may have a profound **antiviral** effect upon the **respiratory system**. It also has **strong antibacterial, anticatarrhal**, and **antiseptic** properties.

Myrtle—is a **decongestant** of the **respiratory system**. It may help **improve oxygenation** and work as an **expectorant** in **discharging mucus**. It is **antiseptic, antibacterial, euphoric**, and **elevating**.

Pine—may help **dilate** and **open** the **respiratory system**, particularly the **bronchial tract**. It may also help **improve circulation throughout** the **lungs**.

Marjoram—is **relaxing, calming**, and **appeasing** to the **muscles** that constrict and sometimes contribute to **headaches**. As an **antispasmodic**, it may help relieve spasms in the **respiratory system**.

Eucalyptus radiata—may have a profound **antiviral** effect upon the **respiratory system**. It may also help reduce **inflammation** of the **nasal mucous membrane**.

Eucalyptus citriodora—is **antiviral**, **anti-infectious**, and **anti-inflammatory**.

Lavender—is an oil that has traditionally been known to **balance** the **body** and to work wherever there is a need. It may help promote **consciousness, health, love, peace**, and a general sense of **well-being**.

Cypress—is **anti-infectious, mucolytic, antiseptic, lymphatic decongestant, refreshing**, and **relaxing**. It may help improve **lung circulation** as well as help relieve other **respiratory problems**.

Tsuga—it is **grounding** and **uplifting** at the same time. It **opens** and **dilates** the **respiratory system** for better oxygen exchange.

Peppermint—is **antiseptic, antispasmodic**, and **anti-inflammatory**. It is **soothing, cooling**, and **dilating** to the **system**.

Body System(s) Affected: The oils in this blend may help it be effective for dealing with various problems related to the **Respiratory System**.

Aromatic Influence: RC is very beneficial when diffused to **decongest** and **relieve allergy-type** symptoms such as **coughs, sore throat**, and **lung congestion**.

Application: **Diffuse**. Dilute with V-6 Oil and **massage** on the **chest, back**, and **feet**. It can be used as a **compress** over the **chest** and **back**. Put on **sinuses** and **nasal passages** (put oil on a Q-tip and rub on inside of **nasal passages**). Rub around **ears, feet, neck**, and **throat**. Apply to **Vita Flex points** on **body**. It can be exchanged and alternated effectively with Raven.

Companion Oils: Apply Raven on feet and RC on throat and chest, alternate morning and night. Run hot steaming water in sink; put Raven, RC, and wintergreen in water; put towel over head, and **inhale** to open sinuses for **flu, colds.** or **pneumonia**. Also use Thieves.

Frequency: Physical; approximately 75 MHz.

Release™

This is a powerful blend for enhancing the **release** of **memory trauma** from the cells of the liver, where anger and hate emotions are stored. The frequency of the oils in Release may aid in the **letting go** of **negative emotions** so one can progress in a more effective and efficient way. It helps to **release frustration**.

Single Oils Contained in This Blend:

Ylang Ylang—may help **balance** the **male-female energies** so one can move closer towards being in **spiritual attunement** and be able to focus their thoughts, filtering out the ever-present garbage. It brings back feelings of **self-love, confidence, joy**, and **peace**.

Lavandin—is an **antifungal**, an **antibacterial**, a **strong antiseptic**, and a **tissue regenerator**.

Geranium—may help with **hormonal balance, liver** and **kidney functions**, and the **discharge** of **toxins** from the **liver** that keep us from having balance. Geranium **opens** the **liver chakra** (solar plexus). It may help **dilate** the **biliary ducts** for **liver detoxification**. It may also help foster **peace, well-being**, and **hope**.

Sandalwood—like frankincense—is high in sesquiterpenes, which were discovered to **increase** the amount of **oxygen** around the **pineal** and **pituitary glands**, thus helping to **improve** one's **attitude**. It **alleviates depression** and assists in the removal of **negative programming** from the cells of the body. It helps one **accept others** with an open heart, while diminishing one's own egocentricity.

Blue Tansy—may help **cleanse** the **liver** thereby helping to release **anger** and **negative emotions**.

Carrier Oil Contained in This Blend: Olive oil.

Body System(s) Affected: The oils in this blend may help it be effective for dealing with various problems related to **Emotional Balance**.

Application: Apply over **liver** or as a **compress**. Put on **ears**, bottoms of **feet**, and especially on **Vita Flex points** on **feet**. Wear as a **perfume or cologne**.

Companion Oils: Put Valor on **feet** first, then put Harmony (for balance) on **feet**, JuvaFlex on **feet**, and Release on **liver**; rotate the oil used each day.

Frequency: Emotional; approximately 102 MHz.

Relieve It™

The pepper oil and other deep penetrating oils in this blend make it effective for the relief of **deep tissue pain**. This extraordinary blend, with its high **anti-inflammatory** action, seems to go beyond **PanAway** in some pain applications, especially when alternated with PanAway and/or helichrysum. It may also help with **sciatica** and **arthritic pain.** (Try wintergreen too!) **PanAway** is more for **bone pain**.

Single Oils Contained in This Blend:

Spruce—**grounds** the **body**, creating the **balance** and the **opening** necessary to **receive** and to **give**. It may help **dilate** the **bronchial tract** to **improve** the **oxygen exchange**. It also helps one release **emotional blocks**.

Pepper, Black—may help **stimulate** the **endocrine system** and **increase energy**. It is an **anti-inflammatory** and was traditionally used for **rheumatoid arthritis**. It may also help **increase cellular oxygenation**.

Hyssop—was used by Moses during the Lord's Passover in Egypt (Exodus 12). It has **anti-inflammatory** and **antispasmodic** properties. It may also have the ability to **open** up the **respiratory system** and **discharge toxins** and **mucus**.

Peppermint—is **antiseptic**, **antispasmodic**, and **anti-inflammatory**. It is **soothing**, **cooling**, and **dilating** to the **system**.

Body System(s) Affected: The oils in this blend may help it be effective for dealing with various problems related to **Muscles and Bones**.

Application: Apply on location and anywhere there is **deep tissue pain**.

Safety Data: ***Can be irritating to sensitive skin. Use with caution during pregnancy. Use with caution if susceptible to epilepsy or high blood pressure.***

Companion Oils: PanAway is a great companion to Relieve It, especially when there is **bone pain**. Other companion oils may include Aroma Siez, Melrose, cypress, and helichrysum.

Frequency: Very Low (Physical); approximately 56 MHz.

RutaVaLa™

(Also available as a roll-on)

Although the Ruta graveolens herb itself, or water extracts from the herb, can have negative effects at very high doses, the steam distilled essential oil of Ruta is composed primarily of ingredients that are generally regarded as safe (GRAS) according to the FDA. Ruta oil is not only very **relaxing** to the body and mind but also **rebalancing** to the energy levels of the body. When coupled with valerian and lavender, both of which are well known for their **sedative** properties, this blend becomes both **relaxing** and **revitalizing** to the entire body, while **calming** stressed nerves and inducing a better quality of **sleep**.

Single Oils Contained in This Blend:

Ruta graveolens—was used historically for **nervous afflictions** and **hysterics**. The steam distilled essential oil is composed primarily of ingredients that are generally regarded as safe (GRAS) by the FDA. Aromatically, it is very **relaxing** and increases drowsiness.

Valerian—has a powerful sedative effect. It is also **antispasmodic, depressant** to the central nervous system, and somewhat **hypnotic**. It may help minimize the shock, the feeling of anxiety, and the stress that accompanies traumatic situations.

Lavender—is an oil that has traditionally been known to **balance** the **body** and to work wherever there is a need. It has **antispasmodic** and **analgesic** properties. It helps to relieve **sore muscles,** eases **tension** and **stress**, and promotes general **healing**. Lavender also reducees cortisol.

Body System(s) Affected: The oils in this blend may help it be effective for dealing with various problems related to the **Nervous System** and to **Emotional Balance**.

Application: **Diffuse** or inhale 1–2 drops every hour or as needed. Dilute heavily for topical application.

Safety Data: ***Avoid using on skin without dilution. Avoid use during pregnancy. Avoid exposure to direct sunlight for up to 12 hours after use.***

Companion Oils: Peace & Calming, White Angelica, and clary sage.

Sacred Mountain™

The predominance of conifer oils in this blend creates a feeling of **protection, empowerment**, and **grounding**. This blend may help one find **security** and **sacredness** within **oneself**. In addition, it is **antibacterial** and very **soothing** to the **respiratory system**.

Single Oils Contained in This Blend:

Spruce—**grounds** the **body**, creating the **balance** and the **opening** necessary to **receive** and to **give**. It also helps one release **emotional blocks**. It was used by the Lakota Indians to enhance their communication with the Great Spirit.

Ylang Ylang—may help **balance** the **male-female energies** so one can move closer towards being in **spiritual attunement** and be able to focus their thoughts, filtering out the ever-present garbage. It brings back feelings of **self-love, confidence, joy,** and **peace**.

Fir—may help create a feeling of **grounding, anchoring** and **empowerment**.

Cedarwood—was used traditionally by the North American Indians to enhance their potential for **spiritual communication**. It may help **open** the **pineal gland**.

Body System(s) Affected: The oils in this blend may help it be effective for dealing with various problems related to **Emotional Balance**.

Aromatic Influence: The aroma of this blend of oils creates a feeling of **strength, empowerment, grounding**, and **protection**.

Application: Diffuse. Apply to solar plexus, brain stem, crown of head, back of neck, behind ears, thymus, and wrists. Wear as perfume or cologne.

Safety Data: *Can be irritating to sensitive **skin**.*

Frequency: High (Spiritual); approximately 176 MHz.

Comments: The three conifer oils have been traditionally used by the North American Indians symbolically to represent the umbrella they create in protecting the earth and bringing energy in from the universe. At night, the animals in the wild lie under the trees for the protection, recharging, and rejuvenation the trees bring to them.

SARA™

The oils in this blend produce a beautiful fragrance that may allow one to relax into a mental state whereby they may be able to release and let go of negative emotions and the memory of traumatic experiences. Although created specifically for relief from the memory trauma of sexual and/or ritual abuse, it may also work well for other traumatic experiences.

Single Oils Contained in This Blend:

Ylang Ylang—may help balance the male-female energies so one can move closer towards being in spiritual attunement and be able to focus their thoughts, filtering out the ever-present garbage. It brings back feelings of self-love, confidence, joy, and peace.

Geranium—may help with hormonal balance, liver and kidney functions, and the discharge of toxins from the liver that keep us from having balance. Geranium opens the liver chakra (solar plexus). It may help dilate the biliary ducts for liver detoxification. It may also help foster peace, well-being, and hope by promoting the release of negative memories.

Lavender—is an oil that has traditionally been known to balance the body and to work wherever there is a need. It may help promote consciousness, health, love, peace, and a general sense of well-being.

Orange—brings peace and happiness to the mind and body and joy to the heart, which feelings provide emotional support to help one overcome depression.

Blue Tansy—may help cleanse the liver and calm the lymphatic system.

Cedarwood—was used traditionally by the North American Indians to enhance their potential for spiritual communication. It may help open the pineal gland.

Rose—has a beautiful fragrance and contains the highest frequency of any oil. It may help enhance the frequency of every cell, which could help bring balance and harmony to the body. It is thought by some to produce a magnetic energy that attracts love and enhances the frequency of self-love, bringing joy to the heart.

White Lotus—was traditionally used by the Egyptians for spiritual, emotional, and physical applications. It has a euphoric fragrance that lifts and stabilizes the emotions, creating a powerful sense of emotional, physical, and spiritual well-being.

Carrier Oil Contained in This Blend: Almond oil.

Body System(s) Affected: The oils in this blend may help it be effective for dealing with various problems related to Emotional Balance.

Aromatic Influence: The aroma of this blend of oils creates a feeling of peace and freedom to move forward in life with joy.

Application: Apply over energy centers, on Vita Flex points, and on temples, nose, and areas of abuse.

Companion Oils: Forgiveness, Hope, Inner Child, Inspiration, Joy, Magnify Your Purpose, 3 Wise Men, Trauma Life, Valor, White Angelica.

Frequency: Emotional; approximately 102 MHz.

Comments: One individual muscle tested positive for this oil for the purpose of overcoming the emotions related to having a twin brother die early in gestation but remain in the womb until full-term delivery.

SclarEssence™

This blend was formulated to support the **hormones** and to increase estradiol and testosterone levels. When taken as a dietary supplement, it may also help improve **digestion**, reduce **bloating**, and help balance the body's pH.

Single Oils Contained in This Blend:

Clary Sage—is beneficial for **regulating cells** and **balancing** the **hormones**. It may help with **menstrual cramps, PMS**, and **premenopause** symptoms. It may also help with **circulatory problems**.

Peppermint—is an **anti-inflammatory** to the **prostate** and **nerves**. It is **soothing** to the **stomach, cooling**, and **dilating** to the **system**.

Sage Lavender—has been shown to increase both estradiol and testosterone levels. It may help **harmonize** and **balance** the **emotions** and reduce **stress-related** conditions. It may also help decongest the **liver**.

Fennel—may help **improve digestive function** by **supporting** the **liver**. It may also help **balance** the **hormones**.

Body System(s) Affected: **Hormonal** and **Digestive Systems**.

Oral Use As Dietary Supplement: *Put 1–20 drops in a capsule. Ingest 1 capsule daily as needed.* ***Not recommended for children.***

Sensation™

Because of the incredibly beautiful aromas of ylang ylang, rosewood, and jasmine, this blend is extremely **uplifting, refreshing**, and **arousing**. It is beneficial for **skin problems** of any kind, as it is very nourishing and hydrating to the skin.

Single Oils Contained in This Blend:

Rosewood—is **soothing** to the **skin, appeasing** to the **mind, relaxing** to the **body**, and creates a feeling of **peace** and **gentleness**.

Ylang Ylang—may help **balance** the **male-female energies** so one can move closer towards being in **spiritual attunement** and be able to focus their thoughts, filtering out the ever-present garbage. It brings back feelings of **self-love, confidence, joy**, and **peace**.

Jasmine—is very **uplifting** to the **emotions**; it may produce a feeling of **confidence, energy, euphoria**, and **optimism**.

Body System(s) Affected: The oils in this blend may help it be effective for dealing with various problems related to the **Hormonal System** and to **Emotional Balance**.

Aromatic Influence: Because the aroma of this blend of oils is so **uplifting** and **arousing**, it creates a feeling of **excitement** and **romance**, which may help move one to new heights of **self-expression** and **awareness**.

Application: Apply on **location**, use for **massage**, and add to your Sensation Bath and Shower Gel. May also be used with a **compress** over the abdomen or just worn as a **cologne** or **perfume**.

Companion Oils: Awaken, Dream Catcher, Into the Future, Joy, Live with Passion

Frequency: Physical and Emotional; approximately 88 MHz.

Stress Away™

(Essential Oil Roll-On)

Those suffering from chronic **stress** tend to have **weaker immune systems**, to be more suceptible to **cardiovascular disease**, and to experience more **premature cell aging**. This portable blend is specially formulated to help relieve everyday **stresses** and **tensions** so that you can **sleep better** at night and live a healthier and happier life.

Single Oils Contained in This Blend:

Copal (or Copaiba)—is extremely high in β-caryophyllene, which has been well documented for its **anti-inflammatory** actions. It has traditionally been used for **muscle aches and pains**, **stiffness**, and **nervous exhaustion**. It helps to **elevate the mood** and **lift depression**, and may amplify the effects of the other essential oils in the blend.

Lime—has a fresh, lively fragrance that is **stimulating** and **refreshing**. It helps one overcome **exhaustion**, **depression**, and **listlessness**.

Cedarwood—may be **calming** and may help to eliminate **nervous tension**.

Ocotea—may help with **emotional balance**.

Lavender—is relaxing and promotes **health** and a general sense of **well-being**.

Other Ingredients Contained in This Blend: Vanilla.

Body System(s) Affected: The oils in this blend may help it to be effective in dealing with problems related to **Emotional Balance** and **Immune System** functioning.

Application: Apply to the **wrists**, **temples**, **neck**, or other desired areas of the body.

Safety Data: ***Consult a physician before using this blend if you are pregnant, nursing, taking medication, or suffering from a medical condition. Do not apply to areas of sensitive tissues. Not for children under six years old.***

Surrender™

Most of the single oils in this blend are **calming**, **relaxing**, and **balancing** to the emotions, making it effective for those with **dominant personalities** who at times may become **unfocused** or **overbearing**. By **balancing** the **emotions**, **clearing** the **mind**, and reducing feelings of **anxiety** and **stress**, this blend may help such individuals recover **equilibrium** and calm **inner strength**.

Single Oils Contained in This Blend:

Lavender—is an oil that has traditionally been known to **balance** the **body** and to work wherever there is a need. It may help promote **consciousness**, **health**, **love**, **peace**, and a general sense of **well-being**.

Roman Chamomile—eliminates some of the emotional charge of **anxiety**, **irritability**, and **nervousness**. Because it is **calming** and **relaxing**, it can combat **stress**.

German Chamomile—can dispel **anger**, stabilize the **emotions**, and help release emotions liked to the past. It may also help to **soothe** and **clear** the **mind** creating an atmosphere of **peace** and **patience**.

Angelica—is referred to by the German people as the "oil of angels." It may help one **release** and **let go** of **negative feelings**.

Mountain Savory—has **immune-stimulant, antimicrobial**, and **antiparasitic** properties. It is also a powerful **energizer** and **motivator**.

Lemon—promotes **health, healing, physical energy**, and **purification**. Its fragrance is **invigorating, enhancing**, and **warming**.

Spruce—**grounds** the **body**, creating the **balance** and the **opening** necessary to **receive** and to **give**. It may help **dilate** the **bronchial tract** to **improve** the **oxygen exchange**. It also helps one release **emotional blocks**.

Body System(s) Affected: The oils in this blend may help it be effective for dealing with various problems related to the **Nervous System** and to **Emotional Balance**.

Aromatic Influence: May help to reduce **anxiety** and calm **nervousness** and **irritability**. It may also help to **balance** the **emotions** and **clear** the **mind**.

Application: Apply on the **forehead**, along the **rim** of the **ears**, at the **nape** of the **neck**, on the **chest**, and on the **solar plexus**. May also be added to **bathwater**.

Safety Data: *Because of some of the oils contained within this blend, it should be used with caution by individuals who are* **pregnant**. *Repeated use could possibly result in* **skin irritation**.

Companion Oils: Clarity, Forgiveness, Grounding, Peace & Calming, Sacred Mountain

Frequency: Physical and Emotional; approximately 98 MHz.

The Gift™

This unique blend combines several essential oils from plants that were used anciently in the desert lands of the Middle East to help protect and heal wounds and to help support the immune system.

Single Oils Contained in This Blend:

Frankincense—has **anti-inflammatory** and **antiseptic** properties that promote **wound healing**. Frankincense was also use anciently along with spikenard to help **regenerate** and **repair tissue**.

Balsam Fir—has **antiseptic** properties and is often used to help heal **wounds** and for **DNA repair**.

Jasmine—has **antispasmodic** properties and may help relieve **pain** and **nervous exhaustion**.

Galbanum—is **antiviral, antispasmodic**, and **antiseptic**, and may help relieve **pain** and **muscle spasms**.

Myrrh—is highly regarded for its **anti-infectious** and **anti-inflammatory** properties. It is also **soothing** to the skin and often used to help heal **wounds**.

Cistus—is **antimicrobial** and can also help stop **bleeding**.

Spikenard—is **antifungal, antibacterial, anti-inflammatory, and regenerative**. It was used anciently along with frankincense to help **regenerate** and **repair tissue**.

Body System(s) Affected: The oils in this blend may help it be effective for dealing with various problems related to the **immune system, skin,** and **muscles and bones**

Application: Apply 1–2 drops on **wounds** or on bandages covering wounds. Apply on bottoms of **feet, temples**, or **neck**. Add 1–2 drops to warm **bathwater. Diffuse**

Safety Data: *Because of some of the oils contained within this blend, it should be used with caution by individuals who are* **pregnant**. *Repeated use could possibly result in* **skin irritation**.

Companion Oils: ImmuPower, Thieves.

Thieves®

The highly antiviral and antiseptic properties of the single oils contained in this blend help protect the body from the onset of **flu, candida, colds**, etc. It may also help with **sinusitis, bronchitis, pneumonia, coughs, strep, sore throats, periodontal (gum) disease, teething, cold sores, canker sores, bruises, cuts, infection, slivers, and splinters** (pulls to surface). It is considered **antiplague**, as it was used by thieves in England to protect them from the plague when stealing from the sick and dying.

Single Oils Contained in This Blend:

Clove—is **antibacterial, antifungal, anti-infectious, antiparasitic**, a **strong antiseptic, antiviral**, and an **immune stimulant**. It may influence **healing** and help create a feeling of **protection** and **courage**.

Lemon—promotes **health, healing, physical energy**, and **purification**. Its fragrance is **invigorating, enhancing**, and **warming**. It is an **antiseptic** and is great for the **respiratory system**.

Cinnamon Bark—is part of the formula the Lord gave Moses (Exodus 30:22-27). It has very specific purposes: (1) it is a **powerful purifier**, (2) it is a powerful **oxygenator**, and (3) it **enhances** the action and the activity of **other oils**. It may have a **stimulating** and **toning** effect on the whole body and particularly on the circulatory system. It is **antibacterial, antifungal, anti-infectious, anti-inflammatory, antimicrobial, antiparasitic, antiseptic, antispasmodic, antiviral, astringent, immune-stimulant, sexual stimulant**, and **warming**.

Eucalyptus radiata—may have a profound **antiviral** effect upon the **respiratory system**. It also has **strong antibacterial, anticatarrhal**, and **antiseptic** properties.

Rosemary cineol—may help **balance heart function, energize** the **solar plexus**, and **reduce mental fatigue**. It may **improve circulation** and help **stimulate** the **nerves**. It is **antiseptic** and **anti-infectious**.

Body System(s) Affected: The oils in this blend may help it be effective for dealing with various problems related to the **immune system**.

Aromatic Influence: Diffuse this blend of oils periodically for 20–25 minutes at a time to help protect the body against the onset of **flu, colds**, and **viruses**.

Application: Massage bottom of **feet, throat, stomach**, and **intestines**. Dilute one drop of Thieves in 15 drops of V-6 Oil and massage the **thymus** to stimulate the **immune system** and massage **under** the **arms** to stimulate the **lymphatic system**. It is best applied to the bottom of the feet as it may be caustic to the skin. **Always dilute with V-6 Oil.**

Safety Data: ***Repeated use can result in extreme contact sensitization. Can cause extreme skin irritation. Use with caution during pregnancy.***

Companion Oils: Put ImmuPower on the **throat** and Thieves on the **feet**; then alternate by putting Thieves on the **throat** and ImmuPower on the **feet**. You can also alternate ImmuPower with Exodus II.

Frequency: Emotional and Spiritual; approximately 150 MHz.

Comments: Studies conducted by Weber State University (Ogden, UT) in 1997 showed the antibacterial effectiveness of this blend (Thieves) against airborne microorganisms. One study showed a 90% reduction in the number of Gram-positive *Micrococcus luteus* organisms after diffusing Thieves for 12 minutes. After diffusing Thieves for a total of 20 minutes, there was a 99.3% reduction. Another study with the Gram-negative *Pseudomonas aeruginosa* showed a kill rate of 99.96% after just 12 minutes of diffusion.

3 Wise Men™

The highly spiritual nature of the oils in this blend allow it to **open** the **crown chakra** and facilitate the release of negative emotions. This blend brings a sense of **grounding** and **uplifting** through **memory recall**. It also keeps negative energy and negative emotions from reattaching to the body.

Single Oils Contained in This Blend:

Sandalwood—like frankincense—is high in sesquiterpenes, which were discovered to **increase** the amount of **oxygen** around the **pineal** and **pituitary glands**, thus helping to **improve** one's **attitude**. It **alleviates depression** and assists in the removal of **negative programming** from the cells of the body. It helps one **accept others** with an open heart, while diminishing one's own egocentricity.

Juniper—evokes feelings of **health**, **love**, and **peace** and may help to **elevate** one's **spiritual awareness**.

Frankincense—contains sesquiterpenes, which may help **oxygenate** the **pineal** and **pituitary glands**. As one of the ingredients for the holy incense, frankincense was used anciently to help **enhance** one's **communication with the Creator**. It was considered a prize possession and was given to Christ at his birth by the three wise men. It may help **promote** a **positive attitude**.

Spruce—**grounds** the **body**, creating the **balance** and the **opening** necessary to **receive** and to **give**. It also helps one release **emotional blocks**. It was used by the Lakota Indians to enhance their communication with the Great Spirit.

Myrrh—is part of the formula the Lord gave Moses (Exodus 30:22-27). It promotes **spiritual awareness** and is a **true gift** (one of the gifts that was brought for the Christ child). When we **open** our **hearts** and **minds** to receive the gifts, they will be given.

Carrier Oil Contained in This Blend: Almond oil.

Body System(s) Affected: The oils in this blend may help it be effective for dealing with various problems related to **Emotional Balance**.

Aromatic Influence: **Diffusing** this blend of oils may help to create a feeling of **reverence** and heightened **spiritual consciousness**.

Application: Apply to the **crown** of the **head** in a clockwise motion to create an energy of opening and releasing, followed by receiving the energy of the oils to **fill** the **new void**. Put on **neck**, **eyebrow**, **solar plexus**, and **thymus** (clockwise). Wear as **perfume** or **cologne**.

Companion Oils: Frankincense, myrrh, sandalwood, juniper, and spruce.

Frequency: Physical; approximately 72 MHz.

Comments: When all or any of the companion oils are combined with 3 Wise Men, a sense of **grounding** and **upliftment** come through the release of memory recall. In addition, when the oil is placed on the crown, it elevates one's spiritual consciousness.

Tranquil™

(Essential Oil Roll-On)

This blend contains a combination of essential oils that are highly regarded for their **calming** and **relaxing** properties. These oils have been formulated to ease **tension** and **anxiety**, reduce **restlessness**, and to **stabilize** and **balance** the body, both **physically** and **emotionally**. Because this blend is offered as a roll-on, it provides a no-mess application in just about any situation. With the small, steel ball applicator, it delivers a precise amount of oil with no runs or drips and no need to rub it in with a finger.

Single Oils Contained in This Blend:

Lavender—is an oil that has traditionally been known to **balance** the **body** and to work wherever there is a need. It has **antispasmodic** and **analgesic** properties. It helps to relieve **sore muscles,** eases **tension** and **stress**, and promotes general **healing**.

Cedarwood—was used traditionally by the North American Indians to enhance their potential for **spiritual communication**. It may help **open** the **pineal gland**. With one of the highest concentrations of **sesquiterpenes**, it is **calming** and **relaxing** to both mind and body.

Roman Chamomile—is **anti-inflammatory** and **antispasmodic**. It is **calming** and **relaxing** and helps to relieve **muscle tension** and **stress**.

Carrier Oils Contained In This Blend: Fractionated coconut oil and virgin coconut oil.

Body System(s) Affected: The oils in this blend may help it be effective for dealing with various problems related to the **Nervous System** and to **Emotional Balance**.

Aromatic Influence: This blend of oils is perfect for **calming** the **nerves** or **emotions** at the end of a long day or in times of stress. It may help one **relax** before going to bed. By helping the body relax, more blood is able to circulate to the brain, allowing **goals** and **dreams** to be visualized more vividly and accurately.

Application: Apply liberally to **temples**, back of **neck,** or **wrists** as needed.

Companion Oils: Lavender (add to feet for **insomnia**).

Transformation™

Many of the oils in this blend are powerfully **energizing** and **stimulating** to the **conscious mind,** allowing for the **support** necessary to make changes, especially **mental** and **emotional changes**.

Single Oils Contained in This Blend:

Lemon—promotes **health, healing, physical energy**, and **purification**. Its fragrance is **invigorating, enhancing**, and **warming**.

Peppermint—is **anti-inflammatory** to the **nerves**. It has a **soothing** and **cooling effect** on **headaches**. It is **purifying** and **stimulating** to the **conscious mind**.

Clary Sage—may calm and enhance the **dream state**, helping to bring about a feeling of **euphoria**.

Sandalwood—like frankincense—is high in sesquiterpenes, which were discovered to **increase** the amount of **oxygen** around the **pineal** and **pituitary glands**, thus helping to **improve** one's **attitude**.

Idaho Blue Spruce— **grounds** the body, creating the feeling of **balance** necessary to receive and to give.

Sacred Frankincense—contains sesquiterpenes, which may help **oxygenate** the **pineal** and **pituitary glands**. As one of the ingredients for the holy incense, frankincense was used anciently to help **enhance** one's **communication with the Creator**. It may help **promote** a **positive attitude**.

Cardamom—is **uplifting, refreshing**, and **invigorating**. It may be beneficial for **clearing confusion**.

Palo Santo—has a wonderfully **calming**, **soothing** aroma with a **powerful energy**. It may help to increase **spiritual awareness** and focus **meditation** while **clearing** the space of **negative energy**.

Ocotea—has a wonderful cleansing property and may aid with inflammation.

Body System(s) Affected: The oils in this blend may help it be effective for dealing with various problems related to **Emotional Balance**.

Aromatic Influence: When diffused or worn as a perfume, this blend of oils may help **stimulate** one's mind and **strengthen** one's resolve when dealing with difficult decisions, especially when related to a change in **attitude** or a change in one's **belief system**.

Application: **Diffuse**, or apply to the **forehead** ("third eye" chakra) and over the **heart**, helping to unite the heart and mind.

Companion Oils: Hope, Humility, Into the Future.

Trauma Life™

Many of the oils in this blend are powerfully **calming** and **grounding**, helping **purge** the **stress** and **uproot** the **traumas** that are often at the heart of our physical fatigue and overburdened immune systems. Others of the oils in this blend are **spiritually uplifting**, bringing us closer to our **Creator** and helping us to see our **trials** from the **proper perspective**. Sometimes, physical and mental difficulties are a result of unreleased trauma. For example, our one-year-old daughter would continually babble until one day she fell down a flight of stairs. Although she was not physically hurt from the fall, we soon noticed that the babbling had stopped. One application of this blend brought back the constant babbling.

Single Oils Contained in This Blend:

Frankincense—contains sesquiterpenes, which may help **oxygenate** the **pineal** and **pituitary glands**. As one of the ingredients for the holy incense, frankincense was used anciently to help **enhance** one's **communication with the Creator**. It may help **promote** a **positive attitude**.

Sandalwood—like frankincense—is high in sesquiterpenes, which were discovered to **increase** the amount of **oxygen** around the **pineal** and **pituitary glands**, thus helping to **improve** one's **attitude**.

Valerian—has a powerful sedative effect. It is also **antispasmodic**, **depressant** to the central nervous system, and somewhat **hypnotic**. It may help minimize the shock, the feeling of anxiety, and the stress that accompanies traumatic situations.

Lavender—is an oil that has traditionally been known to **balance** the **body** and to work wherever there is a need. It may help promote **consciousness**, **health**, **love**, **peace**, and a general sense of **well-being**.

Davana—is **anti-infectious** and may stimulate the **endocrine system** and improve **hormonal balance**.

Spruce—**grounds** the **body**, creating the **balance** and the **opening** necessary to **receive** and to **give**. It may help **dilate** the **bronchial tract** to **improve** the **oxygen exchange**. It also helps one release **emotional blocks**.

Geranium—may help with **hormonal balance**, **liver** and **kidney functions**, and the **discharge** of **toxins** from the **liver** that keep us from having balance. Geranium **opens** the **liver chakra** (solar plexus). It may help **dilate** the **biliary ducts** for **liver detoxification**, which may help one let go of **anger** and **negative emotions**.

Helichrysum—may help **cleanse** the **blood** and improve **circulatory functions**. It is **anticatarrhal** in structure and nature. As a powerful **anti-inflammatory**, it may even help reduce inflammation in the meninges of the brain. On a spiritual level, it may help one **let go of angry feelings** that prevent one from forgiving and moving forward.

Limette (*Citrus hystrix*)—is very high in aldehydes and esters, making it very **sedating** and **calming**.

Rose—possesses the highest frequency of any oil. It may help **enhance** the **frequency** of every cell, which could help bring **balance** and **harmony** to the body. It is thought by some to produce a magnetic energy that attracts **love** and enhances the frequency of **self-love**, bringing **joy** to the heart.

Body System(s) Affected: The oils in this blend may help it be effective for dealing with various problems related to **Emotional Balance**.

Aromatic Influence: When diffused, this blend of oils may help promote the **calming** and **balancing** effect that is necessary in overcoming **trauma**.

Application: Best when applied to the **spine** using the Raindrop Technique. It is also beneficial when placed on the bottoms of the **feet**, on the **chest**, behind the **ears**, on the nap of the **neck**, or in the center of the **forehead** ("third eye" chakra).

Companion Oils: Peace & Calming, Joy, Hope, Into the Future.

Frequency: Physical and Emotional; approximately 92 MHz.

Valor™

This blend has been used to help **empower** the **physical** and **spiritual bodies**. It helps us **overcome fear** and **opposition** so we can stand tall during adversity. It may help build **courage, confidence**, and **self-esteem**. It brings a feeling of **calmness, peace,** and **relaxation**. It may be used in place of Peace & Calming for **hyperactivity** and **attention deficit disorder** in **children**. It has been found beneficial in helping to **align** the **physical structure** of the **body, relieving pain** along the **spine**. It also **balances** and **aligns electrical energies** within the **body**. It is best applied with six drops on each foot or massaged in along the spine using the Raindrop Technique. Valor has been touted as a **chiropractor** in a bottle. It has improved **scoliosis** in as little as 30 minutes, though this should not be considered normal. Some individuals require several months of application before any improvement is seen. *Valor has also been shown to change anaerobic mutated cells back to their aerobic natural state.*

Oil Blends

Single Oils Contained in This Blend:

Spruce—**grounds** the **body**, creating the **balance** and the **opening** necessary to **receive** and to **give**. It may help **dilate** the **bronchial tract** to **improve** the **oxygen exchange**. It also helps one release **emotional blocks**.

Rosewood—is **soothing** to the **skin, appeasing** to the **mind, relaxing** to the **body**, and creates a feeling of **peace** and **gentleness**.

Blue Tansy—may help **cleanse** the **liver** and **calm** the **lymphatic system** to help rid oneself of **anger** and promote a feeling of **self-control**.

Frankincense—contains sesquiterpenes, which may help **oxygenate** the **pineal** and **pituitary glands**. As one of the ingredients for the holy incense, frankincense was used anciently to help **enhance** one's **communication with the Creator**. It may help **promote** a **positive attitude**.

Carrier Oil Contained in This Blend: Almond oil.

Body System(s) Affected: The oils in this blend may help it be effective for dealing with various problems related to **Muscles and Bones, Skin**, the **Nervous System**, and **Emotional Balance**.

Aromatic Influence: This blend of oils may help **balance** the **electrical energies** in the body. **Diffuse** wherever and whenever possible.

Application: It **works best** on the **bottoms** of the **feet**. Put six drops of Valor on **bottoms** of **feet**. Put Valor on **heart, throat chakra, wrists,** and **solar plexus** from **neck** to **thymus**. To **balance left** and **right brain**, put Valor on **left fingers** and rub on **right temple** or put Valor on **right fingers** and rub on **left temple or cross arms** and rub **Vita Flex points** on bottom of **feet**. To **relieve pain** along the **spine**, apply Valor to **Vita Flex points** on **feet** and on **spine** using the **raindrop technique**. Wear as **perfume** or **cologne**.

Companion Oils: **Balance** with Valor and **protect** with White Angelica.

Frequency: **Very low** to balance and align the physical body; aligns the skeletal system; approximately 47 MHz.

Comments: This blend is the most important oil in any application. It helps balance electrical energies within the body, giving courage, confidence, and self-esteem. Most importantly, it builds the bridge between the body and the oils allowing higher frequency oils to raise the frequency of the body thus promoting physical, emotional, and spiritual well-being. (*Refer to the Vita Flex Therapy part of the Science and Application section of this book for the importance of using this blend and how to use it to balance the body's energy*).

Valor™

(Essential Oil Roll-On)

This is the same blend of essential oils as listed above in a base of fractionated coconut oil and virgin coconut oil. Because this blend is offered as a roll-on, it provides a no-mess application in just about any situation. With the small, steel ball applicator, it delivers a precise amount of oil with no runs or drips and no need to rub it in with a finger.

White Angelica™

This unique blend of 10 different oils helps create a frequency field to **ward off** the **bombardment** of **negative energy**. It is important for use in **emotional cleansing**. It may help **increase** the **aura** around the body, bringing a delicate sense of **strength** and **protection** and a greater **awareness** of **one's potential**. It may also help with **anger, depression, headaches** (especially when flying), **hemorrhoids, circulation**, and **lowering high blood pressure**.

Single Oils Contained in This Blend:

Bergamot—is **soothing** to the **endocrine system** and to the **hormones**. It may **uplift** and **calm** the **emotions** and help relieve **anxiety, stress**, and **tension**.

Geranium—may help with **hormonal balance, liver** and **kidney functions,** and the **discharge** of **toxins** from the **liver** that keep us from having balance. Geranium **opens** the **liver chakra** (solar plexus). It may help **dilate** the **biliary ducts** for **liver detoxification**, which may help one let go of **anger** and **negative emotions**.

Myrrh—is part of the formula the Lord gave Moses (Exodus 30:22-27). It promotes **spiritual awareness** and is a **true gift** (one of the gifts that was brought for the Christ child). When we **open** our **hearts** and **minds** to receive the gifts, they will be given.

Sandalwood—like frankincense—is high in sesquiterpenes, which were discovered to **increase** the amount of **oxygen** around the **pineal** and **pituitary glands**, thus helping to **improve** one's **attitude**. It **alleviates depression** and assists in the removal of **negative programming** from the cells of the body.

Rosewood—may help bring a synergism to all the oils. It is **soothing** to the **skin, appeasing** to the **mind, relaxing** to the **body**, and creates a feeling of **peace** and **gentleness**.

Ylang Ylang—may help **balance** the **male-female energies** so one can move closer towards being in **spiritual attunement** and be able to focus their thoughts, filtering out the ever-present garbage. It brings back feelings of **self-love, confidence, joy,** and **peace**.

Spruce—**grounds** the **body**, creating the **balance** and the **opening** necessary to **receive** and to **give**. It also helps one release **emotional blocks**.

Hyssop—was used by Moses during the Lord's Passover in Egypt (Exodus 12). It has **anti-inflammatory** and **antiviral** properties. It may have the ability to **open** up the **respiratory system** and **discharge toxins** and **mucus**. It may also stimulate **meditation** and promote **centering**.

Melissa—is powerful as an **antiviral** agent, yet it is very gentle and very delicate because of the nature of the plant. It has the ability to work with and enhance the gentle aspects of the human body. It is **calming** and **uplifting** and may help to **balance** the **emotions**. It may also help to remove **emotional blocks** and **instill** a **positive outlook** on **life**.

Rose—possesses the highest frequency of any oil. It may help **enhance** the **frequency** of every cell, which could help bring **balance** and **harmony** to the body. It is thought by some to produce a magnetic energy that attracts **love** and enhances the frequency of **self-love**, bringing **joy** to the heart.

Carrier Oil Contained in This Blend: Almond oil.

Body System(s) Affected: The oils in this blend may help it be effective for dealing with various problems related to **Emotional Balance**.

Aromatic Influence: The aroma of this blend of oils may be a tremendous aid in times of **meditation**.

Application: Apply on **shoulders, crown, chest**, behind the **ears,** and on **neck, forehead**, and **wrists**. Add to **bathwater**. Wear as **perfume** or **cologne**.

Safety Data: ***Avoid exposure to direct sunlight for 3 to 6 hours after use.***

Companion Oils: **Balance** with Valor and **protect** with White Angelica. Use with Inspiration, Awaken, and Sacred Mountain to create a feeling of wholeness in the realm of one's own spirituality and oneness with the **Creator**. When the heart is stressed, use Joy and Aroma Life with White Angelica.

Frequency: Physical and Emotional; approximately 89 MHz.

A Great Help for Alzheimer's Disease

When my mother who has Alzheimer's came to live with us, she didn't sleep at night but was up cleaning out drawers, slamming doors, and being generally noisy all night. We were introduced to Young Living Oils and started putting Peace & Calming in a cool mist vaporizer 3–4 times during the day in the living area where she spent her time. In two weeks, she began sleeping ALL NIGHT!!! We've continued using a variety of oils (lavender, Brain Power, lemon, Clarity), and she is now in better health than she's been in 20 years. She still has Alzheimer's, but her mood is mostly stabilized.

-Submitted by E. Pinar (July 2004)

Personal Care Products

These product names are all trademarks of Young Living Essential Oils, and although these product names appear throughout other sections of this book without the trademark symbol, they still refer to these same trademarked products.

A•R•T® Skin Care System (Age-Refining Technology)

This revolutionary set of three synergistic skin care products (Day Activator, Gentle Foaming Cleanser, and Night Reconstructor) provides a complete system for unprecedented protection and restoration of the skin. These products utilize the following ingredients/technologies to provide a superior skin care system: 1) Two innovative enzymes (photolyase and endonuclease) for advanced DNA repair; 2) A revolutionary peptide complex to enhance the production of collagen I, III, IV, and fibroconectin for softening the skin and smoothing wrinkles; 3) Wolfberry seed oil, which contains essential fatty acids like linoleic acid, gamma-linoleic acid (GLA), and oleic acid for intense moisturizing and conditioning of the skin; and 4) Advanced delivery technologies like Laminar Phase Technology (for a highly efficient application and protective barrier) and Liposome Technology (to more quickly deliver greater amounts of ingredients to lower levels of the skin). Then add to all of that the cleansing, stimulating, and regenerative properties of therapeutic-grade essential oils, and these products have no equals currently on the market.

A•R•T® Beauty Masque

This unique mask combines the soothing properties of orchid petals with the gentle cleansing and toning effects of essential oils to nourish, fortify, and soothe the skin.

Ingredients: Aqua (water), *Aloe barbadensis* extract, *Eucommia ulmoides* extract, *Polygonum cuspidatum* root extract, *Torenia concolor* whole plant extract, *Phalaenopsis orchid* flower extract, *Boswellia carteri* resin extract, *Carthamus tinctorius* flower extract, *Angelica polymorpha sinensis* root extract, glycosphingo-lipids, xanthan gum, *Tremella fuciformis* polysaccharide, phenoxyethanol, ethylhexylglycerin, *Vanilla planifolia* (vanilla) absolute.

Essential Oils:

Copaiba—is extremely high in β-caryophyllene, which has been well documented for its anti-inflammatory actions. It has traditionally been used for muscle aches and pains, stiffness, and nervous exhaustion. It helps to elevate the mood and lift depression and may amplify the effects of the other essential oils in the blend.

Lime—has a fresh, lively fragrance that is stimulating and refreshing. It helps one overcome exhaustion, depression, and listlessness.

Cedarwood—may be calming and may help to eliminate nervous tension.

Ocotea—has antibacterial and cleansing properties and may help with emotional balance.

Lavender—is relaxing and promotes health and a general sense of well-being. It is often used to help soothe sensitive or irritated skin.

Suggested Use: Apply on the face 3–4 times per week after washing with ART Gentle Foaming Cleanser.

Body System(s) Affected: **Skin.**

Caution: For external use only. As with any cosmetic, if you are currently being treated for any skin condition, consult a medical professional before using.

A•R•T® Creme Masque

This exquisite masque combines essential oils with oat kernel extracts and hyaluronic acid to help the skin naturally retain moisture, increase turgidity, and decrease the appearance of wrinkles—helping to promote the skin's ability to maintain a full, youthful appearance.

Ingredients: Water, caprylic/capric triglycerides, dicaprylyl carbonate, hydroxypropyl starch phosphate, sorbitol, squalane, cetearyl olivate, sorbitan olivate, *Aloe barbadensis* leaf juice, *Avena sativa* (oat) kernel extract, maltodextrin, panthenol, sodium hyaluronate, vanilla essential oil 16x, coconut alkanes, coco-caprylate/caprate, *Camellia oleifera* leaf extract, pectin, glycerin, cetyl palmitate, sorbitan palmitate, tocopheryl acetate, *Cucumis sativus* (cucumber) fruit extract, xanthan gum, caprylyl glycol, phenoxyethanol, sodium ascorbyl phosphate, sodium gluconate, soy lecithin, hexylene glycol.

Essential Oils:

Vetiver—is often used to promote skin health and clarity and has sedative and calming properties.

Davana—is often used to help soothe rough, dry, and chapped skin.

Roman Chamomile—has soothing properties and is often used to help with dry skin and rashes.

Ylang Ylang—is calming to the nervous system and has sedative properties.

Geranium—is often used to help soothe dry and sensitive skin and to promote healthy skin tissue. It may also help balance sebum in the skin.

Ocotea—has anti-inflammatory, disinfectant, and pain-relieving properties.

Jasmine (absolute)—is often used to help alleviate problems with dry, irritated, or sensitive skin.

Suggested Use: Apply cream on face; leave on for 20 minutes for a quick therapy or overnight for deep moisturizing.

Body System(s) Affected: **Skin.**

Caution: As with any cosmetic, if you are currently being treated for any skin condition, consult a medical professional before using.

A•R•T® Day Activator

This unique, light-bodied, water-based, anti-aging day cream utilizes the innovative photolyase enzyme. This enzyme, powered by visible light, repairs DNA segments in cells that have been damaged by UV radiation. It is quickly absorbed and perfect for wearing underneath makeup and sunscreen to help protect, repair, and build healthy, vibrant skin.

Ingredients: Deionized water, pentylene glycol, glycerin, glyceryl stearate, betaine, cetearyl alcohol, caprylic/capric triglycerides, Ningxia wolfberry (*Lycium barbarum*) seed oil, meadowfoam seed oil and shea butter, *Aloe barbadensis* leaf juice, phenoxyethanol, chlorphenesin, xanthan gum, sodium stearoyl lactylate, carbomer, tetrahexyldecyl ascorbate, tocopheryl acetate, polysorbate 20, squalane, dimethicone, benzoic acid, dipotassium glycyrrhizinate, sodium hyaluronate, *Camellia oleifera* extract, German chamomile (*Chamomilla recutita*) oil (as listed below), retinyl palmitate, sodium PCA, *Chlorella vulgaris* extract, algae extract and mugwort (*Artemisia vulgaris*) extract, plankton extract, micrococcus lysate, palmitoyl oligopeptide, palmitoyl tetrapeptide-3, lecithin, grape (*Vitis vinifera*) seed extract, sandalwood (*Santalum album*) oil, and frankincense (*Boswellia carterii*) oil (as listed below).

Essential Oils:

German Chamomile—has been found to help open the liver, increase liver function and secretion, and support the pancreas. It neutralizes allergies and increases the ability of the skin to regenerate.

Sandalwood—helps strengthen the lymphatic systems, revitalizes the skin, and has been shown to increase blood oxygenation for increased skin cell regeneration.

Frankincense—is high in sesquiterpenes, helps deliver oxygen to the pineal and pituitary glands, improves hGH production, increases leukocyte production, and has been shown to inhibit elastase (the enzyme that breaks down elastin). It has also been shown to increase lipid synthesis for higher cell volume.

Suggested Use: Apply in the morning after cleansing. Using fingertips, massage a generous amount of Day Activator over face and neck regions as needed. Suitable for all skin types.

Body System(s) Affected: **Skin.**

Caution: As with any cosmetic, if you are currently being treated for any skin condition, consult a medical professional before using. For external use only. Keep out of reach of children. Store in a cool, dry place.

A•R•T® Gentle Foaming Cleanser

This unique foaming cleanser gently removes dirt, oil, and makeup from the skin and, unlike so many other commercial products, leaves the skin feeling clean, fresh, hydrated, and soft.

Ingredients: Deionized water, sodium cocoyl glutamate, sodium methyl cocoyl taurate, sodium lauroamphoacetate, decyl glucoside, pure therapeutic-grade essential oils (as listed below), *Aloe barbadensis* leaf juice, tocopheryl acetate, glycerin, cetyl hydroxyethylcellulose, benzoic acid, sorbic acid, sodium hydroxide, *Ginkgo biloba* leaf extract, *Camellia oleifera* leaf extract, retinyl palmitate, citric acid, phenoxyethanol, and chlorphenesin.

Essential Oils:

Frankincense—is high in sesquiterpenes, helps deliver oxygen to the pineal and pituitary glands, improves hGH production, increases leukocyte production, and has been shown to inhibit elastase (the enzyme that breaks down elastin). It has also been shown to increase lipid synthesis for higher cell volume.

Sandalwood—helps strengthen the lymphatic systems, revitalizes the skin, and has been shown to increase blood oxygenation for increased skin cell regeneration.

Lavender—is balancing and calming. It works wherever there is a need and is useful for any type of skin condition.

Lemon—helps promote leukocyte formation and is antiseptic.

Melissa—is a powerful antiviral agent, yet it is very gentle and very delicate because of the nature of the plant. It has the ability to work with and enhance the gentle aspects of the human body. It is anti-inflammatory and energizing.

Suggested Use: With wet hands, massage gently over face. Rinse thoroughly. To be used twice daily, for a refreshing cleanse in the morning and for a thorough cleanse at night. Suitable for all skin types. Store in a cool, dry place.

Body System(s) Affected: Skin.

Caution: As with any cosmetic, if you are currently being treated for any skin condition, consult a medical professional before using.

A•R•T® Night Reconstructor

This unique medium-bodied, water-based, anti-aging night moisturizer utilizes the innovative endonuclease enzyme. This critical enzyme is powered by the energy in your body to cut out damaged DNA segments, reproduce the correct segments from the complimentary strands, and re-insert the new segments into the cell's DNA structure. With pure therapeutic-grade essential oils and superior moisturizing agents, it also provides maximum hydration to the skin during sleep.

Ingredients: Deionized water, pentylene glycol, glycerin, glyceryl stearate, betaine, Ningxia wolfberry (*Lycium barbarum*) seed oil, cetearyl alcohol, meadowfoam seed oil and shea butter, *Aloe barbadensis* leaf juice, phenoxyethanol, chlorphenesin, xanthan gum, sodium stearoyl lactylate, carbomer, tetrahexyldecyl ascorbate, tocopheryl acetate, polysorbate 20, squalane, dimethicone, benzoic acid, dipotassium glycyrrhizinate, sodium hyaluronate, *Camellia oleifera* extract, German chamomile (*Chamomilla recutita*) oil (as listed below), retinyl palmitate, sodium PCA, *Chlorella vulgaris* extract, algae extract and mugwort (*Artemisia vulgaris*) extract, micrococcus lysate, palmitoyl oligopeptide, palmitoyl tetrapeptide-3, lecithin, grape (*Vitis vinifera*) seed extract, sandalwood (*Santalum album*) oil, and frankincense (*Boswellia carterii*) oil (as listed below).

Essential Oils:

German Chamomile—has been found to help open the liver, increase liver function and secretion, and support the pancreas. It neutralizes allergies and increases the ability of the skin to regenerate.

Sandalwood—helps strengthen the lymphatic systems, revitalizes the skin, and has been shown to increase blood oxygenation for increased skin cell regeneration.

Frankincense—is high in sesquiterpenes, helps deliver oxygen to the pineal and pituitary glands, improves hGH production, increases leukocyte production, and has been shown to inhibit elastase (the enzyme that breaks down elastin). It has also been shown to increase lipid synthesis for higher cell volume.

Suggested Use: Apply in the evening after cleansing. Using fingertips, massage a generous amount of Night Reconstructor over face and neck regions as needed. Suitable for all skin types.

Body System(s) Affected: Skin.

Caution: As with any cosmetic, if you are currently being treated for any skin condition, consult a medical professional before using. For external use only. Keep out of reach of children. Store in a cool, dry place.

A•R•T® Purifying Toner

Although the Purifying Toner is not packaged with the other three products as part of the A·R·T Skin Care System, this remarkable formulation of ingredients is a necessary addition to any skin care regimen, and the results are greatest when all four products are used together. The Purifying Toner not only cleanses the skin by removing any unwanted oil, dirt, and impurities that tend to accumulate there, but it also energizes and refreshes the skin's surface, thereby working to restore or maintain a firm, healthy-looking complexion. The added essential oils of frankincense, sandalwood, lemon, and peppermint, along with the plant extracts of lavender and melissa, help to smooth and soften skin, enhance pH balance, minimize oily shine, and reduce the appearance of pores.

Ingredients: Deionized water, SD alcohol 38-B (denatured with peppermint oil), pentylene glycol (derived from coconut and palm for moisture retention), Witch Hazel (*Hamamelis virginiana*) distillate extract, glycerin (from coconut and vegetable sources), pure therapeutic-grade essential oils (as listed below), *Camellia oleifera* leaf extract, grape (*Vitis vinifera*) seed oil, *Aloe barbadensis* leaf juice, retinyl palmitate, allantoin, and polysorbate-20.

Essential Oils:

Frankincense—is high in sesquiterpenes, helps deliver oxygen to the pineal and pituitary glands, improves hGH production, increases leukocyte production, and has been shown to inhibit elastase (the enzyme that breaks down elastin). It has also been shown to increase lipid synthesis for higher cell volume.

Sandalwood—helps strengthen the lymphatic systems, revitalizes the skin, and has been shown to increase blood oxygenation for increased skin cell regeneration.

Lemon—helps promote leukocyte formation and is antiseptic.

Lavender—is balancing and calming. It works wherever there is a need and is useful for any type of skin condition.

Melissa—is a powerful antiviral agent, yet it is very gentle and very delicate because of the nature of the plant. It has the ability to work with and enhance the gentle aspects of the human body. It is anti-inflammatory and energizing.

Peppermint—enhances the effect of the other oils, produces cooling and soothing sensations, invigorates the skin, and helps with nerve regeneration.

Suggested Use: After cleansing, sweep Purifying Toner over face with a cotton ball. Can be used in the morning and again in the evening. For best results, apply the A·R·T Day Activator or Night Reconstructor cream over the Purifying Toner.

Body System(s) Affected: **Skin** (suitable for all skin types).

Caution: As with any cosmetic, if you are currently being treated for any skin condition, consult a medical professional before using. For external use only. Keep out of reach of children. Store in a cool, dry place.

A•R•T® Renewal Serum

This serum combines essential oils, herbal extracts, and orchid petals in a rich blend that helps to nourish and moisturize the skin.

Ingredients: Aqua (water), condensed herbal extracts: *Speranskia tuberculata* whole plant, *Eucommia ulmoides* bark, *Glycine tomentella* root, *Astragalus mongholicus* root, *Polygonum cuspidatum* root, *Phalaenopsis amabilis* (orchid) flower; condensed herbal extracts II: *Torenia concolor* whole plant, *Commiphora myrrha* resin, *Boswellia carteri* resin, *Spatholobus suberectus* stem, *Angelica polymorpha sinensis* root, *Liquidambar formosana* dried fruit, *Crocus sativus* flower, *Chamomilla recutita* flower, niacinamide, hydrolyzed oat protein, phenoxyethanol, *Tremella fuciformis* polysaccharide, sodium hyaluronate, ascorbyl glucoside, ethylhexylglycerin, hydrogenated lecithin, essential oil blend (as listed below).

Essential Oils:

Coriander—is often used to help alleviate skin problems such as oily skin, blackheads, and other impurities. It also has anti-inflammatory and antioxidant properties.

Ylang Ylang—is calming to the nervous system and has sedative properties. It has also been used to help with various skin conditions.

Bergamot—has analgesic, anti-inflammatory, and sedative properties. It is often used to help with skin conditions such as acne, boils, oily complexion, eczema, scabies, and wounds.

Jasmine—is often used to help alleviate problems with dry, irritated, or sensitive skin.

Geranium—is often used to help soothe dry and sensitive skin and to promote healthy skin tissue. It may also help balance sebum in the skin.

Suggested Use: Apply on critical areas of the face twice daily after washing with ART Gentle Foaming Cleanser. Use with ART Beauty Masque and ART Creme Masque.

Body System(s) Affected: **Skin.**

Caution: As with any cosmetic, if you are currently being treated for any skin condition, consult a medical professional before using.

Animal Scents™ Pet Ointment

Instead of harmful chemicals and antibiotics, give your pet the same natural ingredients and powerful germ-fighting essential oils that you've come to rely on. This products is a wonderful blend of wholesome herbs and essential oils designed for helping your pet heal from minor skin irritations, cuts, and scrapes. It sure seems to work great on humans as well.

Ingredients: Mink oil, lecithin, beeswax, lanolin, sesame seed oil, wheat germ oil, pure therapeutic-grade essential oils (as listed below), carrot seed oil (rich in beta carotene; helps to reduce wrinkles and dryness), and rose hip seed oil (helps reduce scarring and prevent premature aging of the skin).

Essential Oils:

Rosewood—is antiseptic, antibacterial, tissue regenerative, soothing to the skin, and increases skin elasticity.

Palmarosa—stimulates new cell growth, regulates oil production, moisturizes, and speeds healing.

Geranium—improves blood flow, regenerates tissue and nerves, cleans oily skin, and may even liven up pale skin.

Patchouli—helps digest toxic material. It tones and tightens skin and helps prevent wrinkles.

Balsam Fir—is a rich source of the antioxidant limonene which has been shown to help relieve overworked and tired muscles and joints.

Myrrh—is soothing to the skin. It is used for chapped and cracked skin and wrinkles.

Melaleuca alternifolia—is tissue regenerative and helps promote the healing of wounds.

Suggested Use: Clean the affected area. Apply as needed. If using additional essential oils, apply oils prior to application of Animal Scents Pet Ointment.

Body System(s) Affected: **Skin.**

Animal Scents™ Pet Shampoo

Stop bathing your pet in chemical-laden products. This product gives you natural ingredients mixed with essential oils to pamper your pet. It also helps with healing their cuts and scratches.

Ingredients: Demineralized water; saponified oils of coconut and olive, pure therapeutic-grade essential oils (as listed below), vegetable gum, aloe vera, and rosemary extract.

Essential Oils:

Citronella—is a natural deodorant and insect repellent. It is also good for oily skin.

Lavandin—is antifungal, antibacterial, strongly antiseptic, and tissue regenerative.

Lemon—helps promote leukocyte formation and is antiseptic.

Geranium—improves blood flow, regenerates tissue and nerves, cleans oily skin, and may even liven up pale skin.

Spikenard—is antibacterial and antifungal and helps with staph infections.

Suggested Use: Pour a small amount of Animal Scents Shampoo into palm, and rub gently between hands. Massage thoroughly into pet's wet coat. Lather. Rinse thoroughly. Repeat if necessary.

Body System(s) Affected: **Skin.**

Precautions: Animal Scents' Shampoo is highly concentrated. If necessary, dilute with water.

AromaGuard® Deodorants

This is one of the most unique deodorant products on the market today. Made with natural ingredients (no toxic aluminum salts or propylene glycol) and bacteria-fighting essential oils, these deodorants will help keep your skin clean and fresh while not interfering with the body's natural cooling system. This formulation is also clean and evaporative, with no sticky residue.

Ingredients: Coconut (*Cocos nucifera*) oil, white beeswax, pure vegetable esters (34 and 40 from palm kernel and coconut oils), zinc oxide, tocopherols (vitamin E), and pure therapeutic-grade essential oils as follow:

Mountain Mint Essential Oils:

Clove—is antibacterial, antifungal, anti-infectious, antiparasitic, a strong antiseptic, antiviral, and an immune stimulant. It may influence healing and help create a feeling of protection and courage.

Lemon—helps promote leukocyte formation and is antiseptic.

Peppermint—enhances the effect of the other oils, produces cooling and soothing sensations, invigorates the skin, and helps with nerve regeneration.

Rosemary cineol—is highly anti-infectious. It is antifungal, antibacterial, and good for various skin conditions.

Eucalyptus radiata—has strong antibacterial and antiseptic properties.

White Fir—is antiseptic and anti-inflammatory. It helps create a feeling of grounding, anchoring, and empowerment.

Meadow Mist Essential Oils:

Lemon—helps promote leukocyte formation and is antiseptic.

Geranium—can be used on almost any kind of skin. It is cleansing, refreshing, astringent, and a mild skin tonic. It is used to balance the hyposecretion of androgens or estrogens that frequently occurs during menopause.

Rosemary cineol—is highly anti-infectious. It is antifungal, antibacterial, and good for various skin conditions.

Rosewood—is antiseptic, antibacterial, tissue regenerative, soothing to the skin, and increases skin elasticity.

Lavender—is balancing and calming. It works wherever there is a need and is useful for any type of skin condition.

Melaleuca alternifolia—is tissue regenerative and helps promote the healing of wounds.

Melaleuca quinquenervia—is powerfully antifungal, antiviral, and antibacterial. It may help protect against radiation and is a strong tissue regenerator.

Clove—is antibacterial, antifungal, anti-infectious, antiparasitic, a strong antiseptic, antiviral, and an immune stimulant. It may influence healing and help create a feeling of protection and courage.

Suggested Use: After bath or shower, apply 3–4 light strokes of AromaGuard to underarms.

Body System(s) Affected: **Skin.**

Precautions: Test skin first for sensitivity. Note: The authors of this book use these deodorants, and when first beginning to use them, the Mountain Mint deodorant would produce an itchy rash under the arms. The Meadow Mist would not produce the rash. After a few weeks of using the Meadow Mist product, the application of Mountain Mint would not produce the rash and has not since. It seems, therefore, that when switching from chemical-laden commercial products to these deodorants, a cleansing process is required, and the Meadow Mist product is recommended for the first while.

Bath & Shower Gel Base

By using saponified coconut and olive oils, the resulting soap is vegetable-based with more than 50 percent moisturizers. Add to that liquid aloe vera extract for for additional moisturizing effects and rosemary extract for its antioxidant properties, and you have a soap that doesn't just clean but also nourishes the skin. *Add your favorite oils to create your own fragrance or therapeutic action.*

Ingredients: Water, saponified coconut (*Cocus nucifera*) oil, saponified olive (*Olea europaea*) oil, vegetable glycerin, guar (*Cyamopsis tetragonoloba*) gum, aloe vera (*Aloe barbadensis*) leaf juice, jojoba (*Simmondsia chinensis*) seed oil, and rosemary (*Rosmarinus officinalis*) leaf extract.

Boswellia™ Wrinkle Cream

Ingredients: Deionized water, dimethyl sulfone, goat cream, Ningxia wolfberry (*Lycium barbarum*) seed oil, glyceryl stearate, caprylic/capric triglyceride, shea butter (*Butyrospermum parki*), stearic acid, stearyl alcohol, sodium PCA, sodium hyaluronate, allantoin, grape (*Vitis vinifera*) seed extract, calendula (*C. officinalis*) flower extract, panthenol (vitamin B5), tocopheryl acetate (vitamin E), retinyl palmitate (vitamin A), lecithin, dipalmitoyl hydroxproline, phenoxyethanol, beta-sitosterol, linoleic acid, tocopherol, sodium ascorbate, mannitol, and pure therapeutic-grade essential oils (as listed below).

Essential Oils:

Geranium—improves blood flow, regenerates tissue and nerves, cleans oily skin, and may even liven up pale skin.

Ylang Ylang—balances the secretion of sebum (a waxy oil produced by the skin). It is energizing and uplifting.

Myrrh—is soothing to the skin. It is used for chapped and cracked skin and wrinkles.

Frankincense—is high in sesquiterpenes. It helps deliver oxygen to the pineal and pituitary glands, improves hGH production, and increases leukocyte production.

Sandalwood—helps strengthen the lymphatic systems and revitalizes the skin.

Instructions: Apply directly to skin. Boswellia Wrinkle Cream is a collagen builder. Used daily, it will help minimize and prevent wrinkles. Put a small amount in hand, emulsify, and apply to face and neck using upward strokes.

Body System(s) Affected: **Skin.**

Cel-Lite Magic™ Massage Oil

Ingredients: Fractionated coconut (*Cocos nucifera*) oil (distilled from pure coconut oil; odorless and colorless; never goes rancid; more readily absorbed by the skin; easily washes out of clothes and sheets with no staining), grape (*Vitis vinifera*) seed oil (antioxidant; rich in bioflavonoids; helps maintain pH balance), wheat (*Triticum vulgare*) germ oil (high in vitamins E, B and lecithin; natural antioxidant; reduces scar tissue and stretch marks; preservative for other base oils), sweet almond (*Prunus amygdalus dulcis*) oil (nourishes the skin; reduces friction for smoother application), organic olive (*Olea europaea*) oil (moisturizing agent), and pure therapeutic-grade essential oils (as listed below).

Essential Oils:

Grapefruit—is excellent for fluid retention and cellulite elimination. It is a diuretic, detoxifier, and a stimulant of the lymphatic system. It is important as an antidepressant.

Cypress—is mucolytic, astringent, diuretic, and lymphatic decongestant. It reduces cellulite and strengthens connective tissue.

Cedarwood—is astringent and diuretic. It helps reduce oily secretions.

Juniper—is a cleanser, detoxifier, and diuretic. It helps the body release fluids.

Clary Sage—is astringent. It is good for cell regulation, cholesterol, and dry skin.

Suggested Use: Shake well before using. Massage on location.

Warning: Avoid eye contact. If contact occurs, rinse thoroughly with water. For external use only. Keep out of reach of children.

Body System(s) Affected: **Skin**.

Cinnamint™ Lip Balm

Ingredients: Coconut (*Cocos nucifera*) oil, beeswax, sweet almond (*Prunus amygdalus dulcis*) oil, jojoba (*Simmondsia chinensis*) seed oil, Ningxia wolfberry (*Lycium barbarum*) seed oil, *Rosa canina* fruit oil, pure therapeutic-grade essential oils (as listed below), tocopherol, and tocopheryl acetate (vitamin E).

Essential Oils:

Peppermint—enhances the effect of the other oils, produces cooling and soothing sensations, invigorates the skin, and helps with nerve regeneration. It also enhances digestion and increases endurance.

Orange—contains over 91% d-Limonene (which helps to promote normal cell life cycles).

Spearmint—brings soothing relief to dry skin.

Cinnamon Bark—is a powerful purifier and a powerful oxygenator. It enhances the action and the activity of the other oils, while its warming action balances the cooling effect of the mint oils to bring comfortable relief to dry, chapped lips.

Instructions: To soften and moisturize lips, apply Cinnamint Lip Balm as often as needed.

Body System(s) Affected: **Skin**.

ClaraDerm™

This product, packaged in a spray bottle, is a blend of essential oils that are most soothing and nourishing to the skin. Designed to be used topically on skin that is stressed before and after childbirth, these oils help to relieve skin irritation and itching and may also improve skin elasticity.

Ingredients: Pure therapeutic-grade essential oils (as listed below) in a base of fractionated coconut oil.

Essential Oils:

Myrrh—is soothing to the skin. It is used for chapped and cracked skin and wrinkles.

Melaleuca alternifolia—is tissue regenerative and helps promote the healing of wounds.

Lavender—is balancing and calming. It works wherever there is a need and is useful for any type of skin condition.

Frankincense—is high in sesquiterpenes. It helps deliver oxygen to the pineal and pituitary glands, improves hGH production, and increases leukocyte production.

Roman Chamomile—helps increase the regenerative ability of the skin. It is a blood cleanser.

Helichrysum—may help cleanse the blood and improve circulatory functions. It is anticatarrhal in structure and nature.

Suggested Use: Spray topically on location.

Body System(s) Affected: **Skin.**

Dragon Time™ Bath & Shower Gel

This product was specially designed for the relief of those monthly aches and pains.

Ingredients: Water, saponified coconut (*Cocus nucifera*) oil, saponified olive (*Olea europaea*) oil, vegetable glycerin, guar (*Cyamopsis tetragonoloba*) gum, aloe vera (*Aloe barbadensis*) leaf juice, pure therapeutic-grade essential oils (as listed below), jojoba (*Simmondsia chinensis*) seed oil, and rosemary (*Rosmarinus officinalis*) leaf extract.

Essential Oils:

Mandarin—is good for skin problems, stretch marks, nervous tension, and restlessness.

Geranium—helps balance the hormones. It is tissue and nerve regenerative.

Rosewood—is antiseptic, antibacterial, tissue regenerative, and soothing to the skin.

Fennel—helps balance the hormones.

Marjoram—is an antispasmodic and is relaxing, calming, and appeasing.

Lavender—helps balance body systems.

Sage—contains estriol and has estrogen-like properties. It is believed to contain elements that contribute to the secretion of progesterone.

Clary Sage—helps balance the hormones. It is a tonic to the reproductive system.

Lemon—helps promote leukocyte formation. It helps brighten a pale, dull complexion by removing the dead skin cells.

Jasmine—has a deeply penetrating effect on the skin. It produces a feeling of confidence, energy, euphoria, and optimism.

Roman Chamomile—helps increase the regenerative ability of the skin. It is a blood cleanser.

Bergamot—is sedative and helps to relieve anxiety, stress, and tension.

Ylang Ylang—is stimulating and helps to balance male-female energies.

Palmarosa—stimulates new cell growth, regulates oil production, and moisturizes.

Blue Tansy—calms the lymphatic system and promotes a feeling of self-control.

Body System(s) Affected: **Emotional Balance, Hormonal System, Skin.**

Dragon Time™ Massage Oil

Ingredients: Fractionated coconut (*Cocos nucifera*) oil (distilled from pure coconut oil; odorless and colorless; never goes rancid; more readily absorbed by the skin; easily washes out of clothes and sheets with no staining), grape (*Vitis vinifera*) seed oil (antioxidant; rich in bioflavonoids; helps maintain pH balance), wheat (*Triticum vulgare*) germ oil (high in vitamins E, B and lecithin; natural antioxidant; reduces scar tissue and stretch marks; preservative for other base oils), sweet almond (*Prunus amygdalus dulcis*) oil (nourishes the skin; reduces friction for smoother application), organic olive (*Olea europaea*) oil (moisturizing agent), and pure therapeutic-grade essential oils (as listed below).

Essential Oils:

Lavender—helps balance body systems.

Fennel—helps balance the hormones.

Clary Sage—helps balance the hormones and is a tonic to the reproductive system.

Sage—contains estriol and has estrogen-like properties. It is believed to contain elements that contribute to the secretion of progesterone.

Ylang Ylang—stimulates adrenal glands and helps balance male/female energies.

Yarrow—is anti-inflammatory, antiseptic, and excellent for menstrual problems.

Jasmine—helps relieve menstrual pains and is good for uterine disorders.

Warning: Shake well before using. Avoid eye contact. If contact occurs, rinse thoroughly with water. For external use only. Keep out of reach of children.

Body System(s) Affected: **Emotional Balance, Hormonal System, Skin.**

Essential Beauty™ Serums

Since ancient times, essential oils have been used in numerous skin care treatments. Even in our modern cosmetic and skin care products, essential oils are utilized for their potent therapeutic benefits. However, these serums are unique in the cosmetic and skin care industries, as they combine potent blends of pure essential oils that target specific skin care needs with a proprietary vegetable oil complex to nourish and protect the skin without overdrying or clogging the pores.

Ingredients: The following is a partial list of ingredients that are common between all three blends: Coconut (*Cocos nucifera*) oil, jojoba (*Simmondsia chinensis*) oil, avocado (*Persea gratissima*) oil (rich in vitamin E and lutein; lutein absorbs UV light to protect skin from sun damage), rosehip (*Rosa rubiginosa*) seed oil (rich in omega-3 essential fats; improves texture and natural moisture balance), lecithin, tocopherol, and Ningxia wolfberry (*Lycium barbarum*) seed oil (helps moisturize outer dermal layers). In addition to these ingredients are the specific essential oils listed under each blend below.

How to Use: For best results, incorporate the use of the A·R·T skin care products in the following three steps.

Step 1: Thoroughly clean the skin with A·R·T Gentle Foaming Cleanser.

Step 2: Sweep the A·R·T Purifying Toner over the face with a cotton ball.

Step 3: Spot apply the desired Essential Beauty Serum to the problem areas on the face and neck regions before moisturizer, sun block, or makeup is applied. If preferred, add 3–5 drops of the serum to the A·R·T Day Activator or Night Reconstructor creams, mix well, and spread evenly over the face. Serums should be applied in the morning and again in the evening.

Body System(s) Affected: **Skin.**

Warning: For external use only. Store in a cool, dark place.

Essential Beauty™ Serum – Acne-Prone Skin Blend

This particular serum contains pure therapeutic-grade essential oils specifically blended together to help remove compacted keratin and sebum from pores and follicles that can contribute to breakouts. The unique vegetable oil complex, listed above in the common description under ingredients, creates a protective lipid layer that hydrates and moisturizes the skin. Some of the essential oils also help provide continued antioxidant activity and cell protection.

Essential Oils:

Eucalyptus staigeriana—is anti-inflammatory, analgesic, and a powerful antispasmodic. It is soothing and relaxing to skin and muscles.

Melaleuca alternifolia—has powerful anti-inflammatory and antimicrobial effects; research has shown it to be very effective in combating acne.

Cedarwood—is rejuvenating, refreshing, antiseptic and beneficial to the skin.

Manuka (*Leptospermum scoparium*)—is powerfully antimicrobial and antifungal. Studies show that it has more antioxidant activity than *Melaleuca alternifolia*. It relaxes the nerves, activates skin cells, and helps to regenerate outer skin layers.

Thyme—contains 46% thymol—one of the most potent natural antimicrobial substances known. It is also antifungal and antiseptic and has been used medicinally in France for dermatitis, psoriasis, and candida.

Essential Beauty™ SERUM – Dry Skin Blend

This particular serum contains pure therapeutic-grade essential oils specifically blended together to help remove compacted keratin and sebum from pores and follicles that can contribute to poor skin clarity. The unique vegetable oil complex, listed above in the common description under ingredients, creates a protective lipid layer that hydrates and moisturizes the skin. Some of the essential oils also help provide continued antioxidant activity and cell protection.

Essential Oils:

Cedarwood—is rejuvenating, refreshing, antiseptic, and beneficial to the skin.

Blue Cypress (*Callitris intratropica*)—is an abundant source of sesquiterpenes.

Lavender—works wherever there is a need; it is useful for any type of skin condition.

Myrrh—is soothing to the skin. It is used for chapped and cracked skin and wrinkles.

Clove—is antibacterial, antifungal, anti-infectious, and a strong antiseptic

Sandalwood—revitalizes the skin and helps to repair DNA and reverse the signs of sun damage.

Evening Peace™ Bath & Shower Gel

This gel is perfect for that evening bath or shower to help you relax after a very stressful day.

Ingredients: Water, saponified coconut (*Cocus nucifera*) oil, saponified olive (*Olea europaea*) oil, vegetable glycerin, guar (*Cyamopsis tetragonoloba*) gum, pure therapeutic-grade essential oils (as listed below), aloe vera (*Aloe barbadensis*) leaf juice, jojoba (*Simmondsia chinensis*) seed oil, and rosemary (*Rosmarinus officinalis*) leaf extract.

Essential Oils:

Lemongrass—helps stimulate the agents in the tissue to rejuvenate and reconnect.

Rosemary cineol—is highly anti-infectious and good for various skin conditions.

Sandalwood—helps strengthen the lymphatic systems and revitalizes the skin.

Geranium—helps balance the hormones and is tissue and nerve regenerative.

Rosewood—is antiseptic, antibacterial, tissue regenerative, soothing to the skin, and increases skin elasticity.

Lemon—helps promote leukocyte formation. It helps brighten a pale, dull complexion by removing dead skin cells.

Blue Tansy—calms the lymphatic system and promotes a feeling of self-control.

Jasmine—has a deeply penetrating effect on the skin. It produces a feeling of confidence, energy, euphoria, and optimism.

Roman Chamomile—is calming and relaxing. It helps increase the regenerative ability of the skin and is a blood cleanser.

Bergamot—is sedative and helps to relieve anxiety, stress, and tension.

Ylang Ylang—is stimulating and helps to balance male-female energies.

Palmarosa—stimulates new cell growth, regulates oil production, and moisturizes.

Clary Sage—helps balance the hormones and is a tonic to the reproductive system.

Body System(s) Affected: **Emotional Balance, Skin.**

Genesis™ Hand & Body Lotion

The essential oils in this product are beneficial for feeding, nurturing, and hydrating the skin. It is excellent for rough, dry skin, wrinkles, and premature aging. It works well after a shower or bath to help seal in moisture.

Ingredients: Deionized water, dimethyl sulfone, glycerin, glyceryl stearate, stearic acid, sodium hyaluronate, sorbitol, *Rosa canina* fruit oil, shea butter (*Butyrospermum parkii*), wheat germ (*Triticum bulgaare*) oil, kukui (*Aleurites moluccana*) nut oil, lecithin, safflower (*Carthamus tinctorius*) oil, apricot (*Prunus armeniaca*) oil, tocopheryl acetate (vitamin E), retinyl palmitate (vitamin A), jojoba (*Simmondsia chinensis*) seed oil, sesame (*Sesamum indicum*) seed oil, aloe vera (*Aloe barbadensis*) leaf juice, grape (*Vitis vinifera*) seed extract, ascorbic acid (vitamin C), pure therapeutic-grade essential oils (as listed below), calendula (*C. officinalis*) flower extract, *Chamomilla recutita* (Matricaria) extract, *Camellia oleifera* leaf extract, St. John's wort (*Hypericum perforatum*) extract, *Fucus vesiculosus* extract, and *Ginkgo biloba* extract.

Essential Oils:

Rosewood—is antiseptic, antibacterial, and tissue regenerative. It is soothing to the skin and increases elasticity.

Palmarosa—stimulates new cell growth, regulates oil production, moisturizes, and speeds healing.

Geranium—can be used on almost any kind of skin. It is cleansing, refreshing, astringent, and a mild skin tonic. It is used to balance the hyposecretion of androgens or estrogens that frequently occurs during menopause.

Jasmine—has a deeply penetrating effect on the skin. It produces a feeling of confidence, energy, euphoria, and optimism.

Lemon—helps promote leukocyte formation and is antiseptic.

Roman Chamomile—helps increase the regenerative ability of the skin. It is a blood cleanser.

Bergamot—helps to relieve anxiety, stress, and tension and helps balance the hormones.

Ylang Ylang—is stimulating and helps to balance male-female energies. May also contain patchouli.

Instructions: Dispense in hand, and apply directly to skin.

Body System(s) Affected: Skin.

Warning: Avoid eye contact. If contact occurs, rinse thoroughly with water.

Grapefruit Lip Balm

Ingredients: Coconut (*Cocos nucifera*) oil extract, beeswax, jojoba (*Simmondsia chinensis*) seed oil, sweet almond (*Prunus amygdalus dulcis*) oil, pure therapeutic-grade essential oils (as listed below), wolfberry (*Lycium barbarum*) seed oil, rosehip (*Rosa rubiginosa*) seed oil, vitamin E (*Tocopherol*), and *Tocopheryl acetate*.

Essential Oils:

Grapefruit—is light and refreshing and does not have the photosensitivity that the other citrus oils have.

Instructions: To soften and moisturize lips, apply Grapefruit Lip Balm as often as needed.

Body System(s) Affected: Skin.

KidScents® Bath Gel

This shower gel has a neutral pH, perfect for young skin. It is gentle, mild, and safe. It contains all-natural ingredients and therapeutic-grade essential oils with no mineral oils, synthetic perfumes, artificial colorings, or toxic ingredients.

Ingredients: Deionized water, decylpolyglucose, vegetable glycerin, sorbitol, dimethyl sulfone, *Anthemis nobilis* flower extract, aloe vera (*Aloe barbadensis*) leaf juice, panthenol, tocopheryl acetate (vitamin E), PG-hydroxyethylcellulose cocodimonium chloride, *Echinacea purpurea* extract, grape (*Vitis vinifera*) seed extract, *Quillaja saponaria* bark extract, *Saponaria officinalis* extract, kiwi (*Actinidia chinensis*) seed oil, jojoba (*Simmondsia chinensis*) seed oil, lemon (*Citrus medica limonum*) seed extract, *Orbignya oleifera* seed oil, Dimethicone PEG-8 meadowfoamate, pure therapeutic-grade essential oils (as listed below), hyaluronic acid, wheat (*Triticum vulgare*) germ oil, hydrolyzed keratin, linoleic acid, and linolenic acid.

Essential Oils:

Cedarwood—is rejuvenating, refreshing, antiseptic, and beneficial to the skin. It is astringent and diuretic and helps reduce oily secretions.

Geranium—can be used on almost any kind of skin. It is cleansing, refreshing, astringent, and a mild skin tonic.

Instructions: Apply a small amount of KidScents Bath Gel to a washcloth or directly to the skin. Rub gently, and then rinse.

Common Sense Caution: While KidScents products contain no harmful ingredients, store out of reach of children to prevent messy spills. Children do not like soap in their mouth or eyes. Use with gentle care.

KidScents® Lotion

This is an extraordinarily gentle and safe lotion with the ideal pH for moisturizing, softening, and protecting young skin. It contains all-natural ingredients and pure therapeutic-grade essential oils with no mineral oils, synthetic perfumes, artificial colorings, or toxic ingredients.

Ingredients: Deionized water, MSM (methylsulfonylmethane), glyceryl stearate, stearic acid, glycerin, grape (*Vitis vinifera*) seed extract, sodium hyaluronate, sorbitol, rose (*Rosa rugosa*) hip oil, shea butter, mango (*Mangifera indica*) butter, wheat germ oil, kukui (*Aleurites moluccana*) nut oil, lecithin, safflower

(*Carthamus tinctorius*) oil, apricot (*Prunus armeniaca*) kernal oil, almond (*Prunus amygdalus dulcis*) oil, tocopheryl acetate (vitamin E), retinyl palmitate (vitamin A), jojoba (*Buxus chinensis*) oil, sesame (*Sesamum indicum*) oil, *Calendula officinalis* extract, chamomile (*Anthemis nobilis*) extract, orange (*Citrus aurantium dulcis*) blossom extract, St. John's Wort (*Hypericum perforatum*) extract, algae (*Gellidiela acerosa*) extract, aloe vera (*Aloe barbadensis*) gel, ascorbic acid (vitamin C), *Ginkgo biloba* extract, and pure therapeutic-grade essential oils (as listed below).

Essential Oils:

Cedarwood—is rejuvenating, refreshing, antiseptic, and beneficial to the skin.

Western Red Cedar—is antibacterial, antiseptic, and calming.

Rosewood—is antiseptic, antibacterial, tissue regenerative, soothing to the skin, and increases skin elasticity.

Geranium—improves blood flow, regenerates tissue and nerves, cleans oily skin, and may even liven up pale skin.

Instructions: Apply KidScents Lotion liberally to the skin.

Common Sense Caution: While KidScents products contain no harmful ingredients, store out of reach of children to prevent messy spills. Children do not like lotion in their mouth or eyes. Use with gentle care.

KidScents® Shampoo

This shampoo contains the finest natural ingredients for gently cleansing young, delicate hair. It is perfectly pH-balanced and contains all-natural ingredients and pure therapeutic-grade essential oils with no mineral oils, synthetic perfumes, artificial colorings, or toxic ingredients.

Ingredients: Deionized water, decylpolyglucose, MSM (methylsulfonylmethane), Roman chamomile (*Anthemis nobilis*) extract, aloe vera (*Aloe barbadensis*) gel, panthenol, tocopheryl acetate (vitamin E), coneflower (*Echinacea purpurea*) extract, kukui (*Aleurites moluccana*) nut oil, jojoba (*Buxus chinensis*) oil, citrus seed extract, grape (*Vitis vinifera*) seed extract, dimethicone copolyol meadowfoamate, pure therapeutic-grade essential oils (as listed below), hyaluronic acid, wheat (*Triticum aestivum*) germ oil, keratin, linoleic acid, and linolenic acid.

Essential Oils:

Tangerine—is calming to the nervous system. It is also a decongestant of the lymphatic system.

Lemon—promotes leukocyte formation and helps remove dead skin cells.

Blue Tansy—helps cleanse the liver and promote a feeling of self-control.

Instructions: Apply a small amount of KidScents Shampoo to the hair. Lather, and then rinse.

Common Sense Caution: While KidScents products contain no harmful ingredients, store out of reach of children to prevent messy spills. Children do not like shampoo in their mouth or eyes. Use with gentle care.

KidScents® Tender Tush™

This product is a mild, soothing, and gentle ointment designed to protect and nourish young skin and promote healing. It contains all-natural ingredients and pure therapeutic-grade essential oils with no mineral oils, synthetic perfumes, artificial colorings, or toxic ingredients. It is particularly useful for diaper rash and other skin irritations.

Ingredients: Coconut (*Cocos nucifera*) oil, cocoa (*Theobroma cacao*) butter, beeswax, wheat germ oil, olive (*Olea europaea*) oil, almond (*Prunus amygdalus dulcis*) oil, and pure therapeutic-grade essential oils (as listed below).

Essential Oils:

Sandalwood—helps strengthen the lymphatic systems and revitalizes the skin.

Rosewood—is antiseptic, antibacterial, tissue regenerative, soothing to the skin, and increases skin elasticity.

Roman Chamomile—helps increase the regenerative ability of the skin and is a blood cleanser.

Lavender—is balancing and calming. It works wherever there is a need and is useful for any type of skin condition.

Cistus—has antibacterial, anti-infectious, and antiviral properties. Because it is high in oxygenating molecules, it may assist the auto-immune system and may help strengthen the immune system.

Blue Tansy—may help cleanse the liver and calm the lymphatic system to help rid one of anger and promote a feeling of self-control.

Frankincense—is anti-inflammatory, high in sesquiterpenes, and helps deliver oxygen to the pineal and pituitary glands. It improves hGH production and increases leukocyte production.

Instructions: Apply liberally to the skin on the bottom or wherever it is needed.

Common Sense Caution: While KidScents products contain no harmful ingredients, store out of reach of children to prevent messy spills. Children do not like ointments in their mouth or eyes. Use with gentle care.

Body System(s) Affected: **Skin**.

KidScents® Slique™ Toothpaste

This new formulation combines Slique essential oil blend with Thieves essential oil blend in a completely safe and natural alternative to other commercial toothpastes. This toothpaste is fluoride free and contains all-natural ingredients and pure therapeutic-grade essential oils with no synthetic dyes or flavorings.

Ingredients: Deionized water, virgin coconut oil, baking soda, calcium carbonate, sunflower lecithin, vegetable glycerin, xanthan gum, xylitol, pure therapeutic-grade essential oils (as listed below), stevia-rebaudioside A (*stevia rebaudiana*).

Essential Oils:

Grapefruit—has natural disinfectant properties. It may also help reduce cravings and hunger.

Tangerine—is often used to help with digestive issues and has a calming influence.

Spearmint—has antibacterial and anti-inflammatory properties and may help soothe the digestive system.

Lemon—has cleansing and antiseptic properties.

Ocotea—was used traditionally for digestive support. It may help reduce swelling, and it has antibacterial properties.

Thieves—is a proprietary blend of clove, lemon, cinnamon bark, *Eucalyptus radiata*, and rosemary essential oils that has been documented to be highly antibacterial and antimicrobial in nature.

Instructions: Brush teeth and gums thoroughly morning and night.

Common Sense Caution: Use only a pea-size amount and do not swallow. Use with gentle care.

LavaDerm™ Cooling Mist

This Cooling Mist provides wonderful relief to any type of burn, from the lightest sunburn to the most serious 3rd degree burn. It quickly cools and hydrates the skin and speeds healing and tissue regeneration.

Ingredients: Deionized water, aloe vera (*Aloe barbadensis*) gel, lavender (*Lavandula angustifolia*) essential oil, and ionic trace minerals.

Instructions: Mist directly on area of concern as often as needed to keep the skin cool and promote regeneration.

Body System(s) Affected: **Emotional Balance, Skin**.

Lavender Bath & Shower Gel

This gel is perfect for a relaxing and rejuvenating bath or shower to help you unwind at the end of a busy day.

Ingredients: Water, sodium methyl cocyl taurate, sodium lauroamphoacetate, lauramidopropyl betain, sea salt, hydroxypropyl methylcellulose, pure therapeutic-grade essential oils (as listed below), Ningxia wolfberry (*Lycium barbarum*) fruit extract, p-anisic acid, rosemary (*Rosmarinus officinalis*) extract, kelp (*Laminaria digitata*) extract, sodium astrocaryum murmururate, algae (*Chlorella vulgaris*) extract, citric acid (vitamin C), levulinic acid, sorbic acid, and phytic acid.

Essential Oils:

Lavender—helps balance body systems.

Myrrh—has an uplifting fragrance. It is nourishing and rejuvenating to the skin.

Lemon—helps promote leukocyte formation and helps brighten a pale, dull complexion by removing dead skin cells.

Davana—is anti-infectious and is soothing to rough, dry, or chapped skin.

Body System(s) Affected: **Emotional Balance, Skin**.

Lavender® Foaming Hand Soap

This product provides the ultimate protection and nourishment in a luxurious, foaming hand soap. Its gentle and cleansing properties allow for frequent use without drying out the skin.

Ingredients: Water, decyl glucoside, cocamidopropyl hydroxysultaine, levulinic acid, sorbic acid, p-anisic acid, phytic acid, cetyl hydroxyethylcelulose, *Ginkgo biloba* leaf extract, green tea (*Camellia sinensis*) leaf extract, tocopheryl acetate (vitamin E), retinyl palmitate (vitamin A), aloe vera (*Aloe barbadensis*) leaf juice, and citric acid.

Essential Oils:

Lavender—helps balance body systems.

Lemon—helps promote leukocyte formation and helps brighten a pale, dull complexion by removing dead skin cells.

Myrrh—has an uplifting fragrance. It is nourishing and rejuvenating to the skin.

Common Sense Caution: Not for internal use. Avoid contact with eyes. If contact occurs, flush eyes liberally with clean, cool water for several minutes. If redness or irritation occurs, discontinue use. If symptoms persist contact your physician.

Body System(s) Affected: **Emotional Balance, Skin**.

Lavender Hand & Body Lotion

This is a wonderfully moisturizing lotion, with several pure therapeutic-grade essential oils to help nourish and repair dry, cracked, rough skin.

Ingredients: Deionized water, glycerin, cetearyl alcohol, sandalwood (*Santalum album*) wood extract, *Phellodendron ameurense* bark extract, barley (*Hordeum distichon*) extract, sodium stearoyl lactylate, glyceryl stearate, pure therapeutic-grade essential oils (as listed below), Ningxia wolfberry (*Lycium barbarum*) seed oil, Ningxia wolfberry (*Lycium barbarum*) fruit extract, *Astrocaryum murumuru* seed butter, rosemary (*Rosmarinus officinalis*) leaf extract, kelp (*Laminaria digitata*), algae (Chlorella vulgaris), p-anisic acid, hydrolyzed silk, aloe vera (*Aloe barbadensis*) leaf extract, Vitamolive (Soliance)/olive fruit oil, tocopherol (vitamin E), beeswax, xanthan gum, levulinic acid, sorbic acid, and phytic acid.

Essential Oils:

Lavender—is balancing and calming. It works wherever there is a need and is useful for any type of skin condition.

Myrrh—is soothing to the skin. It is used for chapped and cracked skin and wrinkles.

Lemon—helps promote leukocyte formation and is antiseptic.

Davana—is antibacterial and antifungal. It is soothing and relaxing to skin and nerves.

Instructions: Use as needed to moisturize dehydrated skin.

Body System(s) Affected: **Emotional Balance, Skin.**

Lavender Lip Balm

Ingredients: Coconut (*Cocos nucifera*) oil, beeswax, jojoba (*Simmondsia chinensis*) seed oil, sweet almond (*Prunus amygdalus dulcis*) oil, Ningxia Wolfberry (*Lycium barbarum*) seed oil, rosehip (*Rosa rubiginosa*) seed oil, pure therapeutic-grade essential oils (as listed below), tocopherol, and tocopheryl acetate (vitamin E).

Essential Oils:

Lavender—is balancing and calming. It works wherever there is a need and is useful for any type of skin condition.

Instructions: To repair and moisturize lips, apply as often as needed.

Body System(s) Affected: **Skin.**

Lavender Rosewood Moisturizing Soap™

Contains oils that nourish the skin while their fragrance is calming and relaxing.

Ingredients: Saponified palm (*Elaeis guineensis*) oil, saponified coconut (*Cocos nucifera*) oil, saponified olive (*Olea europaea*) fruit oil, vegetable gylcerin, pure therapeutic-grade essential oils (as listed below), Ningxia wolfberry (*Lycium barbarum*) seed oil, oat (*Avena sativa*) kernel meal, jojoba (*Simmondsia chinensis*) seed oil, aloe vera (*Aloe barbadensis*) leaf juice, and rosemary (*Rosmarinus officinalis*) leaf extract.

Essential Oils:

Lavender—helps balance body systems.

Rosewood—is antiseptic, antibacterial, tissue regenerative, soothing to the skin, and increases skin elasticity.

Lavender Volume Conditioner™

This is a fabulous, nourishing, volumizing rinse that utilizes vitamins, amino acids, MSM, and essential oils to support and feed fine hair.

Ingredients: Natural vegetable fatty acid base (saponified coconut oil), MSM, quinoa (*Chenopodium quinoa*) extract, milk protein, phospholipids, hydrolyzed soya protein, retinyl palmitate (vitamin A), ascorbic acid (vitamin C), stearamidopropyl diethylamine lactate, tocopherol (vitamin E), rosemary (*Rosmarinus officinalis*) extract, amino acids cysteine and cysteine 8 methionine, glycoprotein (glycogen and mucopolysaccharides), hydrolyzed wheat protein, grape (*Vitis vinifera*) seed extract, panthenol (vitamin B5), cetyl triethylmonium dimethicone copolyol phthalate, meadow (*Dimethicone copolyol meadowfoamate*) seed oil, acetamide MEA, dimethiconol panthenol, keratin, linoleic acid, linolenic acid, hyaluronic acid, sorbitol, wheat germ oil, dimethiconol cysteine, jojoba (*Simmondsia chinensis*) oil, guar gum, pure therapeutic-grade essential oils (as listed below), Ningxia wolfberry (*Lycium barbarum*) seed oil, and phytantriol.

Essential Oils:

Lavender—is balancing and calming. It works wherever there is a need and is useful for any type of skin condition.

Clary Sage—is astringent and good for cell regulation, cholesterol, and dry skin.

Lemon—helps promote leukocyte formation and is antiseptic.

Jasmine—has adeeply penetrating effect on the skin. It produces a feeling of confidence, energy, euphoria, and optimism.

Instructions: Apply Lavender Volume Conditioner through the hair. Leave on hair for a few seconds for light conditioning or for several minutes for deep conditioning. Rinse well. *For maximum benefit, leave on 2 to 5 minutes.*

Lavender Volume Shampoo™

As this shampoo is formulated for the gentle cleansing of fine hair, it makes an excellent shampoo for babies and children.

Ingredients: Coconut oil, olive oil, decyl polyglucose, MSM, deionized water, meadow (*Dimethicone copolyol meadowfoamate*) seed oil, vegetable protein (wheat, oat, and soya), lemon (*Citrus medica limonum*) extract, sugar maple (*Acer sacchrinum*) extract, orange (*Citrus aurantium dulcis*) extract, aloe vera (*Aloe barbensis*) gel, alpha-tocopheryl acetate (vitamin E), retinyl palmitate (vitamin A), ascorbic acid (vitamin C), guar gum, pure therapeutic-grade essential oils (as listed below), almond (*Prunus amygdalus dulcis*) glyceride, panthenol (vitamin B5), soapwort (*Saponaria officinalis*) extract, dimethyl lauramine oleate, cetyl triethylmonium dimethicone copolyol phthalate, grape (*Vitis vinifera*) seed extract, acetamide MEA, dimethiconol panthenol, keratin, linoleic acid, linolenic acid, hyaluronic acid, sorbitol, wheat germ oil, dimethiconol cysteine, jojoba (*Simmondsia chinensis*) oil, inositol, and niacin.

Essential Oils:

Lavender—is balancing and calming. It works wherever there is a need and is useful for any type of skin condition.

Clary Sage—is astringent and good for cell regulation, cholesterol, and dry skin.

Lemon—helps promote leukocyte formation and is antiseptic.

Jasmine—has a deeply penetrating effect on the skin. It produces a feeling of confidence, energy, euphoria, and optimism.

Instructions: Wet hair thoroughly. Apply a small amount of Lavender Volume Shampoo. Massage thoroughly into hair and scalp. Rinse well. Repeat if desired. *For maximum benefit, leave on 2 to 5 minutes.*

Lemon Sandalwood Cleansing Soap™

This soap contains oils that deep clean and revitalize the skin with an invigorating fragrance.

Ingredients: Saponified palm (*Elaeis guineensis*) oil, saponified coconut (*Cocos nucifera*) oil, saponified olive (*Olea europaea*) fruit oil, vegetable gylcerin, pure therapeutic-grade essential oils (as listed below), Ningxia wolfberry (*Lycium barbarum*) seed oil, oat (*Avena sativa*) kernel meal, jojoba (*Simmondsia chinensis*) seed oil, aloe vera (*Aloe barbadensis*) leaf juice, and rosemary (*Rosmarinus officinalis*) leaf extract.

Essential Oils:

Lemon—helps promote leukocyte formation and helps brighten a pale, dull complexion by removing dead skin cells.

Sandalwood—helps strengthen the lymphatic systems and revitalizes the skin.

Melaleuca Geranium Moisturizing Soap™

This soap contains oils that are antiseptic and revitalizing to the skin with a calming fragrance.

Ingredients: Saponified palm (*Elaeis guineensis*) oil, saponified coconut (*Cocos nucifera*) oil, saponified olive (*Olea europaea*) fruit oil, vegetable gylcerin, Ningxia wolfberry (*Lycium barbarum*) seed oil, oat (*Avena sativa*) kernel meal, jojoba (*Simmondsia chinensis*) seed oil, pure therapeutic-grade essential oils (as listed below), *aloe vera* (*Aloe barbadensis*) leaf juice, and rosemary (*Rosmarinus officinalis*) leaf extract.

Essential Oils:

Melaleuca—is antifungal, antiseptic, antibacterial, and tissue regenerative.

Geranium—can be used on almost any kind of skin. It is cleansing, refreshing, and astringent.

Melaleuca ericifolia—is very gentle and non-irritating to the skin. It is well suited for youth and others who may be more sensitive to the oils.

Vetiver—is antispasmodic and locally warming. It is good for arthritis, muscular rheumatism, and sprains.

Morning Start™ Bath & Shower Gel

This gel is perfect for an invigorating bath or shower, to physically and emotionally prepare you for another hectic day. Due to the deep penetrating, cleansing action of the oils in this product, Morning Start may actually help dissolve and wash away oil and grease from the skin.

Ingredients: Water, saponified coconut (*Cocus nucifera*) oil, saponified olive (*Olea europaea*) oil, vegetable glycerin, guar (*Cyamopsis tetragonoloba*) gum, pure therapeutic-grade essential oils (as listed below), *aloe vera* (*Aloe barbadensis*) leaf juice, jojoba (*Simmondsia chinensis*) seed oil, and rosemary (*Rosmarinus officinalis*) leaf extract.

Essential Oils:

Lemongrass—helps stimulate the agents in the tissue to rejuvenate and reconnect.

Rosemary cineol—is highly anti-infectious and is good for various skin conditions.

Juniper (both *J. osteosperma* and *J. scopulorum*)—evokes feelings of health and peace and elevates one's spiritual awareness

Peppermint—is invigorating to the skin and may also help with nerve regeneration.

Body System(s) Affected: **Emotional Balance, Skin.**

Morning Start Moisturizing Soap™

Patterned after the popular Bath and Shower Gel, this soap is uplifting and energizing.

Ingredients: Saponified palm (*Elaeis guineensis*) oil, saponified coconut (*Cocos nucifera*) oil, saponified olive (*Olea europaea*) fruit oil, vegetable gylcerin, pure therapeutic-grade essential oils (as listed below), Ningxia wolfberry (*Lycium barbarum*) seed oil, oat (*Avena sativa*) kernel meal, jojoba (*Simmondsia chinensis*) seed oil, *aloe vera* (*Aloe barbadensis*) leaf juice, and rosemary (*Rosmarinus officinalis*) leaf extract.

Essential Oils:

Lemongrass—helps repair connective tissue: it helps stimulate the agents in the tissue to rejuvenate and reconnect. It is also good as an insect repellent.

Rosemary cineol—is highly anti-infectious. It is antifungal, antibacterial, and good for various skin conditions.

Juniper (both *J. osteosperma* and *J. scopulorum*)—evokes feelings of health, love, and peace and may help to elevate one's spiritual awareness.

Orange Blossom Facial Wash™

Ingredients: Deionized water, MSM (methylsulfonymethane), Ningxia wolfberry (*Lycium barbarum*) seed oil, pure therapeutic-grade essential oils (as listed below), decyl polyglucose, mixed fruit acid complex, hydrolyzed wheat protein, citric acid, calendula extract, chamomile extract, rosebud extract, orange blossom extract, St. John's wort extract, algae, aloe vera gel, kelp extract, *Ginkgo biloba* extract, grape seed extract, and dimethyl lauramine oleate.

Essential Oils:

Lavender—is balancing and calming. It works wherever there is a need and is useful for any type of skin condition.

Patchouli—helps digest toxic material. It tones and tightens skin and helps prevent wrinkles.

Lemon—helps promote leukocyte formation and helps brighten a pale, dull complexion by removing dead skin cells.

Rosemary verbenon—is milder than rosemary cineol and better suited for skin care.

Instructions: Apply warm water to the face to moisten skin. Apply wash directly to the face, and gently massage in a gentle circular motion to create a lather. Rinse thoroughly, and gently pat dry. For best results, use Orange Blossom Facial Wash twice daily. Follow up with Sandalwood Moisture Cream to promote younger and healthier-looking skin.

Body System(s) Affected: **Skin**.

Ortho Ease™ Massage Oil

Ingredients: Fractionated coconut (*Cocos nucifera*) oil (distilled from pure coconut oil; odorless and colorless; never goes rancid; more readily absorbed by the skin; easily washes out of clothes and sheets with no staining), grape (*Vitis vinifera*) seed oil (antioxidant; rich in bioflavonoids; helps maintain pH balance), wheat (*Triticum vulgare*) germ oil (high in vitamins E, B and lecithin; natural antioxidant; reduces scar tissue and stretch marks; preservative for other base oils), sweet almond (*Prunus amygdalus dulcis*) oil (nourishes the skin; reduces friction for smoother application), organic olive (*Olea europaea*) oil (moisturizing agent), and pure therapeutic-grade essential oils (as listed below).

Essential Oils:

Wintergreen—is locally warming and contains methyl salicylate. It has a cortisone-like action that helps to reduce inflammation in the joints and tissue.

Juniper—is antispasmodic and helps reduce muscle aches/pains.

Peppermint—enhances the effect of the other oils. It is high in natural menthol, for a wonderful mentholatum-type of sensation.

Eucalyptus globulus—is wonderful as an anti-inflammatory agent.

Lemongrass—helps repair connective tissue: when combined with marjoram, it helps stimulate the agents in the tissue to rejuvenate and reconnect.

Marjoram—is a powerful muscle relaxant and anti-inflammatory. It is relaxing and soothing to cartilage tissue.

Thyme—is anti-inflammatory, antifungal, antiseptic, and antiviral.

Eucalyptus radiata—is wonderful as an anti-inflammatory agent.

Vetiver—is antispasmodic and locally warming. It is good for arthritis, rheumatism, and sprains.

Clary Sage—helps balance the hormones and is a tonic to the reproductive system.

Warning: Avoid eye contact. If contact occurs, rinse thoroughly with water. For external use only. Keep out of reach of children.

Body System(s) Affected: **Muscles and Bones, Skin**.

Ortho Sport™ Massage Oil

This massage oil is an enhanced version of Ortho Ease, super-charged for the more demanding athlete or sportsman.

Ingredients: Fractionated coconut (*Cocos nucifera*) oil (distilled from pure coconut oil; odorless and colorless; never goes rancid; more readily absorbed by the skin; easily washes out of clothes and sheets with no staining), grape (*Vitis vinifera*) seed oil (antioxidant; rich in bioflavonoids; helps maintain pH balance), wheat (*Triticum vulgare*) germ oil (high in vitamins E, B and lecithin; natural antioxidant; reduces scar tissue and stretch marks; preservative for other base oils), sweet almond (*Prunus amygdalus dulcis*) oil (nourishes the skin; reduces friction for smoother application), organic olive (*Olea europaea*) oil (moisturizing agent), and pure therapeutic-grade essential oils (as listed below).

Essential Oils:

Wintergreen—is locally warming. It contains methyl salicylate and has a cortisone-like action that helps to reduce inflammation in the joints and tissue.

Peppermint—enhances the effect of the other oils. It is high in natural menthol, for a wonderful mentholatum-type of sensation.

Oregano—is a powerful antimicrobial agent and is anti-inflammatory and locally warming.

Eucalyptus globulus—is wonderful as an anti-inflammatory agent.

Elemi—is a very powerful anti-inflammatory agent. It is similar to helichrysum as a topical anesthetic.

Vetiver—is antispasmodic and locally warming. It is good for arthritis, rheumatism, and sprains.

Lemongrass—helps repair connective tissue: when combined with marjoram, it helps stimulate the agents in the tissue to rejuvenate and reconnect.

Thyme—is anti-inflammatory, antifungal, antiseptic, and antiviral.

Warning: Avoid eye contact. If contact occurs, rinse thoroughly with water. For external use only. Keep out of reach of children.

Body System(s) Affected: **Muscles and Bones**.

Peppermint Cedarwood Moisturizing Soap™

This soap contains oils that purify and invigorate the skin with a calming fragrance.

Ingredients: Saponified palm (*Elaeis guineensis*) oil, saponified coconut (*Cocos nucifera*) oil, saponified olive (*Olea europaea*) fruit oil, vegetable gylcerin, pure therapeutic-grade essential oils (as listed below), Ningxia wolfberry (*Lycium barbarum*) seed oil, oat (*Avena sativa*) kernel meal, jojoba (*Simmondsia chinensis*) seed oil, *aloe vera* (*Aloe barbadensis*) leaf juice, and rosemary (*Rosmarinus officinalis*) leaf extract.

Essential Oils:

Peppermint—invigorates the skin and enhances the effects of cedarwood.

Cedarwood—is rejuvenating and refreshing. It is antiseptic and beneficial to the skin.

Prenolone™/Prenolone+™

Moisturizing Cream

This cream utilizes natural pregnenolone (called the "Master Hormone" because it is a precursor to all the other hormones produced within the body including progesterone, estrogen, and testosterone) and a small amount of natural progesterone (derived from soy) to replenish and soften dry or irritated skin. With the help of the essential oils that are included in this formulation, the pregnenolone is quickly and efficiently transferred to the cellular level where it can be converted into the appropriate hormone that the body needs at that particular time. Unlike many natural progesterone creams, there is not the need to regulate the use of this cream as the body can eliminate what is not needed without any side effects. Also, unlike other natural hormone creams, this one can also be used by men. Similar natural hormone creams have been found to help with the following: wrinkles, libido (restores), blood sugar levels (normalizes), cell oxygen levels (restores), bone density (improves), weight control (helps use fat for energy), zinc and copper levels (normalizes), blood clotting (normalizes), thyroid action, breast cancer and fibroids (protects against), headaches, asthma, backaches, infertility, hair loss, depression, hypoglycemia, inflammation, exhaustion, insomnia, arthritis, and more. **The regular Prenolone contains all the same ingredients as Prenolone+ without the addition of DHEA.**

Ingredients: Deionized water, MSM (methylsulfonymethane), caprylic/capric triglyceride, sorbitol, lecithin, pregnenolone, Ningxia wolfberry (*Lycium barbarum*) seed oil, shea butter, glyceryl stearate, aloe vera gel, sodium PCA, stearic acid, calendula extract, Roman chamomile extract, rosebud extract, green tea extract, St. John's wort extract, *Ginkgo biloba* extract, grapeseed extract, algae extract, DHEA (only in Prenolone+), tocopheryl acetate and linoleate (vitamin E), pure therapeutic-grade essential oils (as listed below), hydrolyzed wheat protein, locust bean gum, ionic trace minerals, organic flax seed oil, wheat germ oil, allantoin, wild yam, eleuthero (*Eleutherococcus senticosus*) extract, blue cohosh, black cohosh, kelp, retinyl palmitate (vitamin A), progesterone from soybean extract, and ascorbic acid (vitamin C).

Essential Oils:

Ylang Ylang—is stimulating and helps to balance male-female energies.

Clary Sage—helps balance the hormones and is a tonic to the reproductive system.

Geranium—can be used on almost any kind of skin. It is cleansing, refreshing, astringent, and a mild skin tonic. It is used to balance the hyposecretion of androgens or estrogens that frequently occurs during menopause.

Bergamot—helps to relieve anxiety, stress, and tension and helps to balance the hormones.

Fennel—helps balance the hormones.

Sage—contains estriol and has estrogen-like properties. It is believed to contain elements that contribute to the secretion of progesterone.

Yarrow—is anti-inflammatory, antiseptic, and excellent for menstrual problems.

Instructions: Apply ¼ to ½ tsp. one to two times daily for 21 continuous days. Discontinue use for 7 days, and then repeat. Massage cream thoroughly into soft tissue areas of the body (inside thigh, stomach, breasts, etc.) until absorbed. Individual needs may vary.

Body System(s) Affected: **Emotional Balance, Hormonal** and **Nervous Systems, Muscles and Bones, Skin**.

Warning: Application is intended for external use. If pregnant or under a doctor's care, consult your physician. Keep in a cool, dry place. Do not expose to excessive heat. Keep out of the reach of children.

Companion Products: FemiGen (an herbal complex for supporting the female reproductive system), Dragon Time oil blend, Thyromin (for thyroid support).

Progessence™ Cream

This cream contains natural progesterone (derived from soy), MSM, and wolfberry oil to moisturize and nourish dry skin. With the help of the essential oils that are included in this formulation, the progesterone is quickly and efficiently transferred to the cellular level where it can be utilized by the body. The progesterone contained in this product may help it to lower cholesterol levels, reduce the risk of heart attacks or stroke, normalize sleeping, and help to decrease the symptoms of menopause (such as hot flashes, migraines, and night sweats). Natural hormone creams like this one have been found to help with the following: wrinkles, libido (restores), blood sugar levels (normalizes), cell oxygen levels (restores), bone density (improves), weight control (helps use fat for energy), zinc and copper levels (normalizes), blood clotting (normalizes), thyroid action, breast cancer and fibroids (protects against), headaches, asthma, backaches, infertility, hair loss, depression, hypoglycemia, inflammation, exhaustion, insomnia, arthritis, and more.

Ingredients: Deionized water, MSM, caprylic/capric triglyceride, sorbitol, Ningxia wolfberry (*Lycium barbarum*) seed oil, shea butter, glyceryl stearate, aloe vera gel, sodium PCA, stearic acid, calendula extract, chamomile extract, rosebud extract, orange blossom extract, St. John's wort extract, *Ginkgo biloba* extract, grapeseed extract, algae extract, tocopheryl acetate and linoleate (vitamin E), hydrolyzed wheat protein, locust bean gum, allantoin, lecithin, kelp, retinyl palmitate (vitamin A), ascorbic acid (vitamin C), lecithin, progesterone (from soybean extract), pure therapeutic-grade essential oils (as listed below), eleuthero (*Eleuthero coccus senticosus*), trace mineral complex, organic flax seed oil, wheat germ oil, wild yam extract, black cohosh, and blue cohosh.

Essential Oils:

Geranium—can be used on almost any kind of skin. It is cleansing, refreshing, astringent, and a mild skin tonic. It is used to balance the hyposecretion of androgens or estrogens that frequently occurs during menopause.

Fennel—helps balance the hormones.

Yarrow—is anti-inflammatory, antiseptic, and excellent for menstrual problems.

Sage—contains estriol and has estrogen-like properties. It is believed to contain elements that contribute to the secretion of progesterone.

Instructions: Apply ¼ to ½ tsp. one to two times daily for 21 continuous days. Discontinue use for 7 days and repeat. Massage cream thoroughly into soft tissue areas of the body (inside thigh, stomach, etc.) until absorbed. Individual needs may vary.

Body System(s) Affected: Emotional Balance, Hormonal and Nervous Systems, Muscles and Bones, Skin.

Warning: Application is intended for external use. If pregnant or under a doctor's care, consult your physician. Keep in a cool, dry place. Do not expose to excessive heat. Keep out of the reach of children.

Companion Products: FemiGen (an herbal complex for supporting the female reproductive system), Dragon Time oil blend, Thyromin (for thyroid support).

Progessence™ Plus Serum

This unique progesterone serum contains natural, fully-developed progesterone derived from wild yams that has been super-micronized to enhance skin penetration. It has been paired with frankincense, bergamot, and peppermint essential oils that contain key constituents that further enhance penetration of this progesterone into the deeper layers of the skin where it can be picked up by the blood vessels and transported throughout the body. The progesterone contained in this product may help it to lower cholesterol levels, reduce the risk of heart attacks or stroke, normalize sleeping, and help to decrease the symptoms of menopause (such as hot flashes, migraines, and night sweats). Natural progesterones use may help with the following: wrinkles, libido (restores), blood sugar levels (normalizes), cell oxygen levels (restores), bone density (improves), weight control (helps use fat for energy), zinc and copper levels (normalizes), blood clotting (normalizes), thyroid action, breast cancer and fibroids (protects against), headaches, asthma, backaches, infertility, hair loss, depression, hypoglycemia, inflammation, exhaustion, insomnia, arthritis, and more.

Ingredients: Pure therapeutic-grade essential oils (as listed below), capric/caprylic triglycerides (fractionated coconut oil), vitamin E, USP progesterone (P4 progesterone from wild yam extract).

Essential Oils:

Copaiba—can help relieve inflammation and has a soft, balsamic aroma that can help to elevate the mood and lift feelings of depression.

Frankincense—contains high levels of α-pinene, which may help enhance penetration of hormones through the skin[1].

Cedarwood—has a warm, woody aroma that is calming and can help relieve nervous tension.

Bergamot—contains high levels of d-Limonene, which has been found in various studies to enhance penetration of lipophilic drugs through the skin[2].

Peppermint—contains high levels of menthol to help enhance penetration of progesterone through the skin[3].

Rosewood Leaf—is antifungal and is soothing to the skin.

Clove—has high antioxidant properties.

Instructions: For use by women only. Apply 2–4 drops twice a day over the corotid arteries in the neck and 1–2 drops along the forearms twice a day for enhanced effects. Apply 1–2 drops as needed on temples for menstrual headaches. Application at night may help aid sleep.

Body System(s) Affected: Emotional Balance, Hormonal and Nervous Systems, Muscles and Bones, Skin.

Warnings: Application is intended for external use. If pregnant or under a doctor's care, consult your physician. Do not use if taking a contraceptive containing progesterone or proscribed progestins. Do not use before taking a hot shower or bath.

Companion Products: FemiGen (an herbal complex for supporting the female reproductive system), Dragon Time oil blend, Thyromin (for thyroid support).

Protec™

Protec™ is designed for topical use only; it should never be taken orally. This formula was designed to accompany the night-long retention enema. It helps buffer the prostate from inflammation, enlargement, and tumor activity. It is also suitable for women as a night-long retention douche.

Ingredients: Grape (*Vitis vinifera*) seed oil (antioxidant; rich in bioflavonoids; helps maintain pH balance), wheat (*Triticum vulgare*) germ oil (high in vitamins E, B and lecithin; natural antioxidant; reduces scar tissue and stretch marks; preservative for other base oils), sweet almond (*Prunus amygdalus dulcis*) oil (nourishes the skin; reduces friction for smoother application), organic olive (*Olea europaea*) oil (moisturizing agent), and pure therapeutic-grade essential oils (as listed below).

Essential Oils:

Frankincense—is antitumoral and anti-inflammatory. It is good for prostate problems.

Myrrh—is anti-inflammatory and antiseptic. It helps to decongest the prostate gland.

Sage—contains estriol and has estrogen-like properties. It may help improve estrogen and progesterone-testosterone balance.

Cumin—is antibacterial, antispasmodic, and has some antitumoral properties.

Instructions: For the retention enema or douche, use ½ to 1 oz. and hold all night long for 21 consecutive nights. If irritation occurs, discontinue use for three days before restarting.

Body System(s) Affected: **Hormonal System**.

Regenolone™

Moisturizing Cream

This cream utilizes natural pregnenolone (called the "Master Hormone" because it is a precursor to all the other hormones produced within the body including progesterone, estrogen, and testosterone) and a small amount of natural progesterone (derived from soy) to replenish and soften dry or irritated skin. With the essential oils that are included, this product may be effective in promoting the regeneration of damaged nerves and tissues.

Ingredients: Deionized water, MSM, pure therapeutic-grade essential oils (as listed below), caprylic/capric triglyceride, sorbitol, lecithin, pregnenolone, Ningxia wolfberry (*Lycium barbarum*) seed oil, shea butter, glyceryl stearate, aloe vera gel, sodium PCA, stearic acid, calendula extract, Roman chamomile extract, rosebud extract, green tea extract, St. John's wort extract, *Gingko biloba* extract, grapeseed extract, algae extract, tocopheryl acetate and linoleate (vitamin E), hydrolyzed wheat protein, locust bean gum, trace minerals, flax seed, wheat germ oil, allantoin, wild yam, eleuthero (*Eleuthero coccus senticosus*), kelp, retinyl palmitate (vitamin A), black and blue cohosh extracts, progesterone, and ascorbic acid (vitamin C).

Essential Oils:

Wintergreen—has a cortisone-like action that helps to reduce inflammation in the tissues. It contains methyl salicylate.

Peppermint—is invigorating to the skin, soothing and relaxing to tired muscles, and may also help with nerve regeneration.

Douglas Fir—is calming to tired and overworked joints and very soothing to sore muscles.

Oregano—is a powerful antimicrobial. It is anti-inflammatory and locally warming.

Instructions: Apply ⅛ to ¼ tsp. on location as needed. Individual needs may vary. May be best not to use more than 5 times a day.

Body System(s) Affected: **Hormonal** and **Nervous Systems, Muscles and Bones, Skin**.

Warning: Application is intended for external use. If pregnant or under a doctor's care, consult your physician. Keep in a cool, dry place. Do not expose to excessive heat. Keep out of the reach of children.

Companion Oils: Oregano, thyme, Dragon Time, Mister.

Companion Products: Prenolone/Prenolone+, Thyromin (for thyroid support).

Relaxation™ Massage Oil

Ingredients: Fractionated coconut (*Cocos nucifera*) oil (distilled from pure coconut oil; odorless and colorless; never goes rancid; more readily absorbed by the skin; easily washes out of clothes and sheets with no staining), grape (*Vitis vinifera*) seed oil (antioxidant; rich in bioflavonoids; helps maintain pH balance), wheat (*Triticum vulgare*) germ oil (high in vitamins E, B and lecithin; natural antioxidant; reduces scar tissue and stretch marks; preservative for other base oils), sweet almond (*Prunus amygdalus dulcis*) oil (nourishes the skin; reduces friction for smoother application), organic olive (*Olea europaea*) oil (moisturizing agent), and pure therapeutic-grade essential oils (as listed below).

Essential Oils:

Tangerine—is sedating and calming to the nervous system. It is also a diuretic and a decongestant of the lymphatic system.

Lavender—is sedative. It balances body systems and promotes a general sense of well-being.

Peppermint—is purifying and stimulating to the conscious mind. It is anti-inflammatory and helps with nerve regeneration.

Spearmint—acts as an antidepressant by relieving mental strain and fatigue and by lifting one's spirits.

Rosewood—is appeasing to the mind and relaxing to the body.

Ylang Ylang—is antidepressant, calming, and relaxing. It may help balance male/female energies.

Warning: Shake well before using. Avoid eye contact. If contact occurs, rinse thoroughly with water. For external use only. Keep out of reach of children.

Body System(s) Affected: **Emotional Balance, Skin**.

Rose Ointment™

This ointment dramatically improves the effectiveness of other essential oils that are applied for skin conditions. When applied on top of oils such as PanAway, lavender, helichrysum, and Melrose, this product seals in the volatile constituents of the essential oils, increasing their effectiveness by prolonging their contact with the skin. It also helps maintain the natural pH balance of the skin, conserve its acid mantle, and balance the drying effect that some essential oils may have on the skin.

Ingredients: Mink oil (nurture and regenerate the skin), lecithin (natural dispersing agent; used in place of sodium lauryl sulfate), beeswax (used as the thickening and stabilizing agent), lanolin (taken from sheep wool; excellent for skin care), sesame (*Sesamum indicum*) seed oil (high in linoleic acid; maintains pH balance of the skin), wheat (*Triticum vulgare*) germ oil, pure therapeutic-grade essential oils (as listed below), and rosehip (*Rosa canina*) seed oil (helps reduce scarring and premature aging).

Essential Oils:

Rosewood—is tissue regenerative. It is soothing to the skin and increases elasticity.

Palmarosa—stimulates new cell growth, regulates oil production, moisturizes, and speeds healing.

Patchouli—is used for protection against UV radiation and for tissue regeneration. It helps tighten loose skin and prevent wrinkles.

Myrrh—helps to heal chapped or cracked skin and reduce inflammation.

Carrot seed—is a natural phytonutrient that is rich in beta carotene. It helps to reduce wrinkles and dryness.

Melaleuca—is tissue regenerative and helps promote the healing of wounds.

Rose otto—brings balance and harmony by enhancing the frequency of every cell.

Instructions: Apply directly to skin.

Body System(s) Affected: **Skin**.

Sacred Mountain Moisturizing Soap™

For Oily Skin

This soap contains extra abrasives to remove dead skin cells and contains oils that are antiseptic, purifying, and calming.

Ingredients: Saponified palm (*Elaeis guineensis*) oil, saponified coconut (*Cocos nucifera*) oil, saponified olive (*Olea europaea*) fruit oil, vegetable gylcerin, pure therapeutic-grade essential oils (as listed below), Ningxia wolfberry (*Lycium barbarum*) seed oil, oat (*Avena sativa*) kernel meal, jojoba (*Simmondsia chinensis*) seed oil, *aloe vera* (*Aloe barbadensis*) leaf juice, and rosemary (*Rosmarinus officinalis*) leaf extract.

Essential Oils:

Spruce—helps to open and release emotional blocks.

Ylang Ylang—is stimulating and helps to balance male-female energies.

Balsam Fir—is antiseptic and helps create a feeling of grounding, anchoring, and empowerment.

Cedarwood—is rejuvenating and refreshing. It is antiseptic and beneficial to the skin.

Sandalwood Moisture Cream™

Ingredients: Deionized water, MSM, caprylic/capric triglyceride, sorbitol, goat's cream, Ningxia wolfberry (*Lycium barbarum*) seed oil, rosehip seed oil, shea butter, glyceryl stearate, pure therapeutic-grade essential oils (as listed below), sodium PCA, algae extract, stearic acid, allantoin, lecithin, *Ginkgo biloba* extract, grapeseed extract, calendula extract, chamomile extract, rosebud extract, orange blossom extract, St. John's wort extract, aloe vera gel, kelp, retinyl palmitate (vitamin A), tocopheryl acetate (vitamin E), ascorbic acid (vitamin C), locust bean gum, hydrolyzed wheat protein, sodium hyaluronate, and tocopheryl linoleate (vitamin E).

Essential Oils:

Rosewood—is skin cell regenerative, soothing to the skin, and promotes elasticity. It is appeasing to the mind and relaxing to the body.

Sandalwood—helps strengthen the lymphatic systems and revitalizes the skin.

Lavender—is balancing and calming. It works wherever there is a need and is useful for any type of skin condition.

Myrrh—is soothing to the skin. It is used for chapped and cracked skin and wrinkles.

Rosemary verbenon—is milder than rosemary cineol and better suited for skin care.

Instructions: For best results, use Sandalwood Moisture Cream after cleansing and toning the face and neck to promote younger, healthier skin. Put small amount in hand, emulsify, and apply to face and neck using upward strokes.

Body System(s) Affected: **Skin**.

Satin Facial Scrub™ (Mint)

As a gentle exfoliating scrub designed for **normal skin**, Mint Satin Facial Scrub gently eliminates layers of dead skin cells with a revolutionary formula of jojoba beads and other natural ingredients. It can be used as a drying face mask to draw impurities from the skin. Peppermint essential oil is added to soothe and refresh the skin.

Ingredients: Deionized water, glycerin, caprylic/capric triglyceride, jojoba (*Buxus chinensis*) wax beads, MSM (methylsulfonylmethane), sorbitol, glyceryl stearate, peppermint essential oil (as listed below), aloe vera (*Aloe barbadensis*) gel, stearic acid, algae (*Gellidiela acerosa*) extract, rosemary (*Rosmarinus officinalis*) extract, chamomile (*Anthemis nobilis*) extract, tocopheryl acetate (vitamin E), retinyl palmitate (vitamin A), sodium PCA, shea butter, grape (*Vitis vinifera*) seed extract, zinc oxide, mango (*Mangifera indica*) butter, ascorbic acid (vitamin C), sodium hyaluronate, tocopheryl linoleate (vitamin E), allantoin, hydrolyzed wheat protein, and hydrolyzed soy protein.

Essential Oils:

Peppermint—is invigorating to the skin and may also help with nerve regeneration.

Instructions: Apply warm water to the face to moisten the skin. Apply scrub directly to the face, and gently massage in a circular motion, creating a lather. Rinse thoroughly, and gently pat dry. May also be mixed with Orange Blossom Facial Wash for a milder scrub. Mix ½ tsp. of both in palm of hand before applying. Use four or five times weekly, depending on need.

Body System(s) Affected: **Skin**.

Sensation™ Bath & Shower Gel

The sensual fragrance of this bath gel is a wonderful addition to those romantic evenings.

Ingredients: Water, saponified coconut (*Cocus nucifera*) oil, saponified olive (*Olea europaea*) oil, vegetable glycerin, guar (*Cyamopsis tetragonoloba*) gum, aloe vera (*Aloe barbadensis*) leaf juice, pure therapeutic-grade essential oils (as listed below), jojoba (*Simmondsia chinensis*) seed oil, and rosemary (*Rosmarinus officinalis*) leaf extract.

Essential Oils:

Rosewood—is antiseptic, antibacterial, tissue regenerative, soothing to the skin, and increases skin elasticity.

Ylang Ylang—is stimulating and helps to balance male-female energies.

Jasmine—has a deeply penetrating effect on the skin. It produces a feeling of confidence, energy, euphoria, and optimism.

Body System(s) Affected: **Emotional Balance, Hormonal System, Skin**.

Sensation™ Hand & Body Lotion

Ingredients: Deionized water, dimethyl sulfone (MSM), glyceryl stearate (vegetable based), stearic acid, sodium hyaluronate, sorbitol, *Rosa canina* fruit oil, shea butter (*Butyrospermum parkii*), mango (*Mangifera indica*) seed butter, wheat (*Triticum vulgare*) germ oil, kukui (*Aleurites moluccana*) nut oil, lecithin, safflower (*Carthamus tinctorius*) oil, apricot (*Prunus armeniaca*) kernel oil, sweet almond (*Prunus amygdalus dulcis*) oil, tocopheryl acetate (vitamin E), retinyl palmitate (vitamin A), jojoba (*Simmondsia *chinensis*) seed oil, sesame (*Sesamum indicum*) seed oil, pure therapeutic-grade essential oils (as listed below), aloe vera (*Aloe barbadensis*) leaf juice, grape (*Vitis vinifera*) seed extract, ascorbic acid (vitamin C), *Camellia oleifera* leaf extract, St. John's wort (*Hypericum perforatum*) extract, *Fucus vesiculosus* extract, and *Ginkgo biloba* leaf extract.

Essential Oils:

Rosewood—is antibacterial, tissue regenerative, soothing to the skin, and increases elasticity.

Ylang Ylang—is stimulating and helps to balance male-female energies.

Jasmine—is deeply penetrating. It produces a feeling of confidence, energy, and optimism.

Instructions: Dispense in hand, and apply directly to skin.

Warning: Avoid eye contact. If contact occurs, rinse thoroughly with water. For external use only. Keep out of reach of children.

Sensation™ Massage Oil

Ingredients: Fractionated coconut (*Cocos nucifera*) oil (distilled from pure coconut oil; odorless and colorless; never goes rancid; more readily absorbed by the skin; easily washes out of clothes and sheets with no staining), grape (*Vitis vinifera*) seed oil (antioxidant; rich in bioflavonoids; helps maintain pH balance), wheat (*Triticum vulgare*) germ oil (high in vitamins E, B and lecithin; natural antioxidant; reduces scar tissue and stretch marks; preservative for other base oils), sweet almond (*Prunus amygdalus dulcis*) oil (nourishes the skin; reduces friction for smoother application), organic olive (*Olea europaea*) oil (moisturizing agent), and pure therapeutic-grade essential oils (as listed below).

Essential Oils:

Rosewood—is skin cell regenerative, soothing to the skin, and promotes elasticity. It is appeasing to the mind and relaxing to the body.

Ylang Ylang—balances the secretion of sebum (a waxy oil produced by the skin). It is energizing and uplifting.

Jasmine—has a deeply penetrating effect on the skin. It produces a feeling of confidence, energy, euphoria, and optimism.

Warning: Shake well before using. Avoid eye contact. If contact occurs, rinse thoroughly with water. For external use only. Keep out of reach of children.

Body System(s) Affected: **Emotional Balance, Hormonal System**.

Thieves® AromaBright™ Toothpaste

This all-natural toothpaste was specially formulated with no artificial or synthetic ingredients, no preservatives, no dyes, and no fluoride. It was designed to help lessen tooth sensitivity and to create an environment in the mouth that is unfavorable to harmful bacteria.

Ingredients: Water, calcium carbonate, *Cocos nucifera* (coconut) oil, sodium bicarbonate, glycerin (vegetable), xylitol, xanthan gum, *Mentha piperita* (peppermint) oil, *Mentha spicata* (spearmint) leaf oil, *Eugenia caryophyllus* (clove) bud oil, *Ocotea quixos* (ocotea) leaf oil, *Cinnamomum verum* (cinnamon) bark oil, *Citrus limon* (lemon) peel oil, *Eucalyptus radiata* leaf oil, *Rosmarinus officinalis* (rosemary) leaf oil, *Stevia rebaudiana* leaf extract, lecithin (sunflower).

Essential Oils:

Peppermint—is used as a natural flavoring and a breath-freshening agent.

Spearmint—has a natural breath-freshening action.

Thieves—is a proprietary blend of clove, lemon, cinnamon bark, *Eucalyptus radiata*, and rosemary essential oils that has been documented to be highly antibacterial and antimicrobial in nature.

Ocotea—has antibacterial and anti-inflammatory properties.

Thieves® Cleaning Products

These new antiseptic products utilize the documented bacteria-killing power of the Thieves oil blend. Throw away those chemical-laden cleaning products and fight those germs with these powerful, natural products.

Ingredients:

Thieves® Household Cleaner: Proprietary suspension base of safe surfactants (wetting agents) and Thieves essential oil blend.

Thieves® Spray: Pure grain alcohol, deionized water, Thieves essential oil blend, fractionated coconut oil, and soy lecithin.

Thieves® Wipes: Pure grain alcohol, deionized water, Thieves essential oil blend, fractionated coconut oil and soy lecithin.

Suggested Use: Follow label directions.

Body System(s) Affected: **Immune System**.

Precautions: Keep out of reach of children. Not recommended for use on infants or sensitive areas of the body.

Thieves® Cleansing Soap™

This soap contains oils that are high in antiseptic properties.

Ingredients: Saponified palm (*Elaeis guineensis*) oil, saponified coconut (*Cocos nucifera*) oil, saponified olive (*Olea europaea*) fruit oil, vegetable gylcerin, pure therapeutic-grade essential oils (as listed below), Ningxia wolfberry (*Lycium barbarum*) seed oil, oat (*Avena sativa*) kernel meal, jojoba (*Simmondsia chinensis*) seed oil, *aloe vera* (*Aloe barbadensis*) leaf juice, and rosemary (*Rosmarinus officinalis*) leaf extract.

Essential Oils:

Clove—is antibacterial, antifungal, anti-infectious, antiparasitic, a strong antiseptic, antiviral, and an immune stimulant. It may influence healing and help create a feeling of protection and courage.

Lemon—helps promote leukocyte formation and helps brighten a pale, dull complexion by removing dead skin cells.

Cinnamon Bark—is antibacterial, antifungal, anti-infectious, anti-inflammatory, antimicrobial, antiparasitic, antiseptic, antispasmodic, antiviral, astringent, immune-stimulant, sexual stimulant, and warming.

Eucalyptus radiata—has strong antibacterial, anticatarrhal, and antiseptic properties.

Thieves® Dental Floss

Now with twice the essential oil power, this revolutionary, antimicrobial, essential-oil-fortified dental floss has been double saturated with essential oils. This product rounds out the Thieves line of dental products and provides a powerful germ-fighting product that can be easily carried and used on a daily basis, no matter where you may be.

Ingredients: Pure therapeutic-grade essential oils (as listed below), soy wax, beeswax, and nylon.

Essential Oils:

Thieves—is a proprietary blend of clove, lemon, cinnamon bark, *Eucalyptus radiata,* and rosemary essential oils that has been documented to be highly antibacterial and antimicrobial in nature.

Peppermint—is used as a natural flavoring and a breath-freshening agent.

Thieves® Dentarome™/Dentarome Plus™ Toothpaste

This is a revolutionary, antimicrobial, essential-oil-fortified toothpaste. It is an all-natural toothpaste that includes a highly antimicrobial blend of pure plant-derived essential oils. It contains no sugar, saccharine, sodium lauryl sulfate, or synthetic chemicals, colors, or preservatives of any kind. This formula was tested at Weber State University and found to have potent antimicrobial properties against a wide range of oral microbes including *streptococcus oralis, streptococcus pneumoniae, bramunella catarrhalis, and candida albicans.* Other studies confirm the plaque-fighting and antimicrobial attributes of the essential oils included in Thieves Dentarome and Dentarome Plus, including one study published in the *International Journal of Food Microbiology* that found the essential oils of thyme, clove, and cinnamon to exhibit antimicrobial effects. Another study listed peppermint as one of the most potent essential oils against plaque-causing elements. **The added thymol and eugenol in Dentarome Plus are derived from pure thyme (*Thymus vulgaris*) and clove (*Eugenia caryophyllata*) oils and enhance its antimicrobial potency.**

Ingredients:

Baking Soda—a mild abrasive and fast-acting cleansing agent.

Deionized Water—added for consistency.

Vegetable Glycerin—used as a moistener.

Xanthum Gum—a natural thickener.

Ionic Minerals—added as a nutritional supplement that, together with the essential oil of wintergreen, helps to strengthen teeth.

Thymol & Eugenol—added to Dentarome Plus for more powerful antiseptic and antimicrobial effects. Thymol is derived from thyme oil (*Thymus vulgaris*) and eugenol is derived from clove oil (*Eugenia caryophyllata*).

Stevioside—a natural, intensely sweet extract from a tropical plant native to South America.

Essential Oils:

Wintergreen—is used here to help strengthen teeth. It is also antimicrobial in nature.

Peppermint—is used as a natural flavoring and a breath-freshening agent.

Thieves—is a proprietary blend of clove, lemon, cinnamon bark, *Eucalyptus radiata,* and rosemary essential oils that has been documented to be highly antibacterial and antimicrobial in nature.

Thieves® Dentarome Ultra™ Toothpaste

This product contains a revolutionary formula of all-natural, edible ingredients. Created to be gentle on teeth enamel, the calcium carbonate and zinc oxide in this toothpaste are substantially smaller in particle size than in other popular commercial toothpastes. Add to that the germ- and cavity-fighting power of the pure therapeutic-grade essential oils and other ingredients, and this toothpaste is ultimate in dental care.

Ingredients: Calcium carbonate, essential oil concentrate containing peppermint essential oil and Thieves essential oil blend, zinc oxide, deionized water with papain, xylitol, vegetable glycerine, essential oil base (thymol from *Thymus vulgaris*, *Eucalyptus globulus*, and methyl salycilate from wintergreen), xanthum gum, zinc citrate, lecithin, and stevioside.

Essential Oils:

Peppermint—is used as a natural flavoring and a breath-freshening agent.

<u>**Thieves**</u>—is a proprietary blend of clove, lemon, cinnamon bark, *Eucalyptus radiata*, and rosemary essential oils that has been documented to be highly antibacterial and antimicrobial in nature.

Thyme—contains 46% thymol—one of the most potent antimicrobial substances known.

Eucalyptus—contains eucalyptol. It is also known as 1,8-cineol.

Wintergreen—is used here to help strengthen teeth. It is also antimicrobial in nature.

Thieves® Foaming Hand Soap

This is the ultimate in protection and nourishment in a luxurious, foaming hand soap. This product is dermatologist tested and provides antimicrobial protection with lemon and orange essential oils as well as the Thieves blend of essential oils and skin conditioning benefits with aloe vera, gingko biloba, and vitamin E. It is gentle to allow for frequent use without drying out the skin.

Ingredients: Deionized water, decyl glucoside, cocamidopropyl hydroxysultaine, pure therapeutic-grade essential oils (as listed below), *Aloe barbadensis* leaf juice, tocopheryl acetate (vitamin E), *Ginkgo biloba* leaf extract, retinyl palmitate (vitamin A), *Camellia sinensis* leaf extract, cetyl hydroxyethylcellulose, citric acid, phenoxyethanol, caprylyl glycol, ethylhexylglycerin, and hexylene glycol.

Essential Oils:

<u>**Thieves**</u>—is a proprietary blend of clove, lemon, cinnamon bark, *Eucalyptus radiata*, and rosemary essential oils that has been documented to be highly antibacterial and antimicrobial in nature.

Lemon—helps promote leukocyte formation and is antiseptic.

Orange—contains over 91% d-Limonene (which helps to promote normal cell life cycles).

Caution: Not for internal use. Avoid contact with eyes. If contact occurs, flush eyes liberally with clean, cool water for several minutes. If redness or irritation occurs, discontinue use. If symptoms persist, contact your physician.

Thieves® Fresh Essence Plus™ Mouthwash

This is the ultimate oral rinse, formulated with antimicrobial, pure therapeutic-grade essential oils that naturally contain compounds that have been clinically proven to kill microbes that can cause bad breath, plaque, and periodontal diseases like gingivitis. It is formulated with a patented liposome technology (using soy-derived lecithin), which binds the essential oils to the mucus membrane inside the mouth to provide long-lasting germ-killing and breath-freshening protection. As an all-natural product, it contains **no dyes, no alcohol, no saccharin, and no synthetic flavors or preservatives**.

Unlike some commercially-available products that contain just the active constituents of eucalyptol and menthol, Thieves Fresh Essence Plus Mouthwash uses the entire essential oil. The complete oil exhibits far stronger antimicrobial power than its active constituents alone. From his research on the essential oil of eucalyptus, Jean Valnet, M.D., made the following statement: "The antiseptic properties of the essences of eucalyptus were much more powerful than those of its principle constituent, eucalyptol." The whole oil is also safer because it contains a natural balance of elements that make it relatively harmless to human tissue.

Ingredients: Deionized water, peppermint floral water, melissa floral water, colloidal silver, pure therapeutic-grade essential oils (as listed below), lecithin, polysorbate 80, steviocide (a naturally sweet plant extract), and tocopherol (vitamin E).

Essential Oils:

Peppermint—contains natural menthol.

Thieves—is a proprietary blend of clove, lemon, cinnamon bark, *Eucalyptus radiata*, and rosemary essential oils that has been documented to be highly antibacterial and antimicrobial in nature.

Spearmint—is used as a natural flavoring and a breath-freshening agent.

Vetiver—is high in sesquiterpenes. It is fixative and helps stabilize essential oils.

Instructions: Rinse mouth with one tablespoon or capful of Thieves Fresh Essence Plus for 30–60 seconds or as needed. Store at room temperature.

Thieves® Waterless Hand Purifier

This product is a completely natural alternative to all the other chemical-laden, waterless hand sanitizer products currently on the market.

Ingredients: Denatured ethanol SD-38B (denatured with peppermint essential oil), water, *Aloe barbadensis* leaf, vegetable glycerin, Thieves essential oil blend (as listed below), and hydroxylpropyl cellulose.

Essential Oils:

Thieves—is a proprietary blend of clove, lemon, cinnamon bark, *Eucalyptus radiata*, and rosemary essential oils that has been documented to be highly antibacterial and antimicrobial in nature.

Instructions: Apply a nickel-sized amount to the palm of the hand, and rub until completely absorbed. Use as often as necessary.

Caution: ***Flammable. Keep away from fire or open flame.*** Not for internal use. Keep out of reach of children. Do no use on or near the face. Avoid contact with eyes. If contact occurs, flush eyes liberally with clean, cool water for several minutes. If symptoms persist, contact your physician.

V-6™ Enhanced Vegetable Oil Complex

This new formulation of mixing oil contains the same nourishing oils but with an increased shelf life and virtually no color or odor. Food Grade.

Ingredients: Fractionated coconut (*Cocos nucifera*) oil (distilled from pure coconut oil; odorless and colorless; never goes rancid; more readily absorbed by the skin; easily washes out of clothes and sheets with no staining), organic sesame (*Sesamum indicum*) seed oil (high in linoleic acid; contains vitamins, minerals, amino acids, lecithin, and natural vegetable proteins; moisturizing; easily absorbed into the skin), grape (*Vitis vinifera*) seed oil (antioxidant; rich in bioflavonoids; helps maintain pH balance), sweet almond (*Prunus amygdalus dulcis*) oil (nourishes the skin; contains natural vitamin D; reduces friction for smoother application), wheat (*Triticum vulgare*) germ oil (high in vitamins E, B and lecithin; natural antioxidant; reduces scar tissue and stretch marks; preservative for other base oils), sunflower (*Helianthus annuus*) seed oil (contains natural vitamin E; antioxidant; suitable for a variety of skin types), organic olive (*Olea europaea*) oil (moisturizing agent).

Directions: Suggested blending is 15–30 drops of essential oil to 1 oz. mixing oil. V-6 Enhanced Vegetable Oil Complex is good for mixing massage oils, creating your own blends and formulas, for cooking and making salad dressings, etc.

Valor Moisturizing Soap™

This soap contains the oil blend of Valor, which is soothing and nourishing to the skin with a balancing and calming fragrance.

Ingredients: Vegetable gylcerin, saponified palm (*Elaeis guineensis*) oil, saponified coconut (*Cocos nucifera*) oil, saponified olive (*Olea europaea*) fruit oil, jojoba (*Simmondsia chinensis*) seed oil, Ningxia wolfberry (*Lycium barbarum*) seed oil, pure therapeutic-grade essential oils (as listed below), oat (*Avena sativa*) kernel meal, aloe vera (*Aloe barbadensis*) leaf juice, and rosemary (*Rosmarinus officinalis*) leaf extract.

Essential Oils:

Spruce—grounds the body, creating the balance and the opening necessary to receive and to give. It may help dilate the bronchial tract to improve the oxygen exchange. It helps one release emotional blocks.

Rosewood—is soothing to the skin, appeasing to the mind, relaxing to the body, and creates a feeling of peace and gentleness.

Blue Tansy—may help cleanse the liver and calm the lymphatic system to help rid one of anger and promote a feeling of self-control.

Frankincense—contains sesquiterpenes, which may help oxygenate the pineal and pituitary glands. It may help promote a positive attitude.

Wolfberry Eye Cream™

Ingredients: Deionized water, MSM, caprylic/capric triglyceride, sorbitol, vegetable glycerin, glyceryl stearate, goat's cream, Ningxia wolfberry (*Lycium barbarum*) seed oil, avocado oil, shea butter, kukui nut oil, rosehip seed oil, hydrocotyl extract, pure therapeutic-grade essential oils (as listed below), echinacea extract, sodium PCA, almond oil, jojoba oil, mango butter, sodium hyaluronate, cucumber extract, green tea extract, tocopherol acetate (vitamin E), soy protein, wheat protein, retinyl palmitate (vitamin A), allantoin, witch hazel extract, horse chestnut extract. lecithin, dipalmitoyl hydroxyproline, phenoxyethanol, beta-sitosterol, linoleic acid, sodium ascorbate, mannitol, ascorbyl palmitate, ascorbic acid (vitamin C), citric acid,

Essential Oils:

Lavender—works wherever there is a need; it is useful for any type of skin condition.

Rosewood—is skin cell regenerative, soothing to the skin, and promotes elasticity. It is appeasing to the mind and relaxing to the body.

Roman Chamomile—helps increase the regenerative ability of the skin. It is a blood cleanser.

Frankincense—is high in sesquiterpenes, helps deliver oxygen to the pineal and pituitary glands, improves hGH production, and increases leukocyte production.

Geranium—improves blood flow, regenerates tissue and nerves, cleans oily skin, and may even liven up pale skin.

Instructions: Apply a tiny amount of Wolfberry Eye Cream under eye area and on the eyelid before bed. Repeat in morning if desired.

Endnotes

Note: *This list contains summaries of research articles referenced in this section. For the full article reference, please see Research References in the appendix of this book. Please note that much of this research is still preliminary and is meant as an educational reference to guide further research and study. It should not be used to attempt to diagnose or prescribe any medical condition. Consult with a certified medical professional with regard to any medical condition.*

1. Limonene, alpha- and beta-pinene, and myrcene demonstrated an ability to increase permeation of other essential oil compounds through the skin (Schmitt et al., 2009).

   Niaouli oil was found to enhance permation of the hormone estradiol through hairless mouse skin in vitro, while the main terpene compounds found in niaouli oil (1,8 cineole, alpha-pinene, alpha-terpineol, and d-Limonene) were also found to increase permeation, but not to the extent of the whole oil (Monti et al., 2002).

2. d-Limonene was found to promote the highest penetration of a hydrophilic drug across the skin of horses at the lowest concentration tested (5%) of several known penetration-enhancing substances (Ferrante et al., 2009).

   Limonene was found to be an effective skin penetration enhancer for the drug haloperidol (Lim et al., 2006).

3. The use of propylene glycol combined with menthol was found to be a useful enhancer for the transdermal absorption of propofol (Yamato et al., 2009).

SUPPLEMENTS

This section contains product information about the authors' favorite nutritional supplements. Most of this information was obtained from the product labels. The essential oils in these products act as catalysts to deliver oxygen and nutrients through the cell walls while assisting the body in the removal of toxic waste.

When taking supplements, it is important to give the body a rest one or two days a week. Taking supplements only five or six days out of the week gives the body time to regain its own balance and allow its own healing powers to operate rather than rely solely on the supplements being taken. These supplements are usually dissolved and assimilated by the body within a couple hours, so the effectiveness of the supplements can be increased by taking them throughout the day instead of all at once.

An approximate frequency is indicated for some of the supplements. However, please keep in mind that there are many variables involved in determining frequency. Consequently, these numbers may be difficult to duplicate and appear here only as a general point of reference.

These product names are all trademarks of Young Living Essential Oils, and although these product names appear throughout other sections of this book without the trademark symbol, they still refer to these same trademarked products.

AlkaLime®

AlkaLime® is a precisely-balanced, acid-neutralizing mineral formulation designed to combat yeast and fungus overgrowth and to preserve the body's proper pH balance—the cornerstone of health. This specially-designed alkalizing mineral powder contains an array of high-alkaline biochemic cell salts and other yeast/fungus-fighting elements such as citric acid and essential oils. By boosting blood alkalinity, yeast and fungus are deprived of the acidic terrain they require to flourish. The effectiveness of other essential oils is enhanced when the body's blood and tissues are alkaline.

Ingredients: Sodium (sodium bicarbonate, sodium phosphate, sodium sulfate), calcium (calcium carbonate, calcium phosphate, calcium sulfate), magnesium (magnesium phosphate), potassium (potassium bicarbonate, potassium chloride, potassium phosphate, potassium sulfate), organic lemon powder, pure therapeutic-grade essential oils (as listed below), citric acid, tartaric acid, stevia, silica.

Essential Oils:

Lemon—helps promote leukocyte formation; helps to dissolve cholesterol and fats.

Lime—helps remove dead skin cells; tightens skin and connective tissue. Lemon and lime both become alkaline when absorbed by the body.

Suggested Use: Take one rounded teaspoon in 4 to 6 oz. of distilled or purified water. **Mix only with water.** Drink immediately. For best results, drink one hour before or after eating. To balance pH, take one to three times per day one hour before meals or before retiring. As an antacid, AlkaLime may be taken as needed. Otherwise, an ideal time to take AlkaLime would be prior to bedtime.

Body System(s) Affected: **Cardiovascular** and **Digestive Systems, Muscles and Bones**.

Companion Products: Essentialzyme, Life 5 (probiotic), Mineral Essence, MultiGreens.

Companion Oils: Valor, 3 Wise Men, Harmony, Forgiveness, Joy, Present Time, Release, Inner Child, Grounding, Hope, SARA, White Angelica, Di-Gize, Purification, Thieves, peppermint, and spearmint.

AlkaLime may help reduce the following signs of acid-based yeast and fungus dominance: fatigue/low energy, unexplained aches and pains, overweight conditions, low resistance to illness, allergies, unbalanced blood sugar, headaches, irritability/mood swings, indigestion, colitis/ulcers, diarrhea/constipation, urinary tract infections, rectal/vaginal itch.

Allerzyme™

Allerzyme™ is a vegetable enzyme complex designed to provide some relief from occasional symptoms such as fullness, pressure, bloating, gas, pain, and/or minor cramping that occur after eating. It may also help combat allergies, fermentation, fatigue, and irritable bowel syndrome. Allerzyme contains a powerful combination of sugar-splitting and starch-splitting enzymes, as well as a small amount of fat-digesting and protein-digesting enzymes, that help to promote proper digestion for people with sensitive stomachs.

Ingredients: Amylase, bromelain, peptidase, protease, invertase, phytase, lipase, lactase, cellulase, alpha-galactosidase, malt diastase, plantain (sulfite-free), pure therapeutic-grade essential oils (as listed below), vegetable cellulose, deionized water, barley sprout powder, and silica.

Essential Oils:

Tarragon—may help reduce anorexia, dyspepsia, flatulence, intestinal spasms, nervous and sluggish digestion, and genital urinary tract infection.

Ginger—is warming, uplifting, and empowering; it helps reduce feelings of nausea and motion sickness.

Peppermint—is purifying and stimulating to the conscious mind, anti-inflammatory, and helps with nerve regeneration. It also enhances digestion and increases endurance.

Juniper—is antispasmodic; it also helps reduce muscle aches/pains.

Fennel—is antiparasitic. It promotes the removal of toxic wastes and may break up fluids and toxins and cleanse the tissues.

Lemongrass—helps repair connective tissue. It helps stimulate the agents in the tissue to rejuvenate and reconnect. It helps regulate the parasympathetic nervous system and strengthen vascular walls.

Patchouli—protects against UV radiation and promotes tissue regeneration. It helps tighten loose skin and prevent wrinkles.

Anise—may help calm and strengthen the digestive system.

Suggested Use: Take 1–2 capsules three times daily just prior to all meals. Can also be sprinkled on food or in beverages.

Body System(s) Affected: Digestive and Respiratory Systems.

Companion Products: ComforTone, JuvaTone, Life 5 (probiotic), Sulfurzyme, and Power Meal.

Companion Oils: Di-Gize and JuvaFlex.

Warning: Do not give this product to children under 12 years of age, except under the supervision of a doctor. If symptoms persist, discontinue use of this product and consult your physician. Keep in a cool, dry place. Do no expose to excessive heat or direct sunlight. If pregnant or under a doctor's care, consult your physician before using.

Balance Complete™

(Daily Superfood Energizer + Nutritive Cleanse)

This product is power-packed with an optimal balance of nutrients from a wide variety of superfoods. Also included is a unique blend of fibers, called V-Fiber™, that delivers 11 grams of heart-healthy fiber per serving. This cutting-edge blend of soluble and insoluble fibers provides optimal viscosity for more bulk, improved elimination of fats, more absorption of toxins, less gas and bloating, better colon health, better appetite satisfaction, and incredible blood sugar balance. Not only is it a nutritional, balanced, and complete meal, it is also delicious, naturally sweet, and low glycemic as well.

Ingredients: V-Fiber Proprietary Blend (larch polysaccharides (a pre-biotic that nurtures friendly flora in the intestines), Ningxia Wolfberry (*Lycium barbarum*) fruit, brown rice bran, guar gum, konjac, xanthan gum, chicory root fiber extract (FOS - also known as inulin fiber, a pre-biotic that nurtures friendly flora in the intestines), and sodium alginate), whey protein concentrate (from New Zealand; is ultra-bioactive, non-denatured and certified grass-fed, hormone-free, antibiotic-free, and chemical-free), nonfat dry milk, virgin coconut oil (medium chain triglycerides), natural vanilla flavor, fructose, lecithin, calcium (tricalcium phosphate), phosphorus, Proprietary Enzyme Complex (lactase, lipase, bromelain, papain, and amylase), xylitol, magnesium oxide, barley grass, neohesperidin derivative (flavor from natural citrus), cinnamon bark powder, mixed carotenoids (vitamin A), lo han kuo extract, cream flavor, barley grass juice, aloe vera, vitamin C (ascorbic acid), mixed tocopherols (vitamin E), vitamin B3 (niacinamide), zinc oxide, selenium (selenomethionine), beta-carotene, molybdenum citrate, vitamin B5 (pantothenic acid from calcium pantothenate), vitamin B6 (pyridoxine HCl), chromium amino nicotinate, vitamin B1 (thiamine HCl), vitamin B2 (riboflavin), vitamin D3 (cholecalciferol), vitamin B12 (methylcobalamin), folic acid, orange (*Citrus sinensis*) rind essential oil, biotin, and iodine.

Suggested Use: Add two scoops (1.76 oz. or 50 g) of Balance Complete to 8 oz. cold water. May be mixed with rice, almond, or other milk. Shake, stir, or blend until smooth. For added flavor, add fruit or essential oils. **For daily health maintenance**, replace your least nutritious meal with Balance Complete. **For weight management programs**, replace two daily meals with Balance Complete

5-Day Nutritive Cleanse: Young Living recommends that the following be used to replace all three meals each day for a total of five days: Digest + Cleanse (1 softgel 30–60 minutes before the Balance Complete shake), Balance Complete (1 shake as directed on label), 3 oz. of NingXia Red (to help enhance detoxification while maintaining energy levels), and an extra 8–12 oz. of water. Continue drinking water between meals so that you consume a total number of ounces that is equal to half your body weight in ounces (i.e.: 200 lbs = 100 oz. of water each day). Note: If gas and bloating cause discomfort, add Essentialzyme to each meal. If you have a high metabolism, or if you experience excessive hunger, add a snack of raw fruits or vegetables 1–2 hours after each meal.

Body System(s) Affected: **Digestive System**.

Companion Products: Combine with NingXia Red, Longevity capsules, and Omega Blue (all 4 of these products make up the Core Essentials Complete program and work well together). Also Digest + Cleanse and Essentialzyme.

BLM™

Protect your mobility by providing your bones and joints with the proper nutritional support. This product synergistically combines some of the most potent ingredients known. It is available in both powder and capsule form.

Ingredients: **Manganese citrate** (catalyst to synergize ingredients), potassium chloride, glucosamine sulfate (helps formation of cartilage), **type II collagen** (from chickens - joint-supporting proteoglycans, also contains cartilage matrix glycoprotein (CMGP), which can help reduce oxidative damage to joints), **MSM** (sulfur - restores flexibility to cell membranes, slows breakdown of cartilage), pure therapeutic-grade essential oils (as listed below), gelatin, and rice flour. **The powder form** contains peppermint essential oil and rice bran instead of the gelatin and rice flour. All other ingredients are the same.

Essential Oils:

Balsam Fir—is a rich source of the antioxidant limonene, which has been shown to help relieve overworked and tired muscles and joints.

Wintergreen—contains 99% methyl salicylate, which gives it cortisone-like properties. It may be beneficial for arthritis, rheumatism, tendinitis, and any other discomfort that is related to the inflammation of bones, muscles, and joints.

Clove—is an antioxidant that has one of the highest ORAC (oxygen radical absorbent capacity) scores. It helps preserve the integrity of fatty acids and has been used as a numbing agent in dentistry.

Suggested Use:

Capsules: If you weigh **less than 120 lbs**, take 1 capsule three times a day. If you weigh **between 120 and 200 lbs**, take 1 capsule four times a day. If you weigh **more than 200 lbs**, take 1 capsule five times a day.

Powder: If you weigh **less than 120 lbs**, take 1/4 teaspoon three times a day. If you weigh **between 120 and 200 lbs**, take 1/4 teaspoon four times a day. If you weigh **more than 200 lbs**, take 1/4 teaspoon five times a day. Powder can be taken with water, soy, or rice milk. Allow 4–8 weeks of daily use before expecting noticeable results.

Body System(s) Affected: **Muscles and Bones**.

Blue Agave

This product is an organically-grown, kosher-certified sweetener that is sweeter than table sugar with fewer calories. Because it is scientifically proven to have a low glycemic index (currently at 11), it becomes the sweetener of choice for diabetics and hypoglycemics who need to control their blood sugar levels. It also helps to support normal intestinal function.

Ingredients: *Agave tequilana.*

Suggested Use: Can be used in beverages and food recipes as a sugar replacement. Because Agave is sweeter than table sugar, use only 3/4 the amount of Agave as table sugar. It also makes a delicious replacement for honey in sandwiches and on toast. Can also be used like honey on cereals and in beverages.

Companion Products: Manna Bars and Power Meal.

Body System(s) Affected: **Hormonal System**, **Muscles and Bones**.

ComforTone™

ComforTone™ is an herbal formula with bentonite, apple pectin, and herbal extracts that may relieve constipation, enhance colon function, and dispel parasites and toxins. The addition of essential oils may enhance the flavor as well as the activity of the herbs contained in this formula. This products was designed as a cleanser for any type of bowel irregularity.

Ingredients: Chamomile (*Matricaria recutita*) flower extract (4:1 ratio in 50% ethyl alcohol and 50% distilled water), cascara sagrada (*Frangula purshiana*) bark, psyllium (*Plantago ovata*) seed, barberry (*Berberis vulgaris*) bark, burdock (*Arctium lappa*) root, fennel (*Foeniculum vulgare*) seed, garlic (*Allium sativum*) bulb, echinacea (*E. purpurea*) root, bentonite, diatomaceous earth, ginger (*Zingiber officinale*) root, apple pectin, licorice (*Glycyrrhiza glabra*) root, cayenne (*Capsicum annuum*) fruit, pure therapeutic-grade essential oils (as listed below), and gelatin.

Essential Oils:

Tarragon—may help reduce anorexia, dyspepsia, flatulence, intestinal spasms, nervous and sluggish digestion, and genital urinary tract infection.

Ginger—is warming, uplifting, and empowering; it helps reduce feelings of nausea, and motion sickness.

Tangerine—is sedating and calming to the nervous system. It is also a diuretic and a decongestant of the lymphatic system.

Rosemary cineol—helps balance heart function, stimulates nerves, and decongests the liver.

Anise—may help calm and strengthen the digestive system.

Peppermint—is purifying and stimulating to the conscious mind, anti-inflammatory, and helps with nerve regeneration. It also enhances digestion and increases endurance.

Mugwort (*Artemisia vulgaris*)—has been used to help calm nerves.

German Chamomile—has been found to help open the liver, increase liver function and secretion, and support the pancreas.

Suggested Use: Start with two to five capsules first thing in the morning (½ hour before breakfast) and two to five capsules just before bed. Drink eight to ten 8 oz. glasses of *purified or distilled water per day for best results. If you get cramps, skip the next morning or day, and start up again with two capsules in the morning and two in the evening. After starting ComforTone, you may cut back, but don't stop taking it completely or all the toxins that have been pulled out of the system will go back into the system. Take at least one in the morning and one in the evening, but don't stop once you start. ComforTone can be taken every day without becoming addictive. For maximum results, use with JuvaTone and Essentialzyme.* **Caution**: *Do not take ComforTone at the same time as JuvaTone! When taken together, possible reactions include bloating, gas, and diaphragm and chest pains (heartburn or acid reflux). If a reaction occurs,* *Di-Gize* or *JuvaFlex* applied around the navel or center of the spine has helped. It is best to take ComforTone and JuvaTone at least one hour apart from each other.

Safety Data: ***This product contains Cascara sagrada bark. Read and follow directions carefully. Women who are pregnant or nursing and others who have a medical condition should not use this product except under the direction of a physician. Children under 12 should not use this product. Discontinue use and consult a physician if you have or develop abdominal pain, diarrhea, nausea, or vomiting. Do not exceed recommended dosage. Not for long-term use. Not to be used as a weight-loss product.***

Body System(s) Affected: **Digestive** and **Immune Systems**.

Comments: ComforTone may be used to get rid of parasites. It breaks up the encrustation along the colon wall and relaxes spasms that may occur. Use Di-Gize when there is nausea. If constipation is increased with five ComforTone, increase the water intake (or a spasm in the colon may cause more constipation) and decrease or stop taking ICP. If a person has a history of chronic constipation, don't start ICP and

Supplements

ComforTone at the same time. Start ComforTone until the system is open, and then start ICP with ten glasses of water per day. One woman was paralyzed by surgery and had to have a colonic two times a day. When she started taking ComforTone, she was able to have natural bowel movements.

Frequency: Approximately 43 MHz.

Companion Supplements: Essentialzyme and ICP, JuvaTone, Chelex, ParaFree.

Companion Oils: Di-Gize (use with hot compress on abdomen or rub on feet), JuvaFlex, Purification, Release, Thieves.

CortiStop™

(Women's)

This product is formulated specifically for women and is designed to modulate the production of cortisol (the "death" hormone) in the body, thereby helping to maintain the natural balance and harmony of other important substances like estrogen and progesterone. The negative effects of high amounts of cortisol are also diminished as it provides nutrients that influence glandular balance.

Ingredients: Pregnenolone (promotes glandular balance, improves energy, and reduces stress), l-a-lyso-phosphatidylcholine (Epikuron 100E) (blocks cortisol production), l-a-phosphatidyl choline (LECI-PC 35P) (blocks cortisol production), Black cohosh (*Actaea racemosa*) root extrat (has estrogen-like functions; helps with hot flashes and other menopausal problems), DHEA (derived from wild yam (*Dioscorea villosa*) root—estrogen precursor, shown to enhance memory and increase muscle strength and lean body mass), pure therapeutic-grade essential oils (as listed below), magnesium stearate, silicon dioxide, and gelatin.

Essential Oils:

Fleabane (*Conyza canadensis*)—is a rare essential oil studied by Daniel Pénoël, M.D., for its ability to stimulate the pancreas and liver and counteract retarded puberty. It is a mood enhancer and a promoter of hGH.

Clary Sage—helps balance the hormones and is a tonic to the reproductive system.

Fennel—helps balance the hormones.

Frankincense—is antitumoral and anti-inflammatory, and it increases activity of leukocytes. It also enhances the function of the pituitary and hypothalamus.

Peppermint—is purifying and stimulating to the conscious mind, anti-inflammatory, and helps with nerve regeneration. It also enhances digestion and increases endurance.

Suggested Use: Take one capsule before retiring. If desired, for extra benefits, take another capsule in the morning before breakfast. Use daily for 8 weeks. Discontinue use for 2–4 weeks before resuming.

Precautions: Keep in a cool, dry place. Keep out of reach of children. If pregnant or under a doctor's care, consult your physician before using.

Comments: The natural pro-hormone activity of this formulation has led to restriction of use by some athletic organizations.

Body System(s) Affected: **Hormonal System**.

Companion Products: Manna Bars, NingXia Red, PD 80/20, Power Meal, Prenolone/Prenolone+, Super C, Wolfberry Crisp Bars.

Detoxzyme™

Detoxzyme™ is a vegetable enzyme complex designed to promote detoxification of the body and to support and maintain a healthy intestinal environment. Because it combines essential oils with enzymes that are meant to digest starches, sugars, proteins, and fats, it may also provide relief of occasional symptoms such as fullness, pressure, bloating, gas, pain, and/or minor cramping that occur after eating. By facilitating the optimal absorption of nutrients from foods and supplements, the aging process is delayed and energy levels enhanced.

Ingredients: Amylase, invertase, protease, glucoamylase, bromelain, phytase, lipase, cellulase, lactase, alpha-galactosidase, pure therapeutic-grade essential oils (as listed below), rice bran, cumin seed extract, vegetable cellulose, deionized water, and silica.

Essential Oils:

Cumin—is antibacterial, antispasmodic, and has some antitumoral properties.

Anise—may help calm and strengthen the digestive system.

Fennel—is antiparasitic and promotes the removal of toxic wastes. It may break up fluids and toxins and cleanse the tissues.

Suggested Use: Take 2–3 capsules three times daily between meals. This product may be used in conjunction with a cleansing/detoxifying program. Can be sprinkled on food or in beverages.

Body System(s) Affected: **Digestive** and **Immune Systems**.

Companion Products: ComforTone, JuvaTone, Sulfurzyme, Life 5, and Power Meal.

Companion Oils: Di-Gize and JuvaFlex.

Warning: Do not give this product to children under 12 years of age except under the supervision of a doctor. If symptoms persist, discontinue use of this product and consult your physician. Keep in a cool, dry place. Do not expose to excessive heat or direct sunlight. If pregnant or under a doctor's care, consult your physician before using.

Comments: This formula contains trace minerals that can help to detoxify the body and assist in the reduction of cholesterol and triglycerides. It also helps to open the gallbladder duct, cleanse the liver, and regulate pH levels, thereby reducing acidification, which helps to prevent candida and yeast overgrowth as well as parasite colonization and infestation. It may also help provide relief from diarrhea, constipation, heartburn, and food allergies.

Digest + Cleanse™

(A "Purely Oils" supplement—oil blend in softgels)

This particular supplement is not just another coated peppermint oil supplement. It is a specifically formulated blend of therapeutic-grade essential oils, all of which have been scientifically proven to soothe gastrointestinal upset and support healthy digestion. This product is ideal for anyone who either deals with bowel discomfort and digestive upsets or who could use such a wonderful product to assist them with their cleansing program.

Ingredients: Pure therapeutic-grade essential oils (as listed below), coconut (*Cocus nucifera*) meat oil [virgin], coconut (*Cocus nucifera*) meat oil [fractionated] (contains capric acid which has been shown to inhibit the growth of three strains of candida), gelatin, glycerin, and aqueous coating solution (oleic acid, sodium alginate, medium-chain fatty acids, ethylcellulose, and stearic acid).

Essential Oils:

Peppermint—is antispasmodic and anti-inflammatory and soothing, cooling, and dilating to the system. It also enhances digestion and increases endurance.

Caraway—has been clinically shown to soothe the bowels, improve elimination, and ease digestive discomfort and nausea.

Lemon—contains over 65% d-Limonene (which helps to promote normal cell life cycles), helps promote leukocyte formation, and helps to dissolve cholesterol and fats. It helps to promote a sense of well-being, while alkalizing and cleansing the digestive and lymphatic systems.

Ginger—helps reduce/alleviate feelings of nausea, motion sickness, and vomiting. Along with fennel and anise, it helps to stimulate digestion, reduce gas and bloating, and create an unfriendly environment for parasites.

Fennel—is a diuretic. It may break up fluids and toxins and cleanse the tissues.

Anise—may help calm and strengthen the digestive system.

Suggested Use: Take one capsule once daily with food or as needed.

Body System(s) Affected: **Digestive System**.

Companion Products: Combine with NingXia Red and Balance Complete to make up Young Living's 5-day Nutritive Cleanse Program. Use daily with Omega Blue and Longevity capsules.

Companion Oils: Longevity

Precautions: Keep in a cool, dry place. Do not expose to excessive heat or direct sunlight. If pregnant or under a doctor's care, consult your physician before using.

EndoGize™

This product was specially formulated to support a healthy and balanced endocrine system in women. It is purported to help support the endocrine system in men as well.

Ingredients: Vitamin B6 (pyridoxine HCl), zinc (zinc aspartate), *Eurycoma longifolia* root extract, ashwaganda (*Withanaia somenifera*) root, muira puama (*Ptychopetalum olacoides*) root, l-arginine, epimedium (*Epimedium grandiflorum*) leaf, *Tribulus terrestris* fruit, DHEA (3 beta-hydroxyandro-5-en-17-one), phosphatidylcholine, lecithin (soy), black pepper (*Piper nigrum*) fruit extract, amylase 5000 FCC, validase AFP protease, cellulase 4000, glucoamylase, proprietary blend of pure therapeutic-grade essential oils (as listed below), gelatin, and rice flour.

Essential Oils:

Ginger—helps reduce/alleviate feelings of nausea, motion sickness, and vomiting. Along with fennel and anise, it helps to stimulate digestion, reduce gas and bloating, and create an unfriendly environment for parasites.

Myrrh—is anti-inflammatory and antiseptic. It has high levels of sesquiterpenes and is the second highest ranking substance on the ORAC scale behind clove essential oil.

Cassia—has been used historically for digestive, kidney, and reproductive complaints.

Clary Sage—helps balance the hormones and is a tonic to the reproductive system.

Fleabane (*Conyza canadensis*)—is a rare essential oil studied by Daniel Pénoël, M.D. for its ability to stimulate the pancreas and liver and counteract retarded puberty. It is a mood enhancer and a promoter of hGH

Suggested Use: Take 1 capsule twice daily. Use daily for four weeks. Discontinue for two weeks before resuming.

Body System(s) Affected: **Digestive** and **Hormonal Systems**.

Companion Products: CortiStop (Women's), Exodus, FemiGen (female), MultiGreens, Prenolone/Prenolone+, Progessence, ProGen (male), Super B, Super Cal, Thyromin, Ultra Young+.

Companion Oils: Dragon Time, EndoFlex, Lady Sclareol, Mister, SclarEssence, spearmint (hormone-like), ylang ylang.

Precautions: Keep in a cool, dry place. Do not expose to excessive heat or direct sunlight. Do not use if pregnant or lactating. Intended for adult use only. Keep out of reach of children. If you are taking other medications or have a medical condition, consult your healthcare practitioner prior to use.

Essentialzyme™

Essentialzyme™ is a high-quality enzyme complex that may improve and aid digestion and the elimination of toxic waste from the body. Essentialzyme was formulated to help supply enzymes to people who have difficulty digesting or assimilating food. It helps promote and re-establish proper enzyme balance in the digestive system and throughout the body. It also helps to retard the aging process. The flavor is enhanced with essential oils. It is a **natural antioxidant**.

Ingredients: Pancrealipase, pancreatin, trypsin, betaine HCl, bromelain, thyme leaf powder, carrot powder, alfalfa sprout powder, alfalfa leaf powder, papain, cumin seed powder, pure therapeutic-grade essential oils (as listed below), microcrystalline cellulose, dicalcium phosphate, hydroxypropylcellulose, hydroxypropylmethylcellulose, stearic acid, silicon dioxide, croscarmellose sodium, sodium citrate, sodium carboxymehyl cellulose, dextrin, lecithin, dextrose, peppermint (*Mentha piperita*) leaf.

Essential Oils:

Anise—may help calm and strengthen the digestive system.

Fennel—is a diuretic. It may break up fluids and toxins and cleanse the tissues.

Peppermint—is antispasmodic and anti-inflammatory and soothing, cooling, and dilating to the system. It also enhances digestion and increases endurance.

Tarragon—may help reduce anorexia, dyspepsia, flatulence, intestinal spasms, nervous and sluggish digestion, and genital urinary tract infection.

Clove—is anti-infectious, antiviral, antifungal, and antiparasitic.

Suggested Use: Take one caplet, three times daily between meals. Take Essentialzyme with meals, especially protein meals after 3 p.m., as it will help lessen the burden on the digestive system. Also helps with digestive functions in the liver.

Body System(s) Affected: **Digestive System**.

Companion Products: ComforTone, JuvaTone, Mineral Essence, Life 5, Power Meal.

Companion Oils: Di-Gize, Harmony, JuvaFlex.

Precautions: Keep in a cool, dry place. Do not expose to excessive heat or direct sunlight. If pregnant or under a doctor's care, consult your physician. Do not give this product to children under 12 years of age except under the supervision of a doctor. If symptoms persist, discontinue use of this product and consult your physician.

Essentialzymes-4™

Essentialzymes-4™ is an array of animal and plant enzymes designed to help improve key nutrient digestion, absorption and availability for the body. Essentialzymes-4 was formulated to aid in the breakdown of fats, proteins, fiber, and carbohydrates. It helps promote and re-establish proper enzyme balance in the digestive system and throughout the body. Each capsule set is enhanced by an essential oil blend designed to soothe and calm the stomach.

Plant-Based Enzyme Capsule Ingredients: Riboflavin, protease (3.0, 4.5, 6.0), amylase, cellulase, lipase, peptidase, phytase, bromelain, papain, pure therapeutic-grade essential oils (as listed below), rice flour, gelatin capsule, magnesium stearate, silicon dioxide.

Plant-Based Enzyme Capsule Essential Oils:

Anise—may help calm and strengthen the digestive system.

Ginger—is often used for its calming effect on the stomach and digestive system.

Rosemary—has anti-inflammatory and antispasmodic properties and is often used to help calm a sour stomach.

Tarragon—may help reduce anorexia, dyspepsia, flatulence, intestinal spasms, nervous and sluggish digestion, and genital urinary tract infection.

Fennel—is a diuretic. It may break up fluids and toxins and cleanse the tissues.

Animal-Based Enzyme Capsule Ingredients: Bee pollen powder, pancreatin, lipase, pure therapeutic-grade essential oils (as listed below), rice flour, HPMC capsule, magnesium stearate, silicon dioxide.

Animal-Based Emzyme Capsule Essential Oils:

Ginger—is often used for its calming affect on the stomach and digestive system.

Fennel—is a diuretic. It may break up fluids and toxins and cleanse the tissues.

Tarragon—may help reduce anorexia, dyspepsia, flatulence, intestinal spasms, nervous and sluggish digestion, and genital urinary tract infection.

Anise—may help calm and strengthen the digestive system.

Lemongrass—has anti-inflammatory and analgesic properties and may help improve digestion.

Suggested Use: Take one two-tablet set twice a day with the two largest meals of the day.

Body System(s) Affected: **Digestive System**.

Companion Products: ComforTone, Essentialzyme, JuvaTone, Mineral Essence, Life 5, Power Meal.

Companion Oils: Di-Gize, Harmony, JuvaFlex.

Precautions: Keep in a cool, dry place. Do not expose to excessive heat or direct sunlight. If pregnant or under a doctor's care, consult your physician. For those 12 years of age and older, except under the supervision of a doctor. If symptoms persist, discontinue use of this product and consult your physician.

Estro™ Tincture

Estro™ Tincture is designed with plant-derived phytoestrogens to safely help harmonize the female hormone levels. It works well with Prenolone or Prenolone+.

Ingredients: Extracts of black cohosh (*Cimicifuga racemosa*) root and blue cohosh (*Caulophyllum thalictroides*) root (extracted 1:4 in 47% ethanol), royal jelly, pure therapeutic-grade essential oils (as listed below), and distilled water.

Essential Oils:

Fennel—helps balance the hormones.

Lavender—helps balance body systems.

Clary Sage—helps balance the hormones and is a tonic to the reproductive system.

Suggested Use: Start with 3 half droppers (3 ml), two to three times daily. Increase as needed to as much as three droppers daily. Estro may take as long as four weeks to reach maximum effectiveness.

Body System(s) Affected: **Hormonal System**.

FemiGen™

FemiGen™ is an herbal formula with glandular substances and amino acids that help build and balance the reproductive system and maintain better hormonal balance for developmental years all the way through menopause. When one experiences mood swings, PMS, and symptoms related to menopause, it is an indication that the body is nutritionally out of balance. FemiGen acts as a natural estrogen and helps balance the hormones.

Ingredients: Magnesium (magnesium oxide—11 mg per serving), damiana (*Turnera diffusa*) leaf (blood purifier), *Epimedium sagittatum* aerial parts (detoxifies kidneys), wild yam (*Dioscorea villosa*) root, muira-puama (*Ptychopetalum olacoides*) root (potency wood), ginseng (*Panax quinquefolium*) root, licorice (*Glycyrrhiza glabra*) root extract (extracted 4:1 in 50% ethyl alcohol and 50% distilled water), black cohosh (*Cimicifuga racemosa*) root (30 mg per serving), l-carnitine, dimethyglycine HCl, cramp (*Viburnum opulus*) bark, squaw vine (*Mitchella repens*) aerial parts, l-phenylalanine, l-cystine, l-cysteine HCl, pure therapeutic-grade essential oils (as listed below), and gelatin.

Essential Oils:

Fennel—helps balance the hormones.

Clary Sage—helps balance the hormones and is a tonic to the reproductive system.

Sage—contains estriol and has estrogen-like properties. It is believed to contain elements that contribute to the secretion of progesterone.

Ylang Ylang—stimulates adrenal glands and helps balance male/female energies.

Suggested Use: Take two capsules with breakfast and two capsules with lunch. A maintenance dose of two capsules may be taken three times a day for ten days before a period.

Body System(s) Affected: **Hormonal System**.

Companion Products: Dragon Time Massage Oil.

Companion Oils: Dragon Time, Mister, PanAway, Peace & Calming, Relieve It.

ICP™

This fiber beverage is a unique source of fiber and bulk for the diet, which helps speed the transit time of waste matter through the intestinal tract. The psyllium, oat bran, flax, and rice bran are specifically balanced to eliminate allergy symptoms that people experience when taking psyllium alone. Essential oils enhance the flavor and may help to dispel gas and discomfort. Designed as both a cleanser and a builder, this formula is unsurpassed as an aid in enhancing normal bowel function.

Ingredients: Psyllium seed powder (2.5 g per serving), flax (*Linum usitatissimum*) seed (roto-rooter; strong antioxidant), oat (*Avena sativa*) bran (binds up fat), fennel (*Foeniculum vulgare*) seed (antiparasitic), rice (*Plantago ovata*) bran (roto-rooter), guar gum (*Cyamopsis tetragonoloba*) seed (opens colon), yucca (*Y. schidigera*) root (anticancerous), plant cellulose, flax (*Linum usitatissimum*) seed oil, pure therapeutic-grade essential oils (as listed below), aloe vera (*A. barbadensis*) leaf extract (natural laxative), and enzyme formula (lipase, protease, phytase and peptidase - aids digestion).

Essential Oils:

Anise—is an antispasmodic and relaxant that helps relax the muscles of the colon wall.

Tarragon, Ginger, Lemongrass, and **Rosemary Cineol**—are all antiparasitic by nature and promote the removal of toxic wastes.

Suggested Use: Take five times a week for maintenance (½ cup water, ½ cup apple juice, and one heaping teaspoon (tsp.) of ICP). Take more often for cleansing (start with one heaping teaspoon (tsp.) two to three times a day with carrot juice or other vegetable juices. When things are going well, increase to three teaspoons (tsp.) three times a day). ICP dilutes better in warm water. Drink immediately, as this product tends to thicken quickly when added to liquid. Sprinkle on yogurt, cereal, or other foods. Drink 8 to 16 oz. of fluid per teaspoon. ICP may be added to Power Meal.

Comments: For best results, take ComforTone first and then ICP morning and night. If added to citrus juices, it creates more acid; it is best to use other juices. ICP absorbs toxins so that it can build and improve the wave-like movement of the intestinal walls.

Frequency: Approximately 56 MHz.

Body System(s) Affected: **Cardiovascular** and **Digestive Systems**.

Companion Products: ComforTone, Essentialzyme, JuvaTone, ParaFree, Power Meal.

Companion Oils: Di-Gize, JuvaFlex, Purification, Thieves.

ImmuPro™

ImmuPro is a unique blend of five powerful polysaccharides—natural immune system enhancers that aid in normal immune function and support the body's ability to fight illness. This vegan formula comes in a chewable tablet with a great strawberry taste.

Ingredients: Calcium (as calcium carbonate: 100 mg per serving), zinc (as zinc citrate: 6.8 mg per serving), selenium (as selenomethionine: 68 mcg per serving), copper (as copper chelate: 0.6 mg per serving), Ningxia Wolfberry (*Lycium barbarum*) polysaccharide (185 mg per serving), organic reishi (*Ganoderma lucidum*) mycelia, organic maitake (*Grifola frondosa*) mycelia, organic *Agaricus blazei* mycelia, organic arabinogalactin (larch tree extract), limonene (from orange essential oil), melatonin, organic strawberry powder, fructose, raspberry juice, pure lemon powder, stearic acid or virgin coconut oil, and silica.

Suggested Use: Chew one tablet before retiring. If under stress, chew 2–4 tablets before retiring or one tablet as needed.

Precautions: **May cause drowsiness**. Keep out of reach of children. If pregnant, lactating or under a doctor's care, consult your physician. Keep in a cool, dry place.

Body System(s) Affected: **Immune System**

Companion Products: ImmuneTune, Super C, Exodus, and JuvaTone.

Companion Oils: ImmuPower, Thieves, Exodus II, JuvaFlex, Purification, Release, Valor.

Inner Defense™

This essential oil supplement was specifically designed to boost the body's immune system during times of stress and was formulated with oils that are rich in thymol, carvacrol, and eugenol. These essential oils are encapsulated in easy-to-swallow, liquid softgels that dissolve quickly in the stomach.

Ingredients: Pure therapeutic-grade essential oils (as listed below), virgin coconut oil, gelatin, beeswax, and lecithin.

Essential Oils:

Thieves® Blend, containing the following oils:

Clove—is antibacterial, antifungal, anti-infectious, antiparasitic, a strong antiseptic, antiviral, and an immune stimulant. It helps preserve the integrity of fatty acids.

Lemon—helps to dissolve cholesterol and fats.

Cinnamon Bark—is antifungal, antibacterial, and antiviral.

Eucalyptus radiata—has strong antibacterial, anticatarrhal, and antiseptic properties.

Rosemary cineol—helps balance heart function, stimulates nerves, and decongests the liver.

Oregano—has antibacterial, antifungal, antiviral, and immune-stimulant properties.

Thyme CT Thymol—has been shown in studies to dramatically boost glutathione levels in the heart, liver, and brain. Further studies show that it helps maintain DHA (a nutrient that supports brain function and cardiovascular health) levels in the brain, liver, heart, and kidneys of aging subjects. Because it can also help to prevent the oxidation of fats in the body, it may help to slow the aging process. It is also antifungal and antiviral.

Citronella—has antibacterial, antispasmodic, and anti-inflammatory properties.

Suggested Use: Take 1 capsule daily in the morning, or take 1 capsule 3–5 times daily when stressed. For best results, use Life 5 probiotic 8 hours later.

Body System(s) Affected: **Immune System**

Companion Products: Longevity Capsules, Omega Blue, True Source, Life 5.

Precautions: Keep in a cool, dry place. Do not expose to excessive heat or direct sunlight. Keep out of reach of children. If pregnant or under a doctor's care, consult your physician before using.

JuvaPower™

This food supplement is packed with ingredients that have a dual purpose—to cleanse both the liver and the intestines simultaneously. Many of the ingredients in this supplement are some of the most powerful acid-binding foods. They are packed into this formulation to help support and cleanse the liver by helping to remove acids from the body. Not only does it fortify with optimum nutrition, but it also tastes great. Sprinkle some on a baked potato or some scrambled eggs, and you'll be providing your body with some much needed support for proper digestion.

Ingredients: Rice seed bran, spinach leaf, tomato fruit, beet root, flax seed, oat seed bran, broccoli floret/stalk, cucumber fruit, dill seed, sprouted barley seed, ginger root and rhizome, slippery elm bark, L-taurine, psyllium seed husk, anise seed, fennel seed, aloe vera inner leaf extract, peppermint leaf, and pure therapeutic-grade essential oils (as listed below).

Essential Oils:

Anise—may help calm and strengthen the digestive system.

Fennel—is antiparasitic, promotes the removal of toxic wastes, and may break up fluids and toxins and cleanse the tissues.

Suggested Use: Sprinkle 1 tablespoon on food (i.e., baked potato, salad, rice, eggs, etc.), or add to 4–8 oz. of purified water or rice/almond milk before drinking. Use three times daily for maximum benefits.

Body System(s) Affected: **Digestive System** (especially the **liver**).

Companion Products: ComforTone, JuvaTone, Mineral Essence, Life 5, Power Meal.

Companion Oils: Di-Gize, Harmony, Juva Cleanse, JuvaFlex.

JuvaSpice™

JuvaSpice™ contains all the same ingredients as JuvaPower, spiced up with some potassium, RealSalt®, and cayenne pepper. It is great for adding both nutritional support and flavor to your favorite dishes. Sprinkle some on a baked potato or some scrambled eggs, and you'll be providing your body with some much-needed support for proper digestion.

Ingredients: Rice seed bran, spinach leaf, tomato fruit, beet root, flax seed, oat seed bran, broccoli floret, cucumber fruit, potassium chloride, Redmond RealSalt®, sprouted barley seed, cayenne pepper (*Capsicum annum*) fruit, ginger root and rhizome, slippery elm bark, L-taurine, psyllium seed husk, anise seed, fennel seed, aloe vera inner leaf extract, peppermint leaf, pure therapeutic-grade essential oils (as listed below), aloe vera inner leaf extract, and peppermint leaf.

Essential Oils:

Anise—may help calm and strengthen the digestive system.

Fennel—is antiparasitic, promotes the removal of toxic wastes, and may break up fluids and toxins and cleanse the tissues.

Suggested Use: Sprinkle ⅓–½ teaspoon on food (i.e., baked potato, salad, rice, eggs, etc.), or add to 4–8 oz. purified water or rice/almond milk before drinking.

Body System(s) Affected: **Digestive System** (especially the **liver**).

Companion Products: ComforTone, JuvaTone, Mineral Essence, Life 5, Power Meal.

Companion Oils: Di-Gize, Harmony, Juva Cleanse, JuvaFlex.

JuvaTone™

JuvaTone™ is an amino acid herbal complex with trace minerals and essential oils for enhanced liver function, diminished addictions, and skin improvement in a synergistic suspension isolation process. This product was designed specifically as a cleanser of the liver. The same essential oils that are included in this product are also included in the JuvaFlex oil blend, making it the perfect topically-applied companion to JuvaTone.

Ingredients: Calcium (from calcium carbonate and di-calcium phosphate: 252 mg per serving), copper (as copper citrate: 150 mcg per serving), choline bitartrate (329 mg per serving), dl-methionine (helps recycle glutathione), beet (*Beta vulgaris*) root, inositol, dandelion (*Taraxacum officinale*) root, L-cysteine HCl, alfalfa (*Medicago sativa*) sprouts, Oregon grape (*Berberis aquifolium*) root, parsley (*Petroselinum crispum*) leaves, bee propolis 5x, *Echinacea purpurea* root, pure therapeutic-grade essential oils (as listed below), cellulose, silicon dioxide, magnesium stearate, and cellulose film-coating.

Essential Oils:

Lemon—helps promote leukocyte formation and helps to dissolve cholesterol and fats.

German Chamomile—has been found to help open the liver, increase liver function and secretion, and support the pancreas.

Geranium—is cleansing, refreshing, astringent, and diuretic. It helps support the kidney and bladder functions and helps with stone removal.

Rosemary cineol—helps balance heart function, stimulates nerves, and decongests the liver.

Myrtle—is a decongestant of the respiratory system. It may help improve oxygenation and work as an expectorant in discharging mucus.

Blue Tansy—calms the lymphatic system and promotes a feeling of self-control.

Suggested Use: Take 2 tablets two times daily. Increase as needed up to 4 tablets four times daily. Best when taken between meals. For maximum results, use with ComforTone. **Caution:** *Do not take Com-*

forTone ***at the same time*** *as JuvaTone! When taken together, possible reactions include bloating, gas, diaphragm and chest pains (heartburn or acid reflux). If a reaction occurs, Di-Gize or JuvaFlex applied around the navel or center of the spine has helped.* ***It is best to take ComforTone and JuvaTone at least one hour apart from each other***. Also apply JuvaFlex over the liver, on the spine, or on the feet.

Body System(s) Affected: **Digestive** and **Immune Systems**.

Frequency: Approximately 140 MHz.

Companion Products: ComforTone, Essentialzyme, ICP, ParaFree, Power Meal.

Companion Oils: JuvaFlex, Di-Gize, Forgiveness, Release, Surrender, Thieves.

Comments: People have reported that while using JuvaTone, addictions to coffee, tea, tobacco, sugar, or alcohol are diminished.

K & B™ Tincture

The herbs contained in this supplement, combined with oils, have been traditionally used to help the kidneys and bladder in cases of irregularity, infection, and bed wetting.

Ingredients: Extracts of juniper (*Juniperus communis*) berry, parsley (*Petroselinum crispum*) leaf, uva ursi (*Arctostaphylos u.*) leaf, dandelion (*Taraxacum officinale*) root, and German chamomile (*Matricaria recutita*) flower (extracted 1:4 in 50% ethyl alcohol and 50% water), royal jelly, pure therapeutic-grade essential oils (as listed below), and vegetable glycerin.

Essential Oils:

Geranium—is cleansing, refreshing, astringent, and diuretic. It helps support the kidney and bladder functions and helps with stone removal.

Fennel—is a diuretic and may break up fluids and toxins and cleanse the tissues.

Clove—is anti-infectious, antiviral, antifungal, and antiparasitic.

Roman Chamomile—is a blood cleanser and helps the liver discharge toxins.

Sage—is a diuretic. It contains estriol and has estrogen-like properties. It is believed to contain elements that contribute to the secretion of progesterone.

Juniper—is a cleanser, detoxifier, and diuretic. It helps the body release fluids.

Suggested Use: Take 3 half droppers (3ml) three times daily in distilled water, or as needed. Shake well before using.

Body System(s) Affected: **Digestive System**.

KidScents® Mighty Vites™

This reformulation of a chewable multi-vitamin for kids utilizes nutrient-dense whole food sources. It is now available in both orange cream and mixed berry flavors.

Ingredients: Vitamin A (alpha & beta carotene), vitamin C (ascorbic acid from oranges), vitamin D3 (cholecalciferol), vitamin E (d-alpha tocopheryl acid succinate), Vitamin K (phytonadione), vitamin B1 (thiamine mononitrate), vitamin B2 (riboflavin), vitamin B3 (niacinamide), vitamin B6 (pyridoxal-5-phosphate), folic acid, vitamin B12 (methylcobalamin), biotin, pantothenic acid (d-calcium pantothenate), iodine (potassium iodide), magnesium oxide, zinc yeast complex, selenium yeast complex, copper yeast complex, chromium yeast complex, choline (from soy lecithin), Ningxia Wolfberry (*Lycium barbarum*) fruit, tocotrienois (from natural palm oil), lecithin (soy), malic acid (from apples), olive (*Olea europea*) leaf extract, curcumins (from tumeric rhizome), broccoli (*Brassica oleracea*) floret, barley (*Hordeum vulgare*) grass, MSM (methylsulfonylmethane), spirulina (*S. platensis*) algae, boron (as boron amino acid complex), lutein (from marigold flowers), natural flavors [orange juice powder, cherry juice powder, grape skin powder (30% polyphenols), strawberry juice powder, and other natural flavors], sorbitol, fructose, citric acid, silica, magnesium stearate, and dicalcium phosphate.

Suggested Use: Children 6–12 years old, take three chewable tablets daily. Can be taken before breakfast, lunch, or dinner or in one daily dose.

Body System(s) Affected: **Emotional Balance, Cardiovascular, Immune**, and **Nervous Systems**.

Precautions: Do not exceed recomended dosage. If you are pregnant, nursing, taking medication, or have a medical condition, consult a healthcare practitioner prior to use. Keep in a cool, dry place. Do not expose to excessive heat or direct sunlight.

Life 5™

This product goes way beyond acidophilus with five of the most health-promoting and viable probiotic strains ever combined in a single capsule. Three of these five probiotic strains (the first three listed below) are clinically considered "super strains" for their ability to not only adhere and out-colonize harmful bacteria in the intestines but to also promote and improve the adherence of other friendly bacteria as well. In fact, research has proven that these "super strains" boost immunity, improve nutrient absorption, and relieve bowel distress. Not only is it **safe for children**, but a study at the Wilhelmina Children's Hospital stated that giving probiotic bacteria to children may actually help "prevent allergic disease."

Ingredients: HOWARU™ Rhamnosus (*Ld. rhamnosus*), *Lactobacillus acidophilus* (LA-14), HOWARU™ Bifido (*Bifidobacterium lactis*), *Lactoferrin Streptococcus thermophilus*, *Bifidobacterium bifidum*, microcrystalline cellulose, hydroxypropyl methylcellulose, magnesium stearate, and silica.

Suggested Use: Take 1 capsule every night following a meal or as needed.

Body System(s) Affected: **Digestive System**.

Companion Products: ComforTone, Balance Complete.

Companion Oils: Di-Gize

Precautions: Keep refrigerated. If you are pregnant, nursing, taking medication, or have a medical condition, consult with a healthcare practitioner prior to use.

Longevity™ Capsules

(Longevity oil blend in gel capsules)

This blend of pure therapeutic-grade essential oils, as measured on the ORAC (oxygen radical absorbent capacity) scale, has scored near 150,000! 220 mg of this blend of oils has been placed in gelatin capsules for easier consumption as a dietary supplement. It may help to promote longevity and prevent premature aging. *For the regular oil blend, refer to Longevity in the Blends section of this book.* This blend includes coconut oil (virgin and fractionated) to help disperse the oils more evenly in the body, to help protect against rancidity, to preserve the integrity of the essential oils, and to extend the shelf life. Also, an aqueous coating solution (enteric-type coating produced from seaweed) is applied to the outside of the softgel to help delay the breakdown of the softgel until it has reached the intestines (for optimal absorption and minimal aftertaste).

Ingredients: Pure therapeutic-grade essential oils (as listed below), coconut (*Cocus nucifera*) meat oil [virgin], coconut (*Cocus nucifera*) meat oil [fractionated], gelatin, glycerin, aqueous coating solution (oleic acid, sodium alginate, medium-chain fatty acids, ethylcellulose, and stearic acid), and mixed tocopherols.

Essential Oils:

Thyme CT Thymol—has been shown in studies to dramatically boost glutathione levels in the heart, liver, and brain; further studies show that it helps maintain DHA (a nutrient that supports brain function and cardiovascular health) levels in the brain, liver, heart, and kidneys of aging subjects.

Because it can also help to prevent the oxidation of fats in the body, it may help to slow the aging process. It is also antifungal and antiviral.

Orange—is rich in compounds noted for their stress-reducing effects, lipid-soluble traits, and antioxidant properties that enhance vitamin absorption.

Clove—has one of the highest ORAC (oxygen radical absorbent capacity) scores of any known substance. It is antibacterial, antifungal, anti-infectious, antiparasitic, a strong antiseptic, antiviral, and an immune stimulant. It helps preserve the integrity of fatty acids. Clove may also influence healing and help improve memory.

Frankincense—is antitumoral and anti-inflammatory. It increases the activity of leukocytes for healthy immune function and supports cell regeneration. It also enhances the function of the pituitary and the hypothalamus.

Suggested Use: Take one softgel capsule, once daily with food or as needed.

Body System(s) Affected: **Cardiovascular, Immune, and Nervous Systems; Skin**.

Companion Products: Combine with NingXia Red, Omega Blue, and Balance Complete (all 4 of these products make up the Core Essentials Complete program and work well together). Also Manna Bars, Power Meal, and Wolfberry Crisp Bars.

Companion Oils: Longevity

Precautions: Keep out of reach of children. Keep in a cool, dry place. Do not expose to excessive heat or direct sunlight. If pregnant or under a doctor's care, consult your physician.

Majestic Essence™ Handcrafted Dark Chocolates

This exquisite dark chocolate is handcrafted from organic cacao that has been dried in the shade and roasted at low temperatures to allow the cacao's natural enzymes and antioxidants to remain intact. Flavanols, like epicatechin, found in natural chocolate have been studied for their ability to prevent vascular diseases such as arteriosclerosis (Schroeter et al., 2006; Balzer et al., 2008). These natural flavanols are often destroyed by the high temperatures and alkalinization processes used to create most commercial chocolate. Majestic Essence chocolate is mildly sweetened with natural yaccon (yacón) root, which contains inulin—an indigestible sugar that has an extremely low glycemic index. Inulin is considered a prebiotic food that promotes the growth of beneficial digestive bacteria and has also been found to enhance calcium absorption and bone mineralization in adolescents (Abrams et al., 2005). Each chocolate has also been supplemented with boswellic acid—a constituent of frankincense resin that has been studied for its anti-inflammatory, anticancerous, and gastroprotective properties.

Ingredients: Cocoa liquor, yaccon, cocoa butter, pure, therapeutic-grade essential oils (as listed below), boswellic acid, additional ingredients as listed below for some varieties.

Peppermint Chocolates:

Essential Oils:

Peppermint—is antibacterial, anti-inflammatory (prostate and nerves), antiseptic, antispasmodic, antiviral, and invigorating.

Peppermint with Almond Chocolates:

Essential Oils:

Peppermint—is antibacterial, anti-inflammatory (prostate and nerves), antiseptic, antispasmodic, antiviral, and invigorating.

Additional Ingredients: Almonds.

Thieves Chocolates:

Essential Oils:

Cassia—is antibacterial, antifungal, and antiviral.

Clove—is antibacterial, antifungal, anti-infectious, antiparasitic, a strong antiseptic, antiviral, and an immune stimulant.

Lemon—promotes health, healing, physical energy, and purification. It is an antiseptic and is great for the respiratory system.

Cinnamon—is antibacterial, antifungal, anti-infectious, anti-inflammatory, antimicrobial, antiparasitic, antiseptic, antispasmodic, antiviral, astringent, immune-stimulant, and warming.

Eucalyptus radiata—may have a profound antiviral effect upon the respiratory system. It also has strong antibacterial, anticatarrhal, and antiseptic properties.

Rosemary—may help balance heart function, energize the solar plexus, and reduce mental fatigue. It may improve circulation and help stimulate the nerves. It is antiseptic and anti-infectious.

Ishpingo (*Ocotea quixos*)—was included for its unique exotic flavor.

Chili Chocolates:

Essential Oils:

Lime—is stimulating and refreshing, helping to overcome negativity. It also has antibacterial and antiviral properties.

Nutmeg—helps support the adrenal glands for increased energy. It also helps with digestive problems and has anti-inflammatory and antiparasitic properties.

Black Pepper—is stimulating and may help increase cellular oxygenation.

Additional Ingredients: Chili powder.

Christmas Spirit Chocolates:

Essential Oils:

Orange—is antiseptic and antidepressant. It may help encourage a positive outlook on life, bringing peace and happiness to the mind and body.

Cinnamon—may have a stimulating and toning effect on the whole body and particularly on the circulatory system. It may also help bring about feelings of joy. It is antiseptic, antibacterial, and antiviral.

Spruce—grounds the body, creating the balance and opening necessary to receive and to give. This oil is warming, healing, uplifting, and soothing. It may also help relieve anxiety and act as an antiseptic.

Frankincense Chocolates:

Essential Oils:

Peppermint—is antibacterial, anti-inflammatory (prostate and nerves), antiseptic, antispasmodic, antiviral, and invigorating.

Clove—is antibacterial, antifungal, anti-infectious, antiparasitic, a strong antiseptic, antiviral, and an immune stimulant.

Additional Ingredients: Almonds. This variety also contains approximately 100 mg of boswellic acid (20 times the amount contained in each of the other varieties of chocolates).

Suggested Use: Enjoy 1/2 bar or 1 nugget as a beneficial snack.

Body System(s) Affected: **Digestive, Cardiovascular, Immune,** and **Nervous Systems**.

Allergens: Some varieties contain raw almonds—manufactured on equipment that processes tree nuts.

Master Formula Hers™

This high-potency, time-released multi-vitamin and mineral supplement was formulated specifically for women with betaine HCl and significantly higher amounts of vitamin E, vitamin B3, vitamin B12, magnesium, chromium, and choline. It has been found to reduce the symptoms of PMS as well as increase energy levels in general. This product was designed to help build and feed the reproductive system, and because of the specific ingredients, it may also help women who have had an hysterectomy. It is a **natural antioxidant.**

Ingredients: Vitamin A (retinyl palmitate: 10,000 IU per serving), vitamin C (calcium ascorbate: 400 mg per serving), vitamin D3 (cholecalciferol: 400 IU per serving), vitamin E (d-alpha tocopheryl acetate: 150 IU per serving), vitamin B1 (thiamin HCl: 14 mg per serving), vitamin B2 (riboflavin: 17 mg per serving), vitamin B3 (niacinamide: 33 mg per serving), vitamin B6 (pyridoxine HCl: 27 mg per serving), folic acid (600 mcg per serving), vitamin B12 (cyanocobalamin: 150 mcg per serving), biotin (300 mcg per serving), vitamin B5 (d-calcium pantothenate: 230 mg per serving), calcium (from calcium carbonate and pantothenate: 513 mg per serving), iodine (from Atlantic kelp: 195 mcg per serving), magnesium (from magnesium oxide: 464 mg per serving), zinc (zinc sulfate: 10 mg per serving), amino acid complex from hydrolyzed rice/soy protein [including: selenium (200 mcg per serving), copper (400 mcg per serving), manganese (2 mg per serving), chromium (200 mcg per serving), and molybdenum (5 mcg per serving)], potassium (potassium chloride: 156 mg per serving), choline (as non-GMO lecithin: 200 mg per serving), inositol, PABA (para amino benzoic acid: 1 mg per serving), betaine HCl (1 mg per serving), citrus bioflavonoid complex (from inner pulp and peels of orange, lemon and grapefruit), lemon (*Citrus limon*) essential oil, Ningxia Wolfberry (*Lycium barbarum*) fruit polysaccharide, fractionated coconut oil, vegetable cellulose, magnesium stearate, dicalcium phosphate, vegetable sterols, and silicon dioxide.

Suggested Use: For slow metabolism, four to six tablets daily. For fast metabolism, six to eight tablets daily. Take half of the daily amount before breakfast and half after dinner.

Body System(s) Affected: **Emotional Balance; Cardiovascular, Immune**, and **Nervous Systems**.

Note: Free of allergens. Contains no artificial flavors, preservatives, sugar, cornstarch, corn, wheat, yeast, or soy products.

Safety Data: If pregnant or under a doctor's care, please consult your physician before using.

Frequency: Approximately 88 MHz.

Companion Products: Be-Fit, Estro, FemiGen, MultiGreens.

Companion Oils: Dragon Time, Mister (more estrogen-like oils—may be better for women who have had an hysterectomy), Abundance, Harmony, Joy, Magnify Your Purpose.

Master Formula His™

This high-potency, time-released multi-vitamin and mineral supplement, designed specifically for men, includes all the vitamins and minerals contained in Master Formula Hers, with more vitamin B1, B2, zinc, and molybdenum. It also contains montmorillonite, alfalfa sprouts, and rutin. This product was designed to build and feed the male reproductive organs. Is is a **natural antioxidant**.

Ingredients: Vitamin A (retinyl palmitate: 10,000 IU per serving), vitamin C (calcium ascorbate: 400 mg per serving), vitamin D3 (cholecalciferol: 400 IU per serving), vitamin E (d-alpha tocopheryl acetate:

126 IU per serving), vitamin B1 (thiamin HCl: 27 mg per serving), vitamin B2 (riboflavin: 33 mg per serving), vitamin B3 (niacinamide: 66 mg per serving), vitamin B6 (pyridoxine HCl: 27 mg per serving), folic acid (600 mcg per serving), vitamin B12 (cyanocobalamin: 100 mcg per serving), biotin (300 mcg per serving), vitamin B5 (d-calcium pantothenate: 230 mg per serving), calcium (from calcium carbonate and pantothenate: 560 mg per serving), iodine (from Atlantic kelp: 195 mcg per serving), magnesium (from magnesium oxide: 80 mg per serving), zinc (zinc sulfate: 36 mg per serving), amino acid complex from hydrolyzed rice/soy protein [including: selenium (200 mcg per serving), copper (320 mcg per serving), manganese (2 mg per serving), chromium (100 mcg per serving), and molybdenum (100 mcg per serving)], potassium (potassium chloride: 104 mg per serving), choline (as non-GMO lecithin: 115 mg per serving), PABA (para amino benzoic acid: 1 mg per serving), citrus bioflavonoid complex (from inner pulp and peels of orange, lemon and grapefruit), trace minerals (as montmorillonite), alfalfa sprouts, rutin, inositol (2.5 mg per serving), lemon (*Citrus limon*) essential oil, Ningxia Wolfberry (*Lycium barbarum*) fruit polysaccharide, fractionated coconut oil, vegetable cellulose, magnesium stearate, dicalcium phosphate, vegetable sterols, and silicon dioxide.

Suggested Use: For slow metabolism, take four to six tablets daily. For fast metabolism, take six to eight tablets daily. Take half of the daily amount before breakfast and half after dinner.

Body System(s) Affected: **Emotional Balance, Cardiovascular, Immune**, and **Nervous Systems**.

Note: Free of allergens. Contains no artificial flavors, preservatives, sugar, cornstarch, corn, wheat, yeast, or soy products.

Frequency: Approximately 86 MHz.

Companion Products: Be-Fit, Manna Bars, Mineral Essence, MultiGreens, NingXia Red, ProGen, Power Meal, Sulfurzyme, Wolfberry Crisp Bars.

Companion Oils: Mister, Envision, Magnify Your Purpose, Sacred Mountain.

MegaCal™

Calcium is important for proper health: 98% of the calcium in the body is found in the bones and 1% in the teeth. The other 1% supports these crucial metabolic functions: steady heartbeat, muscle contraction, transmission of nerve impulses, and blood clotting. If this last 1% is not available from one's diet, it is pulled from the bones, creating osteoporosis. Current statistics indicate that 25 million American women and 5 million American men are affected by osteoporosis, showing just how difficult it has become to obtain enough calcium and other minerals through diet alone.

MegaCal differs from other calcium supplements (Super Cal, described in this book, and other popular Coral Calcium supplements) as shown on the following page. This particular product is formulated into a time-released mineral complex and is ideal for those who already have adequate calcium levels due to high consumption of dairy products. It may help alleviate osteoporosis and muscle cramps and support normal thyroid function.

Ingredients: Vitamin C (25 mg per serving), calcium (lactate, glycerophosphate, carbonate and ascorbate: 205 mg per serving), magnesium (citrate, sulfate and carbonate: 187 mg per serving), zinc (gluconate: 326 mcg per serving), manganese (sulfate: 320 mcg per serving), fractionated coconut oil, xylitol, and lemon (*Citrus limon*) rind essential oil.

Suggested Use: Take 1 teaspoon daily mixed in 1 cup of water or juice one hour after meals (or medications) or before retiring.

Body System(s) Affected: **Cardiovascular System, Muscles and Bones, Nervous System**.

Precautions: ***Do NOT feed to dogs.*** Keep out of reach of children. Keep in a cool, dry place. Do not expose to excessive heat or direct sunlight. If pregnant or under a doctor's care, consult your physician.

	MegaCal™	SuperCal™	Coral Calcium
Calcium per serving	205 mg	242 mg	1300 mg
Type of calcium	Lactate pentahydrate, carbonate, glycerophosphate, ascorbate	Citrate	Carbonate
Calcium to magnesium ratio	1:1	2:1	30:1
Additional minerals/nutrients	Magnesium (carbonate, citrate, and sulfate), zinc gluconate, manganese sulfate, xylitol, vitamin C	Magnesium citrate, zinc citrate, potassium citrate, boron (sodium borate)	Magnesium, potassium, zinc, selenium, 60 other micronutrient minerals

Mineral Essence

Mineral Essence contains over 60 organic, ionic trace minerals perfectly blended with royal jelly and essential oils to enhance bio-availability, provide antimicrobial protection, and significantly improve oxygenation to the cells. Mineral Essence differs from other colloidal mineral products on the market in that the ingredients are an ionic, electrolyte solution of minerals and trace minerals. The fluids of the body are largely ionic solutions and every body process is dependent on ions. Calcium, potassium, sodium, chloride, and copper ions are some key ions that participate in the body's electrical events. Potassium is the major positive ion inside the cell. Sodium is the major positive ion found in the fluid outside the cell. Ionic chlorine is the most abundant negative ion. The minerals and trace minerals in an ionic solution like Mineral Essence are balanced and in associations such as ion pairs, which keep them from being reactive.

In contrast, colloidal minerals are a suspension of tiny non-soluble mineral and trace mineral particles in water. Most colloidal minerals are held in suspension by their tiny size and/or a static electrical charge. Colloids do not dissolve into true solutions and are not capable of passing through a semipermeable membrane (such as a cell wall). True colloidal minerals suspended in a aqueous solution are not capable of conducting electricity and are not associated with bio-electric activity in the body.

The physical opposite of a colloid is a crystalloid. The minerals from Utah's inland sea (the Great Salt Lake) used in Mineral Essence are ionic and are electrolytes; thus, they are capable of conducting electrical energy in the body. The full spectrum of minerals and trace minerals found in Mineral Essence would form perfect crystals if all liquid were removed. When blended with essential oils, Mineral Essence becomes the most bio-available mineral product on the market.

To demonstrate how blending trace minerals with essential oils increases their bio-availability, a group of volunteers consumed a teaspoon of liquid trace minerals without any essential oils. Each volunteer experienced diarrhea within 24 hours. Within days, the same volunteers were given double the dosage of the same liquid trace minerals, but this time blended with essential oils. No diarrhea symptoms were experienced. This was due to the fact that the liquid trace minerals, blended with essential oils, were delivered more efficiently and utilized by the body's cells, or in other words made more bio-available.

In the July 1996 issue of *Young Living Essential Edge*, an article entitled "Sunburn Relief" contained the following information. "Dr. Alex Schauss, a prominent mineral researcher, has discovered that burns are painful because certain trace minerals are depleted from the skin and surrounding tissue. If the trace minerals are replenished to the affected area, then the pain will subside almost immediately.... We have had many who have topically applied Mineral Essence directly on the sunburn or burn and received instant pain relief as the healing process began...."

The minerals shown in the table below are in descending order according to the best testing information available. Several independent lab results for Mineral Essence were compared for this approximation. **NOTE:** Some people may wonder if it is safe to consume trace minerals that have trace elements of mercury, arsenic, lead, etc., in such a product. Dr. Alex Schauss explains that our bodies possess the same chemical makeup as sea water. In fact, sea water has been used many times for blood transfusions when plasma was not available. Products created in nature, like sea water, have many elements. Some of these elements, if separated and taken in larger quantities, can be dangerous to our health. When these same elements are synergistically blended by the Creator, we have a totally different product than the sum of the individual elements. Dr. Schauss suggests we consume sea water for its mineral content each day, for sea water provides the perfect balance of trace mineral intake that our body needs for optimum health.

Oxygen	Bismuth	Holmium
Hydrogen	Selenium	Lutetium
Chloride	Cesium	Rhenium
Magnesium	Molybdenum	Samarium
Sulfur	**Xenon	Terbium
Potassium	Lead	Thulium
Sodium	Arsenic	Ytterbium
Boron	Tungsten	Platinum
Lithium	Thorium	Dysprosium
Calcium	Tin	Erbium
Carbon	Thallium	Neodymium
Silicon	Mercury	Praseodymium
Phosphorus	Titanium	Yttrium
Fluorine	Hafnium	Zirconium
Nitrogen	Gold	Cerium
**Argon	Barium	Cobalt
Iron	Lanthanum	Niobium
Zinc	Cadmium	Gallium
Bromine	Uranium	Rubidium
Manganese	**Helium	Tantalum
Copper	Silver	Germanium
Chromium	Strontium	Aluminum
**Krypton	Iodine	Vanadium
Tellurium	Scandium	**Radon
Nickel	Beryllium	***Noble gases never tested for or not*
**Neon	Europium	*found, but are present in sea water*
Antimony	Gadolinium	*according to CRC Press.*

Ingredients: Ionic liquid mineral complex (as listed in the previous chart) and pure therapeutic-grade essential oils (as listed below) in a base of royal jelly and honey.

Essential Oils:

Lemon—helps promote leukocyte formation and helps to dissolve cholesterol and fats.

Cinnamon Bark—is a powerful purifier and a powerful oxygenator; it enhances the action and the activity of the other oils; it is antifungal, antibacterial, and antiviral.

Peppermint—enhances the effect of other oils. It is cooling and soothing. It aids digestion.

Suggested Use: Shake well before using and refrigerate after opening. Take 5 half-droppers (1 ml each) morning and evening or as needed as a mineral supplement. May be added to 4–8 oz. of distilled/purified water or juice before drinking.

Body System(s) Affected: **Emotional Balance; Cardiovascular, Hormonal, Immune**, and **Nervous Systems; Muscles and Bones**.

Companion Products: KidScents Mighty Mist/Vites, Master Formula His/Hers, Power Meal, Sulfurzyme, Wolfberry Crisp Bars.

Companion Oils: Citrus Fresh, Envision, Gathering, Harmony, Valor.

Allergens: This product contains royal jelly, which may cause allergic reactions.

MultiGreens™

MultiGreens™ is a high-protein, high-energy chlorophyll formula that helps the body maintain a high energy level. This reformulation of a long-time favorite called VitaGreen contains ingredients that may aid in cleansing the blood and supporting the immune system. Barley grass and spirulina have been reported to help balance blood sugar levels, alleviating that tired, run-down feeling. Because it is high in chlorophyll, it may help support the thyroid, the digestive system, and strengthen and stimulate muscle development. According to European research, the essential oils in this formula may enhance immune function. It is a **natural antioxidant**.

Ingredients: Choline bitartrate (108 mg per serving), bee pollen, barley (*Hordeum vulgare*) grass juice concentrate, spirulina (*Spirulina platensis*), eleuthero (*Eleutherococcus senticosus*) root, alfalfa (*Medicago sativa*) leaf/stem concentrate, Pacific kelp (*Laminaria digitata*) whole thallus, pure therapeutic-grade essential oils (as listed below), amino acid complex (L-arginine, L-cystine, L-tyrosine), and gelatin.

Essential Oils:

Rosemary cineol—helps balance heart function, stimulates nerves, and decongests the liver.

Lemon—helps promote leukocyte formation and helps to dissolve cholesterol and fats.

Lemongrass—helps repair connective tissue. When combined with marjoram, it helps stimulate the agents in the tissue to rejuvenate and reconnect.

Melissa—is a powerful antiviral agent, yet it is very gentle and very delicate because of the nature of the plant. It has the ability to work with and enhance the gentle aspects of the human body. It is anti-inflammatory and energizing.

Suggested Use: For slow metabolism, take three capsules once or twice daily. For fast metabolism, take four capsules once or twice daily. Best taken 1 hour before meals. For stomach sensitivity, take with meals.

Body System(s) Affected: **Cardiovascular, Digestive, Immune**, and **Nervous Systems, Muscles and Bones**.

Companion Products: Be-Fit, JuvaTone, NingXia Red, Power Meal, Sulfurzyme, Thyromin, Wolfberry Crisp Bars.

Companion Oils: Abundance, Awaken, En-R-Gee, Envision, JuvaFlex, Live with Passion, Magnify Your Purpose, Motivation, Release, Valor.

Frequency: Approximately 76 MHz.

Comments: Because it works so well for promoting pH (Alkaline/Acid) balance and for regulating blood sugar levels, this should be considered a mainstay for individuals with type 'O' blood.

NingXia Nitro™

This revolutionary product combines 40 mg of natural caffeine with B vitamins and the Nitro Alert oil blend to help boost energy, alertness, and cognitive function. It also contains a special form of D-ribose that has been researched for its ability to help increase energy and endurance, while protecting cells from oxidative stress and counteracting any jitteriness from caffeine.

Ingredients: Water, Nitro juice blend concentrate (cherry, kiwi, blueberry, acerola, bilberry, black currant, raspberry, strawberry, cranberry), coconut nectar, Nitro Energy Blend (D-ribose, green tea extract, choline bitartrate, maltodextrin, B3, B12, B6, mulberry leaf extract, Korean ginseng extract, folic acid, potassium iodide), maltodextrin, natural flavors, stevia, pectin, xanthan gum, Nitro Alert oil blend, potassium iodide.

Essential Oils:

Nitro Alert—is an oil blend specially formulated with essential oils that are often used to help boost energy and mental alertness. It includes vanilla, chocolate, *Yerba mate*, spearmint, peppermint, nutmeg, and black pepper oil in a base of wolfberry seed oil.

Suggested Use: Take one tube with 2–4 oz. of NingXia Red or water as needed. Do not consume more than two tubes per day.

Body System(s) Affected: Cellular Function, Digestive System.

Safety Data: ***Consult with a medical professional before using if pregnant or nursing or if taking medication for any health condition. Use with caution if sensitive to caffeine.***

Companion Products: NingXia Red.

Companion Oils: peppermint, black pepper, nutmeg.

NingXia Red®

This new formulation of NingXia Red boosts its already high antioxidant levels, increases the amount of pure, therapeutic grade essential oils, and tastes even better than before! NingXia Red also boasts a low glycemic index, using natural stevia extract and fruit juices as mild sweeteners.

Ingredients: Whole NingXia wolfberry (*Lycium barbarum*) puree, blueberry (*Vaccinium corymbosum*) juice, plum (*Prunus domestica*) juice, cherry (*Prunus avium*) juice, aronia (*Aronia melanocarpa*) juice, pomegranate (*Punica granatum*) juice, grape (*Vitis vinifera*) seed extract, pure therapeutic-grade essential oils (as listed below), water, tartaric acid, natural blueberry flavor, pure vanilla extract, malic acid, pectin, sodium benzoate/potassium sorbate, natural stevia extract.

Essential Oils:

Orange—contains over 91% d-limonene (which helps to promote normal cell life cycles). It is rich in compounds noted for their stress-reducing effects.

Yuzu—contains up to 80% d-limonene. Yuzu oil has also been studied for its anti-inflammatory effects.

Lemon—contains over 65% d-limonene. It helps promote leukocyte formation, and it helps to dissolve cholesterol and fats.

Tangerine—contains up to 80% d-limonene. It is also often used to help soothe the digestive system.

Suggested Use: Take 1–2 fluid ounces twice daily or as needed. Shake well before using, and refrigerate after opening.

Body System(s) Affected: Immune System. Also targeted effects to Liver Function, Eye Health, and Energy Levels.

Companion Products: Manna Bars, Power Meal, Ultra Young+.

Companion Oils: En-R-Gee, EndoFlex, Envision, JuvaFlex, Magnify Your Purpose, Longevity, and Valor.

NingXia Wolfberries, Dried

Enjoy the antioxidant and nutritional benefits of the Ningxia Wolfberry in your cereal, salad, trail mix, baked goods, and more. These dried berries are loaded with nutrients and proteins and are considered one of the healthiest fruits that nature has to provide.

Ingredients: Whole dried Ningxia wolfberries (*Lycium barbarum*).

Suggested Use: Use 1/2 cup of dried berries as desired

Body System(s) Affected: **Digestive** and **Immune Systems, Muscles and Bones.**

Omega Blue™

(Pure Fish Oil + Omega Enhance™)

Omega Blue™ is specially formulated to help you to have better skin, better joints, less inflammation, and better eyesight. This particular supplement is one of the most natural and bio-available fish oils on the market for several reasons. First is the source of the fish oil: the fish oil in this product is harvested from small fish (sardine, anchovy, and mackerel) that grow wild in pristine waters. This initially helps to reduce the amount of toxins (mercury, lead, PCBs and dioxins) that have to be removed through processing. Next is the processing itself: a unique, proprietary process that uses non-molecular distillation helps to maintain the naturally occurring balance of EPA (eicosapentaenoic acid) and DHA (docosahexaenoic acid). This is necessary to help reduce rancidity and minimize the "fishy" flavor of the oil. EPA should represent about 14–18% of the fish oil and DHA should be 8–12%. The total amount of fish oil in this product is 1.65 grams, while EPA is measured at 265 mg (about 16%) and DHA is measured at 182 mg (about 11%). Another thing that makes this product so unique is the addition of the proprietary Omega Enhance blend of essential oils shown below. This powerful blend of oils helps to protect the fragile omega-3 fatty acids by increasing the stability of the fish oil by a minimum of 10 times throughout its entire life cycle (from preparation, through storage in the softgel, all the way through metabolism within the body). Finally, a unique aqueous solution coating (enteric-type coating derived from seaweed) helps to protect the fish oil from oxidation and also helps to ensure that it is released in the intestines for up to 3 times the omega-3 absorption with no "fishy" aftertaste.

Ingredients: Fish oil, pure therapeutic-grade essential oils (as listed below), gelatin, glycerin, and aqueous coating solution (oleic acid, sodium alginate, medium-chain fatty acids, ethylcellulose, and stearic acid).

Essential Oils:

Lemongrass—helps repair connective tissue: it helps stimulate the agents in the tissue to rejuvenate and reconnect. It enhances omega-3's cardiovascular protection. It helps regulate the parasympathetic nervous system and strengthen vascular walls. It has also been clinically shown to help maintain normal, healthy cholesterol levels.

Myrrh—is anti-inflammatory and antiseptic. It has high levels of sesquiterpenes and is the second highest ranking substance on the ORAC scale, behind clove essential oil.

Clove—has one of the highest ORAC (oxygen radical absorbent capacity) scores of any known substance. It is antibacterial, antifungal, anti-infectious, antiparasitic, a strong antiseptic, antiviral, and an immune stimulant. It helps preserve the integrity of fatty acids. Clove may also influence healing and help improve memory. Studies show that when it is combined with fish oil, it reduces inflammation an additional 30%.

German Chamomile—has been found to help open the liver, increase liver function and secretion, and support the pancreas. It promotes digestion and has strong antioxidant and anti-inflammatory properties.

Suggested Use: Take one softgel three times daily or as needed.

Body System(s) Affected: **Cardiovascular and Nervous Systems**.

Companion Products: Use daily with Digest + Cleanse and Longevity capsules. Combine with NingXia Red, Longevity capsules, and Balance Complete (all 4 of these products make up the Core Essentials Complete program and work well together).

Precautions: Keep in a cool, dry place. Do not expose to excessive heat or direct sunlight.

OmegaGize³™

OmegaGize³™ combines three powerful ingredients—fish oil, vitamin D3, and CoQ10—in one powerful package. The Gize³ fish oil used in these capsules contains high levels of the omega-3 fatty acids DHA and EPA, which have been studied for their abilities to promote healthy brain and nervous system functions, cardiovascular health, and immune functions. Vitamin D plays an important role in bone health and strength and helps modulate hormone secretion and immune function. Coenzyme Q10 (or CoQ10) is a substance that plays a critical role in the electron transport chain that helps create cellular energy. It has been studied for its ability to help promote healthy brain, nerve, and cardiovascular functions. These three ingredients are combined with a special essential oil blend to help promote stability and enhance antioxidant and anti-inflammatory effects.

Ingredients: Fish oil, rice tocotrienols, CoQ10 Kaneka™, vitamin D (cholecalciferol), mixed carotenoids, gelatin (tilapia), silicon dioxide, purified water.

Essential Oils:

Clove—has one of the highest ORAC (oxygen radical absorbance capacity) scores of any known substance. It is antibacterial, antifungal, anti-infectious, antiparasitic, a strong antiseptic, antiviral, and an immune stimulant. It helps preserve the integrity of fatty acids. Clove may also influence healing and help improve memory. Studies show that when it is combined with fish oil, it reduces inflammation an additional 30%.

German Chamomile—has been found to help open the liver, increase liver function and secretion, and support the pancreas. It promotes digestion and has strong antioxidant and anti-inflammatory properties.

Spearmint—has antibacterial and anti-inflammatory properties.

Suggested Use: Take 2 capsules twice daily.

Body System(s) Affected: **Cardiovascular and Nervous Systems.**

Companion Products: Combine with NingXia Red, True Source, Longevity capsules, and Balance Complete as part of your daily health regimen.

Precautions: Consult with a physician before using if pregnant or nursing.

ParaFree™

With virtually everyone in the world having parasites of one form or another, there is a tremendous need for a product like this that utilizes the antiparasitic properties of essential oils to help combat this worldwide problem.

Ingredients: Organic sesame (*Sesamum indicum*) seed oil, organic olive (*Olea europaea*) oil, pure therapeutic-grade essential oils (as listed below), gelatin, glycerin, and deionized water.

Essential Oils:

Cumin (*Cuminum cyminum*)—is antiparasitic, antispasmodic, and enhances immune function.

Anise—is antiparasitic, anti-inflammatory, and promotes better digestion.

Fennel—is antiparasitic and supports digestive and pancreatic functions.

Laurel (*Laurus nobilis*)—is antiseptic, antibacterial, antiparasitic, and antiviral. It is a diuretic and a fungicide. It is a digestive for the stomach. It is a purifier and helps with loss of appetite.

Vetiver—is antiseptic, anti-inflammatory, calming, grounding, and locally warming. It helps with muscular rheumatism, arthritis, anxiety, insomnia, depression, oily skin, and acne.

Melaleuca—is antifungal, antiseptic, and antibacterial.

Nutmeg—supports adrenal glands, is anti-inflammatory, and stimulates immune function.

Clove—is antiparasitic.

Idaho Tansy—is highly regarded for its worm-expelling properties.

Thyme—is anti-inflammatory, antifungal, antiseptic, and antiviral.

Suggested Use: Take four softgels two times daily. For best results, take for 21 days and then rest 7 days. Cycle may be repeated three times. Take on an empty stomach for maximum results.

*** Better results may be obtained when using ParaFree with ComforTone and ICP to help break up and remove the plaque and incrustation from the system.

Body System(s) Affected: **Digestive** and **Immune Systems**.

Safety Data: ***Do not take during pregnancy. Many of the oils contained in this product are contraindicated for pregnancy.***

Comments: Since contraindications do exist, one would be well advised to review the safety data in the **appendix** of this book. For additional information, review the books Essential Oil Safety—A Guide for Health Care Professionals by Robert Tisserand and Tony Balacs and Aromatherapy for Health Professionals by Shirley and Len Price.

PD 80/20™

This dietary supplement provides the nutrients necessary to support internal health and bodily functions, as well as memory and mental acuity.

Ingredients: Pregnenolone (640 mg per serving), DHEA (160 mg per serving), rice flour, and gelatin.

Body System(s) Affected: **Emotional Balance, Hormonal System, Muscles and Bones, Cardiovascular** and **Immune Systems**.

Companion Products: Essentialzyme, Life 5, MultiGreens, and Sulfurzyme (capsules or powder).

Companion Oils: Clary sage, Dragon Time, and fennel.

Power Meal™

Power Meal™ is a complete vegetarian protein drink mix containing Ningxia Wolfberry (high in protein and amino acids), MSM (with high-powered, immune-supporting, super-antioxidant properties), and Siberian ginseng. Power Meal is designed as a high-protein, vitamin-rich meal replacement containing a large spectrum of vitamins, trace minerals, and amino acids. Power Meal provides the body with the tools to build lean muscle tissue while providing a vital source of organic sulfur, which is an important facet of proper cellular metabolism and organ function.

Whether used as a meal replacement or as a filling and nutritious snack, Power Meal can help serve as an excellent weight management tool. Free of fats, sugars, and synthetic ingredients, Power Meal provides most of the building blocks the body requires for regeneration and maintenance.

The protein-rich formula of Power Meal, when combined with exercise, can help the body build lean muscle tissue that is the foundation of a lean physique and an important element of weight control. Because muscle burns 22 times as many calories as fat, the addition of muscle tissue can significantly accelerate metabolism and contribute to a more slender body. Because muscle tissue weighs more than adipose (fat) tissue, the addition of muscle mass to the body may not always be accompanied by weight loss–even though body fat may have dropped substantially.

Ingredients: Rice protein concentrate, rice bran and germ, Ningxia Wolfberry (*Lycium barbarum*) fruit, fructose, natural vanilla flavoring, apple (*Malus domestica*) fruit, chicory root fiber extract (FOS), medium-chain triglycerides, calcium (tri-calcium phosphate), soy lecithin (food for the brain), guar gum, magnesium oxide, natural orange flavor, methylsulfonylmethane (MSM—regenerates nerve tissue; detoxifies liver), xanthan gum, lo han kuo extract, cinnamon (*Cinnamomum verum*) bark, lipase (digests fats), protease 4.5, ginkgo biloba extract, protease 3.0, vitamin E (mixed tocopherols), manganese gluconate (antioxidant; regulates blood sugar levels; increases cellular energy), ginger (*Zingiber officinale*) root, choline bitartrate, eleuthero (*Eleutherococcus senticosis*) root, PABA, zinc (from z. lactate), vitamin C (ascorbic acid), protease 6.0, phytase, vitamin A (beta-carotene), talin, betaine HCl, peptidase, white pepper, niacin (vitamin B3), selenium (from selenomethionine), clove (*Syzygium aromaticum*) flower bud, alpha-lipoic acid, vitamin A (from mixed carotenoids), kelp (*Laminaria digitata*), nutmeg (*Myristica fragrans*) seed, fennel (*Foeniculum vulgare*) seed, copper (from c. gluconate), pantothenic acid (from calcium pantothenate - vitamin B5), neohesperidin derivative (flavor from natural citrus), lycopene, pure therapeutic-grade essential oils (as listed below), cardamon (*Elettaria cardamomum*) seed, vitamin B6 (from pyridoxine HCl), thiamine HCl (vitamin B1), riboflavin (vitamin B2), lutein, chromium (from c. aminonicotinate), zeaxanthin, astaxanthin, cholecalciferol, folic acid, biotin (helps cell growth and fatty acid production), and vitamin B12 (from methylcobalamin).

Essential Oils:

Orange—is rich in compounds noted for their stress-reducing effects.

Lemon—helps promote leukocyte formation and helps to dissolve cholesterol and fats.

Grapefruit—is excellent for fluid retention and cellulite. It is a diuretic, a detoxifier, and a stimulant of the lymphatic system. It is important as an antidepressant.

Anise—is antiparasitic, anti-inflammatory, and a promoter of better digestion.

Fennel—is antiparasitic and supports digestive and pancreatic functions.

Nutmeg—supports adrenal glands, is anti-inflammatory, and stimulates immune function.

Suggested Use: Take 2 full scoops with 8 to 12 oz. of pure water or juice. Use as a meal alternative or dietary supplement. For added flavor, mix one serving (2 scoops) with rice or almond milk *(the authors enjoy mixing this with Rice Dream—a brown rice beverage)*. For children under 12, use 1 scoop (½ serving).

Body System(s) Affected: **Cardiovascular, Digestive**, and **Immune Systems, Muscles and Bones**.

Precautions: If pregnant or under a doctor's care, consult your physician. Keep in a cool, dry place. Do not expose to sunlight.

Companion Products: Be-Fit, Master Formula His/Hers, ComforTone, Essentialzyme, ICP, Manna Bars, MultiGreens, NingXia Red, Thyromin, Wolfberry Crisp Bars.

Companion Oils: Abundance, Citrus Fresh, EndoFlex, Envision, Live with Passion, Magnify Your Purpose.

Prostate Health™

These softgels contain an essential oil blend that is combined with saw palmetto extract and pumpkin seed oil, which have demonstrated an ability to support health and proper function of the male prostate gland. The essential oils contained in this supplement have been chosen specifically for their anti-inflammatory constituents and properties.

Ingredients: Saw palmetto (*Serenoa repens/serrulata*) extract, pumpkin seed oil, pure therapeutic-grade essential oils (as listed below), non-GMO modified cornstarch, carrageenan, glycerin, sorbitol, purified water.

Essential Oils:

Geranium—contains estriol and has estrogen-like properties. It may help improve estrogen and progesterone-testosterone balance.

Fennel—is a diuretic and may break up fluids and toxins and cleanse the tissues.

Lavender—is anti-inflammatory and sedative. It balances body systems and promotes a general sense of well-being.

Myrtle—is anti-inflammatory and is a decongestant of the respiratory system. It may help improve oxygenation and work as an expectorant in discharging mucus.

Peppermint—is anti-inflammatory and helps with nerve regeneration. It also enhances digestion and increases endurance.

Suggested Use: Take one capsule twice daily.

Body System(s) Affected: **Hormonal System**.

Companion Products: Be-Fit, Exodus, Master Formula His, MultiGreens, Protec tincture, Power Meal, Sulfurzyme.

Companion Oils: Exodus, Live with Passion, Magnify Your Purpose, Mister, Valor.

Pure Protein Complete™

(Ultra-Bioactive Whey Protein)

This product is meant for those interested in a high-protein diet as part of a fitness or weight-loss program. It is unique among protein drinks that exist commercially. For one thing, it contains a proprietary blend of proteins (see ingredients below). This ultra-clean protein blend comes from New Zealand and is certified grass-fed, hormone-free, antibiotic-free, and chemical-free. It is also prepared with a gentle filtering process that does not denature amino-acids and maintains ultra-bioactivity. These different proteins all metabolize at different rates, which helps to reduce muscle breakdown and provides for better protein synthesis. This sustained protein metabolism helps to maintain stable blood sugar levels, which has been shown to reduce food cravings. Each serving provides 20 grams of this proprietary protein blend, which is supported by a specialized enzyme blend, a low-glycemic carbohydrate matrix, and lots of complementary vitamins and minerals.

Ingredients: Pure Protein Complete Proprietary Protein Blend (whey protein concentrate, sweet whey, milk protein concentrate, nonfat dry milk, and whey protein isolate), Proprietary Carbohydrate Matrix (chicory root fiber extract (FOS), natural vanilla flavor, fructose, guar gum, xanthan gum, xylitol, cellulose, lo han kuo extract, and *Stevia rebaudiana* leaf extract), lecithin, Proprietary Enzyme Complex (lactase, papain, bromelain, amylase, lipase, and bioperine), magnesium oxide, tri-calcium phosphate, mixed carotenoids, vitamin C (ascorbic acid), potassium citrate, vitamin E (natural mixed tocopherols), zinc gluconate, vitamin B3 (niacin), beta carotene, vitamin B5 (calcium pantothenate), neohesperidin derivative (flavor from natural citrus), vitamin B6 (pyridoxine HCl), vitamin B2 (riboflavin), vitamin B1 (thiamine HCl), orange (*Citrus sinensis*) rind essential oil, chromium nicotinate, vitamin D3 (cholecalciferol), vitamin B12 (methylcobalamin), folic acid, biotin, potassium iodide, and sodium selenite.

Suggested Use: Add two scoops to 8 oz. cold water. May be mixed with rice, almond, or other milk. Shake, stir, or blend until smooth. For added flavor, add fruit or essential oils.

Body System(s) Affected: **Muscles and Bones**.

Companion Products: Balance Complete, Digest + Cleanse, Essentialzyme, Longevity capsules, NingXia Red, and Omega Blue.

Rehemogen™ Tincture

This formula contains herbs that were used by Chief Sundance to clean the blood, fight free radicals, and give support to the blood cells and immune system.

Ingredients: Pure therapeutic-grade essential oils (as listed below), extracts of red clover blossom, licorice root, poke root, peach bark, Oregon grape root, stillingia, sarsparilla, cascara sagrada, prickly ash bark, burdock root, buckthorn bark, and royal jelly. Extracted in a 1:4 ratio of grain alcohol and water.

Essential Oils:

Roman Chamomile—is a blood cleanser and helps the liver discharge toxins.

Rosemary cineol—helps balance heart function, stimulate nerves, and decongest the liver.

Thyme—is anti-inflammatory, antifungal, antiseptic, and antiviral.

Melaleuca—is antifungal, antiseptic, antibacterial, and tissue regenerative.

Suggested Use: One to three droppers (25–75 drops) three times daily in distilled water or as desired.

Body System(s) Affected: **Cardiovascular** and **Digestive Systems**.

SleepEssence™

This supplement is uniquely formulated as a natural solution to help promote healthy sleeping patterns. With a combination of lavender, vetiver, valerian, *Ruta graveolens*, and the hormone melatonin (which is naturally produced in the body to regulate the sleep/wake cycle), SleepEssence calms stressed nerves, increases relaxation, and prepares the body for a peaceful night's rest. This supplement is also rich in the sesquiterpene khusinol, which has been found to be twice as effective as lavender at promoting relaxation. Sleep Essence comes in a softgel capsule for easy swallowing. Sleep Essence is not intended to be used on a daily basis or for weeks or months at a time, but rather it is intended to be used for small periods of time when your body needs sleep the most.

Ingredients: Pure therapeutic-grade essential oils (as listed below), melatonin, lecithin, coconut (*Cocus nucifera*) meat oil, carageenan, glycerin, modified cornstarch, and sorbitol.

Essential Oils:

Lavender—is sedative, soothing, and may help with insomnia and stress-reduction.

Vetiver—is calming and sedative. It may be helpful in dealing with insomnia and stress.

Valerian—may help with insomnia, restlessnes, tension, and sleep disturbances.

Mandarin—is sedative and may help with insomnia and nervous tension.

Rue (Ruta graveolens)—is relaxing and promotes sleep.

Suggested Use: Take 1–2 softgel capsules 30–60 minutes before going to bed.

Body System(s) Affected: **Emotional Balance, Cardiovascular System, Digestive System, Endocrine System, and Muscles and Bones.**

Precautions: If pregnant or under a doctor's care, consult your physician before using this supplement. Do not operate heavy machinery for 10 hours after taking SleepEssence. This product is not recommended for long-term use or for use in conjunction with echinacea.

Slique™ Bar: Tropical Berry Crunch

This unique snack bar blends exotic fruits, nuts, and other natural ingredients to help increase feelings of fullness and satiation between meals. This bar contains the essential nutrition from baru nuts, goldenberries, and wolfberries, with lots of protein and fiber, a special essential oil blend, and a potato skin extract that helps trigger the release of cholecystokinin in the body to help curb hunger cravings and promote a feeling of fullness.

Ingredients: Baru nuts, almonds, honey, chicory root inulin, dates, coconut, cocao nibs, goldenberries, Bing cherries, wolfberries (*Lycium barbarum*), quinoa crisps, chia seeds, potato skin extract, sea salt, vanilla (*Vanilla planifolia*) essential oil, sunflower lecithin, orange (*Citrus aurantium dulcis*) peel oil, cinnamon (*Cinnamomum verum*) bark oil.

Essential Oils:

Vanilla—is calming and balancing to the emotions and contains vanillin, which may help reduce cravings.

Orange—has calming and balancing properties and may help soothe the digestive system.

Cinnamon—is uplifting and may help balance blood sugar levels.

Suggested Use: Eat one bar between meals with 12 oz. of water.

Body System(s) Affected: **Digestive System**.

Companion Products: Slique Slim Caps, Slique Tea, Slique Gum, NingXia Red.

Companion Oils: Slique Essence.

Slique™ Essence

Oils contained in this blend have been studied for their abilities to help reduce cravings and appetite, helping to support weight management by promoting a lower level of calorie consumption.

Single Oils Contained in This Blend:

Grapefruit—has been studied for its ability to affect the **autonomic nervous system** and to **reduce appetite**. It also has a **balancing** and **uplifting** aroma.

Tangerine—is often used to help with **digestive issues** and has a **calming** influence.

Spearmint—may help **soothe** the **digestive system**.

Lemon—is often used to help cleanse the **lymphatic system** and to help **dissolve cellulite**. It also has been studied for its ability to reduce **stress**.

Ocotea—was used traditionally for **digestive support**. It may help reduce **swelling** and—in conjunction with proper exercise and healthy eating—may help enhance **weight loss** by helping to balance the pituitary and endocrine systems.

Other Ingredients: Stevia (*Stevia rebaudiana*) leaf extract.

Body System(s) Affected: The oils in this blend may help it be effective for dealing with various problems related to the **Digestive System** and to **Emotional Balance**.

Aromatic Influence: May help to reduce **cravings** and feelings of **hunger**, while promoting **uplifting** and **energizing** feelings.

Application: Add 2–4 drops to your beverage before drinking throughout the day, or inhale the aroma of this blend directly to help reduce feelings of hunger.

Safety Data: ***Because of some of the oils contained within this blend, it should be used with caution by women who are pregnant.***

Supplements

Slique™ Gum

This unique gum combines frankincense resin (which was traditionally chewed to help aid oral health) with peppermint and spearmint essential oils and xylitol, which has been studied for its beneficial oral health properties.

Ingredients: Frankincense resin (*Boswellia frereana*), gum base, isomalt, sorbitol, natural flavors, calcium stearate, natural sweeteners, colors (red cabbage juice and turmeric), essential oil blend (as indicated below), xylitol.

Essential Oils:

Peppermint—is often used to help aid in digestion and has anti-inflammatory and antispasmodic properties.

Spearmint—may help **soothe** the **digestive system**.

Suggested Use: Chew before or after meals as a snack alternative.

Body System(s) Affected: **Digestive System**.

Companion Products: Slique Slim Caps, Slique Tea, Slique Bar.

Companion Oils: Slique Essence.

Slique™ Slim Caps

This amazing product combines two different types of capsules to enhance feelings of fullness and to help support efficient metabolism, working to reduce cravings and feelings of hunger. One type of capsule includes soluble fiber from multiple sources that can expand in the stomach, creating a sensation of fullness. The other capsule contains essential oils with high citral contents, combined with pomegranate seed oil and coconut oil, to help increase metabolic activities in the body.

Ingredients: Citral Caps: fractionated coconut oil, gelatin, pomegranate seed oil (70% punicic acid), silicon dioxide, water; Konjac Caps: konjac powder (glucomannan fiber), microcrystalline cellulose, ocotea leaf fines, fucoxanthin 10%, crosscarmellose sodium, magnesium stearate, silicon dioxide, water

Essential Oils:

Lemongrass—has high citral content and is often used to help reduce cholesterol. It is also used for its sedative properties.

Lemon Myrtle— has high citral content and is often used for its calming, sedative properties.

Idaho Balsam Fir—has diuretic properties and may help reduce swelling. It is also sedative and appeasing.

Suggested Use: Take capsules before meals twice a day with cold water.

Body System(s) Affected: **Hormonal System**.

Companion Products: Slique Gum, Slique Tea, NingXia Red, Slique Bar.

Companion Oils: Slique Essence.

Slique™ Tea

This is a natural tea high in flavonoids and polyphenols, which have been studied for their abilities to aid with obesity, cardiovascular diseases, inflammation, arthritis, and other health concerns. This tea combines ocotea, oolong, and raw Ecuadorian cacao (which contains active vitamin C) with boswellia frankincense powder and proprietary vanilla essential oil for a unique, healthy drink alternative to sugar-filled beverages.

Ingredients: Jade oolong tea, inulin (a prebiotic), ocotea leaf (*Ocotea quixos*), Ecuadorian cacao powder, vanilla essential oil, frankincense powder (*Boswellia sacra*), natural stevia extract.

Essential Oils:

Vanilla—is calming and balancing to the emotions and contains vanillin, which may help reduce cravings.

Suggested Use: Drink with meals, before or after workouts, or any other time.

Body System(s) Affected: **Hormonal System**.

Companion Products: Slique Bar, Be-Fit, NingXia Red, Slique Tea, Slique Gum.

Companion Oils: Slique Essence, or any essential oil or blend desired to enhance the benefits and for a unique flavor.

Stevia Extract™

This dietary supplement may effectively regulate blood sugar. It is a helpful aid to people who have diabetes and hypoglycemia. After hypoglycemics ingest Stevia, blood sugar rises and their energy levels and mental activities increase rapidly. It may also lower elevated blood pressure while not affecting normal blood pressure. It may inhibit the growth and reproduction of some bacteria and other infectious organisms, including the bacteria that causes tooth decay and periodontal (gum) disease. Individuals using Stevia have reported a lower incidence of colds and flu. Individuals who have tried using Stevia as a mouthwash or added to toothpaste have seen significant improvements in the treatment of periodontal disease.

It is a wonderful aid in weight loss and weight management because it contains no calories, and research indicates that it significantly increases glucose tolerance and inhibits glucose absorption. People who ingest Stevia daily often report a decrease in their desire for sweets and fatty foods. It may also improve digestion and gastrointestinal function, soothe upset stomachs, and help speed recovery from minor illnesses.

When applied to the skin, it effectively softens the skin and smooths out wrinkles while helping to heal various skin blemishes, acne, seborrhea, dermatitis, and eczema. People have reported that when Stevia is used on cuts and wounds, there is more rapid healing without scarring. **(Information obtained from United American Industries, Inc.)**

Ingredients: *Stevia rebaudiana* leaf extract and filtered water.

Suggested Use: Use as desired, for supplementing food and/or beverages.

Body System(s) Affected: **Cardiovascular, Digestive**, and **Immune Systems**.

Companion Products: Essentialzyme, Mineral Essence, MultiGreens, Thyromin.

Companion Oils: JuvaFlex, Thieves.

Sulfurzyme™

Sulfurzyme™ is a unique combination of Methylsulfonylmethane (MSM; the protein-building compound found in breast milk) and *Lyceum barbarum* (the Ningxia Wolfberry Powder) that together create a bold new concept in reviving the immune system, supporting almost every major body function, and forestalling an array of degenerative conditions. Of particular importance is MSM's ability to equalize water pressure inside of the cells—a considerable benefit for those plagued with bursitis, arthritis, and tendinitis. It also activates enzymes, helps the body assimilate vitamins, and metabolizes carbohydrates.

Sulfurzyme may help reduce the following signs of sulfur deficiency: poor nail and hair growth, falling hair, eczema, dermatitis, poor muscle tone, acne/pimples, gout, rheumatism, arthritis, weakening of nervous system (MS, Parkinson's, Lou Gehrig's, and Alzheimer's disease), constipation, impairment of mental faculties, lowered libido.

Comments: Sulfur metabolism requires nutritional balance. It takes calcium to metabolize sulfur, magnesium to metabolize calcium, potassium to metabolize magnesium, phosphorus to metabolize potassium, etc. The list goes on! That is why wolfberry is contained in this product; it contains all of the necessary components for sulfur to be metabolized. *(Refer to the Wolfberry Crisp Bar at the end of this section for more information on the benefits of the Ningxia Wolfberry.)*

Capsule Form:

Ingredients: MSM (methylsulfonylmethane: 1.6 g per serving), Ningxia Wolfberry (*Lycium barbarum*) fruit: 200 mg per serving, and gelatin.

Suggested Use: Take 2 capsules two times daily or as needed one hour before or after meals.

Powder Form:

Ingredients: MSM (methylsulfonylmethane: 1.2 g per serving), FOS (frustooligosaccharides), Ningxia Wolfberry (*Lycium barbarum*) fruit: 155 mg per serving, and stevioside (*Stevia rebaudiana*) leaf.

Suggested Use: Mix ½ tsp. with juice or distilled water and take twice daily, one hour before or after meals.

Body System(s) Affected: **Immune** and **Nervous Systems, Muscles and Bones, Skin**.

Companion Products: ComforTone, Essentialzyme, ICP, Master Formula His/Hers, Ortho Ease and Ortho Sport Massage Oils, Power Meal, Ultra Young+.

Companion Oils: En-R-Gee, Envision, Magnify Your Purpose, PanAway, Valor.

Super B™

A B-complex is necessary for the delivery of the essential nutrients needed to support the body's cells, particularly under times of stress when assimilation is most difficult. Although research has shown that mega-doses of B vitamins are not healthy, it has been noted that the diets of many Americans do not provide the recommended amount of B vitamins that are essential for normal functions of immune response. B vitamins included in this formula are B1, B2, B3, B6, and B12 (no essential oils are present in this formula). When all of these B vitamins are combined in the stomach, it causes instant fermentation resulting in stomach upset. To alleviate this problem, this product utilizes a synergistic suspension isolation to provide the release of specific vitamins when necessary so that they can all work together in their separate stages of isolation. This product was designed to help build the body. It is a **natural antioxidant**.

Ingredients: Thiamin HCl (vitamin B1: 25 mg per serving), Riboflavin (vitamin B2: 25 mg per serving), Niacin (vitamin B3 (as nicotinic acid): 100 mg per serving), Vitamin B6 (as pyridoxine HCl: 25 mg per serving), Folic Acid (400 mcg per serving), Vitamin B12 (as cyanocobalamin: 100 mcg per serving), Biotin (150 mcg per serving), Magnesium oxide (25 mg per serving), Zinc gluconate (5 mg per serving), Selenium yeast (50 mcg per serving), PABA (para amino benzoic acid: 25 mg per serving), dicalcium phosphate, cellulose, magnesium stearate and stearic acid.

Suggested Use: One half to one tablet daily, preferably with a meal and not on an empty stomach.

Body System(s) Affected: **Cardiovascular** and **Nervous Systems, Muscles and Bones**.

Safety Data: ***If taken on an empty stomach, one may experience a niacin flush.***

Comments: If a niacin flush occurs, try one drop of peppermint in 20 drops of V-6 Mixing Oil for a full-body massage. This may help the body cool down quickly.

Frequency: Approximately 63 MHz.

Super C™

Research has shown that physical stress, alcohol, smoking, and medication can lower the blood levels of this essential vitamin. When citrus fruits are not readily available, diets may not contain enough vitamin C. Super C is properly balanced with rutin, bioflavonoids, and minerals to work synergistically, balancing the electrolytes and increasing the absorption rate of the vitamin C. Without bioflavonoids, vitamin C has a hard time getting inside the cell, and without proper electrolyte balance and minerals, it will not stay there for long. The essential oils contained in this product not only enhance the flavor, but they all have high levels of bioflavonoid activity. This product was designed to help build up the body.

Ingredients: Vitamin C (ascorbic acid), calcium carbonate, zinc gluconate, manganese sulfate, potassium chloride, citrus bioflavonoids, rutin, cayenne pepper (*Capsicum annuum*) fruit, pure therapeutic-grade essential oils (as listed below), dicalcium phosphate, cellulose, stearic acid, magnesium stearate, and vegetable food-grade coating.

Essential Oils:

Orange—is rich in compounds noted for their stress-reducing effects.

Tangerine—is sedating and calming to the nervous system. It is also a diuretic and a decongestant of the lymphatic system.

Grapefruit—is excellent for fluid retention and cellulite. It is a diuretic, detoxifier, and stimulant of the lymphatic system. It is important as an antidepressant.

Lemon—helps promote leukocyte formation and helps to dissolve cholesterol and fats.

Lemongrass—helps repair connective tissue: when combined with marjoram, it helps stimulate the agents in the tissue to rejuvenate and reconnect.

Suggested Use: For reinforcing immune strength, take two tablets daily. For maintenance, take one tablet daily. Best when taken before meals.

Body System(s) Affected: **Immune** and **Respiratory Systems**.

Companion Products: Exodus, ImmuneTune, MultiGreens, Rehemogen.

Companion Oils: Citrus Fresh, Exodus II, ImmuPower, Motivation, Thieves, Valor.

Frequency: Approximately 80 MHz.

Super C Chewable™

The vitamin C provided in this unique product is enhanced by that of the acerola cherry, a tropical fruit that contains up to 4.5% vitamin C. The addition of citrus bioflavonoids increases vitamin C's support of the immune system while increasing capillary and connective tissue strength. Now you can have one of nature's most powerful antioxidants in a natural, delicious, chewable form.

Ingredients: Vitamin C (ascorbic acid: 117 mg per serving), acerola cherry (*Malpighia glabra*) fruit extract, citrus bioflavonoids from lemon (*Citrus limon*), pure therapeutic-grade essential oils (as listed below), silica and vegetable-grade lubricant (sugar cane and palm oil).

Essential Oils:

Lemon—helps promote leukocyte formation and helps to dissolve cholesterol and fats.

Orange—is rich in compounds noted for their stress-reducing effects.

Suggested Use: Take 1 tablet 3 times daily as needed.

Body System(s) Affected: **Muscle and Bone, Immune System**.

Precautions: A study published in 2002 suggested that the acerola cherry can cause an allergic reaction similar to that caused by latex. If you have experienced such a reaction to latex, you may want to choose a different vitamin C supplement.

Super Cal™

Super Cal™ is formulated with calcium, potassium, and magnesium citrate (which is easier for the body to utilize) specifically for proper electrolyte balance, hormonal balance, and muscle and bone development. It is a **natural antioxidant**. This product is ideal for those on a vegetarian diet or diets that are restricted in calories or high in carbonated beverages. It was designed to help build the body. *Refer to the chart shown under MegaCal in this same section for a comparison of SuperCal to MegaCal and to other popular coral calcium supplements.*

Ingredients: Calcium citrate (242 mg per serving), magnesium citrate (119 mg per serving), zinc citrate (30 mg per serving), potassium citrate (60 mg per serving), boron (sodium borate: 1mg per serving), pure therapeutic-grade essential oils (as listed below), gelatin, stearic acid, and cellulose.

Essential Oils:

Marjoram—is a powerful muscle relaxant. It is anti-inflammatory and relaxing and is soothing to cartilage tissue.

Wintergreen—contains 99% methyl salicylate, which gives it cortisone-like properties. It may be beneficial for arthritis, rheumatism, tendinitis, and any other discomfort that is related to the inflammation of bones, muscles, and joints.

Lemongrass—helps repair connective tissue: when combined with marjoram, it helps stimulate the agents in the tissue to rejuvenate and reconnect.

Myrtle—is a decongestant to the respiratory system. It may help improve oxygenation and work as an expectorant in discharging mucus.

Suggested Use: Take two capsules right before each meal or as needed.

Body System(s) Affected: **Emotional Balance, Cardiovascular** and **Nervous Systems, Muscles and Bones**.

Companion Products: Essentialzyme, Ortho Ease and Ortho Sport Massage Oils, Power Meal, Sulfurzyme.

Companion Oils: Grounding, Harmony, PanAway, Valor.

Frequency: Approximately 78 MHz.

Thieves® Lozenges

Freshen your breath and soothe your sore throat while fighting bacteria with these natural lozenges. This lozenge is made from natural ingredients, including the sweeteners of sorbitol (derived from fruit and shown not to contribute to tooth decay) and xylitol (shown to inhibit plaque growth). The essential oils of lemon, orange, and peppermint provide natural flavoring and germ-fighting ability, especially when combined with the essential oil blend of Thieves.

Ingredients:

Hard Lozenges: Maltitol, lemon (*Citrus limon*) essential oil, Thieves® (a blend of clove, lemon, cinnamon, *Eucalyptus radiata*, and rosemary essential oils), peppermint (*Mentha piperita*) essential oil, pectin, and stevioside (*Stevia rebaudiana*).

Soft Lozenges: Xylitol, sorbitol, orange (*Citrus aurantium*) essential oil, Thieves® (a blend of clove, lemon, cinnamon, *Eucalyptus radiata*, and rosemary essential oils), peppermint (*Mentha piperita*) essential oil, cellulose, silicon dioxide, and vegetable-grade lubricant (sugar cane and palm oil).

Suggested Use: Dissolve 1 lozenge in mouth as needed.

Body System(s) Affected: **Immune System** and **Oral Hygiene**.

Precautions: Keep out of reach of children. Swallowing lozenges whole may cause choking.

Thyromin™

For nourishing the thyroid, balancing metabolism, and reducing fatigue, this product is a combination of specially-selected glandular nutrients, herbs, amino acids, and essential oils. All are grade A quality and are perfectly balanced to bring about the most beneficial biological and nutritional support to the thyroid. This product was not only designed to help build up the body but also to help lay a solid foundation for the healthy functioning of the many organs, tissues, and cells that are effected by the thyroid. It is a **natural antioxidant**.

Ingredients: Vitamin E (d alpha tocopheryl acid succinate: 200 IU per serving), iodine (derived from kelp: 100 mcg per serving), potassium (citrate: 30 mg per serving), parsley (*Petroselinum crispum*) leaf powder, bovine adrenal and pituitary extracts (20 mg each per serving), CoQ10, L-cystine, L-cysteine HCl, pure therapeutic-grade essential oils (as listed below), gelatin, carrageenan, magnesium carbonate, and magnesium stearate.

Essential Oils:

Peppermint—is purifying and stimulating to the conscious mind, anti-inflammatory, and helps with nerve regeneration. It also enhances digestion and increases endurance.

Spearmint—may balance and increase metabolism. It helps burn up fats and toxins in the body and aids digestion.

Myrtle—is a decongestant to the respiratory system. It may help improve oxygenation and work as an expectorant in discharging mucus.

Myrrh—is anti-inflammatory and antiseptic. It helps to decongest the prostate gland.

Suggested Use: One to two capsules daily, immediately before going to sleep.

Body System(s) Affected: **Hormonal System**.

Companion Products: Essentialzyme, FemiGen, JuvaTone, Mineral Essence, MultiGreens (enhances effect of Thyromin; take together for greater effect), Ultra Young+.

Companion Oils: EndoFlex, Clarity, En-R-Gee, JuvaFlex, Magnify Your Purpose.

Frequency: Approximately 52 MHz.

Comments: Thyromin can replace thyroid medication. If currently using thyroid medication, work with your health care professional before starting Thyromin to ensure that the thyroid medication is properly regulated/reduced. For those that are not on thyroid medication but wonder if their thyroid is working properly, here is a simple way to find out. Take your **basal cell temperature** with a mercury thermometer upon awakening first thing in the morning, even before you go to the bathroom or get out of bed. Put the thermometer under your arm pit and rest for 10 minutes. If it reads below 97.6° F (36.5° C) then your thyroid is low (hypothyroidism) and Thyromin may help. Start out with one capsule each night at bedtime and check your temperature in a couple of days. If it is not up to 97.6° F, add one more capsule, *but take it in the morning*. Continue adding more capsules and checking your basal cell temperature until it reads 97.6° F. *Alternate the additional capsules between morning and evening so that half of the number of capsules taken each day are immediately before bed and the other half are in the morning after rising*. Follow the directions on the bottle.

True Source™

This product is a unique blend of vitamins, minerals, antioxidants, and phytonutrients in their natural, synergistic, whole-food form. In fact, the colors of each capsule attest to the vibrancy of each of their contents. The green capsule gets its color from such ingredients as barley grass, spirulina, and chlorella. The purple-colored capsule is from pomegranate, dark grape, and wolfberry, while curcumin (curry) colors the yellow capsule. This nutrient-dense supplement may provide aid to many different areas of the body including eyes, heart, blood pressure, blood sugar, bones, joints, muscles, skin, and hair.

Ingredients:

Green Capsule: Vitamin A (alpha and beta carotene), vitamin C (ascorbic acid), vitamin D (cholecalciferol), vitamin E (mixed tocopherols), vitamin K (phytonadione), vitamin B1 (thiamin mononitrate), vitamin B2 (riboflavin), vitamin B3 (niacinamide), vitamin B6 (pyridoxine HCl), vitamin B6 (pyridoxal-5-phosphate), folic acid, vitamin B12 (methyl cobalamin), biotin (as biotin yeast), pantothenic acid (as calcium pantothenate), iodine (as potassium iodide), magnesium oxide, zinc (from zinc yeast complex), selenium (from selenium yeast complex), copper (from copper yeast complex), chromium (from chromium yeast complex), broccoli (*Brassica oleracea*) aerial parts, *Spirulina platensis* algae, chlorella algae, barley grass, orange (*Citrus sinensis*) fruit, MSM, olive (*Olea europaea*) leaf extract, Ningxia Wolfberry (*Lyceum barbarum*) fruit polysaccharides, l-leucine, tocotrienols (from natural palm oil), coral calcium, boron amino acid complex, lutein (from marigold flowers).

Purple Capsule: Vitamin A (alpha and beta carotene), vitamin C (ascorbic acid), vitamin D (cholecalciferol), vitamin E (mixed tocopherols), vitamin K (phytonadione), vitamin B1 (thiamin mononitrate), vitamin B2 (riboflavin), vitamin B3 (niacinamide), vitamin B6 (pyridoxine HCl), vitamin B6 (pyridoxal-5-phosphate), folic acid, vitamin B12 (methyl cobalamin), biotin yeast, pantothenic acid (as calcium pantothenate), iodine (as potassium iodide), magnesium oxide, zinc (from zinc yeast complex), selenium (from selenium yeast complex), copper (from copper yeast complex), chromium (from chromium yeast complex), broccoli (*Brassica oleracea*) aerial parts, pomegranate (40% ellagic acid), grape (*Vitis vinifera*) skin extract, resveratrol (from *Polygonum cuspidatum*), orange (*Citrus sinensis*) fruit, MSM, olive (*Olea europaea*) leaf extract, Ningxia Wolfberry (*Lyceum barbarum*) fruit polysaccharides, l-leucine, citrus flavonoids (from tangerine extract), tocotrienols (from natural palm oil), boron amino acid complex, lutein (from marigold flowers).

Yellow Capsule: Vitamin A (alpha and beta carotene), vitamin C (ascorbic acid), vitamin D (cholecalciferol), vitamin E (mixed tocopherols), vitamin K (phytonadione), vitamin B1 (thiamin mononitrate), vitamin B2 (riboflavin), vitamin B3 (niacinamide), vitamin B6 (pyridoxine HCl), vitamin B6 (pyridoxal-5-phosphate), folic acid, vitamin B12 (methylcobalamin), biotin (as biotin yeast), pantothenic acid (as calcium pantothenate), iodine (as potassium iodide), magnesium (as magnesium oxide), zinc (from zinc yeast complex), selenium (from selenium yeast complex), copper (from copper yeast complex), chromium (from chromium yeast complex), lecithin (choline), barley grass, orange (*Citrus sinensis*) fruit, curcumin (root and rhizome) extract, MSM (methylsulfonylmethane), olive (*Olea europaea*) leaf extract, Ningxia Wolfberry (*Lyceum barbarum*) fruit polysaccharides, l-leucine, citrus flavonoids (from tangerine extract), tocotrienols (from natural palm oil) , boron (as boron amino acid complex), lutein (from marigold flowers).

Other Ingredients: Gelatin, maltodextrin, silica, rice flour, mannitol, alginate, arabic gum, pea starch, modified food starch, sucrose, sodium ascorbate, dextrin, soy bean oil, and glucose.

Nutrient Content Totals in all three capsules together: vitamin A: 333.34 IU, vitamin C (from oranges): 20mg, vitamin D: 220 IU, vitamin E: 6.67 IU, vitamin K: 33.6 mcg, vitamin B1: .57mg, vitamin B2: .87mg, vitamin B3: 11.7mg, vitamin B6 (pyridoxine HCl): 2 mg, vitamin B6 (pyridoxal-5-phosphate): .67 mg, folic acid: 233.34 mcg, vitamin B12: 3.34mg, biotin: 100 mcg, pantothenic acid (vitamin B5):

2.67mg, Iodine: 55mcg, magnesium: 16.67mg, zinc: 1.67mg, selenium: 30 mcg, copper: .134 mg, chromium: 6.67 mcg

Suggested Use: Take one of each color capsule daily. Capsules can be taken separately or combined together in a single daily dose.

Body System(s) Affected: **Cardiovascular** and **Immune Systems, Muscles and Bones,** and **Skin and Hair**.

Companion Products: Balance Complete, NingXia Red, Longevity capsules, Omega Blue, Life 5

Ultra Young+™

This spray neutriceutical utilizes a unique nutrient delivery system through **oral mucosa absorption** (directly into the bloodstream through the dense network of blood vessels lining the mucus membrane inside the mouth). The advantages of this type of delivery system are protection from rapid first-pass metabolism by the liver and up to ten times the amount of nutrients being delivered to the system compared to the pill or capsule form of the same ingredients. Ultra Young+ is **not** a human growth hormone (hGH or somatotrophin) supplement. This unique product is formulated in such a way as to allow the body to use the hGH it produces naturally. Also, because low blood sugar levels are the key to hGH conversion and assimilation at the cellular level, Ultra Young+ contains Ningxia Wolfberry extract for its insulin–like action. *(Refer to the Wolfberry Crisp Bar at the end of this section for more information on the benefits of the Ningxia Wolfberry.)* This product also contains DHEA (*dehydroepiandrosterone*), which is normally produced in the adrenal gland and is a precursor to many important hormones. Like growth hormone, DHEA production steadily declines after the age of 20.

Ingredients: Vitamin A (beta-carotene: 33 IU per serving), vitamin E (d-alpha-tocopheryl acetate: 15 IU per serving), niacin (vitamin B3: 3 mg per serving), vitamin B6 (385 mcg per serving), zinc (as zinc proteinate: 5 mg per serving), selenium (as selenium yeast proteinate: 15 mcg per serving), L-arginine, *Vicia faba* leaf extract, pure therapeutic-grade essential oils (as listed below), DHEA (2.5 mg per serving), grape (*Vitis vinifera*) seed/skin extract, wolfberry (*Lycium barbarum*) fruit polysacharrides, L-ornithine, pyroglutamate, L-glutamine, L-glycine, L-lysine, GABA (gamma amino butyric acid), *Ginkgo biloba* leaf extract, stevia (*S. rebaudiana*) leaf extract, MSM (methylsulfonymethane), eleuthero (*Eleutherococcus senticosus*) root extract, bee pollen, ginger (*Zingiber officinale*) root extract, inosine, octacosanol, deionized water, pure grain alcohol (5% by volume), vegetable glycerin, hydrolyzed vegetable protein, natural raspberry flavor, essential trace mineral complex and potassium sorbate.

Essential Oils:

Sandalwood—helps strengthen the cardiovascular and lymphatic systems and increases oxygen levels around the pineal and pituitary glands.

Fleabane (*Conyza canadensis*)—is a rare essential oil studied by Daniel Pénoël, M.D., for its ability to stimulate the pancreas and liver and to counteract retarded puberty. It is a mood enhancer and a promoter of hGH.

Suggested Use: Three sprays, two to three times a day for six consecutive days; no sprays on the seventh day (this gives the body the opportunity to continue to generate its own supply of hGH). Vial contains approximately 30 servings (on average, 9 sprays per day). Shake gently before using.

Instructions On Use: Spray Ultra Young+ directly on inside cheeks and on roof of mouth. Avoid swallowing for one to two minutes. Spray upon waking, between meals, and/or just before retiring. Avoid spraying on the tongue, because this generates saliva, promotes swallowing, and reduces its effectiveness. (Comment: It is most effective when given time to penetrate the mucus membranes of mouth and directly enter the blood stream.) Ultra Young+ is best used two to four hours before or after meals with no snacking in between because high blood sugar levels reduce its effectiveness.

Body System(s) Affected: **Hormonal** and **Immune Systems**.

Companion Supplements: Be-Fit, JuvaTone, Manna Bars, Mineral Essence, MultiGreens, NingXia Red, Power Meal, Sulfurzyme, Thyromin, Wolfberry Crisp Bars.

Companion Oils: Frankincense, lavender, Abundance, En-R-Gee, EndoFlex, Envision, Joy, JuvaFlex, Live with Passion, Magnify Your Purpose, Release, Valor.

—More Information on the Human Growth Hormone (hGH)

Benefits:

1. Reverses aging of the thymus gland, a part of our immune system.
2. Dramatically raises levels of cytokines, interleukin 1 & 2, and tumor necrosis factor, all of which play a central role in the human immune system.
3. Improves fat-to-lean ratios.
4. Reverses heart disease.
5. Boosts bone formation.
6. Firms and tightens skin by activating the production of skin proteins, collagen, and elastin.
7. Increases energy.
8. Lifts depression.
9. Restores deep sleep.

Supplementation is not enough: Taking a growth hormone (hGH) supplement is not the answer, since research shows that most people continue to produce ample amounts of the human growth hormone well into their advanced years. The problem is not a lack of hGH but the inability of the liver to convert it to IGF-1. IGF-1 is responsible for actually carrying out the actions of the chemical message sent by hGH. Without a properly functioning liver, IGF-1 conversion does not take place and hGH has a limited effect in the body. This is why Ultra Young+ contains ingredients that dramatically facilitate the conversion of hGH to IGF-1 in the liver—ingredients such as amino acids, the essential oil of *Conyza canadensis*, zinc, vitamin B6, Ningxia Wolfberry extract, and more.

Ultra Young+ contains the anterior pituitary peptide isolate because it is a combination of all hormones secreted by the pituitary gland. Although hGH is the most important, the other hormones must be supplemented to help buffer and activate the effects of hGH. Without them, the body is being stimulated on only one level, a one-sided approach that is inherently abnormal.

Tips for maximizing Ultra Young's benefits:

1. Exercise. Rigorous exercises like running or weight lifting increase hGH levels.
2. Fasting. Extended periods (4 to 8 hours or more) of low blood sugar increase hGH levels and cell receptivity to hGH.
3. Thyroid, pancreas, and liver support. For Ultra Young+ to work at its best, the liver needs to be supported and the thyroid and pancreas need to be functioning normally. For best results, take one to two Thyromin and two to four JuvaTone a day with Ultra Young+.
4. Use lavender and frankincense. These oils are principle ingredients in supplements that support the pituitary. Because essential oils have the same lipid structure as the cell membrane, they have an unmatched ability to penetrate cell walls and transport hormones into the cells.

Wolfberry Crisp™ Bar

The Wolfberry Crisp™ Bar is a delicious and nutritious whole-food bar, made with the Ningxia Wolfberry and other nutrient-packed natural ingredients. With over 15 grams of protein per serving, this bar makes an ideal meal replacement.

Ingredients: Protein complex with soy (isolated soy protein, rice flour, malt and salt) and whey (rice flour, whey protein isolate, whey protein concentrate and calcium carbonate), organic blue agave (*Agave tequilana*) nectar, raw almond butter, Ningxia Wolfberry (*Lycium barbarum*) fruit, raw pumpkin seeds, raw cashews, raw walnuts, unsweetened carob chips (carob powder, nonfat milk powder, whey powder, fractionated palm kernal oil, and soy lecithin), pure vanilla (*Vanilla planifolia*) bean extract, and natural banana flavoring.

Suggested Use: Eat one bar as desired for a meal replacement or high-energy snack.

Body System(s) Affected: **Digestive** and **Immune Systems, Muscles and Bones**.

Companion Products: Be-Fit, ComforTone, Essentialzyme, ICP, JuvaPower, JuvaSpice, KidScents Mighty Mist/Vites, Manna Bars, Master Formula His/Hers, MultiGreens, NingXia Red, Thyromin.

Companion Oils: Abundance, Citrus Fresh, EndoFlex, Envision, Juva Cleanse, Live with Passion, Magnify Your Purpose.

—Benefits of the Ningxia Wolfberry

A group of research scientists from Natural Science University in Beijing, China, discovered a village in Inner Mongolia. Some of the people of the village were 120 or 130 years old and had no signs of cancer, arthritis, AIDS, or lupus. They lived predominately on the wolfberry and vegetables from their gardens. This prompted research into the amazing benefits of the wolfberry. The wolfberry is over 12% protein by weight, has 18 amino acids (6 times higher in proportion than bee pollen), 21 trace minerals, 6 essential fatty acids, vitamins B1, B2, B6, C, and E, calcium, betaine, polyphenols (including a range of carotenoids), and fiber. *(For more information on the amazing research and powerful benefits of the Ningxia Wolfberry, refer to the book, Discovery of the Ultimate Superfood)* The following is a sample of some of the amazing benefits of the Ningxia Wolfberry.

Possibly Supports the Immune System: According to scientific research in China, the wolfberry contains compounds known as *lycium polysaccharides*, which have been studied for their effects on immune function. One study involving cancer patients found that the wolfberry triggered an increase in both *lymphocyte transformation rate* and *white blood cell count* (measures of immune function). In another study, it was shown to increase *phagocytosis* (another index of immune function). Yet another study showed that the consumption of wolfberry led to a strengthening of immunoglobulin A levels (a part of our immunity).

A Powerful Antioxidant: In one clinical study of individuals who consumed wolfberries, *superoxide dismutase (SOD)* levels in the blood increased 48% while *hemoglobin* increased 12%. Even better, *lipid peroxide* levels dropped 65%.

Possibly Inhibit Tumor Growth: From July 1982 to January 1984, the Ningxia Institute of Drug Inspection conducted a clinical experiment using multi-index screening. They concluded the following: The fruits and pedicels of the wolfberry were effective in increasing white blood cells, protecting the liver, and relieving hypertension. The alcoholic extract of wolfberry fruits inhibited tumor growth in mice by 58%, and the protein of wolfberry displayed an insulin-like action that was effective in promoting fat decomposition and reducing blood sugar.

Possibly Reverse Aging: A clinical experiment by the Ningxia Institute of Drug Inspection (Register No. 870306, from October 1982 to May 1985) studied the effects of wolfberry on the blood of aged volunteers. The results were published by the State Scientific and Technological Commission of China, and the authors concluded that the wolfberry caused the blood of older people to **noticeably revert to a younger state**.

Great Potential for High Performance Gains: Wolfberry has a high concentration of the branched-chain amino acid *L-leucine*. Inside the body, L-leucine is converted into a powerful compound called HMB (beta-hydroxy beta-methylbutyrate). According to Richard Passwater, Ph.D., a noted researcher in the field of health-maintenance, "HMB showed that it lowered total and LDL cholesterol levels in blood and helped strengthen the immune system while building muscles and burning body fat. This news is certainly of interest to body builders and other athletes, but it may also become of interest to cancer, AIDS, and muscular dystrophy patients."

Yacon Syrup

Extracted from the tubers of yacon plants grown in the Andes mountains of South America, this low-calorie sweetener is a natural alternative that can be used in a manner similar to honey or maple syrup. This syrup has also been touted for its ability to sweeten with no glycemic index and contains 21 amino acids, 18 minerals, and vitamin C.

Ingredients: Yacon syrup (*Smallanthus sonchifolius*).

Suggested Use: Use in cooking in the same way that you would substitute honey for sugar (approximately 3/4 cup for 1 cup of sugar, reducing liquids).

Body System(s) Affected: Digestive System.

Companion Products: Slique Tea, Stevia Extract.

Notes & New Products

Use this section to write your own notes and information on new products.

Personal Guide

Application Notes and Explanations

1. Next to each oil or blend listed in this section is a symbol (or symbols) that indicates the recommended application method(s) of that oil for the specific condition.

   A: **Aromatic** means that the oils are inhaled through the mouth and nose. This could include inhaling the aroma of the oil directly from the bottle or inhaling the aroma of the oil after it has been applied to the hands or to another material, such as a tissue or a cotton wick. It could also mean breathing in the vapor or mist of an oil that has been diffused or sprayed into the surrounding air.

   T: **Topical** means that the oils are applied directly to the skin, hair, or other surface of the body. This can be through massage, bath, direct application of the oils, or application of the oils within a cream, lotion, bath gel, or soap. While many oils can be applied neat (without dilution), others may need to be diluted with V-6 Oil or with another vegetable or carrier oil before topical application, especially in cases of young or sensitive skin. Refer to the Single Oil section of this book for recommended dilutions.

   I: **Internal** means that the oils are taken orally as a dietary supplement. This is done either by adding the oil to a food or beverage that is then consumed or by swallowing a capsule with the oil inside.

   Specific application instructions are usually listed for each condition, and further detailed information on application techniques can be found in the Science & Application section of this book.

2. Oils and application recommendations are color-coded as **Primary Recommendations** (listed in order of highest recommendation to lowest recommendation when research and consensus between essential oil experts warrants such an ordering) and **Other Recommendations** (listed alphabetically). It is not necessary to use all of the oils listed. Try one oil at a time. If you do not see a change soon, try a different one. What one person needs may be different from what another person needs. (Hint: Use kinesiology testing to determine which oils are right for you.)

3. A subscripted "F" (i.e. $_{F}$clary sage) means the oil has been used medicinally in France.

4. *Neat* means to apply the oil without diluting it with a vegetable oil.

5. If essential oils get into your eyes by accident or if they burn the skin a little, do not try to remove the oils with water. Water will only drive the oils deeper into the tissue. It is best to dilute the essential oils with a pure vegetable oil.

6. The FDA has approved some essential oils for internal use and given them the following designations: GRAS (Generally Regarded As Safe for human consumption), FA (Food Additive), or FL (FLavoring agent). *These designations are listed in the Single Oil Summary Information chart in the Appendix of this book under Safety Data.*

7. Using some oils such as lemon, orange, grapefruit, mandarin, bergamot, angelica, etc. before or during exposure to direct sunlight or UV rays (tanning beds, etc.) may cause a rash, pigmentation, or even severe burns. These oils are designated as photosensitive (PH) or extremely photosensitive (PH*) in the Single Oil or Blend Summary Information in the Appendix of this book. It is best to check the safety data for the oils to be used and then either dilute the oils and test on a small area or avoid their use altogether.

8. Caution should be used with oils such as clary sage, sage, and fennel during pregnancy. These oils contain active constituents with hormone-like activity and could possibly stimulate adverse reactions in the mother, although there are no recorded cases in humans.
9. Particular care should be taken when using cinnamon bark, lemongrass, oregano, and thyme—as they are some of the strongest and most caustic oils. It is best to dilute them with a pure vegetable oil.
10. In this document, several homemade blends are suggested. However, this is done with great hesitancy. Some of the blends listed come from individuals who may not be experts in the field of essential oils and aromatherapy. Rather than mix the oils together, it may be better to **layer the oils**; that is, apply a drop or two of one oil, rub it in, and then apply another oil. If dilution is necessary, a pure vegetable oil can be applied on top.
11. When someone is out of electrical balance, try the following:
    A. Place a drop or two of Harmony in one hand, and then rub the palms of both hands together in a clockwise motion.
    B. Place one hand over the thymus (heart chakra) and the other hand over the navel.
    C. Take 3 deep breaths and switch hands; then take 3 more deep breaths. (Refer to Allergies in this section for more information).
12. Less is often better; use 1–3 drops of oil and no more than 6 drops at a time. Stir and rub on in a clockwise direction.
13. When applying oils to **infants** and to **small children**, dilute 1–2 drops of pure essential oil with ½–1 teaspoon (tsp.) of a pure vegetable oil (V-6 Oil). If the oils are used in the bath, always use a bath gel base as a dispersing agent for the oils. See **Babies/Children** for more information about the recommended list of oils for babies and children.
14. The body absorbs oils the fastest through inhalation (breathing) and second fastest through application to the feet or to the ears. Testing on the thyroid, heart, and pancreas showed that the oils reached these organs in three seconds. Layering oils can increase the rate of **absorption**.
15. When an oil causes **discomfort,** it is because it is pulling toxins, heavy metals, chemicals, poisons, parasites, and mucus from the system. Either stop applying the oils for a short time, to make sure your body isn't eliminating (detoxifying) too fast, or dilute the oils until the body catches up with the releasing. Toxins go back into the system if they cannot be released.
16. When the cell wall thickens, oxygen cannot get in. The life expectancy of a cell is 120 days (4 months). Cells also divide, making duplicate cells. If the cell is diseased, new diseased cells will be made. When we stop the **mutation** of the diseased cells (create healthy cells), we stop the disease. Essential oils have the ability to penetrate and carry nutrients through the cell wall to the nucleus and improve the health of the cell.
17. Each oil has a **frequency**, and each of our organs and body parts has a frequency. The frequency of an oil is attracted by a like frequency within the body. Lower oil frequencies become a sponge for negative energy. The frequency is what stays in the body to maintain the longer-lasting effects of the oil.

    Low frequencies can make physical changes in the body.

    Middle frequencies can make emotional changes in the body.

    High frequencies can make spiritual changes in the body.

    A. Average frequency of the human body during the day time is between 62 and 68 Megahertz (MHz). Bone frequency is 38 to 43 MHz. Frequencies from the neck down vary between 62 and 68 MHz.
    B. Spiritual frequencies range from 92 to 360 MHz.

18. *Use extreme caution when diffusing cinnamon bark* because it may burn the nostrils if you put your nose directly next to the nebulizer of the diffuser.

19. When traveling by air, you should always have your oils hand-checked. X-ray machines may interfere with the frequency of the oils. *See Comments under Asthma for a discussion on plastic nasal inhalers for using oils on the airplane instead of taking the bottles of oil.*

20. Keep oils away from the light and heat, although they seem to do fine in temperatures up to 90 degrees. If stored properly, they can maintain their maximum potency for many years.

The following information will be useful to those who are familiar with the art and technique of blending. (*See the Science and Application section of Reference Guide for Essential Oils for more information.*)

1st—The Personifier oils (1–5% of blend) have very sharp, strong, and long-lasting fragrances. They also have dominant properties with strong therapeutic action.

> **Oils in this classification may include the following:** Angelica, cardamom, German chamomile, cinnamon, cistus, clary sage, clove, coriander, ginger, helichrysum, mandarin, neroli, nutmeg, orange, patchouli, peppermint, petitgrain, rose, spearmint, tangerine, tarragon, wintergreen, ylang ylang

2nd—The Enhancer oil (50–80% of blend) should be the predominant oil as it serves to enhance the properties of the other oils in the blend. Its fragrance is not as sharp as the personifier's and is usually of a shorter duration.

> **Oils in this classification may include the following:** Basil, bergamot, Roman chamomile, black cumin, cajeput, cedarwood, dill, eucalyptus, frankincense, galbanum, geranium, grapefruit, hyssop, jasmine, lavender, lemon, lemongrass, lime, marjoram, melaleuca (tea tree), melissa, myrtle, orange, oregano, palmarosa, patchouli, petitgrain, ravensara, rose, rosemary, sage, spruce, thyme, wintergreen

3rd—The Equalizer oils (10–15% of blend) create balance and synergy among the oils contained in the blend. Their fragrance is also not as sharp as the personifier and is of a shorter duration.

> **Oils in this classification may include the following:** Basil, bergamot, cedarwood, Roman chamomile, cypress, fennel, fir, frankincense, geranium, ginger, hyssop, jasmine, juniper, lavender, lemongrass, lime, marjoram, melaleuca (tea tree), melissa, myrrh, myrtle, neroli, oregano, pine, rose, rosewood, sandalwood, spruce, tarragon, thyme.

4th—The Modifier oils (5–8% of blend) have a mild and short fragrance. These oils add harmony to the blend.

> **Oils in this classification may include the following:** Angelica, bergamot, cardamom, coriander, eucalyptus, fennel, grapefruit, hyssop, jasmine, lavender, lemon, mandarin, melissa, myrrh, neroli, petitgrain, rose, rosewood, sandalwood, tangerine, ylang ylang.

The Science and Application section of the Reference Guide for Essential Oils contains more information on the art of blending. In that same section, another method of blending explains how to use "notes (top, middle, and base notes)" to help determine how different single oils are to be blended together. It also includes an odor intensity chart that further assists in the blending process. Refer to that section for more details and instructions on blending.

There are some tools that make blending much easier and much more enjoyable. Abundant Health offers dispensing syringes with corresponding caps called Adapta-Caps™ that fit on your 15 ml bottles (caps are available for other size bottles as well) and allow for accurate, measured dispensing of the oils. There are even 1 ml syringes with drop markings for easy blend creations. Look for these dispensing tools at www.AbundantHealth4u.com under Glass and Plastic Products.

Abandoned: *See also Emotions.*

Oils—ATAcceptance, ATForgiveness, ATValor.

A—Diffuse into the air. Inhale directly or applied to a tissue or a cotton wick.

T—Dilute, and use as massage oil. Apply to auricular emotional points.

Abscess: *See also Antifungal, Antibacterial, Infection, or Oral Conditions: Abscess.*

> *I had an abscess tooth. The dentist and the specialist he referred me to insisted I have a root canal. I used 3 to 4 drops of Thieves in a glass of water to gargle with. Then I used a mixture of half Thieves and half olive oil and rubbed this on both sides of my gums on the infected area. I then used the Dentarome Plus toothpaste. It has been 2 months and my mouth is fine.*
> ***-Submitted by K. Ernst***

Oils—TAThieves, TAmelaleuca, Tthyme, TAPurification, Tbergamot, Telemi, Tfrankincense, Tgalbanum, TAlavender, TAMelrose, Tmyrrh, TRoman chamomile, Twintergreen.

Blend #1—**Dilute equal parts** Roman chamomile, lavender, and melaleuca (tea tree) in V-6 Oil, and apply on location.

Supplements—Life 5 (probiotic), Super B.

***Comments—Some sources recommend a nontoxic diet and an increase in liquid intake.

—Mouth

Oils—T$_F$Lavender.

T—To reduce swelling, pain, inflammation, and to draw out toxins, it may help to apply the oil(s) with a hot compress. Put Thieves on a rolled up gauze, and place over abscess to pull out the infection.

A—Diffuse into the air.

Absent Minded: *See also Memory.*

Oils—ARosemary[1], Apeppermint[2], Asage lavender[3], ABrain Power, AClarity, Abasil, Acardamom, Afrankincense, Alemongrass, AM-Grain, Asandalwood.

Supplements—Mineral Essence, MultiGreens, Omega Blue, OmegaGize[3], Power Meal, Sulfurzyme, True Source (whole food multi-nutrient), Ultra Young+.

A—Diffuse into the air. Inhale directly or applied to a tissue or a cotton wick.

Abundance:

Oils—ATAbundance, ATcinnamon bark, ATAcceptance, ATbergamot, ATcypress, ATHarmony, ATGathering.

—Attracts

Oils—ATAbundance, ATcinnamon bark.

—Money

Oils—ATGinger, ATpatchouli.

***Comments—One waitress demonstrated her luck when she wore Abundance and Harmony together; she received a whopping $120.00 tip! Who knows, it may work for you too!

A—Diffuse into the air.

T—Wear oil as perfume or cologne.

Abuse:

Abuse is the harmful treatment or use of something or someone. Abuse has many different forms: physical, sexual, verbal, spiritual, psychological, etc. Abuse in all of its forms often has long-lasting negative effects on the person or thing abused.

Oils—TA SARA (releases memory and trauma of sexual or ritual abuse), TA Trauma Life, TA Release, TA melissa, TA Acceptance, TA Brain Power, TA Citrus Fresh, TA Christmas Spirit, TA geranium, TA Forgiveness, TA Grounding, TA Harmony, TA Hope, TA Humility, TA Inner Child, TA Joy, TA lavender, TA Peace & Calming, TA 3 Wise Men, TA sandalwood, TA Surrender, T Tranquil (roll-on), TA Valor, TA ylang ylang.

Supplements—Power Meal, Super B, Super C / Super C Chewable.

—By Father

Oils—AT Sacred Mountain (empowers self), AT Forgiveness, AT lavender.

—By Mother

Oils—Forgiveness, geranium, lavender.

***Comments—*Refer to the page on Auricular Emotional Therapy in the Science & Application section of this book for the points where oils can be applied.*

—Feelings of Revenge

Oils—T Forgiveness (around navel), T Present Time (on thymus), T Surrender (on sternum over heart), T Tranquil (roll-on).

—Protection or Balance

Oils—T Harmony (over thymus; on energy centers/chakras), T White Angelica (on shoulders).

—Sexual/Ritual

Oils—T Forgiveness (around navel), T Release (liver Vita Flex point on feet; under nose), T SARA (over area of abuse), TA Harmony, TA Joy, TA Present Time, TA sage, TA 3 Wise Men, TA Trauma Life, TA Valor, and TA White Angelica.

—Espousal

Oils—TA Release, TA Forgiveness, TA Valor, TA Acceptance, TA Envision, TA Joy, TA Trauma Life.

—Suicidal

Oils—T Hope (on rim of ears), TA Brain Power, TA melissa, TA Present Time.

T—Apply 1 drop in area indicated, or apply 1 drop of the desired oils on each chakra to allow blocked emotions to come out. Apply to auricular emotional points. Dilute, and use as massage oil.

A—Diffuse into the air. Inhale directly.

Accidents: *See Emotions.*

Oils—AT Trauma Life.

A—Diffuse into the air. Inhale directly.

T—Apply 1 drop of the desired oils on each chakra to allow blocked emotions to come out. Apply to auricular emotional points. Dilute, and use as massage oil.

Aches/Pains: *See Pain*

Acidosis: *See also Alkaline and pH Balance.*

Oils—I Lemon, TI Thieves (dissolves and digests acid in the interstitial tissues), T myrrh, IT peppermint.

I—Add 1 drop to 8 oz. rice milk or other beverage and drink. Add 3–5 drops oil to 3–5 drops V-6 Oil in capsule, and swallow.

T—Dilute, and apply 1 drop of the desired oils on location. Add 3–5 drops to 1 Tbs. V-6 Oil, and massage on location. Apply to Vita-Flex points.

Supplements—AlkaLime (acid-neutralizing mineral), Balance Complete, JuvaPower (loaded with acid-binding foods), Life 5 (probiotic) Mineral Essence, MultiGreens (for alkaline/acid balance), Power Meal.

******Comments***—Cancer and candida need an acid condition in order to thrive and spread. In acidic conditions, the oils will neutralize the acid but are consumed in the process and are not able to perform their physiological functions. Increase your use of the oils and take other measures to reduce acid levels in the body. The body can only heal in an alkaline state.

Acid-Forming Foods—Avoid meat, dairy products, whole wheat or rye bread, coffee, tea, wine, beer, root beer, cider, yeast products, soy sauce, cold cereals, potato chips, etc.

Neutralizing Foods—Raw apple cider vinegar is an acid neutralizer. Add a few drops of Thieves to 2 oz. of raw apple cider vinegar and drink in the morning and evening to help reduce acid levels in the body.

Acidosis is a condition of over-acidity in the blood and body tissues. When the body loses its alkaline reserve, pleomorphic virus, bacteria, yeast, and fungus take over and cause degenerative diseases such as, diabetes, cancer, AIDS, arteriosclerosis, arthritis, osteoporosis, chronic fatigue, etc.

Symptoms of acidosis *may include frequent sighing, insomnia, water retention, recessed eyes, rheumatoid arthritis, migraine headaches, abnormally low blood pressure, and alternating constipation and diarrhea.*

Causes of acidosis *may include improper diet, kidney, liver, and adrenal disorders, emotional disturbances, fever, and an excess of niacin, vitamin C, and aspirin.*

Oxygen *reduces the acidity of the blood. All essential oils contain oxygen. We like to flavor our water with 1-2 drops of lemon or peppermint oil. Lemon has the ability to counteract acidity in the body. The citric acid found in lemons is neutralized during digestion, giving off carbonates and bicarbonates of potassium and calcium, which helps maintain the alkalinity of the system.*

Acne: *See also Hormonal Imbalance, Scarring, Skin, and Stress.*

▸▸*Acne is a deep blockage of a skin pore by dead skin cells, tiny hairs, and oil secreted by the sebaceous glands located near the hair follicles in the face, neck, and back. This blockage causes red, irritating blemishes (pimples) on the skin (most commonly found on the oil-producing parts of the body such as the face, chest, back, upper arms, and back of neck).*

Oils—ᵀMelaleuca (tea tree)[4], ᵀ$_F$German chamomile, ᵀ$_F$juniper, ᵀ$_F$lavender, ᵀ$_F$rosewood, ᵀMelrose, ᵀbergamot, ᵀcedarwood, ᵀClarity (on temples), ᵀclary sage, ᵀclove, ᵀeucalyptus, ᵀ*Eucalyptus radiata*, ᵀfrankincense, ᵀGentle Baby, ᵀgeranium, ᵀImmuPower (pimples in ears), ᵀlemon, ᵀlemongrass, ᵀmarjoram, ᵀmyrtle, ᵀpatchouli, ᵀpetitgrain, ᵀPurification, ᵀRaven, ᵀravensara, ᵀRC, ᵀrosemary, ᵀsage, ᵀsage lavender, ᵀsandalwood, ᵀSensation, ᵀspearmint, ᵀthyme, ᵀvetiver, ᵀyarrow.

Personal Care—Essential Beauty Serum - Acne-Prone Skin Blend, A·R·T Skin Care System, Prenolone/Prenolone+, Progessence/Progessence Plus, Rose Ointment, Sensation Massage Oil.

Supplements—ComforTone, Digest + Cleanse, ICP, Essentialzyme, Essentialzymes-4, JuvaTone, and Sulfurzyme. Cleansing the colon may help (*See Cleansing*).

Acne *is often a result of seborrhea (an overproduction of fat from the sebaceous glands), which can oftentimes be traced back to a hormonal imbalance. Stress is another reason for increased sebum production. Consequently, it may be of help to use oils that balance the hormones and reduce stress.*

Essential oil treatments combined with a good diet (lots of vegetables and lots of water), exercise, and increased lymphatic and circulatory flow, will allow the toxic wastes to leave the body as the oxygen and nutrients reach the skin in greater proportions.

One of the best ways to release toxins through the skin is to sweat. Chamomile, hyssop, juniper, lavender, rosemary, and thyme contain sudorific properties and may facilitate the sweating process. The antibacterial and anti-inflammatory oils may assist in the healing process.

—Adult Onset

Adult-onset acne affects many men and women at some point in their adult lives. Possible causes are thought to be hormones, cosmetic products, stress, and increased bacteria. Women often experience increased breakouts with the onset of menstruation each month.

Personal Care—Prenolone/Prenolone+, Progessence/Progessence Plus if the acne stems from a hormonal imbalance.

—Cellular Regenerative

When an injury occurs to the skin, such as the irritation caused by acne, scar tissue will form if the cells are unable to regenerate (replace) themselves.

Oils—**T**Palmarosa, **T**rosewood.

—Healing

Oils—Use antibacterial and anti-inflammatory oils like **T**melaleuca (tea tree)[4], **T**Melrose, **T**geranium, and **T**rosewood.

—Infectious

Oils—**T**Clove.

—Menstrual

Premenstrual or mid-menstrual cycle acne may be helped by balancing the hormones.

Personal Care—Prenolone/Prenolone+, Progessence/Progessence Plus.

Supplements—CortiStop (Women's), FemiGen, Super B.

—Rosacea (Acne Rosacea)

Oils—**T**Lavender. Dilute with V-6 Oil and apply daily after washing face with Orange Blossom Facial Wash and before applying Sandalwood Moisture Cream. Can also add extra lavender oil to Sandalwood Moisture Cream.

Personal Care—Essential Beauty Serum - Acne-Prone Skin Blend, Orange Blossom Facial Wash, Sandalwood Moisture Cream.

***Rosacea** is a chronic, acne-like condition of the facial skin that typically first appears as a flushing or subtle redness on the cheeks, nose, chin or forehead that comes and goes. Left untreated, the condition progresses and the redness becomes more persistent, bumps and pimples appear, and small dilated blood vessels may become visible. In some cases the eyes may be affected, causing them to be irritated and bloodshot and, according to some doctors, even blindness can occur. In the more advanced cases, the nose becomes red and swollen from excess tissue. Currently, this condition can only be controlled.*

—Toxin Release

Oils—Use sudorific oils like **T**chamomile, **T**hyssop, **T**juniper, **T**lavender, **T**rosemary, and **T**thyme to help promote sweating.

T—Apply one of the above oils on location; or try putting about 10 drops of an oil into a small spray bottle with distilled water, and mist your face several times a day.

ADD/ADHD (Attention Deficit Disorder/Attention Deficit Hyperactive Disorder):

See also Hyperactivity.

Attention Deficit Disorder or Attention Deficit/Hyperactive Disorder is a psychological condition characterized by inattentiveness, restlessness, and difficulty concentrating. Although most individuals exhibit all of these symptoms at some point, ADD is characterized by a frequency and duration of these symptoms that are inappropriate to an individual's age.

Oils—**TA**Lavender[6], **TA**Citrus Fresh, **T**RutaVaLa, **T**Tranquil (roll-on), **TA**ledum.

Blend Ideas—Lavender with basil (on crown), Harmony, or Peace & Calming; Basil with Clarity; Frankincense with Valor. Apply 1–3 drops of any of these blends on the bottoms of the feet and on the spine; Diffuse.

Supplements—NingXia Red (provides a full range of vitamins, trace minerals, amino acids, and essential fatty acids), Omega Blue (absolutely necessary), OmegaGize[3], Allerzyme (aids the digestion of sugars, starches, fats, and proteins), Digest + Cleanse, Mineral Essence.

*****Comments**—Avoid sweeteners such as sugar and corn syrup. Eliminate caffeine and food additives from diet. Individuals who have ADD often have high aluminum toxicity.

—Chelating Agent

Oils—**T**Helichrysum.

—Sleeping

Oils—**A**Peace & Calming or **A**Gentle Baby.

T—Dilute 3–5 drops of oil in 1 Tbs. V-6 Oil and use as a massage oil. Add 1–2 drops to warm bathwater (or combine with 1/4 cup bath salts and add to warm bathwater) and bathe.

A—Diffuse into the air.

Addictions:

▸▸*An addiction is an obsession, compulsion, or extreme psychological dependence that interferes with an individual's ability or desire to function normally. Common addictions include drugs, alcohol, coffee, tobacco, sugar, video games, work, gambling, money, explicit images, compulsive overeating, etc.*

Oils—**TA**Acceptance, **TA**JuvaFlex, **TA**bergamot (helps with over indulgences), **TA**Peace & Calming, **TA**Purification, **TA**calamus (tobacco), **TA**GLF.

Supplements—JuvaTone, Digest + Cleanse, Mineral Essence, Super C / Super C Chewable.

Recipe #1—This recipe has worked for individuals who are trying to break addictions. Use JuvaPower, JuvaTone, ComforTone, JuvaFlex and Acceptance together.

—Alcohol (to stop drinking):

Oils—**TA**Purification, **TA**Peace & Calming. Do not use clary sage and alcohol together; it may result in nightmares. For professional assistance, contact the local chapter of Alcoholics Anonymous.

—Alcoholism

▸▸*Alcoholism is an extreme dependence on alcohol that interferes with an individual's social, physical, and mental health.*

Oils—**AT**Rosemary, **AT**fennel, **AT**juniper (Alternative Medicine—A Definitive Guide, p. 492). Can also use **AT**Acceptance, **AT**elemi, **AT**Forgiveness, **AT**GLF, **AT**helichrysum, **AT**Joy, **AT**JuvaFlex, **AT**lavender, **AT**Motivation, **AT**orange, **AT**Roman chamomile, **AT**rosemary verbenon, **AT**Transformation, **AT**Surrender.

Supplements—Work on cleaning out the colon and liver with JuvaPower/JuvaSpice, Balance Complete or the Cleansing Trio, Digest + Cleanse, and JuvaTone or the Master Cleanser (*See Cleansing*). Mineral Essence, Power Meal, Thyromin.

—Coffee

Oils—**AT**Bergamot, **AT**calamus.

—Drugs

Oils—TACumin[6], TAPeace & Calming, TAPurification, TAgrapefruit (withdrawal), TAbasil, TAbergamot, TAeucalyptus, TAfennel, TAlavender, TAmarjoram, TAnutmeg, TAorange, TARoman chamomile, TAsandalwood, TAwintergreen.

Supplements—Super C / Super C Chewable (at least 250 mg per day).

—Smoking/Tobacco

Oils—ABlack pepper[7]. Use Recipe #1 above. Applying either clove or Thieves to the tongue before lighting up helps remove the desire to smoke. Calamus may also help.

***Comments—*One individual used JuvaTone to break a habit of smoking 2 ½ packs of cigarettes a day for 20 years. It only took him 3–5 days!*

—Sugar

Oils—TDill (on wrists to help remove addiction to sweets), TAPurification, TAPeace & Calming.

Supplements—Allerzyme (aids the digestion of sugars, starches, fats, and proteins), Cleansing Trio (ComforTone, Essentialzyme, Essentialzymes-4, and ICP).

—Withdrawal

Oils—ATGrapefruit, TAcumin, Tdill (to the wrists helps reduce the sweating that often accompanies withdrawal), TAlavender, TAmarjoram, TAnutmeg, TAorange, TAsandalwood.

T—Apply to temples and to Vita Flex points on the feet. Apply to stomach, abdomen, liver area, and feet.

A—Diffuse into the air. Inhale directly or applied to tissue or a cotton wick.

Addison's Disease: *See Adrenal Glands: Addison's Disease.*

Adenitis: *See also Lymphatic System.*

▸▸ *Adenitis is an acute or chronic inflammation of the lymph glands or nodes. Drink a lot of water to help remove the toxins from the body.*

Oils—TRosemary, Tpine, Tsage. Could also try Tgarlic or Tonion.

T—Dilute as recommended, and apply on location.

Adrenal Glands: *See also Endocrine System, Lupus, Thyroid.*

▸▸ *The adrenal glands are two small glands located on top of the kidneys. The inner part of the adrenal gland, called the medulla, is responsible for producing adrenalin, a hormone that helps control blood pressure, heart rate, and sweating. The outer part of the adrenal gland, called the cortex, is responsible for producing corticosteroids, hormones that help control metabolism and help regulate inflammation, water levels, and levels of electrolytes such as sodium and potassium. Nutmeg displays properties similar to these hormones. When the adrenal glands are working properly, it is easier to correct low thyroid function.*

Oils—TNutmeg (increases energy; supports adrenal glands), TEndoFlex, TEn-R-Gee, TForgiveness, TJoy.

Blend #1—Add 3 drops clove, 4 drops nutmeg, and 6 drops rosemary to 1 tsp. V-6 Oil. Apply 4–5 drops of this mixture to kidney areas, and cover with a hot compress. Also apply 1–2 drops of mixture to Vita Flex kidney points on the feet, and work in with fingers using the Vita Flex technique.

—Addison's Disease:

»» *Addison's disease is an autoimmune disease where the body's own immune cells attack the adrenal glands and either severely limit or completely shut down the production of the adrenal cortex hormones. Extreme fluid and mineral loss are the life-threatening results.*

Oils—ᵀNutmeg (increases energy; supports adrenal glands), ᵀEn-R-Gee, ᵀEndoFlex, ᵀJoy, ᵀsage (combine with nutmeg).

Supplements—Sulfurzyme (shown to slow or reverse autoimmune diseases), EndoGize, ImmuPro, Master Formula His/Hers, Mineral Essence (help supplement mineral loss), MultiGreens, Super B.

—Cushing's Disease

»» *Cushing's disease is characterized by an overabundance of corticosteroids (such as cortisol) in the body—typically caused by over-production of these steroids by the adrenal glands. This overproduction can be caused by a growth in the adrenal glands or by a tumor in the thyroid, causing production of too much corticotropin (the hormone that stimulates production of corticosteroids in the adrenal gland). This syndrome can also be caused by taking artificial cortisone or cortisone-like substances. Symptoms of excessive corticosteroids include weight gain, muscle loss and weakness, bruising, and osteoporosis.*

Oils—ᵀLemon, ᵀbasil, ᵀForgiveness, ᵀImmuPower, ᵀJoy, ᵀThieves.

Supplements—ImmuPro, Inner Defense.

—Schmidt's Syndrome *See also Addison's Disease above.*

»» *This syndrome refers specifically to an auto-immune disorder that causes Addison's disease in combination with decreased thyroid function.*

Oils—ᵀNutmeg (increases energy; supports adrenal glands), ᵀEn-R-Gee, ᵀEndoFlex, ᵀJoy, ᵀsage (combine with nutmeg).

Supplements—Sulfurzyme (shown to slow or reverse autoimmune diseases), EndoGize, ImmuPro, Inner Defense, Master Formula His/Hers (3 times a day), Mineral Essence (help supplement mineral loss), MultiGreens, Super B (after each meal), Thyromin (first thing in morning), True Source (whole food multi-nutrient).

—Stimulant

Oils—ᵀ$_F$Basil, ᵀ$_F$sage, ᵀrosemary, ᵀclove, ᵀgeranium, ᵀpine.

—Strengthen

Oils—ᵀSpruce (black), ᵀpeppermint.

—Underactive Adrenals *See Addison's Disease.*

Supplements—Thyromin (1–4 tablets daily. *See Suggested Use under Thyromin in the Supplements section of the Reference Guide for Essential Oils*), Master Formula His/Hers, Mineral Essence, MultiGreens, Super B.

T—Apply as a warm compress over kidney area. Dilute as recommended, and apply on location or on Vita-Flex points on the feet.

Aftershave: *See also Skin.*

Oils—ᵀAwaken (can be used instead of aftershave lotion), ᵀValor.

Comments—Try adding Awaken to Sandalwood Moisture Cream, Lavender Hand & Body Lotion, Sensation Hand & Body Lotion, or Genesis Hand & Body Lotion as an aftershave.

T—Dilute with V-6 Oil and apply on skin. *See Comments above for additional applications.*

Personal Care—Genesis Hand & Body Lotion, Sensation Hand & Body Lotion, Sandalwood Moisture Cream, Lavender Hand & Body Lotion, KidScents Lotion (soothes and rehydrates the skin—and smells great too), Prenolone/Prenolone+, Rose Ointment.

Agent Orange Poisoning:

Agent Orange is a toxic herbicide that was used to defoliate areas of the forest during the Vietnam War.

Oils—ᵀGLF or ᵀJuvaFlex (over liver), ᵀEndoFlex (over adrenal glands/kidneys).

T—Apply 1–2 drops to areas indicated above with a hot compress.

Bath—Add 1 cup Epsom salts and 4 oz. of food grade hydrogen peroxide to warm bathwater.

Supplements—Balance Complete, ComforTone, Digest + Cleanse, EndoGize, Essentialzyme, Essentialzymes-4, ICP, ImmuPro, Thyromin.

Recipe #1—3 drops EndoFlex on throat, feet (under big toes and on kidney Vita Flex point). Also across the back over the kidneys. After 90 days, start the Cleansing Trio (ComforTone, Essentialzyme, and ICP), and continue using it for one year.

Recipe #2—1 ImmuPro three times a day, 2 Thyromin at bedtime. After 90 days, start the Cleansing Trio (ComforTone, Essentialzyme, and ICP), and continue for one year.

Aging: *See also Wrinkles.*

Oils—ᴵThyme[8], ᴵLongevity, ᵀcarrot, ᵀfrankincense, ᵀrosehip, ᵀrosewood, ᵀsandalwood.

Supplements—NingXia Red, Longevity Capsules, Ningxia Wolfberries (dried), True Source (whole food multi-nutrient).

I—Add 1–3 drops to an empty capsule with 1–3 drops V-6 Oil, and swallow.

T—Dilute as recommended, and apply on skin.

—MOISTURIZERS

Personal Care—A·R·T Skin Care System (builds collagen, repairs DNA damage, and smooths wrinkles), Boswellia Wrinkle Cream, Essential Beauty Serums (Dry & Acne-Prone Skin Blends), Satin Facial Scrub—Mint, Prenolone/Prenolone+, Progessence/Progessence Plus, Rose Ointment, Sandalwood Moisture Cream, Sensation Hand & Body Lotion, Wolfberry Eye Cream.

Supplements—Wolfberry Crisp Bars *(Refer to the Wolfberry Crisp Bar in the Supplements section of the Reference Guide for Essential Oils for more information on the benefits of the Ningxia Wolfberry)*, Essentialzyme, Essentialzymes-4, Mineral Essence (antioxidant).

Agitation: *See Calming: Agitation.*

AIDS: *See also Antiviral.*

Acquired immune deficiency syndrome (AIDS) is a disease of the human immune system. AIDS progressively inhibits the effectiveness of the immune system, leaving the human body susceptible to both infections and tumors. AIDS is caused by the human immunodeficiency virus (HIV), which is acquired by direct contact of the bloodstream or mucous membrane with a bodily fluid (such as blood, breast milk, vaginal fluid, semen, and preseminal fluid) containing HIV.

Oils—ᵀᴬHelichrysum[9], ᵀᴬcumin (supports immune system; inhibits HIV virus), ᵀᴬThieves, ᵀᴬBrain Power, ᵀᴬcistus, ᵀᴬExodus II, ᵀᴬImmuPower, ᵀᴬlemon, ᵀᴬnutmeg, ᵀᴬValor.

T—Apply to thymus and to bottoms of feet.

A—Diffuse into the air.

Supplements—Balance Complete, Cleansing Trio (ComforTone, Essentialzyme, and ICP), Digest + Cleanse, ImmuPro, Inner Defense, Mineral Essence, MultiGreens, NingXia Red, Power Meal (contains wolfberry which is an immune stimulator), Super B, Super C / Super C Chewable, Thyromin, True Source (whole food multi-nutrient), Ultra Young+.

***Comments—Refer to the chapter entitled "How to Use—The Personal Usage Reference" in the Essential Oils Desk Reference under "AIDS" for specific oil blend and supplement recommendations.

Airborne Bacteria: *See also Antibacterial.*

Oils—ACinnamon bark, Amountain savory, Aoregano, AThieves, Alemongrass[10], Ageranium[10], Afir, Abalsam fir, APurification.

A—Diffuse into the air.

Air Pollution:

Oils—APurification, AThieves, Alemon (sterilize air), AAbundance, AChristmas Spirit, Acypress, Aeucalyptus, Afir, Agrapefruit, AImmuPower, Alavender, Alime, Arosemary.

—Disinfectants

Oils—APurification, A$_F$lemon, Aeucalyptus, Aclove, Acitronella, Agrapefruit, Apeppermint, Asage, Aspruce, Awintergreen.

A—Diffuse into the air.

> *Diffusing essential oils in the home or workplace is one of the best ways to purify our environment. The antiviral, antibacterial, and antiseptic properties of the oils, along with the negative ions and oxygenating molecules that are released when essential oils are diffused, all help to reduce chemicals, bacteria, and metallics in the air.*
>
> *Cinnamon bark, mountain savory, oregano, and Thieves were all tested by Weber State University and were shown to kill 100% of the airborne bacteria present. This was all done by diffusing the oils into the atmosphere.*
>
> *(KID-Radio with Lance Richardson and D. Gary Young, March 5, 1996)*

Alcoholism: *See Addictions: Alcohol.*

Alertness:

Oils—ATPeppermint[11], ITAsage lavender[12], TAbasil, TACitrus Fresh, TAClarity, TAlemon, TArosemary. Apply to temples and to bottoms of feet.

A—Diffuse into the air. Inhale directly or applied to a tissue or a cotton wick.

T—Apply 1–2 drops to temples and to bottoms of feet.

I—Add 1–2 drops to an empty capsule, and swallow.

Alkaline: *See Acidosis, pH Balance.*

Alkali-Forming Foods—Dark green and yellow vegetables, sprouted grains, legumes, seeds, nuts, essential fats (omega-3 and 6), and low sugar fruits like avocados and lemons.

Personal Care—Genesis Hand & Body Lotion balances pH on the skin.

Supplements—AlkaLime, JuvaPower (contains many acid-binding foods), Life 5 (probiotic), Mineral Essence, MultiGreens (helps normalize blood pH levels), Omega Blue and

> ***Alkaline*** *refers to a substance or solution that has a pH of 7.0 or above. The optimum pH for our blood and body tissues is about 7.2 (The use of saliva and urine test strips will show a much lower pH level due to the protein present in the solution. Saliva and urine tests from a healthy body should be about 6.6 to 6.8).*
>
> *The body heals best when it is slightly alkaline. To keep the blood and body tissue at an optimum pH, avoid acid-forming food. See* Acidosis. *Make sure your food intake is 80 percent alkaline, and drink plenty of water.*

OmegaGize[3] (loaded with omega-3 fatty acids of EPA and DHA), Power Meal (predigested protein).

Alkalosis: *See pH Balance.*

▸▸ *Alkalosis refers to a condition where the blood and intestinal tract becomes excessively alkaline. Slight alkalinity is important for a healthy body, but excessive alkalinity can cause depression, fatigue, and sickness.*

Oils—[TI]Anise, [TI]Di-Gize, [TI]ginger, [TI]tarragon.

Supplements—Digest + Cleanse, Essentialzyme, Essentialzymes-4, Life 5 (probiotic), Mineral Essence, MultiGreens (helps normalize blood pH levels), Power Meal (pre-digested protein), Sulfurzyme.

T—Apply 1–2 drops to Vita Flex points on feet.

I—Add 1–2 drops to an empty capsule, and swallow.

Allergies:

▸▸ *An allergy is a damaging immune system response to a substance that does not bother most other people. Allergy symptoms vary greatly, but common allergic responses include itching, swelling, runny nose, asthma, and sneezing.*

Oils—[T]Melaleuca[13], [T][F]lavender[14], [A]peppermint[15], [T][F]patchouli, [T]elemi (rashes), [T]eucalyptus, [T]Harmony, [T]ledum, [T]*Melaleuca ericifolia*, [T]*Melaleuca quinquenervia*, [TA]melissa (skin and respiratory), [T]ImmuPower, [T]Raven, [T]RC, [T]Roman chamomile, [T]spikenard.

***Comments—According to the Essential Oils Desk Reference, "Rub three drops [Harmony] on sternum, breathing deeply" (EDR–June 2002).

Supplements—AlkaLime, ComforTone, ICP fiber beverage (beneficial when there is an allergy to psyllium), ImmuPro, Mineral Essence, Super C / Super C Chewable, Super Cal.

Recipe #1—Apply 1 drop of peppermint on the base of the neck two times a day. Tap the thymus (located just below the notch in the neck) with pointer and index fingers (energy fingers). Diffuse peppermint. For some individuals, the use of peppermint oil has eliminated the need for allergy shots!

Recipe #2—Apply 1 drop of RC and 1 drop of Raven on the base of the neck two times a day. Tap on thymus; massage chest and back with 5 drops Raven, 5 drops RC, and 2 tsp. V-6 Oil. Diffuse RC and Raven.

Recipe #3—For allergy rashes and skin sensitivity, D. Gary Young applies 3 lavender, 6 Roman chamomile, 2 myrrh, and 1 peppermint on location.

—Antihistamine

▸▸ *An antihistamine is a substance that inhibits the effects of histamine. Histamine is a chemical released as a result of an allergic reaction, causing sneezing, itching, increased mucus, swelling, wheezing, cramps, and burning.*

Oils—[TA]Melaleuca[13], [TA]lavender[14], [TA]Roman chamomile.

—Coughing

Oils—[A]Purification.

—Hay Fever

▸▸ *Hay fever, also known as allergic rhinitis, is an allergic reaction to airborne allergens: pollen, pet dander, dust mites, etc.*

Oils—[AT]Lavender[14], [AT]Roman chamomile, [AT]Cajeput, [AT]eucalyptus, [AT]Juva Cleanse, [AT]rose.

—Psychological Allergies (In the Mind)

Recipe #4—Put Harmony on feet, neck, navel, or in your shoes for one to five days.

—To Oils

Put one drop of the oil to which there is an allergy reaction on a cotton ball, and place it in the allergic person's shoe. Add a drop each day until the allergy to that particular oil is gone. Since allergies often indicate an electrical imbalance, try the following:

A. Place a drop or two of Harmony in one hand; then rub the palms of both hands together in a clockwise motion.

B. Place one hand over the thymus (heart chakra) and the other hand over the navel.

C. Take three deep breaths and switch hands; then take three more deep breaths.

Oils—[T]Harmony (helps open the energy meridians and balance the bioelectric field of the body).

T—Apply 1–2 drops to sinuses or to Vita Flex points.

A—Diffuse into the air. Inhale directly or applied to a tissue or a cotton wick.

If you have a reaction to the oils, it is only a reaction to all of the chemicals you have been dumping into your body throughout the years. The oils are merely reacting with the toxins in the subdermal tissues and beginning their removal. ***Cleanse the body!***

Alone (feeling): *See also Emotions.*

Oils—[AT]Acceptance, [AT]Valor.

A—Diffuse into the air. Inhale directly or applied to a tissue or a cotton wick.

T—Dilute, and use as massage oil. Apply to auricular emotional points.

Alopecia Areata: *(Inflammatory hair loss disease) See Hair: Loss.*

Aluminum Toxicity: *See also Alzheimer's Disease, Attention Deficit Disorder.*

Oils—[IT]Juva Cleanse.

I—Add 1–2 drops to an empty capsule, and swallow.

T—Dilute with V-6 Oil, and massage over spine.

Aluminum is one of the most abundant elements on Earth; therefore, we are constantly exposed to it. Some estimate that an average person consumes between three and ten milligrams of aluminum every day. Aluminum toxicity *may contribute to the cause of colic, rickets, kidney and liver dysfunction, speech and memory problems, osteoporosis, and Alzheimer's disease.*

Alzheimer's Disease: *See also Brain, Memory, Pineal Gland, Pituitary Gland.*

▸▸ *Alzheimer's is a progressive and fatal disease that attacks and kills brain cells, causing a loss of memory and a loss of other intellectual capacities. Alzheimer's is most commonly diagnosed in individuals over the age of 65. As the disease progresses, sufferers often experience mood swings, long-term memory loss, confusion, irritability, aggression, and a decreased ability to communicate.*

Supplements—Omega Blue, OmegaGize[3], Cleansing Trio (ComforTone, Essentialzyme, and ICP), Digest + Cleanse, JuvaTone, PD 80/20, Power Meal, Sulfurzyme, True Source (whole food multi-nutrient).

***Comments—*The gingko biloba that is found in Power Meal has been shown to help improve memory loss, brain function, depression, cerebral and peripheral circulation, oxygenation, and blood flow.*

Autopsies have revealed that victims of ***Alzheimer's disease*** *have four times the normal amount of aluminum in the nerve cells of their brain.*

Prevention: *Use glass, iron, or stainless steel cookware. Avoid products containing aluminum, bentonite, or dihydroxyaluminum. Some of these products are aluminum cookware, foil, antacids, baking powders, buffered aspirin, most city water, antiperspirants, deodorants, beer, bleached flour, table salt, tobacco smoke, cream of tartar, Parmesan and grated cheeses, aluminum salts, douches, and canned goods.*

—Blood-Brain Barrier

›› *The blood-brain barrier is the body's filtering mechanism that allows necessary substances, such as blood, to freely enter the brain and spine, while preventing other substances, such as certain drugs, from entering. Studies have shown that sesquiterpenes can pass the blood-brain barrier.*

Oils—Oils that are high in sesquiterpenes include cedarwood, vetiver, sandalwood, black pepper, patchouli, myrrh, ginger, German chamomile, spikenard, galbanum, and frankincense. Some essential oil blends containing some of these oils include: 3 Wise Men, Acceptance, Brain Power, Forgiveness, Gathering, Harmony, Inspiration, Into the Future, Transformation, and Trauma Life. Apply to temples and to bottoms of feet; diffuse.

*****Comments**—*Oils that pass through the blood-brain barrier cannot carry unwanted substances with them.*

—Brain Function

Oils—[A]Sage[16], [A]Clarity.

Supplements—Omega Blue, OmegaGize[3].

—Emotions

Oils—[A] Peace & Calming, [AT]3 Wise Men (crown), [AT]Acceptance, [A]cypress.

A—Diffuse into the air. Inhale directly.

T—Dilute as recommended, and apply over brain stem on back of neck. Dilute with V-6 Oil, and use for massage.

Amino Acids:

> ***Amino acids** have the ability to neutralize and to help eliminate free radicals in the body's system.*

Oils—[A]Lavender.

A—Diffuse into the air. Inhale directly or applied to a tissue or a cotton wick.

Supplements—Pure Protein Complete (has a complete array of ultra-bioactive amino acids), NingXia Red (18 amino acids in whole food form), Cleansing Trio (ComforTone, Essentialzyme, and ICP), FemiGen, JuvaTone, KidScents MightyVites, Master Formula His/Hers, Mineral Essence, Power Meal, Thyromin.

Amnesia: *See Memory.*

Analgesic: *See Pain.*

Anemia:

›› *Anemia is a condition marked by a decreased number of red blood cells or by a deficiency of hemoglobin in the blood. The most common signs of anemia are fatigue, pallor, physical weakness, poor concentration, and shortness of breath on exertion. Anemia is most common in infants and in small children and is often caused by a deficiency of iron in the diet.*

Oils—[T][F]Lemon, [T]carrot, [T]ImmuPower, [T]Juva Cleanse, [T]lavender.

T—Apply to bottoms of feet and to stomach.

—Food

Oils—Flavor water with a drop of lemon.

Supplements—Rehemogen tincture (10 drops twice a day) and JuvaTone together help raise blood cell count.

Anesthesia: *See Pain:Anesthesia, Pain:Analgesic.*

Aneurysm: *See also Blood, Cardiovascular System.*

▸▸ *An Aneurysm is a swelling or dilation of a blood vessel in the area of a weakened blood vessel wall.*

Oils—**TA**Cypress (strengthens the capillary walls and increases circulation), **TA**Aroma Life (chelates plaque), **TA**helichrysum, **TA**frankincense, **TA**Idaho tansy.

T—Apply to temples, heart, and Vita Flex heart points.

A—Diffuse into the air. Inhale directly.

Blend #1—5 frankincense, 1 helichrysum, and 1 cypress. **Diffuse**.

Herbs—Cayenne pepper, garlic, hawthorn berry.

Personal Care—Cel-Lite Magic dilates blood vessels for better circulation.

Supplements—Cleansing Trio (ComforTone, Essentialzyme, and ICP), Sulfurzyme, Super C / Super C Chewable, True Source (whole food multi-nutrient).

Anger: *See also Calming, Liver.*

Oils—**AT**Lavender[17], **AT**ylang ylang[18], **TA**rose[19], **TA**melissa[20], **T**Tranquil (roll-on), orange, **AT**Peace & Calming, **AT**Australian Blue, **AT**bergamot, **AT**cedarwood, **AT**cypress, **AT**Forgiveness, **AT**frankincense, **AT**geranium, **AT**German chamomile, **AT**Grounding, **AT**Joy, **AT**Harmony, **AT**helichrysum, **AT**Hope, **AT**Humility, **AT**Inspiration, **AT**lemon, **AT**mandarin, **AT**marjoram, **AT**myrrh (soothes), **AT**myrtle, **AT**petitgrain, **AT**Present Time, **AT**Release, **AT**Roman chamomile, **AT**Sacred Mountain, **AT**sandalwood, **AT**Surrender, **AT**Trauma Life, **AT**Valor.

***Comments—Refer to the Emotional Release part of the Science and Application section of the Reference Guide for Essential Oils.

—Calms Anger

Oils—**AT**Peace & Calming, **T**Tranquil (roll-on), **AT**Australian Blue, **AT**Inspiration, spruce, **AT**Trauma Life.

—Cleansing After Argument and Physical Fighting

Oils—**AT**Eucalyptus.

—Cleanse the Liver

Oils—(Anger is stored in the liver) **AT**JuvaFlex, **AT** F geranium (cleanses and detoxifies the liver), **AT**GLF, **AT**grapefruit (liver disorders).

—Dispels Anger

Oils—**AT**Ylang ylang[18], **T**Tranquil (roll-on).

—For Communication Without Anger

Oils—**AT**Roman chamomile.

—Lessens Anger

Oils—**AT**Myrrh.

—Overcome

Oils—**AT** F Cedarwood, **AT**bergamot, **AT**Release, **AT**Roman chamomile.

—Releases Locked Up Anger and Frustration

Oils—**AT**Release (together with JuvaFlex), **AT**Surrender, **AT**Transformation, **AT**Valor, **AT**Roman or German chamomile, **AT**Sacred Mountain, **AT**sandalwood.

Supplements—JuvaTone, Thyromin, Super B.

Blend #1—4 drops lavender, 3 geranium, 3 rosewood, 3 rosemary, 2 tangerine, 1 spearmint, 2 Idaho tansy, 1 German chamomile, and 1 oz. V-6 Oil. Apply to back of neck, wrist, and heart.

A—Diffuse into the air. Inhale directly or applied to a tissue or a cotton wick.

T—Dilute, and massage onto the skin. Apply to temples or auricular emotion points.

Angina: *See Cardiovascular System.*

Animals:

Only 1–2 drops of oil is all that is necessary on animals as they respond much more quickly to the oils than do humans. V-6 Oil can be added to extend oil over larger areas and to heavily dilute the essential oil for use on smaller animals, especially cats.

Personal Care—Animal Scents Pet Shampoo, Animal Scents Pet Ointment. Other alkaline shampoos without chemicals are good for animals.

Supplements—Ningxia Red to help support the liver and enhance energy and healing. BLM (added to their food; can help speed the healing of bones), Power Meal, and Sulfurzyme.

I have a large brown tabby cat that was limping bad, so I took him to the vet. The vet said he had a knee injury (he compared it to a football player's injured knee–"cruciate ligament rupture") and said it would need surgery. He wanted me to bring my cat back in a week to see his son (who is also a vet) to make arrangements for the surgery. Later, using V-6 as my carrier oil and combining it with a couple drops of lavender oil, I rubbed my cat from the bottom of the paw up to his hip area. The next day I could see an improvement, and by the time I took him back to the vet he was walking on his leg with only a slight limp. The vet said he would heal nicely on his own and there would be no need for surgery. Today he walks, runs, and is even now jumping with no problems.

-Submitted by M. Rynicki

—Bleeding

Oils—THelichrysum, Tgeranium.

T—Dilute, and apply on location.

—Bones (Pain)

Oils—TPanAway, Twintergreen, Tlemongrass, Tspruce.

T—Dilute, and apply on location.

Personal Care—Ortho Ease or Ortho Sport Massage Oils.

Supplements—BLM (added to their food; can help speed the healing of bones), Power Meal and Sulfurzyme.

—Calm

Oils—ATLavender, ATPeace & Calming, TTranquil (roll-on), ATCitrus Fresh, ATRoman chamomile (for horses, add to feed), ATTrauma Life. Dilute well for cats.

A—Diffuse into the air.

T—Dilute, and apply on back.

—Cancer

–Skin

Oils—TFrankincense, Tcumin.

T—Dilute, and apply on location.

—Cats

Valerie Worwood says that you can treat a cat like you would a child (see Babies). Dilute oils heavily with V-6 Oil. Avoid melaleuca.

Comments—*Cat physiology is so different from other animals and from humans that oils should be used with extreme caution on cats. In fact, melaleuca (or tea tree oil) should never be used on a cat as death can result. Some cases exist where a blend of oils containing melaleuca has killed cats.

—Colds and Coughs

Oils—[T]Eucalyptus, [T]melaleuca (not for cats).

T—Apply on fur or on stomach.

—Cows

Recipe #1—For scours, use 5 drops Di-Gize on stomach (can mix with V-6 Oil to cover a larger area); repeat 2 hours later.

—Cuts and Sores

Oils—[T]Melrose (not on cats).

T—Apply 1 drop on location. Work in with finger.

—Dogs

***Comments—There was a dog that walked with its head down and its tail between its legs. Valor was put on its feet and 3 Wise Men and Joy on its crown. The next day its head was up, and it was happy.

–Anxiety/Nervousness

Oils—[T]Lavender, [T]Peace & Calming, [T]Tranquil (roll-on), [T]valerian, [T]Valor.

T—Rub 1–2 drops between hands, and apply to muzzle, between toes, on top of feet to smell when nose is down, and on edges of ears.

–Arthritis

Oils—[T]Copaiba.

Blend #1—A blend of rosemary, lavender, and ginger diluted with V-6 Oil.

Personal Care—Ortho Ease Massage Oil applied to arthritic areas.

Supplements—Add Sulfurzyme (powder) or vitamin C to their food.

–Bone Injury

Oils—[T]Wintergreen.

T—Apply 1 drop on location. Work in with finger.

Personal Care—Ortho Ease Massage Oil on injury.

Supplements—Add Sulfurzyme (powder) and BLM in food.

One Saturday in February, my husband woke me up by yelling from the living room for me to bring my oils and any oil books I had at hand to him immediately. Our dog, Buddy, (a mutt from the pound, age approx. 7+ years) was lying on the floor, and all of his muscles were completely seized up and tensed to the point where we couldn't move any part of his body. I had most of my oils in my large case and the Higley Reference Guide at my side. I put 4 or 5 drops of lavender oil in my husband's hand and he put that on Buddy's paws, ears, and all over his back and legs—anywhere he was tense that we could reach. We followed the lavender with Peace & Calming, Valor, and frankincense, applied the same way. Those four were the oils I was drawn to by instinct. We massaged him and continued to stroke and pet him during and after the application of oils, and after about 10 minutes he was able to get up and go to the door to go outside and run around. In between applying oils I looked up the info on animals as well as the info on seizures and strokes (we weren't sure what kind of episode he was having), just to make sure my instincts were near to on target (which they were). We had plans to travel about an hour out of town to visit with family, and we kept Buddy with us the whole day just to be sure he was ok. When I tell this story to other people they tell me about how their dog(s) had seizures and had to be put on steroids and eventually

I went to visit my son in Ft. Lauderdale, FL . . . and was also happy to see his dog, Luna, who I've known for 7 years, since she was a puppy. I could tell she was in pain, as she was not as active as usual and was limping. My son, Jason, told me that she is part German Shepherd—a breed that is prone to hip dysplasia. It broke my heart to see her in such pain. Jason had been giving her various vitamins and other supplements for several months, without much success. I myself have had success with Sulfurzyme for an arthritic knee, and I asked if he would like to try that for Luna. We began to give her 1/4 tsp. twice a day with her meals. Within two days, we began to see a change. My son was amazed! As the two weeks passed while I was visiting, we saw a huge change. She was running like her old self, and you could sense that the pain was almost (if not totally) gone. Within a month, Jason told me that she was now even jumping up on furniture, which she was unable to do when we started with the Sulfurzyme. That was 18 months ago, and Luna is still taking Sulfurzyme . . . and still doing great!

–Submitted by Linda Griffith
Dixon, New Mexico

–Chewing On Furniture

Supplements—Mineral Essence (helps satisfy mineral deficiency).

–Digestion

Supplements— Essentialzymes-4, Essentialzyme.

–Heart Problems

Oils—ᵀPeppermint

T—Apply on paws.

Recipe #1—Myrtle, ravensara, and Thieves on back using Raindrop Technique with warm wet pack.

–Limping

Supplements—Sulfurzyme (powder with food).

–Pain and Stress

***Comments—Do Raindrop Technique. (*The video "Essential Tips for Happy, Healthy Pets" demonstrates this technique on a dog and a horse.*) This technique helps relieve stress on the back, shoulders, and legs and also raises immune function and protects against illness.

–Sleep

Oils—ᵀLavender (on paws), ᵀPeace & Calming (on stomach).

T—Apply on indicated areas.

–Stroke

Oils—ᵀBrain Power (on head), ᵀfrankincense (on brain stem area/back of neck), ᵀValor (on each paw).

T—Apply on indicated areas.

–Ticks and Bug Bites

Recipe #2—Apply 1 drop Purification directly on live tick. Can also be applied to untreated tick wound and worked in with finger.

–Travel Sickness

Oils—ᵀPeppermint.

T—Dilute with V-6 Oil, and rub on stomach. Also helps calm stomachaches.

–Traumatized

Oils—ᴬTrauma Life.

A—Rub 1–2 drops between hands, and cup over nose and mouth for dog to inhale.

—Earache

Blend #2—1 drop Melrose or a blend of 1 drop melaleuca (tea tree), 1 drop lavender, and 1 drop Roman chamomile diluted in V-6 Oil. Put in ear, and rub around the ear.

—Ear Infections

Oils—ᵀImmuPower, ᵀPurification (helps ward off insects too).

T—Dip cotton swab in oil, and apply to inside and front of ear.

—Fleas

Oils—ᵀCitronella, ᵀMelrose, ᵀIdaho tansy, ᵀeucalyptus, ᵀlemongrass, ᵀpine.

T—Add 1–2 drops of oil to shampoo.

Blend #3—Combine eucalyptus, orange, citronella, and cedarwood. Add blend to distilled water in a spray bottle, shake well, and mist over entire animal.

—Hemorrhaging

Oils—ᵀCistus (stops internal bleeding)

I—Take 1-2 drops orally.

—Horses

–Anxiety/Nervousness

Oils—ᵀPeace &Calming.

T—Rub 1–2 drops between hands, and apply to nose and on front of chest, knees, and tongue.

–Flies

Oils—ᵀIdaho tansy.

T—Add 1–5 drops to 1 oz. water in a small spray bottle, and mist over animal to keep flies away.

–Hoof Rot

▸▸ *Hoof Rot is a hoof infection commonly found in cattle, sheep, horses, and goats. Hoof Rot attacks the area between the two toes and begins to literally rot away the animal's hoof. This infection is identified by a swelling of the skin between the claws of the hoof and by a foul odor. If not treated, Hoof Rot can easily be spread to other animals.*

Blend #4—Blend Roman chamomile, thyme, and melissa in V-6 Oil, and apply on location.

I have a 21 year old gelding who was diagnosed with "kidney colic" back in January. He would be down one day, up the next, down the next, up for several days, down again, etc. He would show all the general signs of colic but was also wanting to urinate frequently, passing little or nothing. This went on for about four weeks, and the vet thought he probably was trying to pass kidney stones. Since it was happening so often, I was wanting something to give him for the pain instead of using Banamine so much. I had used marjoram, clary sage, and lavender successfully on an intestinal colic, so I tried them; but they just didn't work as well on the kidneys. So I tried JuvaFlex, and the results were dramatic! Four drops over each kidney, with or without a warm compress, would get him up and back to eating and drinking in 10–20 minutes. The pain-killing effects would last from 2–4 hours and seemed to be cumulative. After I had done this for two separate "episodes," the symptoms went away completely. I don't know if the stones dissolved or if he passed them, but he's been pain free for six months.

-Submitted by Jan Early
Tallahassee, Florida

–Infection

Oils—ᵀMelrose, ᵀThieves.

T—Dilute, and apply on location.

–Injuries

***Comments—Do Raindrop Technique. (*The video "Essential Tips for Happy, Healthy Pets" demonstrates this technique on a dog and a horse.*) When a frisky race horse took a fall and was unable to walk, application of the oils using the Raindrop Technique brought the horse out of it in a matter of days.

–Leg Fractures

Recipe #2—Apply ginger and V-6 Oil. Wrap the leg with a hot compress. Massage leg after the fracture is healed with a blend of rosemary and thyme with V-6 Oil. This may strengthen the ligaments and prevent calcification.

–Muscle Tissue/Ligaments

Blend #5—Equal parts lemongrass and lavender on location; wrap to help regenerate torn muscle tissue.

–Saddle Sores

Oils—ᵀMelrose

T—Apply on location.

Personal Care—Rose Ointment.

–Wounds

Oils—[T]Helichrysum, [T]Melrose

T—Dilute as recommended, and apply on location.

Personal Care—Rose Ointment.

—Infection

Oils—[T]Di-Gize, [T]ImmuPower.

T—Apply on the paws.

—Parasites

Oils—[T]Lavender, [T]Di-Gize, [T]Cedarwood.

T—Rub on paws to release parasites.

Supplements—ParaFree.

—Snake Bites (Venomous Wounds)

***Comments—Do Raindrop Technique. (The video "Essential Tips for Happy, Healthy Pets" demonstrates this technique on a dog and a horse.)

> *One couple had a horse that got kicked in the flank, creating a large wound. The Vet treated the wound and gave her some medication. Unfortunately, the wound became reinfected and worsened to the point that the horse almost died. The Vet came over and reopened the wound and flushed out nearly two gallons of blood clots. However, the Vet had no medication with him and would not be able to deliver any more for a couple of days. So, the wife put 15 drops of Thieves in about ¼ cup of olive oil, and while the husband held open the horse's mouth, she poured the oil down its throat. This was repeated 3 or 4 times, and within just a few days the horse was fully recovered.*

Anorexia: *See Eating Disorders: Anorexia.*

Anthrax: *See also Antibacterial.*

▸▸ *Anthrax is a serious, sometimes deadly, infectious disease caused by the bacteria Bacillus anthracis. The disease has three main forms: cutaneous anthrax (the bacteria enter through a cut or sore on the body), gastrointestinal anthrax (the bacteria enter by eating improperly cooked meat from an infected animal), and inhalation anthrax (caused by inhaling anthrax bacteria spores). Symptoms vary with each form.*

Oils—[IAT]$_F$Thyme.

I—Add 2–3 drops to an empty capsule with 2–3 drops V-6 Oil; swallow.

A—Diffuse into the air.

T—Dilute, and apply on location.

Antibacterial:

▸▸ *The term antibacterial refers to anything that kills bacteria or that limits its ability to grow or to reproduce.*

Oils—Oils high in thymol (a phenol), such as [TA]$_F$thyme[21] and [T]mountain savory, tend to be highly antibacterial. Other effective antibacterial oils include [TAI]Thieves (annihilates bacteria), [T]melaleuca[22], [TA]$_F$cinnamon bark[23], [TA]lemongrass[24], [T]peppermint[25], [T]$_F$oregano[26], [T]lemon myrtle[27], [T]$_F$basil[28], [TA]$_F$clove[29], [T]$_F$spearmint[30], [TA]plectranthus oregano, [TA]Purification, [T]$_F$rosemary[31], [T]$_F$cypress, [TA]$_F$rosewood, [TA]rose[32], [T]pink pepper[33], [A]RC, [TA]micromeria, [A]geranium[34], [T]bergamot, [T]cassia, [T]cedarwood, [TA]citronella, [TA]Christmas Spirit, [TA]Citrus Fresh, [T]clary sage, [T]copaiba, [T]Egyptian Gold, [TA]eucalyptus, [T]Evergreen Essence, [TA]fir, [T]grapefruit, [T]Idaho tansy, [TA]juniper, [T]lavender, [TA]lemon, [T]marjoram, [T]*Melaleuca ericifolia*, [T]neroli, [T]ocotea, [T]palmarosa, [T]petitgrain, [TA]pine, [AT]ravensara, [T]Roman chamomile, [T]Sacred Mountain, [T]tarragon, [T]valerian, [T]western red cedar.

> *Dr. Terry Friedmann, MD, would often recommend the following* ***Essential Oil Antibiotic Regimen****:*
>
> *In a "00" capsule put 12 drops of Thieves, 6 drops of oregano, and 2 drops of frankincense. Ingest one capsule every 4 hours for 3 days, then every 8 hours for 4 days.*

*****Comments**—See the "Single Oil Property Chart" in the Appendix of this book for additional antibacterial oils and their strengths.

—AIRBORNE

Oils—[A]Cinnamon bark,[A]mountain savory, [A]oregano, [A]Thieves, [A]lemongrass[24], [A]fir, [A]Purification.

—CLEANSING

Oils—[TA]Purification.

—INFECTION

Oils—[T]Nutmeg (fights).

> *Research at Weber State University has shown that out of 67 oils tested, 66 of them were powerful antibacterial agents. Oregano, cinnamon bark, mountain savory, ravensara, and peppermint were all more powerful as antibacterial agents than penicillin or ampicillin. Thieves was shown to be 60 percent higher in activity against bacteria, germs, and antimicrobial action than either ampicillin or penicillin!*
>
> *(KID-Radio with Lance Richardson and D. Gary Young, March 5, 1996)*

—MRSA (*METHICILLIN RESISTANT STAPHYLOCOCCUS AUREUS*)

Oils—[T]Melaleuca[22], [T]oregano[26], [T]geranium[34], [T]lemon myrtle[27], [T]cinnamon bark, [T]peppermint[30], [T]spearmint[30], [T]lemongrass, [T]clove, [T]*Eucalyptus radiata*, [T]grapefruit, [T]lavender, [T]mountain savory, [T]orange, [T]patchouli, [T]thyme.

—PREVENTS GROWTH OF

Oils—[T]Melrose.

—STAPH INFECTION *See also MRSA above.*

▸▸ *Staph infection is any of a number of infections caused by Staphylococcus bacteria. These condition can vary from mild skin infections to severe and life-threatening blood and respiratory illnesses.*

Recipe #1—Use oregano and hyssop; alternate with oregano and thyme to relieve the pain.

Oils—[T]Helichrysum, [T]lavender, [T]Purification.

*****Comments**—Black pepper or peppermint may make it more painful.

T—Apply on location, liver area, or bottoms of feet

A—Diffuse into the air.

I—Add oils to 00 capsule; swallow.

Antibiotic: *See Antibacterial.*

Anticancerous: *See Cancer: ANTICANCEROUS.*

Anticatarrhal: *See also Congestion.*

▸▸ *Catarrh is an excessive buildup of mucus in the nose or throat.*

Oils—[TA]Eucalyptus[35], [TA]$_F$cypress, [TA]$_F$fir, [TA]$_F$helichrysum (discharges mucus), [TA]Thieves (dissolves excess mucus), [TA]RC, [TA]Raven, [TA]black pepper, [TA]cajeput, [TA]cistus, [TA]dill, [TA]elemi, [TA]frankincense, [TA]ginger, [TA]hyssop (opens respiratory system and discharges toxins and mucous), [TA]jasmine, [TA]myrrh, [TA]onycha (benzoin), [TA]ravensara, [TA]rosemary.

T—Apply on lung area, feet, around nose, and Vita Flex lung points

A—Diffuse into the air.

*****Comments**—See the "Single Oil Property Chart" in the Appendix of this book for additional anticatarrhal oils and their strengths.

Anticoagulant: *See Blood: ANTICOAGULANT.*

Antidepressant: *See Depression: Antidepressant.*

Antifungal:

»*Antifungal refers to any substance that kills or inhibits the growth, metabolism, function, or reproductive ability of fungi. Fungi are a broad range of organisms such as yeast, mold, and mushrooms. While many fungi are safe and beneficial, some create mycotoxins, which are chemicals that can be toxic to plants and animals, including humans. Examples of fungi that can be detrimental to humans include black mold, candida, and ringworm.*

> *I had developed a* ***fungus*** *on my big toenails. The fungus was bad enough that the white, thick toenail was making shoes painful. I went to a podiatric doctor. The doctor removed the inside edge of the left big toenail down to the nail bed. He then prescribed some medicine that was $80 a tube to get rid of the rest. It continued to get worse and was spreading all over the nails and was headed for the rest of the nail beds. I decided to use Animal Scents Ointment on my toes 3 times a day. Now my nails are normal and the thickness is gone.*
>
> ***–Submitted by K. Ernst***

Oils—$^{TA}_{F}$Melaleuca[36], ^{TAI}Thieves, $^{TA}_{F}$cinnamon bark[37], $^{TA}_{F}$clove[38], $^{IAT}_{F}$oregano[39], $^{T}_{F}$thyme[40], ^{T}pink pepper[41], ^{T}lemon myrtle[42], $^{T}_{F}$spearmint, $^{T}_{F}$rosewood, ^{TA}lemon[43], ^{T}mountain savory[44], ^{T}carrot[45], ^{T}Melrose, ^{TA}micromeria, ^{T}Abundance, ^{T}cajeput, ^{T}Egyptian Gold, ^{T}fennel, ^{T}geranium, ^{TA}ImmuPower, ^{TA}juniper, ^{T}lavender, ^{TA}lemongrass, ^{T}mandarin, ^{TA}*Melaleuca ericifolia*, ^{T}palmarosa, ^{T}RC, ^{T}Raven, ^{T}Roman chamomile, ^{T}rosemary verbenon, ^{TA}sage.

***Comments—See the "Single Oil Property Chart" in the Appendix of this book for additional antifungal oils and their strengths.

Blend #1—2 myrrh and 2 lavender. Rub on location.

Supplements—AlkaLime (designed to combat yeast and fungus overgrowth and to preserve the body's proper pH balance), Essentialzyme, Essentialzymes-4, Life 5 (probiotic), Digest + Cleanse (contains coconut oil with capric acid, which has been shown to inhibit the growth of three different strains of *Candida*), Balance Complete, MultiGreens, Super C / Super C Chewable, Thyromin.

***Comments—Refer to the chapter entitled "How to Use—The Personal Usage Reference" in the Essential Oils Desk Reference under "Fungal Infections" for some excellent blends and tips for combating systemic fungal infections.

—Athlete's Foot

»*Athlete's foot (tinea pedis) is a fungal infection that develops on the skin of the feet. This infection causes itching, redness, and scaling of the skin, and in severe cases it can cause painful blistering or cracking of the skin.*

Oils—$^{T}_{F}$Melaleuca[46], ^{T}cajeput, ^{T}cypress, ^{T}*Eucalyptus citriodora*, ^{T}geranium, ^{T}lavender, ^{T}myrrh, ^{T}thyme.

Blend #2—Combine 2 oz. of Genesis Hand & Body Lotion with 10 drops thyme, 10 drops lavender, and 10 drops melaleuca. Rub on feet.

—Candida *See also: Acidosis, Alkaline, Blood, Diet,Food, Thyroid, pH Balance.*

»*Candida refers to a genus of yeast that are normally found in the digestive tract and on the skin of humans. These yeast are typically symbiotically beneficial to humans. However, several species of Candida, most commonly Candida albicans, can cause infections such as vaginal candidiasis or thrush (oral candidiasis) that cause localized itching, soreness, and redness (see Vaginal:Candida for further application methods). In immune system–compromised individuals, these infection-causing species of Candida can spread further, leading to serious, life-threatening complications.*

> ***Candida*** *is caused by the fermentation of yeast and sugar, antibiotics, thyroid shut down, stress, chlorinated water, etc. When there is Candida there is usually hypoglycemia and hypothyroidism. It is usually a digestive problem; putrefaction in the system causes Candida overgrowth. Candida is a natural fungus in the stomach; we need some, but it becomes a problem when there is an overgrowth. Yeast is not the problem; the problem is the fermentation of the yeast. The fermentation exists because of a mineral imbalance and an enzyme imbalance in the digestive system. The enzymes needed for digestion are secreted by the thyroid, so it is necessary to support both the thyroid and the digestive system. Also, maintaining a slightly alkaline state in the blood and body can help to slow the overgrowth of Candida.*

Oils—$^{T}_{F}$Melaleuca[36] (dilute with V-6 Oil for body massage), $^{T}_{F}$lavender[47], ^{IT}oregano[39], ^{TAI}Thieves, ^{T}clove[38], ^{T}lemon myrtle[42], ^{T}mountain savory[44] (dilute with V-6 Oil; can be hot), ^{AT}peppermint[48], ^{T}cinnamon bark, $^{T}_{F}$eucalyptus, $^{T}_{F}$rosewood, $^{T}_{F}$spearmint, $^{T}_{F}$spruce, ^{TA}micromeria, ^{T}bergamot, ^{T}Di-Gize, ^{T}EndoFlex, ^{T}ImmuPower, ^{T}laurel, ^{T}marjoram, ^{T}*Melaleuca quinquenervia*, ^{T}Melrose (+ rosemary), ^{T}ocotea, ^{T}palmarosa (skin), ^{T}rose, ^{T}rosemary, ^{T}tarragon (prevents fermentation), ^{T}thyme.

Supplements—Life 5 (probiotic, prevents overgrowth), Allerzyme (aids the digestion of sugars, starches, fats, proteins), AlkaLime (combats yeast and fungus overgrowth and preserves the body's proper pH balance), Balance Complete, ComforTone, Detoxzyme (helps maintain and support a healthy intestinal environment), Digest + Cleanse, EndoGize, Essentialzyme (increases digestion), Essentialzymes-4, ICP, Mineral Essence, MultiGreens (balances the alkaline/acid condition in the body and provides chlorophyll and oxygen), ParaFree, Power Meal (vegetable protein), Super C / Super C Chewable, Thyromin (to help the thyroid).

–Digestive Candida

Oils—^{T}Di-Gize (hot compresses over abdomen; in a retention enema at night), ^{T}ImmuPower, ^{T}Thieves.

–Vaginal Candida

Oils—$^{T}_{F}$Melaleuca[36], ^{IT}oregano[39], $^{T}_{F}$thyme[40], $^{T}_{F}$myrrh, $^{T}_{F}$bergamot, ^{T}geranium, ^{T}patchouli, ^{T}rosemary, ^{T}spikenard.

Blend #3—2 Tbs. garlic oil, 8 drops lavender, 8 drops melaleuca, 1 ml (1 softgel) vitamin E oil. Apply to irritated area.

Supplements—AlkaLime, Life 5 (probiotic). Yogurt, mixed with a little bit of water and some probiotic powder, may be applied directly to relieve the pain associated with candida.

*****Comments**—*Focus on the underlying problem of system-wide yeast infection. Also, refer to the chapter entitled "How to Use—The Personal Usage Reference" in the Essential Oils Desk Reference under "Fungal Infections" for some excellent blend recipes for dealing with vaginal yeast infections.*

—Fungal Infections

Oils—^{T}Melaleuca, ^{T}*Eucalyptus citriodora*, ^{T}geranium, ^{T}patchouli.

—Mold

▸▸ *Mold are a type of microscopic multi-cellular fungi that grow together to form filaments. Mold is found throughout the world and can survive in extreme conditions. While most mold does not adversely affect humans, an over-abundance of mold spores can cause allergies or other problems within the respiratory system. Additionally, some types of mold produce toxins that can be harmful to humans or to animals.*

Oils—^{AT}Purification, ^{AT}Thieves.

–Toxic Black

Oils—^{TA}Thieves (on feet, as rectal implant, with Raindrop Technique on back).

*****Comments**—One young boy had toxic black mold infection. His parents gave him a rectal implant of 8 ml myrrh, 2 ml oregano, 5 ml *Melaleuca alternifolia*, and 5 ml *Eucalyptus globulus*. They followed up with Thieves, as described above, to help clear him of the infection.

—Prevents Growth Of

Oils—^{T}Melrose (two times a day for seven days), ^{TA}Purification.

—Ringworm

▸▸ *Ringworm (or tinea) is a fungal infection of the skin that can cause itching, redness, and scaling of the skin. The name comes from the ring-shaped patches that often form on the skin.*

Oils—[T]Melaleuca, [T]<u>Melrose</u>, [T]peppermint, [T]thyme, [T]<u>Purification</u>, [T]geranium, [T]lavender, [T]myrrh, [T]<u>RC</u>, [T]<u>Raven</u>, [T]rosemary verbenon.

Blend #1—2 drops lavender, 2 drops melaleuca, and 2 drops thyme, or ,

Blend #2—3 drops melaleuca, 2 drops peppermint, and 3 drops spearmint. Apply 1–2 drops of blend (#s 1 or 2 above) or <u>Melrose</u> on ringworm 3 times a day for 10 days. Then mix 30 drops of melaleuca (tea tree) or <u>Melrose</u> with 2 Tbs. V-6 Oil, and use daily until ringworm is gone.

> *My friend's eight-month-old little boy had a **ringworm** the size of a quarter on his head. After putting lavender neat on it several times, it started to go away; and after a few more times, it was gone altogether. Shortly after that he got a **tick** in his head, and by putting peppermint right on the back of the tick that nasty thing backed right out. I guess [the tick] could not breath. Whatever it was, it got the tick out without us trying to pull it out and perhaps getting only part of the critter out.*
>
> ***-Submitted by V. Frierdich***

Personal Care—Rose Ointment, Ortho Ease, Ortho Sport Massage Oils.

—Thrush *See Candida, above.*

T—Dilute as recommended, and apply on location or on bottoms of feet. Apply on location with a hot compress.

A—Diffuse into the air.

I—Place oils in empty 00 capsule; swallow.

Antihemorrhaging: *See Blood: Hemorrhaging.*

Antihistamine: *See Allergies: Antihistamine.*

Anti-infectious: *See Infection: Anti-infectious. See also Antibacterial, Antifungal, Antiviral.*

Anti-inflammatory: *See also Antioxidant.*

Oils—Oils high in carvacrol (a phenol), like [T]oregano, [T]mountain savory, and [T]thyme, are very effective as anti-inflammatory agents. Other effective oils include [T]frankincense[49], [TA]melaleuca[50], [TA]eucalyptus[51], [T]<u>PanAway</u>, [T]<u>Deep Relief</u> (roll-on), [T][F]lavender[52], [T][F]myrrh[53], [T][F]German chamomile[54], [T]copaiba, [T]<u>Relieve It</u>, [TI][F]wintergreen[55], [AT]dorado azul, [T][F]spruce, [TA]eucalyptus blue, [T][F]tarragon, [T][F]patchouli, [T][F]Roman chamomile, [T]ocotea[56], [TIA]peppermint[57], [T]balsam fir, [T]black pepper, [T]blue cypress, [T]blue tansy, [TI]calamus (gastrointestinal), [T]caraway, [T]citronella, [T]clove, [T]coriander, [T]cypress, [T]elemi (breast and uterus), [T]helichrysum[57], [TA]hyssop (of the pulmonary), [T]juniper, [T]lemongrass, [T]melaleuca, [T]onycha (benzoin), [T]palo santo, [T]<u>Peace & Calming</u>, [T]petitgrain, [T]ravensara, [T]spearmint, [T]spikenard, [T]tangerine.

T—Apply on location and on brain stem area (*this helps stop pain and reduces the production of noradrenaline and cortisol).*

I—Place oils in empty 00 capsule, and swallow.

A—Diffuse into the air.

***Comments—One study showed that oils that inhibit the production of nitric oxide (NO) could greatly reduce the resulting inflammation and tissue damage. The six oils which showed the greatest percentage of NO inhibition were oregano, nutmeg, lemongrass, *Melaleuca ericifolia*, dill, and peppermint.

***Comments—*See the "Single Oil Property Chart" in the Appendix of this book for additional anti-inflammatory oils and their strengths.*

Personal Care—Ortho Sport Massage Oil.

Supplements—According to Dr. David Hill, "Inflammation and oxidation go hand-in-hand." NingXia Red and Longevity Capsules on a daily basis are a powerful combination to help fight oxidation and inflammation system-wide. Also, Omega Blue and OmegaGize[3] contain clove oil and fish oil, which have been shown to work together to reduce inflammation by up to 30%! Majestic Essence Chocolates contain high levels of boswellic acids that have demonstrated an ability to alleviate inflammation[49]. Slique Tea contains flavinoids and polyphenols which have been studied for their abilities to fight inflammation.

***Comments—Refer to the chapter entitled "How to Use—The Personal Usage Reference" in the Essential Oils Desk Reference under "Inflammation" for some excellent blend recipes.

Antimicrobial: *See also Antibacterial, Antifungal, Antiviral.*

Oils—ᵀ*Melaleuca ericifolia* (powerful), ᵀmelissa (shown in lab tests to be effective against *Streptococcus haemolyticus*), ᵀcinnamon bark, ᵀlemongrass, ᵀcypress, ᵀrosemary, ᵀthyme, ᵀAbundance, ᵀhelichrysum, ᵀjasmine, ᵀlavender, ᵀmyrrh, ᵀpalmarosa, ᵀpine, ᵀrosewood, ᵀsage.

T—Apply on location

***Comments—See the "Single Oil Property Chart" in the Appendix of this book for additional antimicrobial oils and their strengths.

Antioxidant:

> ***Antioxidants*** *create an unfriendly environment for free radicals. They can help prevent mutations, work as free radical scavengers, prevent fungus, prevent oxidation in the cells, and help to oxygenate the cells.*

Oils—TAClove[59], ITAthyme[60], TArosemary[61], TApeppermint[62], TAmelaleuca[63], TAhelichrysum[64], TAfir[65], TAlemon[66], Acinnamon bark, TDi-Gize, TAExodus II, TAfrankincense, TAhyssop, TAImmuPower, TAJuvaFlex, ILongevity (take as a dietary supplement to promote longevity), TAMelrose, onycha (benzoin), TAoregano, TAPanAway, TAPurification, TAravensara, TARC, TARelieve It, TARoman chamomile, TAThieves.

T—Dilute as recommended, and apply on location or on Vita Flex points on feet.

A—Diffuse into the air. Inhale directly.

I—Place oils in empty 00 capsule; swallow.

Supplements—NingXia Red (tested at Brunswick Laboratories with S-ORAC score of 363 per oz. The next closest "functional drink" competitor was tested at 8.6), Longevity Capsules (contains clove oil, which has the highest known ORAC score, and thyme oil, which increases antioxidant levels in heart, liver, & kidneys and doubles antioxidant activity in the entire body), Ningxia Wolfberries (dried), Essentialzyme, Essentialzymes-4, JuvaTone, Majestic Essence Chocolates, Master Formula His/Hers, Mineral Essence, MultiGreens, Super C / Super C Chewable, Super B, True Source (whole food multi-nutrient), Wolfberry Crisp Bars (*Refer to the Wolfberry Crisp Bar in the Supplements section of the Reference Guide for Essential Oils for more information on the benefits of the Ningxia Wolfberry*).

Antiparasitic: *See Parasite: Antiparasitic.*

Antirheumatic: *See also Arthritis: Rheumatoid.*

›› *Rheumatism is an older term used to describe many different painful conditions of the muscles, tendons, bones, and joints. Common rheumatic disorders include rheumatoid arthritis, osteoarthritis, lupus, tendinitis, and fibromyalgia.*

Oils—ᵀWintergreen, ᵀeucalyptus, ᵀjuniper, ᵀonycha (benzoin), ᵀoregano, ᵀrosemary, ᵀthyme.

T—Dilute as necessary, and apply on location.

***Comments—See the "Single Oil Property Chart" in the Appendix of this book for additional antirheumatic oils and their strengths.

Antiseptic: *See also Antibacterial, Antifungal, Antiviral.*

▸▸*An antiseptic is a substance applied on a surface that kills or inhibits the growth of disease-causing microorganisms.*

Oils—^{T}Di-Gize (all oils in this blend are antiseptic), $^{T}_{F}$pine (pulmonary, urinary, hepatic), $^{T}_{F}$thyme, $^{T}_{F}$oregano, $^{T}_{F}$peppermint, $^{T}_{F}$cedarwood, ^{T}Purification, ^{T}cinnamon bark, ^{T}melaleuca, $^{T}_{F}$fir, $^{T}_{F}$sage, $^{T}_{F}$sandalwood, $^{T}_{F}$spearmint, $^{T}_{F}$myrtle (skin), $^{T}_{F}$nutmeg (intestinal), $^{T}_{F}$patchouli, ^{T}bergamot, ^{T}citronella, ^{T}clove, ^{T}copaiba, ^{T}cumin, ^{T}elemi, ^{T}eucalyptus, ^{T}Evergreen Essence, ^{T}fennel, ^{T}balsam fir, ^{T}frankincense, ^{T}lavender, ^{T}lemon, ^{T}mandarin, ^{T}marjoram, ^{T}Melrose, ^{T}mountain savory, ^{T}mugwort, ^{T}orange, ^{T}onycha (benzoin), ^{T}ravensara, ^{T}Roman chamomile, ^{T}rosemary cineol, ^{T}rosemary verbenon, ^{T}thyme linalol, ^{T}western red cedar, ^{T}ylang ylang.

T—Apply on location.

***Comments—Most oils can be used as antiseptics. See the "Single Oil Property Chart" in the Appendix of this book for additional antiseptic oils and their strengths.

Personal Care—Rose Ointment (apply over oils to increase antiseptic properties and to extend effectiveness).

Supplements—Super C / Super C Chewable.

Antisexual:

Oils—$^{AT}_{F}$Marjoram (helps balance sexual desires).

A—Diffuse into the air. Inhale directly or applied to hands, tissue, or a cotton wick.

T—Dilute with V-6 Oil and massage into skin.

Antispasmodic:

▸▸*An antispasmodic is an agent that is used to reduce or prevent muscle spasms, cramps, and convulsions.*

Oils—$^{TI}_{F}$Basil, $^{TI}_{F}$peppermint[67], $^{T}_{F}$lavender[68], $^{T}_{F}$German chamomile, $^{IT}_{F}$Roman chamomile (relaxes spastic muscles of the colon wall), $^{TI}_{F}$rosemary, $^{T}_{F}$sage, $^{T}_{F}$marjoram, ^{T}mugwort[69], $^{T}_{F}$spruce, ^{T}anise, ^{T}calamus, ^{T}citronella, ^{T}cumin, ^{TI}fennel, ^{T}helichrysum, ^{T}mandarin, ^{T}petitgrain, ^{T}RutaVaLa, ^{T}spearmint, ^{T}spikenard, ^{TI}tarragon, ^{T}valerian, ^{T}ylang ylang.

***Comments—See the "Single Oil Property Chart" in the Appendix of this book for additional antispasmodic oils.

T—Apply on location. Dilute, and massage on location.

I—Add 2–5 drops to an empty capsule with 2–5 drops V-6 Oil; swallow.

Antitumoral: *See Tumors: Antitumoral. See also Cancer.*

Antiviral:

▸▸*Antiviral refers to a substance that is able to inhibit or stop the development, function, or replication of an infection-causing virus. A virus is a tiny microorganism that can only grow and replicate by living on a host cell. Viruses are responsible for causing numerous human infections and diseases.*

Oils—^{TA}Melissa[70] oil has shown some of the strongest antiviral activity. Oils high in limonene (a monoterpene), like ^{TA}grapefruit, ^{TA}orange, ^{TA}tangerine, ^{TA}palo santo, ^{AT}eucalyptus blue, ^{TA}mandarin, and ^{TA}lemon, may be effective antiviral agents. Other effective antiviral oils include ^{TA}helichrysum[71], $^{TA}_{F}$melaleuca[72], [TA]$_{F}$clove[73], [AT]Thieves (diffuse with extra cinnamon bark to help fight viral conditions), [TA]$_{F}$cinnamon bark, [T]lemon myrtle[74], [TA]manuka[75], [TA]peppermint[76], [TA]$_{F}$ravensara (viral infection), [TA]$_{F}$oregano, [TA]$_{F}$thyme, [TA]$_{F}$rosewood, [A]RC, [TA]myrrh (both internally and externally—reported 75% effective), [TA]Abundance, [TA]blue cypress (especially for HPV), [TA]bergamot, [TA]clary sage, [TA]cypress, [TA]Egyptian Gold, [TA]*Eucalyptus radiata*, [TA]galbanum, [TA]geranium, [TA]hinoki, [TA]hyssop, [TA]Idaho tansy, [TA]ImmuPower, [TA]juniper, [TA]lavender, [TA]*Melaleuca quinquenervia* (viral and fungal infection), [TA]mountain savory, [TA]palmarosa, [TA]pine, [TA]sandalwood, [TA]tarragon.

***Comments—(Viruses often hibernate along the spine) **Do the Raindrop Technique!** Dr. J. C. Lapraz found that viruses cannot live in the presence of cinnamon oil. However, because of its high phenol content, it must be diluted before being applied to the skin. See the "Single Oil Property Chart" in the Appendix of this book for additional antiviral oils and their strengths.

Recipe #1—Massage ImmuPower and oregano along the spine.

When my friend contracted the ***West Nile virus*** *from a mosquito bite last summer, her neck became stiff, and she had swelling in her ears and behind her ears at the base of her brain. She was in great pain and her ears felt "full" all of the time. We applied an oil blend from Young Living Oils called Thieves. She placed the oil at the base of her head and down both sides of her neck and jaw area. This gave her relief from the intense pain in her neck and reduced the swelling in her ears and head. She also drank a couple of drops of the Thieves oil blend in fluids several times a day. She continued doing this for at least a month while she fought this disease. We both agree this probably kept her from more serious complications due to the severity of the illness. We also believe it kept her out of the hospital.*

-Submitted by C. Ness

Supplements—ImmuPro, Inner Defense, Thieves Lozenges, Life 5 (probiotic), ParaFree.

—Airborne Viruses

Recipe #2—ImmuPower on throat and chest, Thieves on feet. Diffuse.

—Asthma *See Asthma.*

—Ebola Virus

Oils—This virus cannot live in the presence of [TA]cinnamon bark or [TA]oregano.

—Epstein–Barr Virus *See Epstein–Barr.*

***Comments—Strengthen immune system, ensure proper thyroid function, and work on hypoglycemia. Use ImmuPower, Thieves.

Supplements—Inner Defense, ImmuPro, NingXia Red, Wolfberry Crisp Bars.

—Respiratory

Oils—[A]*Eucalyptus radiata* (diffuse with Thieves; add spruce to push lower in lungs).

—Spine

Blend #1—5 drops oregano and 5 drops thyme. Put on bottoms of the feet and up the spine using the Raindrop Technique.

—Viral Disease *See also Childhood Diseases*

▸▸*A viral disease is any of a large number of diseases caused by a virus. The list of viral diseases includes AIDS/HIV, chicken pox, adenovirus, Epstein-Barr virus, hepatitis, herpes, measles, meningitis, Ebola virus, and many others.*

Oils—[AT]Cinnamon bark.

Supplements—Inner Defense, ImmuPro, ParaFree, Super C/Super C Chewable, True Source (whole food multi-nutrient).

–Infection

Oils—[TA]Melaleuca, [TA]oregano, [AT]ravensara, [TA]thyme, [TA]cajeput.

Blend #2—Mix one drop each of lavender, orange, and spruce, and apply to chest. Then put 10 drops of frankincense in a cap full of Evening Peace Bath Gel; add to bath as a bubble bath, and soak.

T—Dilute as recommended, and apply on location or to the Vita Flex points on the bottoms of the feet. Apply along the spine.

A—Diffuse into the air. Inhale oil directly or applied to hands, tissue, or a cotton wick.

Anxiety: *See also Calming.*

Anxiety is the body's way of preparing itself to deal with a threat or to deal with future stressful events. While this response is normal, and happens as part of the body's natural response to stress, this response can also happen at inappropriate times or too frequently, as in the case of anxiety disorders. Anxiety can include both physical and mental symptoms such as fear, nervousness, nausea, sweating, increased blood pressure and heart rate, feelings of apprehension or dread, difficulty concentrating, irritability, restlessness, panic attacks, and many others.

Oils—**AT**Lavender[77], **AT**orange[78], **AT**lemon[79], **TA**Roman chamomile[80], **AT**valerian[81], **AT**melissa[82], **AT**copaiba[83], **AT** F ylang ylang, **AT**basil, **AT**bergamot, **AT**cedarwood, **AT**clary sage, **AT**cypress, **AT**Evergreen Essence, **AT**frankincense[84], **AT**geranium, **AT**hyssop, **AT**jasmine, **AT**juniper, **AT**lime, **AT**marjoram, **TA**onycha (combine with rose for massage), **AT**patchouli, **AT**pine, **AT**Release, **AT**rose, **AT**sandalwood, **AT**Surrender, **AT**tangerine, **AT**tsuga (grounding).

—Panic

Panic is a sudden overwhelming feeling of fear and anxiety that tends to dominate a person's thoughts, leading to wild, irrational, and unthinking behavior.

Oils—**AT**Lavender[77], **AT**Roman chamomile[80], **AT**ylang ylang, **AT**Awaken, **AT**bergamot, **AT**fir, **AT**balsam fir, **AT**frankincense, **AT**Gathering, **AT**Harmony, **AT**marjoram, **AT**myrrh, **AT**rosemary, **AT**sandalwood, **AT**spruce, **AT**thyme, **AT**Valor, **AT**White Angelica, **AT**wintergreen.

A—Diffuse into the air. Inhale directly or applied to hands, tissue, or a cotton wick.

T—Dilute in V-6 Oil, and massage into the skin. Dilute as recommended, and apply to back of neck, temples, or Vita Flex points on the feet. Apply to auricular emotional points. Add 1–2 drops to 1/4 cup bath salts or to 1 Tbs. bath and shower gel, and dissolve in warm bathwater.

Apathy: *See also Depression.*

Oils—**A**Joy, **A**Transformation, **A**Valor, **A**orange, **A**peppermint, **A**frankincense, **A**geranium, **A**Harmony, **A**Highest Potential, **A**Hope, **A**jasmine, **A**marjoram, **A**rose, **A**rosemary, **A**rosewood, **A**sandalwood, **A**3 Wise Men, **A**thyme, **A**White Angelica, **A**ylang ylang.

A—Diffuse into the air. Inhale directly or applied to hands, tissue, or a cotton wick.

Aphrodisiac:

Oils—**AT** F Sandalwood, **AT**rose, **A**Idaho blue spruce, **AT**Sensation, **AT**Lady Sclareol, **A**cinnamon bark, **AT**clary sage, **AT**ginger, **AT**jasmine, **AT**patchouli, **AT**neroli, **AT**ylang ylang.

Personal Care—Sensation Bath & Shower Gel, Sensation Massage Oil, Sensation Hand & Body Lotion.

*An Aphrodisiac is a substance used to stimulate feelings of love or sexual desire. Many books of aromatherapy tout the **aphrodisiac** qualities of a number of oils. Perhaps an aphrodisiac to one individual may not be to another. The most important factor is to find an oil that brings balance to the mind and body. A balanced individual is more likely to extend love.*

A—Diffuse into the air. Wear as perfume or cologne.

T—Dilute in 1 Tbs. V-6 Oil, and use as massage oil. Add 1–2 drops to 1/4 cup bath salts or to 1 Tbs. bath and shower gel, and dissolve in warm bathwater.

Apnea:

Apnea is the cessation of breathing. During sleep, periods of apnea can occur for a few seconds before breathing resumes. May be due to irregular heartbeats, high blood pressure, obesity, or damage to the area of the brain responsible for controlling respiration.

Oils—TValor (on feet), AClarity (diffuse), ATBrain Power, ARaven, ARC.

A—Inhale directly or applied to hands, tissue, or a cotton wick. Diffuse into the air.

T—Dilute as recommended, and apply to Vita Flex points on the feet.

Supplements—MultiGreens, Super B, Thyromin.

Recipe #1—Try 3 MultiGreens twice per day, 1 Super B three times per day with meals, and 1 Thyromin before bed.

Appetite:

—Loss Of

Oils—TA FBergamot, TA Fnutmeg, TAginger, TAspearmint, TAcalamus, TAcardamom, TAhyssop, TAlemon, TAmyrrh, TAorange.

T—Apply to stomach, bottoms of feet.

A—Diffuse into the air.

Supplements—ComforTone, Essentialzyme, Essentialzymes-4.

—Suppressant

Oils—TASlique Essence.

Supplements—Slique Bar, Slique Tea, Slique Gum, Slique Slim Caps.

Argumentative: *See also Calming.*

Oils—ATPeace & Calming, ATylang ylang, ATorange, TTranquil (roll-on), ATRoman chamomile, ATHarmony, ATAcceptance, ATcedarwood, ATeucalyptus, ATfrankincense, ATHope, ATHumility, ATjasmine, ATJoy, ATthyme, ATTransformation, ATTrauma Life, ATValor.

A—Inhale directly. Diffuse into the air.

T—Apply to auricular emotional points. Dilute in V-6 Oil, and apply as massage oil.

Arms-flabby:

Oils—TCypress, Tfennel, Tjuniper, Tlavender.

T—Dilute in V-6 Oil, and massage into skin on location.

Arterial Vasodilator: *See Arteries: Vasodilator. See also Cardiovascular System.*

Arteries:

Oils—TAAroma Life, TAlavender, TAMelrose.

T—Dilute as recommended, and apply to carotid arteries in neck, over heart, and to reflex points on the feet.

A—Diffuse into the air. Inhale directly or applied to hands.

Personal Care—Cel-Lite Magic and drink Chamomile Tea.

Supplements—Cleansing Trio (ComforTone, Essentialzyme, and ICP).

—ARTERIOSCLEROSIS *See Also Cardiovascular System:* ATHEROSCLEROSIS.

▸▸*Arteriosclerosis is a hardening, stiffening, or loss of elasticity of the arteries that occurs over time as the artery walls experience excessive pressure.*

Oils—**T**Aroma Life, **T**$_F$cedarwood, **T**lemon[85] (increase white and red blood cells), **T**ginger, **T**juniper, **T**rosemary, **T**thyme, **T**wintergreen.

T—Apply to heart and Vita Flex points on feet.

–BLOOD CLOTS *See also Blood:* CLOTS

Oils—**I**Ocotea[86], **I**fennel[87], **IT**clove[88], **T**balsam fir, **T**grapefruit, **T**helichrysum.

Supplements—In addition to vitamins E and C, all supplements containing essential oils should help increase the supply of oxygen in the blood stream. Rehemogen (tincture) together with JuvaTone may help build blood and hemoglobin platelets (raise cell count); also True Source (whole food multi-nutrient).

I—Place 2–3 drops in an empty capsule with V-6 Oil; swallow.

T—Dilute as recommended, and apply to carotid arteries, over heart, and to Vita Flex points on the feet.

—STRENGTHENS

Oils—**TA**Aroma Life

T—Dilute as recommended, and apply to carotid arteries in neck, over heart, and to reflex points on the feet.

A—Diffuse into the air. Inhale directly or applied to hands.

—VASODILATOR

▸▸*A vasodilator is a substance that causes a blood vessel to dilate (increase in diameter) through the relaxation of the endometrial cells lining the vessel walls. This gives the blood more room to flow and lowers the blood pressure.*

Oils—**T**Eucalyptus[89], **T**rosemary[89], **T**$_F$marjoram, **T**Aroma Life.

T—Apply to carotid arteries in neck, over heart, and to Vita Flex points on feet.

Arteriosclerosis: *See Arteries:* ARTERIOSCLEROSIS.

Arthritis: *See also Acidosis.*

▸▸*Arthritis is the painful swelling, inflammation, and stiffness of the joints*

Oils—**TA**Frankincense[90], **TA**$_F$rosemary[91], **TA**$_F$marjoram[91], **TA**Aroma Siez, **TA**PanAway, **TA**$_F$spruce, **TA**$_F$cypress, **TA**wintergreen (drains toxins that cause pain), **TA**fir (has cortisone-like action), **TA**Aroma Life, **TA**basil,**TA**cedarwood, **TA**clove, **TA**eucalyptus[91], **TA**balsam fir, **TA**ginger, **TA**Harmony (with Valor), **TA**helichrysum, **TA**hyssop, **TA**Idaho tansy, **TA**ImmuPower, **TA**lavender, **TA**Melrose, **TA**nutmeg, **TA**onycha (benzoin), **TA**palo santo, **TA**Peace & Calming, **TA**peppermint, **TA**pine, **TA**Purification, **TA**Roman chamomile, **TA**sage lavender, **TA**Valor, **TA**white fir (has cortisone-like action).

T—Apply oils on location.

A—Diffuse into the air.

Blend #1—Combine 1 oz. Ortho Ease with 25 drops wintergreen, 12 drops cypress, 9 drops Roman chamomile, and 3 drops juniper. Massage on location.

Blend #2—Combine Ortho Ease with wintergreen alone, and apply on location.

Blend #3—Wintergreen with PanAway.

Personal Care—Ortho Ease Massage Oil, Prenolone/Prenolone+, Progessence/Progessence Plus, Regenolone.

Supplements—AlkaLime, BLM, Mineral Essence, MultiGreens, NingXia Red, Power Meal (contains wolfberry), Slique Tea, Sulfurzyme (contains wolfberry), Super C / Super C Chewable, Super Cal, Thyromin (improves thyroid function and energy levels).

—Arthritic Pain

Oils—[T]Wintergreen, [T]PanAway, [T]palo santo, [T]spruce, [T]ginger.

T—Dilute as recommended, and apply on location.

—Osteoarthritis

›› *Osteoarthritis is a degenerative arthritis where the cartilage that provides lubrication between the bones in a joint begins to break down, becoming rough and uneven. This causes the bones in the joint to wear and create rough deposits that can become extremely painful.*

Detoxify with cypress, fennel, and lemon. Massage affected joints with rosemary, chamomile, juniper and lavender (Alternative Medicine—A Definitive Guide, p. 537).

Oils—[T]Wintergreen, [T]eucalyptus, [T]basil, [T]lavender, [T]lemon, [T]marjoram, [T]thyme.

T—Dilute as recommended, and apply on location.

—Rheumatoid Arthritis

›› *Rheumatoid arthritis: Rheumatoid arthritis is arthritis caused by inflammation within the joint, causing pain and possibly causing the joint to degenerate.*

Oils—[TA]$_F$Spruce, [TA]$_F$marjoram, [TA]$_F$cypress, [TA]PanAway, [TA]$_F$pine, [TA]$_F$nutmeg, [TA]$_F$lemon, [TA]$_F$bergamot, [TA]$_F$ginger, [TA]angelica, [TA]black pepper, [TA]cajeput, [TA]cinnamon bark, [TA]coriander, [TA]eucalyptus, [TA]fennel, [TA]fir, [TA]balsam fir, [TA]galbanum, [TA]geranium, [TA]hyssop, [TA]juniper, [TA]lavender, [TA]oregano (chronic), [TA]palo santo, [TA]Peace & Calming, [TA]peppermint, [TA]Roman chamomile, [TA]rosemary, [TA]tarragon, [TA]thyme, [TA]wintergreen.

T—Dilute as recommended, and apply on location.

A—Diffuse into the air.

Personal Care—Prenolone/Prenolone+, Progessence/Progessence Plus, Regenolone.

Blend #4—Combine 2 oz. of Ortho Ease with 7 drops wintergreen, 6 drops ginger, 19 drops eucalyptus, 6 drops juniper, 8 drops marjoram, and 3 drops peppermint. Rub on location.

Ashamed: *See Emotions.*

Oils—[AT]Acceptance, [AT]Forgiveness, [AT]Valor.

A—Diffuse into the air. Inhale directly or applied to hands, tissue, or a cotton wick.

T—Apply to auricular emotional points.

Assault: *See Emotions.*

Oils—[AT]Trauma Life.

A—Diffuse into the air. Inhale directly or applied to hands, tissue, or a cotton wick.

T—Apply to auricular emotional points.

Assimilating Food:

Supplements—Enzyme products: Allerzyme (aids the digestion of sugars, starches, fats, and proteins), Detoxzyme (helps maintain and support a healthy intestinal environment), Essentialzyme, Essentialzymes-4. Also Balance Complete, Digest + Cleanse, Power Meal (predigested protein), and Super B.

Asthma: *See Respiratory System.*

»*Asthma is a disease that causes the lung's airways to narrow, making it difficult to breathe. Episodes (or attacks) of asthma can be triggered by any number of things, including smoke, pollution, dust mites, and other allergens. Asthma causes reoccurring periods of tightness in the chest, coughing, shortness of breath, and wheezing.*

Oils—AT F Eucalyptus[92], AT F peppermint[93], AT F frankincense (on crown), AT Raven (diffuse), AT RC (some people use RC or Raven instead of inhaler), AT dorado azul, AT rose[94], AT F thyme[92], AT F lemon, AT F marjoram, AT F oregano, AT F pine, AT F sage, AT cajeput, AT calamus, AT clary sage, AT cypress, AT Evergreen Essence, AT fir, AT hyssop, AT laurel, AT lavender, AT mugwort[95], AT myrrh, AT myrtle, AT onycha (benzoin), AT ravensara, AT rose, AT rosemary, AT sage AT lavender, AT tsuga (opens respiratory tract).

A—Avoid steam inhalation. Drop on pillow or diffuse into the air.

T—Dilute as necessary, and apply over lungs and throat.

Recipe #1—May insert RC and Raven with 1 tsp. V-6 Oil in rectum. **Or** Raven rectally with RC on chest and back. Reverse each night. **Or** *Eucalyptus radiata* and frankincense in rectum.

*****Comments**—**Plastic nasal inhalers** work very well for breathing in the essential oils. Nasal inhaler blanks (empty inhalers) are available from Abundant Health to fill with your choice of oil. Just saturate an absorbent wick with the essential oil or blend, insert wick into the inhaler blank, and plug the end. Then just unscrew the cap, place inhaler next to or inside each nostril, and breathe deeply. Replace the cap to prevent evaporation. These are great to take on airplanes instead of the messy, bulky oil bottles.

Blend #1—Combine 10 drops cedarwood, 10 drops eucalyptus, 2 drops Roman chamomile, and 2 oz. water. Put on hanky and inhale. Can also be used to gargle.

Blend #2—Combine 10 drops Raven, 5 drops hyssop, and 2 tsp. V-6 Oil. Massage on spine and chest.

Personal Care—Prenolone/Prenolone+.

Supplements—Super C / Super C Chewable, Thyromin.

*****Comments**—Do a colon and liver cleanse with either the Master Cleanser (see Cleansing) or with the Cleansing Trio supplements (ComforTone, ICP, Essentialzyme) and JuvaTone.

—Attack

Oils—A RC or A Raven.

A—Just smelling from the bottle has stopped attacks.

Recipe #1—3 Wise Men on crown, Raven on throat, RC on lungs, Thieves on feet, ImmuPower on spine. May insert RC and Raven with V-6 Oil in rectum, **or** Raven rectally with RC on chest and back; reverse each night.

Recipe #2—Inhale or diffuse bergamot, eucalyptus, hyssop, lavender, or marjoram. Try frankincense for calming. (*Alternative Medicine—The Definitive Guide*, p. 824).

Recipe #3—Apply frankincense to the crown, RC on the throat and chest, and Raven on the back. Then inhale the aroma of the oils from your hands.

Astringent:

▸▸*An astringent is a substance that controls bleeding by causing the body's tissues and vessels to contract.*

Oils—^T^Lemon, ^T^onycha (benzoin).

T—Dilute as necessary, and apply on location.

Athletes Foot: *See Antifungal: Athlete's Foot.*

Attention Deficit Disorder: *See ADD. See also Hyperactivity.*

Aura:

Oils—^AT^White Angelica, ^AT^Awaken, ^AT^Joy, ^AT^Sacred Mountain.

—Increase Aura Around Body

Oils—^AT^White Angelica (use with Awaken and Sacred Mountain).

—Protection Of

Oils—^AT^White Angelica.

—Strengthen

Oils—^AT^White Angelica.

A—Wear as perfume or cologne. Diffuse into the air.

T—Dilute as necessary, and apply on chakras.

Autism:

▸▸*Autism is a developmental disorder that impairs the normal development of communication, sociality, and human interaction.*

—Reduce Anxiety/Fear

Blend #1—Bergamot, geranium, and clary sage. Layer or dilute in V-6 Oil for a massage.

—Stimulate the Senses

Blend #2—Basil, lemon, peppermint, and rosemary. Layer or dilute in V-6 Oil for a massage.

***Comments—Make sure that no negativity exists when the oils are used because the autistic child will make those associations when the oil is used again.

Autoimmune System: *For Autoimmune diseases, see AIDS, Grave's Disease, Hashimoto's Disease, and Lupus.*

Oils—^AT^ImmuPower, ^AT^cistus.

A—Diffuse into the air.

T—Dilute as necessary, and apply to Vita Flex points on the feet. Dilute with V-6 Oil, and massage into skin.

Supplements—ImmuPro, MultiGreens, NingXia Red, Sulfurzyme (helps mitigate effects of autoimmune diseases), Thyromin, True Source (whole food multi-nutrient).

Avoidance: *See Emotions.*

Oils—^AT^Magnify Your Purpose, ^AT^Motivation.

A—Diffuse into the air. Inhale directly or applied to hands, tissue, or a cotton wick.

T—Apply to auricular emotional points.

Awake: *See also Alertness.*

—Jet Lag *See Jet Lag*

—Staying Awake While Driving

Blend #1—Clarity and En-R-Gee together. Diffuse.

Awaken the Mind, Spirit:

Oils—ATAwaken, ATmyrrh.

A—Diffuse into the air. Inhale directly or applied to hands, tissue, or a cotton wick.

T—Apply to auricular emotional points.

Awaken the Past:

Oils—ATCypress.

A—Diffuse into the air. Inhale directly or applied to hands, tissue, or a cotton wick.

T—Apply to auricular emotional points.

Awareness:

—Greater Awareness of Ones Potential

Oils—ATBelieve, ATInto the Future, ATWhite Angelica.

—Increases Sensory System

Oils—ATAwaken, ATwintergreen.

—Opens Sensory System

Oils—ATPeppermint, ATwintergreen.

—Revitalizes

Oils—ATLemongrass.

—Self

Oils—ATAcceptance, ATBelieve.

—Spiritual

Oils—ATBelieve, ATfrankincense, ATInspiration (enhances spiritual mood), ATmyrrh, AT3 Wise Men.

A—Diffuse into the air. Inhale directly or applied to hands, tissue, or a cotton wick.

T—Apply to auricular emotional points. Dilute with V-6 Oil, and massage into skin.

Babies: *See Children/Infants.*

Back:

Oils—TPanAway, TEndoFlex, TRelieve It, TValor (aligns; a chiropractor in a bottle), Tthyme (for virus in spine), Twintergreen, Tbasil, Tblack pepper, Tcypress, Teucalyptus, Tgeranium, Tginger, Tjuniper, Tlavender, Toregano, Tpeppermint, TRoman chamomile, Trosemary, Tsage, Ttangerine.

Supplements—BLM, EndoGize.

—Calcified (spine)

▸▸ *Calcification occurs when calcium builds up in tissue and causes the tissue to harden. As people age, calcification can cause the ligaments of the spine to thicken and harden, making the spinal canal narrow, creating pressure on the spinal nerve.*

Oils—ᵀPanAway, ᵀrosemary, ᵀgeranium.

Personal Care—Ortho Ease Massage Oil (combine with PanAway on spine).

Supplements—Super C / Super C Chewable.

I was about 8½ hours into a 10 hour round trip drive and my back started to seize up. I have an old muscle injury, and I knew I was in trouble. I had my oils on the seat next to me and grabbed my PanAway at a stoplight and poured it in my hand. I was in a hurry. I had planned on putting on about 5 drops, but the oil was warm, and I think I ended up with about 20 in my hand. Rather than waste it, I put it all on my lower back and sat back in my seat. Within a few minutes my spine did a complete correction starting at the base and going up to the back of my head. I felt each click as it ran up my spine. Needless to say, my back no longer hurt, and I had no stiffness when I finally got out of the car!

-Submitted by Andrea Safford
Warrenton, Virginia (July 2004)

—Deteriorating Discs

▸▸ *Deteriorating disc disease occurs as people age and their spinal discs begin to deteriorate. As deterioration progresses, movement becomes restricted and pain in the neck and back increases. Although most commonly associated with aging, disc deterioration can be caused by back injuries as well.*

Recipe #1—Do raindrop therapy with just the application of the oils, none of the working along the spine.

Personal Care—Ortho Ease Massage Oil.

Supplements—BLM, Super C / Super C Chewable.

—Herniated Discs

▸▸ *A herniated disc is caused when one of the discs of the spine is damaged and either bulges or breaks open. When the herniated disc presses on a nerve, it causes pain in the buttock, thigh, and calf. Herniated discs can be caused by spinal injuries or by the wear and tear that come with age as the discs begin to dry out.*

Oils—ᵀValor (3 drops on location may help relieve pressure) ᵀPanAway, ᵀRelieve It, (massage up disc area three times to help with pain), ᵀcypress (strengthens blood capillary walls, improves circulation, powerful anti-inflammatory), ᵀblack pepper, ᵀpeppermint.

Recipe #2—Do raindrop therapy with just the application of the oils, none of the working along the spine.

Blend #1—Lemongrass with Idaho tansy; then marjoram with balsam fir or frankincense to help repair the damage.

Personal Care—Ortho Ease Massage Oil.

Supplements—BLM, Super C / Super C Chewable.

—Low Back Pains

Oils—ᵀDeep Relief (roll-on), ᵀsandalwood.

Recipe #3—Rub Valor on top and bottoms of feet, Di-Gize on colon, and Ortho Ease up the back. Massage cypress up the disc area three times. Cypress strengthens blood capillary walls, improves circulation, and is a powerful anti-inflammatory. Use helichrysum to increase circulation, decongest, and reduce inflammation and pain. Use peppermint to stimulate the nerves (may need to dilute with Ortho Ease). Layer basil, Aroma Siez, Relieve It, and spruce.

Supplements—BLM

—Muscular Fatigue

Oils—ᵀMarjoram, ᵀrosemary, ᵀclary sage, ᵀlavender.

—PAIN

Oils—ᵀDeep Relief (roll-on), ᵀValor, ᵀPanAway.

Personal Care—ᵀOrtho Sport Massage Oil.

Blend #2—5 to 10 drops each of rosemary, marjoram, and sage **or**

Blend #3—5 to 10 drops each of lavender, eucalyptus, and ginger **or**

Blend #4—5 to 10 drops each of peppermint, rosemary, and basil.

Recipe #4—Apply PanAway and Valor on the shoulders. If the individual being worked on is lying on their stomach, the person applying the oils to the shoulders should cross their arms so the electrical frequency is not broken (right to right etc.). Apply the following oils **up** the spine, one at a time, using a probe on each vertebra if possible; stroke with fingers, feathering gently in 4" strokes three times for each oil: Peppermint (excites the back), cypress (anti-inflammatory), Aroma Siez, Relieve It, and spruce. Follow the procedure with a hot compress. The blends above have also been used with success. Follow the same stroking procedure, and dilute the blends with a little V-6 Oil for a massage.

Supplements—BLM.

—SCOLIOSIS

›› *Scoliosis is an abnormal sideways curvature of the spine. Scoliosis can cause back pain and uneven shoulders or hips. Severe cases of scoliosis can be disabling.*

Recipe #5—May be caused by a virus. **Do the Raindrop Technique!**

***COMMENT—The videos listed in the Bibliography are highly recommended for a professional visual presentation of the Raindrop Technique.

Blend #5—8 drops basil, 12 drops wintergreen, 5 drops cypress, 10 drops marjoram, and 2 drops peppermint.

–CORRECT

Oils—Do the following (a variation of the Raindrop Technique) every 7 to 10 days for a minimum of 8 times to help get rid of **scoliosis**:

1. Rub Valor on feet.
2. Apply oregano and thyme using the Raindrop Technique up the spine.
3. Apply **blend #5** (shown above) along the spine. Push or pull in the direction that the spine needs to be strengthened. Knead fingers clockwise three times. Then work two fingers up the spine with the other hand on top of the hand that is doing the kneading (do this three times).
4. Apply Aroma Siez and marjoram on the muscles on each side of the spine. Apply warm wet towel to back, and have individual lay on their back.
5. Work the Vita Flex areas down the leg to the feet with basil, wintergreen, cypress, and peppermint in V-6 Oil.
6. Work the spine Vita Flex areas on the feet; then give feet a mild pull.
7. Put one hand under the chin and the other hand at the back of the neck. Have the person receiving the massage breathe in and out as you gently rock and pull the neck in time with their breathing.
8. Take towel off. If the back gets too hot during massage, apply V-6 Oil.
9. Measure the spine to see how much it has changed.

—STIFFNESS

Oils—[T]Marjoram, [T]Valor.

***Comments—Do the Raindrop Technique.

Personal Care—Ortho Sport Massage Oil.

—VIRUSES ALONG SPINE *See Also Antiviral*

Recipe #6—Layer *Eucalyptus radiata*, ImmuPower, oregano, and Ortho Ease on spine. Viruses tend to hibernate along the spine.

T—Dilute as necessary, and apply along the spine, on affected muscles, or on reflex points on the feet. Do the Raindrop Technique. Dilute in V-6 Oil, and massage into muscles on the back or along the spine. Apply as a hot compress over the affected area.

Bacteria: *See Antibacterial.*

Balance:

Oils—[TA]Valor, [TA]frankincense (balances electrical field), [TA]vetiver (is shown to have a balancing effect on the whole body when applied to the brain stem), [TA]Acceptance, [TA]Aroma Siez, [TA]Awaken, [TA]cedarwood, [TA]Harmony, [TA]Mister, [TA]palo santo, [TA]Roman chamomile, [TA]ylang ylang.

—BALANCE MALE/FEMALE ENERGIES

Oils—[TA]Acceptance, [TA]ylang ylang.

—CHAKRAS

Oils—[TA]Harmony, [TA]Valor.

—EMOTIONAL

Oils—[TA]Envision.

—ELECTRICAL ENERGIES

Oils—[TA]Valor, [TA]frankincense, [TA]Harmony.

—FEELING OF

Oils—[TA]Envision, [TA]spruce.

—HARMONIC BALANCE TO ENERGY CENTER

Oils—[TA]Acceptance, [TA]Harmony.

Supplements—Master Formula His/Hers.

T—Dilute as necessary, and apply on location. To balance energies, start by applying 3–6 drops Valor on the bottom of each foot. Some may be applied to the neck and shoulders if desired. When working on someone else, place the palms of the hands on the bottom of each foot (left hand to left foot and right hand to right foot), and hold for 5 to 15 minutes. If working on yourself, perform the Cook's Hookup by lifting the right foot and placing the right ankle on top of the left knee in cross-legged fashion. Next place the left hand on the right ankle, and cup the front of the ankle with the fingers. Then cross the right hand over the left; and with the right hand, grasp the heel of the right foot (with thumb around the back and fingers cupping the bottom of the heel). Hold this for 5 to 15 minutes. The balancing of the electrical energies can be felt by either a pulse in the hands and feet or by a warming sensation.

A—Inhale directly or applied to the hands. Diffuse into the air.

Baldness: *See Hair: Baldness, Loss.*

Bath:

Oils—While tub is filling, add oils to the water (oils will be drawn to your skin quickly from the top of the water, so use gentle oils like lavender, Roman chamomile, rosewood, sage, ylang ylang, etc). For the most benefit, add 5–10 drops of your favorite essential oil to 1/2 ounce Bath and Shower Gel Base. You can also add 3–5 drops to 1/4–1/2 cup bath or Epsom salts before dissolving in warm bathwater.

Personal Care—Evening Peace, Relaxation, and Sensation Bath and Shower Gels as well as Lavender Rosewood, Sacred Mountain, and Peppermint Cedarwood Moisturizing Soaps are all wonderfully soothing in the evening. Morning Start Bath and Shower Gel as well as Lemon Sandalwood and Thieves Cleansing Soaps are all terrific ways to jump-start your day.

Bed Wetting: *See Bladder: Bed Wetting and Incontinence.*

Belching:

Oils—[T]Di-Gize.

T—Apply to stomach and on Vita Flex points.

Bereavement (Mourning):

Oils—[AT]Basil, [AT]cypress.

A—Diffuse into the air. Inhale directly or applied to hands, tissue, or a cotton wick.

T—Apply to auricular emotional points.

Betrayed (Feeling): *See also Emotions.*

Oils—[AT]Acceptance, [AT] Forgiveness, [AT]Transformation, [AT]Valor.

A—Diffuse into the air. Inhale directly or applied to hands, tissue, or a cotton wick.

T—Apply to auricular emotional points.

Birthing: *See Pregnancy.*

Bites: *See also Insect.*

Oils—[T]Basil, [T]cinnamon bark, [T]lavender, [T]lemon, [T]sage, [T]thyme (all have antitoxic and antivenomous properties). Can also try fresh [T]garlic oil.

—Allergic

Oils—[T]Purification.

—Bees and Hornets

Recipe #1—Remove the stinger; apply a cold compress of Roman chamomile to area for several hours or for as long as possible. Then apply 1 drop of Roman chamomile three times a day for two days. Idaho tansy may also work.

—Gnats and Midges

Recipe #2—Lavender; or 3 drops thyme in 1 tsp. cider vinegar or lemon juice. Apply to bites to stop irritation.

—Insect

Oils—[T]Cajeput, [T]patchouli.

—Mosquito

Oils—[T]Helichrysum, [T]lavender.

—Snake

Oils—[T]Basil, [T]patchouli.

—Spiders, Brown Recluse, Bee Stings, Ants, Fire Ants

Oils—[T]Basil (neutralizes), [T]Purification, [T]thyme, [T]cinnamon bark, [T]lavender, [T]lemon, [T]lemongrass, [T]peppermint.

Recipe #3—(For Spiders) 3 drops lavender and 2 drops Roman chamomile in 1 tsp. alcohol. Mix well in clockwise motion, and apply to area three times a day.

—Ticks

Recipe #4—After getting the tick out, apply 1 drop lavender every 5 minutes for 30 minutes.

How to remove:

- Do not apply mineral oil, Vaseline, or anything else to remove the tick, as this may cause it to inject the spirochetes into the wound.
- Be sure to remove the entire tick. Get as close to the mouth as possible, and firmly tug on the tick until it releases its grip. Don't twist. If available, use a magnifying glass to make sure that you have removed the entire tick.
- Save the tick in a jar, and label it with the date, where you were bitten on your body, and the location or address where you were bitten for proper identification by your doctor, especially if you develop any symptoms.
- Do not handle the tick.
- Wash hands immediately.
- Check the site of the bite occasionally to see if any rash develops. If it does, seek medical advice promptly.

—Wasps (are alkaline)

Recipe #5—1 drop basil, 2 drops Roman chamomile, 2 drops lavender, and 1 tsp. cider vinegar. Mix in clockwise motion; put on area three times a day.

Bitterness: *See also Emotions.*

Oils—[AT]Acceptance, [AT]Forgiveness, [AT]Roman chamomile, [AT]Valor.

A—Diffuse into the air. Inhale directly or applied to hands, tissue, or a cotton wick.

T—Apply to auricular emotional points.

Bladder:

▸▸ *The urinary bladder is a hollow organ that collects urine before it is disposed of by urination. The bladder sits on the pelvic floor.*

Oils—[T]EndoFlex

T—Apply over kidneys as a hot compress.

—Bed Wetting and Incontinence

Recipe #1—Before bed, rub cypress mixed with V-6 Oil on abdomen.

—Infection/Cystitis

›› *Cystitis is a bladder infection characterized by urinary burning, urgency, and increased frequency. Other possible symptoms include blood in the urine, pelvic discomfort, and a low-grade fever.*

Oils—IT F Lemongrass, IT Thieves, T F German chamomile, T F spearmint, T F thyme, T basil, T bergamot, T cajeput, T cedarwood, T cinnamon bark, T clove, T eucalyptus, T fennel, T frankincense, T hyssop, T Inspiration, T juniper, T lavender, T marjoram, T onycha (benzoin), T oregano, T pine, T sage, T sandalwood (for 1st stages of bladder infection), T rosewood.

T—Massage or bathe with one of these oils.

I—Add 1 drop lemongrass or 1 drop Thieves to 8 oz. juice or water; drink three times a day.

Supplements—NingXia Red (½ cup followed by a full cup of water has brought relief within 10 minutes when taken at the first sign of discomfort).

***Comments—One individual who had a bladder infection took 1 oz. NingXia Red (followed by 6–8 oz. water) every four hours. They were over the infection in two days.

—Hanging Down

Recipe #3—Valor on feet; 3 drops ravensara and 1 drop lavender on calves (bladder should pull up).

Blame: *See Emotions.*

Oils—AT Acceptance, AT Forgiveness, AT Valor.

A—Diffuse into the air. Inhale directly or applied to hands, tissue, or a cotton wick.

T—Apply to auricular emotional points.

Blister: *(on lips from sun)*

Oils—T Lavender

T—Apply as often as needed. (It should take fever out and return lip to normal.)

Bloating: *See Digestive System: Bloating.*

Blocked (Emotionally): *See Emotions.*

Blood:

›› *Blood is the fluid inside the body that transports oxygen and nutrients to the cells and carries waste away from the cells. It also transports cells involved in the immune and inflammatory response, hormones and other chemical messengers that regulate the body's functions, and platelets that help facilitate the blood clotting necessary to repair damaged blood vessels. Blood is primarily composed of plasma (water with dissolved nutrients, minerals, and carbon dioxide) that carries red blood cells (the most numerous type of cells in blood, responsible for transporting oxygen), white blood cells (cells involved in the immune system and immune response), and platelet cells. Blood is circulated in the body by the pumping action of the heart propelling blood through various blood vessels. Proper and healthy circulation and function of blood throughout the body is critical for health, and even for the sustaining of life.*

Blood Types—Different blood types have different dominating glands.

Type A: more prone to be alkaline pH balanced. Natural vegetarians. A type A child living in the home of a type O parent is affected by parents' programing or conditioning or visa versa. They have problems with their thyroids, may have a tendency to gain weight, and need exercise.

Type AB: may want to be a vegetarian on some days but not on others. Can go either way, like A or O types. They may be affected by either the A or O parent. AB types haven't decided whether to be an A or B type. They may even need more protein than O types.

Type B: down the middle, more balanced. Takes them about 3 years to convert to being a vegetarian.

Type O: more prone to acidic condition in blood. AlkaLime is an acid-neutralizing mineral formulation and may help preserve the body's proper pH balance. Big eaters may need to take more supplements because they are not assimilating the nutrients. If they are not assimilating their food, they eat and get full quick and one hour later they are hungry again. They get more gas because they lack enzyme secretion. They may need **Essentialzyme** for the enzymes, and **Digest + Cleanse** to improve digestion and assimilation of nutrients. They eat more, digest less, but don't gain weight. May take 8 years to totally convert to vegetarian diet. Need more protein; **Pure Protein Complete**, **Vitagreen** and **Power Meal** are mainstays for O types as they are high protein and high energy formulas; nuts and seeds are good too. Nutrients in purest form reduces the need to eat. They have a harder time structuring their diet and they get cold because of poor circulation. If an O type is slender, has high energy, is compulsive in behavior, and/or is a hard worker, they may need as many as 16 MultiGreens and 10 Master Formula His/Hers per day.

—Anticoagulant

▸▸ *An Anticoagulant is a substance that keeps blood from clotting.*

Oils—**TI**Clove[96], **IT**fennel[97], **TA**F helichrysum, **TA**angelica, **TA**cassia, **TA**lavender, **TA**tangerine, **TA**tarragon.

T—Apply on location or on bottoms of feet.

I—Place 1–3 drops of oil in an empty capsule, and ingest up to 3 times per day.

A—Diffuse into the air. Apply oils to hands, and inhale oils from hands cupped over the nose. Inhale oil applied to a tissue or a cotton wick.

—Blood Pressure

–High (hypertension)

> **OILS TO AVOID IF HYPERTENSIVE**
>
> ***Single oils:*** *Hyssop, rosemary, sage, thyme, and possibly peppermint.*
>
> **This list is a compilation of the safety data contained in aromatherapy books written by the following authors: Ann Berwick, Julia Lawless, Shirley & Len Price, Jeanne Rose, Robert Tisserand, and Tony Balacs.*

Oils—**AT**F Ylang ylang[98] (arterial; put in hand, rub palms together, cup over nose, and breathe deeply for 5 minutes and/or put on feet), Aroma Life, **TA**F marjoram[99] (regulates), **TA**eucalyptus[99], **TA**F lavender, **TA**F spearmint, **TA**clary sage, **TA**clove, **TA**balsam fir (lowers), **TA**goldenrod, **TA**lemon, **TA**nutmeg, **TA**wintergreen.

T—Place oils on heart points on left arm, hand, foot, and over heart.

A—Can also smell from palms of hands, diffuse, or place a few drops on a cotton ball and put in a vent. *See Comments under Asthma for a discussion on using* ***plastic nasal inhalers****.*

*****Comments**—Refer to the chapter entitled "How to Use—The Personal Usage Reference" in the Essential Oils Desk Reference under "Blood Pressure, High" for specific product recommendations.

Recipe #1—3 ylang ylang and 3 marjoram in bathwater. Bathe in the evening twice a week.

Blend #1—5 geranium, 8 lemongrass, 3 lavender, and 1 oz. V-6 Oil. Rub over heart and heart Vita Flex points on left foot and hand.

Blend #2—10 ylang ylang, 5 marjoram, 5 cypress, and 1 oz. V-6 Oil. Rub over heart and on heart Vita Flex points on left foot and hand.

–Low

Oils—$^{AT}{}_{F}$Rosemary, ^{AT}Aroma Life, ^{AT}hyssop (raises), ^{AT}pine, ^{AT}ylang ylang.

T—Place oils on heart points on left arm, hand, foot, and over heart.

A—Can also smell from palms of hands, diffuse, or place a few drops on a cotton ball and put in a vent. *See Comments under Asthma for a discussion on using* ***plastic nasal inhalers***.

—Blood Protein

Supplements—MultiGreens.

—Bleeding (Stops)

Oils—^{T}Helichrysum, ^{T}Aroma Life, ^{T}geranium (will increase bleeding first to eliminate toxins and then stop it), ^{T}cistus, ^{T}onycha (benzoin), ^{T}rose. Can also use ^{T}cayenne pepper tincture.

T—Dilute as necessary, and apply on location.

***Comments—Some have found that taking 14 capsules of helichrysum internally over a 24 hour period, right before surgery, can help prep the blood so that bleeding is reduced. Can also topically apply helichrysum to the surgical location before surgery.

—Broken Blood Vessels

Oils—^{T}Helichrysum, ^{T}grapefruit.

T—Dilute as necessary, and apply on location.

***Comments—One woman had some blood vessels break in her brain, which effected her short-term memory, concentration, focus, and emotions. She used the oils of Clarity, basil, rosemary, peppermint, and cardamom. Not only did her blood vessels heal, but her concentration, awareness, focus, and self-esteem increased.

—Build

Recipe #1—Rehemogen (tincture) together with JuvaTone and Juva Cleanse may help build blood and hemoglobin platelets (raise cell count).

—Cholesterol

▸▸ *Cholesterol is a soft, waxy substance found in the bloodstream and in all of the body's cells. The body requires some cholesterol to function properly, but high levels of cholesterol narrow and block the arteries and increase the risk of heart disease.*

Oils—^{TI}Helichrysum (regulates), ^{IT}dill[100].

T—Dilute as necessary, and apply on heart Vita Flex points on the feet.

I—Add 3–5 drops essential oil to 3–5 drops V-6 Oil in an empty capsule; swallow.

—Cleansing

Oils—$^{T}{}_{F}$Helichrysum, ^{T}Juva Cleanse, ^{T}Roman chamomile.

T—Dilute as necessary, and apply to bottoms of feet.

Supplements—MultiGreens, Rehemogen Tincture (purifier).

—Clots

▸▸ *Blood Clots occur as a natural bodily defense to repair damaged blood vessels and to keep the body from losing excessive amounts of blood. However, clotting can become dangerous if an internal blood clot breaks lose in the circulatory system and blocks the flow of blood to vital organs.*

Oils—**TI**Clove[96], **IT**fennel[97], **TA** $_F$helichrysum, **TA**balsam fir (reduces pressure), **TA**grapefruit.

T—Apply on location or on bottoms of feet.

I—Place 1–3 drops of oil in an empty capsule; ingest up to 3 times per day.

A—Diffuse into the air. Apply oils to hands, and inhale oils from hands cupped over the nose. Inhale oil applied to a tissue or a cotton wick.

Recipe #2—Balsam fir, helichrysum, and cistus together (both topically and internally 3–4 times per day) help to dissolve blood clots.

—**Hemorrhaging** *See also Female Specific Conditions: Hemorrhaging.*

Oils—**T**Helichrysum, **T**cistus, **T**rose. Can also use **T**cayenne pepper.

T—Dilute as necessary, and apply on location or on bottoms of feet.

—**Low Blood Sugar** *See also Hypoglycemia*

When the level of glucose in the blood drops below its normal level, this is called "low blood sugar" or "hypoglycemia." Since glucose is such an important source of energy for the body, low blood sugar can result in light-headedness, hunger, shakiness, anxiety, weakness, confusion, nervousness, difficulty speaking, and anxiety.

Oils—**TI**Thieves (balances blood sugar), **T**cinnamon bark, **T**clove, **T**thyme.

T—Dilute as necessary, and apply on location or on bottoms of feet.

I—Place 1–3 drops of oil in an empty capsule; ingest.

Supplements—AlkaLime, Mineral Essence, MultiGreens (balances blood sugar).

—**Sticky**

Oils—**IT**Clove[101], **IT**thyme (inhibits blood platelet aggregation)

I—Place 1–3 drops of oil in an empty capsule; ingest.

T—Dilute as necessary, and apply on location or on bottoms of feet.

Supplements—Longevity Capsules (contains both clove and thyme oils)

—**Stimulates**

Oils—**IT**Peppermint[102], **IT** $_F$lemon (helps with the formation of red and white blood cells).

I—Place 1–3 drops of oil in an empty capsule; ingest.

T—Dilute as necessary, and apply on location or on bottoms of feet.

—**Vasodilator**

A vasodilator is a substance that causes a blood vessel to dilate (increase in diameter) through the relaxation of the endometrial cells lining the vessel walls. This gives the blood more room to flow and lowers the blood pressure.

Oils—**T**Eucalyptus[89], **T**rosemary[89], **T** $_F$marjoram, **T**Aroma Life, **T**lemongrass.

T—Apply to carotid arteries in neck, over heart, and to Vita Flex points on feet.

—**Vessels** *See also Arteries, Cardiovascular System, Capillaries, Veins*

Oils—**T**Aroma Life, **T**cypress (strengthens the capillary walls and increases circulation), **T**lemongrass (vasodilator).

T—Dilute as necessary, and apply on location or on bottoms of feet.

Supplements—Cel-Lite Magic dilates blood vessels for better circulation.

Body Systems: *See Bones, Cardiovascular System, Digestive System, Emotions, Hormonal System, Immune System, Muscles, Nervous System, Respiratory System, Skin.*

—BALANCE

Oils—**AT**Valor, **AT**Harmony, **AT**Joy, **AT**lavender, **AT**spruce.

—CONTROL

Oils—**AT**Cedarwood.

—ODORS

Oils—**AT**Purification (obnoxious odors), **AT**sage.

—STRENGTHEN VITAL CENTERS

Oils—**AT**Oregano.

—SUPPORT

Oils—**AT**Fir, **AT**ledum, **AT**Valor.

A—Inhale directly or applied to cupped hands.

T—Dilute as necessary, and apply to Vita-Flex points on feet or to auricular points. Dilute with V-6 Oil, and use as massage oil.

Boils:

▸▸*A boil is a skin infection that forms in a hair follicle or oil gland. The boil starts as a red, tender lump that after a few days forms a white or yellow point in the center as it fills with pus. Boils commonly occur on the face, neck, armpits, buttock, and shoulders and can be very painful.*

Oils—**T**Melaleuca[103], **T**Melrose, **T**Purification, **T**bergamot, **T**clary sage, **T**frankincense, **T**galbanum, **T**Gentle Baby, **T**lavender, **T**lemon, **T**lemongrass, **T**Raven, **T**ravensara, **T**RC, **T**Roman chamomile.

Personal Care—Rose Ointment.

***Comments—One individual put lemon oil on a sore that looked like a boil. The next day it turned black, puss came out, and it got smaller and finally disappeared.

> *I have suffered from large boils on the tops of my legs for about 30 years, and nobody could help me get rid of them. Last fall I counted 12 boils. I started using Lavender and did the Master Cleanser, lemonade cleanse. On the third day, my boils opened and ran freely. This was in January of this year. Now I only occasionally get them, and they are many times smaller than before. I know if I continue the regimen, they will eventually leave altogether.*
>
> ***-Submitted by K. Ernst (July 2004)***

Bonding: *See Emotions.*

Oils—**AT**Gentle Baby.

A—Diffuse into the air. Inhale directly or applied to hands, tissue, or a cotton wick.

T—Apply to auricular emotional points.

***Comments—Use Release or other oils listed under Emotional Release in the Science and Application section of the Reference Guide for Essential Oils to help release emotional connections to one who has passed on. Also, to help children create good bonds with others, tell them about the person when working with the oils.

Bones:

Oils—**T**Wintergreen, **T**PanAway (bone pain), **T**spruce, **T**cedarwood, **T**cypress, **T**fir, **T**juniper, **T**lavender, **T**lemongrass, **T**marjoram, **T**peppermint, **T**Relieve It, **T**sandalwood.

Supplements—BLM, Super Cal, Mineral Essence, Power Meal, Sulfurzyme, True Source (whole food multi-nutrient).

—Bone Spurs

▸▸ *A bone spur (osteophyte) is a bony projection formed on a normal bone. Bone spurs form as the body tries to repair itself by building extra bone in response to continued pressure, stress, or rubbing. Bone spurs can cause pain if they rub against soft tissues or other bones.*

> *One lady had a heel spur flare up one evening, so she took a bath with birch and cypress before retiring. The next morning, the pain was a little better. She then put 6 drops birch, 6 drops cypress, and, on top of that, 5 drops RC on a cotton pad and applied it to her heel. In 10 minutes all pain was gone, and even after four days the pain had not returned.*

Oils—ᵀWintergreen, ᵀcypress, ᵀmarjoram, ᵀRC (dissolves).

—Broken (Heal)

Recipe #1—Wintergreen and cypress (before bed); helichrysum, oregano, and Valor (in morning). Frankincense and balsam fir can also be used internally and externally.

Blend #1—9 drops wintergreen, 8 drops each of spruce, white fir, and helichrysum, and 7 drops clove (good when inflammation is causing the pain).

Blend #2—Equal parts lemongrass, clove, *Eucalyptus radiata*, and *Melaleuca alternifolia* (tea tree). Has been used to heal an infected bone fracture in as little as 3 months.

Personal Care—Ortho Ease mixed with lavender, lemongrass, and PanAway. Ortho Sport with juniper, lemongrass, and marjoram (apply over broken bones).

Supplements—BLM and Super Cal.

—Bruised

Oils—ᵀHelichrysum, ᵀRelieve It, ᵀPanAway.

—Cartilage

▸▸ *Cartilage is a type of connective tissue in the body that provides structure and support for other tissues without being hard and rigid like bone. Unlike other connective tissues, cartilage does not have blood vessels. Cartilage is found in many areas of the body, including the joints, ears, nose, bronchial tubes, and intervertebral disks.*

Oils—ᵀSandalwood (regenerates), ᵀwhite fir (pain from inflammation).

—Degeneration

Recipe #1—Apply Ortho Ease and then peppermint.

Supplements—Super C / Super C Chewable.

—Development

Supplements—Ultra Young+ (may help boost bone formation), Super C / Super C Chewable, True Source (whole food multi-nutrient).

—Osteomyelitis *See also Antibacterial*

▸▸ *Osteomyelitis is a bone infection usually caused by bacteria. The infection often starts in another area of the body and then spreads to the bone. Symptoms include fever, pain, swelling, nausea, drainage of pus, and uneasiness. Diabetes, hemodialysis, recent trauma, and IV drug abuse are risk factors for osteomyelitis.*

Recipe #2—Equal parts lemongrass, clove, *Eucalyptus radiata*, and *Melaleuca alternifolia* (tea tree), either blended together or applied individually, on the direct topical location.

****Comments**—Osteomyelitis is infection in the bones. Often, the original site of infection is elsewhere in the body and spreads to the bone by the blood. Bacteria or fungus may sometimes be responsible for osteomyelitis.

—Osteoporosis *See also Hormonal Imbalance*

Osteoporosis is a disease characterized by a loss of bone density, making the bones extremely fragile and susceptible to fractures and breaking. Osteoporosis is significantly more common in women then in men, especially after menopause; but the disease does occur in both genders.

Studies and clinical experience by Dr. John R. Lee indicate that bone mass can be reversed (regained) by as much as 41% with the use of Natural Progesterone. For information on Dr. Lee's book, see Hormonal Imbalance.

Oils—TPanAway, Twintergreen, Tclove, Tspruce, Tthyme, Tgeranium, Tpeppermint, TAroma Siez, Tchamomile (Roman and German), Tcypress, Tfennel, fir (cortisone-like action), Tginger, Thyssop, Tlemon, Tnutmeg, Toregano, TPeace & Calming, Tpine, TRelieve It, Trosemary.

Supplements—Super Cal, BLM, FemiGen, PD 80/20, Prenolone/Prenolone+, Progessence/Progessence Plus.

—Pain

Oils—TPanAway, Twhite fir, Twintergreen.

—Rotator Cuff (sore) *See also Shoulder*

The rotator cuff is the group of muscles and tendons that encircles and supports the arm at the shoulder joint.

Oils—TWintergreen (bone), Tlemongrass (torn or pulled ligaments), TPanAway, Tpeppermint (nerves), Twhite fir (inflammation), TRelieve It, Tspruce.

T—Dilute as necessary, and apply on location or on Vita Flex points on the feet.

Boredom:

Oils—AAwaken, AMotivation, AValor, ABelieve, Acedarwood, Acypress, ADream Catcher, Afir, Afrankincense, AGathering, Ajuniper, Alavender, Apepper, ARoman chamomile, Arosemary, Asandalwood, Aspruce, Athyme, Aylang ylang.

A—Diffuse into the air. Inhale directly.

Bowel: *See Digestive System.*

Boxed in (Feeling):

Oils—ATPeace & Calming, ATValor, TTranquil (roll-on).

A—Diffuse into the air. Inhale directly or applied to hands, tissue, or a cotton wick.

T—Apply to auricular emotional points.

Brain:

The Brain is the central part of the nervous system. It is responsible for processing sensory stimuli and directing appropriate behavioral responses to each stimulus, or set of stimuli. The brain also stores memories and is the center of thought.

Oils—ATLavender[104], ATlemon[105], ATlemongrass, ATAroma Life, ATblue cypress (improves circulation), ATclary sage (opens brain, euphoria), ATsacred frankincense, ATcypress, ATdorado azul (stimulates hypothalamus), ATgeranium, ATspearmint, ATTransformation, True Source (whole food multi-nutrient)

Supplements—Longevity Capsules (contains thyme oil, which helps preserve omega-3s in the brain; and contains clove oil, which helps to protect the neurons), Omega Blue or OmegaGize[3] (contain pure fish oil with naturally occurring ratios of EPA and DHA)

—ACTIVATES RIGHT BRAIN.

Oils—ATBergamot, ATgeranium, ATgrapefruit, AThelichrysum, ATRoman chamomile, ATwintergreen.

—BROKEN BLOOD VESSELS *See Blood: BROKEN BLOOD VESSELS.*

—CEREBRAL (BRAIN)

Oils—AT FNutmeg.

—CONCUSSION *See Concussion*

—FOOD

Recipe #1—Omega-3 fatty acids found in Flax Seed Oil and Sesame Oil (taken internally).

*The **blood-brain barrier** is the barrier membrane between the circulating blood and the brain that prevents certain damaging substances from reaching brain tissue and cerebrospinal fluid. The American Medical Association (AMA) determined that if they could find an agent that would pass the blood-brain barrier, they would be able to heal **Alzheimer's, Lou Gehrig's, Multiple Sclerosis, and Parkinson's disease**. In June of 1994, it was documented by the Medical University of Berlin, Germany and Vienna, Austria that **sesquiterpenes have the ability to go beyond the blood-brain barrier. High levels of sesquiterpenes** are found in the essential oils of cedarwood, vetiver, sandalwood, black pepper, patchouli, myrrh, ginger, vitex, German chamomile, spikenard, galbanum, and frankincense. Some blends containing these oils include: 3 Wise Men, Acceptance, Brain Power, Forgiveness, Gathering, Harmony, Inspiration, Into the Future, and Trauma Life (refer to Single Oil Chart in the Appendix for other blends that contain these oils).*

—INJURY

Oils—ATSacred frankincense/frankincense[106], ATValor, ATpeppermint[107], ATlemon[108].

—INTEGRATION

Oils—ATValor, AThelichrysum (increases neurotransmitter activity), ATclary sage, ATcypress, ATgeranium, ATlemongrass, ATspearmint.

—NEUROLOGICAL INJURY (BREAKDOWN OF MYELIN SHEATH)

›› *The myelin sheath is an insulating layer of protein and fatty substances that forms around nerves (including those in the brain), increasing the speed of nerve impulses. Damage to the myelin sheath interrupts these nerve impulses and can cause diseases such as multiple sclerosis, peripheral neuropathy, central pontine myelinolysis, and other neurological diseases.*

Oils—ATPeppermint[107], ATfrankincense, ATlemongrass, ATValor.

—OXYGENATE

Oils—AEucalyptus[109], Arosemary[109], Ablack pepper[110], TAhelichrysum, TAsandalwood, TAblue cypress.

Recipe #2—3 drops each of helichrysum and sandalwood once or twice a day on the back of neck, temples, and behind ears down to jaw. Also blue cypress.

—TUMOR *See Cancer: BRAIN*

Oils—TAFrankincense[111], TAValor.

A—Diffuse into the air. Inhale directly or applied to a tissue or a cotton wick.

T—Dilute as recommended, and rub onto the brain stem area, back of neck, temples, behind ears down to jaw, or on reflex points on the feet. Apply as a cold compress.

Breast: *See also Cancer: BREAST, Pregnancy/Motherhood: LACTATION.*

Oils—TClary sage, Tgeranium, Tcypress, Telemi (inflammation), Tfennel, Tlemongrass, Tsage, Tspearmint, Tvetiver.

Personal Care—ClaraDerm, Prenolone/Prenolone+/Progessence/Progessence Plus (for tenderness and swelling).

—ENLARGE AND FIRM

Oils—TClary sage, Tfennel, Tsage, TSclarEssence.

Blend #1—Equal parts vetiver, geranium, and ylang ylang.

Personal Care—A·R·T Purifying Toner (to tone and tighten skin)

—LACTATION *See Pregnancy/Motherhood.*

—MASTITIS (BREAST INFECTION) *See also Antibacterial*

Oils—TCitrus Fresh (with lavender), TExodus II, Tlavender, Ttangerine.

Blend #2—Equal amounts of lavender and tangerine. Dilute with some V-6 Oil, and apply to breasts and under arms twice a day.

—MILK PRODUCTION *See Pregnancy/Motherhood.*

—SORE NIPPLES

Oils—TRoman chamomile.

Personal Care—Animal Scents Pet Ointment

—STRETCH MARKS

Oils—TGentle Baby.

T—Dilute as necessary, and apply on location or on Vita Flex points on the feet.

Breath(ing): *See Respiratory System.*

Bronchitis: *See also Respiratory System.*

▸▸ *Bronchitis is a disease of the respiratory system, marked by inflamed and narrowed bronchial tubes. Symptoms include coughing, breathlessness, and thick phlegm. Bronchitis occurs in two forms: Acute (lasting six weeks or less) and Chronic (reoccurring frequently over two or more years).*

Oils—ATEucalyptus[112], AT*Eucalyptus radiata*[112], ATFthyme[113], TBreathe Again, AITThieves, ATFfir (obstructions of bronchi), ATFmelaleuca, ATRC, ATRaven, ATravensara, ATFpeppermint, ATFpine, ATFcedarwood, ATFrosemary, ATFclary sage, ATFcypress, ATFmarjoram, ATFspearmint, ATFmyrtle, ATAbundance, ATbasil, ATbergamot, ATcajeput, ATclove, ATelemi, ATfrankincense, ATginger, AThinoki, ATImmuPower, ATlavender, ATledum, ATlemon, AT*Melaleuca ericifolia*, ATmyrrh, ATnutmeg, ATonycha (benzoin), ATRoman chamomile, ATrose, ATsage lavender, ATsandalwood, ATtsuga (opens respiratory tract), ATwintergreen.

Blend #1—10 drops cedarwood, 10 drops eucalyptus, 2 drops Roman chamomile, and 2 oz. water. Put on hanky and inhale. Blend can also be added to water for gargling.

Blend #2—Clove, cinnamon bark, melissa, and lavender (Alternative Medicine—The Definitive Guide, p. 55).

***Comments—Refer to the chapter entitled "How to Use—The Personal Usage Reference" in the Essential Oils Desk Reference under "Bronchitis" for specific oil blend and supplement recommendations.

Recipe #1—According to Dr. Daniel Pénoël, bronchitis can be broken down into three separate areas, each of which should be considered separately. Following are the three areas and the specific blends recommended by Dr. Pénoël:

Inflammation—Mix equal portions of *Eucalyptus citriodora* and lemongrass. Apply 36 drops per foot to the sinus and lung Vita Flex points. Add to V-6 Oil, and apply over the chest.

Infection—Mix 1 tsp. melaleuca, 25 drops palmarosa or geranium, 3 drops peppermint, 1 drop thyme. Apply 3–6 drops per foot to the sinus and lung Vita Flex points. Add to V-6 Oil, and apply over the chest.

Accumulation of Fluids (mucus)—Mix 25 drops each of *Eucalyptus dives*, peppermint, and dill. Apply 3–6 drops per foot to the sinus and lung Vita Flex points.

—Chronic

Oils—ATEucalyptus[112], AT F ravensara, AT F sage, AT F sandalwood, AT F oregano, ATelemi, ATlaurel.

—Children

Oils—ATEucalyptus[112], ATmelaleuca, ATlavender, AT*Melaleuca ericifolia*, ATRoman chamomile, ATrosemary, ATthyme (CT linalol).

—Clear Mucus

Oils—ATEucalyptus[112], ATonycha (benzoin), ATThieves, ATbergamot, ATsandalwood, and ATthyme (*Alternative Medicine—The Definitive Guide*, p. 824).

***Comments—*Diffusing the oils is a great way to handle a respiratory problem.*

A—Diffuse the oils into the air. Inhale directly or from a tissue or a cotton wick. *See Comments under Asthma for a discussion on using* ***plastic nasal inhalers***.

T—Dilute as necessary, and rub on chest. Add 2–3 drops to water; gargle.

I—Add 1–2 drops to 8 oz.; drink. Add 3–5 drops to an empty capsule with 3–5 drops V-6 Oil; swallow.

Bruises:

▸▸*A bruise is a tissue injury that results in blood capillaries breaking and spilling blood into the tissue. This can cause swelling, soreness, and a visible discoloration when the bruise is near the skin.*

Oils—THelichrysum, Tgeranium, TPanAway, Tfennel, Tangelica, Thyssop, Tlavender, TMelrose, TThieves.

T—Dilute as necessary, and apply on location.

***Comments—Refer to the chapter entitled "How to Use—The Personal Usage Reference" in the Essential Oils Desk Reference under "Bruising" for some excellent blend recipes and supplement recommendations.

Bugged (Feeling): *See Emotions.*

Oils—ATAcceptance, ATForgiveness, ATPeace & Calming, ATValor.

A—Diffuse into the air. Inhale directly or applied to hands, tissue, or a cotton wick.

T—Apply to auricular emotional points.

Bugs (Repel): *See Bites and Insect: Repellent.*

Bulimia: *See Eating Disorders: Bulimia.*

Bumps:

Oils—TFrankincense, TMelrose, TPanAway, TPeace & Calming.

T—Dilute as necessary, and apply on location.

Bunions: *See Bursitis: Bunions.*

Burdens: *See Emotions.*

Oils—ATAcceptance, ATHope, ATRelease, ATTransformation, ATValor.

A—Diffuse into the air. Inhale directly or applied to hands, tissue, or a cotton wick.

T—Apply to auricular emotional points.

Burns:

A burn is an injury to tissue (often the skin) caused by heat, chemicals, or radiation. Minor burns are painful and red, while more serious burns can blister, cause swelling, and char or destroy the skin and underlying tissues. Minor burns can be treated by immersing them in cool water, while more serious burns require medical treatment.

*Dr. Alex Schauss, a prominent mineral researcher, has discovered that **burns** are painful because certain trace minerals are depleted from the skin and surrounding tissue. If the trace minerals are replenished to the affected area, then the pain will subside almost immediately. Many people have received instant pain relief when Mineral Essence was either taken internally or topically applied on the sunburn or burn.*

Oils—$^{T}_{F}$Lavender (cell renewal), ^{T}ravensara (healing), ^{T}tamanu (mix with helichrysum), ^{T}eucalyptus, ^{T}geranium, ^{T}helichrysum, ^{T}Idaho tansy, ^{T}melaleuca, ^{T}peppermint, ^{T}Roman chamomile, ^{T}rosehip.

Personal Care—LavaDerm Cooling Mist (soothing and cooling for all burns), Lavender Hand & Body Lotion (moisturizes and promotes healing).

Supplements—Mineral Essence (can be taken internally and applied topically).

Blend #1—Put 3 drops of lavender in some Lavender Hand & Body Lotion, and apply. This is effective for pain, healing, peeling, and sunburns.

Blend #2—10 drops German chamomile, 5 drops Roman chamomile, and 10 drops lavender. Mix together, and add 1 drop to each square inch of burn after it has been soaked in ice water. If you don't have the chamomile, lavender will do great. Can top with LavaDerm Cooling Mist to keep skin cool and moist.

—Cleansing

Oils—^{T}Melrose.

—Infected

Oils—^{T}Purification.

—Pain

Blend #1 (above)

Supplements—Mineral Essence (apply topically).

—Healing *See Scarring.*

Oils—^{T}Rosehip.

Blend #1 (above)

Blend #3—Ravensara or geranium mixed with helichrysum.

René Maurice Gattefossé, PhD, a French cosmetic chemist who coined the phrase "Aromatherapy," severely burned his hand in a laboratory accident. The continual application of lavender oil soothed the pain, nullified the effects of gas gangrene, and healed his hand without a scar.

—Peeling

Blend #1, Blend #2 (both shown above).

—Sunburn *See Sunburn.*

—Sun Screen

Oils—$^{T}_{F}$Helichrysum, ^{T}tamanu.

T—Dilute as necessary, and apply on location. Place 2–3 drops with 1 oz. distilled water in a misting spray bottle, shake well, and mist on location.

Bursitis:

▸▸ *Bursitis is the inflammation of the fluid-filled sack located close to joints that provides lubrication for tendons, skin, and ligaments rubbing against the bone. Bursitis is caused by infection, injury, or diseases such as arthritis and gout. Bursitis causes tenderness and pain, which can limit movement.*

Oils—**T**PanAway, **T**Aroma Siez, **T**cypress, **T**cajeput, **T**ginger, **T**hyssop, **T**juniper, **T**onycha (benzoin), **T**Roman chamomile.

Blend #1—Apply 6 drops of marjoram on shoulders and arms; wait 6 minutes. Then apply 3 drops of wintergreen; wait 6 minutes. Then apply 3 drops of cypress.

Personal Care—Ortho Ease, Ortho Sport.

Supplements—BLM

—Bunions

▸▸ *Bunions are bursitis located at the base of a toe, often caused by constrictive footwear.*

Oils—**T**Aroma Siez, **T**M-Grain, **T**cypress, **T**carrot, **T**German chamomile, **T**juniper.

Blend #2—6 drops eucalyptus, 3 drops lemon, 4 drops ravensara, and 1 drop wintergreen in 1 oz. V-6 Oil. Apply a couple drops of this blend directly on area of concern as often as desired.

T—Dilute as necessary, and apply on location.

Calcium: *See Hormonal Imbalance.*

Supplements—Allerzyme (aids the digestion of sugars, starches, fats, and proteins), Digest + Cleanse, Super Cal, Mineral Essence.

According to Dr. John R. Lee, processed food, carbonated soft drink, caffeine, high protein, sugar, and salt consumption all contribute to increased calcium deficiency in the human body (Burton Goldberg Group, Alt. Med., The Definitive Guide, pp 773-4). Sulfur cannot be metabolized if there is a calcium deficiency. This can cause poor nail and hair growth, falling hair, eczema, dermatitis, poor muscle tone, acne, pimples, gout, rheumatism, arthritis, and a weakening of the nervous system.

Calluses: *See Skin: Calluses.*

Calming:

Oils—**AT**Peace & Calming, **AT**lavender[114], **AT**ylang ylang[115], **T**Stress Away, **AT**rose[116], **AT**Citrus Fresh, **AT**melissa[117], **AT**orange[118], **AT**F cedarwood, **AT**hinoki, **AT**yuzu, **AT**hong kuai, **AT**bergamot, **AT**sacred frankincense, **A**clary sage, **AT**Gentle Baby, **AT**jasmine, **AT***Melaleuca ericifolia*, **AT**myrrh, **AT**onycha (benzoin), **AT**Release, **AT**Surrender, **AT**tangerine, **AT**Trauma Life, **AT**western red cedar.

Supplements—SleepEssence (short-term only).

—Agitation

Oils—**AT**Lavender[114], **AT**rose[116], **AT**ylang ylang[115], **AT**F bergamot, **AT**Peace & Calming, **AT**Trauma Life (calms), **AT**cedarwood, **AT**clary sage, **AT**Forgiveness, **AT**frankincense, **AT**geranium, **AT**Harmony, **AT**Joy, **AT**juniper, **AT**marjoram, **AT**myrrh, **AT**rosewood, **AT**sandalwood, **AT**Transformation, **AT**Valor.

—Hyperactivity

Oils—**AT**Lavender[119], **AT**Peace & Calming (gets them off Ritalin), **AT**Citrus Fresh, **AT**RutaVaLa, **AT**Valor (sometimes works better than Peace & Calming) **AT**Roman chamomile, **AT**Trauma Life (calming).

***Hyperactivity** may indicate a trace mineral deficiency. Get off Prozac and Ritalin and use Mineral Essence. It is interesting to note that 48 out of 49 death row inmates were tested and found to be deficient in the same trace minerals.*

Supplements—ComforTone, Essentialzyme, Essentialzymes-4, ICP, Mineral Essence, healthy diet.

—Sedative

▸▸ *A sedative is a calming or sleep-inducing agent*

Oils—**AT**Lavender[120], **AT**Peace & Calming, **AT**RutaVaLa, **T**Tranquil (roll-on), **AT**bergamot, **AT**Citrus Fresh[121], **AT**valerian[122], **AT**neroli, **AT**angelica, **AT**cedarwood, **AT**clary sage, **AT**coriander, **AT**cypress, **AT**elemi, **AT**frankincense, **AT**geranium, **AT**hyssop, **AT**jasmine, **AT**juniper, **AT**lemongrass, **AT**melissa, **AT**marjoram, **AT**onycha (benzoin), **AT**orange, **AT**patchouli, **AT**Roman chamomile, **AT**rose, **AT**sandalwood, **AT**tangerine, **AT**Trauma Life, **AT**vetiver (nervous system), **AT**ylang ylang. Use intuition as to which one may be best for the given situation. In addition, check the safety data for each of the oils in the Appendix of this book.

***Comments—*Refer to Blend #3 under Insomnia for a blend of oils that can either be taken internally in water or applied to the back of the neck to help relax the body.*

A—Diffuse into the air. Inhale directly, or apply to hands, tissue, or a cotton wick, and inhale.

T—Dilute as recommended, and apply 1–2 drops to back of neck, temples, chest, shoulders, wrist, back, or reflex points on the feet. Dilute in V-6 Oil, and massage into the back, shoulders, neck, or arms.

Cancer: *See Chemicals, Tumors, Radiation.*

▸▸ *Cancer can be any of many different conditions where the body's cells duplicate and grow uncontrollably, invade healthy tissues, and possibly spread throughout the body. It is estimated that 95% of cancers result from damage to DNA during a person's lifetime rather than from a preexisting genetic condition (American Cancer Society, 2008). The most important factor leading to this DNA damage is DNA mutation. DNA mutation can be caused by radiation, environmental chemicals we take into our bodies, free radical damage, or DNA copying or division errors. If the body is working properly, it can correct these mutations either by repairing the DNA or by causing the mutated cell to die. When the DNA mutation is severe enough that it allows the cell to bypass these controls, however, the mutated DNA can be copied to new cells that continue to replicate and create more and more new cells uncontrollably, leading to a cancerous growth within an individual.,*

Oils—**AIT**Frankincense[123] (combine with ledum and take internally), **ATI**sandalwood[124], **AT**lavender[125], **TAI**rosemary[126], **AT**caraway[127], **ATI**lemongrass[128], **AIT**clove[129], **AT**basil[130], **TIA**geranium[131], **ATI**clary sage[132], **T**orange[133], **TA**myrrh[134], **TA**$_F$tarragon, **T**Di-Gize (rub on feet and stomach), **TA**ImmuPower (put on throat and all over feet, three times a day), **TA**Melrose (cancer sores, fights infection), **TA**Juva Cleanse, **TA**rose, **TA**sage.

> *When the cell wall thickens, oxygen cannot get in. The life expectancy of a cell is 120 days (4 months). Cells also divide, making duplicate cells. If the cell is diseased, new diseased cells will be made. When we stop the mutation of the diseased cells (create healthy cells), we stop the disease. Essential oils have the ability to penetrate and carry nutrients through the cell wall to the nucleus and improve the health of the cell.*

***Comments—Since it is very important to maintain a positive attitude while healing, it may be helpful to address the emotions using Acceptance, Believe, Envision, Forgiveness, Gathering, Gratitude, Hope, Joy, Live with Passion, and/or ravensara (*refer to the emotional therapies in the Science and Application section of the Reference Guide for Essential Oils*). One of the most common emotions cancer patients have to deal with is anger or a pattern of resentment. Others are fear, judgement, and doubt. Doubt limits God and restricts His ability to work miracles in our lives. Praying for all those with cancer can help release these emotions. Also, work on recognizing why cancer was chosen.

***Comments—All conifer oils have great value in fighting cancers, while balsam fir and white fir have more specific actions.

***Comments—Oils high in limonene (like grapefruit, tangerine, orange, palo santo, mandarin, fleabane, and lemon) have been shown to be effective in fighting cancer.

***Comments—Refer to the chapter entitled "How to Use—The Personal Usage Reference" in the Essential Oils Desk Reference under "Cancer" for some excellent blend recipes, supplement recommendations, and cleansing and maintenance programs for many different kinds of cancer.

*****Important Notice:** Health care professionals are emphatic about avoiding heavy massage when working with cancer patients. Light massage may be used, but never over the trauma area. Also, the information in this section should not be perceived as a cure for cancer. Always consult with your health care professional.

Supplements—Cleansing Trio (ComforTone, Essentialzyme, and ICP), AlkaLime (acid-neutralizing mineral formulation), Balance Complete, Digest + Cleanse, ImmuPro, Inner Defense, MultiGreens, NingXia Red (nutrient powerhouse), NingXia Wolfberries (dried), Power Meal, Sulfurzyme, Super C / Super C Chewable, True Source (whole food multi-nutrient), Wolfberry Crisp Bars (*Refer to the Wolfberry Crisp Bar in the Supplements section of the Reference_Guide for Essential Oils for more information on the benefits of the Ningxia Wolfberry*).

There must be an acid condition in the body for cancer to thrive and spread. See pH Balance. Power Meal contains predigested proteins and helps the body move towards an alkaline balance. AlkaLime combats yeast and fungus overgrowth and helps preserve the body's proper pH balance.

Cancer cells also have a very low frequency.

*****Comments**—One lady who was receiving chemotherapy treatments for cancer of the spleen used Di-Gize to promote elimination through the colon. Her doctors wondered why her chemotherapy treatments had not made her sick. When she felt any discomfort (light nausea or cramps in the descending colon), she rubbed 4–6 drops of Di-Gize on her abdomen, and within 10 minutes all discomfort stopped.

The following are recipes that some individuals have used successfully:

Recipe #1—For the first month, supplement with the following: 6 MultiGreens three times a day, 6 Super C / Super C Chewable three times a day, and 1 ImmuPro three times a day. After remission, apply ImmuPower on the spine three times a day. Do a *light* full body massage with 6 clove and 15 frankincense in 1 oz. V-6 Oil.

Recipe #2—Supplement with the following: Cleansing Trio (ComforTone, Essentialzyme, and ICP), 12 Super C / Super C Chewable, and 9 MultiGreens. Drink ½ gallon of carrot juice each day. Eliminate white flour, white sugar, and red meat from the diet. Rub Thieves on the feet, and do a *light* full body massage with frankincense.

Recipe #3—Supplement with the following: 1 Master Formula His/Hers, 2 MultiGreens, 6 Super C / Super C Chewable. Do a *light* full body massage with frankincense, clove, and V-6 Oil. Apply ImmuPower to the spine and feet twice a day.

—Bone

Oils—**T**Frankincense

Recipe #1—Cleansing Trio (ComforTone, Essentialzyme, and ICP) for a week, then JuvaTone was added for six days, then Super B was added morning and evening. Other vitamin supplements included Super C / Super C Chewable, MegaCal, and Super Cal. All processed foods were eliminated, and a strict vegetarian diet was followed, including 8 glasses of water each day. Birch was applied on location for pain. Frankincense and lavender were applied on the feet.

—Brain

Frankincense contains sesquiterpenes which allow it to go beyond the blood-brain barrier. Sesquiterpenes are also found in many of the emotional blends. ImmuPower builds the immune system. Clove is antiparasitic and antitumoral.

Oils—**AT**Frankincense[135], **AT**myrrh[136], **AT**clove

The following are recipes that some individuals have used successfully:

Recipe #4—*Light* massage daily on spine with 1 oz. V-6 Oil, 15 drops frankincense, and 6 drops clove. Rub brain stem area with ImmuPower. Diffuse 15 drops frankincense and 6 drops clove for ½ hour three times a day.

Recipe #5—Diffuse frankincense 24 hours a day, and massage the brain stem area with frankincense.

—Breast

Oils—TARosemary[137], TAlavender[138], TAfrankincense, TAclove.

Supplements—FemiGen.

Personal Care—Progessence/Progessence Plus.

***Comments—Often there is an emotional issue of self-worth that must be dealt with as well.

—Cervical

Oils—TAFrankincense, TAgeranium, TAclove, TAcypress, TAlavender, TAlemon.

—Colon

Oils—ITALavender[139], TAgeranium[140], TAfrankincense[141], TAlemongrass[140].

Supplements—ICP (fiber beverage that helps prevent), Super Cal (studies have shown that taking calcium supplements at night helps protect the colon from polyps and cancer).

—Diet

Fast 21 days (*See Fasting or Cleansing*); then have soup. *See Diet.*

—Heart

Supplements—HRT

*One woman had **cancer of the heart,** which literally ate a hole in the heart. She took the tincture HRT, and the tissue of her heart regenerated and the cancer disappeared!*

***JuvaTone** and **Rehemogen** build blood and hemoglobin platelets One individual had total **liver regeneration** by using JuvaTone, Rehemogen, and JuvaFlex.*

—Liver

Oils—TAFrankincense[142] (hot compress over liver), TAlemongrass[143], TAlavender[144], TAGLF, TAJuvaFlex, TAJuva Cleanse, TAmyrrh.

Supplements—JuvaTone was formulated to fight cancer in the liver.

—Lung

Oils—TAFrankincense (rub on chest, or add 15 drops to 1 tsp. V-6 Oil for nightly retention enema), TAlavender[145].

Blend #1—15 drops frankincense, 5 drops clove, 6 drops ravensara, 4 drops myrrh, and 2 drops sage. This blend can be mixed with 1 tsp. V-6 Oil if it is too strong. It is best when inserted into rectum.

—Lymphoma

▸▸ *Lymphoma is a cancer of the lymphatic system (part of the immune system). Hodgkin's' disease is a form of lymphoma, and lymphomas are generally classified in two categories: Hodgkin lymphoma and non-Hodgkin lymphomas.*

Nodes or small tumors in neck and groin. Cleanse liver.

Blend #2—10 drops frankincense, 5 drops myrrh, and 3 drops sage. Mix with small amount of V-6 Oil, and apply daily over nodes or tumor areas and rectally. Every other day, apply frankincense neat.

–Hodgkin's Disease

▸▸ *Hodgkin's disease (or Hodgkin's lymphoma) is a type of cancer that affects lymphocytes (white blood cells). It can cause enlarged lymph nodes and cause fever, sweating, fatigue, and weight loss.*

Oils—TClove (Apply to liver, kidney, and Vita Flex points on feet).

—Lymphoma Stage 4 (bone marrow)

Extreme fatigue: eat vegetables and fruits; no meat.

Oils—TImmuPower (on the spine).

Recipe #6—Life 5 (probiotic), Cleansing Trio (ComforTone, Essentialzyme, and ICP), 6 Super C / Super C Chewable three times a day, 6 MultiGreens three times a day. After remission, continue one more month; then reduce amounts for maintenance.

—Melanoma *See also Corns, Warts.*

>> *Melanoma is the most serious type of skin cancer. It is a malignant tumor that affects the melanocytes (the cells that produce the pigment melanin that colors our skin, hair, and eyes) in our skin. Melanoma often manifests itself in the forms of moles—new moles or ones that already exist. It can be spotted by noticing changes in the moles such as symmetry, edges, color, and size. Melanoma can be cured if treated early; but if it spreads, it can cause death.*

Oils—TI Sandalwood[146], T frankincense[147], T lavender.

Aloha! I have been using essential oil for many years, resulting in many amazingly wonderful results. One of the best took place when a dear friend was being consumed by cancer. She was in stage 4 for 4 years—amazing in itself. RC and frankincense were used the most. When she was put into the hospice, with only days left, the oils were still used, and she remained in the hospice for another year and a half. Others at the hospice got sick with colds and flu, including the workers, but my friend never got any of the passing bugs... Amazing to say the least, but this was a true testimonial to the antiviral and antibiotic effects of the oils.

-Submitted by Yvonne Vnuk-Nielsen
Kailua, Hawaii (July 2004)

—Ovarian

Oils—T ImmuPower (on spine three times a day).

Blend #3—15 drops frankincense, 6 drops geranium, and 5 drops myrrh in ½ tsp. V-6 Oil; alternate: one night in vagina (tampon to retain), next in rectum.

Recipe #7—6 FemiGen a day, 8 Super C / Super C Chewable a day. Those with "A" type blood should take 8 MultiGreens a day while those with "O" type blood should take 12 or more a day; MultiGreens is a mainstay, it is a predigested protein and helps maintain an alkaline balance.

—Prostate

Oils—T Anise (blend with frankincense, fennel, ImmuPower, Mister, sage, and/or yarrow). I Juva Cleanse.

T—Apply to posterior scrotum, ankles, lower back, and bottoms of feet.

I—Add 3–5 drops to empty capsule; swallow.

Personal Care—Protec was designed to accompany the night-long retention enema. It helps buffer the prostate from inflammation, enlargement, and tumor activity.

Recipe #1—Diffuse ImmuPower. Do a spinal massage and Vita Flex on the feet with ImmuPower. Blend 5 drops frankincense, 15 drops Mister, and 2 tsp. V-6 Oil together **or** 15 drops ImmuPower with 2 tsp. V-6 Oil. Insert and retain in the rectum throughout the night.

Case History #1—A 71-year-old man had prostate cancer and bone metastasis. After three weeks of using frankincense, sage, myrrh, and cumin in rectal implants, he was free of cancer.

—Throat

Oils—TA Frankincense, TA lavender.

—Uterine

Oils—TA Geranium, TA ImmuPower.

Blend #4—2–5 drops cedarwood **or** 2–5 drops lemon **or** 2–5 drops myrrh in 1 tsp. V-6 Oil.

Personal Care—Progessence/Progessence Plus.

T—Dilute as necessary, and apply 1–5 drops on location and on Vita Flex points on the feet and hands. Apply as a warm compress over affected area.

A—Diffuse into the air. Inhale oil directly or applied to hands, tissue, or a cotton wick.

I—Add 3–5 drops of oil in an empty capsule; swallow

Candida: *See Antifungal: Candida*

Cankers: *See Acidosis.*

Canker sores are small, round sores that develop in the mouth, typically inside the lips and cheeks or on the tongue.

Oils—TThieves, Tmelaleuca, TAustralian Blue, Tchamomile (both German and Roman), TEnvision, Thyssop, Tlaurel, TMelrose, Tmyrrh, Toregano, Tsage lavender.

T—Dilute as necessary, and apply on location.

Blend #1—Sage with clove and lavender.

Blend #2—Sage with Thieves.

> ***Canker sores*** *are occasionally associated with Crohn's disease, which affects the bowels. Deficiencies of iron, vitamin B12, and folic acid have been linked to this disease in some people. Stress and allergies are usually the cause of open sores in the mouth. To avoid getting canker sores, it is important to have a body chemistry that is balanced in minerals, acidity, and alkalinity (Prescription for Nutritional Healing, p. 126).*

Supplements—Inner Defense, AlkaLime (combats yeast and fungus overgrowth and preserves the body's proper pH balance), ImmuPro, Mineral Essence, MultiGreens.

Capillaries: *See also Cardiovascular System.*

Capillaries are the small, thin blood vessels that allow the exchange of oxygen and other nutrients from the blood to cells throughout the body and allow the exchange of carbon dioxide and other waste materials from these tissues back to the blood. The capillaries connect the arteries (that carry blood away from the heart) and veins (that carry blood back to the heart).

—Broken *See also Bruises*

Oils—TGeranium, Tcypress, Thyssop, Tlime (soothes), TRoman chamomile.

T—Dilute as necessary, and apply on location.

Blend #1—Apply 1 drop lavender and 1 drop Roman chamomile.

Carbuncles: *See also Boils.*

A carbuncle is a swollen, puss-filled lump or mass under the skin, varying from the size of a pea to the size of a golf ball. Carbuncles form in infected hair follicles

Oils—TMelaleuca.

T—Dilute as necessary, and apply on location.

Cardiotonic: *See Cardiovascular System: Heart.*

Cardiovascular System: *See also Arteries, Blood, Capillaries, Veins.*

Oils—TA FOrange (cardiac spasms), TAcypress (strengthens the capillary walls and increases circulation), TAvalerian[148], TAthyme[149], TAanise, TAAroma Life (cardiac spasms), TAcinnamon bark (strengthens), TAclary sage, TAclove, TAEn-R-Gee, TAfleabane (dilates), TAgoldenrod, TAhelichrysum, TAmarjoram, TAonycha (benzoin), TApalmarosa (supports), TAPanAway, TArosemary, TAsandalwood (strengthens), TAtsuga (opens and dilates for better oxygen exchange), TAylang ylang.

Supplements— Omega Blue, OmegaGize[3], FemiGen, ICP, Majestic Essence Chocolates, Mineral Essence, Slique Tea, Super B, Super Cal, True Source (whole food multi-nutrient).

Personal Care—Progessence/Progessence Plus.

—ANGINA

> ***Angina pectoris** is a severe spasmodic pain in the chest that is due to an insufficient supply of blood to the heart.*

Oils—TA F Ginger, ITAvalerian[148], TA F orange (for false angina), TAAroma Life, TAlaurel.

Supplements—True Source (whole food multi-nutrient).

—CIRCULATION

Oils—TA F Cypress, TAeucalyptus[150], TAvalerian[148], TAAroma Life, TAbasil, TAcinnamon bark, TACitrus Fresh, TAclary sage, TAcopaiba (stimulates), TAcumin, TAgeranium, TAhelichrysum, TAhyssop, TAJuva Cleanse, TAnutmeg, TAonycha (benzoin), TAoregano, TApeppermint, TAPeace & Calming, TARC, TArosemary, TAsage lavender, TAthyme, TAwintergreen.

–CAPILLARIES

Oils—TACypress (strengthens the capillary walls, and increases circulation), TAoregano, TAthyme.

–PROMOTES HEALTHY

Oils—TAOnycha (benzoin), TAPanAway.

Personal Care—Cel-Lite Magic dilates the blood vessels for better circulation; may add grapefruit or cypress to enhance. Also Ortho Ease and Ortho Sport.

Supplements—Cleansing Trio (ComforTone, ICP, Essentialzyme), JuvaTone, NingXia Red, Thyromin.

***__Comments__—*Constipation affects circulation. Improving the circulation in the colon and liver improves the circulation in the blood.*

—HEART

Oils—TAAroma Life (on heart and all Vita Flex heart points), TAylang ylang (balances heart function), TAmarjoram, TAgeranium, TAJoy, TAValor (on feet), TACitrus Fresh, TAClarity, TAcypress, TADragon Time, TAfleabane, TAForgiveness, TAGentle Baby, TAginger, TAHarmony, TAHope, TAhyssop, TAlavender, TAMister, TAM-Grain, TAPanAway, TARelieve It, TArosemary, TAWhite Angelica.

> ***HEART PUMP FOR HEART STRESS***
>
> *Using your thumbs, apply pressure in an alternating "pumping" fashion between the following two heart points: (1) on the left hand at the lifeline under the ring finger; and (2) just inside the elbow. Also apply Aroma Life to the chest and to the hand and heart points. And of course, GET HELP FAST!*

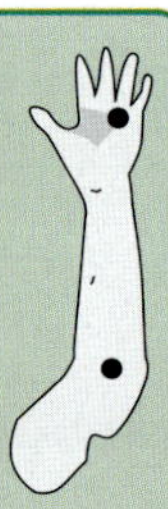

Supplements—Longevity Capsules (contains thyme oil to help preserve omega-3 fatty acids in the heart), Omega Blue, OmegaGize^3, Mineral Essence, NingXia Red, Power Meal, Rehemogen Tincture, Slique Tea, Sulfurzyme, Super B, Ultra Young+ (may help reverse heart disease), True Source (whole food multi-nutrient), Wolfberry Crisp Bars.

–ANGINA *See ANGINA above*

–ARRHYTHMIA

▸▸*Arrhythmia is an irregular heart beat rhythm: the heart either beats too slow, too fast, or in an irregular pattern. Arrhythmia can be a symptom of a larger problem.*

Recipe #1—PanAway on heart and Relieve It on left foot Vita Flex heart point (rotate each application). Goldenrod and lavender are also good. Research done by Dr. Pénoël indicates that ylang ylang may be beneficial in preventing or correcting an irregularity in the force or rhythm of the heart.

–BRINGS JOY TO HEART

Oils—AChristmas Spirit, ACitrus Fresh, AJoy.

C

–Cardiotonic

Oils—TALavender, TAthyme.

Supplements— True Source (whole food multi-nutrient).

–Coronary Artery

Personal Care—Prenolone/Prenolone+, Progessence/Progessence Plus.

***Comments—*Research has shown that natural progesterone protects the coronary artery from going into spasms. Provera, a synthetic progestin, offers no protection from coronary artery spasms. In fact, it promotes the spasm to the point of completely shutting off the flow of blood. This may explain the increase in heart attacks in women 5 to 10 years after menopause, many of whom are on synthetic progestin.*

Supplements—FemiGen, Super B.

–Heart Tissue

Oils—TAMarjoram (has been found to help rejuvenate the smooth muscle tissue of the heart).

–Hypertension (high blood pressure) *See Blood.*

–Large Valve

Oils—TAAroma Life (shortness of breath).

–Palpitations

>> *Palpitations are irregular, pounding, sporadic, or fluttering heart beats. The heart beats are irregular enough that the person becomes aware of them.*

Oils—TAAroma Life, TA$_F$orange, TA$_F$ylang ylang, TAlavender, TAmelissa, TApeppermint.

–Prolapsed Mitral Valve

>> *Mitral valve prolapse (MVP) is a condition where the valve between the upper and lower chambers of the heart does not close correctly, sometimes allowing leakage of blood through the valve opening.*

Oils—TAMarjoram.

–Stimulant

Oils—TACoriander, TAcumin.

–Strengthens Heart Muscle

Oils—TALavender, TAmarjoram, TApeppermint, TArose, TArosemary (Alternative Medicine—A Definitive Guide, p. 722).

–Strengthening

Oils—TACinnamon bark.

Supplements—Wolfberry Crisp Bars.

–Tachycardia *See also Anxiety, Shock, Stress*

>> *Tachycardia is an abnormally rapid resting heart rate, indicating a possible overworking of the heart.*

Oils—TA$_F$Lavender, TA$_F$ylang ylang (smell on tissue or straight from bottle in emergency), TAAroma Life (combine with ylang ylang), TAAustralian Blue, TAgoldenrod, TAIdaho tansy, TAlavender, TAneroli, TAorange, TAPanAway, TARelieve It, TAspikenard.

Supplements—Power Meal, Sulfurzyme, True Source (whole food multi-nutrient), Wolfberry Crisp Bars.

—Phlebitis

>> *Phlebitis is the inflammation of a superficial vein, typically in the legs or groin area. Wearing support hose or a compression bandage over the affected area can help aid in healing.*

Oils—$^{TA}_{F}$Helichrysum (prevents), $^{TA}_{F}$lavender, ^{TA}cypress, ^{TA}geranium, ^{TA}grapefruit, ^{TA}Roman chamomile, ^{TA}Valor.

Recipe #1—Massage toward heart, and wear support hose until healed, possibly two to three months. Use Aroma Life every morning and night. Do the Raindrop Technique on leg.

—Stimulant

Oils—$^{TA}_{F}$Nutmeg, ^{TA}onycha (benzoin), ^{TA}pine.

—Support

Oils—^{TA}Goldenrod.

T—Dilute oils as necessary, and apply oils to area: to carotid arteries, heart, feet, under left ring finger, above elbow, behind ring toe on left foot, and to Vita Flex points on the feet. Add 1–2 drops to bathwater for a bath. Dilute with V-6 Oil, and massage on location or on chest, neck, or feet.

A—Diffuse into the air. Inhale directly or applied to hands, tissue, or a cotton wick.

Carpal Tunnel Syndrome: *See also Inflammation.*

▸▸ *Carpal Tunnel Syndrome is a condition where inflamed carpal ligaments at the wrist press upon the median nerve. Indications include tingling or numbness in the palm or thumb and first three fingers of the hand, weak grip, or impaired finger movement.*

Oils—^{T}Deep Relief (roll-on), ^{T}basil, ^{T}cypress, ^{T}eucalyptus, ^{T}lavender, ^{T}lemongrass, ^{T}marjoram, ^{T}oregano, ^{T}peppermint.

T—Apply oils on location, and either use massage or Vita Flex to work them in.

Recipe #1—First start with basil and marjoram on the shoulder to help release any energy blockages. Then use lemongrass on the wrist and oregano on the rotator cup in the shoulder. Next apply marjoram and cypress on the wrist and then cypress on the neck and down to the shoulder. Lastly, apply peppermint from the shoulder down the arm to the wrist then out to the tips of each finger.

***Comments—Make sure it really is carpal tunnel syndrome, because many people who think they have carpal tunnel syndrome (one report says up to 90%) really have problems with muscles in the neck and shoulder that create similar symptoms.

Blend #1—Layer geranium, balsam fir, juniper, peppermint, and sandalwood on the wrist. Apply several times per day for an extended period to give the nerves time to heal.

Personal Care—Ortho Ease or Ortho Sport Massage Oils. Massage into neck, shoulder, and wrist. Prenolone/Prenolone+ / Progessence/Progessence Plus (on shoulder and wrist).

Supplements—BLM, Mineral Essence, Sulfurzyme, Super Cal.

Cataracts: *See Eyes.*

Catarrh (Mucus): *See Anticatarrhal, Congestion.*

Cavities: *See Oral Conditions.*

Celibacy (vow not to marry):

Oils—^{A}Marjoram.

A—Diffuse into the air. Inhale directly or applied to tissue or to a cotton wick.

Cells:

Oils—All essential oils restore cells to original state. Need to change the RNA and DNA to change the habit.

Supplements—NingXia Red (nutrients promote cellular health).

—DNA (cell chemistry)

>> *DNA is the genetic material of the cell. DNA contains all of the codes that enable the cell to build the materials needed for proper cell structure and function. Mutation of DNA can lead to cell death or to cancer.*

Supplements—Master Formula His/Hers, MultiGreens, Super B, Thyromin.

—Frequency

Oils—ATRose (enhances frequency of every cell, which brings balance and harmony to body).

—Liver

Oils—TAHelichrysum (stimulates cell function).

—Oxygenation

Oils—ATBlack pepper.

—Regulating

Oils—ATClary sage (removes negative programming).

—RNA (cell memory)

>> *Ribonucleic acid (RNA) is a molecule similar to DNA. RNA is transcribed from DNA and is used in the production of proteins, as well as in regulating gene expression of the DNA*

–Stimulates

Oils—ATAbundance.

T—Dilute as necessary, and apply to area of concern. Dilute with V-6 Oil, and massage on location.

A—Diffuse into the air. Inhale directly or applied to cupped hands, tissue, or a cotton wick.

Cellulite: *See also Weight.*

>> *Cellulite refers to deposits of fat under the skin of the thighs, abdomen, and buttocks that cause the skin to appear dimpled.*

Try flavoring 1 gallon of water with 5 drops grapefruit and 5 drops lemon. Adjust to taste, and drink. This may also improve energy levels.

Oils—$^{T}_{F}$Grapefruit, $^{T}_{F}$cedarwood, $^{T}_{F}$rosemary, Tbasil, Tcumin, Tcypress, Tfennel, Tgeranium, Tjuniper, Tlavender, Tlemon, Tlime, Torange, Toregano, Tpatchouli, Trosewood, Tsage, Tspikenard (increases metabolism to burn fat), Ttangerine (dissolves), Tthyme. *Refer to the chapter entitled "How to Use—The Personal Usage Reference" in the Essential Oils Desk Reference under "Cellulite" for some excellent blend recipes and recommendations.*

Supplements—Allerzyme (aids the digestion of sugars, starches, fats, and proteins), Digest + Cleanse, Power Meal (eat for breakfast).

—Attacks Fat and Cellulite

Oils—TGrapefruit, Tbasil, Tlavender, Tlemongrass, Trosemary, Tsage, Tthyme.

Personal Care—Cel-Lite Magic (add grapefruit to increase activity and to dissolve cellulite even faster).

Chakras (Energy Centers): *(Refer to the chart at the end of the Science and Application section of the Reference Guide for Essential Oils.)*

Oils—TA Harmony (apply 1 drop on each chakra to open the energy centers and to balance the electrical field of the chakras, starting at the base chakra located on the coccyx at the end of the spinal column and working up), TA lavender (brings harmony to chakras), TA rosemary (opens chakras), TA sandalwood (affects each chakra differently).

—Unites Head and Heart

Oils—TA Helichrysum.

—Angelic Chakra (#8—located above the crown of the head)

Oils—TA Angelica, TA neroli.

—Crown Chakra (#7)

Oils—TA 3 Wise Men (to replace void with good/positives), TA angelica (links 7-8, 7-1), TA basil, TA cistus, TA frankincense (links 1-7), TA lavender, TA myrrh, TA onycha, TA ravensara, TA rose, TA rosemary, TA rosewood (links 7-1), TA sandalwood (links 7-1), TA spikenard, TA spruce.

–Balance

Oils—TA Highest Potential.

–Open

Oils—TA Forgiveness, TA Harmony.

—Brow Chakra (3rd Eye -#6)

Oils—TA Acceptance, TA Awaken, and TA Dream Catcher (rub on lobe of ear to increase vision and spiritual vision); TA cedar leaf (western red cedar), TA cedarwood, TA clary sage, TA frankincense, TA Harmony, TA helichrysum, TA juniper, TA mugwort, TA palo santo, TA peppermint, TA pine, TA rose, TA rosemary, TA spruce, TA thymes, TA Transformation, TA tsuga.

–Open

Oils—TA Frankincense, TA Harmony.

—Throat Chakra (#5)

Oils—TA Carrot seed, TA chamomile (Roman and German), TA cypress, TA frankincense, TA geranium, TA lavender, TA rose geranium, TA sandalwood, TA spearmint, TA spruce.

–Open

Oils—TA Harmony.

—Heart Chakra (#4)

Oils—TA Bergamot, TA carrot seed, TA cinnamon bark, TA frankincense, TA helichrysum, TA hyssop, TA inula, TA laurel, TA lavandin, TA lavender, TA marjoram, TA melissa, TA neroli, TA onycha, TA oregano, TA pepper (black), TA rose, sage, TA sandalwood, TA spikenard, TA tansy.

–Opens a Closed Heart

Oils—TA Bergamot, TA Harmony.

—Solar Plexus Chakra (#3)

Oils—TA Calamus, TA cardamom, TA carrot seed, TA cedarwood, TA cinnamon bark, TA citronella, TA fennel, TA ginger, TA juniper, TA lemon, TA lemongrass, TA melissa, TA pepper (black), TA peppermint, TA rosemary, TA spikenard, TA thymes (all chemotypes), TA valerian, TA vetiver, TA ylang ylang.

–Open

Oils—TAHarmony.

—Sacral Chakra (Sex/Navel -#2)

Oils—TACassia, TAcinnamon bark, TAclary sage, TAcoriander, TAcypress, TAgeranium, TArose geranium, TAjasmine, TAmyrrh, TAniaouli, TApatchouli, TApetitgrain, TApine, TArose, TAsandalwood, TAtangerine, TAvetiver, TAylang ylang.

–Balance

Oils—TAAcceptance (balances Sacral Chakra which stores denial and sexual abuse), TAsage.

–Open

Oils—TAHarmony.

—Base Chakra (Root -#1)

Oils—TACardamom, TAcarrot seed, TAcedar leaf (western red cedar), TAcedarwood, TAclove, TAfrankincense, TAginger, TAlaurel, TAmyrrh, TAonycha, TApatchouli, TApepper (black), TApeppermint, TAsandalwood, TAvetiver.

–Open

Oils—TAHarmony.

T—Dilute as necessary, and apply on chakras or as indicated. Dilute with V-6 Oil, and massage on chakras.

A—Inhale directly. Diffuse into the air.

Change (Personal): *See also Emotions.*

Oils—ATForgiveness, ATInto the Future, ATJoy, ATMagnify Your Purpose, ATSacred Mountain, AT3 Wise Men, ATTransformation.

A—Diffuse into the air. Inhale directly or applied to hands, tissue, or a cotton wick.

T—Apply to auricular emotional points.

Charley Horse: *See also Muscles: Spasms.*

Oils—TAroma Siez, Tbasil, TDeep Relief (roll-on).

T—Dilute as necessary, and apply on location. Dilute with V-6 Oil, and massage on location.

Personal Care—Prenolone/Prenolone+, Progessence/Progessence Plus.

Cheeks:

Oils—TJasmine.

T—Dilute as necessary, and apply on location. Dilute with V-6 Oil, and massage on location

Blend #1—5 drops Aroma Siez, 3 drops wintergreen, and 3 drops spruce. Work oils between hands in a clockwise motion, and pat on cheeks. Cup hands over nose and inhale.

Personal Care—A·R·T Skin Care System, A·R·T Purifying Toner, A·R·T Beauty Masque.

Chelation: *See also Detoxification: Metals.*

Oils—TAHelichrysum, TAAroma Life, TAcardamom, (powerful chelator and anticoagulant).

Traditional intravenous chelation therapy can cause scar tissue on the vascular walls. These oils, supplements, and tinctures provide a more natural approach to chelation. They may take longer to achieve the same results but with minimal side effects.

T—Dilute as necessary, and apply on feet and on liver area.

A—Diffuse into the air. Inhale directly.

*****Comments**—Drink lots of distilled water.

Personal Care—Cel-Lite Magic.

Supplements—Cleansing Trio (ComforTone, Essentialzyme, and ICP), MultiGreens (use with cardamom), Rehemogen Tincture.

*****Comments**—The apple pectin that is contained in ICP helps remove unwanted metals and toxins from the body.

Chemicals: *See Metals.*

Oils—$^{T}_{F}$Helichrysum.

T—Dilute as necessary, and apply on feet and on liver area.

Chicken Pox: *See Childhood Diseases.*

Chiggers: *See Insect.*

Childbirth: *See Pregnancy/Motherhood.*

Childhood Diseases:

—CHICKEN POX (2 WEEKS)—SLEEP IS VERY GOOD. *See also Antiviral, Shingles.*

›› *Chickenpox is a common childhood illness caused by the virus Varicella zoster (which is also responsible for shingles). Symptoms of chickenpox include mild fever, weakness, and a rash. The rash appears as red spots that form into blisters that eventually burst and then crust over. Chickenpox is highly contagious and can be contracted by anyone, but it is most common in children under the age of 15.*

Oils—^{T}Lavender, ^{TA}melaleuca, ^{T}Australian Blue, ^{A}bergamot, ^{T}eucalyptus, ^{T}Roman chamomile, ^{T}sage lavender.

Bath—(relieves the itching) 2 drops lavender, 1 cup bicarbonate of soda, and 1 cup soda in bath; soak.

Blend #1—5 to 10 drops each of German chamomile and lavender to 1 ounce Calamine lotion. Mix and apply twice a day all over body.

Blend #2—10 drops lavender, 10 drops Roman chamomile, and 4 oz. Calamine lotion. Mix and apply twice a day all over body.

Blend #3—Add enough ravensara to some green clay (from health food store) to form a paste that can be dabbed on the pox to relieve itching.

Diffuse—an antiviral oil (such as lemon), and apply the same oil all over the body twice a day.

—MEASLES

›› *Measles is a viral infection of the respiratory system that causes coughing, runny nose, red eyes, fever, and a rash on the skin.*

Oils—$^{AT}_{F}$Eucalyptus, ^{AT}melaleuca, ^{AT}German chamomile, ^{AT}lavender.

–GERMAN (3 DAY)—USE ANTIVIRAL OILS. *See Antiviral.*

–Rubella

Recipe #1—Sponge down with one of these oils: chamomile (Roman or German), lavender, melaleuca.

—Mumps

▸▸ *Mumps is a viral infection that causes fever, chills, headache, and painful swelling of the saliva glands.*

Oils—[TA]Melaleuca, [TA]lemon, [TA]lavender.

—Whooping Cough

▸▸ *Whooping cough, or pertussis, is a bacterial infection that causes cold-like symptoms, followed by severe coughing fits.*

Oils—[AT][F]Oregano, [AT]basil, [AT]cinnamon bark (diffuse, or dilute well; avoid for children), [AT]clary sage, [AT]cypress, [AT]grapefruit, [AT]hyssop, [AT]lavender, [AT]thyme.

Diffuse—Basil, eucalyptus, lavender, melaleuca, peppermint, Roman chamomile, rose, thyme.

T—Dilute as necessary, and apply on location or on chest, throat, and Vita Flex points. Use a hot compress for deeper penetration. Add 1–2 drops to 1 quart warm water, and use water for a sponge bath.

A—Diffuse into the air.

Children/Infants: *See also Childhood Diseases, Hyperactive.*

Personal Care—KidScents Bath Gel, KidScents Lotion, KidScents Shampoo, KidScents Tender Tush, KidScents Toothpaste.

Supplements—KidScents MightyVites (chewable vitamin tablets), Life 5 (probiotic; for older children), NingXia Red.

—Bonding

Oils—[T]Gentle Baby

T—One drop gently rubbed on baby's feet and another drop or two brushed over mom's hair and aura—open palms skimming body surface, head to foot).

—Colic

▸▸ *Colic is any extended period of crying and fussiness that occurs frequently in an infant. While the exact cause is not known, it has been speculated that the cause may be from indigestion, the build-up of gas, lactose intolerance, or a lack of needed probiotic bacteria in the intestines.*

Oils—[T]Fennel[151], [T]German chamomile[152], [T]melissa[152], [T][F]marjoram, [T]angelica, [T]bergamot, [T]cardamom, [T]carrot (with fennel), [T]coriander, [T]cumin, [T]dill, [T]ginger, [T]orange, [T]peppermint, [T]Roman chamomile, [T]rosemary, [T]spearmint, [T]ylang ylang.

T—Dilute 1–2 drops in 2 Tbs. V-6 Oil, and massage a small amount of this blend gently on stomach and back.

Blend #1—Combine 2 Tbs. almond oil with 1 drop Roman chamomile, 1 drop lavender, and 1 drop geranium. Mix and apply to stomach and back.

***Comments—*Burping the baby and keeping the abdomen warm with a warm water bottle will often bring relief.*

—Common Cold

Oils—[AT]Thyme, [AT]lemon, [AT]cedarwood, [AT]*Melaleuca ericifolia*, [AT]rosemary, [AT]rose, [AT]sandalwood.

A—Diffuse into the air.

T—Dilute 1–2 drops of oil in 2 Tbs. V-6 Oil, and massage a little on neck and chest.

Blend #2—Combine 2 Tbs. V-6 Oil with 2 drops melaleuca (tea tree), 1 drop lemon, and 1 drop rose otto. Massage a little of the blend on the neck and chest.

—Constipation

Oils—TRosemary[153], Tginger, Tmandarin, Torange.

T—Dilute one of the oils in V-6 Oil, and massage stomach and feet.

—Cradle Cap Remedy

Cradle cap is a yellowish scaling of the skin on the head that commonly occurs in young infants. The scaling is yellowish in color and often disappears by the time the infant is a few months old.

Blend #3—Combine 2 Tbs. almond oil with 1 drop lemon and 1 drop geranium or with 1 drop cedarwood and 1 drop sandalwood. Mix and apply a small amount on head.

—Croup

Croup is a viral respiratory infection that causes inflammation of the area around the larynx (voice box) and a distinctive-sounding cough. Often, taking an infant or child outside to breath cool night air can help open the restricted airways, as can humidity.

Oils—ATMarjoram, ATthyme, ATravensara, ATrosewood, ATsandalwood.

A—Diffuse into the air.

T—Dilute 1–2 drops in 2 Tbs. V-6 Oil. Massage.

—Crying

Oils—ATYlang ylang, ATlavender, ATRoman chamomile, ATcypress, ATfrankincense, ATgeranium, AT rose otto.

A—Diffuse into the air.

T—Dilute 1–2 drops in 2 Tbs. V-6 Oil. Massage.

When using essential oils on babies and children, it is always best to ***dilute 1–2 drops of pure essential oil with ½–1 tsp. V-6 Mixing Oil****. If the oils are used in the bath, always use a bath gel base as a dispersing agent for the oils.*

Keep the oils out of children's reach*. If an oil is ever ingested, give the child an oil-soluble liquid such as milk, cream, or half & half. Then call your local poison control center or seek emergency medical attention. A few drops of pure essential oil shouldn't be life-threatening, but for your protection, it is best to take these precautions.*

In Shirley Price's book, Aromatherapy for Babies and Children, she mentions ***twenty oils that are safe for children****. Nineteen of them are oils with the same botanical names as those mentioned in this book. These oils are:*

*Bergamot (Citrus bergamia)**
*Cedarwood (Cedrus atlantica)***
Chamomile, Roman (Chamaemelum nobile),
Cypress (Cupressus sempervirens)
Frankincense (Boswellia carterii)
Geranium (Pelargonium graveolens)
Ginger (Zingiber officinale)
Lavender (Lavandula angustifolia)
*Lemon (Citrus limon)**
*Mandarin (Citrus reticulata)**
Marjoram (Origanum marjorana)
Melaleuca-Tea Tree (Melaleuca alternifolia)
*Orange (Citrus aurantium)**
Rose Otto (Rosa damascena)
*Rosemary (Rosmarinus officinalis)***
Rosewood (Aniba rosaeodora)
Sandalwood (Santalum album)
Thyme (Thymus vulgaris CT linalol)
Ylang Ylang (Cananga odorata)

**These oils are photosensitive; always dilute. To prevent a rash or pigmentation of the skin, do not use citrus oils when exposed to direct sunlight.*

***These oils should never be used undiluted on babies and children.*

Caution: *Do not use synthetic or adulterated oils. Do not use oils with different botanical names until the safety data has been thoroughly reviewed.*

—Diaper Rash

Diaper rash is a red rash of the skin in the diaper area caused by prolonged skin exposure to the moisture and different pH of urine and feces. Often, more frequent bathing of the area and more frequent diaper changes will help alleviate the rash.

Oils—T$_F$Lavender.

T—Dilute 1–2 drops in 2 Tbs. V-6 Oil, and apply a small amount on location.

Blend #4—Combine 1 drop Roman chamomile and 1 drop lavender with V-6 Oil or Genesis Hand & Body Lotion. Apply.

Personal Care—KidScents Tender Tush (formulated specifically for diaper rash), Rose Ointment.

—Digestion (sluggish)

Oils—TLemon, Torange.

T—Dilute 1–2 drops in 2 Tbs. V-6 Oil. Massage on feet and stomach.

—Dry Skin

Oils—TRosewood, Tsandalwood.

T—Dilute 1–2 drops in 2 Tbs. V-6 Oil, and apply a small amount on location.

—Earache

Oils—TMelaleuca, Tlavender, T*Melaleuca ericifolia*, TRoman chamomile, Tthyme (sweet).

T—Put a diluted drop of oil on a cotton ball, and place the cotton ball in the ear; rub a little bit of diluted oil behind the ear.

Blend #5—Combine 2 Tbs. V-6 Oil with 2 drops lavender, 1 drop Roman chamomile, and 1 drop melaleuca. Put a drop on a cotton ball, and put cotton ball in ear; rub oil behind the ear and on the ear Vita Flex feet points.

Other—Garlic oil works great too, but it is stinky!

—Fever

Oils—TLavender, Apeppermint.

T—Dilute in V-6 Oil, and massage baby (back of neck, feet, behind ears, etc.).

A—Diffuse into the air.

—Flu

▸▸ *Flu, or influenza, is a viral infection that affects the respiratory system. Symptoms may include coughing, sneezing, fever, runny nose, congestion, muscle aches, nausea, and vomiting.*

Recipe #1—Cypress, lemon, *Melaleuca ericifolia*. Dilute 1 drop of each in 1 Tbs. bath gel for a bath; diffuse.

—Hiccoughs/Hiccups

Oils—AMandarin.

A—Diffuse into the air.

—Hyperactive

Oils—APeace & Calming, ACitrus Fresh, ATrauma Life.

A—Diffuse into the air.

—Jaundice

▸▸ *Jaundice is a condition where the liver cannot clear the pigment bilirubin quickly enough from the blood, causing the blood to deposit the bilirubin into the skin and whites of the eyes, turning them a yellowish color.*

Oils—TGeranium, Tlemon, Tlime, Tmandarin, Trosemary.

T—Dilute, and apply on the liver area and on the liver Vita Flex feet points.

—Premature

Oils—Since premature babies have very thin and sensitive skin, it is best to avoid the use of essential oils.

—Rashes

Oils—TLavender, TRoman chamomile, Trose, Tsandalwood.

T—Dilute in V-6 Oil, and apply a small amount on location.

—Teeth Grinding

Oils—TLavender, TAPeace & Calming.

T—Dilute, and apply a small amount to feet.

A—Diffuse into the air.

—Teething

Oils—TLavender, TGerman chamomile, Tginger, Tmarjoram, Tmelaleuca.

T—Dilute, and apply a small amount to feet.

—Tonsillitis

›› *Tonsillitis is inflammation of the tonsils, two lymph-filled tissues located at the back of the mouth that help provide immune support. These may become inflamed due to a bacterial or viral infection.*

Oils—TMelaleuca, Tlemon, Tginger, Tlavender, TRoman chamomile.

T—Dilute 1–2 drops in 2 Tbs. V-6 Oil, and apply a small amount to tonsils and to lymph nodes.

—Thrush *See also Antifungal*

›› *Thrush is an oral fungal infection caused by Candida albicans. It causes painful white-colored areas to appear in the mouth.*

Oils—TMelaleuca[154], Tlavender[155], Tthyme[156], Tgeranium, Tlemon, T*Melaleuca ericifolia*, Trosewood.

T—Dilute 1–2 drops essential oil in 2 Tbs. V-6 Oil, and apply a small amount on location.

Blend #3—2 Tbs. garlic oil, 8 drops lavender, 8 drops *Melaleuca ericifolia*, 1 ml (1 softgel) vitamin E oil. Apply to nipples just before nursing, or apply with a clean finger into baby's mouth. Also try Animal Scents Pet Ointment.

***Comments—Besides Gentle Baby listed under Bonding, no other commercial blends are listed in this section because many of them contain oils that are not recommended for babies. The author's admit that they have used many of the commercial blends mentioned in this book on their babies and children with great success and no side effects. We are careful, however, to use only a couple drops at a time, diluted in V-6 Oil, and only for external application. Also, we do not continue applications for any extended period of time.

Chills:

Oils—TGinger, Tonycha (benzoin), Tsage lavender.

T—Dilute as necessary, and apply to bottoms of feet and to solar plexus.

Chlorophyll:

Supplements—MultiGreens.

Cholera: *See also Antibacterial.*

›› *Cholera is a potentially severe bacterial infection of the intestines by the Vibrio cholerae bacteria. This infection can cause severe diarrhea, leading to dehydration that can cause low blood pressure, shock, or death. Rehydration with an oral rehydration solution is the most effective way to prevent dehydration. If no commercially prepared oral rehydration solution is available, a solution made from 1 tsp. salt, 8 tsp. sugar, and 1 liter clean water (with some mashed fresh banana, if available, to add potassium) can work in an emergency.*

Oils—TA FRavensara, TA Frosemary, TAclove.

T—Dilute as necessary, and massage gently over stomach and kidney area.

A—Diffuse into the air. Inhale directly.

Cholesterol:

>> *Cholesterol is an important lipid that comprises part of the cell membrane and myelin sheath and that plays a role in nerve cell function. It is created by the body and can be found in many foods we eat. An imbalance of certain types of cholesterol in the blood has been theorized to play a role in the formation of plaques in the arteries (atherosclerosis).*

Oils—**TI**Lemongrass (clinically shown to help lower cholesterol)[157], **T**$_F$clary sage, **T**$_F$helichrysum (regulates), **AT**lavender[158], **TI**dill[159].

Supplements—MultiGreens, True Source (whole food multi-nutrient).

T—Apply on Vita Flex points, over heart, and along arms.

I—Add 3–5 drops to an empty capsule, and swallow.

A—Diffuse into the air. Inhale directly.

Chorea: *See Saint Vitus' Dance.*

Chronic Fatigue: *See also Acidosis, Hormonal Imbalance.*

>> *Chronic fatigue syndrome refers to a set of debilitating symptoms that may include prolonged periods of fatigue that are not alleviated by rest, difficulty concentrating, muscle and joint pain, headaches, and sore throats that cannot be explained by any other known medical condition. While the exact cause of chronic fatigue syndrome is not known, some have theorized that it is caused by a virus (such as the Epstein-Barr virus) left in the body after an illness.*

> ***Chronic Fatigue*** *is often caused by the Epstein-Barr virus. It may also be a result of chemical and metal toxicity or of conditions of high acidity.*
>
> *Women who are pregnant seldom have Chronic Fatigue Syndrome because of the higher amounts of natural progesterone being produced.*

Oils—**TA**Thieves, **TA**basil, **TA**peppermint, **TA**Clarity, **TA**Di-Gize, **TA**ImmuPower, **TA**lavender, **TA**lemongrass, **TA**rosemary, **TA**Transformation.

T—Dilute as necessary, and apply to sore muscles or joints, to the back, or to the feet. Add 1–2 drops to warm bathwater, and bathe. Combine any of these oils with the Raindrop Technique.

A—Diffuse into the air. Inhale directly or applied to hands, tissue, or to a cotton wick.

*****Comments**—Basil and peppermint are a good combination together.

Supplements—NingXia Red, AlkaLime (acid-neutralizing mineral), Balance Complete (*refer to the 5-Day Nutritive Cleanse program listed under Balance Complete in the Supplements section of the Reference Guide for Essential Oils. This program also uses Digest + Cleanse and NingXia Red to help enhance detoxification while maintaining/increasing energy levels*), Cleansing Trio (ComforTone, Essentialzyme, and ICP), Digest + Cleanse, ImmuPro, Inner Defense, Life 5 (probiotic), Longevity Capsules, Master Formula His/Hers, Mineral Essence, MultiGreens, Power Meal, and Super Cal, True Source (whole food multi-nutrient).

Personal Care—Prenolone/Prenolone+, Progessence/Progessence Plus.

Dr. Friedmann uses the following recipe on his patients:

Recipe #1—1) Use the Cleansing Trio (ComforTone, Essentialzyme, and ICP) to detoxify. 2) Build the body and tissues with Mineral Essence and Master Formula His/Hers. 3) Build the immune system with ImmuPower and ImmuPro.

Cigarettes: *See Smoking.*

Circulation: *See Cardiovascular System: Circulation.*

Circulatory System: *See Cardiovascular System.*

Cirrhosis: *See Liver.*

Clarity of Thoughts:

Oils—^A^Clarity, ^A^rosemary, ^A^Transformation.

A—Diffuse into the air. Inhale directly or applied to hands.

Cleansing: *See also Housecleaning.*

Oils—^TA^Di-Gize (when cramping), ^TA^fennel, ^TA^hyssop, ^TA^juniper, ^A^melaleuca, ^TA^Melrose, ^T^Release (over liver), ^TA^ 3 Wise Men (when trauma—put on liver to let emotions go).

T—Dilute as necessary, and apply on location. Apply over liver area.

Cleansing may help to prevent disease, improve immune function, and make the body stronger. It may also cause an emotional cleansing. DRINK LOTS OF WATER! A child of any age can go on a cleanse. Gary Young suggests that you spend two days cleansing for every year old you are. He recommends that you take ICP and Essentialzyme five days a week and fast once a week on distilled water and lemon juice.

A—Diffuse into the air. Inhale directly or applied to hands, tissue, or a cotton wick.

—Body Cleanse

Supplements—Balance Complete (*refer to the 5-Day Nutritive Cleanse program listed under Balance Complete in the Supplements section of the Reference Guide for Essential Oils. This program also uses Digest + Cleanse and NingXia Red to help enhance detoxification while maintaining energy levels*), Cleansing Trio (ComforTone, Essentialzyme, and ICP), Digest + Cleanse. The oils contained in the Cleansing Trio will push heavy metals into the system; use Sacred Mountain and Peace & Calming to balance the system. If colon is blocked, start with ComforTone to open it. JuvaTone is the final stage of cleansing and can be taken as often as four times a day. Rehemogen Tincture supports the body during a cleanse.

—Cuts

Oils—^T^Elemi, ^T^lavender, ^T^Melrose.

T—Dilute as necessary, and apply on location.

—Master Cleanser or Lemonade Diet

Lemon converts to alkaline in the body. Lemons can be harmful to teeth only when in water that is not distilled because there can be a reaction with the minerals in the water. Toxins are eliminated from the bowels and bladder. Drink 6 to 12 glasses of the lemonade drink daily. When you get hungry, just drink another glass of lemonade. No other food or vitamins should be taken; the lemonade is already a food in liquid form. An herbal laxative tea may be used to help elimination. More details can be found in the book by Tom Woloshyn, The Complete Master Cleanse. It will take 30 days on lemon to change the chemistry in the body. We have to change the DNA and RNA (memory or belief system) to change a habit. Then, do 30 days on carrot juice.

2 Tbs. fresh lemon or lime juice (approx. ½ lemon), 2 Tbs. of grade B maple syrup (grade A is not as rich in nutrients but can be used if grade B is not available). 1/10 tsp. cayenne pepper or to taste (cayenne is a thermal warmer and dilates the blood vessels; also has vitamin A). Combine above ingredients in a 10 oz. glass of distilled water. No substitute sugars. In the case of diabetes, use black strap molasses instead of the maple syrup. Drink between three quarts and a gallon of this lemonade each day with an herbal laxative tea first thing in the morning and

just before retiring for the night. Refer to the book *The Complete Master Cleanse* for more specific details including suggestions and specific instructions for coming off the cleanse.

Closed Minded:

Oils—ATAwaken, ATInspiration.

A—Diffuse into the air. Inhale directly or applied to hands, tissue, or a cotton wick.

T—Apply to auricular emotional points. Dilute with V-6 Oil, and massage into skin.

Clothes:

Recipe #1—Western red cedar. Place a few drops on a cotton ball, and put it in a plastic sack. Leave the sack open so the odor of the oil can do its work without it staining any clothes. Place the bag in a closet or storage box.

Cockroaches: *See Insects: Cockroaches.*

Coffee (Stop Drinking): *See also Addictions. (See the case study on the body's frequency reaction to coffee in the Science and Application section of the Reference Guide for Essential Oils).*

Oils—APeace & Calming, APurification.

A—Inhale directly or applied to the hands. Diffuse into the air.

Supplements—JuvaTone.

Colds: *See also Antiviral, Coughs, Congestion.*

Oils—AT FMelaleuca, AT Flemon, ATThieves, AT Frosemary, ATthyme, ATRaven, ATravensara, ATRC (put a few drops in a box of tissue), Ahinoki, ATangelica, ATAustralian Blue, ATbasil, ATblue cypress (aches and pains), ATcajeput, ATcopaiba, ATeucalyptus (in hot water, breathe deep), ATExodus II, ATfir (aches and pains), ATginger, ATIdaho tansy, ATlavender, ATledum, ATmyrtle, ATonycha (benzoin), ATorange, AToregano, ATpeppermint (relieves nasal congestion), ATpine, ATsage lavender.

It seems that because we live in the South there are a lot of "stuffy noses" in the spring and fall. When I have a client in my business complaining of these types of symptoms, I offer them some oils to sniff for relief. I offer a drop of peppermint first and then a drop of RC blend. Then, if they have used the word "infection," I offer a drop of Thieves blend. I offer one drop of each in the palm of their hand, one at a time. Then I show them how to stir 3 times and cup their hands over the nose and deeply inhale each oil. They are always amazed at the immediate relief.
-Submitted by Pam Jones
Benton, Arkansas (July 2004)

A—Diffuse into the air. Place 1–2 drops in a bowl of hot water, and inhale the vapors. Inhale directly or applied to the hands, tissue, or a cotton wick.

T—Dilute as necessary, and apply 1–2 drops to the throat, temples, forehead, back of neck, sinus area, below the nose, to chest, or to the Vita Flex Points on the feet.

Recipe #1—Apply Raven to the back and RC to the chest with Thieves on the feet. For the next application, rotate Raven and RC. Other oils can be diffused or applied to the forehead, temples, back of neck, and chest. *Refer to the chapter entitled "How to Use—The Personal Usage Reference" in the Essential Oils Desk Reference under "Colds and Flu" for some excellent recipes and supplement recommendations. Also, refer to Comments under Asthma in this book for a discussion on using* **plastic nasal inhalers**.

Blend #1—Mix 6 drops RC and 2 drops ravensara. Apply to the chest, neck, throat, and sinus area. Diffuse, or put 4 drops in a half cup of hot water; then place nose and mouth over the opening of the cup (not in the water) and breathe deeply.

Supplements—Thieves Lozenges.

***Comments—Dr. Pénoël recommends applying a trace of *Melaleuca alternifolia* to the tip of the tongue and swallowing. This works best when done immediately upon noticing a sore throat. Repeat every minute until the throat feels better. Then apply it behind the ears and down under the jaw line. After repeating this a few times (every 5–10 minutes), massage a couple drops on the back of the neck to relieve any blockage.

Cold Sores: *See also Herpes Simplex.*

Oils—ᵀAustralian Blue, ᵀmelaleuca, ᵀmelissa[160], ᵀpeppermint[161], ᵀbergamot[162], ᵀblue cypress, ᵀgeranium, ᵀlavender, ᵀlemon, ᵀMelrose (fights infection), ᵀRC, ᵀRoman chamomile, ᵀThieves.

Colic: *See Children/Infants: Colic.*

Colitis: *See Colon: Colitis.*

Colon: *See also Diverticulitis.*

▸▸ *The colon, or large intestine, is the last part of the digestive system. Its function is to extract water and vitamins created by friendly bacterial flora from the material moving through the digestive system.*

Oils—ᴵᵀDi-Gize, ᴵᵀpeppermint, ᵀcalamus (may help reduce inflammation), ᵀRelease.

Supplements—Balance Complete (*refer to the 5-Day Nutritive Cleanse program listed under Balance Complete in the Supplements section of the Reference Guide for Essential Oils. This program also uses Digest + Cleanse and NingXia Red to help enhance detoxification while maintaining energy levels.*), Cleansing Trio (ComforTone, Essentialzyme, and ICP), Digest + Cleanse, JuvaPower/JuvaSpice, Life 5 (probiotic). *Refer to the Supplements section of the Reference Guide for Essential Oils for specific usages.*

—Colitis

▸▸ *Colitis is inflammation of the large intestine or colon. The exact cause is not known, but it may involve an autoimmune response. Symptoms can include abdominal pain, tenderness, frequent need to expel stools, diarrhea, and possibly bloody stools and fever in the case of ulcerative colitis.*

Oils—ᵀᴬ$_F$Helichrysum (viral), ᵀᴬ$_F$tarragon, ᵀᴬ$_F$thyme (when there is infection), ᵀᴬanise, ᵀᴬcalamus (viral), ᵀᴬclove (bacterial). Redmond clay (from Redmond Minerals 1-800-367-7258) helps clean fecal matter out of pockets in the colon.

Supplements—AlkaLime, Balance Complete (uses 5 different fibers for optimal absorption and cleansing action), Cleansing Trio (ComforTone, Essentialzyme, and ICP), Digest + Cleanse.

—Diverticulitis

▸▸ *Diverticula, sac-like herniations through the muscular wall of the large intestine (colon), are caused by increased pressure in the bowel from constipation. The existence of these sacs that are filled with trapped fecal sludge is called diverticulosis. When they become infected, the rotting feces erodes the surrounding mucosa and blood vessels, and bleeding, rupturing, and infection begins. This is known as diverticulitis.*

Recipe #1—Use Redmond clay (1-800-367-7258) to help remove fecal matter from the pockets. Rub abdomen with cinnamon bark and V-6 Oil. Anise or lavender may also help. Calamus may help with earlier stages of diverticulitis.

Supplements—Balance Complete (*refer to the 5-Day Nutritive Cleanse program listed under Balance Complete in the Supplements section of the Reference Guide for Essential Oils. This program also uses Digest + Cleanse and NingXia Red to help enhance detoxification while maintaining energy levels*), ComforTone to open blocked colon (use daily, increasing dosage by one until bowels are eliminating waste 2–4 times per day), then ICP (fiber beverage) to cleanse colon, and Essentialzyme or Essentialzymes-4, for digestive enzyme support. Digest + Cleanse and JuvaPower/JuvaSpice may also help.

—Polyps *See also Polyps.*

▸▸ *Colon polyps are tumors that arise from the bowel surface and protrude into the inside of the colon. Most polyps eventually transform into malignant cancer tumors.*

***Comments**—Cleanse the colon! Stanley Burroughs' Master Cleanse is an ideal cleansing program which affects the entire body. However, if fecal matter is not being eliminated from the colon 2–3 times per day, it may be necessary to start with ComforTone first until bowel movements are more frequent. Then toxins released during the Master Cleanse can be quickly eliminated from the body. (See MASTER CLEANSER under Cleansing)

Supplements—Cleansing Trio (ComforTone, Essentialzyme, and ICP). *Refer to the Supplements section of the Reference Guide for Essential Oils.*

—Prolapsed Colon—not assimilating

Supplements—Essentialzyme, Essentialzymes-4.

***Comments**—*Stanley Burroughs recommends performing a colon lift and describes the procedure for doing so in his book Healing for the Age of Enlightenment on pages 55 to 59.*

—Spastic (has no peristaltic action)

Supplements—Balance Complete, ComforTone then ICP (fiber beverage).

T—Apply topically with a compress. Dilute as necessary, and apply 1–2 drops on lower abdomen or on Vita Flex points on the feet. Use 1–2 drops in warm bathwater for a bath.

I—Take 2 drops of each in distilled water 1–2 times per day. Use Redmond clay (from Redmond Minerals 1-800-367-7258) to remove fecal matter from pockets in the colon.

A—Diffuse into the air. Inhale directly or applied to the hands, tissue, or a cotton wick.

Coma:

Oils—TAwaken, Tfrankincense, Tsandalwood, TValor, Tblack pepper, Tcypress, THope, Tpeppermint, TSurrender, TTrauma Life.

T—Dilute as necessary, and massage on brain stem area, mastoids (behind ears), temples, and bottoms of feet.

Supplements—Mineral Essence, Ultra Young+.

Comforting:

Oils—ATGentle Baby.

A—Diffuse into the air. Inhale directly or applied to hands, tissue, or a cotton wick.

T—Apply to auricular emotional points. Dilute with V-6 Oil, and massage into skin.

Compassion:

Oils—ATHelichrysum.

A—Diffuse into the air. Inhale directly or applied to hands, tissue, or a cotton wick.

T—Apply to auricular emotional points. Dilute with V-6 Oil, and massage into skin.

Complexion: *See Skin:* COMPLEXION.

Concentration (Poor):

Oils—^A^Lavender[160], ^A^lemon, ^A^peppermint, ^A^Brain Power, ^A^Awaken, ^A^basil, ^A^cedarwood, ^A^Clarity, ^A^cypress, ^A^Dream Catcher, ^A^eucalyptus, ^A^Gathering, ^A^juniper, ^A^myrrh, ^A^orange, ^A^rosemary, ^A^sandalwood, ^A^3 Wise Men, ^A^ylang ylang.

Supplements—Omega Blue, OmegaGize[3]

Concussion: *See also Brain.*

▸▸*A Concussion is a traumatic brain injury that most commonly occurs as a result of a blow to the head. Concussion symptoms include headaches, dizziness, blurred vision, vomiting, disorientation, difficulty focusing attention, ringing in the ears, selective memory loss, etc.*

Oils—^T^Frankincense[161], ^T^cypress.

T—Dilute as necessary, and rub on brain stem and bottoms of feet.

***Comments—One woman had a concussion with headaches and hallucinations. By applying cypress over her brain stem, her headaches left for good.

Confidence:

Oils—^AT^Jasmine, ^AT^Live with Passion, ^AT^sandalwood (self), ^AT^Transformation, ^AT^Valor.

A—Diffuse into the air. Inhale directly or applied to hands, tissue, or a cotton wick.

T—Apply to auricular emotional points. Dilute with V-6 Oil, and massage into skin.

Confusion:

Oils—^AT^Awaken, ^AT^basil, ^AT^Brain Power, ^AT^cedarwood, ^AT^Clarity, ^AT^cypress, ^AT^fir, ^AT^frankincense, ^AT^Gathering, ^AT^geranium, ^AT^ginger, ^AT^Harmony, ^AT^jasmine, ^AT^juniper, ^AT^marjoram, ^AT^peppermint, ^AT^Present Time, ^AT^rose, ^AT^rosemary, ^AT^rosewood, ^AT^sandalwood, ^AT^spruce, ^AT^thyme, ^AT^Transformation, ^AT^Valor, ^AT^ylang ylang.

A—Diffuse into the air. Inhale directly or applied to hands, tissue, a or a cotton wick.

T—Apply to auricular emotional points. Dilute with V-6 Oil, and massage into skin.

Congestion: *See also Anticatarrhal.*

Oils—^AT^Eucalyptus[162], ^AT^*Eucalyptus radiata*, ^AT^RC, ^AT^Di-Gize, ^T^Breathe Again, ^AT^cedarwood, ^AT^coriander, ^AT^cypress, ^AT^Exodus II, ^AT^fennel, ^AT^ginger, ^AT^myrtle (excellent for children), ^AT^Raven, ^AT^rosemary.

Personal Care—Cel-Lite Magic.

Supplements—Cleansing Trio (ComforTone, ICP, Essentialzyme), Digest + Cleanse.

—DECONGESTANT

Oils—^AT^~F~Cypress, ^AT^~F~German chamomile, ^AT^any of the citrus oils, ^AT^juniper, ^AT^melaleuca, ^AT^patchouli.

—EXPECTORANT

Oils—^AT^Eucalyptus[162], ^AT^~F~marjoram, ^AT^~F~ravensara, ^AT^black pepper, ^AT^elemi, ^AT^frankincense, ^AT^helichrysum, ^AT^mugwort, ^AT^pine.

—Mucus

Oils—**AT**Eucalyptus[162], **AT**$_F$cypress, **AT**$_F$rosemary, **AT**helichrysum (discharge), **AT**goldenrod (discharges respiratory mucus), **AT**hyssop (opens respiratory system and discharges toxins and mucus), **AT**mugwort (expels), **AT**onycha (benzoin), **AT**Thieves (dissolves excess mucus).

T—To help discharge mucus, rub oil(s) on chest, neck, back, feet, throat, or lungs.

A—Diffuse oils into the air. Inhale directly or applied to tissue or a cotton wick.

Conjunctivitis: *See Eyes: Conjunctivitis.*

Consciousness:

Oils—**AT**Lavender.

—Open

Oils—**AT**Rosemary.

—Purifying

Oils—**AT**Peppermint.

—Stimulating

Oils—**AT**Peppermint, **AT**Transformation.

A—Diffuse into the air. Inhale directly or applied to hands, tissue, or a cotton wick.

T—Apply to auricular emotional points. Dilute with V-6 Oil, and massage into skin.

Constipation: *See Digestive System.*

Contagious Diseases:

Oils—**AT**$_F$Ginger.

A—Diffuse into the air. Inhale directly or applied to hands, tissue, or a cotton wick.

T—Dilute as necessary, and apply to Vita Flex points on the feet, or over lymph nodes.

Control:

—Of Your Life

Oils—**AT**Cedarwood, **AT**Dream Catcher, **AT**Envision.

—Self

Oils—**AT**Motivation, **A**Roman chamomile.

A—Diffuse into the air. Inhale directly or applied to hands, tissue, or a cotton wick.

T—Apply to auricular emotional points.

Convulsions: *See Seizure: Convulsions.*

Cooling Oils: *See also Temperature: Lower.*

Oils—**TA**Angelica, **TA**citrus oils, **TA**eucalyptus, **TA**lavender, **TA**melaleuca, **TA**mountain savory, **TA**peppermint, **TA**Roman chamomile, **TA**spruce. Other oils that are high in aldehydes and esters can produce a cooling effect.

T—Dilute as necessary, and apply to the skin. Dilute with V-6 Oil to create massage oil, and massage into skin.

A—Diffuse into the air.

Corns: *See Feet: Corns. See also Warts.*

Cortisone:

▸▸ *Cortisone is a type of steroid hormone. It suppresses the immune system and reduces inflammation.*

Oils—[T]$_{F}$Spruce (is like cortisone), [T]EndoFlex, [T]lavender, [T]Relieve It, [T]Roman chamomile, [T]wintergreen.

T—Dilute as necessary, and apply on skin.

Blend #1—Combine 3 drops Roman chamomile, 3 drops lavender, 5 drops spruce, and 1 drop wintergreen, and apply as a natural cortisone.

Supplements— Prostate Health and Thyromin, together with EndoFlex are beneficial for both men and women. The three items together may also help the body produce its own cortisone. Can also try EndoGize.

Coughs:

Oils—[AT]RC, [AT]frankincense, [AT]$_{F}$eucalyptus, [AT]$_{F}$melaleuca, [AT]$_{F}$myrtle (helps remove mucus from lungs), [AT]cedarwood, [AT]angelica, [AT]cajeput, [AT]cardamom, [AT]elemi (unproductive), [AT]fir, [AT]ginger, [AT]hinoki, [AT]jasmine, [AT]juniper, [AT]myrrh, [AT]onycha (benzoin), [AT]peppermint, [AT]pine, [AT]myrrh, [AT]ravensara, [AT]Roman chamomile, [AT]sage lavender, [AT]sandalwood, [AT]Thieves (dissolves excess mucus and reduces inflammation), [AT]thyme.

Supplements—Thieves Lozenges.

—Allergy

Oils—[A]Purification.

—Severe

Oils—[AT]Elemi, [AT]frankincense.

Blend #1—3 drops fir, 3 drops lemon, 2 drops ravensara, and 1 drop thyme.

Blend #2—15 drops Raven, 15 drops RC, 5 drops lemon, and 10 drops Peace & Calming. Rub on chest, throat, and neck. Can also be diffused.

—Smokers

Oils—[AT]Myrtle.

A—Diffuse into the air. Place 1–2 drops in bowl of hot water, and inhale vapors.

T—Dilute as necessary, and apply to throat and chest area.

Courage:

Oils—[A]Clove, [A]fennel, [AT]ginger, [AT]Live with Passion, [AT]Valor (gives).

A—Diffuse into the air. Inhale directly or applied to hands, tissue, or a cotton wick.

T—Apply to auricular emotional points. Dilute with V-6 Oil and massage into skin.

Cradle Cap: *See Children/Infants: Cradle Cap.*

Cramps: *See also Digestive System, Hormonal Imbalance, Menstruation, Muscles, PMS.*

Cramps are sudden, involuntary muscle contractions that often cause severe pain. Abdominal cramps are commonly caused by stress, menstruation, mild food poisoning, and Irritable Bowel Syndrome.

Oils—$^{T}_{F}$Cypress, $^{T}_{F}$marjoram, ^{T}Aroma Siez, $^{T}_{F}$lavender, ^{T}wintergreen, ^{T}basil, ^{T}blue cypress (abdominal), ^{T}clary sage, ^{T}Exodus II, ^{T}galbanum, ^{T}ginger, ^{T}rosemary.

Personal Care—Relaxation Massage Oil.

Supplements—Digest + Cleanse (contains oils proven to soothe gastrointestinal upset).

—Leg Cramps

Oils—^{T}Aroma Siez, ^{T}marjoram, ^{T}basil, ^{T}German chamomile, ^{T}lavender, ^{T}rosemary, ^{T}vetiver.

Personal Care—Ortho Ease, Ortho Sport, or Relaxation Massage Oils, Prenolone/Prenolone+, Progessence/Progessence Plus.

Supplements—BLM, Mineral Essence, Super Cal.

—Menstrual Cramps *See Dysmenorrhea.*

Personal Care—Prenolone/Prenolone+, Progessence/Progessence Plus.

Supplements—FemiGen.

Recipe #1—Take 2 FemiGen three times a day, 10 days before period. Start again two days after cycle. May take up to 6 tablets three times a day.

—Stomach Cramps

Recipe #2—Add 3 drops basil in a capsule with Di-Gize; swallow.

T—Dilute as necessary, and apply on location. Dilute with V-6 Oil to create a massage oil; massage on location. Apply as a warm compress.

Creates Sacred Space:

Oils—^{AT}Sacred Mountain.

A—Diffuse into the air. Inhale directly or applied to hands, tissue, or a cotton wick.

T—Apply to auricular emotional points. Dilute with V-6 Oil, and massage into skin.

Crohn's Disease:

Crohn's disease is a chronic inflammation of part of the intestinal wall that is thought to be caused by an overactive immune response. It can cause abdominal pain, diarrhea, nausea, and loss of appetite.

Oils—^{IT}Peppermint, ^{IT}Di-Gize, ^{IT}basil, ^{T}calamus.

Recipe #1—Do Raindrop Technique on spine with ImmuPower.

Supplements—Sulfurzyme, AlkaLime, Balance Complete, Cleansing Trio (ComforTone, ICP, and Essentialzyme), Digest + Cleanse, Life 5 (probiotic), Mineral Essence, MultiGreens, Power Meal.

***Comments—*Refer to the chapter entitled "How to Use—The Personal Usage Reference" in the Essential Oils Desk Reference under "Crohn's Disease" for a specific regimen of supplements.*

I—Add 2–5 drops to an empty capsule with 2–5 drops of V-6 Oil; swallow.

T—Dilute as necessary, and apply on abdomen or on Vita Flex points on the feet. Dilute with V-6 Oil to create massage oil, and massage over abdomen and on feet.

Crown Chakra: *See Chakras*

Cushing's Disease: *See Adrenal Glands: Cushing's Disease.*

Cuts: *See also Tissue, Wounds.*

Oils—ᵀHelichrysum, ᵀlavender, ᵀmelaleuca, ᵀbasil[163], ᵀhinoki, ᵀcypress, ᵀelemi (infected), ᵀMelrose (rejuvenates tissue), ᵀonycha (benzoin), ᵀpine, ᵀravensara, ᵀRelieve It, ᵀRoman chamomile (healing), ᵀrosewood, ᵀsage lavender, ᵀThieves.

T—Dilute as necessary, and apply on location.

Cystic Fibrosis:

›› *Cystic Fibrosis is an hereditary disease where thick, sticky mucus builds up in the lungs and in the digestive track. Cystic Fibrosis is life-threatening and can result in respiratory failure.*

Recipe #1—Alternate with Thieves, RC, lavender, and myrtle. Apply to brain stem area (back of neck), temples, chest, bottoms of feet. Diffuse. Raven is stronger and can replace myrtle for helping to remove mucus accumulation in the lungs. EndoFlex and helichrysum can also be used with benefit.

Recipe #2—(*Staphylococcus*) Oregano, thyme, and Melrose (up the spine using the Raindrop Technique), then 10 drops lemon, 5 drops melaleuca, and 3 drops frankincense (rub on feet and chest, and diffuse) **or** 10 drops Raven and 5 drops hyssop.

Supplements—EndoGize, Essentialzyme, Essentialzymes-4, Master Formula His/Hers, MultiGreens, all vitamins.

Cystitis (Bladder Infection): *See Bladder: Infection.*

Dandruff: *See Hair: Dandruff.*

Day Dreaming:

Oils—ᴬᵀAwaken, ᴬᵀcedarwood, ᴬᵀClarity, ᴬᵀDream Catcher, ᴬᵀeucalyptus, ᴬᵀGathering, ᴬᵀginger, ᴬᵀHarmony, ᴬᵀhelichrysum, ᴬᵀHighest Potential, ᴬᵀlavender, ᴬᵀlemon, ᴬᵀmyrrh, ᴬᵀpeppermint, ᴬᵀPresent Time, ᴬᵀrose, ᴬᵀrosemary, ᴬᵀrosewood, ᴬᵀSacred Mountain, ᴬᵀsandalwood, ᴬᵀspruce, ᴬᵀ3 Wise Men, ᴬᵀthyme, ᴬᵀValor, ᴬᵀylang ylang.

A—Diffuse into the air. Inhale directly or applied to hands, tissue, or a cotton wick.

T—Apply to auricular emotional points. Dilute with V-6 Oil, and massage into skin.

Death (of Loved One): *See Emotions: LOSS.*

Oils—ᴬᵀTrauma Life.

A—Diffuse into the air. Inhale directly or applied to hands, tissue, or a cotton wick.

T—Apply to auricular emotional points. Dilute with V-6 Oil, and massage into skin.

Debility:

Oils—ᴬᵀ$_F$Nutmeg, ᴬᵀcardamom, ᴬᵀcumin (nervous), ᴬᵀsage lavender.

A—Diffuse into the air. Inhale directly or applied to hands, tissue, or a cotton wick.

T—Dilute with V-6 Oil, and massage into skin.

Decongestant: *See Congestion: Decongestant.*

Defeated: *See Emotions: Defeated.*

Degenerative Disease: *See pH Balance.*

>> *A degenerative disease is a disease where the affected tissues or organs are damaged due to internal mechanisms, and not due to infection. Quite a few different diseases can be categorized as degenerative diseases, including Alzheimer's disease, cancer, Parkinson's disease, atherosclerosis, diabetes, osteoporosis, rheumatoid arthritis, and many others. Support the cells and tissues through proper nutrition, reducing stress, exercising regularly, and eliminating toxins.* *See specific conditions in this guide for lists of oils and other products that can support the body for each condition.*

Oils—ACitrus Fresh, AExodus II, Afrankincense, Alavender, Alemon, Aorange, APurification, Atangerine, ATransformation.

A—These oils are excellent to diffuse in the room. Not only do they purify the air, but they also help deliver needed oxygen to the starving cells. All other essential oils and supplements are beneficial for providing oxygen and nutrients to the cells of the body. *See specific ailments.*

Supplements—NingXia Red (provides a full range of nutrients), Power Meal, True Source (whole food multi-nutrient).

***Comments—A lack of nutrients at the cellular level causes degenerative disease. The general health condition of the body will improve if the necessary nutrients are received by the body at the cellular level. Toxins change the pH of the cell wall, which change significantly reduces the ability of the cell to assimilate nutrients and oxygen. This process is the beginning of cellular starvation, which leads to degenerative disease. We then become hosts to viral and bacterial invasions due to our weakened or compromised immune system. Essential oils are antimicrobial and help our immune systems fight off the ravages of disease. They also have the ability to deliver nutrients to our nutritionally depleted cells. When essential oils are blended with the proper nutrients that the body requires, the essential oils act as the delivery system to take the nutrients directly into the cell and through the compromised cell wall, which has had the pH altered due to chemical toxins in the body. This process allows the body to rebuild and regain its healthful condition and allows the body's immune system to normalize. In addition, essential oils have the highest oxygenating molecules of any known substance. So they deliver oxygen to the cells, which helps in the regeneration process. (Young Living Essential Edge Newsletter —July 1996).

Dehydration:

>> *Rehydration with an oral rehydration solution is the most effective way to prevent dehydration. If no commercially prepared oral rehydration solution is available, a solution made from 1 tsp. salt, 8 tsp. sugar, and 1 liter clean water (with some mashed fresh banana, if available, to add potassium) can work in an emergency.*

Supplements—Mineral Essence.

Delivery: *See Pregnancy: Delivery.*

Denial:

Oils—ATRoman chamomile, ATsage.

—Overcome

Oils—ATAbundance, ATAcceptance, ATAwaken, ATTransformation.

A—Diffuse into the air. Inhale directly or applied to hands, tissue, a or a cotton wick.

T—Apply to auricular emotional points. Dilute with V-6 Oil, and massage into skin.

Dental Infection: *See Oral Conditions: Infection.*

Deodorant:

Oils—[T]Acceptance, [T]Aroma Siez, [T]bergamot, [T]citronella, [T]cypress, [T]Dragon Time, [T]Dream Catcher, [T]EndoFlex, [T]eucalyptus, [T]geranium, [T]Harmony, [T]Joy, [T]lavender, [T]melaleuca, [T]Mister, [T]myrtle, [T]Peace & Calming, [T]RC, [T]Release, [T]White Angelica.

T—Apply oils neat to the skin, or dilute with some V-6 Oil for application under the arms. Also, 2–3 drops of an oil can be added to 4 oz. of unscented talcum powder and 2 oz. of baking soda. Mix this well, and apply under the arms, on the feet, or on other areas of the body.

Personal Care—AromaGuard Deodorants, Dragon Time Bath & Shower Gel, Dragon Time Massage Oil, Evening Peace Bath & Shower Gel, Morning Start Bath & Shower Gel, Relaxation Massage Oil, Lavender Hand & Body Lotion, Sandalwood Moisture Cream. Add a couple drops of one of the oils listed above for additional fragrance.

Deodorizing:

Oils—[A]$_F$Myrtle, [A]Purification, [A]clary sage, [A]myrrh, [A]peppermint, [A]sage, [A]thyme.

A—Diffuse into the air. Add 8–10 drops in 1 tsp. perfumers or grain alcohol (such as vodka), and combine with distilled water in a 1 oz. spray bottle. Spray into the air or on affected surface.

Depletion:

Oils—[AT]Cypress.

A—Diffuse into the air. Inhale directly or applied to tissue or a cotton wick.

T—Dilute with V-6 Oil to create a massage oil, and massage onto the skin.

Depression: *See Diet.*

▸▸ *Depression is a disorder marked by excessive sadness, energy loss, feelings of worthlessness, irritableness, sudden weight loss or gain, trouble sleeping, and loss of interest in activities normally enjoyed. These symptoms can continue for weeks or months if not treated and can destroy an individual's quality of life.*

Oils—[AT]Lemon[164], [AT]$_F$frankincense[165], [A]lavender[166], [AT]Joy (5 drops in palm of non-dominant hand, stir clockwise three times with dominant hand, then apply over heart and breathe in deeply), [A]$_F$bergamot[167], [AT]Valor (helps balance energies), [AT]$_F$ylang ylang, [AT]$_F$rosemary (nervous), [AT]$_F$rosewood, [AT]tangerine[167], [AT]grapefruit[167], [AT]Hope (on ears, especially for emotional clearing), [AT]jasmine, [AT]neroli, [AT]sage (relieves depression), [AT]Sensation, [AT]Acceptance, [AT]basil, [AT]calamus, [AT]clary sage, [AT]EndoFlex (apply often while taking Mineral Essence and Thyromin supplements), [AT]Gathering, [AT]Gentle Baby (on solar plexus), [AT]geranium, [AT]ginger, [AT]Harmony, [AT]Highest Potential, [AT]Inspiration, [AT]juniper (over heart), [AT]M-Grain, [AT]onycha (benzoin), [AT]PanAway, [AT]Live with Passion, [AT]patchouli, [AT]Peace & Calming (back of neck), [AT]pepper (on crown for spirit protection), [AT]ravensara (lifts emotions), [AT]Release, [AT]Roman chamomile, [AT]sandalwood, [AT]Trauma Life.

> ***Depression** can be caused by a calcium deficiency. Stay away from carbonated soft drinks, specifically cola drinks that are high in phosphorus; they leech calcium from the body. Eating heavy protein at night does not give the body enough time to digest the food before going to sleep. The undigested food then ferments, which robs the system of needed oxygen and heightens the sense of depression.*

A—Diffuse into the air. Inhale directly or applied to hands, tissue, or a cotton wick. *See Comments under Asthma for a discussion on using* ***plastic nasal inhalers****.*

T—Dilute with V-6 Oil to create a massage oil, and massage onto the skin. Apply to auricular emotion points.

Personal Care—Sensation Massage Oil, Lemon Sandalwood or Thieves Cleansing Soaps, Prenolone/Prenolone+, Progessence/Progessence Plus, Sensation Bath & Shower Gel.

Supplements—Mineral Essence, NingXia Red (helps raise energy levels), Omega Blue, OmegaGize³, EndoGize, PD 80/20, Thyromin, True Source (whole food multi-nutrient), Ultra Young+ (helps lift depression).

Blend #1—Combine 1–2 drops each of frankincense, 3 Wise Men, and Hope in the palm of your hand; rub hands together clockwise, cup hands over nose and mouth, and breathe deeply.

—ANTIDEPRESSANT

Oils—ATLemon[164], ATbergamot[167], ATorange[167], AT Ffrankincense[165], ATlavender[166], ATJoy, ATAbundance, ATAwaken, ATChristmas Spirit, ATCitrus Fresh, ATDream Catcher, ATelemi, ATgeranium, ATjasmine, ATmelissa, ATMotivation, ATneroli, AТonycha (benzoin) (combine with rose for massage), ATPeace & Calming, ATravensara, ATRoman chamomile, ATrose, ATSacred Mountain, ATsandalwood, AT3 Wise Men, ATValor.

T—Dilute as necessary, and apply to bottoms of feet and over heart.

A—Diffuse into the air.

Supplements—Omega Blue, OmegaGize³

***Comments—See the "Single Oil Property Chart" in the Appendix of this book for additional antidepressant oils and their strengths.

–RECOVERY FROM COMMERCIAL ANTIDEPRESSANTS LIKE PROZAC

Recipe #1—Brain Power, Clarity, Joy, Peace & Calming, and Valor all help repair brain damage from the commercial drugs that inhibit serotonin metabolism. They also stimulate the pineal gland which normally metabolizes 50% of the serotonin in the body. The liver and pancreas are extremely toxic. Cleanse with GLF, JuvaPower, Juva Cleanse, and/or JuvaFlex. Coriander, dill and Thieves help regulate the blood sugar. Frankincense helps prevent cancer (risk of breast cancer increases by 7x with the use of Paxil). Balsam fir helps to decrease the cortisol levels. Also focus on strengthening the smooth muscle tissues (especially heart and intestines) as they are contracted by the drugs.

Supplements— CortiStop (Women's), Digest + Cleanse, JuvaPower/JuvaSpice, Omega Blue, OmegaGize³, Power Meal.

—IMMUNE DEPRESSION

Oils—TA FSpruce.

T—Dilute with V-6 Oil to create a massage oil, and massage onto the skin.

A—Diffuse into the air.

Personal Care Products—Morning Start Bath & Shower Gel, Thieves Cleansing Soap.

Blend #2—5 drops bergamot, 5 drops lavender; diffuse.

Supplements—ImmuPro, Inner Defense, True Source (whole food multi-nutrient).

—POSTPARTUM DEPRESSION (BABY BLUES) *See Pregnancy/Childbirth: Postpartum Depression*

—SEDATIVES *See also Calming*

Oils—ATLavender[168], TAylang ylang[169], ATmelissa[170], ATtarragon[171], ATRutaVaLa (roll-on), ATPeace & Calming, TAvalerian, TTranquil (roll-on), ATbergamot, ATcedarwood, ATclary sage, ATcypress, ATfrankincense, ATgeranium, AThyssop, ATjasmine, ATjuniper, ATmarjoram, AT*Melaleuca ericifolia*, ATmelissa, ATneroli, ATonycha (benzoin), ATpatchouli, ATRoman chamomile, ATrose, ATsandalwood, TStress Away. Use intuition as to which one may be best for the given situation. In addition, check the safety data for each of the oils in the Appendix of this book.

A—Diffuse into the air. Inhale directly or applied to hands, tissue, or a cotton wick. *See Comments under Asthma for a discussion on using* ***plastic nasal inhalers****.*

T—Dilute with V-6 Oil to create a massage oil, and massage onto the skin. Apply to auricular emotion point.

—Suicidal Depression

Recipe #1—Put Valor and then Inspiration on feet, and hold feet for a few minutes until relaxed; this may start to release a past negative memory, which could lead to crying, etc. If not, rub Present Time over thymus and then a drop of Inner Child on their thumb, and have them suck the thumb, pushing the pad of the thumb to the roof of the mouth. Once the emotional release starts, put Grounding on the back of the neck and sternum, and then put Release on the crown of the head; wait for a while, allowing then to deal with the release. After the emotional release has subsided, rub Joy over the heart and Hope on the ears. After they wake up the next morning, apply a couple drops of Gentle Baby on solar plexus and over the heart. Magnify Your Purpose may also be helpful to wear as a perfume/cologne.

Supplements—Thyromin.

—Cleansing the Flesh and Blood of Evil Deities

Oils—ATCedarwood, ATmyrrh.

A—Diffuse into the air.

T—Dilute with V-6 Oil to create a massage oil, and massage onto the skin. Apply to auricular emotion points.

–History

"Breaking the lineage of iniquity." The ancient Egyptians believed that if they didn't clear the body and mind of negative influences before dying, they could not progress into the next life and return to this world to take up the body they had left in the tomb (resurrection).

Deprogramming:

Oils—ATForgiveness, ATInner Child, ATRelease, ATSARA, ATTrauma Life.

A—Diffuse into the air. Inhale directly or applied to tissue or a cotton wick.

T—Apply to chakras. Dilute with V-6 Oil to create a massage oil, and massage onto the skin.

Dermatitis:

See Skin: Dermatitis.

Despair:

Oils—ATLemon, ATlavender, ATJoy, ATAcceptance, ATBelieve, ATcedarwood, ATclary sage, ATfir, ATForgiveness, ATfrankincense, ATGathering, ATgeranium, ATGratitude, ATGrounding, ATHarmony, ATHope, ATlemongrass, ATorange, ATpeppermint, ATrosemary, ATsandalwood, ATspearmint, ATspruce, ATthyme, ATTransformation, ATValor, ATylang ylang.

A—Diffuse into the air. Inhale directly or applied to tissue or a cotton wick.

T—Apply to auricular emotion points. Dilute with V-6 Oil to create a massage oil, and massage onto the skin.

Despondency:

Oils—ATBergamot, ATclary sage, ATcypress, ATGathering, ATgeranium, ATginger, ATHarmony, ATHope, ATInner Child, ATInspiration, ATJoy, ATorange, ATPeace & Calming, ATPresent Time, ATrose, ATrosewood, ATsandalwood, ATTransformation, ATTrauma Life, ATValor, ATylang ylang.

A—Diffuse into the air. Inhale directly or applied to tissue or a cotton wick.

T—Apply to auricular emotion points. Dilute with V-6 Oil to create a massage oil, and massage onto the skin.

Detoxification: *See also Chelation, Cleansing, Housecleaning.*

Oils—T$_F$Helichrysum, T$_F$juniper (detoxifier), TGLF, Trosemary[172], Tdill[173], TJuvaFlex.

T—Apply oils to liver area, intestines, and Vita Flex points on feet.

Supplements—Balance Complete (*refer to the 5-Day Nutritive Cleanse program listed under Balance Complete in the Supplements section of the Reference Guide for Essential Oils. This program also uses Digest + Cleanse and NingXia Red to help enhance detoxification while maintaining energy levels*), Cleansing Trio (ComforTone, Essentialzyme, and ICP), Digest + Cleanse, JuvaTone.

—Metals *See also Chelation*

Oils—TAHelichrysum, TAclove (chelates metal ions), TAJuva Cleanse (helps to remove metals from the body), TAPeace & Calming, TASacred Mountain, TAValor.

T—Dilute as necessary, and apply on feet and on liver area.

A—Diffuse into the air. Inhale directly.

Heavy metals in the system give off toxic gases and can create allergic symptoms and hormonal imbalances. For example, cadmium can create hyperactivity and learning disabilities in children. Cigarette smoke and caffeine all contain cadmium. Ridding the body of heavy metals is extremely important for proper immune function. Cast iron cookware leaves heavy iron deposits in the body. Aluminum cookware leaves aluminum deposits in the body. Glass or Stainless Steel cookware is best.

Supplements— Cleansing Trio (ComforTone, Essentialzyme, and ICP), JuvaTone, Longevity Capsules.

–Pull Out

Recipe #1—Drink distilled water. The absence of minerals in distilled water creates a vacuum-like action that pulls metals and toxins from the body.

Blend #1—Combine 10 drops cypress, 10 drops juniper, and 10 drops lemongrass with 1 oz. V-6 Oil, and massage under arms, over kidneys, and on bottoms of feet.

Blend #2—Add 2–4 drops Thieves and 1–3 drops helichrysum to a rolled gauze, and place between cheek and gums to pull out dental mercury. Leave in one place during the night, and throw away the gauze roll in the morning. The next night, place a new gauze roll with oil in a different place. Continue in a like manner until all areas have been affected. ***Note: Dilute with V-6 Oil for use on very sensitive gums or on children.***

—Toxins

Oils—TAHyssop (opens respiratory system and discharges toxins and mucus), Tlemongrass (helps increase lymphatic circulation for enhanced toxin removal), Tpatchouli (digests toxic wastes), TAfennel, TAfir.

T—Dilute as necessary, and apply on feet and on liver area.

A—Diffuse into the air. Inhale directly.

Supplements—Balance Complete, Cleansing Trio (ComforTone, Essentialzyme, and ICP), Digest + Cleanse. These cleansing products may help remove toxic by-products from the body. Also, take Detoxzyme between meals to break down toxins.

***Comments**—Another way to help remove toxins through the skin is to add 2 cups of apple cider vinegar to warm bathwater, and soak in the tub for 25 minutes.

Diabetes:

>> *Diabetes is a disease characterized by the body's inability to properly produce or use the hormone insulin. Insulin, produced in the pancreas, helps regulate the level of sugars in the blood, as well as the conversion of starches and sugar into the energy necessary for life. Common diabetes symptoms include a frequent need to drink and urinate, blurred vision, mental fatigue, and possibly weight loss (depending on the type). Over time, diabetes can lead to additional complications, such as strokes, heart disease, kidney failure, and even the necessity of removing a limb.*

> ***Caution:** Diabetics should not use angelica. Watch insulin intake carefully; you may have to cut down. Keep your physician informed!*

Oils—TA F Rosemary[174], TA sage[175], TA cumin[176], TA F eucalyptus, TA F geranium, TA F pine, TA F ylang ylang, TA coriander (normalizes glucose levels), TA cypress, TA dill (helps lower glucose levels by normalizing insulin levels and supporting pancreas function), TA fennel, TA ginger, TA hyssop, TA juniper, TA lavender, TA Thieves.

Blend #1—8 drops clove, 8 drops cinnamon bark, 15 drops rosemary, and 10 drops thyme in 2 oz. of V-6 Oil. Put on feet and over pancreas.

Blend #2—5 drops cinnamon bark and 5 drops cypress. Rub on feet and on pancreas.

Supplements—Balance Complete (contains a blend of fibers to help maintain stable blood sugar levels), Cleansing Trio (ComforTone, Essentialzyme, and ICP), Digest + Cleanse, ImmuPro, Inner Defense, Majestic Essence Chocolates (low glycemic chocolate), Mineral Essence, MultiGreens, Power Meal, Pure Protein Complete (contains a blend of proteins and fibers to help reduce spikes and maintain stable blood sugar levels), Stevia, Sulfurzyme (take in morning with vitamin C before breakfast and at bed time), True Source (whole food multi-nutrient), Yacon Syrup.

***Comments**—A seven-year-old girl took 6 MultiGreens a day (balances blood sugar), Bodygize three times a day, and ImmuneTune.

—Pancreas Support

Oils—TA Cinnamon bark, TA fennel, TA geranium.

—Sores (diabetic)

Recipe #1—Do the Raindrop Technique, and put Valor on the Vita Flex points. Also lavender and Melrose.

T—Dilute as necessary, and apply on back, chest, feet, and over pancreas.

A—Diffuse into the air.

Diaper Rash: *See Children/Infants: Diaper Rash.*

Diarrhea: *See Digestive System: Diarrhea.*

Diet: *See Blood, Fasting, Food, and Cleansing.*

>> *Diet is extremely important when trying to correct cancer, hypoglycemia, candida, etc. First, cleanse the body: drink a lot of distilled water; stay away from sugars and meats; eat vegetable protein in the mornings, carbohy-*

drates and starches for lunch, and fruit in the evening. Hydrochloric acid and pepsin are secreted in the morning to help digest protein.

Supplements—Enzyme products: Allerzyme (aids the digestion of sugars, starches, fats, and proteins), Detoxzyme (helps maintain and support a healthy intestinal environment), Digest + Cleanse.

—Post-Diet Saggy Skin

Recipe #1—Combine 8 drops each of sage, pine, lemongrass, and 1 oz. of V-6 Oil. Rub on saggy areas.

Digestive System: *See also Bowel, Colon, Giardia, Hiccoughs/Hiccups, Stomach, Ulcers.*

The human digestive system is the series of organs and glands that process food. The digestive system breaks down food, absorbs nutrients for the body to use as fuel, and excretes as bowel movements the part that cannot be broken down.

> ***Digestive problems** may indicate a mineral deficiency. Use Mineral Essence. Life 5 (probiotic) is necessary when you are detoxifying or on any type of prescription drug; you must feed the intestinal tract. If you have digestion problems, take Life 5 to stop the fermentation process.*

Oils—**IT** F Peppermint[177], **IT**caraway[178], **TI**Di-Gize (acid stomach; aids the secretion of digestive enzymes), **TI** F fennel[179] (sluggish), **T** F lemongrass[180] (purifier), **TI**ginger[181], **TI** F clary sage (weak), **TI** F marjoram (stimulates), **T** F nutmeg (for sluggish digestion; eases), **T** F patchouli (stimulant), **TI** F grapefruit, **TI** F sage (sluggish), **TI**anise (accelerates), **TI**basil, **TI**bergamot, **TI**black pepper, **TI**cardamom (nervous), **T**cinnamon bark, **TI**clove, **TI**coriander (spasms), **TI**cumin (spasms and indigestion), **T**GLF, **T**juniper, **TI**JuvaFlex (supports and detoxifies), **T**laurel, **IT**lemon (indigestion), **TI**mandarin (tonic), **T**myrrh, **T**myrtle, **T**neroli, **T**ocotea, **TI**orange (indigestion), **TI**oregano[182], **TI**rosemary[183], **TI**spearmint, **TI**tangerine (nervous and sluggish), **TI**tarragon (nervous and sluggish).

I—Add the oil(s) to your food. Add 1–5 drops of oil to an empty capsule with 1–5 drops of V-6 Oil; swallow.

T—Dilute as necessary, and rub on stomach or apply as a compress over abdomen.

Diffusion—See Negative Ions for oils that produce negative ions when diffused to help stimulate the digestive system.

Supplements—AlkaLime (combats yeast and fungus overgrowth and preserves the body's proper pH balance), Balance Complete, ComforTone, Digest + Cleanse (contains oils proven to soothe gastrointestinal upset and promote healthy digestion), Essentialzyme, Essentialzymes-4 (enzymes help build the digestive system; take before meals for acid stomach), ICP (helps speed food through digestive system; lower incidence of fermentation), Life 5 (probiotic), Master Formula His/Hers, Mineral Essence, Multi-Greens, NingXia Red, ParaFree, Sulfurzyme. Other enzyme products include: Allerzyme (aids the digestion of sugars, starches, fats, and proteins), Detoxzyme (helps maintain and support a healthy intestinal environment).

—Bloating

Oils—**TA**Di-Gize.

T—Apply to stomach and to Vita Flex points

A—Diffuse into the air.

Supplements—ComforTone.

—Constipation

Constipation is a condition characterized by infrequent or difficult bowel movements. A person is considered constipated if he or she has fewer than three bowel movements a week or if the stools are

> *Poor bowel function may be caused by enzyme deficiency, low fiber, poor bowel tone, not enough liquid in diet, stress, incorrect pH balance, and/or bad diet.*

See pages 25–27 for more detailed application instructions.

hard and difficult to expel. Common causes of constipation include a lack of fiber, dehydration, ignoring the urge to have a bowel movement, depression, medications, large dairy intake, stress, and abuse of laxatives.

Oils—[T][F]Orange, [T]rosemary[183], [T]lemon[183], [T]peppermint[183], [T][F]marjoram, [T]Di-Gize, [T]anise, [T]black pepper, [T]copaiba, [T]fennel, [T]ginger, [T]juniper, [T]patchouli, [T]rose, [T]sandalwood, [T]tangerine, [T]tarragon.

T—Dilute as necessary, and massage clockwise around abdomen and on Vita Flex points (feet & shins).

Supplements—ComforTone, ICP (fiber beverage), AlkaLime, Essentialzymes-4, Essentialzyme, Sulfurzyme, and lots of water. If there is a chronic history of constipation, use ComforTone until the system is open, and then start ICP.

Blend #1—Mix together 6 drops each of orange, tangerine, and spearmint, and rub on lower stomach and colon.

Blend #2—15 drops cedarwood, 10 drops lemon, 5 drops peppermint, and 2 oz. V-6 Oil. Massage clockwise over lower abdomen three times a day, and take supplements.

–Children

Oils—Fruit juices or lots of water. Geranium, patchouli, Roman chamomile, rosemary, tangerine.

—Cramps *See Cramps*

—Diarrhea *See also Acidosis*

›› *Diarrhea is an abnormal increase in the frequency of bowel movements, marked by loose, watery stools. Diarrhea is defined as more than three bowel movements a day. Cases of Diarrhea that last more than two days can become a serious problem and can cause dehydration.*

Oils—[IT][F]Peppermint[184], [IT][F]ginger, [IT][F]geranium, [T][F]melaleuca, [T][F]myrrh, [T][F]sandalwood (obstinate), [T]cardamom, [T]cistus, [T]cumin, [T]myrtle, [T]ocotea, [T]spearmint (not for babies).

Supplements—AlkaLime, Essentialzyme, Essentialzymes-4, Life 5 (probiotic).

–Antispasmodic

Oils—[IT]Peppermint[185], [T]galbanum[186], [T]cypress, [T]eucalyptus, [T]Roman chamomile.

–Children

Oils—[T]Geranium, [T]ginger, [T]Roman chamomile, [T]sandalwood.

–Chronic

Oils—[T][F]Nutmeg, [T][F]orange, [T]Di-Gize (apply over stomach, colon, and VF points), [T]neroli.

–Stress-Induced

Oils—[T]Lavender[187].

I—Place 1–3 drops in an empty capsule; swallow.

T—Dilute as necessary, and apply 1–2 drops on stomach, abdomen, or Vita Flex points on the feet.

—Gas/Flatulence

Oils—[T][F]Ginger, [T][F]lavender, [T][F]tarragon, [T]peppermint, [T]fennel, [T]angelica, [T]anise, [T]bergamot, [T]cardamom, [T]coriander, [T]copaiba, [T]cumin, [T]eucalyptus, [T]juniper, [T]myrrh, [T]nutmeg, [T]onycha (benzoin), [T]Roman chamomile, [T]rosemary, [T]spearmint (not for babies).

T—Dilute as necessary, and apply to large intestine, stomach, abdomen, and Vita Flex points of feet.

—Gastritis *See also Anti-inflammatory*

›› *Gastritis is inflammation of the stomach lining.*

Oils—[TI]Di-Gize, [TI]peppermint, [TI]fennel, [I]lemongrass[180], [T]calamus, [T]laurel, [T]pine, [TI]sage, [T]spikenard, [TI]tarragon, [T]yarrow.

T—Apply over stomach area with hot compress.

I—One drop of oil in rice or almond milk taken as a dietary supplement. Place 1–2 drops in an empty capsule; swallow.

Supplements—AlkaLime, Balance Complete, Cleansing Trio (ComforTone, Essentialzyme, and ICP), Digest + Cleanse, Life 5 (probiotic), Mineral Essence.

—Heartburn

▸▸ *Heartburn is a painful burning sensation in the chest or throat. It occurs as a result of backed up stomach acid in the esophagus. Heartburn can be triggered by certain foods, medication, pregnancy, and alcohol.*

Oils—$^{T}_{F}$Lemon, $^{T}_{F}$peppermint, ^{T}Di-Gize (over stomach and colon), ^{T}cardamom, ^{T}Gentle Baby (over thymus).

T—Dilute as necessary, and apply 1–2 drops to chest or to area indicated.

Blend #1—2 drops lemon, 2 drops peppermint, 3 drops sandalwood, and ½ oz. V-6 Oil. Apply to breast bone. Using palm of hand, massage in a clockwise motion—applying pressure. Do Vita Flex on feet.

Supplements—AlkaLime, Essentialzyme, Essentialzymes-4, JuvaPower/JuvaSpice.

—Indigestion

Oils—$^{T}_{F}$Peppermint, ^{T}ginger, $^{T}_{F}$lavender, $^{T}_{F}$thyme, $^{T}_{F}$grapefruit, $^{T}_{F}$orange (nervous), ^{T}angelica, ^{T}cardamom, ^{T}copaiba, ^{T}coriander, ^{T}cumin, ^{T}GLF, ^{T}goldenrod, ^{T}JuvaFlex, ^{T}laurel, ^{T}myrrh, ^{T}nutmeg, ^{T}tarragon, ^{T}valerian (nervous indigestion).

T—Dilute as necessary, and apply to stomach, intestines, and Vita Flex points on feet.

Supplements—AlkaLime, Balance Complete, Cleansing Trio (ComforTone, Essentialzyme, and ICP), Digest + Cleanse (contains oils proven to soothe gastrointestinal upset and to promote healthy digestion).

—Intestinal Problems *See also Colon*

Oils—$^{TI}_{F}$Basil, $^{TI}_{F}$marjoram, ^{TI}ginger, ^{TI}rosemary, ^{T}cajeput, ^{T}calamus (reduces inflammation and detoxifies), ^{T}patchouli (aids in the digestion of toxic waste), ^{T}tarragon.

Supplements—Digest + Cleanse (helps soothe gastrointestinal upset), Life 5 (probiotic), AlkaLime, Balance Complete, Cleansing Trio (ComforTone, Essentialzyme, and ICP), ParaFree, JuvaTone.

–Antiseptic

Oils—^{T}Nutmeg.

–Cramps

Oils—$^{TI}_{F}$Clary sage, ^{IT}Di-Gize (add 3 drops basil in capsule with Di-Gize), ^{T}blue cypress.

–Flora

Recipe #1—Take **kefir with Life 5** (probiotic) first thing in the morning on an empty stomach to help implant good bacteria in the intestines (yogurt will help maintain good bacteria but not implant it).

Supplements—Life 5 (probiotic), Balance Complete (contains inulin, which helps build intestinal flora).

–Parasites

Oils—^{IT}Oregano[188], ^{T}palmarosa[189], ^{IT}lavender[190], $^{IT}_{F}$bergamot, $^{IT}_{F}$clove, ^{IT}Di-Gize, $^{IT}_{F}$fennel, $^{IT}_{F}$lemon, $^{IT}_{F}$Roman chamomile, ^{IT}ginger (helps to create an unfriendly environment for parasites), ^{IT}peppermint, ^{IT}ravensara.

Supplements—AlkaLime, Cleansing Trio (ComforTone, Essentialzyme, and ICP), Digest + Cleanse (contains oils that create an unfriendly environment for parasites), and ParaFree assist in cleansing the intestinal tract of toxic debris and parasites, which are hosts for many diseases.

–SOOTHE

Oils—TSpearmint.

–SPASM

Oils—T F Tarragon, T F fennel.

T—Dilute as necessary, and apply to stomach, intestines, and Vita Flex points on feet.

I—Place 1–2 drops of oil in an empty capsule, and swallow. Add 1–2 drops of oil to 16 oz. of water, or to 8 oz. rice or almond milk, and drink. Add oils as flavoring to food.

—IRRITABLE BOWEL SYNDROME

Oils—ITPeppermint[191], ITcaraway[192], ITDi-Gize, ITcalamus, TIdaho tansy, Tanise, IJuva Cleanse.

I—Place 1–2 drops of oil in an empty capsule, and swallow. Add 1–2 drops of oil to 16 oz. of water, or to 8 oz. rice or almond milk, and drink. Add oils as flavoring to food

T—Dilute 1–2 drops with V-6 Oil, and apply over abdomen with a hot compress

Recipe #1—Take 2 drops each of calamus, caraway, Di-Gize, and peppermint in distilled water 1–2 times per day.

Blend #1—10–15 drops Di-Gize, 5–6 drops ledum, and 1 drop peppermint in a capsule; take internally. *Abundant Health offers capsules that work well with the oils.*

Supplements—Balance Complete, ComforTone, Digest + Cleanse, (enteric-coated to release in the bowels) ICP (fiber beverage), JuvaPower/JuvaSpice, JuvaTone, Life 5 (probiotic), Majestic Essence Chocolates (contain boswellic acid that can help alleviate IBS), NingXia Red.

—NORMAL FUNCTION OF BOWELS (INTESTINES)

Supplements—Balance Complete (utilizes five different fibers for optimal cleansing power), ComforTone, Digest + Cleanse, ICP (fiber beverage for normal function of bowels).

—PARALYSIS OF BOWELS (INTESTINES)

Supplements—ComforTone, Digest + Cleanse.

***Comments—*One women was paralyzed by surgery and had to have 2 colonics a day. She took ComforTone and then she was able to have natural bowel movements.*

Diphtheria:

Diphtheria is an infectious bacterial (Corynebacterium diphtheriae) disease that causes fever, sore throat, swollen glands, bluish coloration of the skin, bloody liquid drainage from the nose, and a gray covering in the back of the throat that blocks the airways and makes it difficult to breath.

Oils—TAFrankincense, TAgoldenrod.

T—Dilute as necessary, and apply 1–2 drops on throat, sinuses, or Vita Flex points on the feet.

A—Diffuse into the air. Inhale directly or applied to hands.

Disappointment:

Oils—[AT]Clary sage, [AT]Dream Catcher, [AT]eucalyptus, [AT]fir, [AT]frankincense, [AT]Gathering, [AT]geranium, [AT]ginger, [AT]Grounding, [AT]Harmony, [AT]Hope, [AT]Joy, [AT]juniper, [AT]lavender, [AT]orange, [AT]Present Time, [AT]spruce, [AT]thyme, [AT]Valor, [AT]ylang ylang.

A—Diffuse into the air. Inhale directly or applied to tissue or a cotton wick.

T—Apply to auricular emotion points. Dilute with V-6 Oil to create a massage oil, and massage onto the skin.

Discouragement:

Oils—[AT]Bergamot, [AT]cedarwood, [AT]Dream Catcher, [AT]frankincense, [AT]geranium, [AT]Hope, [AT]Joy, [AT]juniper, [AT]lavender, [AT]lemon, [AT]orange, [AT]rosewood, [AT]Sacred Mountain, [AT]sandalwood, [AT]spruce, [AT]Valor.

A—Diffuse into the air. Inhale directly or applied to tissue or a cotton wick.

T—Apply to auricular emotion points. Dilute with V-6 Oil to create a massage oil, and massage onto the skin.

Disinfectant: *See also Antibacterial, Antifungal, Antiviral.*

Oils—[T][F]Lemon, [T]Purification, [T][F]sage, [T]ocotea, [T]grapefruit.

T—Add —2 drops of oil to a wet cloth, and use the cloth to wipe down counters and other surfaces.

A—Diffuse into the air.

Blend #1—Add the following number of drops to a bowl of water (numbers in parenthesis indicate portions for a smaller batch): 10 lavender (2), 20 thyme (4), 5 eucalyptus (1), 5 oregano (1). If using the larger portions, add to a large bowl of water. If using the numbers in the parentheses, add the oils to a small bowl of water. Use blend to disinfect small areas.

Diuretic:

▸▸*A diuretic is a substance that causes the body to increase the rate of urination and fluid elimination.*

Oils—[T][F]Lemongrass, [T][F]rosemary, [T][F]sage, [T][F]cedarwood, [T][F]lavender, [T]tangerine, [T]cardamom, [T]cypress, [T]EndoFlex, [T]fennel, [T]grapefruit (all citrus oils), [T]juniper, [T]lemon, [T]marjoram, [T]mugwort, [T]onycha (benzoin), [T]orange, [T]oregano, [T]valerian.

—Alleviates Fluids

Oils—[T]Tangerine, [T]cypress, [T]fennel.

Blend #1—1 drop fennel, 2 drops cypress, 5 drops tangerine; apply from the top of the foot to the knee.

T—Dilute as necessary, and apply oil(s) to kidney area on back, to bottoms of feet, and on location.

Diverticulitis: *See Colon: Diverticulitis.*

Dizziness:

Oils—[A]Tangerine.

A—Inhale directly or applied to hands.

DNA:

▸▸ *DNA is the genetic material of the cell. DNA contains all of the codes that enable the cell to build the materials needed for proper cell structure and function. Mutation of DNA can lead to cell death or to cancer.*

Oils—ATChamomile (strengthens positive imprinting in DNA).

—Unlock Emotional Trauma in DNA

Oils—ATAcceptance, AT3 Wise Men (instructs DNA to open for discharge of negative trauma), ATsandalwood (unlocks negative programing in DNA and enhances the positive programming in the DNA cell to create a feeling of security and protection).

A—Diffuse into the air. Inhale directly or applied to tissue or a cotton wick.

T—Dilute with V-6 Oil to create a massage oil, and massage onto the skin. Apply to Vita Flex points.

Down Syndrome:

▸▸ *Down syndrome is a genetic disorder that typically results in slower physical and mental development and in distinct facial features. Down syndrome is the single most common human birth defect.*

Oils—TAClarity, TAValor.

T—Apply to bottoms of feet.

A—Diffuse into the air.

Supplements—Master Formula His/Hers, Mineral Essence.

Dream State:

Recipe #1—ATDream Catcher dissipates negative thoughts and helps one hold onto dreams until they become reality. To help enhance the vividness of dreams, try applying cedarwood and valerian to the back of the neck (from the top of the shoulders to the base of the skull), and work the oils in with the Vita Flex technique. *For help with getting to a deep sleep, see Blend #3 under Insomnia.*

—Influences

Oils—ATClary sage (enhances vivid dream recall). ATTransformation.

—Protection From Negative Dreams (that might steal your vision)

Oils—ATDream Catcher (helps one achieve dreams).

A—Diffuse into the air. Inhale directly or applied to tissue or a cotton wick.

T—Apply to auricular emotion points or to back of neck. Dilute with V-6 Oil to create a massage oil, and massage onto the skin.

Drowning in Own Negativity:

Oils—ATGrapefruit (prevent), ATTransformation.

A—Diffuse into the air. Inhale directly or applied to tissue or a cotton wick.

T—Apply to auricular emotion points. Dilute with V-6 Oil to create a massage oil, and massage onto the skin.

Drugs: *See Addictions; Drugs.*

Dying:

Oils—ATAwaken, ATTransformation.

Recipe #1—The following combinations have also been used to help individuals pass on more peacefully into the next life: Frankincense (under the nose) and rose (over the heart), **or** 3 Wise Men (under the nose) and Joy (over the heart).

A—Diffuse into the air. Inhale directly or applied to tissue or a cotton wick.

T—Apply to auricular emotion points. Dilute with V-6 Oil to create a massage oil, and massage onto the skin.

Dysentery: *See also Digestive System: Diarrhea.*

›› *Dysentery is severe, frequent diarrhea, often with blood or mucus, that occurs because of infection by bacteria or amoeba. Dysentery can be fatal, due to dehydration, if left untreated.*

Oils—T F Myrrh, T eucalyptus, T lemon, T Roman chamomile, T black pepper, T cajeput, T cistus, T clove (amoebic), T cypress, T melissa.

T—Dilute as necessary, and apply on abdomen and on bottoms of feet.

Supplements—JuvaPower/JuvaSpice

Dyspepsia: *See Digestive System: Indigestion.*

Ears:

Oils—TA Helichrysum (improves certain hearing losses), TA Purification, TA eucalyptus, TA Melrose (fights infection and earache), TA cumin (deafness following a bad viral flu infection), TA elemi, TA geranium, TA Idaho tansy, TA juniper, TA marjoram, TA valerian (combine with helichrysum for added pain relief), TA Valor, TA vitex.

Instructions to increase and restore hearing—

1. Rub **Valor** on bottoms of feet, especially on the 2 smallest toes, and on the smallest fingers of the hand.
2. For each ear, layer 2 drops of **helichrysum**, **Purification**, **juniper**, and **peppermint** (in that order) around the inside (not deep) and back of ear, on the mastoid bone (behind ear), along the bottom of the skull around to the back of the head, and down the brain stem area.
3. Then do the following ear adjustment:
    1. Pull one ear **up** and then the other ear up—10 times each side; 20 times total.
    2. Pull one ear **back** and then the other back—5 times each side; 10 times total.
    3. Pull one ear **down** and then the other down—5 times each side; 10 times total.
    4. Pull one ear **forward** and then the other forward—5 times each side; 10 times total.
    5. Then make one quick pull with fingers in each direction (up/back/down/forward).
4. Rub **geranium** all around back and front of ear.
5. (Optional) Rub 2 drops **ravensara** around base of both ears.

—Earache

Recipe #1—1 drop of either basil, Melrose, or ImmuPower. Can also try 1 drop each of helichrysum and valerian together. Put the drop in your hand, and soak a small piece of cotton (small enough to fit snugly in the ear) in the oil. Place the piece of cotton in the ear, and apply the leftover oil on both the front and back of the ear with a finger.

Supplements—JuvaPower/JuvaSpice.

—Earache In Animals

Recipe #1—(Not cats) 1 drop Melrose on cotton swab, and then swab around in well of ear.

Do not put oils directly into ear canal.

—Hearing In A Tunnel

Oils—TA Purification, TA ravensara.

—Infection

Recipe #2—ImmuPower, melaleuca, Melrose (inside well of ear; down and around ear on the outside and under chin). Purification (inside well of ear), *Melaleuca ericifolia* and lavender (all around outside of ear). Can also try myrrh and rosemary cineol together.

> ***Ear infections*** *can be caused by food allergies!*
>
> ***Caution:*** *When working on the ears, do not put the oils directly into the ear canal. Apply only 1–2 drops of oil to the ear by rubbing on the inside, outside, and on the mastoid bone directly behind the ear.*

—Inflammation

Oils—TA Eucalyptus, TA palo santo.

—Pimples (in ears)

Oils—TA ImmuPower.

—Tinnitus

▸▸ *Tinnitus is a ringing or other audible noise in the ears caused by ear infection, wax buildup, or a block in the Eustachian tube.*

Oils—TA Helichrysum (rub on inside and outside of ears, along mastoid bone behind ear), TA juniper.

T—Dilute as necessary, and apply on surface of the ear (not inside the ear canal) and behind the ear on the mastoid bone. Place 1 drop of oil on a cotton swab, and swab around the ear canal.

A—Diffuse into the air.

Eating Disorders:

—Anorexia

▸▸ *Anorexia is a psychological disorder where a person becomes obsessed with body size and weight, often depriving him or herself of food to avoid gaining weight.*

Oils—TA F Tarragon, TA grapefruit, TA Citrus Fresh, TA angelica, TA Christmas Spirt, TA coriander, TA Purification, TA Melrose, TA Valor.

T—Dilute as necessary, and apply to stomach and bottoms of feet.

A—Diffuse into the air. It may also help to diffuse antidepressant oils.

***Comments—*Some studies have shown that people suffering from anorexia have a tendency to have lower levels of zinc.*

Supplements—Mineral Essence.

–Antidepressants

Oils—AT Lemon[164], AT lavender[166], AT bergamot[167], AT Citrus Fresh[167], AT Acceptance, AT basil, AT clary sage, AT neroli, AT Roman chamomile, AT ylang ylang AT coriander, AT grapefruit.

A—Diffuse into the air.

T—Dilute with V-6 Oil to create a massage oil, and massage onto skin.

—Bulimia

>> *Bulimia is a disorder categorized by periods of overeating, or binging, followed by periods of self-induced vomiting, fasting, or abuse of laxatives and diuretics to purge the body of the food or to compensate for the overeating.*

Oils—[T]Citrus Fresh, [T]grapefruit.

T—Apply to stomach and bottoms of feet.

—OVEREATING

>> *Overeating is eating too much food for the body. It can include binging (eating so much at one time that the stomach is overly filled and uncomfortable or painful), or chronic overeating (eating more than the body needs over a long period of time). Consistently overeating can lead to obesity and other health problems.*

Oils—[A]Grapefruit[193], [A]lemon[193], [A]ginger, [A]peppermint, [A]spearmint.

A—Diffuse into the air. Inhale directly or applied to hands, tissue, or a cotton wick.

Eczema: *See Skin: Eczema.*

Edema: *See also Hormonal Imbalance, Inflammation.*

>> *Edema is swelling caused by the abnormal accumulation of fluids in a tissue or body cavity. This can be caused by an allergic reaction, inflammation, injury, or as a signal of problems with the heart, liver, or kidneys.*

Oils—[TI][F]Grapefruit, [T][F]cypress (alleviates fluids), [T][F]lemongrass, tangerine (alleviates fluids), [T]fennel (breaks up fluids), [T]juniper, [T]geranium, [T]ledum, [T]rosemary.

Blend #1—1 drop fennel, 2 drops cypress, 5 drops tangerine. Apply from the top of the foot to the knee.

—ANKLES

Blend #2—5 drops cypress, 3 drops juniper, and 10 drops tangerine, or use equal parts of cypress and tangerine. Apply from ankles to knees and on Vita Flex bladder points on feet.

—DIURETIC *See Diuretic*

Oils—[T][F]Lemongrass, [T][F]rosemary, [T][F]sage, [T][F]cedarwood, [T][F]lavender, [T]tangerine, [T]cardamom, [T]cypress, [T]EndoFlex, [T]fennel, [T]grapefruit (all citrus oils), [T]juniper, [T]lemon, [T]marjoram, [T]mugwort, [T]onycha (benzoin), [T]orange, [T]oregano, [T]valerian.

***Comments—For water retention in the legs, Dr. Friedmann would rub tangerine, cypress, and juniper on inside of ankle(s) and leg(s) and on the kidney and heart Vita Flex points. He also had his patients inhale the oils as they were rubbed on.

T—Dilute as necessary, and apply 1–2 drops on location.

I—Add 1–2 drops to 8 oz. of water; drink every 3 hours.

Elbow: *See Tennis Elbow.*

Electrical Problems in the Body: *See Balance for methods of balancing the electrical energies of the body.*

Oils—[TA]Valor, [TA]frankincense, [TA]Harmony.

T—Dilute as necessary, and apply to back and to bottoms of feet.

A—Diffuse into the air. Inhale directly or applied to hands.

Electrolytes:

›› *Electrolytes are chemicals in the body, such as salts and minerals, needed for proper body functioning.*

—Balancing

Oils—ᴵCitrus Fresh (increases absorption of vitamin C).

I—Add 1–2 drops to empty capsule; swallow.

Supplements—Super C / Super C Chewable, Mineral Essence.

Emergency Oils:

Oils—Start with the Everyday Oils collection (frankincense, lemon, lavender, peppermint, Purification, PanAway, Peace & Calming, Thieves, and Valor), then add to that cistus and helichrysum (for bleeding and tissue repair), then oregano, balsam fir, and sandalwood (for DNA repair and any tissue damage).

The following oils are recommended by Dr. Daniel Pénoël as ones that everyone should have with them for any emergency:

Melaleuca (*alternifolia*)—Colds, coughs, cuts, sore throat, sunburn, wounds.

Ravensara—Powerful antiviral and antiseptic. Respiratory problems, viral infections, wounds.

Peppermint—Analgesic (topical pain reliever) for bumps and bruises. Also for fever, headache, indigestion, motion sickness, nausea, nerve problems, spastic colon, vomiting.

Basil—Earache, fainting, headaches, spasms (can substitute fennel), poisonous insect or snake bites, malaria.

Lavender—Burns (mix with melaleuca), leg cramps, herpes, heart irregularities, hives, insect bites and bee stings, sprains, sunstroke. *If in doubt, use lavender!*

Geranium—Bleeding (increases to eliminate toxins, then stops; can substitute cistus), diarrhea, liver, regenerates tissue and nerves, shingles.

Helichrysum—Bruises, bleeding (stops on contact), hearing, pain, reduce scarring, regenerate tissue.

*****Comments**—*Dr. Pénoël also recommends including Melaleuca ericifolia because it is more suited to children then Melaleuca alternifolia, and also elemi because it has similar properties to frankincense and myrrh but is less expensive.*

Emotions: *See Emotional Release in the Science and Application section at the beginning of the Reference Guide for Essential Oils. Also, refer to the Auricular Emotional Therapy chart in that same section for points on the ears where the oils can be applied.*

Oils—ᴬᵀAcceptance, ᴬᵀAroma Siez, ᴬᵀAwaken (supports spiritual emotions), ᴬᵀCitrus Fresh and ᵀᴬspruce (on the chest and breathe in Sacred Mountain), ᴬcypress (healing), ᴬᵀEnvision (support and balance), ᴬᵀbalsam fir (balancing), ᴬᵀGathering (to help with feelings and thoughts), ᴬᵀgeranium (women), ᴬᵀGerman chamomile (stability), ᴬᵀgoldenrod (relaxing and calming), ᴬᵀGratitude, ᴬᵀHumility, and ᴬᵀForgiveness (to help with forgiveness), ᴬᵀlavender (men), ᴬᵀmelissa (supports mind and body), ᴬᵀLive with Passion (balancing, uplifting, strengthening, and stabilizing), ᴬᵀpalo santo, ᴬᵀravensara (lifts emotions), ᴬᵀRelease (soothing), ᴬᵀrose (brings balance and harmony to the body), ᴬᵀsage lavender (improves

> *For* **Emotions**, *see other topics such as:* Abuse, Agitation, Anger, Anxiety, Apathy, Argumentative, Boredom, Concentration (Poor) Confusion, Daydreaming, Despair, Despondency, Disappointment, Discouragement, Fear, Frustration, Grief/Sorrow, Guilt, Irritability, Jealously, Mood Swings, Obsessiveness, Resentment, Restlessness, and Shock.
>
> *For more information on using essential oils to help release stored emotions, read Releasing Emotional Patterns using Essential Oils by Carolyn Mein.*
>
> *For some exciting information about how emotions and feelings affect one's physical health, you may want to read Karol K. Truman's books, Feelings Buried Alive Never Die ... and Healing Feeling from Your Heart.*

mood), AT Surrender (calming and balancing), AT 3 Wise Men, AT Transformation, AT Trauma Life, AT valerian (helps replace emotions), AT White Angelica (balances and protects), AT white lotus.

Blend #1—Layer the oils listed below. Wait 10 minutes between each oil to allow the emotions to be released more gently. The individual releasing the emotions should shut their eyes and should have no sounds, music, or candles in the room to distract them. They need to shut down their senses to get into their subconscious deep seated emotions. Breathe synergistically with their breathing.

1. Rub Valor on feet. If there are 2 helpers, have one person hold the individual's feet (your right hand to their right foot, left to left; cross arms if necessary) during the entire procedure. Be sure not to break the energy.
2. Rub Peace & Calming on navel, feet, and on the forehead (from left to right).
3. Put Harmony on each chakra in clockwise direction, on wrists, on shoulders, and on inside ankles.
4. Put 3 Wise Men on crown.

Personal Care—Evening Peace or Sensation Bath & Shower Gel; Relaxation or Sensation Massage Oil; Sacred Mountain, Lavender Rosewood, or Peppermint Cedarwood Moisturizing Soaps; Prenolone/Prenolone+, Progessence/Progessence Plus, Sensation Hand & Body Lotion.

—Acceptance (self-acceptance)

Oils—AT Acceptance, AT Forgiveness, AT Joy, and AT Transformation.

—Anger and Hate

Oils—T Joy (apply to pituitary Vita Flex points on feet and hands), T Release, and T Valor (layer these three oils on the anger or hate auricular ear point). AT Acceptance, AT Forgiveness, AT helichrysum (with deep-seated anger for strength to forgive), AT Humility.

—Balance

Oils—AT Australian Blue, AT balsam fir, AT Forgiveness, AT frankincense, AT geranium, AT Grounding, AT Harmony, AT Hope, AT Inner Child, AT Joy, AT juniper, AT lavender, AT onycha (combine with rose for massage), AT orange, AT Present Time, AT Release, AT Roman chamomile, AT sage lavender, AT sandalwood, AT SARA, T Stress Away, AT 3 Wise Men, AT Transformation, AT Trauma Life, AT Valor, AT vetiver, AT White Angelica.

Personal Care—Prenolone/Prenolone+, Progessence/Progessence Plus.

—Blocks

Oils—AT Cypress, AT frankincense, AT Harmony, AT helichrysum, AT Release (over liver), AT sandalwood, AT spearmint, AT spikenard, AT spruce, AT 3 Wise Men, AT Trauma Life, and AT Valor (help to release emotional blocks). AT Acceptance (can help one accept the change).

—Burdened (Bearing Burdens of the World)

Oils—T Release and T Valor (layer these two oils on the specific ear point). AT Acceptance.

—Childhood Issues

Oils—T SARA (apply to the heart point on the ears).

–Fear (relating to Childhood Issues)

Oils—T Gentle Baby, T Highest Potential, T Inner Child, T SARA.

–Father or Mother

Oils—T Gentle Baby and/or T Inner Child.

—Clearing

The emotions of the mind are the most elusive part of the human body. People are extremely handicapped emotionally and are continually looking for ways to clear these negative emotions. Many of the emotional blends referred to in this book were created from the research of the ancient Egyptian rituals of clearing emotions. They were created with the intent of helping people overcome the trauma of emotional and physical abuse enabling them to progress and achieve their goals and dreams. The Egyptians took three days and three nights to clear emotions. In order to create a very peaceful setting, they would put the person in a room with 10–12 inch thick walls of solid cement and close the door so there would be no sight or sound.

Oils——ATForgiveness, ATGrounding, ATHarmony (use Hope when emotional clearing), ATInner Child, ATJoy, ATjuniper, ATPresent Time, ATRelease (massage a couple drops on both ears for a general clearing), ATSARA, AT3 Wise Men, ATValor, ATWhite Angelica.

***Comments—For some simple instructions on how to do emotional clearing, refer to the page on Emotional Release in the Science and Application section of the Reference Guide for Essential Oils. Another good reference for information on clearing negative emotions is the book, Releasing Emotional Patterns by Carolyn L. Mein, D.C.

—Coldness (emotional)

Oils—ATMyrrh, ATylang ylang.

—Confidence

Oils—ATEnvision, ATHighest Potential, ATjasmine (euphoria), ATLive with Passion.

—Defeated

Oils—ATAcceptance, ATcypress, ATfir, ATForgiveness, ATInspiration, ATJoy, ATjuniper, ATspruce, AT3 Wise Men, ATValor.

—Depression *See also Depression*

Oils—Most of the single oils and blends help with depression as they tend to lift by raising one's frequency. Some of the best include ATChristmas Spirit, ATCitrus Fresh, ATGentle Baby, ATHighest Potential, ATHope, ATJoy, ATPeace & Calming, ATValor, and ATWhite Angelica. Use whichever blend(s) work best for you. Other oils that may be good to use include ATHumility, ATInner Child, ATlavender, ATSARA, and ATTransformation.

Supplements—Omega Blue, OmegaGize[3].

—Emotional Trauma

Oils—ATSandalwood, ATTrauma Life.

—Expression (self-expression)

Oils—TMotivation and TValor (for courage to speak out—TJoy may be added to encourage enjoying life to its fullest). Take deep breaths to help express oneself.

—Excessive

Oils—TSurrender (apply to the **self-expression** point on the ears).

—Focused

Oils—TRelease, then TAcceptance or TGathering (layer oils on the **self-expression** point on the ears).

—Lost Identity

Oils—TAInner Child (apply to the **self-expression** point on the ears).

—Eyes *See Eyes for oils that help with eyesight.*

—Vision of Goals

Oils—TBelieve, TDream Catcher, TAcceptance, AT3 Wise Men (layer on the **eyes & vision** point on the ears). ATEnvision, ATInto the Future.

—Father

Oils—TALavender. Another oil that may be helpful to layer on top of lavender is Thelichrysum, especially when deep-seated anger is present.

–Childhood Issues

Oils—TAGentle Baby, TAInner Child.

–Male Abuse

Oils—[T]Helichrysum and [TA]lavender (layer oils on the **father** point on the ears).

–Sexual Abuse

Oils—[T]Lavender, [T]Release, and [T]ylang ylang (layer oils on the **father** point on the ears). [TA]SARA.

—Fear

Oils—[T]Valor, [T]Release, and [T]Joy (layer on the **fear** point on the ears). [TA]Acceptance, [TA]Harmony, [TA]Highest Potential.

–Childhood Issues

Oils—[TA]Gentle Baby, [TA]Inner Child, [TA]SARA.

–Future

Oils—[TA]Into the Future.

—Female Issues *See Mother, below.*

—Grief

Oils—[TA]Bergamot (apply to the **heart** point on the ears), [A]tangerine (increases optimism and releases emotional stress).

—Heart (Broken or Heavy Heart): *Refer to both Grief and Loss as well.*

Oils—[T]Acceptance, [T]Forgiveness, and [T]Joy (layer oils on the **heart** point on the ears). [TA]Release, [TA]Transformation, [TA]Valor.

—Loss (eases the feeling)

Oils—[TA]Joy, [TA]Sensation, [TA]tangerine (stability).

—Male Issues: *See Father, above.*

—Mind (open)

Oils—[T]3 Wise Men (apply to the **open the mind** point on the ears as well as to the crown of the head and the navel). [TA]Acceptance, [TA]Believe, [TA]Clarity, [TA]frankincense, [TA]Gathering, [TA]Magnify Your Purpose, [TA]Motivation, [TA]Release, [TA]sandalwood, [TA]Transformation.

—Mood Elevation Protocol

Recipe #1—Valor (one drop on each wrist; hold wrists together), Harmony (one drop on solar plexus), Joy (one drop over the heart), White Angelica (one drop on hands—rub hands together; then brush through hair, over the face, shoulders, and chest, and down the legs).

—Mother

Oils—[T]Geranium (apply to the **mother** point on the ears), [TA]Inner Child, [TA]SARA.

–Abandonment

Oils—[T]Geranium, [T]Acceptance, and [T]Forgiveness (layer oils on the **mother** point on the ears).

–Sexual Abuse

Oils—[T]Geranium and [T]ylang ylang (layer oils on the **mother** point on the ears).

—Overwhelmed

Oils—[T]Acceptance and [T]Hope (layer on the **overwhelmed** point on the ears), [TA]Grounding, [TA]Valor.

—Pity (self-pity)

Oils—[T]Acceptance (apply to the **self-pity** point on the ears). [TA]Forgiveness, [TA]Joy.

–Courage (to move beyond feeling)

Oils—TRelease then TValor (layer on the **self-pity** point on the ears).

–Painful (Can feel like heaviness in the chest)

Oils—TPanAway (apply to the **self-pity** point on the ears).

—Protection From Negative Emotions

Oils—TMagnify Your Purpose (empowering and uplifting), Tgrapefruit, THighest Potential, Tpalo santo, T3 Wise Men (release), TWhite Angelica. Apply oils to the forehead and over the heart.

—Rejection

Oils—TForgiveness and TAcceptance (layer on the rejection point on the ears). TAGrounding, TAValor.

–From Father

Recipe #2—Use lavender first then Forgiveness and Acceptance. Layer on the **rejection** point on the ears.

–From Mother

Recipe #3—Use geranium first then Forgiveness and Acceptance. Layer on the **rejection** point on the ears.

—Release

Oils—TA FRoman chamomile.

—Stress *See also Anxiety*

Oils—TABelieve, TAclary sage, TAEvergreen Essence, TALive with Passion, TASurrender.

—Suicidal

Oils—TAGathering, TAHope, TAJoy, TALive with Passion, TARelease, TATrauma Life.

—Sympathy & Guilt

Oils—TJoy and TInspiration (layer on the **sympathy & guilt** point on the ears). TARelease, TAPanAway, TAAcceptance.

—Uplifting

Oils—TAValor (on feet), TADream Catcher, TAEn-R-Gee, TAGratitude, TAHighest Potential, TAlemon, TAorange, TATransformation, TAwintergreen.

—Vision *See Eyes.*

A—Diffuse into the air. Wear as a perfume or cologne. Inhale directly or applied to hands, tissue, or a cotton wick. *See Comments under Asthma for a discussion on using **plastic nasal inhalers**.*

T—Apply to the specific auricular emotion points (*See Auricular Emotion Chart in the Science and Application chapter of this book for point locations*), or to area(s) indicated above. Apply behind ears and across forehead. Dilute with V-6 Oil to create a massage oil, and massage onto the skin.

Emphysema: *See also Blend #5 under Respiratory System.*

›› *Emphysema is a chronic pulmonary disease where airflow is restricted through the lungs due to destruction (typically caused by airborne toxins such as those in cigarette smoke) of the wall of the alveoli (small air sacs in the lungs where oxygen and carbon dioxide is exchanged with the blood). This destruction of the alveolar wall causes the alveoli to collapse when air is expelled from the lungs, trapping air inside.*

Oils—ATEucalyptus, TARaven (hot compress on chest), AT*Eucalyptus radiata*, ATExodus II.

Recipe #1—May use Raven rectally; RC on chest and back. Reverse each night. Thieves on feet; ImmuPower on spine.

Blend #1—Equal parts rosemary cineol, lemon, and peppermint. Diffuse.

A—Diffuse into the air.

T—Dilute as necessary, and apply to chest and back. Apply as a warm compress on chest.

Empowerment:

Oils—ATMagnify Your Purpose, ATSacred Mountain, ATTransformation.

A—Diffuse into the air. Inhale directly or applied to tissue or a cotton wick.

T—Apply to auricular emotion points. Dilute with V-6 Oil to create a massage oil, and massage onto the skin.

Endocrine System: *See Adrenal Glands, Thyroid, Pituitary Gland, Lupus, etc.*

›› *The adrenal glands, pituitary gland, thyroid gland, parathyroid glands, thymus gland, pineal gland, pancreas, ovaries, and testes are all a part of the endocrine system. The endocrine glands secrete hormones, transmitted via the bloodstream, which are responsible for regulating growth, metabolism, enzyme activity, and reproduction. Essential oils may either act as hormones or stimulate the endocrine glands to produce hormones. This production of hormones has a regulating effect on the body.*

Oils—AT FRosemary, ATcinnamon bark, ATblack pepper, ATdill, ATEndoFlex, ATsage lavender.

A—Diffuse into the air. Inhale directly or applied to tissue or a cotton wick.

T—Dilute as necessary, and apply 1–2 drops on the reflex points on the feet, lower back, thyroid, liver, kidneys, gland areas, the center of the body, or both sides of the spine and clavicle area. Dilute with V-6 Oil to create a massage oil, and massage onto skin.

Personal Care—Prenolone/ Prenolone+, Progessence/Progessence Plus.

Supplements— EndoGize,Thyromin and FemiGen (women) or Prostate Health (men), Power Meal (pre-digested protein).

Endometriosis: *See Hormonal Imbalance.*

›› *Endometriosis is the growth of endometrial tissue in abnormal locations, such as on the ovaries or in the peritoneal (abdominal) cavity.*

Oils—TGeranium, Tcypress, Tclary sage, Teucalyptus, TMelrose (hot compress on abdomen), Tnutmeg, TThieves (on feet).

T—Dilute as necessary, and apply on lower abdomen or on feet. Apply as a warm compress. Place 1–2 drops in warm bathwater, and bathe.

Personal Care—Prenolone/ Prenolone+, Progessence/Progessence Plus, ClaraDerm (spray).

Supplements—Cleansing Trio (ComforTone, Essentialzyme, and ICP), Digest + Cleanse, Super C / Super C Chewable, FemiGen.

Recipe #1—Combine bergamot, lavender, and clary sage, and use with a hot compress over the abdomen **or** add 2 drops of each to 1 Tbs. V-6 Oil, and insert into the vagina; use a tampon to retain overnight. This may help rebuild the normal tissue.

Endurance:

—Physical

Oils—ABalsam fir (inhale from hands), TEn-R-Gee (on feet), ATpeppermint (cooling).

A—Inhale directly or applied to hands, tissue, or a cotton wick. *See Comments under Asthma for a discussion on using plastic nasal inhalers.*

T—Dilute as necessary, and apply on skin.

Supplements— NingXia Nitro, Power Meal, Pure Protein Complete.

Energy:

Oils—ATFFir, ATEn-R-Gee, ATValor (balances), ATpeppermint, ATAbundance, ATAwaken, ATbasil (when squandering energy), ATblack pepper, ATClarity, ATcypress, ATEnvision (balances), ATeucalyptus (builds), ATHope, ATJoy, ATjuniper, ATlemon, ATlemongrass, ATMotivation, ATmyrtle (supports adrenal glands to increase energy), ATnutmeg (increases), Aorange, ATpalo santo, ATrosemary, Athyme (gives energy in times of physical weakness and stress), ATWhite Angelica.

Personal Care—Morning Start Bath & Shower Gel or Lemon Sandalwood Cleansing Soap gives you a fresh start with a surge of energy.

Supplements—NingXia Red, NingXia Nitro, MultiGreens (gives energy), Master Formula His/Hers (Multi-Vitamin), Mineral Essence, Thyromin, Super B.

—Electrical Energy (frequency)

Oils—ATForgiveness (high frequency), ATrose.

—Increase

Oils—ATEn-R-Gee, ATpeppermint, ATBrain Power, ATClarity, ATeucalyptus, ATgrapefruit, ATpalo santo, ATrosemary.

Diffusion—*See Positive Ions for oils that produce positive ions when diffused to help increase energy.*

Supplements—Ultra Young+.

—Integrates Energy for Equal Distribution

Oils—ATPatchouli.

—Magnetic

Oils—ATAbundance, ATJoy (enhances and attracts magnetic energy of prosperity and joy around the body).

—Negative

Oils—ATWhite Angelica (frequency protects against bombardment of), ATginger, ATjuniper (clears negative energy), ATpalo santo (clears).

—Physical

Oils—ACinnamon bark, Alemon, ATbergamot, Apatchouli.

—Sexual

Oils—ATLady Sclareol, Aylang ylang (influences).

A—Inhale directly or applied to hands. Diffuse into the air.

T—Dilute with V-6 Oil to create massage oil, and massage into muscles. Place 1–2 drops in warm bathwater, and bathe. Dilute as necessary, and apply 1–2 drops on temples, back of neck, liver area, or feet.

Energy Centers: *See Chakras.*

Enlightening:

Oils—AHelichrysum.

A—Diffuse into the air. Inhale directly or applied to hands, tissue, or a cotton wick.

Enteritis:

▸▸ *Enteritis is inflammation of the small intestine, usually caused by consuming food or drink contaminated with bacteria or a virus. Symptoms include abdominal pain, severe diarrhea, and loss of appetite.*

Oils—**T**Cajeput.

T—Apply on abdomen or on Vita Flex points on the feet.

Enzymes:

▸▸ *Enzymes are proteins that facilitate the acceleration of natural chemical processes within the body.*

Recipe #1—Fresh carrot juice has one of the largest concentrations of enzymes. Drink 8 oz. per day. Add apple and lemon to help with detoxification.

Supplements—Enzyme products: Allerzyme (aids the digestion of sugars, starches, fats, and proteins), Detoxzyme (helps maintain and support a healthy intestinal environment).

Epilepsy: *See Seizure: Epilepsy.*

Epstein-Barr: *See also Antiviral, Chronic Fatigue, Hypoglycemia, Mononucleosis.*

Oils—**TA**ImmuPower, **TA**Thieves, **TA**eucalyptus.

Recipe #1—Do **Raindrop Technique** on spine with the addition of ImmuPower.

Supplements—AlkaLime, ComforTone, Essentialzyme, Essentialzymes-4, ICP, ImmuPro, Inner Defense, JuvaPower/JuvaSpice, JuvaTone, Mineral Essence, MultiGreens, Super C / Super C Chewable, Thyromin, True Source (whole food multi-nutrient).

Equilibrium:

Oils—**AT**Surrender (emotional), **AT**ylang ylang.

—Nerve

Oils—**AT**Petitgrain.

A—Diffuse into the air. Inhale directly or applied to tissue or a cotton wick.

T—Dilute as necessary, and apply on location. Dilute with V-6 Oil to create a massage oil, and massage onto the skin.

Essential Oils:

Essential oils function as a **catalyst** to deliver nutrients to starving cells.

—Sensitive to Skin (caustic, high in phenols, may need to dilute)

Oils—Cinnamon bark, clove, fennel, grapefruit, lemon, nutmeg, orange, oregano, peppermint. Test the oil first in a small, sensitive area. If irritation occurs, dilute with 1 drop of above oil to 20 drops lavender, or mix 1:4 with V-6 Oil.

Estrogen:

▸▸ *Estrogens are hormones produced by the ovaries that regulate the development of female characteristics and the menstrual cycle in females.*

Oils—TAClary sage, TASclarEssence, and TAMister help the body produce estrogen. TAAnise (increases).

T—Dilute as necessary, and apply on the lower abdomen. Dilute in V-6 Oil, and use as massage oil.

A—Diffuse into the air. Inhale directly or applied to hands, tissue, or a cotton wick.

***Comments—Some sugar sweeteners block estrogen. Honey goes into the bloodstream quickly, which affects the pancreas and the production of estrogen.

Personal Care—Prenolone/Prenolone+ (pregnenolone is the master hormone; it is used to balance estrogen and progesterone, whichever is needed).

Supplements—2 FemiGen three times a day, ten days before period. Start again two days after cycle. May take up to 6 tablets three times a day. CortiStop (Women's) can also help increase estrogen levels by lowering cortisol levels. 1 dropper of Estro Tincture three times a day in water

Euphoria:

Oils—AClary sage, Ajasmine.

A—Inhale directly or applied to hands, tissue, or a cotton wick. Diffuse into the air.

Exhaustion: *See also Energy.*

Recipe #1—First, work with one or more of the following nervous system oils to calm and relax: Bergamot, clary sage, coriander, cumin, elemi, frankincense, lavender, pine, sage lavender. Secondly, use basil, ginger, grapefruit, lavender, lemon, Roman chamomile, rosemary, sandalwood, or Transformation.

Expectorant: *See Congestion: Expectorant.*

Expression (Self Expression):

Oils—ATHelichrysum, ATInto the Future, ATJoy (when unable to express physically), ATMotivation, ATRaven, ATRC, ATTransformation, ATValor.

A—Diffuse into the air. Inhale directly or applied to tissue or a cotton wick.

T—Apply to self expression auricular emotion point. Dilute with V-6 Oil to create a massage oil, and massage onto the skin.

Eyes:

Oils—TCarrot (is good around eye area), Tlemongrass (improves eyesight), Tcypress (also helps circulation), Tlemon, T*Eucalyptus radiata*, Tfennel, Tfrankincense, TGerman chamomile, Tlavender, Tsandalwood.

> ***NEVER PUT OILS DIRECTLY IN THE EYES!***
>
> *Be careful when applying oils near the eyes. Be sure to have some V-6 Mixing Oil handy for additional dilution if irritation occurs. Never use water to wash off an oil that irritates.*

Recipe #1—Thieves on feet (especially 2 big toes), M-Grain on thumb prints, layer Mister, Dragon Time, and EndoFlex on Vita Flex points, ankles, and pelvis.

Base Oils (good blends of)—Almond or hazelnut.

Supplements—NingXia Red (provides a significant amount of minerals and carotenoids that protect against eyesight deterioration. *See Comments below*), Power Meal, Sulfurzyme, True Source (whole food multi-nutrient), Wolfberry Crisp Bars.

*****Comments**—According to the book Discovery of the Ultimate Superfood, "The Ningxia wolfberry is rich in two eye-protecting carotenoids—zeaxanthin and lutein—that are absolutely essential for protecting vision from the free radical damage, protein destruction, and blindness that occur with age."

Eye Drop Recipe—Combine 5 parts distilled water, 2 parts honey, and 1 part apple cider vinegar (do not use white vinegar). Mix together, and store in a bottle. Does not need to be refrigerated. This special eye drop formula is found in Stanley Burroughs' book, *Healing for the Age of Enlightenment* and has proven over the years to be superior to most commercial eye drops. These drops have been successful for helping to clear glaucoma, cataracts, spots, film, and growths of various kinds. Apply drops one at a time to each eye several times a day until condition has cleared.

—Cataracts

▸▸*A cataract is a clouding of the normally transparent lens of the eye. This clouding results in blurry vision, seemingly faded colors, double vision, glare, and difficulty seeing at night. Over time, the clouding can increase and lead to severe vision problems.*

Blend #1—8 drops lemongrass, 6 drops cypress, and 3 drops eucalyptus. Apply around the eye area two times a day. Don't get in the eyes.

—Dry-Itchy

Oils—**A**Melaleuca (in humidifier).

—Conjunctivitis (Pink Eye)

▸▸*Conjunctivitis is an inflammation or infection of the membranes covering the whites of the eyes (conjunctiva) and the inner part of the eyelids. Swelling, redness, itching, discharge, and burning of the eyes are common symptoms. Frequent causes include allergies, bacterial or viral infection, contact lenses, and eye drops.*

Oils—**AT***Eucalyptus radiata*, **AT**jasmine.

A—Diffuse oils into the air.

T—Dilute as necessary, and apply oils to Vita Flex points on the feet or to temples.

—Eye Lid Drop (or Drooping Eyelids)

▸▸*A drooping eyelid is characterized by an excessive sagging of the upper eyelid. Drooping can be present at birth as a result of underdeveloped eyelid muscles, or it can occur with aging. Drooping eyelids can cause visual impairment if they droop enough to partially cover the eye.*

Blend #2—1 drop Aroma Life, 1 drop helichrysum, 5 drops lavender.

Blend #3—Helichrysum and peppermint (don't get in the eyes).

Personal Care—Cel-Lite Magic (around eyes).

Supplements—3 MultiGreens four times a day. After massaging Vita Flex points, eat two whole oranges a day with the white still on the orange. It is very important to eat all the white you can plus Super C / Super C Chewable, ComforTone, and ICP (fiber beverage) after meals.

Vita Flex Points—Fingers, toes, and around the eyes.

—Glaucoma

Supplements—Essentialzyme/Essentialzymes-4 (to help relieve stress on the pancreas, if congested), Sulfurzyme (to help regulate the fluid pressure in the eye), Super C / Super C Chewable, Super B, True Source (whole food multi-nutrient).

> *I have had glaucoma for several years and have had my eye drop prescription changed numerous times because of rising pressure. I used a mixture of one third clove, one third lemon, and one third olive oil and rubbed it on my face above and below my eyes. The last time I was at the doctor, my pressure was 14. It was the lowest pressure I have had since I was diagnosed.*
> ***-Submitted by K. Ernst (July 2004)***

 See pages 25-27 for more detailed application instructions.

—Improve Vision

Oils—[T]Frankincense, [T]juniper, [T]lemongrass, [T]Dragon Time, [T]EndoFlex, [T]Mister, [T]M-Grain, [T]sandalwood, [T]Thieves.

******Comments**—According to Dr. Mercola, just about any oil can be used if it is consistently rubbed around each eye for several minutes twice a day. This must be continued for at least 3 weeks before any improvement can be seen. He recommends using frankincense and lavender.

Blend #4—10 drops lemongrass, 5 drops cypress, and 3 drops *Eucalyptus radiata* in 1 oz. V-6 Oil. Apply around eyes morning and night to improve eyesight. Can also be applied to Vita Flex eye points on fingers and toes and also on the ears *(refer to the Auricular Emotional Therapy chart in the Science & Application section of this book for the Eyes and Vision point on the ears).*

Blend #5—5 drops lemongrass, 3 drops cypress, and 2 drops eucalyptus in 1 oz. of V-6 Oil. Apply as a blend, or layer the oils on the eye area (not in eyes).

*****Comments**—*One individual who was not able to see color and who had no peripheral vision rubbed frankincense on his eyelids and just above his eyebrows. Soon thereafter he was able to see color, and his peripheral vision returned.*

—Iris, Inflammation Of

▸▸ *The iris is the colored part of the eye that regulates the amount of light entering the eye through the pupil. When the iris becomes inflamed, it results in a condition called iritis. Iritis is normally related to a disease or infection in another part of the body, but it can also be caused by injury to the eye. Symptoms of iritis include blurred vision, pain, tearing, light sensitivity, red eye, and a small pupil size.*

Oils—[T]Eucalyptus.

—Retina (bleeding)

Blend #6—5 drops tangerine, 5 drops orange, and 5 drops grapefruit. Mix, and apply 2 drops on fingers and toes. Massage Vita Flex points two times a day or more. Diffuse, and let vapor mist around eye. Rub Cel-Lite Magic around the eyes too. Then eat two whole oranges a day with the white still on the orange. Eat all of the white you can.

Supplements—Super C / Super C Chewable.

—Retina (strengthen)

▸▸ *The retina is a layer of nerves lining the back of the eye. The retina is responsible for sensing light and then sending impulses (via the optic nerve) back to the brain so that visual images can be formed.*

Oils—[T]Cypress, [T]lemongrass, [T]helichrysum, [T]juniper, [T]lavender, [T]peppermint, [T]sandalwood.

Blend #7—5 drops juniper, 3 drops lemongrass, 3 drops cypress. Rub on brain stem twice a day.

—Spiritual Eyes (3rd eye, brow chakra) *See also Chakras*

Oils—[T]Acceptance, [T]Awaken, [T]Dream Catcher.

T—Rub oil on earlobe to increase both physical and spiritual vision.

—Swollen Eyes

Blend #1—Cypress and helichrysum. Lavender (antiseptic) is also safe around eyes. If swollen eyes are due to allergies, try putting peppermint on the back of the neck.

T—Caution: Never put essential oils directly in the eyes! Be careful when applying oils near the eyes. Be sure to have some V-6 Oil handy for additional dilution if irritation occurs. Dilute as necessary, and apply oils to feet, Vita Flex eye points, thumbs, ankles, pelvis, eye area (not in eyes), and eyebrows.

A—Diffuse into the air.

Facial Oils: *See also Skin.*

Oils—TMyrrh, Tpatchouli, Tsandalwood, Tvetiver. *Refer to the Personal Care Products section of the Reference Guide for Essential Oils for many other beneficial skin care products.*

Personal Care—Essential Beauty Serums (Dry & Acne-Prone Skin Blends).

—Broken Capillaries

Oils—TCypress, Tgeranium, Thyssop, TRoman chamomile.

—Dehydrated

Oils—TGeranium, Tlavender.

—Disturbed

Oils—TGeranium, Tlavender, TRoman chamomile, Tclary sage, Thyssop, Tjuniper, Tlemon, Tpatchouli, Tsandalwood.

—Dry

Oils—TGeranium, TGerman chamomile, Trosemary, Thyssop, Tlemon, Tpatchouli, Tsandalwood.

—Energizing

Oils—TBergamot, Tlemon.

—Hydrating

Oils—TGeranium, Tlavender, Tcypress, Tfennel, Thyssop, Tlemon, Tpatchouli, Tsandalwood.

—Normal

Oils—TGeranium, Tlavender, Tlemon, TRoman chamomile, Tsandalwood.

—Oily

Oils—TLemon, Torange, Tcypress, Tfrankincense, Tgeranium, Tjasmine, Tjuniper, Tlavender, Tmarjoram, Tpatchouli, TRoman chamomile, Trosemary.

—Revitalizing

Oils—TCypress, Tfennel, Tlemon.

—Sensitive

Oils—TGeranium, TGerman Tchamomile, Tlavender.

T—Dilute as necessary, and apply to face (avoiding eyes), back of neck, behind ears, or Vita Flex points on the feet.

Fainting: *See also Shock.*

▸▸ *Fainting is a temporary loss of consciousness caused by a momentary disruption of blood flow to the brain. Fainting can result from standing in one place too long, coughing very hard, fear, emotional trauma, heavy bleeding, or severe dehydration. Fainting can sometimes be a symptom of a more serious condition.*

Oils—APeppermint, Arosemary, ATrauma Life, Ablack pepper[194], Anutmeg, Abasil, ABrain Power, AClarity, Alavender, Aneroli, Aspearmint.

A—Inhale directly.

Faith:

Oils—ATHope (increases), ATTransformation (for anchoring and stabilizing new-found faith).

A—Diffuse into the air. Inhale directly or applied to tissue or a cotton wick.

T—Apply to crown chakra or to auricular emotion point. Dilute with V-6 Oil to create a massage oil, and massage onto the skin.

Fasting:

>> *Fasting is the avoidance of solid foods altogether, while liquid consumption ranges between nothing (complete avoidance of all liquids as well) and fresh juices, with just water being somewhere in the middle.* ***Complete avoidance fasting (no food or liquid) should only be done when you are feeling good,*** *while fasting on fresh juices can be very healing when sick. The Master Cleanser lemonade fast (*see Cleansing*) is one of the most beneficial juice fasts. While it takes 30 days on this cleanse to change the chemistry in the body (such as eliminating the need or desire for animal proteins), very effective health results can be achieved after only 10 days. To enhance the effectiveness of the change in body chemistry, the 30 day lemon juice fast can be followed by a carrot juice fast for another 30 days. MultiGreens may be taken two times a day for two weeks but should then be stopped so changes can be made at the cellular level; protein prevents this change. When a mother fasts, the breast-fed baby gets the benefits as well (the mammary glands filter the toxins so they are not harmful to the baby).*

Fat: *See also Cellulite, Diet, and Weight.*

Ultra Young+ may help stimulate the pituitary for increased production of the human growth hormone. This hormone is one of the most powerful side effect–free agents for rejuvenating the body, restoring lean body mass, and reducing fat.

Bath (**attack fat**)—Add 6 drops of the following blend to the bathwater, and soak in tub.

Blend #1—8 drops grapefruit, 5 drops cypress, 4 drops lavender, 4 drops basil, and 3 drops juniper.

Supplements—Allerzyme (aids the digestion of sugars, starches, fats, and proteins), Balance Complete, Digest + Cleanse, Power Meal (eat for breakfast as a meal replacement), Ultra Young+ (improves fat-to-lean ratios by stimulating production of the human growth hormone).

***Comments—Eat more grapefruit to dissolve fat faster. Also, trans fats replace essential fatty acids in the brain and are highly acidic. Remove trans fats from diet!

Father (Problems With):

Oils—TA Acceptance, TA lavender, TA Valor.

T—Apply to father auricular emotion point. Dilute with V-6 Oil to create a massage oil, and massage onto the skin.

A—Diffuse into the air. Inhale directly or applied to tissue or a cotton wick.

Fatigue: *See also Energy.*

Oils—TA F Ravensara (muscle), TA F rosemary (nervous), TA F thyme (general) TA En-R-Gee, TA clove, TA pine.

Supplements—NingXia Red.

—Mental

Oils—TA Basil, TA lemongrass, TA Clarity, TA Peace & Calming.

Blend #1—Basil and lemongrass together are a good combination. Apply on temples, back of neck, and feet. Diffuse.

—Overcoming

Recipe #1—Thyme or En-R-Gee on spine, wait a few minutes, then Awaken all over the back and spine; **or** En-R-Gee on feet and Awaken on temples and cheeks.

—Physical *See Energy*

Oils—TA Clarity, TA Peace & Calming.

Supplements—AlkaLime (acid-neutralizing mineral formulation), MultiGreens, Omega Blue, OmegaGize[3], Power Meal, Sulfurzyme, Thyromin, Wolfberry Crisp Bars.

T—Dilute as necessary, and apply on liver or on feet. Dilute with V-6 Oil, and apply as a body massage.

A—Diffuse into the air. Inhale directly or applied to hands.

Fatty Deposits: *See also Cellulite, Fat, Weight.*

—Dissolve

Supplements— Allerzyme (aids the digestion of sugars, starches, fats, and proteins), Balance Complete (contains a mix of 5 different kinds of fibers to help cleanse the digestive system), Digest + Cleanse, Master Formula His/Hers, MultiGreens, Power Meal.

Fear: *See also Anxiety, Calming.*

> *Fear causes the blood vessels to tighten, restricting the amount of oxygen and nutrients that can reach the cells.*

Oils—**AT**Bergamot, **AT**clary sage, **AT**cypress, **AT**fir, **AT**geranium, **AT**Highest Potential, **AT**Hope, **AT**juniper, **AT**marjoram, **AT**Motivation (releases emotional and physical fears), **AT**myrrh, **AT**orange, **AT**Present Time, **AT**Roman chamomile, **AT**rose, **AT**sandalwood, **AT**spruce, **AT**Valor, **AT**White Angelica, **AT**ylang ylang.

A—Diffuse into the air. Inhale directly or applied to tissue or a cotton wick.

T—Apply to auricular emotion points. Dilute with V-6 Oil for massage onto the skin.

Feet:

Oils—**T**Lemon, **T**lavender, **T**Roman chamomile, **T**fennel, **T**pine (excessive sweating).

—Calluses

Oils—**T**Melrose, **T**oregano

—Club Foot

Oils—**T**Ginger (see below), **T**rosemary (see below), **T**lavender, **T**Roman chamomile.

***Comments—Do not use ginger or rosemary on babies *except* for treating for club foot.

—Corns

Oils—**T**Clove, **T**carrot, **T**Citrus Fresh, **T**grapefruit, **T**lemon, **T**myrrh, **T**peppermint, **T**Roman chamomile, **T**tangerine.

T—Apply 1 drop of oil directly on corn.

> *Stanley Burroughs touts clove oil as being wonderful for corns, skin cancer, and warts. He suggests using your finger to apply a small amount of clove oil directly on warts or corns. After a short time, use an emery stick to scrape off the top of the wart or corn and apply the oil again. Repeat several times daily until wart or corn disappears. The same technique can be used for skin cancer. (Healing for the Age of Enlightenment, p. 104.)*

—Odor

Recipe #1—Mix 1 Tbs. baking powder with 2 drops of sage, and put in a plastic bag. Shake and eliminate lumps with a rolling pin and put in shoes. Rub calamus on feet.

T—Dilute as necessary, and apply on location. Dilute with V-6 Oil, and massage on location.

Female Specific Conditions: *See also Hormonal Imbalance, Infertility, Ovaries, Pregnancy/ Motherhood, Uterus.*

Oils—**TA**Mister (during time of month when you are out of sorts), **TA**clary sage, **TA**anise, **TA**Sacred Mountain (female balance).

Supplements—Master Formula Hers, MultiGreens, FemiGen, Prenolone/Prenolone+, Progessence/Progessence Plus.

—ABNORMAL PAP SMEARS

Recipe #1—Add 10 drops ImmuPower and 5 drops frankincense to 1 Tbs. V-6 Oil, and insert into vagina. Use tampon to retain overnight. Take Master Formula Hers to support nutrient level. May continue daily for as long as necessary.

—BALANCE FEMALE HORMONES

Oils—TAYlang ylang, TAbergamot, TAsage lavender.

Personal Care—Dragon Time Bath & Shower Gel for that time of month that leaves women with lower back pain, stress, and sleeping difficulties. Pour between 1 tsp. and 1 oz. of the gel in water while filling your tub.

Supplements—One week after the cycle, take Master Formula Hers four times a day and 6 Multi-Greens a day. CortiStop (Women's) can also help reduce cortisol levels and balance hormones.

—HEMORRHAGING *See also Hemorrhaging.*

Recipe #2—Combine 10 drops helichrysum with 1 tsp. V-6 Oil, and massage on ankles, lower back, and stomach.

—HOT FLASHES

A hot flash is a sudden, intense feeling of heat in the face and upper body, often accompanied by an increased heart rate, sweating, dizziness, headache, weakness, or anxiety. Hot flashes are generally associated with the symptoms of menopause and premenopause.

Oils—T FPeppermint, Tclary sage (estrogen), TEndoFlex, Tbergamot (estrogen), Tfennel, TDragon Time, TMister (estrogen—works for women in Canada).

T—Apply these oils on the ankles at the ovary and uterus Vita Flex points.

Blend #1—If hypoglycemic, use Aroma Siez with M-Grain. Apply over ovaries, pelvis, ankles, bottoms of feet.

*****Comments**—Some women have had success using a drop of EndoFlex under their tongue three times a day. Be cautious as it contains nutmeg and an overdose could cause problems.

Personal Care—Prenolone/Prenolone+, Progessence/Progessence Plus.

Supplements—CortiStop (Women's), EndoGize, FemiGen, Mineral Essence.

—INFECTION

Oils—TA FBergamot (general), TAMelrose, TAfrankincense

*****Comments**—You may mix the oils listed above and insert in vagina at night; may alternate with the blend below.

Blend #2—8 drops juniper, 8 drops melaleuca, and 8 drops Purification. Put in water and douche **or** add 3 drops of each to 1 tsp. V-6 Oil, and insert at night using a tampon to retain.

Blend #3—8 drops juniper, 8 drops lavender, and 8 drops Melrose. Alternate with Blend #1, and follow same instructions.

—INFERTILITY (FEMALE) *See also Fertility.*

Oils—TClary sage, TSclar-Essence, Tcypress, Tfennel, Tgeranium, Tmelissa, Tnutmeg, TRoman chamomile, Tthyme.

Recipe #3—Before the cycle, rub 10 drops Dragon Time around ankles, lower back, and lower stomach. During the cycle, rub 4 drops basil in the same places as before.

Personal Care—Prenolone/Prenolone+, Progessence/Progessence Plus.

Supplements—FemiGen, Master Formula Hers.

—Menopause *See also Hormonal Imbalance*

Menopause is the permanent ending of a female's menstruation and fertility. For most American women, Menopause occurs around age 51 and is often recognized by hot flashes, irregular periods, vaginal dryness, mood swings, difficulty sleeping, thinning hair, abdominal weight gain, and decreased fertility.

Oils—$^{T}_{F}$Cypress, $^{T}_{F}$lavender, $^{T}_{F}$orange, $^{T}_{F}$fennel, $^{T}_{F}$sage, ^{T}Roman chamomile, ^{T}angelica, ^{T}basil, ^{T}bergamot, ^{T}cardamom, ^{T}clary sage, ^{T}Dragon Time (add V-6 Oil and use in douche, enema, or in rectum), ^{T}EndoFlex (on throat, parathyroid, and thyroid), ^{T}geranium, ^{T}jasmine, ^{T}Mister, ^{T}neroli, ^{T}nutmeg (balances hormones), ^{T}rose, ^{T}rosemary, ^{T}SclarEssence, ^{T}thyme.

Personal Care—Add between 1 tsp. and 1 oz. of Dragon Time Bath & Shower Gel to bath while filling tub with water. Soaking helps relieve lower back pain, stress, and sleeping difficulties that are associated with a woman's cycle. Dragon Time Massage Oil.

Supplements—Progessence/Progessence Plus, CortiStop (Women's), EndoGize, FemiGen, PD 80/20, Prenolone/ Prenolone+.

***__Comments__—The possibility for heart attacks in women increases by 5–10% following menopause.

–Pre-Menopause

Oils—$^{T}_{F}$Clary sage, $^{T}_{F}$fennel, ^{T}sage lavender (helps raise hormone levels naturally), ^{T}EndoFlex, ^{T}lavender, ^{T}Mister, ^{T}nutmeg (balances hormones), ^{T}SclarEssence, ^{T}tarragon.

—Menstruation *See Also Endometriosis, Hormonal Imbalance*

Menstruation, also known as a woman's "period," is the regular shedding of the uterus lining and vaginal discharge of blood when a woman is not pregnant. A woman's period lasts between two and seven days and reoccurs on an average of every 28 days.

–Amenorrhea

Oils—$^{T}_{F}$Basil, ^{T}Dragon Time, ^{T}carrot, ^{T}cistus, ^{T}clary sage, ^{T}fennel, ^{T}hyssop, ^{T}juniper, ^{T}lavender, ^{T}marjoram, ^{T}myrrh, ^{T}peppermint, ^{T}Roman chamomile, ^{T}rose, ^{T}rosemary, ^{T}sage, ^{T}sage lavender.

***Amenorrhea** is the absence of menstruation. The oils listed are those which induce menstrual flow (emmenagogic).*

***Emmenagogue** is an agent that induces or hastens menstrual flow. Many of these oils should be avoided during pregnancy. Please see* Pregnancy *for safety data.*

***Dysmenorrhea** is painful menstruation. Apply one or more of these oils to the abdomen. It may also help to use a hot compress. Each of us has different body chemistries, so if one oil doesn't work, try a different one.*

***Menorrhagia** is abnormally heavy or extended menstrual flow. It may also refer to irregular bleeding at any time. This situation may be a sign of a more serious condition, so please see your doctor.*

–Dysmenorrhea

Oils—$^{T}_{F}$Tarragon, ^{T}clary sage (followed by basil), ^{T}lavender, ^{T}cypress, ^{T}peppermint, ^{T}Dragon Time, ^{T}EndoFlex, ^{T}fennel, ^{T}jasmine, ^{T}juniper, ^{T}marjoram, ^{T}Roman chamomile, ^{T}rosemary, ^{T}sage, ^{T}sage lavender, ^{T}yarrow.

Bath & Shower Gels—Add 1 tsp.–1 oz. Dragon Time Bath & Shower Gel to bath while filling tub with water. Soaking helps relieve lower back pain, stress, and sleeping difficulties that are associated with a woman's cycle.

–General Care

Blend #4—Before and during cycle, combine 10 drops Dragon Time with 4 drops basil, and rub around ankles, lower back, and lower stomach.

I have been using Young Living Essential Oils for a little over a year now. Since then, my health has improved somewhat. I decided to stop using birth control pills on Labor Day of 2003, due to being sick from them most of the time and wanting to try something else. I started putting EndoFlex on the bottom of my feet on the endocrine reflex areas. I also continued receiving colonics twice a month and eating cultured vegetables. Between the EndoFlex, colonics, and cultured vegetables, my periods have become more regular and less painful. A friend of mine who's also using EndoFlex on her feet has said that her hot flashes have stopped since she's been using EndoFlex.

-Submitted by Christie Krajewski
Batesville, Arkansas (July 2004)

Personal Care—Dragon Time Massage Oil (uncomfortable days and irregularity). PD 80/20, Prenolone/Prenolone+, or Progessence/Progessence Plus may help to regulate the hormones which should alleviate many of the problems associated with menstruation. *See Hormonal Imbalance.*

Supplements—One week after the cycle, take Master Formula Hers four times a day and 6 MultiGreens a day. Also EndoGize, FemiGen (for PMS).

–IRREGULAR

Oils—$^{T}_{F}$Sage, $^{T}_{F}$peppermint, $^{T}_{F}$rosemary, ^{T}clary sage, ^{T}fennel, ^{T}lavender, ^{T}melissa, ^{T}Roman chamomile, ^{T}rose.

–MENORRHAGIA

Oils—^{T}Cypress, ^{T}geranium, ^{T}Roman chamomile, ^{T}rose.

–SCANTY

Oils—^{T}Lavender, ^{T}peppermint, ^{T}jasmine, ^{T}melissa. *See also oils listed under Amenorrhea.*

—OVARIES *See Ovaries.*

—PMS (Premenstrual Syndrome) *See also Hormonal Imbalance.*

›› *Premenstrual syndrome (PMS) is a group of symptoms such as irritability, anxiety, moodiness, bloating, breast tenderness, headaches, and cramping that occur in the days or hours before menstruation begins and then disappear once menstruation begins. PMS is thought to be caused by the fluctuation in hormones during this time, or by the way progesterone is broken down by the body. Caffeine intake from beverages or chocolate is also thought to enhance PMS symptoms.*

Oils—$^{TA}_{F}$Clary sage, $^{TA}_{F}$tarragon, ^{TA}fennel[195], ^{TA}angelica, ^{TA}anise, ^{TA}bergamot, ^{TA}Exodus II, ^{TA}geranium, ^{TA}grapefruit, ^{TA}jasmine, ^{A}lavender, ^{TA}nutmeg, ^{TA}Peace & Calming, ^{TA}Roman chamomile.

Personal Care—Dragon Time Massage Oil, Progessence/Progessence Plus, Prenolone/Prenolone+.

Supplements—FemiGen, Master Formula Hers, MultiGreens, Omega Blue, OmegaGize³, Wolfberry Crisp Bars.

–Apathetic-Tired-Listless

Oils—^{TA}Geranium, ^{TA}grapefruit, ^{TA}bergamot, ^{TA}fennel, ^{TA}Roman chamomile.

Personal Care—Dragon Time Bath & Shower Gel.

Blend #5—10 drops Dragon Time and 4 drops basil. Rub blend on ankles, lower back, and lower stomach. Use before and during cycle.

–IRRITABLE

Oils—^{TA}Bergamot, ^{TA}clary sage, ^{TA}nutmeg, ^{TA}Roman chamomile.

Blend #5—Before and during cycle, combine 10 drops Dragon Time with 4 drops basil, and rub on ankles, lower back and lower stomach.

Supplements—NingXia Red, Omega Blue, OmegaGize³, PD 80/20, Prenolone/Prenolone+, Progessence/Progessence Plus, Wolfberry Crisp Bars. One week after the cycle, take Master Formula Hers four times a day and 6 MultiGreens a day. Also FemiGen (for PMS)—take 2 FemiGen three times a day before period, and start again two days after cycle.

–VIOLENT AGGRESSIVE

Oils—^{TA}Bergamot, ^{TA}geranium, ^{TA}nutmeg.

Supplements—Omega Blue, OmegaGize³.

–WEEPING-DEPRESSION

Oils—[TA]Bergamot, [TA]clary sage, [TA]geranium, [TA]nutmeg.

Supplements—Omega Blue, OmegaGize[3].

—Postpartum Depression *See Pregnancy/Motherhood: Postpartum Depression*

—Reproductive System

Supplements—[TA]FemiGen (may help build and balance the reproductive system and help maintain better hormonal balance for developmental years all the way through menopause).

T—Dilute as necessary, and apply to the abdomen, lower back, groin, shoulders, or Vita Flex points on the feet. Dilute with V-6 Oil for massage oil, and massage on abdomen, lower back, and shoulders. Apply as a warm compress to the abdomen. Add 1–2 drops to 2 tsp. olive oil, insert into vagina, and retain overnight with a tampon.

A—Diffuse into the air. Inhale directly or applied to hands.

Fertility: *See also Female Specific Conditions, Male Specific Conditions.*

Oils—[T]Clary sage, [T]Mister, [I]SclarEssence (taken as a dietary supplement to help raise estradiol and testosterone levels), [T]bergamot, [T]Dragon Time, [T]fennel, [T]geranium, [T]melissa, [T]sage, [T]Sensation, [T]yarrow.

T—Apply on reproductive Vita Flex areas on feet, particularly around front of ankle, in line with ankle bone, on each side of ankle under ankle bone, and up along the Achilles tendon. Women: on lower back and on lower abdomen near pubic bone. Can also dilute with V-6 Oil and use as vaginal retention implant. Men: on lower abdomen near pubic bone, on area between scrotum and rectum, and as a rectal implant (diluted with V-6 Oil).

I—Add 2–4 drops to an empty capsule with 2–4 drops V-6 Oil, and swallow.

Personal Care—Prenolone/Prenolone+, Progessence/Progessence Plus, Protec (as rectal or vaginal implant).

Supplements—AlkaLime, Balance Complete (*refer to the 5-Day Nutritive Cleanse program listed under Balance Complete in the Supplements section of the Reference Guide for Essential Oils. This program also uses Digest + Cleanse and NingXia Red to help enhance detoxification while maintaining energy levels*), Digest + Cleanse, Ultra Young+, MultiGreens. FemiGen (women), Prostate Health (men), True Source (whole food multi-nutrient).

***Comments—An accumulation of petrochemicals in the body can cause sterility in both men and women. Do the **MASTER CLEANSER** (See Cleansing) for 10 to 20 days consecutively. After coming off the cleanse, focus on alkaline-ash foods. When the body is acidic, it can be hard to conceive.

Fever:

▸▸ *Fever is an increase of the body's core temperature, typically in response to an infection or injury. A fever is the body's natural response to help enhance the immune system's ability to fight the infection.*

Oils—[ITA][F]Peppermint (reduces), [I][F]lemon or lime (reduces), [TA][F]eucalyptus, [I]clove, [TA]basil, [TA]bergamot, [TA]fennel (breaks up), [TA]fir, [TA]ginger, [T]ImmuPower (rub on spine), [TA]lavender, [TA]ledum, [TA]melaleuca, [TA]rosemary cineol, [TA]sage lavender, [TA]spearmint (not on babies).

Personal Care—Cinnamint Lip Balm.

Supplements—AlkaLime, MineralEssence, Super C / Super C Chewable.

—To Cool the System

Oils—[IA]Clove, [ITA]peppermint, [TA]bergamot, [TA]*Eucalyptus radiata*.

—To Induce Sweating

My daughter, Haley, at age 18 was ill one Sunday, and later in the evening she was feeling quite worse. When we checked, she had a fever of 105 degrees. I filled a gel capsule with 10 drops of clove oil and had her take it with some water. In ½ an hour I checked her temperature again, and it was down to 102. I gave her 5 more drops in another capsule, and in another ½ hour her fever was totally gone!

-Submitted by Sally Donahue
Wilsonville, Oregon (July 2004)

Oils—[ITA]Peppermint, [TA]lavender, [T]Roman chamomile, [T]rosemary, [T]basil, [T]cypress, [T]fennel, [T]melaleuca.

I—Add 1 or 2 drops to 8 oz. rice milk or water, and sip slowly.

T—Dilute as necessary, and apply to bottoms of feet or to spine.

A—Diffuse into the air.

Fiber:

There are two kinds of fiber: soluble fiber is important for absorbing toxins and removing them from the body; insoluble fiber is important for scrubbing the intestines to remove any buildup of waste material. Viscosity is the balance between soluble and insoluble fiber. A blend of different fibers provides for maximum viscosity, which equals optimal absorption and cleansing capabilities. Fiber also helps to slow and balance the absorption of sugars and fats, thereby balancing blood sugar levels. Research has shown that balancing blood sugar levels can extend life expectancy by up to 50%.

Supplements—Balance Complete (contains a blend of 5 different fibers for maximum viscosity), Cleansing Trio (ComforTone, Essentialzyme, and ICP).

Fibrocysts: *See Hormonal Imbalance.*

Fibroids: *See also Hormonal Imbalance.*

›› *Fibroids are noncancerous growths of muscle and connective tissue in the uterus. Fibroids can be painful and may affect fertility and pregnancy*

Oils—[T]Frankincense, [T]helichrysum, [T]cistus, [T]EndoFlex, [T]Idaho tansy, [T]lavender, [T]oregano, [T]pine, [T]Valor.

T—Put 3 drops of either oil in douche. Also apply to Vita Flex points of feet.

Personal Care—Cel-Lite Magic, Protec.

Supplements—AlkaLime, EndoGize, Essentialzyme, Essentialzymes-4, Power Meal, Thyromin, Ultra Young+, MultiGreens.

Fibromyalgia: *See also Acidosis, Hormonal Imbalance.*

›› *Fibromyalgia is long-term localized or generalized aches, pain, or tenderness in the muscles, ligaments, or other soft tissue that can interfere with normal movement, sleep, or other activities. There is no known cause of fibromyalgia, and many different factors may contribute to the development of this condition. Some have suggested eliminating refined sugar or lowering the body's pH level. Others have recommended stretching, reducing stress, exercises, massage, or better sleep.*

Recipe #1—May need to detoxify the liver. ImmuPower; massage with PanAway, adding wintergreen & spruce for an additional cortisone response. It may be helpful to use some anti-inflammatory oils like helichrysum, lavender, myrrh, patchouli, rosemary, rosewood, spruce, thyme, or wintergreen.

Blend #1—Combine 2 drops cinnamon bark, 10 drops eucalyptus, 10 drops ginger, 6 drops nutmeg, 10 drops peppermint, and 3 drops rosemary with 2 Tbs. V-6 Oil, and massage chest and back once a day.

Personal Care—Ortho Ease or Ortho Sport Massage Oils (for full body); do Raindrop Technique.

Supplements—NingXia Red, Sulfurzyme, Allerzyme (aids the digestion of sugars, starches, fats, and proteins), AlkaLime (combat yeast and fungus overgrowth and preserve the body's proper pH balance), Balance Complete (high in fiber to absorb toxins and clean the intestinal tract), Digest + Cleanse, JuvaTone, Life 5 (probiotic), Mineral Essence, MultiGreens, PD 80/20, Power Meal, Super

C / Super C Chewable, Super Cal (no more than 1 per day, because of the poor ability to utilize minerals), Thyromin, True Source (whole food multi-nutrient).

***Comments—Dr. Bernard Jensen suggested that people with fibromyalgia should eliminate all refined sugars from their diet. *Refer to the chapter entitled "How to Use—The Personal Usage Reference" in the Essential Oils Desk Reference under "Fibromyalgia" for an excellent supplement regimen.*

Fibrositis: *See Fibromyalgia.*

Finger:

—Mashed

Recipe #1—Geranium (for the bruising), helichrysum (to stop the bleeding), lavender (to help everything), lemongrass (for tissue repair), and PanAway (for the pain). Layer oils on location.

Flatulence: *See Digestive System: Gas/Flatulence.*

Flu: *See Influenza.*

Fluids: *See Edema or Diuretic.*

Focus:

Oils—ABrain Power (during strenuous mental activity), Alavender[196], AGathering (for greater focus), ABelieve, AClarity, AHighest Potential, ASurrender (balancing; clears the mind).

A—Diffuse into the air. Inhale directly or applied to hands.

Supplements—Omega Blue, OmegaGize[3], Sulfurzyme.

Food: *See pH Balance.*

Oils—Use basil for soups and stuffing. Use cinnamon bark, clove, orange, tangerine, and thyme for flavorings.

The body secretes pepsin, protease, and hydrochloric acid in the morning for the digestion of protein. If you eat fruit in the morning, you have almost instant putrefaction (fermentation). Subacid fruits (like strawberries) are the only fruits that can be eaten with protein.

*** COMMENTS—According to the Essential Oils Desk Reference, "They are so concentrated that only 12 drops of an essential oil is equivalent to a full 1–2 oz. bottle of dried herbs. For a recipe that serves 6–10 people, add 1–2 drops of an oil, and stir in after cooking and just before serving so that the oil does not evaporate" (EDR-June 2002; Ch. 4; Other Uses; Cooking). Refer to that same section in the Essential Oils Desk Reference for more ideas on cooking with essential oils.

—Breakfasts

Recipe #1—Proteins (meat, fish, eggs), mixed grains, sunflower seeds, nuts, Power Meal, and Pure Protein Complete. Fruit in the morning will cause candida overgrowth, hypoglycemia, and dysfunction of the thyroid gland. Take Essentialzymes-4 to help with the digestion, especially when animal protein has been eaten. Also, 8 oz. of carrot juice per day with apple and lemon helps detoxify the body and provides necessary enzymes.

—Lunch

Recipe #2—Eat salads and complex carbohydrates like rice, beans, soup, steamed vegetables, bread (Jack Sprout Bread is good) that is toasted (reduces gluten content), baked potatoes, yams, and squash.

—AFTER 3:00 PM

Recipe #3—Refrain from eating animal proteins. Power Meal is predigested proteins and can be eaten with fruit. Foods that are easier on the digestive system at night are fruit, soups, lightly steamed vegetables, and salads.

—ASSIMILATION OF

Supplements—Enzyme products: Allerzyme (aids the digestion of sugars, starches, fats, and proteins), Detoxzyme (helps maintain and support a healthy intestinal environment), Digest + Cleanse, Essentialzyme/Essentialzymes-4 (multiple enzyme products).

Buttered Basil Garlic Melt

1 loaf cheese bread or any artisan bread, cut into 1 inch slices
1/2 stick butter
1/2 teaspoon garlic powder
4 drops basil essential oil
Sliced mozzarella cheese

Melt butter; then add garlic powder, and stir well. Add basil oil; mix well. With a large unused paint brush, brush on butter mixture until saturated. Cover sliced bread with slices of cheese, and bake at 350° until golden brown.
Yummmmmie! Even my Baby loved it.

-Submitted by Jill Burk
Saginaw, Michigan (July 2004)

—FIBER

Supplements—Balance Complete, ICP (fiber beverage).

—OIL

Supplements—V-6 Oil (six different vegetable oils) is excellent for cooking and for making salad dressings.

—SUGAR SUBSTITUTE

Supplements—Stevia, Yacon Syrup.

Food Poisoning:

›› *Food poisoning refers to the effects on the digestive tract of pathogenic organisms—or the toxins they produce—that are ingested into the body in food. Symptoms of food poisoning can include stomach pain, cramps, diarrhea, nausea, and vomiting.*

Oils—[I]Thieves, [I]tarragon, [I]Exodus II, [I]patchouli, [I]rosemary cineol.

I—Place 2–5 drops in an empty capsule with 2–5 drops V-6 Oil, and swallow.

Recipe #1—Flavor a cup of water with 6 drops Di-Gize, swish around in mouth, and swallow.

Supplements—Detoxzyme, Essentialzyme, Essentialzymes-4,.

Foot: *See Feet.*

Forehead:

Oils—[T]Jasmine.

T—Apply 1 drop to forehead.

Forgetfulness: *See Memory.*

Forgive (and Forget):

Oils—[TA]Acceptance, [TA]Forgiveness, [TA]3 Wise Men, [TA]Transformation, [TA]Valor, [TA]White Angelica.

A—Diffuse into the air. Inhale directly or applied to tissue or a cotton wick.

T—Apply to auricular emotion points. Dilute with V-6 Oil to create a massage oil, and massage onto the skin.

***Comments—It has been said that "the conscious thought to forgive quells the fear response in the amygdala."

Formaldehyde:

Oils—**T**Purification (removes).

T—Dilute as necessary, and apply to feet. Massage into the skin.

Fortifying:

Oils—**TA**Cypress.

T—Dilute with V-6 Oil to create massage oil, and massage into the skin.

A—Diffuse into the air. Inhale directly or applied to hands.

Freckles:

Oils—**T**Idaho tansy.

T—Mix 2–3 drops with lotion, and spread over face. Can be used two or three times per week.

Free Radicals: *See also Antioxidant.*

Free radicals are highly reactive molecules with at least one unpaired electron. The unpaired electron can cause harm to the body as it tries to take electrons from another molecule to make itself more stable, subsequently causing disease formation.

—Eliminate

Oils—**I**Longevity

I—Dilute 1 drop in 4 oz. soy or rice milk; drink. Place 2–5 drops in an empty capsule with 2–5 drops V-6 Oil; swallow.

Supplements—Longevity Capsules and NingXia Red help eliminate and prevent the buildup of free radicals.

Frigidity: *See also Libido, Sex Stimulant.*

Oils—**TA** $_F$Clary sage, **TA** $_F$ylang ylang (helps balance male/female energies), **TA**Lady Sclareol, **TA**Chivalry, **TA**jasmine, **TA**nutmeg (overcome frigidity and impotence), **TA**rose.

T—Dilute with V-6 Oil to create massage oil, and massage into the skin.

A—Diffuse into the air. Wear as perfume or cologne. Inhale directly or applied to the hands.

Supplements—Prenolone/Prenolone+, Progessence/Progessence Plus.

Frustration:

Oils—**TA**Acceptance, **TA**clary sage, **TA**frankincense, **TA**Gathering, **TA**ginger, **TA**Hope, **TA**Humility, **TA**juniper, **TA**lavender, **TA**lemon, **TA**orange, **TA**peppermint, **TA**Present Time, **TA**Roman chamomile, **TA**spruce, **TA**3 Wise Men, **TA**thyme, **TA**Valor, **TA**ylang ylang.

A—Diffuse into the air. Inhale directly or applied to tissue or a cotton wick.

T—Apply to auricular emotion points. Dilute with V-6 Oil to create a massage oil, and massage onto the skin.

See pages 25–27 for more detailed application instructions.

Fungus: *See Antifungal: Fungus.*

Gallbladder:

»» *The gallbladder is a small sac that stores extra bile from the liver until it is needed to help with digestion in the small intestine. The gallbladder is located just below the liver.*

Oils—T F Geranium, T F German chamomile, TI JuvaFlex (stimulates), TI Juva Cleanse, T Forgiveness, T **GLF**, T juniper, T lavender, T Release, T rosemary (supports), T Surrender (over liver & pancreas).

Recipe #1—Take 2 capsules JuvaFlex - AM, 2 Juva Cleanse - PM.

Supplements—Essentialzyme, Essentialzymes-4, Sulfurzyme (aids bile secretion and magnifies effects of vitamins).

—Infection In

Oils—T F Helichrysum.

—Stones

»» *Gallstones are formed by cholesterol that has crystallized from the bile stored in the gallbladder. These stones can sometimes block the duct that comes from the gallbladder or the small opening from the common hepatic duct that allows bile to flow into the small intestine. This can result in pain and can lead to more serious complications, such as infections or jaundice.*

Oils—T F Nutmeg, T geranium, T grapefruit, T juniper, T Juva Cleanse, T lime, T rosemary, T wintergreen.

T—Dilute as necessary, and apply over gallbladder area (can use a hot compress) and on Vita Flex points on feet.

I—Place 2–5 drops in empty capsule, and swallow.

Gangrene:

»» *Gangrene is the localized decay of body tissue caused by a loss of blood to that area. Gas gangrene is caused by bacteria invading a deep wound that has lessened the blood supply or cut it off entirely. The bacteria create gases and pus in the infected area, causing severe pain and accelerating decay of the tissue.*

Oils—T Lavender (used by Dr. Gattefossé to recover from gas gangrene), T Thieves, T ImmuPower, T cistus, T elemi, T Exodus II, T Melrose, T mountain savory, T ravensara, T thyme.

Supplements—ImmuPro, Inner Defense, Super C / Super C Chewable.

Gas: *See Digestive System: Gas/Flatulence.*

Gastritis: *See Digestive System: Gastritis.*

General Tonic:

Oils—TA F Spruce, TA grapefruit, TA lemon, TA mountain savory.

T—Dilute with V-6 Oil to create massage oil, and massage onto the skin. Dilute as necessary, and apply to bottoms of feet.

A—Diffuse into the air.

Genitals:

Oils—T F Clary sage.

T—Apply 1–2 drops on location or on Vita Flex points on the feet.

Gentleness:

Oils—[A]Rosewood.

A—Diffuse into the air. Inhale directly or applied to tissue or a cotton wick.

Germs: *See also Antibacterial, Antifungal, Antiviral.*

—Airborne

Oils—[A]Fir.

—Germicidal

Oils—[AT]$_F$Lemon, [A]RC.

A—Diffuse into the air.

T—Dilute as necessary, and apply on location. Add 2–5 drops to a small bowl of water, and use water on a cloth to wipe intended areas.

Gingivitis: *See Oral Conditions: Gingivitis.*

Glandular System: *See also Endocrine System.*

Oils—[T]$_F$Sage, [T]Egyptian Gold, [T]blue cypress (may help stimulate the amygdala, pineal gland, pituitary gland, and hypothalamus), [T]spearmint, [T]spruce.

T—Dilute as necessary, and apply on location or on the Vita Flex points on the feet.

Supplements— Prostate Health (male) or FemiGen (female) for glandular nutrients.

Glaucoma: *See Eyes: Glaucoma.*

Goiter: *See also Endocrine System, Lymphatic System, Thyroid: Hyperthyroidism.*

▸▸ *Goiter is a condition where the thyroid gland grows larger than is normal, often causing the neck and larynx to enlarge as well. This enlargement can cause a cough and make it difficult to breathe and to swallow. Goiter is often caused by an iodine deficiency in the body, but it can have other causes as well.*

Recipe #1—Cleanse the lymphatic system. Balance the endocrine system with EndoFlex and EndoGize.

Gout:

▸▸ *Gout is the painful inflammation of a joint caused by a buildup of uric acid crystals deposited in the joint. Uric acid is formed during the natural breakdown of dead tissues in the body. An excess of uric acid in the bloodstream can lead to the formation of crystals in the joints or kidneys (kidney stones). Some good ways to prevent the formation of uric acid crystals include maintaining a healthy body weight (which leaves less body tissue to be broken down), exercising, and drinking plenty of water.*

Oils—[T]$_F$Fennel, [IT]$_F$lemon, [T]PanAway, [T]wintergreen, [T]pine, [T]basil, [T]calamus, [T]geranium, [T]hyssop, [T]Juva Cleanse, [T]JuvaFlex, [T]nutmeg, [T]onycha (benzoin), [T]thyme, [T]yarrow.

T—Dilute as necessary, and apply on location. Dilute with V-6 Oil to create a massage oil, and massage on location.

I—Add 1–2 drops to 8 oz. water, and drink.

Recipe #1—Cleanse with the **Master Cleanser** program(*See Cleansing*), and drink lots of fluids (water, juices, etc.).

Personal Care—Ortho Ease and Ortho Sport Massage Oils.

Supplements—Balance Complete, Cleansing Trio (ComforTone, Essentialzyme, and ICP), Digest + Cleanse, JuvaTone, Mineral Essence, MultiGreens, Sulfurzyme, Super C / Super C Chewable, Super Cal, Thyromin.

***Comments—Refer to the chapter entitled "How to Use—The Personal Usage Reference" in the Essential Oils Desk Reference under "Gout" for some excellent blend recipes and supplement recommendations.

Grave's Disease: *See also Thyroid: Hyperthyroidism.*

▸▸ *Graves' disease is an autoimmune disease caused by an abnormally-shaped protein stimulating the thyroid to make and secrete more hormones. This can cause an enlargement of the thyroid, bulging eyes, increased heart rate, high blood pressure, and anxiety.*

Oils—TALemongrass, TAblue tansy, TAEndoFlex, TAmyrrh, TAspruce.

T—Dilute as recommended, and apply on thyroid area or on reflex points on the feet.

A—Diffuse into the air.

Supplements—EndoGize, ImmuPro, Inner Defense, Mineral Essence, MultiGreens, Sulfurzyme (helps mitigate the effects of autoimmune diseases), Thyromin, True Source (whole food multi-nutrient).

Grief/Sorrow:

Oils—ATBergamot (turns grief into joy), ATclary sage, ATeucalyptus, ATForgiveness, TAGentle Baby (massage whole body), ATHope, TAJoy (over the heart), ATjuniper, ATlavender, ATPresent Time, ATRelease, ATRoman chamomile, TASacred Mountain (back of the neck), T3 Wise Men (rub on crown), ATTransformation, ATValor (on the feet), TAWhite Angelica (on the forehead or shoulders).

A—Diffuse into the air. Inhale directly or applied to tissue or a cotton wick.

T—Apply to auricular emotion points. Dilute with V-6 Oil to create a massage oil, and massage onto the skin.

Grounding:

Oils—ATGrounding, ATfir, ATHope, ATJoy, ATpatchouli, ATspruce, AT3 Wise Men, ATtsuga.

—Feeling Of

Oils—ACypress.

A—Diffuse into the air. Inhale directly or applied to tissue or a cotton wick.

T—Apply to auricular emotion points or on sacral chakra. Dilute with V-6 Oil to create a massage oil, and massage onto the skin.

Guilt:

Oils—ATAcceptance, ATAwaken, ATcypress, ATForgiveness, ATfrankincense, ATGathering, ATgeranium, ATHarmony, ATInner Child, ATInspiration, ATjuniper, ATlemon, ATmarjoram, ATPeace & Calming, ATPresent Time, ATRelease, ATRoman chamomile, ATrose, ATsandalwood, ATspruce, ATthyme, ATValor, ATWhite Angelica.

A—Diffuse into the air. Inhale directly or applied to tissue or a cotton wick.

T—Apply to auricular emotion points. Dilute with V-6 Oil to create a massage oil, and massage onto the skin.

Gulf War Syndrome:

Oils—ATExodus II.

A—Diffuse into the air.

T—Dilute with V-6 Oil to create a massage oil, and massage onto the skin. Apply to Vita Flex points on the feet.

Gum Disease: *See Oral Conditions: Gum Disease.*

Gums: *See also Oral Conditions: Gingivitis, Gum Disease.*

Oils—TMyrrh (infection), Tlavender, TMelrose (fights infection), TRoman chamomile, Tsage lavender (infection).

T—Dilute as necessary, and apply 1–2 drops on location with a cotton ball or a cotton swab. Mix 1–2 drops with 4 oz. water, and use as a mouth-rinse.

Personal Care—Thieves Dentarome/Dentarome Plus Toothpaste, Thieves Fresh Essence Plus Mouthwash, KidScents Toothpaste (for children).

—Surgery on Gums

***Comments—For one individual, helichrysum was applied with a Q-tip every 15 minutes to kill the pain. No other pain killer was used.

Habits: *See also Addictions.*

Oils—ATAcceptance, ATlavender, ATTransformation.

A—Diffuse into the air. Inhale directly or applied to tissue or a cotton wick.

T—Dilute with V-6 Oil to create a massage oil, and massage onto the skin.

***Comments—To break bad habits, you need to change the DNA and RNA. Sandalwood and frankincense help with this.

Hair: *Refer to the Personal Care Products section of this book for a list of ingredients and more details on chemical-free shampoos and conditioners.*

***Comments—Refer to the chapter entitled "How to Use—The Personal Usage Reference" in the *Essential Oils Desk Reference* under "Hair and Scalp Problems" for some excellent blend recipes.

—Baldness *See also Loss below*

Recipe #1—Apply 2–3 drops each of cedarwood, lavender, rosemary, and sage oil on location and on bottoms of feet before bedtime and/or in the morning after washing with Lavender Volume products shown below.

Personal Care—Lavender Volume Shampoo and Lavender Volume Conditioner together.

Supplements—Sulfurzyme may help if the hair is falling due to a sulfur deficiency.

—Beard

Oils—TLemon, Trosemary, Tcypress, Tlavender, Tthyme.

—Body

Oils—TCedarwood (gives the hair shaft more body, more strength, and more life), Ttamanu.

—Children

Personal Care—Lavender Volume Shampoo with Lavender Volume Conditioner or KidScents Shampoo.

—Color

Recipe #1—(keep light) Apply 1 drop chamomile, 1 drop lemon, and 1 quart of water. Rinse hair.

—Damaged (perms, color-treated, bleached)

Oils—TTamanu.

Personal Care— KidScents Shampoo.

—Dandruff *See also Antifungal*

Dandruff is a scalp condition characterized by the excessive shedding of dead skin cells. A small amount of flaking on the scalp is normal as old skin cells die off and fall away; but dandruff results when the amount of dead skin cells becomes excessive and visible.

Oils—TFRosemary, TFlavender, Twintergreen, Tmelaleuca, Tbasil, Tcedarwood, Tcypress, Tpatchouli, Tsage, Tsage lavender, Tthyme, Tvalerian.

Personal Care—KidScents Shampoo, Lavender Volume Shampoo, Lavender Volume Conditioner.

—Dry

Oils—TGeranium, Tsandalwood, Tlavender, Trosemary, Twintergreen.

—Estrogen Balance

Estrogen is a steroid hormone that causes the development of female characteristics such as breasts and larger hips, that helps with calcium uptake and balance, and that plays many other important roles. Estrogen also helps hair to grow faster and to stay on the head longer. If estrogen levels fall, hair loss can quickly result.

Recipe #2—Clary sage in Lavender Volume Shampoo and Lavender Volume Conditioner helps promote estrogen balance in the membrane tissue around the hair follicle. This serves to balance testosterone levels and to prevent the thickening of the tissue around the follicle that results in hair loss.

Blend #1—1 drop lavender and 6 drops patchouli in 2–5 oz. Lavender Volume Shampoo.

Blend #2—Mix together 2 drops cinnamon bark, 4 drops cypress, 4 drops geranium, 2 drops juniper, 5 drops lavender, and 3 drops rosemary. Then put one drop of the blend into ¼ tsp of water, and rub on bald area and on entire scalp. A gentle night treatment.

Personal Care—Lavender Volume Shampoo and Lavender Volume Conditioner (with clary sage—*see Recipe #2 above*).

Supplements—ComforTone, Essentialzyme, Essentialzymes-4, MultiGreens, Super B (stress), Thyromin.

—Fragile Hair

Oils—TClary sage, Tlavender, Tthyme, TRoman chamomile, Tsandalwood, Twintergreen.

Personal Care—KidScents Shampoo, Lavender Volume Shampoo, and Lavender Volume Conditioner.

—Greasy

Oils—TPetitgrain.

—Growth (stimulate)

Oils—TThyme[197], Trosemary[197], Tlavender[197], Tcedarwood[197], Tylang ylang (promotes), Tbasil, Twestern red cedar, Tcypress, Tgeranium, Tginger, Tgrapefruit, Thyssop, Tlemon, Tsage.

Personal Care—Lavender Volume Shampoo and Lavender Volume Conditioner.

Supplements—Sulfurzyme. A deficiency in sulfur can result in hair loss or poor hair growth.

—Itching

Oils—[T][F]Peppermint (skin), [T]lavender.

—Loss *See also* Baldness *above*

Oils—[T][F]Rosemary[197], [T][F]lavender[197], [T][F]cedarwood[197], [T]thyme[197], [T][F]ylang ylang, [T]clary sage, [T]cypress, [T]laurel (after infection), [T]lemon, [T]Roman chamomile, [T]sage, [T]sage lavender, [T]wintergreen.

–Alopecia Areata (inflammatory hair loss disease)

Oils—[T]Thyme[197], [T]rosemary[197], [T]lavender[197], [T]cedarwood[197].

> *In males, hair loss can often be blamed on heredity, hormones (high levels of testosterone), and aging. Other reasons for hair loss may include poor circulation, hypertension, acute illness, surgery, radiation, scarlet fever, syphilis, stress, sudden weight loss, iron deficiency, diabetes, hypothyroidism, drugs, poor diet, and vitamin deficiency.*
>
> *Avoid hair products that are not natural on the hair. Avoid chlorinated swimming pools or polluted seas. Chemical products may also leave a residue buildup which can cause hair loss. Correcting a hormonal imbalance or hypertension (dilate blood vessels and stimulate cell division) may help.*

T—Add any or all of these oils to jojoba and grapeseed carrier oils, and massage into scalp daily.

Personal Care—Lavender Volume Shampoo and Lavender Volume Conditioner.

Supplements—Sulfurzyme, Super B, Thyromin.

***Comments—*Refer to the chapter entitled "How to Use—The Personal Usage Reference" in the Essential Oils Desk Reference under "Hair Loss" for some excellent blend recipes.*

—Silky and Shiny

Oils—[T]Tamanu.

Personal Care—KidScents Shampoo.

—Split Ends

Personal Care—KidScents Shampoo.

T—Apply 1–2 drops of oil to hands, and massage into hair and scalp before bath or shower; then shampoo and rinse hair as normal. Add 1–2 drops of oil to 2 Tbs. of an unscented shampoo or shower gel, and use to shampoo hair.

Halitosis: *See Oral Conditions: Halitosis.*

Hands: *See also Skin.*

Oils—[T]Geranium, [T]lemon, [T]sandalwood, [T]eucalyptus, [T]lavender, [T]patchouli, [T]rosemary.

—Dry

Oils—[T]Geranium, [T]patchouli, [T]sandalwood.

Personal Care—Genesis Hand & Body Lotion, Rose Ointment.

—Neglected

Oils—[T]Geranium, [T]lemon, [T]patchouli.

—Tingling In

Recipe #1—Lemongrass in Genesis Hand & Body Lotion.

T—Dilute as necessary, and apply 1–2 drops to hands. Dilute 1–2 drops in 1 Tbs. almond or olive oil, and use as massage oil to massage into hands.

Hangovers:

Oils—TALemon, TAgrapefruit, TAfennel, TAlavender, TArose, TArosemary, TAsandalwood.

T—Add 3–4 drops to warm bathwater, and bathe. Dilute as recommended, and apply 1–2 drops to back of neck or over liver. Dilute with V-6 Oil to create massage oil, and massage onto back and neck.

A—Inhale directly or applied to hands, tissue, or a cotton wick. Drop 1–2 drops in a bowl of hot water, and inhale vapors. Diffuse into the air.

Supplements—Super C / Super C Chewable.

Happiness:

Oils—ATChristmas Spirit, ATJoy.

A—Diffuse into the air. Inhale directly or applied to tissue or a cotton wick.

T—Apply to auricular emotion points. Dilute with V-6 Oil to create a massage oil, and massage onto the skin.

Harmony in Body Systems:

Oils—ATAcceptance, Aclove, ATgeranium (harmonizing), ATHarmony, ATInspiration, ATLady Sclareol (women), ATRoman chamomile.

Personal Care—Sensation Hand & Body Lotion. Sensation Massage Oil creates an exotic arousal and increases sexual desire. The fragrance creates a peaceful and harmonious feeling that is helpful in easing relationship stress. Relaxation Massage Oil also creates a peaceful and harmonious feeling.

—Of Mind and Body

Oils—ATRelease.

A—Diffuse into the air. Inhale directly or applied to tissue or a cotton wick.

T—Apply to auricular emotion points or to chakras. Dilute with V-6 Oil to create a massage oil, and massage onto the skin.

Harshness:

Oils—ATJasmine.

A—Diffuse into the air. Inhale directly or applied to tissue or a cotton wick.

T—Apply to auricular emotion points. Dilute with V-6 Oil to create a massage oil, and massage onto the skin.

Hashimoto's Disease: *See also Thyroid: HYPERTHYROIDISM.*

»*Hashimoto's disease is an autoimmune disorder where the immune system attacks the thyroid, causing it to swell up and become irritated. Possible symptoms include abnormal fatigue, weight gain, muscle pain and stiffness, a hoarse voice, prolonged menstrual bleeding, constipation, a feeling of tightness in the throat, sensitivity to cold, dry skin, and depression.*

Oils—TALemongrass, TAEndoFlex, TAmyrrh, TAblue tansy, TAspruce.

T—Dilute as necessary, and apply over thyroid area or to Vita Flex points on the feet.

A—Diffuse into the air. Inhale oil applied to hands.

Supplements—Thyromin, ImmuPro, EndoGize, Inner Defense, Mineral Essence, MultiGreens, Sulfurzyme (helps mitigate effects of autoimmune diseases), True Source (whole food multi-nutrient).

Hate:

Oils—ATAcceptance, ATForgiveness, ATRelease.

A—Diffuse into the air. Inhale directly or applied to tissue or a cotton wick.

T—Apply to auricular emotion points. Dilute with V-6 Oil to create a massage oil, and massage onto the skin.

Hay Fever: *See Allergies: Hay Fever.*

Headaches:

> *Clarity may cause headaches when chemicals or metals are in the brain. To break this blockage, put Aroma Life or helichrysum on arteries in the neck.*

Oils—TA FPeppermint[198], TAAroma Siez, TAM-Grain, TA Frosemary, TDeep Relief (roll-on), TAbasil, TAAroma Life (massage on arteries in neck), TAcalamus, TAcardamom, TAClarity, TAclove, TAcumin, TAeucalyptus, TADragon Time, TAfrankincense, TAGentle Baby, TAlavender, TAmarjoram, TAMister, TARelieve It, TAsage lavender.

*****Comments**—According to the Essential Oils Desk Reference, "For headaches, put one drop [Thieves] on tongue and push tongue against the roof of the mouth." (EDR-June 2002; Ch. 8; Thieves; Application) Also, refer to the chapter entitled "How to Use—The Personal Usage Reference" in the Essential Oils Desk Reference under "Headaches" for some excellent blend recipes and supplement recommendations for several different types of headaches.

—Cold/Flu Headaches

Oils—TACumin.

—Emotional Headaches

Oils—TAJoy.

—Menstrual Migraines *See also Hormonal Imbalance*

»*Many women find that their migraine headaches are closely related to their menstrual cycles, occurring when their estrogen and progesterone levels are at their lowest.*

Oils—TASage lavender.

—Children's Migraines

Blend #1—5 drops Roman chamomile, 10 drops grapefruit, 5 drops peppermint, 3 drops rosemary, and 4 oz. V-6 Oil for children under age seven, or 2 oz. V-6 Oil for children over age seven.

—Migraine Headaches

»*A migraine is a severe and painful type of headache. Symptoms of migraines include throbbing pain accompanied by nausea, vomiting, and heightened sensitivity to light. Migraines can be triggered by stress, anxiety, sleep or food deprivation, bright lights, loud noises, and hormonal changes.*

> *My husband has been bothered by migraine headaches for much of his adult life. Doctors have treated this condition with various medications—all with their own bag of side effects. So one day I decided to have him try peppermint oil, a drop on each temple. To his amazement, the headache was gone in seconds, and the cooling feel of the peppermint gave him a feeling of energy and revitalization.*
>
> ***-Submitted by Kathleen Mueller, Menomonee Falls, WI (July 2004)***

Oils—TAM-Grain, TA Fpeppermint[198], TA Fbasil, TA Feucalyptus, TAPanAway, TDeep Relief (roll-on), TAAroma Siez, TAcumin, TAGerman chamomile, TAgrapefruit, TAlavender, TAmarjoram, TAPeace & Calming, TARelieve It, TARelease, TARoman chamomile, TAspearmint, TAvalerian, TAwintergreen, TAylang ylang.

*****Comments**—May be caused by problems in the colon. Cleanse the colon using supplements.

H

Supplements—AlkaLime (if caused from acidosis), Balance Complete, Cleansing Trio (ComforTone, Essentialzyme, and ICP), Digest + Cleanse. Do not use ComforTone and JuvaTone together (*See ComforTone in the Supplements section of the Reference Guide for Essential Oils*).

Personal Care—Progessence/Progessence Plus.

—Stress (Tension) Headaches

▸▸ *Stress headaches (or tension headaches) are the most common type of headache. Tension headaches are characterized by dull, constant pressure or pain (usually on both sides of the head). Tension headaches can last from thirty minutes to several days and tend to come back when a person is under stress.*

Oils—TAM-Grain, TDeep Relief (roll-on), TARoman chamomile.

—Sugar Headaches

Oils—TAThieves (for low blood sugar headaches).

Supplements—Allerzyme (aids the digestion of sugars, starches, fats, and proteins), AlkaLime, Digest + Cleanse, Mineral Essence.

T—Dilute as recommended, and apply to temples, back of neck, and forehead

A—Diffuse into the air.

Healing:

Oils—TThe Gift, Tfrankincense, ATPanAway, ATmelaleuca, Aclary sage, TAcceptance, Tclove, Tcypress, Aeucalyptus, ATHumility, Alemon, ATsage.

T—Dilute with V-6 Oil to create a massage oil, and massage on location, on feet, or on back and neck.

A—Diffuse into the air.

Recipe #1—Combinations of sandalwood, frankincense, and lavender or frankincense and balsam fir (add myrrh if dealing with infection) have been used to help heal after surgery or major injuries. Also, combine the following oils (ratio in drops) in a 5 ml bottle: 20 valerian, 5 vetiver, 2 helichrysum, 1 clove, 1 peppermint. Applying several drops of this blend to the brain stem area (cervical vertebrae on back of neck) before surgery has been shown to maintain normal white blood cell counts during surgery, thereby speeding recovery by up to 30%. Any of these combinations may be used both internally and externally.

Health:

Oils—AAbundance, Alavender, Alemon.

A—Diffuse into the air.

Supplements—Balance Complete, Cleansing Trio (ComforTone, Essentialzyme, and ICP), Digest + Cleanse, Longevity Capsules, NingXia Red, Omega Blue/OmegaGize[3] (omega-3 essential fatty acids). The following is a recommended daily regimen to help maintain and promote optimal health: NingXia Red and Longevity Capsules (for optimal antioxidant support), Omega Blue (to support cell membranes and optimal brain function), and Balance Complete (to replace the least nutritional meal; for nutritional support, toxin removal, and healthy elimination).

—Promotes

Oils—AEucalyptus, Ajuniper.

A—Diffuse into the air. Inhale directly or applied to hands, tissue, or a cotton wick.

Hearing: *See Ears.*

Heart: *See Cardiovascular System: Heart.*

Heartburn: *See Digestive System: Heartburn.*

Hematoma: *See also Bruise.*

A hematoma is a collection of blood outside of the blood vessels. The most common form of a hematoma is a bruise. Hematomas can also form into hard, blood-filled sacs that look like welts and can move to different locations. These often dissolve on their own.

Oils—$^{T}_{F}$Helichrysum, ^{T}Aroma Life, ^{T}German chamomile.

T—Dilute as necessary, and apply on location.

Hemorrhaging: *See also Blood: Hemorrhaging, Female Specific Conditions: Hemorrhaging.*

Hemorrhaging is excessive or uncontrollable blood loss.

Oils—^{T}Helichrysum, ^{T}rose, ^{T}ylang ylang.

T—Massage around ankles, lower back, and stomach. Cayenne pepper may also help.

Hemorrhoids:

Hemorrhoids are swollen, twisted veins that occur in the rectum or anus. They are caused by increased pressure within the veins, often due to pregnancy, frequent lifting, or constipation.

Oils—$^{T}_{F}$Cypress, $^{T}_{F}$clary sage, $^{T}_{F}$patchouli, $^{T}_{F}$peppermint, $^{T}_{F}$sandalwood, ^{T}Aroma Life, ^{T}basil, ^{T}frankincense, ^{T}helichrysum, ^{T}juniper, ^{T}myrrh.

T—Dilute as necessary, and apply 1–2 drops on location. Mix 1–2 drops with 1 tsp. V-6 Oil, and apply using a rectal syringe.

Recipe #1—Put cypress and helichrysum inside and on location.

Hepatitis: *See Liver: Hepatitis.*

Hernia:

A hernia is the protrusion of a tissue or organ through tissue or muscle outside of the body cavity in which it is normally contained. There are several different types of hernias, and the symptoms vary with each type.

—Hiatal Hernia

A hiatal (hiatus) hernia is when a portion of the stomach protrudes through the diaphragm into the chest cavity above. This can cause pain, acid reflux, and heartburn. This type of hernia can be caused by a birth defect or may be brought on by heavy lifting, stress, or being overweight.

Oils—^{T}Basil, ^{T}peppermint, ^{T}cypress, ^{T}fennel, ^{T}geranium, ^{T}ginger, ^{T}hyssop, ^{T}lavender, ^{T}rosemary, ^{T}vitex.

Recipe #1—Drink water. Put the first two fingers of each hand just below the sternum (under center of rib cage), press in firmly, and brush down quickly and firmly. This can also be done after raising up on toes and while dropping down on heels to more firmly emphasize the effect.

Supplements—Essentialzyme/Essentialzymes-4 before meal, ComforTone, ICP (fiber beverage) after meal.

—Incisional Hernia

An incisional hernia is caused by a protrusion through scar tissue from an abdominal wound or incision that has not healed correctly.

Oils—[T]Basil, [T]helichrysum, [T]lemongrass, [T]geranium, [T]ginger, [T]lavender, [T]lemon, [T]melaleuca.

—Inguinal Hernia

»*An inguinal hernia is when the intestines protrude into the inguinal canal (a small opening that leads from the abdominal cavity into the groin area). This can sometimes be seen as a bulge in the groin area and is usually painless, but it may become painful if the blood supply to the herniated portion of the intestine is restricted (strangulated).*

Oils—[T]Lemongrass, [T]lavender.

T—Dilute as necessary, and apply oil(s) on location, lower back, and Vita Flex points on feet.

Herpes Simplex:

»*Herpes simplex type 1 and type 2 viruses are the two viruses that cause genital and oral herpes infections. These viruses cause painful outbreaks of blisters and sores to occur in the affected area when the virus is active in the skin or mucus membranes, followed by periods of latency when the virus resides in the nerve cells around the infected area.*

Jean Valnet, MD, a French physician, recommends a blend of lemon and geranium. Tisserand suggests eucalyptus and bergamot. Dr. Wabner says that a one-time application of either true rose oil or true melissa oil led to complete remission of herpes simplex lesions. Apply the oil directly on the lesions at the first sign of an outbreak. (Alternative Medicine—The Definitive Guide, p. 56).

Oils—[T]Peppermint[199], [T]melaleuca[200], [T]helichrysum[201], [T]clove[202], [T][F]lavender, [T][F]ravensara, [T]melissa[203], [T]manuka[204], [T]Australian Blue, [T]blue cypress, [T]bergamot (with *Eucalyptus radiata)*, [T]eucalyptus, [T]geranium, [T]lemon, [T]rose.

Hiccoughs/Hiccups:

Oils—[AT][F]Tarragon, [AT]sandalwood.

A—Diffuse into the air. Inhale directly or applied to hands, tissue, or a cotton wick.

T—Dilute as necessary, and apply to the diaphragm area or to Vita Flex points on the feet.

High Blood Pressure: *See Blood.*

Hives: *See Acidosis, pH Balance.*

»*Hives are itchy patches of inflamed spots on the skin surrounded by redness, typically caused by an allergic reaction or a viral infection.*

Oils—[T]Melaleuca[205], [T]peppermint[206], [T]lavender[207], [T]patchouli (may relieve itching), [T]Roman chamomile.

T—Dilute as necessary, and apply on location. Dilute with V-6 Oil to create a massage oil, and massage on location.

***Comments—Hives may be the result of too much acid in the blood or the result of a niacin flush (vitamin B3 taken on empty stomach).

Supplements—AlkaLime (combat yeast and fungus overgrowth and preserve the body's proper pH balance), MultiGreens, Super Cal (may prevent).

***Comments—One woman broke out in hives over her entire body. She used peppermint oil diluted with V-6 Oil for a body massage; and almost instantly her body cooled off, and the hives diminished until gone.

Hodgkin's Disease: *See Cancer: Lymphoma.*

Hope:

Oils—[AT]Hope (restores).

A—Diffuse into the air. Inhale directly or applied to tissue or a cotton wick.

T—Apply to auricular emotion points. Dilute with V-6 Oil to create a massage oil, and massage onto the skin.

Hormonal Imbalance:

Oils—[AT]SclarEssence, [AT]ylang ylang, [AT]dorado azul, [AT]anise.

A—Diffuse into the air. Inhale directly or applied to tissue or a cotton wick.

T—Dilute as necessary, and apply to Vita Flex points on the ankles, to the lower back, thyroid, liver, kidneys, gland areas, center of the body and along both sides of the spine, or to the clavicle area.

Personal Care—Prenolone/Prenolone+, Progessence/Progessence Plus.

Supplements—FemiGen, Mineral Essence, Sulfurzyme (lowered libido).

Hormonal System: *See also Endocrine System.*.

Oils—[TA]$_F$Spearmint (hormone-like), [TA]ylang ylang, [TA]clary sage, [TA]Acceptance, [TA]Aroma Life, [TA]Clarity, [TA]davana, [AT]dorado azul, [TA]Dragon Time, [TA]EndoFlex, [TA]fennel, [TA]goldenrod, [TA]Gentle Baby, [TA]Mister, [TA]M-Grain, [TA]myrrh, [TA]myrtle, [TA]peppermint, [TA]Relieve It, [TA]sage, [TA]sage lavender, [TA]sandalwood, [TA]SclarEssence.

Personal Care—Dragon Time Massage Oil, Prenolone/Prenolone+, Progessence/Progessence Plus.

Supplements—CortiStop (Women's), EndoGize, Estro Tincture, FemiGen (female), Prostate Health (male), Slique Tea, Thyromin, Ultra Young+.

A hormonal imbalance can cause many problems, including PMS, pre- and post-menopausal conditions, depression, endometriosis, fibromyalgia, fibrocysts, infertility, insomnia, irregular menstrual cycles, lowered libido, menstrual migraines, osteoporosis, ovarian cysts, unexplained first-trimester miscarriages, water retention, etc. Carbonated water can cause hormone deficiency. But most often it is a result of estrogen dominance; that is, not enough progesterone to balance out the amount of estrogen. Estrogen is manufactured in several places of the body, even after menopause, and is also found in much of our food, especially in animal and dairy products. Progesterone is secreted by the corpus luteum, by the placenta, and in small amounts by the adrenal glands. If the ovaries are not functioning properly, have been removed, or if they have atrophied because of menopause or hysterectomy, the woman is undoubtedly estrogen dominant. Therefore, she is a candidate for the problems listed above. One successful approach for the above problems is NATURAL PROGESTERONE (obtained from the Wild Yam or SOY). Two good books to read about natural progesterone are What Your Doctor May Not Tell You About Premenopause and What Your Doctor May Not Tell You About Menopause. Both books were written by John R. Lee, MD.

—Balance

Oils—[TA]$_F$Clary sage, [TA]ylang ylang, [AT]dorado azul, [TA]Mister (creates greater balance), [TA]Legacy, [TA]bergamot, [A]clove, [TA]EndoFlex, [TA]fennel, [TA]geranium, [TA]nutmeg, [TA]sage.

Personal Care—Dragon Time Massage Oil, Prenolone / Prenolone+, Progessence/Progessence Plus.

Supplements—CortiStop (Women's), EndoGize, Estro Tincture, FemiGen (female), Prostate Health (male), MultiGreens, Super B, Super Cal, Thyromin, Ultra Young+.

—Disturbances

Supplements—EndoGize, Prostate Health (male), or FemiGen (female).

—Female

Oils—[TA]Lady Sclareol, [AT]dorado azul (balances estrogen), [TA]Mister (for estrogen).

Supplements—CortiStop (Women's), EndoGize, Estro Tincture, FemiGen, Ultra Young+.

—MALE

Oils—TAMister

Supplements—EndoGize, Prostate Health, Ultra Young+.

—SEXUAL ENERGY

Oils—TAGoldenrod, TALady Sclareol, TAylang ylang.

Supplements—EndoGize.

T—The most common places to apply oils for hormonal balance are on the Vita Flex points on the ankles, on the lower back, thyroid, liver, kidneys, gland areas, on the center of the body and along both sides of the spine, and on the clavicle area. Dilute as necessary, and apply on these areas.

A—Diffuse into the air.

Hot Flashes: *See Female Specific Conditions: Hot Flashes.*

Housecleaning:

—BATHROOMS/KITCHENS

Oils—TFir, Tlemon, Tspruce, or Thinoki for cleaning and disinfecting.

—CARPETS

Oils—TPurification, Tlemon (has been used to remove black shoe polish)

—DISHES

Recipe #1—A couple of drops of Melrose or lemon in the dishwater make for sparkling dishes and a great smelling kitchen.

—FURNITURE POLISH

Oils—TFir, Tlemon, or Tspruce work well for polishing furniture.

—GUM/GREASE

Oils—TLemon (is terrific for dissolving gum and grease).

—LAUNDRY

Oils—TLemon, TPurification.

***Comments—Adding oils to the washer can increase the antibacterial benefits, provide greater hygiene, and make the clothes come out with a fresh, clean smell. A few drops of oil can also be placed on a washcloth and put in the dryer with laundry or added to a bottle of water, shook well, and sprayed into the dryer before drying the laundry.

—MOLD/FUNGUS *See also Antifungal*

Oils—TPurification, TThieves.

T—Put a few drops of oil on your dust cloth; or put 10 drops in a spray bottle of water, and spray as a mist.

Hyperactivity: *See Calming: Hyperactivity.*

Hyperpnea (Abnormal rapid breathing): *See Respiratory System: Hyperpnea.*

Hypertension (High blood pressure): *See Blood.*

Hypoglycemia: *See also Blood: Low Blood Sugar. See also Protein.*

Hypoglycemia is a condition of low levels of sugar in the blood. It is most common in people with diabetes but can be caused by drugs or by a tumor in the pancreas that causes the pancreas to create too much insulin. Symptoms of hypoglycemia can include hunger, sweating, weakness, palpitations, shaking, dizziness, and confusion.

Protein deficiency causes ***hypoglycemia****. Honey enters the blood stream faster than sugar and can cause hypoglycemia. When flu and virus enter the body and mix with problems of hypoglycemia, they can cause candida, Epstein-Barr virus, allergies, etc. There is a progressive deterioration from hypoglycemia. Signs of hypoglycemia include headaches, fatigue, PMS, orneriness, moodiness, weakness, light-headedness, and a lack of hunger in the morning because the body is still digesting its food from the night before.*

Oils—T F Eucalyptus, T Thieves, T cinnamon bark, T clove, T Gentle Baby, T Gratitude, T thyme.

T—Dilute as necessary, and apply over pancreas and on Vita Flex points on the feet.

Supplements—Allerzyme (aids the digestion of sugars, starches, fats, and proteins), AlkaLime, Balance Complete, Digest + Cleanse, MultiGreens, Power Meal, Pure Protein Complete, Stevia, Sulfurzyme, Wolfberry Crisp Bars, Yacon Syrup.

Hysteria:

Oils—AT Lavender[208], TA melaleuca, TA neroli.

T—Dilute as necessary, and apply to heart and to bottoms of feet

A—Diffuse into the air.

Immune System:

The Immune System is the body's defense against disease. The immune system protects the body by identifying and killing bacteria, viruses, parasites, other microorganisms, and tumor cells that would harm the body. The immune system is comprised of several different types of white blood cells (lymphocytes) that recognize, process, or destroy foreign objects; the bone marrow that creates several types of white blood cells; the thymus that creates white blood cells and teaches them to recognize foreign objects and to distinguish them from the body's cells; lymphatic vessels that help transport lymph and white blood cells; and several other organs, such as the lymph nodes, tonsils, spleen, and appendix, that filter out foreign objects and serve as a place for white blood cells to gather, interact, and share information about infections.

Oils—TA Thieves (enhances; massage on feet and body), TA ImmuPower, ITA oregano[209], TA frankincense[210], TA lemon[211], TA Abundance, TA cistus, TA clove, TA cumin, TA Exodus II, TA geranium, TA Idaho tansy, TA lavender, TA ledum (supports), TA melaleuca, TA mountain savory, TA Raven, TA ravensara, TA rosemary (supports), TA thyme (immunological functions), TA white lotus.

Supplements—ImmuPro, Inner Defense, AlkaLime (designed to combat yeast and fungus overgrowth and to preserve the body's proper pH balance), Cleansing Trio (ComforTone, Essentialzyme, and ICP), Digest + Cleanse, Longevity Capsules, Master Formula His/Hers, Mineral Essence, MultiGreens, NingXia Red, NingXia Wolfberries (dried), Power Meal, Super B, Super C / Super C Chewable, Thyromin, Ultra Young+ (may help raise levels of cytokines, interleukin 1 & 2, and tumor necrosis factor), True Source (whole food multi-nutrient), Wolfberry Crisp Bars (*Refer to the Wolfberry Crisp Bar in the Supplements section of the Reference Guide for Essential Oils for more information on the benefits of the Ningxia Wolfberry).*

—Stimulates

Oils—A Thieves (diffuse with clove), TA F oregano[209], TA F frankincense[210], TA ImmuPower, TA F Cinnamon bark, TA F melaleuca, T Breathe Again, T The Gift, TA lavender (for immune system), TA mountain savory.

—Boosting Immune Defense

Oils—[TA]Cumin, [TA]ledum.

T—Dilute as necessary, and apply oil(s) to bottoms of feet, along spine, or under arms. Dilute with V-6 Oil to create massage oil, and massage into the skin.

A—Diffuse into the air for ½ hour at a time.

Impetigo: *See Skin: Impetigo.*

Impotency:

Oils—[T]$_{F}$Clary sage, [TI]$_{F}$clove, [I]SclarEssence (taken internally as a dietary supplement; helps to raise testosterone levels), [T]$_{F}$sandalwood, [TI]Mister, [TI]$_{F}$ginger, [T]goldenrod, [T]jasmine, [T]nutmeg, [T]rose, ylang ylang.

T—Dilute as necessary, and apply to Vita Flex points on the feet, to groin area, or to abdomen.

I—Add 2–4 drops oil to an empty capsule with 2–4 drops V-6 Oil, and swallow.

Supplements— Prostate Health.

Personal Care—Prenolone+.

Incontinence: *See Bladder.*

Indifference:

Oils—[AT]Jasmine.

A—Diffuse into the air. Inhale directly or applied to tissue or a cotton wick.

T—Apply to auricular emotion points. Dilute with V-6 Oil to create a massage oil, and massage onto the skin.

Indigestion: *See Digestive System: Indigestion.*

Infection: *See also Antibacterial, Antifungal, Antiviral.*

Oils—[TA]$_{F}$Cinnamon bark, [TA]Thieves, [TA]$_{F}$clary sage, [TA]$_{F}$bergamot, [TA]$_{F}$pine (severe), [TA]Melrose (prevents growth of all infections), [TA]myrrh (with oregano), [TA]cajeput (urethra), [TA]clove, [TA]cypress, [AT]elemi (chest/bronchial infections), [TA]Idaho tansy, [TA]jasmine (bacterial infection), [TA]juniper, [TA]fennel, [TA]lavender, [TA]lemongrass, [TA]*Melaleuca quinquenervia* (viral), [TA]oregano, [TA]peppermint, [AT]Raven, [TA]ravensara, [TA]rosemary (with myrrh for oral infection), [TA]thyme (urinary infection).

Supplements—Inner Defense.

—Anti-infectious

Oils—[TA]$_{F}$Cinnamon bark, [AT]$_{F}$spruce, [TA]$_{F}$basil, [TA]$_{F}$pine, [TA]$_{F}$thyme, [TA]$_{F}$rosemary, [TA]myrrh (with oregano), [TA]$_{F}$ravensara, [TA]$_{F}$cypress, [TA]Purification, [TA]$_{F}$lavender, [TA]$_{F}$rosewood, [TA]$_{F}$patchouli, [TA]cassia, [TA]clove, [TA]davana, [TA]elemi, [TA]eucalyptus, [TA]hyssop, [TA]Idaho tansy, [TA]marjoram, [TA]melaleuca, [TA]*Melaleuca ericifolia*, [TA]petitgrain, [TA]rose, [TA]Roman chamomile, [TA]spearmint, [TA]spikenard, [TA]tarragon.

***Comments—See the "Single Oil Property Chart" in the Appendix of this book for additional anti-infectious oils and their strengths.

Supplements—Super C / Super C Chewable.

—Infected Wounds

Oils—**T**Frankincense, **T**melaleuca, **T**basil[213], **T**patchouli.

Blend #1 *(to draw infection out)*—1 drop thyme. Apply hot compress twice daily. Mix together 3 drops lavender, 2 drops melaleuca, and 2 drops thyme with 1 tsp. V-6 Oil. After the infection and pus have been expelled, apply a little of the mixture twice daily on the infected area.

Supplements—ImmuPro, Inner Defense, Super C / Super C Chewable.

Infectious Disease:

Oils—**TA**Cinnamon bark, **TA**ImmuPower, **TA**melaleuca, **A**Raven, **A**RC, **TA**thyme (bacterial infection), **TA**bergamot, **TA**clove, **TA**Exodus II, **TA**ginger, **TA**hyssop (viral infections), **TA**juniper (viral infections), **TA**lemon, **TA**myrtle.

T—Dilute as necessary, and apply on location and on bottoms of feet.

A—Diffuse into the air.

***Comments—Dr. Young uses Raven, RC, and ImmuPower together for infectious diseases.

Inferiority (Overcoming):

Oils—**TA**Peppermint, **TA**Transformation.

A—Diffuse into the air. Inhale directly or applied to tissue or a cotton wick.

T—Apply to auricular emotion points. Dilute with V-6 Oil to create a massage oil, and massage onto the skin.

Infertility: *See also Female Specific Conditions, Hormonal Imbalance, Male Specific Conditions.*

Oils—**T**Clary sage, **T**Dragon Time (place on ankles, lower abdomen, and in vagina for women), **T**Mister (for men, place in rectum, across lower back, around and under ankles), **T**geranium, **T**anise, **T**bergamot, **T**cypress, **T**fennel, **T**melissa, **T**nutmeg, **T**Roman chamomile, **T**sage, **T**thyme, **T**yarrow, **T**ylang ylang.

T—Dilute as necessary, and apply as indicated, or apply on Vita Flex points, groin area, or lower abdomen.

***Comments—Feed the thyroid.

Supplements— Prostate Health (male) or FemiGen (female), Prenolone/Prenolone+ / Progessence/Progessence Plus, and 1–3 MultiGreens three times a day.

Inflammation: *See Anti-inflammatory.*

Influenza: *See also Antiviral, Colds, Respiratory System.*

▸▸ *Influenza, commonly referred to as "the flu," is a highly contagious viral infection of the respiratory system. Influenza is marked by a sudden onset of high fever, dry cough, sore throat, muscle aches and pains, headache, fatigue, loss of appetite, nausea, and nasal congestion.*

Oils—**AT**RC, **TA**Raven (apply to thymus area, Vita Flex points on feet, chest, back, and on any place where the flu has settled), **AT**$_F$melaleuca, **AT**$_F$peppermint, **AT**Thieves, **AT**$_F$rosemary, **TA**ImmuPower, **AT**$_F$myrtle, **AT***Eucalyptus radiata*, **T**blue cypress (aches and pains), **AT**clove, **AT**copaiba, **AT**Exodus II, **T**fir (aches and pains), **AT**goldenrod, **AT**ginger, **T**Idaho tansy (on bottoms of feet), **AT**lavender, **AT**ledum, **AT**-*Melaleuca ericifolia*, **AT**onycha (benzoin), **AT**orange, **AT**oregano, **AT**pine, **AT**sage lavender, **AT**thyme, **AT**tsuga.

A—Diffuse into the air

T—Dilute as necessary, and apply to chest, back, neck, sinuses, or Vita Flex points on the feet..

***Comments—According to the Essential Oils Desk Reference, "[Idaho] tansy should be applied topically on stomach and bottom of feet." (EDR-June 2002; Ch. 28; Flu) It may be best to dilute Idaho tansy first in one teaspoon V-6 Oil before topical application.

Bath Recipe #1—2 Tbs. Evening Peace Bath & Shower Gel with drops of the following oils: 1 wintergreen, 20 eucalyptus, 5 frankincense, 3 helichrysum, 15 ravensara, and 6 spruce. Mix together, and put mixture under the faucet while running HOT bathwater. SOAK until cool. Also consider using Thieves Cleansing Soap to wash hands with, especially during cold and flu season.

Supplements—Essentialzyme, Essentialzymes-4, Master Formula His/Hers, ParaFree, Super C / Super C Chewable, True Source (whole food multi-nutrient).

One Sunday after church a friend commented that I looked "exhausted." I thought that strange because I had gotten a good night's sleep. I walked over to a meeting for a mission trip I would be participating in, and an hour later I started getting a headache and felt something happening to my throat. About 30 minutes later, I knew I was coming down with the flu as the headache and sore throat intensified and I started feeling shaky. Fortunately, I had peppermint, oregano and Thieves in my truck; and as soon as I got in, I rubbed several drops of oregano on my feet, rubbed Thieves on my neck and throat, and put several drops of peppermint in my water and started drinking it. By the time I got home, the headache and sore throat had lessened. That evening and for the next several days I took by capsule a combination of lemon, mountain savory, and oregano three times a day. While I could tell my body was fighting an infection (as indicated by my desire to take naps), the oils completely stopped the flu in its tracks, and the headache and sore throat never returned.

-Submitted by Kevin Dunn
Los Angeles, California (July 2004)

Injuries: *See also Cuts, Pain, Scarring, Tissue, Wounds. See also Blend #2 under Pain for pain reduction.*

Oils—TBalsam fir (with frankincense, sandalwood, myrrh, and helichrysum for pain and inflammation), Tcistus (promotes healing of scar tissue), Thelichrysum (reduces scarring and discoloration), TMelrose (regenerates tissue), Tsandalwood (for any DNA repair).

—Sport

Oils—TBalsam fir, Thelichrysum, TMelrose, TPanAway.

Personal Care—Ortho Ease Massage Oil, Ortho Sport Massage Oil.

T—Dilute as necessary, and apply on location.

Inner Knowing:

Oils—ATInner Child (reconnects you with your inner child), ATSARA.

A—Diffuse into the air. Inhale directly or applied to tissue or a cotton wick.

T—Apply to auricular emotion points. Dilute with V-6 Oil to create a massage oil, and massage onto the skin.

Insanity:

Oils—TAHope (ears), TARelease (liver),TA Relieve It.

T—Dilute as necessary, and apply on area indicated or on temples or brain stem area.

A—Inhale directly. Diffuse into the air.

Insect:

—Bites *See also Bites.*

Oils—TIdaho tansy, Tcajeput, Tbergamot.

Dr. Jean Valnet says that basil, cinnamon, garlic, lavender, lemon, onion, sage, savory, and thyme are effective against insect bites because of their antitoxic and antivenomous properties.

Blend #1—Combine 3 drops Roman chamomile, 4 drops eucalyptus, 10 drops lavender, and 1 drop thyme with 1 Tbs. V-6 Oil.

***Comments—*Refer to the chapter entitled "How to Use—The Personal Usage Reference" in the Essential Oils Desk Reference under "Insect Bites" for some excellent blend recipes for bites/stings from different types of insects.*

—CHIGGERS

Oils—ᵀLavender.

—COCKROACHES

Blend #2—Combine 10 drops peppermint and 5 drops cypress in ½ cup of water; spray.

—POISONS FROM BROWN RECLUSE SPIDER OR WASPS

Oils—ᵀBasil (known to neutralize poisons), ᵀPurification (removes poisons from the body).

> *My husband was bitten by a spider on his stomach. The bite swelled with a large blister, and it itched terribly. I used lavender oil—about a drop—on the area. In about 4 hours my husband asked for another application of the "magic oil". My husband has an allergy and reacts to any type of a bite. In fact, he usually has to go to the Dr. and get shots and prescriptions.*
> ***-Submitted by Mary Rynicki (July 2004)***

—INSECTICIDAL

Oils—ᵀCitronella, ᵀpatchouli[214], ᵀclove[215], ᵀlavender[216], ᵀbasil[217], ᵀmelaleuca[218], ᵀpink pepper[219], ᵀrosemary[220].

—ITCHING

Oils—ᵀLavender.

Personal Care—Lavender Hand & Body Lotion (with lavender).

—REPELLENT

Oils—ᵀᴬCitronella[221], ᵀᴬclove[222], ᵀᴬpatchouli[223], ᵀᴬPurification, ᵀᴬlavender[224], ᵀᴬlimette[225], ᵀᴬplectranthus oregano, ᵀᴬmicromeria, ᵀᴬpink pepper[226], ᵀᴬbasil, ᵀᴬbergamot, ᵀᴬcedarwood.

Blend #3—Combine 5 drops lavender, 5 drops lemongrass, 3 drops peppermint, and 1 drop thyme; put on feet, or add to a cup of water and spray on.

Blend #4—Clove, lemon, and orange.

> *My husband was stung by a wasp last year on the inside of the hand. He removed the stinger and asked me to put something on it. I put Purification on it, and the itching stopped. After his shower that evening, I put Purification on it again. The next morning, you couldn't see or even tell that he'd been stung. I've also put Purification on coworkers who have had mosquito/bug bites that itched. After the Purification went on the bites, the itching stopped.*
> ***-Submitted by Christie Krajewski***
> ***Batesville, Arkansas (July 2004)***

Blend #5—Put 5 drops lemon and 5 drops Purification in a little spray bottle of water, and mist on your skin to protect yourself against insects, flies, and mosquitoes. *1 or 2 oz. glass or plastic spray bottles work very well and are small enough to take with you.*

***Comments—Dr. Friedmann came in contact with a person who had bugs growing on her face and scalp. Somehow she was subjected to a fungus to which the bugs were attracted. The bugs established their nest and laid and hatched their eggs on her skin. She had been using many products and was only able to suppress the problem but not correct it. Dr. Friedmann applied Melrose, helichrysum, lavender, and ImmuPower on her thymus. She stopped using all other chemicals, and several weeks later the bugs were almost gone.

T—Dilute as necessary, and apply on location. Dilute with V-6 Oil to create a massage oil, and apply to skin. Add 3–5 drops to 1 oz. water in a small spray bottle, and mist onto the skin.

A—Diffuse into the air. Apply 1–2 drops on a ribbon or string and hang from windows, branches, or vents.

Insomnia:

Oils—[AT][F]Lavender[227] (best when combined with Roman chamomile and dill), [AT]RutaVaLa, [AT]valerian[228], [AT][F]bergamot, [AT]Citrus Fresh, [AT][F]orange, [AT]Peace & Calming, [AT][F]ylang ylang, [AT][F]cypress, [AT][F]marjoram, [AT][F]ravensara, [AT][F]myrtle (for hormone-related insomnia), [AT]angelica, [AT]basil, [AT]clary sage, [AT]lemon, [AT]*Melaleuca ericifolia*, [AT]neroli, [AT]nutmeg (small amount), [AT]petitgrain, [AT]Roman chamomile (small amount), [AT]rosemary, [AT]sandalwood, [AT]Surrender (behind the ears).

Blend #1—Combine 6 drops Citrus Fresh with 6 drops lavender or 6 drops Peace & Calming. Apply blend to big toes, bottoms of feet, 2 drops around navel, and 3 drops on back of neck.

Blend #2—2 drops Roman chamomile, 6 drops geranium, 3 drops lemon, and 4 drops sandalwood. Mix together, and add 6 drops in your bath at bedtime and 5 drops with 2 tsp. V-6 Oil for a massage after bath.

Blend #3—Combine 20 ml valerian, 5 ml vetiver, 2 ml helichrysum, 1 ml clove, and 1 ml peppermint in a 1 oz. dropper bottle. Add several drops (up to 3 droppers full) to 2–3 oz. of water, and drink—followed by ½ tsp. AlkaLime in water.

Supplements—ImmuPro.

***Comments—Refer to the chapter entitled "How to Use—The Personal Usage Reference" in the Essential Oils Desk Reference under "Insomnia" for some excellent blend recipes.

—For Children

–12 months to 5 years

Oils—[AT]Lavender, [AT]Roman chamomile

–5 to 12 years

Oils—[AT]Lavender, [AT]clary sage, [AT]geranium, [AT]*Melaleuca ericifolia*, [AT]ylang ylang (infection).

A—Diffuse into the air. Place 1–2 drops on a pillow or stuffed animal. Add 1–3 drops to 1 oz. distilled water in a spray bottle, and mist into the air.

T—Dilute as necessary, and apply to bottoms of feet or back of neck. Dilute with V-6 Oil to create a massage oil, and massage onto back of legs, feet, and arms. Add 1–2 drops to bathwater, and bathe.

Intestinal Problems: *See Digestive System: Intestinal Problems.*

Invigorating:

Oils—[TA]Wintergreen.

—In Summer

Oils—[TA]Eucalyptus, [TA]peppermint.

T—Dilute in V-6 Oil to create massage oil, and massage onto the skin. Add 1–2 drops to 1 oz. cool distilled water in a spray bottle, and mist onto the skin.

A—Diffuse into the air.

Ions:

—Increase Negative Ions

Oils—When dispersed into the air through a cool-air nebulizing diffuser, the following oils ionize negatively: Bergamot, cedarwood,

> ***Negative ions** are produced naturally by wind and rain. They help stimulate the parasympathetic nervous system, which controls rest, relaxation, digestion, and sleep. However, if you live in an environment with an overabundance of negative ions, such as in the country or by the ocean, you may benefit greatly from diffusing the oils listed under* Positive Ions. *The production of more positive ions can help bring greater balance to the area and provide a more healthy environment.*

citronella, *Eucalyptus citriodora*, grapefruit, lavandin, lavender, lemon, lemongrass, mandarin, orange, patchouli, sandalwood.

—Increase Positive Ions

Oils—When dispersed into the air through a cool-air nebulizing diffuser, the following oils ionize positively: Cajeput, clove, cypress, eucalyptus, frankincense, helichrysum, juniper, marjoram, *Melaleuca quinquenervia*, palmarosa, pine, ravensara, rosemary, thyme, ylang ylang.

***Positive ions** are produced by electronic equipment and are typically found in man-made environments. They help stimulate the sympathetic nervous system, necessary for recovering, strengthening, and energizing. However, an overabundance of positive ions can lead to stress and agitation. The diffusion of the oils listed under* Negative Ions *can help balance the ions and help produce a more stress-free environment.*

Iron:

***Comments—Iron is important for learning. Raisins are a good natural source.

Supplements—Master Formula His/Hers, KidScents MightyVites (chewable).

Irritability: *See also Calming.*

Oils—ATLavender, ATForgiveness, ATHope, ATHumility, ATInspiration, ATmyrrh, ATPresent Time, ATSurrender, ATValor.

A—Diffuse into the air. Inhale directly or applied to hands, tissue, or a cotton wick.

T—Dilute with V-6 Oil to create massage oil, and massage into the skin.

***Comments—All single oils can help **except** eucalyptus, pepper, peppermint, and rosemary.

Supplements—AlkaLime.

Irritable Bowel Syndrome: *See Digestive System: Irritable Bowel Syndrome.*

Itching:

Oils—TPeppermint (ears), Tlavender, TPeace & Calming (ears).

T—Dilute as necessary, and apply on location or on ears.

Blend #1—6 drops lavender and 3 drops rosemary with Lavender Hand & Body Lotion.

Personal Care—Rose Ointment, Lavender Hand & Body Lotion.

Jaundice: *See Liver: Jaundice*

Jealousy:

Oils—ATBergamot, ATeucalyptus, ATForgiveness, ATfrankincense, ATHarmony, ATHumility, ATJoy, ATlemon, ATmarjoram, ATorange, ATrose, ATrosemary, ATSacred Mountain, ATsandalwood, ATthyme, ATValor, ATWhite Angelica.

A—Diffuse into the air. Inhale directly or applied to hands, tissue, or a cotton wick.

T—Apply to auricular emotion points. Dilute with V-6 Oil to create massage oil, and massage into the skin.

Jet Lag:

Jet lag is the disruption of normal sleep patterns experienced while the hypothalamus (the body's internal clock) adjusts to rapid changes in daylight and nighttime hours when flying to different areas of the world. Jet lag can cause tiredness, fatigue, and insomnia during normal sleeping hours. It is recommended to drink lots of fluids and to avoid alcohol or caffeine while flying to help prevent jet lag. Avoiding naps and forcing yourself to stay awake until your normal bedtime the first day can also help the body recover more quickly.

Oils—ᵀValor, ᵀpeppermint, ᵀBrain Power, ᵀeucalyptus, ᵀClarity, ᵀEn-R-Gee, ᵀgeranium, ᵀgrapefruit, ᵀImmuPower (for protection), ᵀlavender, ᵀlemongrass, ᵀPresent Time.

T—Dilute as necessary, and apply to temples, thymus, and bottoms of feet. It is best to not eat heavy foods and to drink as much water as possible.

Supplements—Power Meal, Sulfurzyme, Super C / Super C Chewable.

Joints: *See also Rotator Cuff, Shoulder (Frozen), Tennis Elbow.*

Oils—ᵀWintergreen (discomfort), ᵀspruce (aching), ᵀcajeput (stiff), ᵀbalsam fir (pain from exercising), ᵀDouglas fir (calming to tired and overworked joints), ᵀnutmeg, ᵀRoman chamomile (inflamed).

T—Dilute as necessary, and apply on location or on Vita Flex points on the feet. Dilute with V-6 Oil and massage on location.

Supplements—True Source (whole food multi-nutrient).

******Comments***—Refer to the chapter entitled "How to Use—The Personal Usage Reference" in the Essential Oils Desk Reference under "Joint Stiffness and Pain" for some excellent blend recipes.

Joyous:

Oils—ATJoy, ATAbundance, ATbergamot (turns grief to joy), ATChristmas Spirit, ATCitrus Fresh (brings joy to children), Aorange.

A—Diffuse into the air. Inhale directly or applied to hands, tissue, or a cotton wick.

T—Apply to auricular emotion points. Dilute with V-6 Oil to create massage oil, and massage into the skin.

Kidneys: *See also Diuretic.*

The kidneys are paired organs located just below the rib cage on either side of the spine that function to filter waste and extra water from the blood. The kidneys convert the waste and extra water into urine that is then excreted through urination. The kidneys also play an important role in hormone production.

Oils—ᵀ$_F$Lemongrass (combine with juniper for greater synergistic effect), Ithyme[229], ᵀAroma Life, ᵀcalamus (reduces congestion after intoxication), ᵀclary sage, ᵀEndoFlex, ᵀgeranium, ᵀgrapefruit, ᵀjuniper (for better function of kidneys), ᵀJuvaFlex, ᵀledum (strengthen), ᵀRelease.

T—Apply over kidneys as a hot compress. Dilute as necessary, and apply over kidneys or on Vita Flex points on the feet.

I—Add 1–2 drops to an empty capsule, and swallow. Use as flavoring in food.

***Comments—Drink plenty of distilled water (3–4 quarts each day). When kidneys start producing ammonia, the ammonia can go to the brain—and people have died from that alone. Do the **MASTER CLEANSER** (*See Cleansing*).

Supplements—Longevity Capsules (contains thyme oil to help preserve omega-3 fatty acids in the kidneys), K&B Tincture, EndoGize, MultiGreens (turns blood back to alkaline).

*****Comments**—Refer to the chapter entitled "How to Use—The Personal Usage Reference" in the Essential Oils Desk Reference under "Kidney Disorders" for some excellent blend recipes and supplement recommendations.

—Blockage

Recipe #1—Massage Release and other oils onto the kidney points on the feet twice a day.

Supplements—Cleansing Trio (ComforTone, Essentialzyme, and ICP), JuvaTone (First week: 2 tablets a day; Second week: 3 tablets a day for 90 days).

—Capillaries Being Attacked In Kidneys

Supplements—Need to support the body and cleanse the blood with MultiGreens, Cleansing Trio (ComforTone, Essentialzyme, and ICP).

—Infection In

Oils—ᵀRosemary.

T—Dilute as necessary, and apply to kidneys and to Vita Flex points.

Blend #1—Cypress, marjoram, and Thieves or JuvaFlex. Apply as a hot compress.

Nutrition—Drink one gallon of distilled water and 2 quarts of cranberry juice in a day.

Supplements—Inner Defense, NingXia Red (1–3 oz. followed by 8–10 oz. of water 3 times daily).

—Inflammation (Nephritis)

Oils—ᵀAroma Life, ᵀjuniper, ᵀJuvaFlex.

T—Dilute as necessary, and apply to kidneys and to Vita Flex points.

*****Comments**—Do a colon cleanse (*see Cleansing*).

Nutrition—Drink one gallon of distilled water and 2 quarts of cranberry juice in a day.

Supplements—K&B Tincture, MultiGreens, Power Meal, Rehemogen Tincture, Super C / Super C Chewable.

*****Comments**—*Refer to the chapter entitled "How to Use—The Personal Usage Reference" in the Essential Oils Desk Reference under "Kidney Disorders," subcategory "Inflammation in the Kidneys (Nephritis)," for a very specific regimen of supplements and blends.*

—Muscles That Won't Work In The Kidneys

Oils—ᵀAroma Siez, ᵀEndoFlex.

Blend #2—8 drops fennel and 10 drops juniper.

T—Dilute as necessary, and apply to kidneys and to Vita Flex points.

—Stones

»*A kidney stone is a solid piece of material that forms as chemicals in the urine crystallize and adhere together in the kidney. Small stones may pass through urination without causing pain. Larger stones with sharp edges and corners, however, can cause an extreme amount of pain as they are passed out of the body through the urinary tract.*

Oils—ᵀEucalyptus, ᵀhyssop, ᵀjuniper.

T—Dilute as necessary, and apply to kidneys and to Vita Flex points. Apply as a hot compress over kidney area.

Blend #3—10 drops juniper and 10 drops geranium. Apply as a hot compress over kidneys once a day.

Supplements—After being on the Cleansing Trio (ComforTone, Essentialzyme, andICP) for 10 days, add Super C / Super C Chewable.

Recipe #2—To pass (without edges), drink 4 oz. distilled water with juice from ½ lemon every 30 minutes for 6 hours straight. Then take 2 Tbs. extra light virgin olive oil with the juice from 1 full lemon. Repeat daily until stone passes.

Knee Cartilage Injury:

Blend #1—8 drops clove, 12 drops ginger, and 10 drops nutmeg with 2 oz. V-6 Oil. Massage three times a day. Apply ice for swelling and inflammation. Wrap knee and elevate when sitting. Use the ice method three times a day, and alternate with a hot compress and the oils.

Personal Care—Ortho Ease Massage Oil, Ortho Sport Massage Oil, Regenolone.

Supplements—BLM

Labor: *See also Pregnancy/Motherhood.*

Oils—[T]Gentle Baby, [T]jasmine (pain).

T—Dilute as necessary, and apply on ankles and abdomen.

Lactation (Secretion of breast milk): *See also Pregnancy/Motherhood: Nursing.*

Oils—[T][F]Fennel or [T]basil (increase flow), [T]peppermint (with cold compress—decrease flow).

T—Apply above the breasts on the lymph area, and apply 2–3 drops on the spine, about breast level.

Supplements—PD 80/20, Prenolone/Prenolone+, Progessence/Progessence Plus.

Lactose Intolerance:

›› *Lactose intolerance is the inability of the body to fully digest lactose, a sugar found in milk and in other dairy products. Symptoms of lactose intolerance include abdominal pain and bloating, diarrhea, nausea, and gas.*

Oils—[IT]Lemongrass (reported to help eliminate lactic acid from fermentation of lactose in milk).

I—Add 1–2 drops to 1 tsp. honey, and swallow; or add 1–2 drops to 4 oz. rice or almond milk, and drink. Place 1–2 drops in an empty capsule, and swallow.

T—Dilute as recommended, and apply 1–2 drops on abdomen or on reflex points on the feet.

Supplements—Allerzyme, Essentialzyme, Essentialzymes-4, Life 5 (probiotic), Power Meal.

Laryngitis:

›› *Laryngitis is an inflammation and swelling of the voice box (called the larynx) that causes the voice to sound hoarse or raspy. Laryngitis is most commonly caused by viruses, allergies, or overuse of the voice and will generally go away by itself within two weeks.*

Oils—[AT]Sandalwood, [A]frankincense, [AI]lavender, [AT]thyme, [ATI]Melrose, [AT]jasmine, [AT]ledum, [AT]onycha (benzoin), [AT]sage.

A—Diffuse into the air.

T—Dilute as necessary, and apply to neck and to Vita Flex points on the feet.

I—Add 1–2 drops to 1 tsp. honey, and swallow

Blend #1—Add one drop each of Melrose and lemon to 1 tsp. honey. Swish around in mouth for a couple of minutes to liquefy; then swallow.

Laundry: *See Housecleaning: Laundry.*

Laxative:

Oils—TI Hyssop, T jasmine, TI tangerine.

T—Apply to abdomen with warm compress. Dilute as necessary, and massage on abdomen; or apply to Vita Flex points on the feet.

I—Add 1–2 drops to 8 oz. rice or almond milk, and drink.

Blend #1—Dilute equal parts rosemary, lemon, and peppermint oils[230] in V-6 Oil, and massage on abdomen.

Supplements—Balance Complete, Cleansing Trio (ComforTone, Essentialzyme, and ICP), Digest + Cleanse.

Legs, Restless:

Restless legs are caused by the body dumping acid into the system at night. The following recipe was recommended to counteract this reaction to the over-acidification of the body.

Recipe #1—In the evening before bed, take 1 Tbs of JuvaPower (in almond, rice or soy milk, or water), followed by ½ tsp of AlkaLime in water. Then apply 2–3 drops each of valerian, Roman chamomile, and lavender to the brain stem area (back of neck from shoulders to base of skull), and work them in with the Vita Flex technique.

Leg Ulcers: *See Ulcers: Leg.*

Lethargy:

Oils—AT Jasmine, AT Transformation.

A—Diffuse into the air. Inhale directly or applied to hands.

T—Dilute with V-6 Oil to create massage oil, and massage into skin. Add 1–2 drops to 1 Tbs. bath or shower gel, and use in bath or shower.

Libido (Low): *See also Frigidity, Sex Stimulant.*

Oils—AT Ylang ylang, AT Sensation, AT Dragon Time, AT Live with Passion, AT Mister, AT Joy, AT nutmeg, AT rose, I SclarEssence.

***Comments—Do the MASTER CLEANSER (*See Cleansing*).

Supplements— Progessence/Progessence Plus, PD 80/20, Prenolone/Prenolone+, Sulfurzyme.

—Men *See also Prostate.*

Oils—AT Cinnamon, AT black pepper, AT ginger, AT myrrh, AT pine.

Personal Care—Protec (combine with frankincense to decongest the prostate).

—Women

Oils—AT Jasmine, AT Lady Sclareol, AT clary sage, AT geranium, .

A—Diffuse into the air. Dissolve 8–10 drops in 2 tsp. pure grain or perfumers alcohol, combine with distilled water in a 1 or 2 oz. spray bottle, and spray into the air or on clothes or bed linens.

T—Dilute as necessary, and apply on temples, neck, or wrists. Dilute with V-6 Oil to create a massage oil, and massage into the skin. Combine 1–2 drops with 1/4 cup Epsom salts, and dissolve in warm bathwater for a romantic bath.

I—Place 2–5 drops in an empty capsule, and swallow.

Lice:

Oils—TMelaleuca[231], Tcitronella[232], Tpine (repels), Teucalyptus, Tgeranium, Tlavender, Tlemon, Trosemary.

T—Apply oil(s) to scalp and to bottoms of feet three times a day.

Ligaments: *See also Muscles.*

Oils—TLemongrass (torn or pulled: combine with marjoram to stimulate torn ligaments; combine with basil if torn ligaments produce spasms), TDeep Relief (roll-on), Tpalo santo.

Supplements—BLM

—Torn

Oils—TLemongrass, TPanAway, Twintergreen, Tclove, Thelichrysum, Tmarjoram.

Personal Care—Ortho Sport Massage Oil.

T—Dilute as necessary, and apply on location or on Vita Flex points on the feet.

Lipoma: *See Tumors: Lipoma.*

Lips:

Oils—TGerman chamomile, Tlavender, Tlemon, Tmelaleuca.

T—Dilute as necessary, and apply on lips.

—Dry Lips

Blend #1—Combine 2–5 drops geranium with 2–5 drops lavender, and apply 1–2 drops on lips.

Personal Care—Cinnamint or Lavender Lip Balms

Listlessness: *See also Calming.*

Oils—ATJasmine.

A—Diffuse into the air. Inhale directly or applied to hands.

T—Dilute with V-6 Oil to create massage oil, and massage into skin. Add 1–2 drops to 1/4 cup Epsom salts, and dissolve in warm bathwater before bathing.

Liver:

›› *The liver is the largest internal organ of the body. It is located in the upper abdomen and helps with digestion, produces cholesterol used to make several hormones and cellular membranes, removes waste products and old cells from the blood, and metabolizes harmful substances and toxins into harmless chemicals.*

Oils—TALedum (powerful detoxifier), TAdill[233], TArosemary[234], TAcaraway[233], TAJuvaFlex (detoxification), TAJuva Cleanse, TA$_F$sage (for liver problems), TA$_F$helichrysum, TA$_F$geranium (cleanses and detoxifies the liver), TA$_F$German chamomile, TAthyme[235], TAAcceptance, TAcypress, TADi-Gize, TAfleabane, TAGLF, TAgoldenrod (supports liver function), TAgrapefruit (liver disorders), TAmyrrh, TAPeace & Calming, TAravensara, TAsage lavender (congestion), TRelease (apply to liver and to Vita Flex points), TARoman chamomile, TA3 Wise Men (on crown).

Supplements—JuvaTone, Balance Complete, Digest + Cleanse, Longevity Capsules (contains thyme oil to help preserve omega-3 fatty acids in the liver). Also NingXia Red, Omega Blue, OmegaGize[3], and Power Meal.

*****Comments**—When the liver is toxic, it makes the mind lethargic and slows the emotions. For those who have liver problems, be careful about the oils used and the amounts. Ease into a liver cleanse!

—**Cirrhosis of the Liver**

▸▸ *Cirrhosis is scarring of the liver that occurs as the liver tries to repair damage done to itself. When extensive liver damage occurs, the massive scar tissue buildup makes it impossible for the liver to function. The most common causes of cirrhosis are fatty liver (resulting from obesity or diabetes) and alcohol abuse; but any damage done to the liver can cause cirrhosis.*

Oils—**TA**Frankincense, **TA**myrrh, **TA**geranium, **TA**juniper, **TA**lavender, **TA**Roman chamomile, **TA**rosemary, **TA**rose.

Supplements—JuvaTone, NingXia Red, Super C / Super C Chewable.

—**Cleansing**

Oils—**TA**Juva Cleanse, **TA**clove (increases detoxification), **TA**GLF, **TA**JuvaFlex, **TA**carrot seed, **TA**helichrysum, **TA**geranium, **TA**German chamomile, **TA**ledum (with JuvaTone), **TA**myrrh, **TA**sage lavender.

Supplements—Longevity Capsules, NingXia Red, Sulfurzyme (may help detoxify the liver).

—**Function (improve)**

Recipe #1—GLF, JuvaFlex, goldenrod, and myrrh. Do a compress over the liver, and alternate the oils on the liver Vita Flex points.

Supplements—NingXia Red, Omega Blue, OmegaGize³, Power Meal.

—**Hepatitis** *See also Antiviral*

▸▸ *Hepatitis is any swelling or inflammation of the liver. This can interfere with normal liver functioning and can possibly lead to cirrhosis or cancer over time. The most common cause of hepatitis is from one of the five different forms of hepatitis viruses, but it can also be caused by alcohol consumption, other viruses, or medications. Possible symptoms of hepatitis include diarrhea, jaundice, stomach pain, loss of appetite, dark-colored urine, pale bowel movements, nausea, and vomiting.*

Oils—**TA**GLF, **T**JuvaFlex (over the liver), **I**myrrh (with ledum internally for hepatitis B & C), **TA**cinnamon bark, **TA**cypress, **TA**eucalyptus, **TA**ImmuPower (on spine and liver), **TA**melaleuca, **TA**oregano, **TA**patchouli, **TA**ravensara (viral), **T**Release (on feet and liver), **TA**Roman chamomile, **TA**rosemary, **TA**thyme.

Supplements—NingXia Red.

Recipe #2—The following regimen has been useful: Use the Cleansing Trio (ComforTone, Essentialzyme, and ICP) for 1 week, 4 Life 5 (probiotic) a day, Master Formula His/Hers, 1 MultiGreens a day, 4 Super C / Super C Chewable three times a day. Add JuvaTone on the 3rd day.

*****Comments**—Refer to the chapter entitled "How to Use—The Personal Usage Reference" in the Essential Oils Desk Reference under "Liver," subcategory "Hepatitis," for a specific daily program using supplements and blends.

–**Detoxify Liver**

Oils—**T**Ledum and **TA**JuvaTone together.

–**Viral**

Oils—**I**F Myrrh and **ITA**JuvaFlex, **TA**frankincense[236], **TA**F ravensara, **TA**F rosemary, **TA**GLF, **TA**ledum.

Supplements—Super C / Super C Chewable.

—**Jaundice**

▸▸ *Jaundice is a condition characterized by a yellow appearance of the skin and the whites of the eyes. Jaundice is a result of excessive levels in the blood of a chemical called bilirubin. Bilirubin is a pigment that is made when hemoglobin from old or dead red blood cells is broken down. Jaundice occurs when the liver is unable*

L

to pass bilirubin from the body as fast as it is being produced. Jaundice is often a symptom of other diseases or conditions.

Oils—TA F Geranium, TA GLF, TA Juva Cleanse, TA lemon, TA rosemary, TA sage lavender.

—Regeneration

Supplements—NingXia Red

***Comments—*One individual had total liver regeneration using JuvaTone, Rehemogen, and JuvaFlex.*

—Spots

▸▸ *Liver spots are gray, black, or brown spots that appear on the skin in areas that have had a lot of sun exposure over the years. Liver spots are not harmful, but many people wish to eliminate them for cosmetic reasons.*

Personal Care—Prenolone/Prenolone+, Progessence/Progessence Plus.

—Stimulant for Liver Cell Function

Oils—TA F Helichrysum, TA GLF, TA ledum (combine with JuvaTone).

Supplements—Balance Complete, Cleansing Trio (ComforTone, Essentialzyme, and ICP), JuvaTone (helps increase digestion in the liver), NingXia Red, Omega Blue, OmegaGize³.

T—Dilute as necessary, and apply 1–2 drops over liver area and on Vita Flex points on the feet. Apply along the spine for viral infections, alternating oils. Apply as a hot compress over the liver area.

A—Diffuse into the air. Inhale directly or applied to hands.

I—Add 3–5 drops oil to an empty capsule with 3–5 drops V-6 Oil; swallow.

Longevity:

Oils—A Fennel, IA Longevity.

A—Diffuse into the air. Inhale directly or applied to hands, tissue, or a cotton wick.

I—Add 3–5 drops to an empty capsule; swallow.

Supplements—NingXia Red (whole wolfberry puree), Longevity Capsules (Longevity blend + frankincense in gel caps for internal consumption), Omega Blue/OmegaGize³ (omega-3s).

Loss of Loved One:

Oils—AT Basil, AT cedarwood, A cypress, AT fir, AT Forgiveness, AT jasmine, AT Joy, AT rose, AT spruce, AT Transformation, AT Valor, AT ylang ylang.

A—Diffuse into the air. Inhale directly or applied to hands, tissue, or a cotton wick.

T—Apply to auricular emotion points. Dilute with V-6 Oil to create massage oil, and massage into skin.

Personal Care—Sensation Hand & Body Lotion, Sensation Bath & Shower Gel, Sensation Massage Oil.

Loss of Smell:

Oils—A Basil.

A—Inhale directly. Diffuse into the air.

Lou Gehrig's Disease: *See also Alzheimer's Disease, Brain, Multiple Sclerosis, Parkinson's Disease, Pineal Gland, Pituitary Gland.*

▸▸ *Lou Gehrig's disease (also known as amyotrophic lateral sclerosis) is a progressive and fatal neurological disease that affects nerve cells in the brain and spinal cord. As the disease progresses, motor neurons die, and the brain loses its ability to control muscle movement. Later stages of the disease can lead to complete paralysis. Eventually, control is lost of the muscles needed to breathe, to speak, and to eat.*

Oils—**TA**Cypress (circulation), **TA**Valor, **TA**frankincense, **TA**sandalwood, **TA**Acceptance (may help to oxygenate the pineal and pituitary glands), **TA**Clarity (for brain function), **TA**Egyptian Gold, **TA**Peace & Calming.

*****Comments**—Use the same oils as you would if you were handling Multiple Sclerosis, Alzheimer's, and Parkinson's Disease. Drink distilled water.

T—Dilute as necessary, and apply 1–2 drops on brain stem area, neck, spine, and Vita Flex points on the feet. Add 1–2 drops to 1 Tbs. V-6 Oil, and massage on back, neck, and feet.

A—Diffuse into the air. Inhale directly or applied to hands.

Supplements—Cleansing Trio (ComforTone, Essentialzyme, and ICP), Digest + Cleanse, JuvaPower/JuvaSpice, JuvaTone, Omega Blue, OmegaGize[3], Sulfurzyme.

Love:

Oils—**AT**Forgiveness, **AT**Joy, **AT**juniper, **AT**Lady Sclareol, **AT**lavender, **AT**Sensation, **AT**ylang ylang.

Personal Care—Sensation Massage Oil, Sensation Hand & Body Lotion, Sensation Bath & Shower Gel (contains oils used by Cleopatra to enhance love and to increase the desire to be close to that someone special).

—Attracts

Oils—**AT**Joy.

—Self Love

Oils—**AT**Joy.

A—Diffuse into the air. Inhale directly or applied to hands, tissue, or a cotton wick.

T—Apply to auricular emotion points. Dilute with V-6 Oil to create massage oil, and massage into skin.

Lumbago: *See Back: Lower Back Pain.*

Lungs: *See Respiratory System: Lungs.*

Lupus: *See also Adrenal Glands, Digestive System, Endocrine System, Immune System, Thyroid.*

▸▸ *Lupus is an autoimmune disease that occurs when the immune system begins attacking its own tissues and organs. Lupus can cause pain, damage, and inflammation in the joints, blood vessels, skin, and organs. Common symptoms include joint pain or swelling, fever, muscle pain, and red rashes (often on the face).*

Oils—**TA**Clove, **TA**Joy, **TA**Thieves (every 2 hours on the feet), **TA**Present Time (key oil for lupus), **TA**Valor (always use first on the feet for courage to overcome fear and build self esteem), **TA**Acceptance, **TA**EndoFlex, **TA**ImmuPower (alone has clearedup Lupus).

Bath—Put 30 drops EndoFlex in softened bath gel.

> ***Lupus** is a collagen breakdown that may effect the skin, joints, and other systems of the body. It occurs because of thyroid and adrenal malfunction. The immune system cells malfunction and some of the good immune cells turn and destroy other good immune cells. This attack leads to an allergic reaction. The immune cells go crazy and attack whatever is convenient for them. The endocrine systems are usually affected and may shut down. In order to heal Lupus, it is necessary to cleanse the body, reduce the toxins, increase blood circulation, and nutritionally support the endocrine functions. When this happens, the adrenal glands can secrete the cortisone that is necessary for connective tissue repair and maintenance.*
>
> *To determine whether or not the thyroid needs help, you must monitor your basal cell temperature. Place a mercury thermometer under your arm pit, and leave it there for 10 minutes. If your temperature is below 97.6°, you need to work on the thyroid (See Recipe #2 below).*

Massage—Thieves (every 2 hours on feet).

Personal Care—A·R·T Skin Care System, Regenolone (may help reverse symptoms).

Supplements—Balance Complete, ComforTone, Digest + Cleanse, EndoGize, ICP, and Essentialzyme (cleanses the body of toxins and supports the digestive function), Thyromin (is a main stay for lupus as it feeds and regulates the thyroid), ImmuPro, Inner Defense, MultiGreens (high in chlorophyll; contains melissa, which supports the connective tissue and the immune function), NingXia Red (contains mannose, an essential sugar that helps to prevent infection—lupus patients are all deficient in this), Power Meal (predigested protein that contains wolfberry), True Source (whole food multi-nutrient). Carrot juice is also very supportive.

***__Comments__—Refer to the chapter entitled "How to Use—The Personal Usage Reference" in the Essential Oils Desk Reference under "Lupus" for a specific daily regimen using supplements and blends.

—Adrenal Glands *See also Adrenal Glands*

Recipe #1—Nutmeg has adrenal cortex properties and is contained in EndoFlex. EndoFlex or Blend #1 can be applied over the adrenal gland area using a hot compress. Also, apply on and massage the Vita Flex points.

Blend #1—3 drops clove (rub in), 5 drops nutmeg (rub in), 7 drops rosemary (rub in), and 20 drops V-6 Oil. Apply a hot compress.

Blend #2—30 drops cypress, 30 drops lemongrass, and 30 drops EndoFlex in 4 oz. V-6 Oil. Massage whole body every day.

—Fluid Retention (caused by steroids)

Oils—TAEndoFlex.

—Endocrine System Support *See Endocrine System.*

Oils—TAEndoFlex.

The following is a recipe that has been used for individuals with Lupus:

Recipe #2—If your basal cell temperature is below 97.6° F (36.5° C), you need to work on the thyroid. Take 2 Thyromin at bedtime. If your temperature does not come up in three days, you will need to increase the amount of Thyromin you are taking. Take 1 upon arising along with the 2 at bedtime. When your temperature gets back up to 97.6° F, stop taking the one in the morning. Gradually go off the 2 at night. Check regularly to see that your temperature continues to stay at 97.6° F. In addition, choose one of the following oils to work as a tissue generator: Acceptance, Joy, Present Time, or Valor; apply to Vita Flex points and to thyroid. To support the adrenal glands, use Blend #1. To determine the adrenal area, lay a yard stick across the back from elbow to elbow, and go up 2". Apply ImmuPower on the spine and Vita Flex points. Finally, supplement with Super C / Super C Chewable and 2 Thyromin, or more if needed.

Case History #1—After taking Thyromin in the following manner for two months, one individual was totally free from Lupus: 2 capsules in the morning and 2 in the evening until temperature stayed down for three days; then increased to 3 capsules in the morning and 3 in the evening. Also, oils used included ImmuPower and Valor, among others.

Case History #2—A nurse in a hospital in the East gave ImmuPower to a patient who was leaving the hospital after another serious bout with Lupus. The patient had suffered from Lupus for 22 years, but she felt better very soon after she started using ImmuPower. And no symptoms of Lupus were found in her at all after eight days.

Case History #3—After suffering from systemic lupus for some time, one lady decided there was nothing left to try from the doctors. She turned to the oils and started applying ImmuPower, EndoFlex, and Joy over her thymus and on her feet over the Vita Flex points for the pineal and pituitary glands. She also began taking Thyromin supplements. After only a day and a half of applying EndoFlex to her toes, she began to have some feeling return. After a while (specific time unknown), the "butterfly" on her face disappeared, and blood tests returned "just fine".

Thought Patterns and Emotions—Some feelings you experience may be subconscious or may be patterns that you inherited from your ancestors in the DNA. A feeling of giving up. Feeling that it is better to die than to stand up for one's self. Anger and a need to be punished. Feelings of deep grief. Laughing on the outside, but crying on the inside. Self destructive programming; an internal cannibalism; a loss of self worth. (Remember it may not have begun with you; we carry in our cells the programming of our ancestors for 4 generations back). You may feel one or more of the above. Reprogram your cells by claiming your power, loving and approving of yourself (no judgment). You are free and safe; speak up for yourself freely and easily. Visualize your body healed or healing. Learn the reason you chose this lesson, and learn from it so you can get past it and be healed. Put as little energy as possible into your affliction.

Lyme Disease: *See also Antibacterial, Insect: Repellent.*

Lyme Disease is an inflammatory illness caused by the bite of a tick carrying the bacterium Borrelia burgdorferi. Signs of Lyme disease include flu-like symptoms, joint pain, neurological problems, and a rash.

Oils—^T^Clarity (back of ears), ^T^Joy (over heart), ^TA^RC (on chest), ^T^Sacred Mountain (on back of neck), ^T^Thieves (on feet and thymus), ^T^White Angelica (on forehead).

T—Dilute as necessary, and apply on location indicated.

A—Inhale directly.

Supplements—Cleansing Trio (ComforTone, Essentialzyme, and ICP), Inner Defense.

Lymphatic System: *See also Immune System.*

The lymphatic system is made up of the tissues and organs (bone marrow, thymus, spleen, lymph glands, etc.) that produce and store the cells used to fight infection and disease. The lymphatic system transports immune cells through a fluid called lymph.

Oils—^A^~F~Cypress, ^TA^~F~sage, ^TA^sandalwood (supports), ^TA^Di-Gize, ^TA^JuvaFlex (detoxifying), ^TA^ledum (inflamed lymph nodes), ^TA^tangerine.

—**Balance and Longevity**

Oils—^TA^Aroma Life, ^TA^Mister.

Blend #1—5 drops Roman chamomile, 5 drops lavender, and 5 drops orange in 2 Tbs. V-6 Oil. Apply a few drops of blend, and massage.

—**Cleansing**

Oils—^TA^Lemon, ^TA^lime.

—**Decongestant For**

Oils—^A^~F~Cypress, ^TA^~F~grapefruit, ^TA^Aroma Life, ^TA^Citrus Fresh, ^TA^cumin, ^TA^helichrysum, ^TA^lemongrass, ^TA^myrtle, ^TA^orange, ^TA^rosemary, ^TA^tangerine, ^TA^thyme.

Personal Care—Cel-Lite Magic.

—**Drainage Of**

Oils—^TA^~F~Helichrysum, ^TA^~F~lemongrass.

—**Eliminates Waste Through**

Oils—^TA^~F~Lavender.

L

—Increase Function Of

Oils—[TA]Lemon.

Personal Care——Cel-Lite Magic (stimulates lymph), Relaxation Massage Oil.

Supplements—Master Formula His/Hers, MultiGreens, Power Meal.

T—Dilute as necessary, and apply on neck, arms, thyroid area, and Vita Flex points on the feet. Add 1–2 drops to warm bathwater, and bathe.

A—Diffuse into the air. Inhale directly or applied to the hands.

Lymphoma: *See Cancer: Lymphoma, Hodgkin's Disease.*

Malaria:

Recipe #1—Lemon with honey in water to prevent.

Male Specific Conditions: *See also Aftershave, Impotence, Skin, Sterility.*

Oils—[AT]Awaken.

Personal Care—PD 80/20, Prenolone/Prenolone+, Lavender Hand & Body Lotion (moisturizes skin leaving it soft, silky, and smooth), Sensation Hand & Body Lotion (moisturizes and protects skin with an alluring fragrance). KidScents Lotion makes a great aftershave as it soothes and rehydrates the skin.

—Genital Area

–Infection

Oils—[T]Melaleuca, [T]oregano, [T]eucalyptus, [T]lavender, [T]patchouli.

–Inflammation

Oils—[T]Lavender, [T]Roman chamomile, [T]hyssop.

–Swelling

Oils—[T]Eucalyptus, [T]lavender, [T]rosemary, [T]cypress, [T]hyssop, [T]juniper.

—Hormonal System (male)

Oils—[T]Mister (balances), [T]SclarEssence (increases testosterone levels).

—Infertility (male)

Oils—[T]Basil, [T]clary sage, [T]SclarEssence, [T]cedarwood, [T]sage, [T]thyme.

Supplements—Master Formula His, MultiGreens.

—Jock Itch

Recipe #1—Put 2 drops of either cypress, lavender, melaleuca, or patchouli in 1 tsp. V-6 Oil, and apply to area morning and night; or put 2 drops of any one of these oils in a small bowl of water, and wash and dry area well.

Supplements— Prostate Health, Master Formula His, MultiGreens.

T—Dilute as necessary, and apply on location or on Vita Flex points on the feet. Dilute with V-6 Oil to create massage oil, and massage on location. Add 1–2 drops to warm bathwater, and bathe.

A—Diffuse into the air. Inhale directly or applied to hands, tissue, or a cotton wick.

Massage:

Personal Care—Any of the different Massage Oils; Ortho Ease and Ortho Sport are excellent.

Blend #1—5 drops Roman chamomile, 5 drops lavender, and 5 drops orange with 2 Tbs. V-6 Oil. Apply as a relaxing massage.

***Comments—A simple massage oil can be made by mixing 2–10 drops essential oil with 1 Tbs. of any carrier oil, such as V-6 Oil, jojoba, sweet almond, olive, or sesame.

Measles: *See Childhood Diseases: Measles.*

Medication:

Supplements—Super C / Super C Chewable.

Meditation:

Oils—ATSacred frankincense, ATwestern red cedar, ATDream Catcher (also for sweat lodges), Aelemi, ATGratitude, ATHumility, ATInspiration, Amyrrh, ATRoman chamomile, ATsandalwood, ATSacred Mountain, ATtsuga (uplifting and grounding).

A—Diffuse into the air. Inhale directly or applied to hands, tissue, or a cotton wick.

T—Dilute with V-6 Oil to create massage oil, and massage into skin. Add 1–3 drops to 1/4 cup Epsom salts, and dissolve in warm bathwater for bathing.

Melanoma: *See Cancer: Melanoma.*

Memory:

Oils—TARosemary[237], TAsage lavender[238], TApeppermint[239], TAClarity, TAAroma Life, TAbasil (for poor memory), TAbergamot, TAcalamus, TAclove (memory deficiency), TADragon Time, TAEn-R-Gee, TAGentle Baby, TAginger, TAgrapefruit, TAJoy (of love), TAlavender, TAlemon (improves), TAlemongrass, TAMister, TAmountain savory (may bring back good memories), TAM-Grain, TARelieve It, TArose.

Blend #1—Add a drop of lemongrass to 1–3 drops of Clarity. May be best to dilute with a few drops of V-6 Oil. Apply to forehead, temples, behind ears, and on back of neck. Cup hands over nose and mouth, and breathe deeply.

Blend #2—Add a drop of rosemary to 1–3 drops of M-Grain. Apply as described in Blend #1.

Supplements—True Source (whole food multi-nutrient).

—Amnesia

▸▸ *Amnesia is a condition where a person experiences either complete or partial loss of memory. Most commonly, Amnesia is caused by a head injury. But amnesia can also be caused by traumatic experiences, strokes, brain tumors, exposure to toxic substances, seizures, etc.*

Oils—TARosemary, TAbasil, TAclove.

—Forgetfulness

Oils—TASage lavender, TArosemary, TBrain Power (1 drop under tongue), TAAcceptance (over heart and liver), TAcedarwood, Clarity, TAcypress, TADream Catcher, TAHighest Potential, TAHope, TAfir, TAGathering, TAgeranium, TAjuniper, TAmarjoram, TAmyrrh, TAorange, TAPresent Time, TARoman chamomile, TArose, TAsandalwood, TA3 Wise Men, TArose, TAValor, TAWhite Angelica, TAylang ylang.

Supplements—Omega Blue, OmegaGize[3], Ultra Young+, MultiGreens.

—Improve

Oils—TA$_F$Clove, TAsage lavender, Aclary sage, TAlime.

Blend #3—5 drops basil, 2 drops peppermint, 10 drops rosemary, and 1 oz. V-6 Oil.

—Releases Negative

Oils—[TA]Forgiveness (has high frequencies), [A]geranium, [TA]palo santo, [TA]3 Wise Men.

—Retention

Oils—[TA]Clarity.

—Stimulate

Oils—[TA]Calamus, [A]rosemary.

Blend #4—2 drops blue tansy, 2 drops Roman chamomile, 3 drops geranium, 4 drops lavender, 3 drops rosemary, 3 drops rosewood, 1 drop spearmint, 2 drops tangerine, and 1 oz. V-6 Oil. Apply a few drops of blend to back of neck, wrist, and heart.

T—Wear as a perfume or cologne. Dilute as necessary, and apply to temples.

A—Diffuse into the air. Inhale directly or applied to hands, tissue, or a cotton wick. *See COMMENTS under Asthma for a discussion on using* ***plastic nasal inhalers****. These work well if used while studying material that needs to be remembered (i.e. school exams) and then used again during testing to help recall studied material*[240]*.*

Menopause: *See Female Specific Conditions: Menopause.*

Menstruation: *See Female Specific Conditions: Menstruation.*

Mental: *See also Alertness, Energy, Memory, Brain, Stress.*

Oils—[AT]Brain Power (increases capacity and clarity by dissolving petrochemicals), [AT][F]oregano (mental diseases), [A]Common Sense (clarity and focus), [A]sage (strain), [AT]vitex (unrest).

Supplements—Omega Blue (a powerful blend of EPA and DHA from fish oil, plus essential oils to preserve and support delivery to the brain; critical nutrients for proper brain function), OmegaGize[3], True Source (whole food multi-nutrient).

—Accuracy

Oils—[AT]Clarity, [AT]peppermint. Diffuse or inhale.

—Alertness

Oils—[AT]Clarity, [AT]En-R-Gee, [AT]sacred frankincense, [A]hong kuai.

***Comments—*These oils are good for night driving.*

—Fatigue

Oils—[AT][F]Basil, [AT][F]rosemary, [AT][F]ylang ylang, [AT]sacred frankincense, [AT]Awaken, [AT]Aroma Life, [AT]cardamom, [AT]Clarity,
[AT]Dragon Time, [AT]Gentle Baby, [AT]lemongrass, [AT]Mister, [AT]M-Grain, [AT]Relieve It, [A]sage.

Blend #1—Basil and lemongrass together are a good combination.

—Impairment

Supplements—Sulfurzyme.

—Retardation

Supplements—Can be due to a mineral deficiency. KidScents MightyVites, Mineral Essence.

—Stress

Oils—[AT]Clary sage,[AT]Evergreen Essence, [A]pine, [A]Common Sense, [AT]Surrender, [T]Tranquil (roll-on).

Supplements—ImmuPro.

A—Diffuse into the air. Inhale directly or applied to hands, tissue, or a cotton wick. *See COMMENTS under Asthma for a discussion on using* ***plastic nasal inhalers****.*

T—Wear as a perfume or cologne. Dilute as necessary, and apply to temples.

Metabolism:

—Balance

Oils—[A]Clove, [AT]Valor, [AT]EndoFlex (increases), [AT]spearmint, [AT]oregano.

—Increase (over all)

Oils—[I]Spearmint (add to water, and freeze to emulsify throughout), [AT]eucalyptus blue, [AT]spikenard.

—Lipid

Oils—[T]Hyssop (regulates).

—Strengthen (vital centers)

Oils—[AT]Sage.

Supplements—Thyromin (regulates metabolism), Power Meal.

A—Diffuse into the air. Inhale oil applied to tissue or a cotton wick.

T—Dilute as recommended, and apply 1–2 drops on neck or on bottoms of the feet.

Metals: *See Detoxification: Metals. See also Chelation.*

Mice (Repel):

Oils—[A]Purification.

A—Diffuse into the air. Apply to cotton balls, and place in small openings where mice may enter.

Migraine Headaches: *See Headaches: Migraine.*

Mildew: *See also Antifungal.*

Mildew is a whitish fungus that forms a flat growth on plants and organic material. Mildew attacks clothing, leather, paper, ceilings, walls, floors, shower walls, windowsills, and other places with high moisture levels. Mildew can produce a strong musty odor, especially in places with poor air circulation.

Recipe #1—Place a few drops of Purification in a spray bottle, and spray into the air or directly onto a wall to neutralize mildew.

Mind: *See also Alertness, Brain, Energy, Memory, Mental.*

Oils—[AT]Basil (absentminded), [AT]Believe (stimulates), [AT]Surrender (clearing), [A]Common Sense (soothes and focuses), [AT]western red cedar (powerful effects on subconscious and unconscious mind), [AT]sacred frankincense.

A—Diffuse into the air. Inhale directly or applied to hands, tissue, or a cotton wick. *See COMMENTS under Asthma for a discussion on using* ***plastic nasal inhalers****.*

T—Wear as a perfume or cologne. Dilute as necessary, and apply to temples.

Minerals (deficiency):

Supplements—Cleansing Trio (ComforTone, Essentialzyme, and ICP), Mineral Essence.

Miscarriage: *See Pregnancy/Motherhood.*

Mold: *See Antifungal: Mold.*

Moles:

Oils—^T^Frankincense, ^T^Melrose, ^T^geranium, ^T^lavender.

T—Dilute as necessary, and apply on location.

> *I used a combination of lavender and frankincense on a new **mole** that grew in with a very crusty surface. By the time I was able to have an appointment with my doctor, it had totally disappeared.*
>
> ***–Submitted by Judi Arndt***
> ***Colorado Springs, Colorado (July 2004)***

Moment:

—Being In

Oils—^A^Present Time.

A—Inhale directly or applied to hands. Diffuse into the air.

Mono (Mononucleosis): *See also Antiviral, Chronic Fatigue, Epstein-Barr.*

›› *Mononucleosis is viral disease caused by the Epstein-Barr virus and usually spread through contact with infected saliva, tears, and mucous. Symptoms of this disease include fatigue, weakness, severe sore throat, fever, swollen lymph nodes, swollen tonsils, headache, loss of appetite, and a soft or swollen spleen. Once individuals are exposed to the Epstein-Barr virus, they carry the virus for the rest of their lives.*

Oils—^TA^ImmuPower, ^TA^RC, ^TA^Thieves.

Blend #1—3 drops oregano, 3 drops Thieves, and 3 drops thyme. Rub on feet.

—Infectious

Oils—^TA^~F~Ravensara.

Supplements—Build immune system. Inner Defense, Cleansing Trio (ComforTone, Essentialzyme, and ICP), ImmuPro, Power Meal, Super C / Super C Chewable, True Source (whole food multi-nutrient).

T—Dilute as necessary, and apply on throat and on feet.

A—Diffuse into the air. Inhale directly or applied to the hands.

Mood Swings: *See also Hormonal Imbalance.*

Oils—^A^Clary sage, ^A^Peace & Calming, ^A^lavender, ^A^Valor, ^A^ylang ylang, ^A^Acceptance, ^A^bergamot, ^A^Dragon Time or ^A^Mister, ^A^fennel, ^A^Gathering, ^A^geranium, ^A^Harmony, ^A^jasmine, ^A^Joy, ^A^juniper, ^A^lemon, ^A^peppermint, ^A^Present Time, ^A^rose, ^A^rosemary, ^A^sage, ^A^sage lavender, ^A^sandalwood, ^A^spruce, ^A^Trauma Life, ^A^yarrow.

A—Diffuse into the air. Inhale directly or applied to hands, tissue, or a cotton wick.

***Comments—Can be due to a vitamin B deficiency.

Supplements—AlkaLime (if due to over-acidification), Super B.

Morning Sickness: *See Pregnancy/Motherhood.*

Personal Guide

Mosquitoes: *See also Insect.*

***Comments—Frequent mosquito bites could be due to a vitamin B deficiency.

Supplements—Super B.

Mother (Problems with):

Oils—TAAcceptance, TAgeranium, TAValor.

T—Apply to **mother** auricular emotion point. Dilute with V-6 Oil to create massage oil, and massage into skin. Add 1–3 drops to 1/4 cup Epsom salts, and dissolve in warm bathwater for bathing.

A—Diffuse into the air. Inhale directly or applied to hands, tissue, or a cotton wick.

Motion Sickness: *See also Nausea.*

>> *Motion sickness is a feeling of illness that occurs as a result of repeated movement, such as that experience in a car, on a boat, or on a plane. These motions interfere with the body's sense of balance and equilibrium. The most common symptoms of motion sickness include dizziness, fatigue, and nausea.*

Oils—TA FPeppermint, TAginger, TADi-Gize, TAM-Grain, TAnutmeg,TA spearmint.

T—Apply to feet, temples, and wrists.

A—Inhale directly or applied to hands, tissue, or a cotton wick. Diffuse into the air. *See COMMENTS under Asthma for a discussion on using **plastic nasal inhalers**.*

Recipe #1—Apply a drop or two of Di-Gize to the hands; stir in a clockwise motion, apply behind both ears, rub hands together, cup over nose and mouth, and breathe deeply.

***Comments—According to the Essential Oils Desk Reference, "Mix 4 drops peppermint and 4 drops ginger in 1 ounce V-6 Oil. Rub on chest and stomach before traveling." (EDR–June 2002; Ch. 28; Digestion Problems; Travel Sickness)

Motivation:

—To Move Forward

Oils—ATEnvision (emotional support), ATMagnify Your Purpose (empowering and uplifting), ATMotivation, ATmyrrh, ATLive with Passion.

A—Diffuse into the air. Inhale directly or applied to hands, tissue, or a cotton wick.

T—Dilute with V-6 Oil to create massage oil, and massage into skin.

Supplements—Sulfurzyme.

MRSA (Methicillin Resistant Staphylococcus Aureus): *See Antibacterial: MRSA.*

M

Mucus: *See Congestion: Mucus. See also Anticatarrhal.*

Multiple Sclerosis (M.S.): *See also Myelin Sheath.*

According to D. Gary Young, progesterone is absolutely necessary in manufacturing, building, repairing, and rejuvenating the myelin sheath. Progesterone is naturally produced from pregnenolone.

>> *Multiple sclerosis (MS) is an autoimmune disease in which the immune system attacks and gradually destroys the myelin sheath (which covers and insulates the nerves) and the underlying nerve fibers of the central nervous system. This destruction of the myelin sheath interferes with communication between the brain and the rest of the body. Symptoms of MS include par-*

tial or complete loss of vision, tingling, burning, pain in parts of the body, tremors, loss of coordination, unsteady gait, dizziness, and memory problems.

Oils—**TA**Frankincense, **TA**sandalwood, **TA**peppermint, **TA**Aroma Siez, **TA**Clarity, **TA**cypress, **TA**elemi, **TA**geranium, **TA**helichrysum, **TA**Idaho tansy, **TA**juniper, **TA**oregano, **TA**Peace & Calming, **TA**rosemary, **TA**sage, **TA**thyme, **TA**wintergreen.

T—Dilute as necessary, and apply on spine, back of neck, and feet. Dilute with V-6 Oil to create a massage oil, and massage on back and neck.

A—Diffuse into the air. Inhale directly or applied to hands.

******Comments**—Do the Raindrop Technique.

Personal Care—PD 80/20, Prenolone/Prenolone+, Progessence/Progessence Plus.

Supplements—Cleansing Trio (ComforTone, Essentialzyme, and ICP), ImmuPro, Inner Defense, JuvaPower/JuvaSpice, JuvaTone, Mineral Essence, MultiGreens, Omega Blue/OmegaGize[3] (a powerful blend of EPA and DHA from fish oil plus essential oils to preserve and support delivery to the brain; critical nutrients for proper brain function), Power Meal, Sulfurzyme, Super B, Super C / Super C Chewable, True Source (whole food multi-nutrient).

The following are recipes that have been used successfully:

Recipe #1—Supplement with MultiGreens, Cleansing Trio (ComforTone, Essentialzyme, and ICP), and Super C / Super C Chewable. Blend 10 drops cardamom, 10 drops peppermint, and 10 drops rosemary with 1 oz. V-6 Oil for a full body massage. Finally, diffuse Acceptance and Awaken.

Recipe #2—Supplement with 8 Super Cal, 2 Super B (after breakfast), 6 Super C / Super C Chewable, 6 MultiGreens four times a day, and Master Formula His/Hers. Apply juniper and peppermint, one at a time, on the spine. If the M.S. is in the neck, work up the spine. If it is in the legs, work down the spine. Do a cold compress, and wait for 30 minutes. Remove the compress and repeat again.

Recipe #3—Take 2 droppers full of Mineral Essence morning and evening to conduct the current to reconnect the nerve tissues. Take ½ Super B in the morning and evening with meals for the first week. Then increase the dosage. Use juniper, geranium, and peppermint on the bottoms of the feet and up the legs and spine. Apply oils in the direction of the paralysis. Apply juniper and cypress on the base of the neck; then add Aroma Siez. Next do the Raindrop Technique on the spine using oregano and thyme. Use Peace & Calming and Clarity for brain function and cypress for circulation. Use the Cleansing Trio (ComforTone, Essentialzyme, and ICP) and JuvaTone. Also use Super C / Super C Chewable for six days. Then start on Super B morning and evening with a meal, 6 MultiGreens four times a day.

Blend #1—6 drops juniper, 4 drops sandalwood, 2 drops peppermint, and 12 drops geranium. Mix, and massage into neck, spine, and bottoms of feet.

******Comments**—Avoid hot baths, etc. Heat is the worst thing you can do. If anything, insulate the body with ice packs. Lowering the body temperature with cold packs helps to regenerate the myelin sheath. The person can be kept in the cold packs either for as long as they can stand it or until their body temperature drops 3 degrees. The body temperature must be monitored closely to avoid lowering it too far. This process can be repeated until the person can only stand being in the cold packs for 20 minutes. It is also best to avoid diet foods, especially those that contain aspartame, as it is known to cause MS, brain damage, and other problems.

Mumps: *See Childhood Diseases: Mumps.*

Muscles:

Oils—ᵀMarjoram, ᵀAroma Siez, ᵀpeppermint[241], ᵀwintergreen, ᵀDeep Relief (roll-on), ᵀbasil, ᵀcypress, ᵀbalsam fir, ᵀlavender, ᵀlemongrass, ᵀpalo santo, ᵀValor, ᵀwhite fir.

Personal Care—Ortho Ease Massage Oil, Ortho Sport Massage Oil, Relaxation Massage Oil (these oils are great for all problems associated with muscles).

Supplements—BLM, Mineral Essence, NingXia Red, Power Meal, Pure Protein Complete (the ideal blend of 5 ultraclean, ultrabioactive whey proteins; provides prolonged assimilation for better protein synthesis), Sulfurzyme, Super Cal, Super C Chewable, Wolfberry Crisp Bars (*Refer to the Wolfberry Crisp Bar in the Supplements section of the Reference Guide for Essential Oils for more information on the benefits of the Ningxia Wolfberry*).

*****Comments**—One professional trainer for body builders used Be-Fit, Power Meal, and Wolfberry Bars to increase muscle mass and strength beyond anything he had previously achieved!

—Aches and Pains

Oils—ᵀPanAway, ᵀDeep Relief (roll-on), ᵀwintergreen, ᵀ_F clove, ᵀAroma Siez, ᵀwhite fir (with inflammation), ᵀcopaiba, ᵀblue cypress, ᵀbalsam fir, ᵀDouglas fir, ᵀginger, ᵀhelichrysum, ᵀlavender, ᵀlemongrass (especially good for ligaments), ᵀmarjoram, ᵀnutmeg, ᵀoregano, ᵀpalo santo, ᵀpeppermint, ᵀRelieve It, ᵀRoman chamomile, ᵀrosemary, ᵀspearmint, ᵀthyme, ᵀvetiver.

Supplements—Sulfurzyme.

*****Comments**—*Refer to the chapter entitled "How to Use—The Personal Usage Reference" in the Essential Oils Desk Reference under "Muscles" for some excellent blends to help sore and tight muscles.*

—Anti-Inflammatory *See also Anti-inflammatory*

Oils—ᵀFrankincense, ᵀpeppermint, ᵀDeep Relief (roll-on), ᵀbasil, ᵀbalsam fir, ᵀwhite fir.

*****Comments**—*Refer to the chapter entitled "How to Use—The Personal Usage Reference" in the Essential Oils Desk Reference under "Muscles" for an excellent blend to help reduce inflammation.*

—Cardiac Muscle *See also Cardiovascular System: Heart*

Oils—ᵀᴬMarjoram, ᵀᴬlavender, ᵀᴬrosemary verbenon (helps regulate), ᵀᴬgoldenrod, ᵀᴬneroli, ᵀᴬpeppermint, ᵀᴬrose.

—Cramps/Charley Horses

▸▸ *A muscle cramp or charley horse is the sudden, involuntary contraction of a muscle. Muscle cramps can occur in any muscle in the body, but they usually occur in the thigh, calf, or arch of the foot. Cramps can be caused by excessive strain to the muscle, injury, overuse, dehydration, a lack of necessary salts or minerals, or a lack of blood flow to the muscle. Muscle cramps can happen during or after a physical activity and while lying in bed.*

Oils—ᵀAroma Siez, ᵀmarjoram, ᵀDeep Relief (roll-on), ᵀrosemary, ᵀbasil, ᵀclary sage, ᵀcoriander, ᵀcypress, ᵀgrapefruit, ᵀjasmine, ᴬlavender, ᵀpine, ᵀRoman chamomile, ᵀthyme, ᵀvetiver.

Supplements—BLM, Mineral Essence, Sulfurzyme, Super Cal.

Blend #1—Equal parts rosemary and Aroma Siez. Apply neat; or mix with V-6 Oil, and massage.

—Development

▸▸ *When muscles are stretched or used during exercise, they produce a substance that activates stem cells already present in the tissue. Once these cells are activated, they begin to divide—creating new muscle fiber, and thereby increasing the size and strength of the muscles.*

Oils—ᵀWintergreen (with spruce), ᵀPanAway.

Supplements— MultiGreens (stimulates and strengthens), Power Meal, Pure Protein Complete, Super Cal.

—Fatigue

Oils—ᵀMarjoram, ᵀbalsam fir, ᵀcypress, ᵀDouglas fir, ᵀpeppermint, ᵀAroma Siez, ᵀeucalyptus, ᵀgrapefruit, ᵀravensara, ᵀrosemary, ᵀthyme.

Supplements—Mineral Essence, Super Cal.

—Inflammation: *See Anti-Inflammatory*

—Over-Exercised

Oils—ᵀBalsam fir, ᵀwhite fir (with inflammation), ᵀeucalyptus, ᵀDeep Relief (roll-on), ᵀDouglas fir, ᵀginger, ᵀlavender, ᵀthyme.

Bath—3 drops marjoram and 2 drops lemon in a tub of water. Soak.

Blend #1—Equal parts of eucalyptus, peppermint, and ginger. Mix with V-6 Oil, and massage.

—Rheumatism (Muscular) *See also Fibromyalgia*

Oils—ᵀPalo santo, ᵀrosemary, ᵀthyme.

—Smooth Muscle

Oils—ᵀMarjoram, ᵀrosemary[242], ᵀpeppermint, ᵀbergamot, ᵀblack pepper, ᵀclary sage, ᵀcypress, ᵀfennel, ᵀjuniper, ᵀlavender, ᵀmelissa, ᵀneroli, ᵀRoman chamomile, ᵀsandalwood.

***__Comments__—*Essential oils with high proportions of ester compounds are especially effective.*

—Spasms

Oils—ᵀBasil, ᵀmarjoram, ᵀPanAway, ᵀRoman chamomile, ᵀAroma Siez, ᵀclary sage, ᵀcypress, ᵀlavender, ᵀjasmine, ᵀpeppermint.

Personal Care—Cel-Lite Magic, Ortho Ease Massage Oil.

Supplements—Super Cal.

—Sprains

▸▸*A sprain is an injury to a ligament caused by excessive stretching. The ligament can have little tears in it, or it can be completely torn apart and still be considered a sprain. The most common areas to receive a sprain are the ankle, knee, and wrist. After a person receives a sprain, the area will swell rapidly and be quite painful.*

Oils—ᵀ$_F$Marjoram, ᵀlemongrass, ᵀPanAway, ᵀwhite fir, ᵀAroma Siez, ᵀblack pepper, ᵀclove, ᵀeucalyptus, ᵀginger, ᵀhelichrysum, ᵀIdaho tansy, ᵀjasmine, ᵀlavender, ᵀPeace & Calming, ᵀnutmeg, ᵀpine, ᵀRoman chamomile, ᵀrose, ᵀrosemary, ᵀthyme, ᵀvetiver.

—Stiffness

Oils—ᵀAroma Siez, ᵀPanAway, ᵀDeep Relief (roll-on).

—Tension (especially in shoulders and neck)

Oils—ᵀMarjoram, ᵀAroma Siez, ᵀRelieve It, ᵀpeppermint[241], ᵀDeep Relief (roll-on), ᵀDouglas fir, ᵀhelichrysum, ᵀjuniper, ᵀlavender, ᵀRoman chamomile, ᵀspruce.

Personal Care—Ortho Ease and Ortho Sport Massage Oils, Evening Peace Bath & Shower Gel (relaxes tired, fatigued muscles and helps alleviate tension).

—Tissue

Supplements—Pure Protein Complete and Power Meal (contain a complete amino acid and vitamin profile and have a high level of predigested protein to maintain a good food supply for muscle tissue), BLM, Ultra Young+ (increase production of growth hormone, which increases formation of lean muscle tissue).

***Comments—*Refer to the chapter entitled "How to Use—The Personal Usage Reference" in the Essential Oils Desk Reference under "Muscles" for some excellent blends to help improve circulation in the muscles and to aid in the regeneration of muscle tissue.*

—TONE

Oils—Apply these oils before exercise. ᵀCypress, ᵀwintergreen, ᵀmarjoram, ᵀbasil, ᵀblack pepper, ᵀginger, ᵀgrapefruit, ᵀjuniper, ᵀlavender, ᵀlime, ᵀorange, ᵀpeppermint, ᵀpetitgrain, ᵀpine, ᵀrosemary, ᵀthyme.

Supplements— Pure Protein Complete, Sulfurzyme.

***Comments—*Poor muscle tone may indicate a sulfur deficiency.*

—TORN MUSCLES

Oils—ᵀHelichrysum and ᵀspruce (take pain away—use hot packs), ᵀlemongrass, ᵀginger (circulation), ᵀlemon myrtle.

Personal Care—Ortho Sport Massage Oil.

T—Dilute as necessary, and apply on location. Dilute with V-6 Oil to create a massage oil, and massage into desired muscles. Add 1–2 drops to warm bathwater, and bathe. Apply as hot (or cold for strains or sprains) compress.

A—Diffuse into the air.

Muscular Dystrophy:

▸▸ *Muscular dystrophy is any of several genetic diseases that cause gradual weakening of the skeletal muscles. The most common forms, Duchenne and Becker muscular dystrophies, are caused by a gene defect that inhibits or alters the production of dystrophin, a protein necessary for proper muscle cell structure.*

Oils—ᵀLemongrass, ᵀmarjoram (combine with equal parts lemongrass), ᵀbasil, ᵀrosemary, ᵀAroma Siez, ᵀeucalyptus, ᵀgeranium, ᵀginger, ᵀlavender, ᵀlemon, ᵀorange, ᵀpine, ᵀRelieve It.

Personal Care—Ortho Ease Massage Oil, Ortho Sport Massage Oil.

Supplements—Essentialzyme, Essentialzymes-4, Mineral Essence, MultiGreens, Power Meal, Sulfurzyme, Thyromin, Ultra Young+.

T—Dilute as necessary, and apply on location. Dilute with V-6 Oil to create a massage oil, and massage on location. Add 1–2 drops to warm bathwater, and bathe. Apply as a cold compress.

Myelin Sheath:

▸▸ *The myelin sheath is an insulating layer of protein and fatty substances that forms around nerves (including those in the brain), increasing the speed of nerve impulses. Damage to the myelin sheath interrupts these nerve impulses and can cause diseases such as multiple sclerosis, peripheral neuropathy, central pontine myelinolysis, and other neurological diseases.*

Oils—ᵀImmuPower, ᵀpeppermint, ᵀjuniper, ᵀgeranium

T—Apply with **cold** compress *(remember, **no heat**!).*

Supplements—Omega Blue/OmegaGize[3] (contains DHA, which helps support the myelin sheath), ImmuPro.

Nails:

Oils—TCitrus Fresh, Tlemon (repeated use may help harden), Tmelaleuca[243] (infection), Tfrankincense, Tmyrrh, Teucalyptus, Tgrapefruit, Tlavender, Tlime, Tmelaleuca, Toregano, Tpatchouli, Tpeppermint, Travensara, Trosemary, Tthyme.

T—Dilute as necessary, and apply on nails.

Blend #1—Equal parts frankincense, lemon, and myrrh. Mix with a couple drops of wheat germ oil, and apply 2–3 times per week.

Supplements—Sulfurzyme (helps with growth and removal of ridges and cracks), Mineral Essence, Super Cal.

***Comments—*A deficiency in sulfur can cause poor nail growth.*

Narcolepsy:

▸▸ *Narcolepsy is a disorder that is characterized by sudden and uncontrollable drowsiness and attacks of sleep at unexpected and irregular intervals. It is frequently misdiagnosed as hypothyroidism (insufficient thyroid hormone), hypoglycemia (insufficient blood sugar), epilepsy, or multiple sclerosis. Proper diagnosis requires overnight monitoring with a device used to detect brain waves called an electroencephalograph.*

Oils—ATBrain Power

A—Diffuse into the air. Inhale directly or applied to hands.

T—Apply to the brain stem, neck, and Vita Flex points on the feet.

Supplements—Mineral Essence, MultiGreens, Thyromin, Ultra Young+.

***Comments—*Establishing a routine of strict bedtimes and daytime naps may also help reduce the number of unexpected sleep attacks.*

Nasal: *See Nose.*

Nausea: *See also Motion Sickness, Pregnancy/Motherhood: Morning Sickness, Vomiting.*

Oils—IATGinger[244], A$_F$peppermint, AT$_F$lavender, ATcalamus, ATcardamom, ATclove, TDi-Gize (over stomach and colon), ATjuniper, ATM-Grain, ATnutmeg, ATrosewood, ATspearmint, ATtarragon.

A—Diffuse. Inhale directly. *See COMMENTS under Asthma for a discussion on using plastic nasal inhalers.*

I—Place 2–5 drops in an empty capsule, and swallow.

T—Apply behind ears and on Vita Flex points.

Blend #1—2 drops lavender, 2 drops spearmint, and 2 drops of another oil for your type of nausea. Mix together, and put a little on a cotton ball; inhale three times a day, or diffuse.

Neck:

Oils—TGeranium, Tclary sage, Tlemongrass, Tbasil, Tlemon, Torange, Thelichrysum.

T—Dilute with V-6 Oil to create a massage oil, and massage on neck.

Supplements—BLM.

—Chronic Pain

Oils—TPanAway.

T—Apply to base of big toe.

Negative Ions: *See Ions: Negative.*

Negativity:

Oils—ATSandalwood (removes negative programming from the cells), ATTransformation.

—Breaks Up

Oils—ATDream Catcher, ATForgiveness, ATpalo santo.

—Drowning In Own

Oils—AGrapefruit.

A—Diffuse into the air. Inhale directly or applied to tissue or a cotton wick.

T—Apply to auricular emotion points. Dilute with V-6 Oil to create a massage oil, and massage onto the skin.

Nervous System: *See also Lou Gehrig's Disease, Carpal Tunnel Syndrome, Multiple Sclerosis, Paralysis, Parkinson's Disease*

▸▸ *The nervous system is a network of nerve cells that regulates the body's reaction to external and internal stimuli. The nervous system sends and receives nerve impulses to and from organs and muscles throughout the body. The body relies on these impulses to function. The nervous system is comprised of the* ***central nervous system*** *(the brain and spinal cord) and the* ***peripheral nervous system*** *(all other nerves). The peripheral nervous system is comprised of the* ***somatic nervous system*** *(nerves that connect to the skeletal muscles and sensory nerve receptors in the skin) and the* ***autonomic nervous system*** *(nerves that connect to the cardiac and smooth muscles and other organs, tissues, and systems that don't require conscious effort to control). The autonomic system is divided further into two main parts as well: the sympathetic and parasympathetic nervous systems. The* ***sympathetic nervous system*** *functions to accelerate heart rate, increase blood pressure, slow digestion, and constrict blood vessels. It activates the "fight or flight" response in order to deal with threatening or stressful situations. The* ***parasympathetic nervous system*** *functions to slow heart rate, store energy, stimulate digestive activity, and relax specific muscles. It allows the body to return to a normal and calm state after experiencing pain or stress.*

Oils—TAPeppermint[245] (soothes and strengthens; place on wrists or location of nerve damage), TA$_F$basil (stimulant and for nervous breakdown), TAlavender[246], ATlemon[247], ATgrapefruit[248], ATpepper[248] (stimulant), TAfrankincense[249], TA$_F$sage, TAcopaiba[250], TAlemongrass (for nerve damage; activates), ATRutaVaLa, TAjuniper[251] (better nerve function), TArosemary[252], TAbalsam fir, ATbergamot, ATBrain Power, TAcalamus, TAcedarwood (nervous tension), TAcinnamon bark, TAcumin (stimulant), TADi-Gize, TAgeranium (regenerates nerves), TAginger, Ajasmine (nervous exhaustion), TAmarjoram (soothing), TA-*Melaleuca ericifolia* (nervous tension), TAnutmeg (supports), TAorange, TApalmarosa (supports), ATPeace & Calming, TApetitgrain (reestablishes nerve equilibrium), TApine (stimulant), TAravensara, TARoman chamomile, TAsage lavender, TAsandalwood, TAspearmint, TAspruce (fatigue), TAvalerian (central nervous system depressant), TAvetiver.

Personal Care—Regenolone (helps nerve regeneration).

Supplements—Mineral Essence, Omega Blue, OmegaGize[3], Sulfurzyme, Super B.

—Nervousness *See also Calming*

Oils—ATOrange[254], ATcypress, ATgoldenrod, ATSurrender, ATtangerine.

—Neuralgia

▸▸ *Neuralgia is intense pain felt along the path of a nerve. Neuralgia results from damage or irritation to a nerve. Causes can include certain drugs, diabetes, infections, inflammation, trauma, and chemical irritation.*

Oils—TA$_F$Marjoram, TAeucalyptus[252], TA$_F$Roman chamomile, TAcajeput, TAcedarwood, TAhelichrysum, TAjuniper, TAlavender, TAnutmeg, TApine, TAsage lavender.

—Neuritis

▸▸ *Neuritis is the inflammation of a nerve or of a group of nerves. Neuritis causes pain, poor reflexes, and muscle atrophy.*

Oils—TA F Roman chamomile, TA eucalyptus[252], TA lavender, TA cedarwood, TA clove, TA juniper, TA yarrow.

—Neurological Problems

Oils—Limit the use of oils with high *ketone* content.

*****Comments**—A 4 year old child was in a car accident where she suffered severe brain damage. The surgeon removed part of her brain, which sent her into a coma. After being in a coma for two months, Dr. Friedmann was asked to help her. He used oils that are commonly used for neurological problems. He put Valor on the back of her neck, skull, and feet. He also used Present Time and Awaken. She came out of the coma and started doing physical therapy.

—Neuropathy

▸▸ *Neuropathy is the broad term for any of a series of diseases that adversely affect the nerves or nerve cells. Some forms of neuropathy include peripheral neuropathy (the most common), cranial neuropathy, auditory neuropathy, and optic neuropathy.*

Oils—TA Lemongrass, TA peppermint, TA eucalyptus, TA lavender, TA Roman chamomile, TA Brain Power, TA cedarwood, TA cypress, TA geranium, TA helichrysum, TA juniper, TA JuvaFlex, TA Valor.

Personal Care—PD 80/20, Prenolone/Prenolone+, Progessence/Progessence Plus, Regenolone.

Supplements—Mineral Essence, Sulfurzyme, Super B.

*****Comments**—Refer to the chapter entitled "How to Use—The Personal Usage Reference" in the Essential Oils Desk Reference under "Nerve Disorders," subcategory "Neuropathy," for some excellent blends.

–Pain

Recipe #1—Apply Relieve It, helichrysum, and/or PanAway with a cold compress. Massage with peppermint, juniper, and geranium, and reapply cold compresses.

—Neurotonic

Oils—AT Melaleuca, AT F ravensara, AT thyme.

—Parasympathetic Nervous System

Oils—AT Lavender[246], AT F lemongrass (regulates), AT F marjoram (increases tone of), AT Peace & Calming, T Tranquil (roll-on), AT Valor.

Diffusion—*See Ions: Negative for a list of oils that ionize negatively when diffused to help stimulate the parasympathetic nervous system.*

*****Comments**—See the Autonomic Nervous System chart in the Science and Application section of the Reference Guide for Essential Oils.

—Sympathetic Nervous System

Oils—AT Grapefruit[248], AT black pepper[248], AT fennel[248], AT Brain Power, AT Clarity, AT *Eucalyptus radiata*, AT ginger, AT peppermint.

*****Comments**—Stimulation of certain areas of the Sympathetic Nervous System can be achieved by application of any of the above oils at the appropriate places along the spinal column (*refer to the Autonomic Nervous System chart in the Science and Application section of the Reference Guide for Essential Oils*).

Supplements—Mineral Essence, Power Meal, Sulfurzyme, Super Cal, Ultra Young+.

***Comments—*Stress can create a condition that has been termed as "Sympathetic System Override," where the production of cortisol, adrenalin, and 5HT (serotonin) skyrockets and heavily overloads the lymphatic and cardiovascular systems. Essential oils can help suppress "Sympathetic System Override"; and the following recipe has been used to do just that—and to bring the body back into a parasympathetic state.*

Recipe #2—Apply frankincense to the top of the spine (at the base of the skull), and work it in. This is the "gatekeeper," and it helps prepare the body to more effectively transmit and utilize the oils that follow. Then apply 3–5 drops of each of the following oils, one at a time, up the back of the neck, and work each one in individually: valerian, vetiver, and balsam fir. Other oils can be added, such as Roman chamomile, helichrysum, clove, and peppermint.

—Virus of Nerves

Blend #1—Clove and frankincense.

T—Dilute as necessary, and apply on location, spine, back of neck, or Vita Flex points on the feet. Dilute with V-6 Oil to create a massage oil, and massage on location. Add 1–2 drops to warm bathwater, and bathe.

A—Diffuse into the air. Inhale directly or applied to the hands.

Neuralgia: *See Nervous System: Neuralgia.*

Neuritis: *See Nervous System: Neuritis.*

Neurological Problems: *See Nervous System: Neurological Problems.*

Neuromuscular:

Oils—**T**Roman chamomile, **T**tarragon.

T—Dilute as necessary, and apply on location, spine, back of neck, or Vita Flex points on the feet. Dilute with V-6 Oil to create a massage oil, and massage on location. Add 1–2 drops to warm bathwater, and bathe.

Neuropathy: *See Nervous System: Neuropathy.*

Neurotonic: *See Nervous System: Neurotonic.*

Night Sweats: *See also Hot Flashes and Hormonal Imbalance.*

Oils—**TA**$_F$Sage, **TA**EndoFlex.

T—Dilute as necessary, and apply on temples, forehead, or bottoms of feet. Dilute with V-6 Oil to create a massage oil, and massage on back of neck or spine. Add 1–2 drops to warm bathwater, and bathe.

A—Diffuse into the air. Inhale directly or applied to the hands.

Nose:

Oils—**TA**Melaleuca, **TA**rosemary.

—Bleeding

Oils—**T**Helichrysum, **T**cypress, **T**frankincense, **T**lavender, **T**lemon.

Blend #1—2 drops cypress, 1 drop helichrysum, and 2 drops lemon in 8 oz. ice water. Soak cloth, and apply to nose and to back of neck.

—NASAL MUCUS MEMBRANE

Oils—Both **AT**eucalyptus and **AT**peppermint may help reduce inflammation.

—NASAL NASOPHARYNX

Oils—**AT**Eucalyptus.

—POLYPS *See also Polyps.*

A nasal polyp is an abnormal tissue growth inside the nose. Since nasal polyps are not cancerous, very small polyps generally do not cause any problems. But larger polyps can obstruct the nasal passage and make it difficult to breath or smell and can cause frequent sinus infections. Possible symptoms of polyps include runny nose, decreased sense of smell, decreased sense of taste, snoring, facial pain or headache, itching around the eyes, and persistent congestion.

Oils—**TA**Frankincense, **TA**RC (can be applied to inside of nose with cotton swab), **TA**oregano, **TA**basil, **TA**citronella, **TA**peppermint, **TA**Purification.

***Comments**—A colon and liver cleanse may be helpful. Wintergreen or Valor may also be applied to bridge of nose for possible structural realignment.

***Comments**—Nasal polyps are caused by an overproduction of fluid in the mucous membranes. They are seen with asthma, hay fever, chronic sinus infections, and cystic fibrosis. In fact, one source stated that one out of four people with cystic fibrosis have nasal polyps. They may also be a result of blockages in the brain or of some trauma to the nose in which structural integrity has been compromised. Diet may also be a factor.

T—Dilute as necessary, and apply to exterior of nose (use caution because of close proximity to eyes)

A—Diffuse into the air, and breathe in diffused mist.

Nursing: *See Pregnancy/Motherhood: NURSING.*

Obesity: *See also Diet, Weight.*

Oils—**AI**Grapefruit[254], **A**fennel[248], **AI**orange, **IA**Slique Essence, **A**rosemary, **A**GLF, **A**juniper, **A**Juva Cleanse, **AI**tangerine.

Supplements—Balance Complete, Digest + Cleanse, JuvaPower/JuvaSpice, NingXia Red, Power Meal (eat for breakfast as a meal replacement), Slique Tea, Slique Bar, Slique Gum, Slique Slim Caps, Wolfberry Crisp Bars.

—REDUCE

Oils—**A**Juva Cleanse, **AI**orange, **AI**tangerine.

A—Diffuse into the air. Inhale directly or applied to hands, tissue, or a cotton wick.

I—Add 1 drop to 8–12 oz. of water, and drink.

Obsessiveness:

Oils—**AT**Acceptance, **AT**Awaken, **AT**clary sage, **AT**cypress, **AT**Forgiveness, **AT**geranium, **AT**helichrysum, **AT**Humility, **AT**Inner Child, **AT**Joy, **AT**lavender, **AT**marjoram, **AT**Motivation, **AT**Present Time, **AT**rose, **AT**Sacred Mountain, **AT**sandalwood, **AT**Valor, **AT**ylang ylang.

A—Diffuse into the air. Inhale directly or applied to tissue or a cotton wick.

T—Apply to auricular emotion points. Dilute with V-6 Oil to create a massage oil, and massage onto the skin.

Odors: *See also Deodorant.*

Oils—**AT**Purification (neutralizes and eliminates), **AT**bergamot, **AT**lavender.

Personal Care—AromaGuard Deodorants.

—Body

Oils—**T**Purification (obnoxious odors).

—Controlling

Oils—**AT**Cedarwood.

A—Diffuse into the air. Dissolve 8–10 drops in 1 tsp. perfumers or pure grain alcohol, and combine with distilled water in a 1 oz. spray bottle. Spray into the air or on affected surface.

T—Dilute as necessary, and apply on skin or under arms. Add 2–3 drops to 1 Tbs. baking soda, and apply under the arms, on the feet, or on other areas of the body.

Opening (to receive):

Oils—**A**Fir, **AT**Transformation.

A—Diffuse into the air. Inhale directly or applied to tissue or a cotton wick.

T—Apply to chakras. Dilute with V-6 Oil to create a massage oil, and massage onto the skin.

Opposition:

Oils—**AT**Valor.

A—Diffuse into the air. Inhale directly or applied to tissue or a cotton wick.

T—Apply to auricular emotion points. Dilute with V-6 Oil to create a massage oil, and massage onto the skin.

Oral Conditions: *See also Gums, Teeth.*

Oils—**T**$_F$Rosewood.

T—Dilute as necessary, and swab on location in mouth. Mix 1–2 drops with 4 oz. of water, and use as mouth-rinse. Place 5–6 drops with 1 oz. distilled water in a small spray bottle, and mist into the mouth.

—Abscess

Recipe #1—Apply helichrysum, Purification, or Roman chamomile using a hot compress on face. It may also help to apply one drop of oil to a cotton ball and apply it directly to the abscess. Put Thieves on a rolled-up gauze, and place over abscess to pull out the infection.

Blend #1—Use clove, wintergreen, myrrh, and helichrysum to help with infection.

—Gingivitis

>> *Gingivitis is an inflammation of the gums because of bacteria associated with plaque buildup. When infected with gingivitis, the gums become red and swollen and often bleed during teeth brushing.*

Oils—**T**Thieves, **T**$_F$sage[255], **T**melaleuca[256], **T**Melrose, **T**Forgiveness, **T**Harmony, **T**helichrysum, **T**myrrh, **T**Present Time, **T**rose, **T**rosemary.

T—Dilute as necessary, and apply on throat and gums.

Personal Care—Thieves AromaBright or Dentarome/Dentarome Plus Toothpaste, Thieves Fresh Essence Plus Mouthwash, KidScents Toothpaste (for children).

—**Gum Disease**

▸▸ *Gum disease is an infection of the tissue and bones surrounding the teeth and is caused by a buildup of plaque. Gum disease consists of two parts: first gingivitis and then periodontal disease.*

Oils—[T]Thieves, [T]$_F$melaleuca[256], [T]Melrose (fights infection), [T]Forgiveness, [T]Harmony, [T]myrrh, [T]Present Time, [T]tsuga.

T—Dilute as necessary, and apply on throat and gums.

Personal Care—Thieves AromaBright or Dentarome/Dentarome Plus Toothpaste, Thieves Fresh Essence Plus Mouthwash.

—**Halitosis (Bad Breath)**

Oils—[T]$_F$Peppermint[257], [T]Thieves, [T]$_F$nutmeg, [T]cardamom, [T]lavender.

T—Mix 1–2 drops with 4 oz. of water, and use as mouth-rinse. Combine 5–6 drops with 1 oz. distilled water in a small spray bottle, and mist into the mouth.

> *Don't you just love the feel of clean teeth and fresh breath! Try putting a drop of Thieves on your toothbrush instead of toothpaste. At first it is a little warm, but it sure feels refreshing. If this doesn't work for you, try putting a drop on your toothpaste; or put 10 drops of Thieves in a small spray bottle full of distilled water, and mist it in your mouth before brushing your teeth.*

Supplements—AlkaLime.

Personal Care—Thieves AromaBright or Dentarome/Dentarome Plus Toothpaste, Thieves Fresh Essence Plus Mouthwash, KidScents Toothpaste (for children).

—**Infection**

Oils—[T]Melaleuca, [T]Thieves, [T]clove and [T]frankincense, [T]helichrysum, [T]myrrh.

T—Dilute as necessary, and apply to jaws and gums.

Personal Care—Thieves AromaBright or Dentarome/Dentarome Plus Toothpaste, Thieves Fresh Essence Plus Mouthwash, KidScents Toothpaste (for children).

Osteomyelitis: *See Bones: Osteomyelitis.*

Osteoporosis: *See Bones: Osteoporosis.*

Ovaries: *See also Female Specific Conditions, Hormonal Imbalance.*

Oils—[TA]$_F$Rosemary (regulates), [TA]$_F$myrtle, [TA]Di-Gize, [TA]geranium, [TA] Gratitude.

—**Ovarian Cysts**

Oils—[TA]Basil.

Blend #1—5 drops frankincense and 5 drops Melrose. Mix, and apply to lower back and abdomen. May also consider adding this blend to 2 tsp. of olive oil and, before going to bed, while lying down, inserting blend into vagina and retaining with a tampon throughout the night.

Personal Care—PD 80/20, Prenolone/Prenolone+, Progessence/Progessence Plus, Protec.

Supplements—FemiGen (helps feed the body), Master Formula Hers.

T—Dilute as necessary, and apply on abdomen and on Vita Flex points on the feet. Dilute with V-6 Oil to create a massage oil, and massage onto abdomen and lower back. Add 1–2 drops to 2 tsp. olive oil, insert into vagina, and retain overnight with a tampon.

A—Diffuse into the air. Inhale directly or applied to hands, tissue, or a cotton wick.

Overcome and Release Unpleasant, Difficult Issues in Life:

Oils—**AT**Acceptance, **AT**Release, **AT**Roman chamomile, **AT**SARA, **AT**Transformation, **AT**Trauma Life.

A—Diffuse into the air. Inhale directly or applied to tissue or a cotton wick.

T—Apply to auricular emotion points. Dilute with V-6 Oil to create a massage oil, and massage onto the skin.

Overeating: *See Eating Disorders.*

Overweight: *See Obesity and Weight.*

Overwhelmed:

Oils—**AT**Acceptance, **AT**Hope, **AT**Release, **AT**Valor.

A—Diffuse into the air. Inhale directly or applied to tissue or a cotton wick.

T—Apply to auricular emotion points. Dilute with V-6 Oil to create a massage oil, and massage onto the skin.

Oxygen:

—Oxygenating

Oils—**AT**Sandalwood (increases oxygen around pineal and pituitary glands), **AT**frankincense, **AT**fennel, **AT**fir, **AT**oregano.

All essential oils increase the ability of the body to take oxygen to the cells and to push toxins out. The oils pick up more oxygen and take it to the site of discomfort.

Personal Care—Satin Facial Scrub - Mint (deep cleansing that dispenses nutrients and oxygen).

—Oxygen Exchange

Oils—**AT**Tsuga (increases by opening and dilating respiratory tract).

A—Diffuse into the air. Inhale directly or applied to tissue or a cotton wick.

T—Dilute as recommended, and apply 1–2 drops to forehead, chest, and sinuses.

Pain:

Oils—**T**PanAway, **T**Relieve It, **T**Deep Relief (roll-on), **TA**lavender[258], **T**eucalyptus[259], **A**lemon[260], **T**rosemary[261], **T**clove[262], **T**copaiba[263], **T**laurel[264], **T**blue cypress, **T**balsam fir, **T**sage lavender.

Blend #1—Vetiver & valerian together make a powerful pain killer as do palo santo and frankincense.

Personal Care—Ortho Ease or Ortho Sport (stronger) Massage Oils. These massage oils help seal in and enhance the effectiveness of the single oils or oil blends.

Supplements—Sulfurzyme contains MSM, which has been shown to be very effective in controlling pain, especially in the joints and tissues.

Blend #2—20 drops valerian, 5 drops vetiver, 2 drops helichrysum, 1 drop clove, and 1 drop peppermint. Combine this ratio (in drops) in a 5 ml bottle, and then apply 3–6 drops of this blend on the back of the neck (up the cervical vertebrae—top of shoulders to base of skull), and work oils in with Vita Flex. *Working this into the brain stem helps stop pain and reduces the production of noradrenaline and cortisol.*

—ANALGESIC

»*An analgesic is a substance that acts as a pain reliever.*

Oils—TPanAway, TAlavender[258], Teucalyptus[259], Alemon[260], Trosemary[261], Tclove[262], Tcopaiba[263], Tlaurel[264], Tbergamot, Tgeranium, Thelichrysum, Tlemongrass, Tmarjoram, Tmelaleuca, Toregano, Tpeppermint, TRoman chamomile, Twintergreen.

***Comments**—See the "Single Oil Property Chart" in the Appendix of this book for additional analgesic oils and their strengths.

—ANESTHESIA

»*Anesthesia is an artificially induced insensitivity to pain or other sensation. Anesthesia is commonly used before surgeries and other procedures so that the patient does not feel pain.*

Oils—TPanAway, Tclove[262], Thelichrysum.

***Comments**—One individual applied helichrysum every 15 minutes during gum surgery, and there was no bleeding and no pain. No other anesthetic was used.

—BONE

Oils—TPanAway, Twintergreen, Tspruce, Tcedarwood, Tcypress, Tfir, Thelichrysum, Tjuniper, Tpeppermint, Tsandalwood; Tall the tree oils.

Supplements—Super Cal, True Source (whole food multi-nutrient).

—CHRONIC

Oils—TPanAway (add 1–2 drops wintergreen for extra strength), Twintergreen, Tcypress, Tfir, TRelieve It, Thelichrysum, Tbasil, Tclove, Tcedarwood, Telemi, TIdaho tansy, Tginger, Tjuniper, Tpeppermint, Trosemary cineol, Tsandalwood, Tspruce, Tvalerian.

Blend #2—Equal parts of wintergreen, elemi, and Idaho tansy.

Personal Care—Ortho Ease or Ortho Sport (stronger) Massage Oils.

Supplements—Super Cal.

—GENERAL

Oils—TPanAway, TRelieve It, TDeep Relief (roll-on), TAlavender[258], Teucalyptus[259], Trosemary[261], Twintergreen, TAroma Siez, Tblue cypress, Tbalsam fir, Tfrankincense, Tginger, Thelichrysum, Tmarjoram, TRoman chamomile, Tsage lavender, Twhite fir (pain from inflammation).

—GROWING

Recipe #1—Massage with wintergreen, cypress, and peppermint. Wait 5 minutes, and then apply PanAway or Deep Relief (roll-on). Seal with Ortho Ease.

Personal Care—Ortho Ease Massage Oil.

Supplements—Sulfurzyme, Super Cal.

—JOINTS

Oils—TPanAway, Twintergreen, TDeep Relief (roll-on), Tspruce, Tbalsam fir, Tnutmeg, TRoman chamomile (inflamed).

—MUSCLE

Oils—TAroma Siez, TPanAway, TDeep Relief (roll-on), T$_F$clove[262], Twintergreen, Twhite fir (pain from inflammation), Tbasil, Tbalsam fir, Tginger, Thelichrysum, Tlavender, Tlemongrass (especially good for ligaments), Tmarjoram, Tnutmeg, Toregano, Tpalo santo, Tpeppermint, TRelieve It, TRoman chamomile, Trosemary verbenon, Tsage lavender, Tspearmint, Tspruce (torn muscles), Tthyme, Tvetiver.

—Surgical

Recipe #2—Valerian, vetiver, helichrysum, clove, and peppermint. Balsam fir and frankincense (equal parts); up to 3 droppers full in water 4 times daily. Also GLF, topically and internally, 3–4 times daily.

Blend #3—20 ml valerian, 5 ml vetiver, 2 ml helichrysum, 1 ml clove, 1 ml peppermint. Combine oils in a 1 oz. dropper bottle. In postsurgical experiments, 3 droppers full of this blend have been taken in water (internally) up to 6 times daily for effective pain control.

—Tissue

Oils—**T**PanAway, **T**balsam fir (good for deep tissue pain), **T**Deep Relief (roll-on), **T**Relieve It, **T**helichrysum.

T—Dilute as necessary, and apply on location. Dilute with V-6 Oil to create a massage oil, and massage on location. Apply as a warm compress on affected area. Add 3–5 drops to 1/4 cup Epsom salts, and dissolve in warm bathwater before bathing.

A—Diffuse into the air. Inhale directly or applied to hands.

Painting:

Recipe #1—Add one 15 ml bottle of your favorite essential oil (or oil blend) to any five gallon bucket of paint. Stir vigorously, mixing well, and then either spray paint or paint by hand. This should eliminate the paint fumes and after-smell.

Palpitations: *See Cardiovascular System:Heart.*

Pancreas:

▸▸ *The pancreas is a gland organ located behind the stomach. The pancreas is responsible for producing insulin and other hormones and for producing "pancreatic juices" that aid in digestion.*

Oils—**T** $_F$Cypress (for insufficiencies), **T**rosemary, **TA**RC, **T**coriander, **T**dill, **T**fleabane, **TA**lemon, **T**Raven, **TA**Thieves.

—Pancreatitis

▸▸ *Pancreatitis is the term used to describe pancreas inflammation. Pancreatitis occurs when the pancreatic juices that are designed to aid in digestion in the small intestine become active while still inside the pancreas. When this occurs, the pancreas literally begins to digest itself. Acute pancreatitis lasts for only a short time and then resolves itself. Chronic pancreatitis does not resolve itself but instead gradually destroys the pancreas.*

Oils—**TA**Lemon, **TA**marjoram.

—Stimulant For

Oils—**TA** $_F$Helichrysum, **TA**fleabane.

—Support

Oils—**TA**Cinnamon bark, **TA**EndoFlex, **TA**geranium, **TA**fennel, **TA**coriander.

Supplements—EndoGize, Essentialzyme, Essentialzymes-4, MultiGreens, Stevia, Thyromin, Yacon Syrup.

T—Dilute as necessary, and apply over pancreas area or on Vita Flex points on the feet.

A—Diffuse into the air. Inhale directly or applied to the hands.

Pancreatitis: *See Pancreas: Pancreatitis.*

Panic: *See Anxiety: Panic. See also Calming.*

Paralysis: *See also Nervous System.*

Oils—TAPeppermint, TAlemongrass, TAgeranium, TAValor, TAAwaken, TAcypress, TAginger, TAhelichrysum, TAjuniper, TAnutmeg, TAPurification.

Blend #1—Combine 6 drops cypress, 15 drops geranium, 10 drops helichrysum, 5 drops juniper, 2 drops peppermint, and V-6 Oil. May rejuvenate nerve damage up to 60%. Put on location and on feet.

Supplements—Support the body with MultiGreens, Super B, Master Formula His/Hers, Mineral Essence. When the paralysis starts to reverse, there will be pain; apply PanAway on location and on feet.

T—Dilute as necessary, and apply on location and on feet. Dilute with V-6 Oil to create a massage oil, and massage on location.

A—Diffuse into the air. Inhale directly or applied to the hands.

Parasites: *See also Digestive System, Intestinal Problems.*

▸▸ *A parasite is an organism that grows on or in another organism at the host organism's expense. A parasite cannot live independently and is fed and sheltered by the host organism without making any helpful contribution itself.*

ParaFree was specifically designed to help the body rid itself of parasites. The essential oils contained in this supplement are black cumin, anise, fennel, laurel, vetiver, nutmeg, Melaleuca alternifolia, Idaho tansy, clove, and thyme.

Since this product is to be used orally, and contraindications do exist, one would be well-advised to review the book, Essential Oil Safety—A Guide for Health Care Professionals by Robert Tisserand and Tony Balacs or Aromatherapy for Health Professionals by Shirley and Len Price.

Oils—IT$_F$Oregano[265], T$_F$thyme, TI$_F$fennel, ITDi-Gize, T$_F$tarragon, ITlavender[266], T$_F$cinnamon bark, Tcopaiba[267] (skin), T$_F$Roman chamomile, T$_F$nutmeg, ITlemon, Tanise, Tclove, ITginger, Thyssop, Tlemongrass, Tmelaleuca, Tmountain savory, Tmugwort (blend with thyme), Trosemary, Trosewood, Tspearmint, Tspikenard, Ttangerine, Ttarragon.

***Comments—See the "Single Oil Property Chart" in the Appendix of this book for additional antiparasitic oils and their strengths.

Supplements—Cleansing Trio (ComforTone, Essentialzyme, and ICP), Digest + Cleanse (contains oils that create an unfriendly environment for parasites), ParaFree.

—Intestinal

Oils—IT$_F$Lemon, IToregano[265], IT$_F$Roman chamomile, Travensara.

Supplements—Cleansing Trio (ComforTone, Essentialzyme, and ICP), Digest + Cleanse, ParaFree.

***Comments—*Individuals have passed parasites within 12 hours using Di-Gize on stomach.*

I—Add 2–4 drops oil to an empty capsule with 2–4 drops V-6 Oil, and swallow.

T—Dilute as necessary, and apply oil on stomach, liver, intestines, and Vita Flex points on the feet to help pass parasites. Dilute as necessary, and apply on location

Parasympathetic Nervous System: *See Nervous System: Parasympathetic.*

Parathyroid:

▸▸ *The parathyroid gland is responsible for secreting a hormone necessary for the metabolism of calcium and phosphorus. It is located near or within the posterior surface of the thyroid gland.*

Oils—ᵀEndoFlex.

T—Apply over the thyroid gland at the bottom of the throat or on the parathyroid Vita Flex point on the feet.

Supplements—EndoGize.

Parkinson's Disease: *See Brain, Pineal Gland, Pituitary Gland, and Alzheimer's Disease.*

▸▸ *Parkinson's disease is a progressive neurodegenerative disease marked by impairment of muscle movement and speech. Symptoms of Parkinson's disease include slowed motion, muscle stiffness, difficulty maintaining balance, impaired speech, loss of automatic movements (such as blinking, smiling, and swinging the arms while walking), and hand tremors.*

Cedarwood, vetiver, sandalwood, black pepper, myrrh, patchouli, ginger, German chamomile, spikenard, galbanum, and frankincense all contain sesquiterpenes which have the ability to go beyond the blood-brain barrier. See Pineal Gland *and* Pituitary Gland*.*

Oils—**TA**Clarity (brain function), **T**marjoram, **AT**frankincense, **TA**lavender, **TA**Valor, **AT**Acceptance, **AT**basil, **AT**bergamot, **AT**cypress (circulation), **AT**Gathering (high in sesquiterpenes and in frequency), **AT**geranium, **AT**helichrysum, **AT**juniper, **AT**Juva Cleanse, **AT**lemon, **AT**nutmeg, **AT**orange, **AT**Peace & Calming, **AT**peppermint, **AT**rosemary, **AT**sandalwood, **AT**thyme, **T**Tranquil (roll-on), **AT**vitex.

T—Dilute 5–10 drops oil in 1 Tbs. V-6 Oil, and massage on affected muscles, back, legs, and neck. Dilute as necessary, and apply on base of neck or on Vita Flex points on the feet. Add 3–5 drops to warm bathwater before bathing.

A—Diffuse into the air. Inhale directly or applied to hands, tissue, or a cotton wick.

Supplements—BLM, Cleansing Trio (ComforTone, Essentialzyme, and ICP), JuvaPower/JuvaSpice, JuvaTone, Omega Blue, OmegaGize[3], Power Meal (contains choline, which is beneficial for Parkinson's disease), Sulfurzyme.

The following recipe has been used by Dr. Terry Friedmann of Paradise Valley, Arizona:

Recipe #1—Use the Cleansing Trio (ComforTone, Essentialzyme, and ICP) for one week; then add JuvaTone and 10 MultiGreens along with it. Drink 10 glasses of distilled water daily. Diffuse the oil of helichrysum and frankincense together for one hour at night.

Recipe #2—Apply frankincense to the top of the spine (at the base of the skull), and work it in. Then apply 3–5 drops of each of the following oils, one at a time, up the back of the neck, and work each one in individually: valerian, vetiver, balsam fir, Roman chamomile, and western red cedar. This will help to suppress the override of the sympathetic system and bring about a change in attitude and ability.

—To Prevent

Recipe #1—Keep liver and blood clean with Juva Cleanse, JuvaTone, and the Cleansing Trio (ComforTone, Essentialzyme, and ICP). Massage with helichrysum and sandalwood to help chelate metallics out of the body.

Past:

Oils—**AT**Present Time (helps to bring you into the present so you can go forward), **AT**Transformation.

A—Diffuse into the air. Inhale directly or applied to tissue or a cotton wick.

T—Apply to auricular emotion points. Dilute with V-6 Oil to create a massage oil, and massage onto the skin.

Peace: *See also Calming.*

Oils—ATPeace & Calming, Alavender, ATylang ylang, TTranquil (roll-on), Ajuniper, ATmarjoram, ATRelease, ATTrauma Life.

—Finding

Oils—ATangerine.

—Promote

Oils—ATRoman chamomile.

Supplements—Cleansing Trio (ComforTone, Essentialzyme, and ICP) and JuvaTone.

A—Diffuse into the air. Inhale directly or applied to hands, tissue, or a cotton wick.

T—Dilute with V-6 Oil to create a massage oil, and massage onto the skin. Add 3–5 drops to Epsom or bath salts, and dissolve in warm bathwater before bathing.

Pelvic Pain Syndrome:

›› *Pelvic pain syndrome is characterized by pain in the pelvis area that continues for several months. Symptoms include severe and steady pain, dull aching, a feeling of pressure deep in the pelvis, painful bowel movements, pain during intercourse, and pain when sitting down.*

Oils—TGinger, Tgeranium, Tbergamot, Tclove, Tnutmeg, Tthyme.

T—Place 2–3 drops in warm bathwater, and soak for 10 minutes. Dilute with V-6 Oil to create a massage oil, and massage on location.

Periodontal Disease: *See Oral Conditions:Gum Disease.*

Personal Growth:

Oils—ATTransformation.

—Eliminating Blocked

Oils—ATHelichrysum, ATfrankincense.

A—Diffuse into the air. Inhale directly or applied to tissue or a cotton wick.

T—Dilute with V-6 Oil to create a massage oil, and massage onto the skin.

Personality (Multiple):

Oils—ATInner Child, ATSARA, ATSensation.

A—Diffuse into the air. Inhale directly or applied to tissue or a cotton wick.

T—Apply to auricular emotion points. Dilute with V-6 Oil to create a massage oil, and massage onto the skin.

Perspiration:

Oils—TPurification, TPetitgrain.

T—Dilute as necessary, and apply on location. Combine 3–4 drops oil with 4 oz. unscented talcum powder and 2 oz. baking soda, and apply under the arms, on the feet, or on other areas prone to perspire.

Supplements—Cleansing Trio (ComforTone, Essentialzyme, and ICP).

Pest Troubles: *See also Insect, Mice.*

Oils—[A]Ravensara.

A—Diffuse into the air. Apply to cotton balls or strips of fabric, and place in areas where pests may enter.

pH Balance: *See also Acidosis and Alkalosis.*

Supplements—AlkaLime (combats yeast and fungus overgrowth and preserves the body's proper pH balance), Balance Complete, ComforTone (to help clean out the colon), Digest + Cleanse, Essentialzyme, Essentialzymes-4, JuvaTone (to clean the liver) and Mineral Essence (if body is too alkaline), MultiGreens (brings blood back to an alkaline pH).

Personal Care—Genesis Hand & Body Lotion (balances pH on skin).

> *According to Dr. Robert O. Young in his book, One Sickness, One Disease, One Treatment, "disease is an expression of pH." Dr. Robert Young believes that there is only one disease, which is "the constant over-acidification of the blood and tissues which disturbs the central regulation of the human body, all of which is mainly the result of an inverted way of living and eating." All sickness and disease that leads to death begins with an over-acidification of the blood and tissues and culminates with yeast and fungus. A normal healthy body should have a pH of about 7.2. (The use of saliva and urine test strips will show a much lower pH level due to the protein present in the solution. Saliva and urine tests from a healthy body should be about 6.6 to 6.8.) To maintain this pH, our diet should consist of 80% alkaline foods and 20% acid foods. "In the healing of disease, when the individual is acidic, the higher the ratio of alkaline elements in the diet, the faster will be the recovery."*

Pharyngitis: *See also Rhinopharyngitis.*

›› *Pharyngitis is an inflammation of the back of the throat (the pharynx). Symptoms of pharyngitis include sore throat, fever, skin rashes, muscle aches, headache, joint pain, and swollen lymph nodes.*

Oils—[AT]Goldenrod.

A—Diffuse into the air, and inhale the vapors.

T—Dilute as necessary, and apply to sinuses, neck, and Vita Flex points on the feet.

Phlebitis: *See Cardiovascular System: Phlebitis.*

Pimples: *See Acne.*

Pineal Gland:

›› *The pineal gland is a tiny endocrine gland located close to the center of the brain. It is responsible for producing the hormone melatonin that regulates the sleep/wake cycle. The pineal gland also serves to regulate blood pressure, sexual development, growth, body temperature, and motor function. The pineal gland is also involved in the process of creativity and planning things to do. If the pineal gland is not open, negative emotions will be attracted back to the aura.*

> ***Oils containing sesquiterpenes are especially effective in oxygenating the pineal and pituitary glands.*** *These include cedarwood, vetiver, sandalwood, black pepper, myrrh, patchouli, ginger, German chamomile, spikenard, galbanum, and frankincense (in order of sesquiterpene content). Blends include 3 Wise Men, Acceptance, Brain Power, Forgiveness, Gathering, Harmony, Inspiration, Into the Future, and Trauma Life.*

—Opens and Increases Oxygen

Oils—[A]Frankincense, [A]sandalwood (increases oxygen), [A]3 Wise Men (same frequency as pineal), [A]Acceptance, [A]Brain Power, [A]cedarwood, [A]Forgiveness, [A]Gathering, [A]Harmony, [A]Inspiration, [A]Into the Future, [A]Release, [A]spruce, [A]Transformation, [A]Trauma Life.

A—Inhale directly or applied to hands, tissue, or a cotton wick. Diffuse into the air.

***Comments—*Just smelling the essential oils will increase the oxygen production, particularly around the pineal and pituitary glands, and will help increase the secretion of antibodies, endorphins, and neurotransmitters.*

Pink Eye: *See Eyes: Conjunctivitis.*

Pituitary Gland: *See also Endocrine System.*

›› *The pituitary gland is located at the base of the brain and is considered to be the master gland because its secretions stimulate the other endocrine glands. The pituitary has an anterior and a posterior lobe. The anterior lobe secretes the human growth hormone (stimulates overall body growth), adrenocorticotropic hormone (controls steroid hormone secretion by the adrenal cortex), thyrotropic hormone (stimulates the activity of the thyroid gland), and three gonadotropic hormones (control growth and reproductive activity of the ovaries and testes). The posterior lobe secretes the antidiuretic hormone and oxytocin. The antidiuretic hormone causes water retention by the kidneys. Oxytocin stimulates the mammary glands to release milk and also causes uterine contractions. An overactive pituitary during childhood can cause a child to be extremely tall, while an underactive pituitary can result in the opposite.*

Supplements—Ultra Young+ (a new spray nutraceutical, which contains ingredients that are necessary for stimulating the pituitary gland into producing the human growth hormone (hGH) and allowing the body to utilize it).

—Balances

Oils—ATGeranium, ATylang ylang.

—Increases Oxygen

Oils—AT3 Wise Men, ATfrankincense, ATsandalwood, ATAcceptance, ATBrain Power, ATEgyptian Gold, ATForgiveness, ATGathering, ATHarmony, ATInspiration, ATInto the Future, ATTrauma Life.

A—Inhale directly or applied to hands, tissue, or a cotton wick. Diffuse into the air. Can also rub a couple drops of oil between hands, cup hands over nose and mouth, and breathe deeply *(see Comments under Pineal above).*

T—Apply to the forehead, back of neck, and Vita Flex points on big toes.

Plague: *See also Antibacterial.*

›› *Plague is a potentially deadly bacterial disease that is caused by the Yersinia pestis bacteria, which is transmitted to humans and animals through close contact or through bites from fleas that have previously bitten infected animals. Symptoms include fever, headaches, and extremely swollen and hot lymph nodes. If left untreated, plague can quickly invade the lungs, causing severe pneumonia, high fever, bloody coughing, and death.*

Oils—TA$_F$Clove, TAThieves (annihilates bacteria), TAAbundance.

T—Dilute as necessary, and apply to neck, chest, and Vita Flex points on the feet.

A—Diffuse into the air.

Supplements—Inner Defense.

Pleurisy: *See also Antibacterial, Antiviral, Respiratory System.*

›› *Pleurisy is an inflammation of the moist membrane (pleura) that surrounds the lungs and lines the rib cage. Pleurisy is characterized by a dry cough, chest pain, and difficulty breathing. Viral infection is the most common cause of pleurisy; but bacterial lung infections, chest injuries, and drug reactions are also possible causes.*

Oils—AT$_F$Cypress, AT$_F$thyme.

A—Diffuse into the air.

T—Dilute as necessary, and apply to chest or to Vita Flex points on the feet. Apply to chest with a warm compress.

PMS: *See Female Specific Conditions: PMS.*

Pneumonia: *See also Antibacterial, Respiratory System.*

Pneumonia is an illness characterized by lung inflammation. The lungs are infected by a bacteria, fungus, or virus. The result is a cough, chest pain, difficulty breathing, fever, shaking chills, headache, muscle pain, and fatigue. Pneumonia is a special concern for young children and for individuals over the age of sixty-five. Pneumonia ranges in seriousness from mild to life threatening.

Oils—**AT**RC, **AT**Thieves (on feet), **AT**thyme[268], **AT**cinnamon[268], **AT**oregano[269], **AT**Raven (on back and on feet), **AT**ravensara, **AT**eucalyptus, **AT***Eucalyptus radiata*, **AT**melaleuca, **T**Tranquil (roll-on), **AT**cajeput, **AT**Exodus II, **AT**frankincense, **AT**ImmuPower (on spine), **AT**lavender, **AT**lemon, **AT***Melaleuca ericifolia*, **AT**myrrh.

A—Diffuse into the air. Place 4 drops in 1/2 cup hot water, and inhale steam vapors deeply.

T—Dilute as necessary, and apply to indicated area or to chest, back, and Vita Flex points on the feet. Apply as a warm compress to the chest. Add 2–3 drops to 1 tsp. V-6 or olive oil; then place in rectum, and retain overnight.

Supplements—Inner Defense, Master Formula His/Hers, Ultra Young+.

Recipe #1—One or more of the following can be used with great effect:

1. RC on chest.
2. Put 15 drops of RC in 2 cups of hot water in a bowl; wet towel in the bowl, ring out, and put on chest with a dry towel on top.
3. Put 4 drops of RC or eucalyptus in ½ cup hot water, and inhale steam deeply.
4. Raven in rectum; RC on chest and back (reverse each night).

***Comments—Refer to the chapter entitled "How to Use—The Personal Usage Reference" in the Essential Oils Desk Reference under "Lung Infections - Pneumonia" for some excellent blend recipes and supplement recommendations.

Poison Oak/Ivy:

Poison oak and poison ivy are plants with an oily sap called urushiol that causes an itchy rash when it comes into contact with the skin. Infection by poison oak or poison ivy is recognized by redness and itching of the skin, a rash, red bumps, and later oozing blisters. A rash caused by poison oak or by poison ivy usually lasts from 5–12 days.

Recently I got ***Poison Ivy/Oak*** *for the first time. I looked in my Reference Guide for Essential Oils and decided to use Melrose on my poison ivy. The itching would stop for about 5 minutes and then start up again. I decided to put Purification on, which stopped the itching for maybe an hour or two before it would start up again. Getting desperate, I used Joy and sometimes Harmony (since I had more Harmony) on the poison ivy. The itching would stop for most of the day, and I would forget about having poison ivy. I didn't start the Harmony and Joy until about 3 or 4 days into the poison ivy flare up; but it's now the 6th day, and I'm not itching unless I take a shower or sweat profusely. From this experience with poison ivy, I'm convinced that the presence of rose, rosewood, and palmarosa in Joy and Harmony have all helped in the healing of our "skin conditions." I plan to stock up on Harmony and Joy for future needs.*

-Submitted by Christie Krajewski
Batesville, Arkansas (July 2004)

Oils—**T**Rose, **T**lavender, **T**Joy, **T**Harmony, **T**Melrose, **T**Roman chamomile, **T**rosewood, **T**palmarosa.

T—Dilute as necessary, and apply on location. Dilute with V-6 Oil to make a massage oil, and apply on location.

Personal Care—Rose Ointment.

Pollution: *See also Purification.*

Oils—**AT**Purification.

—Air

Oils—**A**Lemon, **A**peppermint, **AT**Purification.

—Cigarette Smoke

Oils—[A]Purification.

—Water

Oils—[I]Lemon, [I]peppermint, [I]Purification.

A—Diffuse into the air.

I—Add 1–2 drops oil to 8–16 oz. of water; allow to sit for 5 minutes, and then drink.

T—Add 3–5 drops to 1 oz. water in a spray bottle, and mist on location.

Polyps: *See also Colon, Nose: Polyps.*

Oils—[AT]Di-Gize, [AT]Exodus II, [AT]peppermint, [AT]spikenard, and others with strong antibacterial properties (*See Antibacterial*).

Supplements—ComforTone, Essentialzyme, Essentialzymes-4, Master Formula His/Hers, Super Cal.

***Comments—In two separate articles published in 1998, bacterial infection was found to exist when polyps were present. In the case of colorectal (intestinal) polyps, *E. coli* and similar bacteria were found to be adhering to the walls of the large intestine, and even partially penetrating the intestinal mucosa (Gastroenterology 1998; 115: 281-286). In the case of gastric polyps (small growths in the stomach lining), the *Helicobacter pylori* bacteria was found; and when eradicated, the polyps disappeared in 71% of the patients within a 12 to 15 month period (Annals of Internal Medicine 1998; 129: 712-715).

A—Diffuse into the air. Inhale directly or applied to hands, tissue, or a cotton wick.

T—Dilute as necessary, and apply on location.

Positive Feelings:

Oils—[AT]Acceptance, [AT]Abundance, [AT]Envision, [AT]Forgiveness, [AT]Idaho tansy, [AT]Joy, [AT]Motivation, [AT]Live with Passion, [AT]3 Wise Men (releases negative memory/trauma and reinforces positive feelings, which creates greater spiritual awareness).

A—Diffuse into the air. Inhale directly or applied to hands, tissue, or a cotton wick.

T—Apply to auricular emotion points. Dilute with V-6 Oil to create a massage oil, and massage onto the skin. Add 3–5 drops to Epsom or bath salts, and dissolve in warm bathwater before bathing.

Positive Ions: *See Ions: Positive Ions.*

Potassium Deficiency:

Potassium is important for a healthy nervous system and a regular heart rhythm. It works with sodium to control the body's water balance and regulates the transfer of nutrients to the cells.

Supplements—Master Formula His/Hers, Mineral Essence, Thyromin.

***Potassium** is important for a healthy nervous system and a regular heart rhythm. It works with sodium to control the body's water balance and regulates the transfer of nutrients to the cells.*

Potential:

Oils—[AT]Acceptance, [AT]Awaken (realize our highest potential), [AT]Believe (release our unlimited potential), [AT]Gathering, [AT]Transformation, [AT]White Angelica (greater awareness of one's potential).

A—Diffuse into the air. Inhale directly or applied to hands, tissue, or a cotton wick.

T—Apply to auricular emotion points. Dilute with V-6 Oil to create a massage oil, and massage onto the skin.

Power:

Oils—ASacred Mountain, ASurrender (calming and relaxing to dominant personalities), AValor.

A—Diffuse into the air. Inhale directly or applied to hands, tissue, or a cotton wick.

Power Surges: *See Hot Flashes.*

Prayer:

Oils—ATFrankincense, ATInspiration, ATSacred Mountain.

A—Inhale directly or applied to hands, tissue, or a cotton wick. Diffuse into the air.

T—Apply to crown chakra. Dilute with V-6 Oil to create a massage oil, and massage onto the skin.

Pregnancy/Motherhood:

Oils—ATGentle Baby (relieves stress during pregnancy; can also be used by fathers to relieve stress during delivery), ATgeranium, ATylang ylang, ATlavender, ATRoman chamomile, ATjasmine, ATgrapefruit, ATtangerine, ATelemi.

A—Diffuse into the air. Inhale directly or applied to hands, tissue, or a cotton wick.

T—Dilute with V-6 Oil, and massage gently on abdomen, chest, arms, legs, feet, back, or area of concern. Add 1–2 drops to 1/4 cup Epsom salt, and dissolve in warm bathwater before bathing.

Supplements—PD 80/20, Prenolone/Prenolone+, Progessence/Progessence Plus, Thyromin (use before, during, and after).

Personal Care—ClaraDerm (essential oil spray—apply topically to stressed skin before and after childbirth).

—Anxiety/Tension *See also Calming*

Oils—AInto the Future (help let go of fear and trauma), TTranquil (roll-on), APresent Time (help mother focus on giving birth).

A—Diffuse into the air. Inhale directly or applied to hands, tissue, or a cotton wick.

Blend #1—Add 10 drops lavender, 10 drops orange, 2 drops marjoram, 2 drops cedarwood, and 1 drop Roman chamomile to 4 oz. sweet almond oil or to V-6 Oil. Use as a massage oil or in bathwater.

Supplements—PD 80/20, Prenolone/Prenolone+, Progessence/Progessence Plus.

—Baby (Newborn)

Recipe #1—Frankincense (1 drop on the crown for protection), myrrh (on remaining umbilical cord and around navel to protect from infection), Valor (1 drop divided between both feet and 1–2 drops rubbed up spine to help ensure proper alignment).

—Breasts *See also Breasts*

Oils—TFennel (tone), TRoman chamomile (sore nipples).

PREGNANCY SAFETY DATA

Avoid During Pregnancy

Single Oils: *Basil, birch, calamus, cassia, cinnamon bark, hyssop, Idaho tansy, lavandin, rosemary, sage, tarragon.*

Blends: *Di-Gize, Dragon Time, Exodus II, Grounding, Mister.*

Other: *Estro, FemiGen, ParaFree, Protec,*

Use Cautiously During Pregnancy

Single Oils: *Angelica, cedarwood, chamomile (German/blue), cistus, citronella, clary sage, clove bud, cumin (black), cypress, davana, fennel, laurel, marjoram, mountain savory, myrrh, nutmeg, peppermint, rose, spearmint, vetiver, yarrow.*

Blends: *Aroma Siez, Clarity, Harmony, ImmuPower, Relieve It, Thieves.*

Other: *Prenolone/Prenolone+, ComforTone, Essentialzyme, Dragon Time Massage Oil.*

It was very difficult to compile a list of oils and products to be avoided during pregnancy. Each aromatologist has a different opinion. We feel that an oil that is unsafe is an oil that has been adulterated or one that is used improperly. Oils that are diluted, applied externally, and used in moderation should not create a problem. This list is a compilation of the safety data contained in aromatherapy books written by the following authors: Ann Berwick, Julia Lawless, Shirley & Len Price, Jeanne Rose, Robert Tisserand, and Tony Balacs.

T—Dilute 3–5 drops in 1 Tbs. V-6 Oil, and massage on location.

—Conception

Recipe #2—Do a proper cleansing for one year before. You may want to start with the Master Cleanser (See Cleansing for more information).

Supplements—Balance Complete (*refer to the 5-Day Nutritive Cleanse program listed under Balance Complete in the Supplements section of the Reference Guide for Essential Oils. This program also uses Digest + Cleanse and NingXia Red to help enhance detoxification while maintaining energy levels*), Cleansing Trio (especially ComforTone for the colon and ICP for the intestines), Digest + Cleanse, JuvaTone (cleanses liver).

—Constipation *See also Digestive System: Constipation*

Supplements—ComforTone can be taken during pregnancy as long as you do not get diarrhea. Diarrhea can cause cramping which could bring on labor. Essentialzyme, Essentialzymes-4, JuvaTone (helps change genetics in the colon and purge the liver).

—Delivery

Oils—[TA]Lavender (circulation stimulating, calming, antibiotic, anti-inflammatory, antiseptic), [AT]nutmeg (balances hormones, calms the central nervous system, alleviates anxiety, increases circulation, and does good to the blood supply), [T]Valor (Align mother's hips: apply along inside and bottom of each foot; then have someone hold feet—right palm to right foot and left palm to left foot—to balance energy flows. Rub a couple drops along newborn's spine for alignment.), [T]clary sage, [A]Forgiveness, [A]Gentle Baby, [A]Harmony.

T—Dilute as necessary, and apply as indicated or on hips, bottoms of feet, or abdomen. Dilute with V-6 Oil to create massage oil, and massage on hips, bottoms of feet, or abdomen.

A—Diffuse into the air. Inhale directly or applied to hands, tissue, or a cotton wick.

***CAUTION—*Nutmeg is generally nontoxic, nonirritant, and nonsensitizing. However, large doses may cause nausea, stupor, and tachycardia. Use in moderation and with great care during pregnancy. See the safety data about nutmeg in the Appendix of this book.*

–Avoid Episiotomy

Recipe #2—ClaraDerm Spray (spray onto and massage into perineum three times daily), Gentle Baby or geranium (neat or added to olive oil; massage perineum).

Blend #2—8 drops geranium, 5 drops lavender, 1 oz. V-6 Oil. Prepare three weeks before delivery, and rub on perineum three times a day. One week before delivery, prepare the same blend and add 5 drops fennel. Continue applying three times daily.

Diffuse—Hope, Joy, Motivation, Live with Passion, Peace & Calming.

–Uterus

Recipe #2—Tone uterus with 1–3 drops of clary sage around ankles (one woman dilated and had her baby in 1 ½ hours), Dragon Time, fennel, Gathering, sage.

–Transition

Oils—[T]Basil.

T—Dilute as necessary, and apply 1–2 drops to temples, abdomen, or Vita Flex points on feet.

—Early Labor

Oils—[T]Lavender

T—Rub on tummy to stop early labor.

—Energy

Blend #3—Equal portions of Roman chamomile, geranium, and lavender in V-6 Oil.

—HEMORRHAGING

▸▸ *Postpartum Hemorrhaging is excessive bleeding following childbirth. It is commonly defined as losing 500 ml of blood after vaginal birth and 1000 ml of blood after a cesarean birth. Postpartum hemorrhaging generally occurs within 24 hours following the birth and can be life threatening if not stopped.*

Blend #4—Helichrysum and Gentle Baby together on lower back (prevent).

—HIGH BLOOD PRESSURE

▸▸ *High blood pressure can potentially be dangerous in pregnancy. High blood pressure can cause a decreased flow of blood to the placenta, slowing down the baby's growth; premature placenta separation from the uterus, taking away the baby's oxygen and nutrients and causing heavy bleeding in the mother; premature birth; and the risk of future disease.*

Oils—**T**Aroma Life (over heart), **AT**ylang ylang[270].

***Comments—Avoid using hyssop, rosemary, sage, thyme, and possibly peppermint.

T—Dilute as necessary, and apply on area indicated or over heart area and on Vita Flex points.

A—Diffuse into the air or applied to hands, tissue, or a cotton wick.

—KEEP BABY IN BIRTH CANAL

Oils—**T**Gentle Baby.

T—Dilute as necessary, and apply to Vita Flex points on hands and feet.

***Comments—*One mother would rub Gentle Baby on her little fingers and little toes when contracting. Then she would squeeze the sides of her little fingers while someone else squeezed her little toes. This was repeated during contractions until the baby decided to stay in the birth canal.*

—LABOR (DURING)

Oils—**TA**Clary sage (kick labor into gear; some have combined with fennel), **T**Gentle Baby (apply to ankles and hands when labor starts), **A**Into the Future (to help move past fear and trauma), **TA**jasmine (speed up contractions), **A**Present Time (to help focus).

T—Dilute as necessary, and apply on indicated area or on ankles, lower abdomen, or hands.

A—Inhale directly or applied to hands. Diffuse into the air.

Blend #5—**(Use only when ready to deliver.)** 2 oz. V-6 Oil, 8 drops clary sage, 8 drops lavender, 8 drops jasmine. May be useful when trying to induce labor or augment a slow, lazy labor.

–PAIN

Oils—**T**PanAway

T—Apply to lower back and tummy area.

***Comments—*Refer to the chapter entitled "How to Use—The Personal Usage Reference" in the Essential Oils Desk Reference under "Pregnancy" for a wonderful blend to use during labor.*

—LABOR (POST)

Oils—**T**Geranium, **T**lavender.

T—Dilute as necessary, and apply on abdomen, ankles, or bottoms of feet.

***Comments—*Lavender is calming and has a slight analgesic effect. It also stimulates circulation, which is great for both mother and baby, and has anti-inflammatory and antiseptic properties. Geranium is one of the best oils to stimulate circulation, which in turn facilitates easy breathing. It has a contractive effect and helps pull together dilated tissues, so it is healing for the uterus and endometrium after the birth. Ge-*

ranium is also an antidepressant and is known for its uplifting effect (Alternative Medicine—A Definitive Guide, pp. 806-7).

—LACTATION *See* NURSING/LACTATION *below*

—MASTITIS (BREAST INFECTION) *SEE ALSO* ANTIBACTERIAL

▸▸ *Mastitis is a breast infection occurring in women who are breast-feeding. Mastitis causes the breast to become red, swollen, and very painful. Symptoms of mastitis include breast tenderness, fever, general lack of well-being, skin redness, and a breast that feels warm to the touch. Mastitis generally occurs in just one breast, not in both.*

Oils—TLavender, TCitrus Fresh (with lavender), TExodus II, Ttangerine.

T—Dilute as necessary, and apply on location.

Blend #6—Equal amounts of lavender and tangerine. Dilute with some V-6 Oil, and apply to breasts and under arms twice a day.

Supplements—MultiGreens, Power Meal.

—MISCARRIAGE (AFTER)

Oils—TAFrankincense, TAgrapefruit, TAgeranium, TAlavender (may help prevent), TARoman chamomile, Tspruce (2 drops on solar plexus).

T—Dilute with V-6 Oil to create a massage oil, and massage on back, legs, and arms. Add 3–4 drops to warm bathwater before bathing. Apply as indicated.

A—Inhale directly or applied to hands. Diffuse into the air.

Supplements—JuvaTone, Cleansing Trio (ComforTone, Essentialzyme, and ICP).

—MORNING SICKNESS *SEE ALSO* NAUSEA.

▸▸ *Morning sickness is the nauseated feeling accompanying the first trimester of pregnancy for many women. Morning sickness can often include vomiting. For most women, morning sickness begins around the sixth week of pregnancy and ends around the twelfth week. Although it is called "morning" sickness, the symptoms can occur at any time during the day.*

Oils—ITAGinger[271], ITDi-Gize (Sip 1–2 drops in water or apply 1–2 drops around the navel), ATpeppermint, ATcalamus, ATM-Grain.

> **Caution**: *Although Di-Gize is recommended for morning sickness, it contains some oils which some aromatologists strongly discourage using. It may have a lot to do with purity. Use at your own risk. I did, and it worked for me!*

T—Dilute as necessary, and apply on or behind ears, down jaw bone, over stomach as a compress, and on Vita Flex points on feet.

I—Take as indicated; or place 1–3 drops in an empty capsule, and swallow.

A—Inhale directly or applied on hands (rub together and smell); or put a drop on your pillow.

Recipe #3—Can also put 4–6 drops of spearmint in a bowl of boiled and cooled water and place the bowl on floor beside the bed overnight to keep the stomach calm.

Supplements—ComforTone, Essentialzyme, Essentialzymes-4.

—NURSING/LACTATION

Oils—TClary sage (brings in milk production), T$_F$fennel or Tbasil (increases milk production), Tgeranium.

T—Apply above breasts on lymph area and on spine at breast level.

Caution: Fennel should not be used for more than 10 days, as it will excessively increase flow through the urinary tract.

–INCREASE MILK PRODUCTION

Blend #7—7–15 drops fennel and either 7–15 drops geranium or 5–10 drops clary sage. Dilute 1–2 drops of blend in 2 Tbs. V-6 Oil.

Supplements—Master Formula Hers, MultiGreens.

–Decrease Milk Production

Oils—TPeppermint, Tjasmine[272].

T—Apply with cold compress over breasts. Refer to Methods of Application under the Science and Application section of the Reference Guide for Essential Oils for instructions on using cold compresses.

—On Chakras

Oils—TAwaken (after pregnancy).

T—Dilute as necessary, and apply on chakras.

—Placenta

The placenta is the organ responsible for sustaining life in an unborn baby. The placenta attaches to the uterus wall and connects to the mother's blood supply to provide nutrients and oxygen for the fetus. The placenta plays other essential roles as well: It removes waste created by the fetus, triggers labor and delivery, and protects the fetus against infection.

Oils—TBasil (has been used to help retain), Tjasmine (helps expulsion).

T—Dilute as necessary, and apply on lower abdomen and on Vita Flex points on the feet.

—Postpartum Depression (Baby Blues)

Postpartum depression is depression sometimes experienced by mothers shortly after giving birth. New mothers may experience symptoms such as irritableness, sadness, uncontrollable emotions, fatigue, anxiety, difficulty sleeping, thoughts of suicide, hopelessness, and guilt. Postpartum depression is typically thought to result from a hormonal imbalance caused by the pregnancy and childbirth.

> ***Natural Progesterone or Pregnenolone may help prevent postpartum depression.*** *Just before a woman has a baby her body produces about 400 mg of progesterone each day to help hold the placenta in place. When the baby is born, the production of progesterone falls dramatically. The body's inability to produce high doses of progesterone can help induce postpartum depression.*

Oils—ATJoy, ATlavender[273], ATlemon[274], ATgrapefruit, ATPeace & Calming, ATHope, ATValor, ATbasil, ATbergamot, ATclary sage, ATfennel, ATfrankincense, ATgeranium, ATGentle Baby, ATHarmony, ATjasmine, ATmyrrh, ATnutmeg (use in moderation), ATorange, ATpatchouli, ATvetiver, ATWhite Angelica.

A—Diffuse into the air. Inhale directly or applied to hands, tissue, or a cotton wick.

T—Apply to auricular emotion points. Dilute as necessary, and apply to temple or forehead. Dilute with V-6 Oil to create a massage oil, and massage into skin. Add 1–3 drops to warm bathwater before bathing.

Personal Care—Prenolone/Prenolone+, Progessence/Progessence Plus.

Supplements—ImmuPro, Omega Blue, OmegaGize[3].

Some women have had wonderful results with the following recipe:

Recipe #1—Valor first (2–5 drops on each foot; hold to balance energies), Harmony (use finger to dab a small amount onto each energy center [chakra]), Joy (apply a drop between and just above the breasts), and White Angelica (on the crown of the head and over the top of the shoulders).

—Self Love

Oils—TAJoy.

T—Apply to auricular emotion points. Dilute with V-6 Oil to create a massage oil, and massage into skin.

A—Diffuse into the air. Inhale directly.

—Skin Elasticity

Oils—[T]Aroma Life, [T]Clarity, [T]Dragon Time, [T]Gentle Baby, [T]Mister, [T]M-Grain, [T]Relieve It.

Caution: Many of these blends contain oils that many aromatologists feel should be avoided or used with caution during pregnancy (which may have to do with purity). Use at your own risk and with caution.

T—Dilute with V-6 Oil to create a massage oil, and apply on location.

Personal Care—A·R·T Skin Care System, ClaraDerm (essential oil spray—apply topically to stressed skin before and after childbirth).

—Stretch Marks *See also* Skin

Stretch marks are thin purple or red lines on the skin that appear as the skin is rapidly stretched over a short period of time. Many women notice the appearance of stretch marks in the last few months of pregnancy. These marks most often appear on the breasts, stomach, buttocks, thighs and hips. Stretch marks tend to fade over time, but it is difficult to eliminate them completely. The best way to avoid serious stretch marks in pregnancy is to keep the skin well moisturized and as elastic as possible.

Oils—[T]Gentle Baby

T—Dilute as necessary, and apply every day on tummy.

Personal Care—ClaraDerm (essential oil spray—apply topically to stressed skin before and after childbirth).

—Toxemia/Preeclampsia

Preeclampsia, also known as toxemia, is pregnancy-induced high blood pressure. Symptoms include protein in the urine, elevated blood pressure levels, sudden weight gain, blurred vision, abdominal pains in the upper-right side, and swelling in the hands and face.

Oils—[TA]Aroma Life.

T—Dilute with V-6 Oil, and apply on bottoms of feet and on abdomen.

A—Diffuse into the air. Inhale directly or applied to hands, tissue, or a cotton wick.

Pride:

Oils—[AT]Peppermint (dispels).

A—Inhale directly or applied to hands. Diffuse into the air.

T—Apply to auricular emotion points. Apply to crown chakra.

Procrastination:

Oils—[AT]Motivation (easier to take action; gets you out of the mood of procrastination), [AT]Magnify Your Purpose (empowering and uplifting), [AT]Acceptance, [AT]Envision (emotional support).

A—Inhale directly or applied to hands. Diffuse into the air.

T—Apply to auricular emotion points. Dilute with V-6 Oil to create a massage oil, and massage into skin. Apply to crown chakra.

Progesterone:

Oils—[AT]EndoFlex, [AT]Grounding.

A—Inhale directly. Diffuse into the air.

T—Dilute as necessary, and apply to lower abdomen, lower back, or to Vita Flex points on the feet.

***Comments—Progesterone is made from cholesterol and helps to protect against cancer.

Personal Care—PD 80/20, Prenolone/Prenolone+, Progessence/Progessence Plus.

Prosperity:

Oils—AT Abundance, AT bergamot, A cinnamon bark, AT cypress.

A—Inhale directly or applied to hands. Diffuse into the air. Wear as perfume or cologne.

T—Apply to auricular emotion points. Apply to crown and heart chakra. Add 1–3 drops to 1/4 cup Epsom salts, and dissolve in warm bathwater before bathing.

Prostate:

▸▸ *The prostate gland is a small organ just beneath that bladder that is part of the male reproductive system. Its primary function is to create and store fluid that helps nourish and protect the sperm.*

Oils—T Frankincense, T Mister, T Australian Blue, T EndoFlex, T blue cypress, T Gratitude, T helichrysum, T juniper, T Juva Cleanse, T yarrow.

T—Dilute as necessary, and apply to the posterior, scrotum, ankles, lower back, or bottoms of feet. Add 5 drops to 1 Tbs. V-6 Oil or olive oil; insert into rectum, and retain throughout the night.

Personal Care—Progessence/Progessence Plus, PD 80/20, Prenolone/Prenolone+, Protec (designed to accompany the night long retention enema, it helps buffer the prostate from inflammation, enlargement, and tumor activity).

Supplements—Prostate Health (an herbal support for the male glandular system; it may prevent prostate atrophy and malfunction and protect men from prostate cancer), Master Formula HIS.

—Decongestant

Oils—T Mister (decongests prostate and balances hormones), T_F cypress, T_F spruce, T_F myrtle, T ImmuPower, T Di-Gize, T Dragon Time, T myrrh, T sage, T yarrow.

T—Apply oils to inside ankle and heel. ImmuPower on lower spine and in rectum.

Blend #1—Combine 15 drops frankincense and 5 drops Mister with 2 tsp. V-6 Oil. Insert blend into rectum with bulb syringe or pipet, and retain throughout night.

Blend #2—Combine 10 drops frankincense and 10 drops lavender with 2 tsp. V-6 Oil. Insert blend into rectum with bulb syringe, and retain throughout night.

Blend #3—Combine 10 drops frankincense, 5 drops myrrh, and 3 drops sage with 2 tsp. V-6 Oil. Insert blend into rectum with bulb syringe or pipet, and retain through night.

***Comments—*Abundant Health offers dispensing syringes with rectal insertion tips.*

—Enlargement (Benign Prostatic Hyperplasia)

▸▸ *The size of the prostate begins at about the same size as a walnut, but the size increases as a male ages. If the prostate grows too large, it can block passage of urine from the bladder through the urethra. This blockage can lead to an increased risk for developing urinary tract stones, infections, or damaged kidneys.*

Recipe #1—Mix 10 drops of Mister with 1 Tbs. of V-6 Oil; insert in rectum, and retain overnight. May also apply either sage, fennel, or yarrow to posterior, scrotum, ankles, lower back, and bottoms of feet.

—Inflamed/Prostatitis

▸▸ *Prostatitis is an inflamed prostate, typically due to infection. This can cause pain in the lower back and groin area, painful urination, and the need to urinate frequently.*

Oils—ᵀCypress, ᵀlavender, ᵀthyme (Alternative Medicine—A Definitive Guide, p. 742).

T—Dilute as necessary, and apply to the posterior, scrotum, ankles, lower back, or bottoms of feet. Add 5 drops to 1 Tbs. V-6 Oil or olive oil; insert into rectum, and retain throughout the night.

—Strengthen

Supplements—PD 80/20, Prenolone/Prenolone+, Prostate Health, Protec.

—Thought Patterns and Emotions

*****Comments**—The prostate represents the masculine principle. Men's **prostate problems** have a lot to do with low self-worth and with an incorrect belief that as they get older they become less of a man. Ideas may be in conflict about sex, refusing to let go of the past, fearing aging, and feeling like throwing in the towel. They may be feeling inadequate in their sexual role, may be holding onto unpleasant memories of previous relationships, or may be feeling unfulfilled in love.

Prostate Cancer: *See Cancer: Prostate.*

Protection: (from negative influence)

Oils—ᴬClove, ᴬᵀcypress, ᴬᵀfennel (protection from psychic attack), ᴬfir, ᴬᵀfrankincense, ᴬᵀHarmony, ᴬᵀJoy, ᴬᵀpalo santo, ᴬᵀSacred Mountain, ᴬᵀValor, ᴬᵀWhite Angelica.

A—Diffuse into the air. Inhale directly or applied to hands.

T—Dilute as necessary, and apply to temples, forehead, heart, or crown of the head.

Protein:

*****Comments**—Carbonated water prevents the absorption of protein. Protein deficiency causes hypoglycemia.

> *A* ***protein deficiency****, either from the lack of protein intake or from the inability to digest it, creates an acidic pH in the blood. A high acidity level in the blood creates an environment for cell mutation and disease. See* Acidosis.

Supplements—Digest + Cleanse, Essentialzyme, Essentialzymes-4, MultiGreens, Power Meal (predigested protein), Pure Protein Complete, Sulfurzyme (helps digest protein).

Psoriasis: *See also Skin.*

▸▸ *Psoriasis is a skin condition characterized by patches of red, scaly skin. The most commonly affected areas are the elbows, knees, scalp, back, face, palms, and feet. But other areas can be affected as well. Psoriasis does not have a known cure, but there are medications and creams to lessen the symptoms. Psoriasis tends to be less severe in the warmer months.*

Oils—ᵀ$_F$Helichrysum, ᵀ$_F$thyme, ᵀbergamot, ᵀcajeput, ᵀcedarwood, ᵀlavender, ᵀmelaleuca, ᵀpatchouli, ᵀRoman chamomile.

T—Dilute as necessary, and apply on location.

Blend #1—Combine 2–3 drops each of Roman chamomile and lavender for use as an ointment for pH Balance.

Personal Care—A·R·T Skin Care System, Rose Ointment (helps soften cracking skin), Essential Beauty Serum - Dry Skin Blend, Lavender Volume Shampoo and Lavender Volume Conditioner for psoriasis of the scalp.

Supplements—AlkaLime, Balance Complete, Cleansing Trio (ComforTone, Essentialzyme, and ICP), Digest + Cleanse, JuvaPower/JuvaSpice, JuvaTone, Sulfurzyme.

Psychic:

Oils—**A**Cinnamon bark (awareness), **A**fennel (protect from attack), **A**lemongrass.

—Centers

Oils—**A**Elemi (balances, strengthens, fortifies).

A—Diffuse into the air.

Puberty:

Oils—**TA**Fleabane (stimulates retarded puberty).

T—Dilute as necessary, and apply to lower abdomen, lower back, and bottoms of feet.

A—Diffuse into the air. Inhale directly.

Pulmonary: *See Respiratory System: Lungs.*

Purge: *See Cleansing.*

Purification:

Oils—**AT**Purification, **AT**lemon, **AT**Abundance, **AT**Acceptance, **AT**cedarwood, **AT**En-R-Gee, **A**eucalyptus, **A**fennel, **A**lemongrass, **TA**melaleuca, **A**orange, **AT**sage.

—Air

Oils—**A**Lemon, **TA**Hong Kuai (diffuse, or add to a spray bottle of water to deodorize and sterilize the air).

—Cigarette Smoke

Oils—**A**Purification.

—Dishes

Recipe #1—2 drops of Melrose or lemon in the dishwater for sparkling dishes and a great-smelling kitchen.

—Water

Oils—**I**F Lemon, **I**peppermint.

—Clothing

Recipe #2—Adding oils to the washer or dryer decreases bacteria, improves hygiene, and gives clothes a fresh, clean smell.

—Furniture

Recipe #3—A few drops of fir, lemon, or spruce oil on a dust cloth, or 10 drops in a 1 oz. glass or plastic spray bottle filled with distilled water, works well for polishing, cleaning, and disinfecting furniture, kitchens, and bathrooms. You may also consider adding Abundance to increase your abundance. Lemon oil works for dissolving gum and grease. Use Purification for mold and fungus. If you don't have a diffuser, you may want to add 10–12 drops of Purification to 8 oz. of distilled water in a spray bottle, and spray into the air.

A—Diffuse into the air. Add 10–15 drops to 1–2 oz. distilled water in a spray bottle; shake, and mist into the air.

T—Add 3–5 drops to 1 oz. water; soak rag in water, and apply on location. Add 1–2 drops to warm bathwater before bathing. Add 1–2 drops to a bowl of water, and use to soak fruits and vegetables.

I—Add 1–2 drops to 8–16 oz. water; wait 5 minutes, and drink.

Pus: *See also Antibacterial, Infection, and Anti-infectious.*

Oils—Melaleuca is useful in healing pus-filled wounds.

Radiation: *See Cancer.*

›› *Radiation is energy emitted from a source and sent through space or matter. Different forms of radiation can include light, heat, sound, radio, microwaves, gamma rays, or X-rays, among others. While many forms of radiation are around us every day and are perfectly safe (such as light, sound, and heat), frequent or prolonged exposure to high-energy forms of radiation can be detrimental to the body, possibly causing DNA mutation, damaged cellular structures, burns, cancer, or other damage.*

Oils—**IT**Peppermint[275] (gamma), **T**sandalwood[276] (UV), **T**tamanu[277] (UV), **TA***Melaleuca quinquenervia*, **TA**Melrose, **TA**patchouli.

—Computer, TV, Microwave

Recipe #3—Fill a wooden bowl half full of peat moss and half full of hazelnuts. Add 30 drops of Melrose, and then set the bowl on top of the appliance. Using an equipment diode may also help (available from Abundant Health).

Valerie Worwood suggests Recipe #1 below to be used at least two to three weeks before the radiation treatments begin. Don't use it during the treatment, but use it between treatments and for at least a month after your last treatment.

RECIPE #1*—10 drops lavender, 5 drops German chamomile, 5 drops Roman chamomile, 5 drops tagetes, 5 drops yarrow, and 2 tsp. of vinca infused oil. Massage the entire torso, including the back and abdomen and the trauma area. This treatment will not conflict with the doctor's treatment. Note: Vinca is made from periwinkle, which is known to contain alkaloids that in some cases can suppress the cancerous cells. (The Complete Book of Essential Oils & Aromatherapy, pp. 249-50).*

The following Dr. Westlake formula utilizes Bach Flower Remedies to counteract the side effects of cancer patients who have received radiation therapy.

RECIPE #2*—"Mix 3.5 grams of sea salt with 100 ml of distilled water. In a 10 ml dropper bottle, combine 2 drops of each of the following Bach Flower Remedies: Cherry Plum, Gentian, Rock Rose, Star of Bethlehem, Vine, Walnut and Wild Oat. Top off the bottle with the sea salt solution. Take 2 drops 3 to 4 times a day, or add 10 to 15 drops to a bath. People who have been exposed to radiation sources, such as X-rays, cobalt therapy or other medical radiation therapies, or who have been contaminated in an escape from a nuclear power station, or who regularly use office or domestic equipment that gives out low-level radiation, such as color television sets, microwaves, and visual display units, would do well to use this formula in a bath once or twice a week." (Aromatherapy—An A to Z by Patricia Davis, p. 269)*

*****Comments**—*Melrose may help protect the body during radiation treatments if used 10 days before, during, and 10 days after.* **Do not use on the day of radiation treatment***. According to Dr. Pénoël, massage with* Melaleuca quinquenervia *helps to prevent radiation side effects. Remember to keep all massage light and away from trauma area.*

—Radiation Burns

›› *A radiation burn is skin damage due to radiation exposure. Radiation burns include anything from sunburns to burns caused by medical radiation treatments. Radiation burns are generally recognized by their red appearance and can be quite painful.*

Recipe #1.

—Side-Effects

›› *The possible side effects of radiation therapy are numerous and depend, in part, on which area of the body is being treated. Some common side effects include nausea, hair loss (if the head is exposed to radiation), fatigue, low blood count, skin damage, scarring, diarrhea, swelling, and difficulty swallowing. The majority of these side effects will only last for a couple of months after the treatment has been completed. Other side effects, although more rare, can potentially appear six or more months after the treatment has been complet-*

ed. These later side effects may include infertility, secondary cancer, lymphedema (swelling in the arm or leg), joint problems, and mouth problems.

Recipe #2.

—Treatments

*****Comments**—Radiation treatments can produce tremendous toxicity within the liver. Cut down on the use of oils with high phenol content to prevent increasing the liver toxicity.

–Chemotherapy

›› *Chemotherapy is the use of chemical drugs to treat cancer. Chemotherapy attacks rapidly dividing cells, so it can often negatively affect normal cells as well, such as those related to bone marrow, hair, skin, mouth, stomach, and intestines.*

*****Comments**—Because of the greater amounts of toxicity produced, even greater care should be taken to limit the use of oils with high *phenol* content.

—Weeping Wounds From

Oils—^T^Melaleuca, ^T^oregano, ^T^thyme.

Supplements—The apple pectin that is contained in ICP helps remove unwanted metals and toxins. It is also valuable in radiation therapy.

T—Dilute as necessary, and apply on location, bottoms of feet, kidneys, or thyroid.

I—Place 2–3 drops in an empty capsule, and swallow.

A—Diffuse into the air.

Rashes: *See Skin: Rashes.*

Raynaud's Disease:

›› *Raynaud's disease is a condition that causes the arteries supplying blood to the skin to suddenly narrow and inhibit blood circulation. As a result, specific areas of the body feel numb and cool. The most commonly affected areas are the toes, fingers, nose, and ears. During an attack, the skin turns white and then blue. As circulation returns and warms the affected areas, a prickling, throbbing, stinging, or swelling sensation often accompanies it. These attacks are often triggered by cold temperatures and by stress.*

Oils—^TA^Cypress, ^TA^Aroma Life, ^TA^clove, ^TA^fennel, ^TA^geranium, ^TA^helichrysum, ^TA^lavender, ^TA^nutmeg, ^TA^rosemary.

T—Dilute as necessary, and apply on the affected area, carotid arteries, and on Vita Flex points on the feet.

A—Diffuse into the air. Inhale oil directly or applied to hands, tissue, or a cotton wick.

Regenerating:

Oils—^T^Helichrysum, ^T^lavender, ^T^Melrose.

T—Dilute as necessary, and apply on location. Dilute with V-6 Oil to create a massage oil, and massage into skin.

Blend #1—Blend equal parts of Thieves and V-6 Oil, and apply on location.

Supplements—Power Meal, True Source (whole food multi-nutrient).

Rejection:

Oils—^TA^Acceptance, ^TA^Joy.

T—Apply to rejection auricular emotion point. Dilute with V-6 Oil to create a massage oil, and massage into skin.

A—Inhale directly or applied to hands. Diffuse into the air.

Relationships:

Personal Care—Sensation Bath & Shower Gel contains oils used by Cleopatra to enhance love and to increase the desire to be close to that someone special. Sensation Massage Oil creates an exotic arousal and increases sexual desire. The fragrance creates a peaceful and harmonious feeling that is helpful in easing relationship stress. Sensation Hand & Body Lotion.

—Enhancing

Oils—**TA**Lady Sclareol (especially for the woman—best if applied by male partner), **TA**ylang ylang.

—Ending Relationships

Oils—**A**Basil.

T—Dilute with V-6 Oil, and massage onto skin.

A—Diffuse into the air. Inhale directly or applied to hands.

Relaxation:

Oils—**AT**Lavender[278], **T**Tranquil (roll-on), **TA**ylang ylang[279], **A**lemon[280], **T**Stress Away, **AT**Peace & Calming, **A**Citrus Fresh, **TA**rose[281], **AT**clary sage, **AT**frankincense, **AT**Gentle Baby, **AT**geranium, **AT**jasmine, **AT**Roman chamomile, **AT**sandalwood, **AT**Trauma Life (calming).

Supplements—SleepEssence (short-term only).

Personal Care—Relaxation Massage Oil, Evening Peace Bath & Shower Gel.

—Diffusion *See Negative Ions for oils that produce negative ions when diffused to help promote relaxation.*

Oils—**A**Lavender, **A**Peace & Calming.

—Sense Of

Oils—**AT**Ylang ylang.

Blend #1—1 drop bergamot, 2 drops lavender, 2 drops marjoram, and 4 drops rosewood.

A—Diffuse into the air. Inhale directly or applied to hands, tissue, or a cotton wick.

T—Dilute with V-6 Oil to create a massage oil, and massage into skin. Place 3–5 drops in 1/4 cup Epsom salts or other bath salts, and dissolve in warm bathwater before bathing.

Release Negative Trauma:

Oils—**AT**Inspiration, **AT**Release, **AT**Transformation.

A—Diffuse into the air. Inhale directly or applied to hands.

T—Dilute as necessary, and apply to temples, forehead, heart, or crown of the head.

Resentment:

Oils—**AT**Forgiveness, **AT**Harmony, **AT**Humility, **AT**Idaho tansy, **AT**jasmine, **AT**Release, **AT**rose, **AT**White Angelica.

A—Diffuse into the air. Inhale directly or applied to tissue or a cotton wick.

T—Apply to auricular emotion points. Dilute with V-6 Oil to create a massage oil, and massage onto the skin.

Respiratory System: *see also Bronchitis, Pleurisy, Pneumonia.*

Vita Flex points for the bronchial tubes are located between the bones on the tops of the feet. The sinus points are located at the base of the middle three toes on the bottoms of the feet. One of the most effective ways to handle a respiratory problem is by doing rectal implants. There is a nerve that goes from the rectum to the lungs. The oils will travel in this manner in 3 seconds. The next best method is through inhalation.

▸▸ *The Respiratory System's primary purposes are to supply the blood with oxygen, which is then delivered to all parts of the body, and to remove waste carbon dioxide from the blood and eliminate it from the body. The Respiratory system consists of the mouth, nose, and pharynx (through which air is first taken in), larynx (voice box), trachea (airway leading from the larynx to the lungs), bronchi (which branch off from the trachea and go into the lungs), bronchiole (smaller tubes that branch off from the bronchi), alveoli (tiny sacs filled with capillaries that allow inhaled oxygen to be transferred into the blood and carbon dioxide to be expelled from the blood into the air in the lungs), pleura (which covers the outside of the lungs and the inside of the chest wall), and diaphragm (a large muscle at the bottom of the chest cavity that moves to pull air into the lungs (inhale), and to push air out of the lungs (exhale).*

Oils—**AT**RC, **AT**Raven (all respiratory problems), **AT** F eucalyptus[282] (general stimulant and strengthener), **AT***Eucalyptus radiata*, **AT** F peppermint[283] (aid), **AT**eucalyptus blue (infection), **AT** F fir (opens respiratory tract, increases oxygenation, decongests, and balances), **AT** F myrtle, **AT** F spearmint, **T**Breathe Again, **AT**dorado azul, **AT**cinnamon[284], **AT**Thieves (diffuse with *Eucalyptus radiata*; add spruce to help push the oils deeper into the lungs), **AT**Abundance, **AT**anise, **AT**basil (restorative), **AT**bergamot (infections), **AT**cajeput (infections), **AT**clary sage (strengthens), **AT**clove, **AT**Di-Gize, **AT**EndoFlex, **AT**fennel (stimulant), **AT**frankincense, **AT**goldenrod (discharges mucus), **AT**GLF, **AT**helichrysum (relieves), **AT**hyssop (opens respiratory system and discharges toxins and mucus), **AT**JuvaFlex, **AT**ledum (supports), **AT**lemon, **AT**marjoram (calming), **AT**melaleuca, **AT***Melaleuca ericifolia*, **AT**Melrose, **AT**oregano (antiseptic), **AT**pine (dilates and opens bronchial tract), **AT**ravensara, **AT**rosemary verbenon, **AT**Sacred Mountain (soothing), **AT**sage lavender, **AT**spruce (combine with any eucalyptus oils, especially *Eucalyptus polybractea*), **AT**tsuga (dilates and opens tract).

Supplements—Inner Defense, Super C / Super C Chewable.

Recipe #1—Dr. Young alternates the oils of Raven and RC in rectal implants. He uses 20 drops of the oil in 1 Tbs. of V-6 Oil and implants it rectally using a pipet (glass dropper) or a syringe with a rectal insertion tip (*available at Abundant Health*).

Blend #1—3 drops wintergreen, 8 drops eucalyptus, 6 drops fir, 6 drops frankincense, 1 drop peppermint, 10 drops ravensara, and 1 oz. V-6 Oil.

Blend #2—3 drops German chamomile, 10 drops fir, and 5 drops lemon.

—Acute

Oils—**AT**RC and **AT**Raven, **AT**Thieves.

Blend #3—5 drops eucalyptus, 8 drops frankincense, and 6 drops lemon. Add to 1 oz. V-6 Oil for a hot compress on chest, and rub neat (without V-6) on bottoms of feet under toes.

Blend #4—3 tsp. *Eucalyptus radiata* (or any oil from the Myrtaceae botanical family) and 1 tsp. balsam fir (or any conifer oil). Apply to Vita Flex points on the feet; add to V-6 Oil, and apply to chest area; or diffuse.

*My 18-year-old daughter has had **respiratory problems** for years, and finally the doctors put her on inhalers. These helped, but she did not like the way they made her feel. Soon after I started using therapeutic grade essential oils, we began using them on her. After a few weeks, she was off her inhalers and has never needed them since. She has, however, had the occasional upper-respiratory infection, which in the past has always led to a bout with bronchitis and several months of coughing. Now, we apply oils and the infection goes away without bronchitis ever showing up. This has saved vacations and more! We apply the oils to her chest, back, and feet twice a day. The oils we use are hyssop, myrrh, and two Young Living blends—RC and Raven.*

-Submitted by Lauren Martin (July 2004)

Blend #5—10 drops each of *Eucalyptus radiata* and myrrh. Add to 1 Tbs. of V-6 Oil, and insert rectally with a syringe for an overnight retention enema. Works well for all lung conditions, including emphysema, pneumonia, and tuberculosis.

—Breathing

Oils—ATRaven, ATRC (may work instead of an inhaler), ATfrankincense, ATcinnamon bark, ATExodus II, ATginger, AThyssop, ATjuniper, ATmarjoram, ATnutmeg, ATRoman chamomile, ATrosemary, ATthyme.

—Hyperpnea (Abnormal rapid breathing)

Oils—TA$_F$Ylang ylang (lung area and Vita Flex points).

—Lungs

Oils—ATRaven (stronger than RC), AT$_F$eucalyptus, ATRC (diffuse to open lungs and to send oxygen to red blood cells),ATAroma Life, ATBelieve, ATcopaiba (stimulates), ATForgiveness, ATfrankincense (stimulates), AThyssop (diffuse to clear lungs of mucus), ATJoy, ATravensara, AT Thieves.

Blend #5—Equal parts *Melaleuca ericifolia* and either RC or Raven (depending on strength desired). Add to 1 oz. V-6 Oil, and insert into rectum for retention (at least 15 min., if not overnight). Rectal implant is one of the quickest ways toaffect the lungs.

–Pulmonary Artery/Vein

Oils—TAAroma Life, TA$_F$sage, TA$_F$sandalwood, TAcypress, TAeucalyptus, TApine (antiseptic).

The pulmonary is the designated artery conveying blood from the right ventricle of the heart to the lungs or any of the veins conveying oxygenated blood from the lungs to the left atrium of the heart.

—Oxygen

Oils—ATCedarwood, ATfrankincense, ATsandalwood, ATall essential oils.

Personal Care—Satin Facial Scrub - Mint (deep cleansing that dispenses nutrients and oxygen). Mix with Orange Blossom Facial Wash for a milder cleanse.

—Shortness Of Breath

Oils—ATAroma Life.

Blend #1—For shortness of breath due to overexertion (lots of work, no sleep, etc.), add 10 drops each of eucalyptus and peppermint to a basin of lukewarm water. Soak some cloths in this water, and wring them out—leaving them fairly moist. Then wrap the joints (ankles, knees, wrists, elbows, and neck) with the cloths. While relaxing and allowing the compresses to cool the joints, have another person do Vita Flex on the Pineal Gland and Adrenal Gland points on the feet.

A—Diffuse into the air. Inhale directly; or apply to hands, tissue, or a cotton wick, and inhale. Add 3–4 drops to a small bowl of steaming-hot water, and inhale the vapors.

T—Dilute as necessary, and apply to chest, sinuses, neck, or Vita Flex points on the feet. Add 2–3 drops to water, and gargle. Apply to chest as a warm compress.

Restlessness: *See also Calming.*

Oils—ATRutaVaLa, ATlavender, ATPeace & Calming, TTranquil (roll-on), ATorange, ATvalerian, ATAcceptance, ATangelica, ATbasil, ATbergamot, ATcedarwood, ATfrankincense, ATGathering, ATgeranium, ATHarmony, ATInspiration, ATJoy, ATrose, ATrosewood, ATSacred Mountain, ATspruce, ATTrauma Life, ATValor, ATylang ylang.

A—Diffuse into the air. Inhale directly or applied to hands.

T—Dilute with V-6 Oil to create a massage oil, and massage onto the skin. Add 3–5 drops to 1/4 cup bath salts, and dissolve salts in warm bathwater before bathing. Dilute as necessary, and apply to wrists.

Rheumatic Fever:

›› *Rheumatic fever is a complication of strep throat or scarlet fever. It is an inflammatory disease that can cause permanent damage to the heart. Symptoms of rheumatic fever include painful and swollen joints, chest pain, fever, fatigue, the sensation of a pounding heartbeat, shortness of breath, rash, sudden jerky body movements, and unusual displays of emotion. Rheumatic fever is most common in children between ages 5 and age 15.*

Oils—$^{T}_{F}$Tarragon, ^{T}ginger. Both help with pain.

T—Dilute as necessary, and apply on location or on Vita Flex points on the feet.

Rheumatism: *See Muscles, Arthritis.*

Rhinitis:

›› *Rhinitis is inflammation of the nasal mucus membrane. Rhinitis is commonly caused by viral infections and allergies and can be acute (short-term) or chronic (long-term). Symptoms of Rhinitis may include runny nose, sneezing, congestions, and ear problems.*

Oils—^{AT}Basil, ^{AT}sage lavender.

A—Diffuse into the air and inhale mist through nose.

T—Dilute as necessary, and apply to sinuses, sides of nose, or to Vita Flex points on the feet.

Rhinopharyngitis:

›› *Rhinopharyngitis is an inflammation of the mucus membrane and the pharynx. Symptoms include high fever, reduced sense of smell, runny nose, sneezing, and a red, swollen throat. Rhinopharyngitis is the precursor of the common cold.*

Oils—$^{A}_{F}$Ravensara.

A—Diffuse into the air, and inhale mist through nose.

Ringworm: *See Antifungal: Ringworm.*

Romantic Touches:

Oils—^{T}Jasmine, ^{T}Lady Sclareol, ^{T}patchouli, ^{T}Sensation, ^{T}ylang ylang.

T—Dilute with V-6 Oil, and apply a small amount on location.

Personal Care—Sensation Massage Oil, Sensation Bath & Shower Gel, Sensation Hand & Body Lotion.

Rosacea (Acne Rosacea): *See Acne: Rosacea*

Sacredness:

Oils—^{AT}Sacred Mountain (sacred place of protection within self).

A—Inhale directly or applied to hands, tissue, or a cotton wick. Diffuse into the air.

T—Apply to crown chakra. Dilute with V-6 Oil to create a massage oil, and massage onto the skin.

Sadness:

Oils—[AT]Joy (over heart), [AT]Acceptance, [AT]helichrysum, [AT]Inspiration, [T]onycha (combine with rose in V-6 Oil for calming/uplifting massage), [AT]orange (overcome), [AT]3 Wise Men, [AT]Transformation, [AT]Valor.

A—Diffuse into the air. Inhale directly or applied to tissue or a cotton wick. Wear as a perfume or cologne.

T—Apply to auricular emotion points. Dilute with V-6 Oil to create a massage oil, and massage onto the skin.

Saint Vitus' Dance (Chorea):

›› *Chorea is a neurological disorder that is characterized by rapid, irregular, involuntary movements of the body. These movements can affect the hands, feet, neck, trunk, and face. They are irregular and seem to move randomly from one body part to another. The quick movements of the feet and hands are similar to dancing and piano playing.*

Blend #1—5 drops Aroma Siez, 3 drops basil, 6 drops juniper, and 8 drops peppermint.

Sanitation: *See also Antibacterial, Antifungal, Antiviral.*

Oils—[T]Purification, [T]citronella, [T]lemongrass.

T—Add 5–10 drops to a small bowl of water, and use water to clean counters and other surfaces.

Scabies: *See Skin: Scabies.*

Scarring:

›› *Scars are fibrous connective tissue that is used to quickly repair a wound or injury and replace the damaged skin or tissue Scar tissue is often not as strong or as functional as the regular tissue.*

Oils—[T][F]Lavender (burns), [T]helichrysum (reduces), [T]Gentle Baby, [T]rose (prevents), [T]frankincense (prevents), [T]geranium, [T]hyssop (prevents), [T]Melrose, [T]rosehip (reduces).

Personal Care—A·R·T Skin Care System, Lavender Hand & Body Lotion (moisturizes skin and promotes healing).

Blend #1—Equal parts helichrysum and lavender mixed with liquid lecithin.

Blend #2—3 drops rosemary, 15 drops rosewood, and 1¾ oz. hazelnut oil.

Blend #3—6 drops lavender, 3 drops patchouli, 4 drops rosewood, and vitamin E oil.

—Prevent Formation

Oils—[T]Frankincense, [T]helichrysum, [T]rose, [T]hyssop, [T]myrrh, [T]rosehip seed.

Blend #4—5 drops helichrysum, 2 drops patchouli, 4 drops lemongrass, and 3 drops lavender in ¼–½ oz. V-6 Oil.

Blend #5—Equal parts lavender, lemongrass, and geranium.

T—Dilute as necessary, and apply on location.

Schmidt's Syndrome: *See Adrenal Glands: Addison's Disease.*

Sciatica:

▸▸ *The sciatic nerve (the longest nerve in the body) runs from the spinal cord through the buttock and hip area and down the back of each leg. When this nerve is pinched or irritated due to something such as a herniated disc, it can cause pain in the area, numbness and weakness, tingling sensations, or a loss of bladder or bowel control.*

Oils—^{T}Cistus (followed by peppermint), $^{T}_{F}$thyme, $^{T}_{F}$helichrysum, $^{T}_{F}$tarragon (with Idaho tansy—can promote sciatic regeneration), ^{T}peppermint, ^{T}Aroma Life, ^{T}cardamom, ^{T}fir, ^{T}Gentle Baby, ^{T}hyssop, ^{T}M-Grain, ^{T}PanAway, ^{T}Relieve It, ^{T}sandalwood, ^{T}spruce (alleviates pain), ^{T}Valor.

T—Apply over area with a cold compress. Dilute as necessary, and apply on lower back, buttocks, or legs. Dilute with V-6 Oil to create a massage oil, and massage on location.

Recipe #1 Apply one (or more) of the above oils with a cold compress, and lightly massage with Roman chamomile or lavender and wintergreen. Relief can also be obtained by applying Joy and lavender to the bottoms of the feet.

Blend #1—Tarragon, balsam fir, and spearmint (small amount) or tarragon, basil, and peppermint.

Personal Care—Ortho Ease Massage Oil.

Recipe #2—Apply frankincense to the top of the spine (at the base of the skull), and work the oil in. Then apply 3–5 drops of each of the following oils, one at a time, up the back of the neck, and work each one in individually: valerian, vetiver, balsam fir, and tarragon. While working each one into the spine, a glass probe or glass dropper can be used to gently stimulate the tops of each of the vertebrae.

Scoliosis: *See Back: Scoliosis.*

Scrapes: *See also Cuts, Wounds.*

Oils—^{T}Lavender, ^{T}ravensara.

T—Dilute as necessary, and apply on location.

Scurvy:

▸▸ *Scurvy is a disease caused by a deficiency of ascorbic acid (vitamin C). Some results of scurvy are general weakness, anemia, gum disease (gingivitis), skin hemorrhages, spots on the skin (usually the thighs and legs), and bleeding from the mucus membranes.*

Oils—$^{T}_{F}$Ginger.

T—Dilute as necessary, and apply over kidneys, liver, and on corresponding Vita Flex points on the feet.

Supplements—Super C / Super C Chewable.

Security:

Oils—^{AT}Christmas Spirit, ^{AT}Sacred Mountain.

—Creating

Oils—^{AT}Acceptance, ^{AT}Roman chamomile.

—Feeling Of

Oils—^{A}Cypress.

—In the Home

Oils—^{AT}Bergamot.

—Self Secure

Oils—ATOregano.

A—Diffuse into the air. Inhale directly or applied to hands, tissue, or a cotton wick.

T—Dilute with V-6 Oil to create a massage oil, and massage into skin. Apply to auricular emotion points. Add 3–5 drops to 1/4 cup Epsom salts, and dissolve in warm bathwater before bathing.

Sedative: *See Calming: Sedative.*

Seizure:

A seizure is an uncontrolled, abnormal electrical discharge in the brain that may produce physical convulsions, minor physical signs, thought disturbances, or a combination of symptoms. The symptoms depend on what parts of the brain are involved.

—Convulsions

A convulsion is the repeated, rapid contracting and relaxing of muscles resulting in the uncontrollable shaking of the body. Convulsions usually last about 30 seconds to 2 minutes and are often associated with seizures.

Oils—TAClary sage, TAlavender[285], TAValor, TABrain Power, TAneroli, TARoman chamomile.

Supplements—KidScents MightyVites, Mineral Essence, Ultra Young+.

—Epilepsy

Epilepsy is a neurological condition where the person has recurring, unpredictable seizures. Epilepsy has many possible causes, although in many cases the cause is unknown. Possible causes may include illness, injury to the brain, or abnormal brain development.

Oils—TABrain Power, TAclary sage.

Supplements—Cleansing Trio (ComforTone, Essentialzyme, ICP), JuvaPower/JuvaSpice.

OILS TO AVOID IF EPILEPTIC

There are several oils that should not be used if prone to epilepsy. Please see the Appendix for safety data on the oils and products mentioned in this book. For further contraindication information, please consult the following books:

Essential Oil Safety—A Guide for Health Care Professionals by Robert Tisserand and Tony Balacs and Aromatherapy for Health Professionals by Shirley and Len Price.

—Grand Mal

The grand mal seizure, also known as the tonic-clonic seizure, is the most common seizure. The tonic phase last about 10–20 seconds. During this stage, the person looses consciousness and the muscles contract, causing the person to fall down. During the clonic phase, the person experiences violent convulsions. This phase usually lasts less than two minutes.

Recipe #1—Need to support the body. Aroma Siez (apply using the Raindrop Technique up the spine), Brain Power and Peace & Calming (diffuse, and apply around naval), Joy (over the heart), Sacred Mountain (back of neck and crown), and Valor (on feet).

Supplements—Cleansing Trio (ComforTone, Essentialzyme, and ICP), JuvaPower, Omega Blue, OmegaGize[3].

***Comments—Grand Mal seizures can sometimes be caused by zinc and copper imbalance. Mineral Essence provides zinc and copper in both ionic and colloidal form for optimal assimilation.

T—Dilute as necessary, and apply to back of neck and to brain Vita Flex points on bottoms of feet.

A—Inhale directly or applied to hands. Diffuse into the air.

Self Adjustment:

Oils—TA Awaken.

T—Dilute with V-6 Oil to create a massage oil, and massage into skin. Apply to auricular emotion points. Add 3–5 drops to 1/4 cup Epsom salts, and dissolve in warm bathwater before bathing.

A—Diffuse into the air. Inhale directly or applied to hands, tissue, or a cotton wick.

Self Esteem:

Oils—AT Acceptance, AT Forgiveness, AT Joy, AT Valor.

—Build

Oils—AT Joy, AT Transformation, AT Valor.

—Self Love

Oils—TA Joy, TA Valor.

A—Diffuse into the air. Inhale directly or applied to hands, tissue, or a cotton wick.

T—Apply to auricular emotion points. Dilute with V-6 Oil to create a massage oil, and massage into skin. Add 3–5 drops to 1/4 cup Epsom salts, and dissolve in warm bathwater before bathing.

Self Hypnosis:

Oils—A Clary sage, A geranium, A patchouli.

A—Inhale directly or applied to hands. Diffuse into the air.

Self Pity:

Oils—AT Acceptance, AT Motivation, AT Transformation, AT Valor.

A—Diffuse into the air. Inhale directly or applied to hands, tissue, or a cotton wick.

T—Apply to auricular emotion points. Dilute with V-6 Oil to create a massage oil, and massage into skin.

Sensory System (Senses): *See also Awareness.*

Oils—AT Wintergreen.

A—Inhale directly or applied to hands, tissue, or a cotton wick. Diffuse into the air.

T—Dilute with V-6 Oil to create a massage oil, and massage into skin.

Sexual Abuse:

Oils—AT SARA (its fragrance, when inhaled, may enable a person to relax into a mental state such that he or she may be able to let go of the memory trauma of sexual and/or ritual abuse).

A—Inhale directly. Diffuse into the air, and inhale.

T—Apply on auricular emotion points.

Sexually Transmitted Diseases (STD): *See AIDS, Herpes Simplex*

Sexual Stimulant:

Oils—AT Sensation, AT F cinnamon bark (general), AT F ylang ylang (sex drive problems), AT ginger, AT goldenrod, AT rose, AT SclarEssence.

Personal Care—Sensation Bath & Shower Gel (contains oils used by Cleopatra to enhance love and to increase the desire to be close to that someone special), Sensation Massage Oil (creates an exotic arousal and increases sexual desire. The fragrance creates a peaceful and harmonious feeling that helps to ease relationship stress.), PD 80/20, Prenolone/Prenolone+ (for both males and females), Progessence/Progessence Plus (for females only), Sensation Hand & Body Lotion.

Supplements—EndoGize, Master Formula His/Hers, Mineral Essence, MultiGreens.

—AROUSING DESIRE

Oils—ATClary sage, ATLady Sclareol.

—FRIGIDITY *See Frigidity.*

Oils—ATLady Sclareol, ATnutmeg (overcome).

—IMPOTENCE

Oils—ATGoldenrod, ISclarEssence (use capsules to take internally).

—INFLUENCES

Oils—ATLady Sclareol, Apatchouli.

A—Wear as perfume or cologne. Diffuse into the air.

T—Dilute with V-6 Oil to create a massage oil, and massage into the skin. Add 3–5 drops to 1/4 cup Epsom or bath salts, and dissolve in warm water before bathing. Dilute as necessary, and apply on skin.

I—Add 2–3 drops to an empty capsule, and swallow.

Shingles: *See also Antiviral, Childhood Diseases: CHICKEN POX.*

›› *Shingles is an acute viral infection with inflammation of certain spinal or cranial nerves and the eruption of vesicles along the affected nerve path. It usually strikes only one side of the body and is often accompanied by severe neuralgia. Also called herpes zoster. Some say it is necessary to cleanse the liver to eliminate/avoid shingles.*

Dr. Schnaubelt says that his greatest success in helping individuals with shingles came from applying a blend of 50 percent Ravensara aromatica and 50 percent Calophyllum inophyllum (Tamanu). "Drastic improvements and complete remission occur within seven days." (Alternative Medicine—The Definitive Guide, p. 56).

Oils—TAustralian Blue, TFravensara, Tmelaleuca, Teucalyptus, Tblue cypress, Tbergamot, Tgeranium, Tlavender, Tlemon, Ttamanu, TRoman chamomile.

Blend #1—10 drops lavender, 10 drops melaleuca (tea tree), and 10 drops thyme mixed in Genesis Hand & Body Lotion. Rub on feet.

Personal Care—Ortho Sport Massage Oil, PD 80/20, Prenolone/ Prenolone+, Progessence/Progessence Plus.

Supplements—Cleansing Trio (ComforTone, Essentialzyme, and ICP).

—HERPES ZOSTER

Oils—TAustralian Blue, Tmelaleuca (*See Alternative Medicine—The Definitive Guide, p. 972*), Tblue cypress, T*Eucalyptus radiata*, Tbergamot, Tgeranium, Tlavender, TRoman chamomile.

T—Dilute as necessary, and apply on location. Dilute with V-6 Oil to create a massage oil, and massage on location and on bottoms of feet.

Shock: *See also Fainting.*

›› *Shock is a potentially life-threatening condition where the body suffers from severely low blood pressure. This can be caused by low blood volume due to bleeding or dehydration, inadequate pumping of the heart, or dilation of the blood vessels due to head injury, medications, or poisons from bacterial infections. Shock can cause pale or bluish skin that feels cold or clammy to the touch, confusion, rapid breathing, and a rapid heartbeat. Without the needed oxygen being sent to the body's tissues and cells, the organs can shut down and, in severe cases, can lead to death. Shock often accompanies severe injuries or other traumatic situations. A person suffering from shock should be made to lie down with the feet elevated above the head, kept warm, and have the head turned to the side in case of vomiting. Check breathing often, and ensure that any visible bleeding is stopped. Get emergency medical help as soon as possible.*

Oils—**TA**$_F$Peppermint, **TA**$_F$Roman chamomile, **TA**helichrysum, **TA**Aroma Life, **TA**Joy, **TA**Australian Blue, **TA**basil, **TA**Clarity (to keep from going into shock), **TA**Gathering, **TA**Grounding, **TA**Highest Potential, **TA**Inspiration, **TA**melaleuca, **TA**melissa, **TA**myrrh, **TA**neroli, **TA**rosemary, **TA**Valor, **TA**ylang ylang.

T—Dilute as necessary, and apply on back of neck, feet, over heart, or on front of neck.

A—Inhale directly or applied to hands. Diffuse into the air.

Shoulder (Frozen):

Oils—**T**Basil, **T**wintergreen, **T**lemongrass, **T**oregano, **T**peppermint, **T**white fir, **T**Deep Relief (roll-on).

Recipe #1—Begin by applying white fir to shoulder Vita Flex point on foot (same side of body as frozen shoulder) to deal with any inflammation. Work it in with Vita Flex technique. Then check for improvement in pain reduction and/or range of motion (check after each oil to help determine what the problem really was). In a similar manner, apply lemongrass (for torn or pulled ligaments), basil (for muscle spasms), and wintergreen (for bone problems) on the same Vita Flex point on the foot. After applying the oils to the foot and determining which oil(s) get the best results, apply the same oil(s) on the shoulder, and work the oil into the area with Vita Flex. Then apply peppermint (for nerves) and oregano (create thermal reaction to enhance elasticity of muscle and help it to stretch) on the shoulder, and work each one into the area with Vita Flex. Finally, apply white fir to the other shoulder to create balance as the opposite shoulder will compensate for the sore one. Drink lots of water.

T—See Recipe #1 above. Dilute as necessary, and apply on shoulder and on Vita Flex points on the feet.

Personal Care—Regenolone.

Supplements—Sulfurzyme.

Sinuses:

▸▸ *Sinuses are several hollow cavities within the skull that allow it to be more lightweight, while still maintaining strength. These cavities are connected to the nasal cavity through small channels. When the mucous membrane lining these channels becomes swollen or inflamed due to colds or allergies, these channels can become blocked, making it difficult for the sinuses to drain correctly. This can lead to infection and inflammation of the mucous membrane within the sinuses (sinusitis). There are sinus cavities behind the cheek bone and forehead, and near the eyes and nasal cavity.*

Oils—**AT**$_F$Helichrysum, **AT**$_F$myrtle, **T**Breathe Again, **AT**eucalyptus, **AT**peppermint, **AT**RC, **AT**cedarwood, **AT**PanAway, **T**Thieves (on feet).

A—Inhale directly or applied to hands. Diffuse into the air. Place 1–2 drops in a bowl of hot water, and inhale vapors.

T—Dilute as necessary, and apply on sides of nose or on forehead.

***Comments—Eucalyptus and other sinus oils work really well when rubbed on each side of the nose. It seems to clear the sinuses almost immediately.

Sinusitis: *See also Respiratory System.*

Oils—[AT] F Eucalyptus, [AT] F rosemary, [AT] F pine, [T] Breathe Again, [AT] RC, [AT] cajeput, [AT] elemi, [AT] *Eucalyptus radiata*, [AT] fir, [AT] ginger, [AT] *Melaleuca ericifolia*, [AT] myrtle, [AT] peppermint, [AT] ravensara, [AT] sage lavender.

A—Inhale directly or applied to hands. Diffuse into the air. Place 1–2 drops in a bowl of hot water, and inhale vapors.

T—Dilute as necessary, and apply on sides of nose or on forehead.

Skeletal System: *See Bones. See also Scoliosis.*

Skin: *See also Acne, Allergies, Boils, Bruises, Burns, Cancer: Skin, Cuts, Dermatitis, Eczema, Facial Oils, Feet: Corns, Moles, Psoriasis, Wounds, Wrinkles.*

Contact-sensitization is a type of allergic reaction which can occur when a substance comes into contact with the body. A few essential oils applied to the skin may cause sensitization, perhaps only after repeated application (the amount used is not significant). The skin reaction appears as redness, irritation, or vesiculation. A rule of thumb when applying oils to someone is that people with darker hair usually have less sensitive skin while those with blond or red hair are generally more sensitive.

***Single oils:** Bergamot, cassia, cinnamon bark, citronella, clove, fennel, Laurus nobilis, ylang ylang.*

(For a list of possible skin irritants, please see the Appendix of this book.)

▸▸ *The skin is the organ that covers the body, offering the first layer of protection to the internal organs and tissues from exposure to the environment and fungal, bacterial, and other infections. It helps regulate body heat and helps prevent evaporation of water from the body. The skin also carries nerve endings that allow the body to sense touch, heat, and pain. The skin is comprised of three layers. The upper layer is the epidermis, the middle layer is the dermis, and the deeper layer is the hypodermis, or subcutis layer.*

Oils—[T] F Peppermint (itching skin), [T] F melaleuca (healing), [T] F myrtle (antiseptic), [T] sandalwood (regenerates), [T] frankincense, [T] lavender, [T] myrrh (chapped and cracked), [T] Roman and German chamomile (inflamed skin), [T] Acceptance, [T] Aroma Life, [T] cajeput, [T] cedarwood, [T] Clarity, [T] cypress, [T] Dragon Time, [T] Gentle Baby (youthful skin), [T] geranium, [T] helichrysum, [T] Inner Child, [T] jasmine (irritated skin), [T] juniper, [T] ledum (all types of problems), [T] lemon, [T] marjoram, [T] Melrose, [T] Mister, [T] M-Grain, [T] onycha (chapped and cracked), [T] orange, [T] palmarosa (rashes, scaly, and flaky skin), [T] patchouli (chapped; tightens loose skin and prevents wrinkles), [T] Relieve It, [T] rosehip, [T] rosemary, [T] rosewood (elasticity and candida), [T] sage, [T] sage lavender, [T] Sensation, [T] Valor, [T] vetiver, [T] western red cedar (nourishing), [T] ylang ylang.

T—Dilute as necessary, and apply on location. Dilute with V-6 Oil to create massage oil, and massage on location. Add 1–2 drops to 1 tsp. unscented lotion, and apply on location. Add 1–2 drops to bath or shower gel, and apply to the skin.

Personal Care—A·R·T Skin Care System, AromaGuard Deodorants, Boswellia Wrinkle Cream, ClaraDerm, Essential Beauty Serums (Dry, & Acne-Prone Skin Blends), Genesis Hand & Body Lotion (hydrates, heals, and nurtures the skin), Satin Facial Scrub - Mint (eliminates layers of dead skin cells and slows down premature aging of the skin), Orange Blossom Facial Wash combined with Sandalwood Moisture Cream (cleans and moisturizes dry or prematurely aging skin), Prenolone , Progessence/Progessence Plus, Regenolone (helps moisturize and regenerate tissues), Rose Ointment (for skin conditions and chapped skin), Lavender Hand & Body Lotion (moisturizes skin, leaving it feeling soft, silky, and smooth), Sensation Hand & Body Lotion (moisturizes, softens, and protects the skin from weather, chemicals, and household cleaners).

Bar Soaps—Lavender Rosewood Moisturizing Soap, Lemon Sandalwood Cleansing Soap, Peppermint Cedarwood Moisturizing Soap, Sacred Mountain Moisturizing Soap for Oily Skin, Thieves Cleansing Soap.

Bath & Shower Gels—Dragon Time (for women who have lower back pain, stress and sleeping problems due to menstruation), Evening Peace (relaxes tired, fatigued muscles and helps to alleviate tension), Morning Start (dissolves oil and grease), and Sensation (aphrodisiac).

Supplements for Skin—JuvaTone, Sulfurzyme, Ultra Young+ (helps firm and tighten skin by activating the production of skin proteins, collagen, and elastin).

—Aftershave

Recipe #1—Awaken can be used instead of aftershave lotion. Try adding Awaken to Sandalwood Moisture Cream, Lavender Hand & Body Lotion, Sensation Hand & Body Lotion, or Genesis Hand & Body Lotion as an aftershave. KidScents Lotion makes a great aftershave, as it soothes and rehydrates the skin (and smells good too).

—Aging *See also* Wrinkles *below*

Oils—ᵀFrankincense, ᵀpatchouli (prevents wrinkles), ᵀrosehip (retards), ᵀrosewood (slows), ᵀcarrot, ᵀrose.

T—Dilute as necessary, and apply on location. Dilute with V-6 Oil or other carrier oil, such as jojoba, apricot, hazelnut, or sweet almond, to create massage oil, and apply to areas of concern. Add 3–4 drops to 1/4 cup Epsom salts, and dissolve in warm bathwater before bathing.

Personal Care— A·R·T Beauty Masque, Boswellia Wrinkle Cream, Genesis Hand & Body Lotion, Satin Facial Scrub - Mint, PD 80/20, Prenolone/Prenolone+, Progessence/Progessence Plus, Rose Ointment, Sandalwood Moisture Cream.

Supplements—Ultra Young+ (helps firm and tighten skin by activating the production of skin proteins, collagen, and elastin).

S

—Calluses

›› *A callus is a flat, thick growth of skin that develops on areas of the skin where there is constant friction or rubbing. Calluses typically form on the bottoms of the feet, but they can also form on the hands or on other areas of the bodies that are exposed to constant friction.*

Oils—ᵀMelrose and ᵀoregano (calluses on feet), ᵀcarrot, ᵀpeppermint, ᵀRoman chamomile.

T—Dilute as necessary, and apply on location.

*For years, I had been troubled with an **actinic keratosis** on the back of my hand. It had been caused by excessive sun exposure when I was younger. Farmers often get them on their foreheads. My dermatologist said there was no way to get rid of it—unless I wanted to freeze it off with liquid nitrogen. He didn't want to do that because it was over 1/2 inch in diameter, and freezing it would have made a hole in my hand. The growth continued to bother me. It was red, scaly, and itchy. One day, in desperation, I put some "Thieves" blend on it. The Thieves seemed to make it feel better, so I continued to apply it once a day. It is now several months later, and the growth has almost disappeared. I intend to continue using Thieves on it until it is gone. It doesn't bother me anymore, and the redness and itching have disappeared.*

-Submitted by Judy Brown
Geneva, New York (July 2004)

—Chapped/Cracked

›› *Chapped or cracked skin is the result of the depletion of natural oils (sebum) in the skin, leading to dehydration of the skin beneath it. Some common causes for chapped skin include exposure to the cold or wind, repeated contact with soap or chemicals that break down oils, or a lack of essential fatty acids in the body.*

Oils—ᵀMyrrh, ᵀelemi, ᵀdavana, ᵀ onycha (benzoin), ᵀpatchouli.

T—Dilute as necessary, and apply on location. Dilute with V-6 Oil to create a massage oil, and apply on location.

Blend #1—1 drop geranium, 1 drop patchouli, and 1 drop rosemary in Genesis Hand & Body Lotion or Lavender Hand & Body Lotion.

Blend #2—1–3 drops of both onycha (benzoin) and rose in Genesis Hand & Body Lotion, Lavender Hand & Body Lotion (makes a wonderful hand cream), or Rose Ointment. May also add lemon and/or lavender for their additional healing properties.

Personal Care—Cinnamint or Lavender Lip Balms

—**Complexion**

Personal Care—A·R·T Skin Care System

–**Dull**

Oils—T Jasmine, T orange.

–**Oily (Greasy)**

Oils—T Bergamot, T orange, T cajeput, T clary sage, T cypress, T jasmine, T lavender, T lemon, T nutmeg, T ylang ylang.

T—Dilute as necessary, and apply oils to face, neck, and intestines.

—**Dermatitis** *See Eczema/Dermatitis below*

—**Diaper Rash:** *See Children/Infants: Diaper Rash*

—**Disease**

Oils—T Rose, T Melrose.

T—Dilute as necessary, and apply on location.

—**Dry**

Oils—T F Rosewood, T geranium, T lavender, T Gentle Baby, T Roman chamomile, T davana, T jasmine, T lemon, T neroli, T patchouli, T sandalwood.

T—Dilute as necessary, and apply on location. Dilute with V-6 Oil to create massage oil, and massage on location. Add 1–2 drops to 1 tsp. unscented lotion, and apply on location.

Personal Care— A·R·T Renewal Serum, Genesis Hand & Body Lotion (hydrates, heals, and nurtures), Orange Blossom Facial Wash (gently cleanses the skin), PD 80/20, Prenolone/Prenolone+, Progessence, Sandalwood Moisture Cream (hydrates), Lavender Hand & Body Lotion (nourishes and moisturizes), Sensation Massage Oil (silky and youthful skin)

—**Eczema/Dermatitis**

▸▸ *Dermatitis is any inflammation of the upper layers of the skin that results in redness, itching, pain, or possibly blistering. It can be caused by contact with an allergen or irritating substance, fungal infection, dehydration, or possibly another medical condition.*

Oils—T F Helichrysum, T F German chamomile, T F rosewood, T F thyme, T F patchouli, T F juniper, T bergamot, T eucalyptus, T geranium, T hyssop, T lavender, T *Melaleuca ericifolia*, T melissa, T onycha (benzoin), T pine, T sage, T sage lavender.

Supplements—Essentialzyme, Essentialzymes-4, JuvaPower/JuvaSpice, Sulfurzyme.

*****Comments**—Eczema or dermatitis may indicate a sulfur deficiency.

–**Dry**

Oils—T F German chamomile, T bergamot, T geranium, T hyssop, T rosemary.

–**Wet**

Oils—T F German chamomile, T hyssop, T juniper, T lavender, T myrrh.

T—Dilute with V-6 Oil to create a massage oil, and apply on location. Dilute as necessary, and apply oil on location.

—**Facial Mask**

Oils—T Myrrh, T patchouli, T sandalwood, T vetiver.

T—Add 2–3 drops to a facial mask. Can use individually or together. Frankincense is too drying to the skin alone, but it can be combined with any or all of these others.

Personal Care— A·R·T Creme Masque, A·R·T Beauty Masque, Orange Blossom Facial Wash, Satin Facial Scrub - Mint.

—FEEDS SKIN AND SUPPLIES NUTRIENTS

Personal Care—Boswellia Wrinkle Cream, Rose Ointment.

—IMPETIGO

Impetigo is a bacterial skin infection that causes sores and blisters filled with a yellowish fluid. These sores can be itchy and painful and can easily be spread to other areas of the skin or to another person.

Recipe #2—Lavender, myrrh. Boil 4 ounces water; let water cool. Add 5–10 drops lavender, and wash infected skin. You may also use myrrh (cover for an hour). Do hot compress on site.

—ITCHING

Oils—[T]Peppermint, [T]lavender, [T]Peace & Calming.

T—Dilute as necessary, and apply on ears and on location.

Personal Care—ClaraDerm (essential oil spray), Lavender Hand & Body Lotion.

—RASHES

A rash is an area of irritated skin, redness, or red bumps on the body. Rashes may be localized or may cover large patches of the body. A rash may be caused by a chemical or allergen irritating the skin, or as a symptom of another medical condition or infection.

Oils—[T,F]Melaleuca, [T]Melrose, [T]elemi (allergic), [T]hinoki, [T]lavender, [T]palmarosa, [T]Release (on Vita Flex points of feet), [T]Roman chamomile.

T—Dilute as necessary, and apply on location.

If the rash occurs from application of oils to the skin, it may be due to the oils reacting with accumulated synthetic chemicals (toxins) that are trapped in the fatty layers of the skin. Take the following steps: 1) Try diluting the oils first (1–3 drops of oil to ½ tsp. V-6 Oil), 2) reduce the number of oils used with each application (use oils one at a time), 3) reduce the amount of oils (number of drops) used, and 4) reduce the frequency of application (more time between applications). Drinking pure (steam-distilled) water helps promote the elimination of accumulated toxins from the body. Initiating programs to cleanse the bowels and blood will also help remove accumulated toxins and reduce the possible recurrences of the rash. If the rashes persist, discontinue use of the oils and consult your health care professional.

***Comments—Red spots on body may indicate a biotin deficiency; take Super C or Super C Chewable.

Personal Care—KidScents Tender Tush, Rose Ointment.

***Comments—Dr. Friedmann had a patient who had a rash for three years on the side of the face and arms, and the eyes were weeping. The patient had gone to five physicians for treatments and had no success. Dr. Friedmann did the following: 1) Did a culture of the eye and face and determined that the patient had staphylococcus. 2) Had the patient apply Melrose and lavender alternately morning and night. 3) Had the patient take Mineral Essence and Colloidal Essence (a colloidal silver product). After a short period of time, the patient's face and eyes totally cleared up and the arms were healing.

—RINGWORM: *See Antifungal: Ringworm*

—SAGGY SKIN

Blend #1—Combine 8 drops each of sage, pine, and lemongrass with 1 oz. V-6 Oil. Rub on areas.

—SCABIES

Scabies is an infestation of the skin by mites (Sarcoptes scabei) that burrow into the upper layers of the skin, causing small, extremely itchy bumps.

Oils—[T]Thieves (needs to be diluted), [T]melaleuca, [T]lavender and [T]peppermint, [T]bergamot, [T]laurel, [T]pine.

T—Add 5–10 drops to 1 Tbs. V-6 Oil, and apply a small amount on location morning and night.

—**Scarring** *See Scarring*

—**Sensitive**

Oils—[T]Geranium, [T]German chamomile, [T]jasmine, [T]lavender, [T]neroli.

Personal Care—Lavender Hand & Body Lotion.

—**Stretch Marks** *See Stretch Marks*

—**Sunburn** *See Sunburn*

—**Tones**

Oils—[T]Patchouli.

T—Dilute with V-6 Oil to create a massage oil, and massage into the skin.

Personal Care—Cel-Lite Magic, Satin Facial Scrub - Mint, Sandalwood Moisture Cream.

Supplements—Ultra Young+ (helps firm and tighten skin by activating the production of skin proteins, collagen, and elastin).

—**Vitiligo**

▸▸ *Vitiligo is white patches of the skin caused by the death or dysfunction of pigment-producing cells in the area. While the exact cause is unknown, it may be caused by an immune or genetic disorder, or may have a relationship to thyroid problems.*

Vitiligo may be due to a malfunction of the pineal gland and possibly the pituitary gland as well. See Pineal *and* Pituitary *for oils and products that can help oxygenate these glands. Another possible remedy includes daily exposure of the eyes to full-spectrum light without contacts or eyeglasses.*

Oils—[T]Sandalwood, [T]vetiver, [T]frankincense, [T]Melrose, [T]myrrh, [T]Purification, [T]sage.

T—Apply behind ears and to back of neck. Then rub hands together, cup hands over nose and mouth, and breathe deeply. Can also be applied to Vita Flex points relating to the pineal and pituitary glands on the feet and hands.

—**Wrinkles**

Oils—[T]Frankincense, [T]patchouli, [T]lavender, [T]carrot, [T]fennel, [T]geranium, [T]helichrysum, [T]lemon, [T]rosewood, [T]sandalwood, [T]cistus, [T]clary sage, [T]cypress, [T]elemi, [T]galbanum, [T]myrrh, [T]neroli, [T]orange, [T]oregano, [T]rose, [T]rosemary, [T]spikenard, [T]thyme, [T]ylang ylang.

Wrinkles *occur as we mature and as we lose oxygen to the tissues. Essential oils oxygenate the tissues and thereby slow down the premature aging of the skin.*

Blend #1—3 drops lavender, 4 drops geranium, 2 drops patchouli, 6 drops rosewood, and 1 oz. V-6 Oil. Rub on wrinkles in an upward, lifting motion.

Blend #2—1 drop frankincense, 1 drop lavender, and 1 drop lemon. It's like magic for wrinkles. Rub on morning and night around the eyes.

Blend #3—5–10 drops frankincense added to Sandalwood Moisture Cream.

Blend #4—Equal amounts of sandalwood, helichrysum, geranium, lavender, and frankincense. Combine with either Genesis Hand & Body Lotion or Lavender Hand & Body Lotion, and apply to skin.

Personal Care— A·R·T Creme Masque, A·R·T Skin Care System (repairs DNA damage, builds collagen), Boswellia Wrinkle Cream (collagen builder), Essential Beauty Serums (Dry, & Acne-Prone Skin Blends), Rose Ointment, Sandalwood Moisture Cream, Lavender Hand & Body Lotion, Satin Facial Scrub - Mint, Wolfberry Eye Cream. The following three items can be used together to help tone the skin and prevent wrinkles: Orange Blossom Facial Wash, Rose Ointment, Sandalwood Moisture Cream, Lavender Hand & Body Lotion.

Supplements—Essentialzyme, Essentialzymes-4, PD 80/20, Prenolone/Prenolone+, Progessence/Progessence Plus, Thyromin (thyroid function affects the skin), Ultra Young+.

–Prevent

Oils—**T**Gentle Baby and **T**patchouli (prevents and retards).

Personal Care—A·R·T Skin Care System, Boswellia Wrinkle Cream (collagen builder), Essential Beauty Serums (Dry, & Acne-Prone Skin Blends), Satin Facial Scrub - Mint, Wolfberry Eye Cream. The following three items can be used together to help tone the skin and to prevent wrinkles: Orange Blossom Facial Wash, Sandalwood Moisture Cream.

–Smooth

Recipe #3—Add 2 drops frankincense to a little Genesis Hand & Body Lotion or Lavender Hand & Body Lotion, and apply.

Personal Care—A·R·T Skin Care System, Boswellia Wrinkle Cream (collagen builder), Essential Beauty Serums (Dry, & Acne-Prone Skin Blends).

T—Dilute as necessary, and apply on location. Dilute with V-6 Oil or other carrier oil, such as jojoba, apricot, hazelnut, or sweet almond, to create massage oil, and apply to areas of concern. Add 3–4 drops to 1/4 cup bath salts, and dissolve in warm bathwater before bathing.

Sleep:

Oils—**AT**Lavender[286] (on spine), **AT**RutaVaLa, **AT**Peace & Calming, **TA**valerian[287] (disturbances), **T**Tranquil (roll-on), **A**marjoram, **A**Roman chamomile, **T**Stress Away.

A—Diffuse into the air. Apply 1–2 drops to pillow or stuffed animal. Add 2–5 drops to 1 oz. distilled water in a small spray bottle, and mist into the air or on linens before sleeping. *See also Negative Ions for oils that produce negative ions when diffused to help promote sleep.*

T—Dilute as necessary, and apply on area indicated or on back, bottoms of feet, or back of neck. Add 3–4 drops to 1/4 cup Epsom or bath salts, and dissolve in warm bathwater before bathing. Dilute with V-6 Oil to create massage oil, and massage into the skin.

Supplements—SleepEssence, Ultra Young+ (restores deep sleep).

—Animals

Oils—**T**Peace & Calming, **T**Trauma Life.

T—Oils can be used on the paws of animals to help them relax and sleep when in pain.

—Good Nights Sleep

Recipe #1—*See also Insomnia for additional blends.* ¼ cup bath salts and 10 drops geranium or lavender in bath; soak in tub. Bathe with Evening Peace Bath Gel.

—Restless *See also Legs, Restless for recipe*

Oils—**AT**Lavender, **AT**Gathering.

A—Diffuse into the air. Apply 1–2 drops to pillow or stuffed animal.

T—Dilute as necessary, and apply on area indicated or on legs, back, bottoms of feet, or back of neck. Dilute with V-6 Oil to create massage oil, and massage into the skin.

—Sleeping Sickness

▸▸ *Sleeping sickness is swelling of the brain caused by an infection carried by tsetse flies. Symptoms include fever, anxiety, drowsiness, insomnia at night, sweating, mood changes, swollen lymph nodes, and an uncontrollable urge to sleep. Without treatment, this disorder can be fatal.*

Oils—ᵀJuniper, ᵀpeppermint, ᵀPeace & Calming (on big toes, back of neck, and navel), ᵀgeranium, ᵀValor (on feet).

T—Dilute as necessary, and apply on area indicated or on back of neck, lymph nodes, and Vita Flex points on the feet.

Slimming and Toning Oils: *See also Weight.*

Oils—^AI^Grapefruit[288], ^I^sage[289], ^A^lemongrass, ^AI^orange, ^A^basil, ^A^lavender, ^A^rosemary, ^A^thyme.

A—Inhale directly. Diffuse into the air.

I—Add 1 drop to 12–16 oz. of water, and drink. Add 1–2 drops to empty capsule, and swallow.

Slivers (Splinters):

Recipe #1—Mix 10 drops Thieves with 4 Tbs. V-6 Oil, and massage bottoms of feet, armpits, throat, and lower stomach. Put 30 drops of Thieves in bath gel, and use the gel in the shower each day (this helps pull the slivers to gently massage them out) .

Smell, Loss of:

Just smelling the oils helps stimulate the sense of smell. ***To smell the oils,*** *first close the eyes; then hold the left nostril closed, breathe in the smell of the oil through the right nostril, and then breathe out through the mouth. Breathing in the fragrance of the oils in this manner stimulates every endocrine gland in the brain. Next hold the right nostril closed and repeat the process.*

Oils—^A^Basil (helps when loss of smell is due to chronic nasal catarrh), ^A^peppermint.

A—Inhale directly or applied to hands. Diffuse into the air.

—Stimulate Sensory Cortex

Oils—^T^Brain Power.

T—Place under the tongue, behind the ears, and on the forehead. Can also place a couple drops of oil in the hands, rub hands together in a clockwise motion, cup hands over the nose and mouth, and breathe deeply.

***Comments—*According to the Essential Oils Desk Reference, "Massage 1 or 2 drops [of Brain Power] with a finger on the insides of cheeks in the mouth. Doing this 1 or 2 times a day will immediately improve the smell sensory cortex." (EDR-June 2002; Ch. 8; Brain Power; Application)*

Smoking: *See also Addictions: Smoking, Air Pollution, Purification.*

Oils—^A^Black pepper[290], ^A^Purification.

—Cigarette

Oils—^A^Black pepper[290], ^A^Purification.

—Purify Air

Oils—^A^Purification, ^A^lemon.

—Stop Smoking *See also Addictions.*

Oils—^A^Black pepper[290], ^A^clove (removes desire), ^T^Thieves (on tongue before lighting up helps remove desire), ^A^GLF, ^A^Peace & Calming, ^A^Present Time (helps with insecurity), ^A^Purification.

Personal Guide

Supplements—JuvaPower/JuvaSpice, JuvaTone, Super C / Super C Chewable.

***Comments—*One individual used JuvaTone to break a habit of smoking 2½ packs of cigarettes a day for 20 years. Another individual who used JuvaTone went from smoking a pack a day to 1 cigarette in 1½ weeks.*

A—Inhale directly or applied to hands. Diffuse into the air.

T—Apply as indicated.

Snoring:

Oils—**T**RC.

T—Rub on throat before sleeping to help keep the airway open.

Soothing:

Oils—**TA**Gentle Baby, **TA**Roman chamomile, **TA**myrrh, **TA**onycha (benzoin), **AT**Release.

T—Dilute with V-6 Oil, and apply on area of concern or on back, legs, feet, and arms.

A—Diffuse into the air. Inhale directly or applied to hands, tissue, or a cotton wick.

Sores: *See also Antibacterial, Antifungal, Antiviral, Cuts, Wounds.*

Oils—**T**Melaleuca, **T**basil[291], **T**Thieves, **T**pine.

T—Dilute as necessary, and apply on location.

S

Sore Throat: *See Throat.*

Spacing Out:

Oils—**A**Grounding, **A**Acceptance, **A**Present Time, **A**Sacred Mountain.

A—Inhale directly or applied to hands, tissue, or a cotton wick. Diffuse into the air.

Spasms: *See also Digestive System, Muscles, Antispasmodic.*

Oils—**T**Basil, **T**$_F$cypress, **T**Aroma Siez, **T**calamus, **T**Deep Relief (roll-on), **T**jasmine (muscle), **T**lavender (antispasmodic), **T**marjoram (relieves), **T**oregano, **T**Peace & Calming, **T**peppermint, **T**Roman chamomile, **T**spikenard, **T**tarragon, **T**thyme.

—Spasticity

Oils—**T**Cypress, **T**ginger, **T**juniper, **T**lavender, **T**lemon, **T**rosemary, **T**sandalwood.

T—Dilute as necessary, and apply on location of spasm or on Vita Flex points on the feet. Apply as a warm compress over area of concern.

Spina Bifida:

›› *Spina bifida is a birth defect in which the vertebrae of the lower spine do not form correctly, leaving a gap or opening between them. In the most severe cases, this can cause the meninges (the tissue surrounding the spinal cord), or even the spinal cord itself, to protrude through the gap. If the spinal cord protrudes through the gap, it can prevent the nerves from developing normally, causing numbness, paralysis, back pain, and loss of bladder and bowel control and function. This later type often also develops along with a defect in which the back part of the brain develops in the upper neck rather than within the skull, often causing a mental handicap.*

Oils—TAEucalyptus, TAlavender, TARoman chamomile, TAlemon, TAnutmeg, TAorange, TArosemary, TA3 Wise Men.

T—Apply oil(s) to bottoms of feet, forehead, back of neck, along spine.

A—Diffuse into the air.

***Comments—Do the Raindrop Technique.

Spine: *See Back.*

Spiritual:

Oils—ATAwaken, ATBelieve, ATDream Catcher, ATGathering,AT Gratitude, ATHumility, ATInspiration.

—Awareness

Oils—ATAcceptance, ATwestern red cedar, ATcedarwood, ATjuniper, AThinoki, ATmyrrh, ATSacred Mountain, ATspruce, ATTransformation, AWhite Angelica, ATwhite lotus.

—Balancing

Oils—ATJoy, ATInto the Future, ATspruce.

—Increase

Oils—ATBelieve, ATcedarwood (enhances), Afrankincense (opening and enhancing spiritual receptivity), ATGratitude, ATTransformation.

—Inner Awareness

Oils—ATBelieve, ATGratitude, ATInner Child, ATInspiration.

—Meditation

Oils—ATBelieve, ATwestern red cedar, ATfrankincense, ATInspiration, ATtsuga, ATWhite Angelica.

—Prayer

Oils—ATGratitude, ATInspiration, ATWhite Angelica.

—Protection

Oils—T3 Wise Men (on crown and shoulders).

—Purity of Spirit

Oils—ATMyrrh.

—Spiritually Uplifting

Oils—ATBelieve, ATGratitude, ATSacred Mountain, ATTransformation.

A—Inhale directly or applied to hands, tissue, or a cotton wick. Diffuse into the air.

T—Dilute as necessary, and apply on indicated areas or on crown, forehead, or heart.

Spleen:

▸▸ *The spleen is a fist-sized spongy tissue that is part of the lymphatic system. Its purpose is to filter bacteria, viruses, fungi, and other unwanted substances out of the blood and to create lymphocytes (white blood cells that create antibodies).*

Oils—TLaurel, Tmarjoram.

T—Dilute as necessary, and apply over spleen or on Vita Flex points on the feet. Apply as a warm compress over upper abdomen.

Sports: *See Aches/Pains, Bones, Injuries, Muscles, Tissue.*

—Excel In

Oils—TClarity (on forehead), TPeace & Calming (back of neck), TPanAway (injuries), TValor (on feet for courage and confidence), TTranquil (roll-on).

—Injuries

Oils—THelichrysum, TPanAway, TDeep Relief (roll-on), Tlemongrass, TMelrose, TPeace & Calming.

Supplements—BLM

—Track Competition

Oils—IBalsam fir

I—Take 2–3 drops in a capsule before the competition to help reduce muscle soreness afterward.

Blend #1—5 drops basil, 5 drops bergamot, and 2 tsp. V-6 Oil.

Personal Care—Ortho Ease Massage Oil, Ortho Sport Massage Oil. Massage into the muscles to increase oxygen and elasticity in the tissues to prevent the muscles and ligaments from tearing during strenuous exercise. It may also be used after to prevent the muscle from cramping.

Supplements—MultiGreens.

T—Dilute as necessary, and apply on area indicated or on area of concern.

Sprains: *See Muscles: Sprain.*

Spurs, Bone: *See also Bones.*

Oils—TLavender, TRC (dissolves).

T—Apply directly on location.

Stains: *See also Housecleaning.*

Oils—TLemon (removes).

T—Apply 1–2 drops on location.

Staph Infection: *See Antibacterial: Staph Infection, MRSA.*

Sterility:

Oils—TClary sage, $^{T}_{F}$geranium, Trose (wonderful for both men and women), Tjasmine, Tneroli, Tsage lavender, Tsandalwood, TSclarEssence (taken internally, helps increase estradiol and testosterone levels), Trosewood, Tvetiver.

T—Apply several together (or alternate individually) by massage or aromatic bath.

I—Add 1–3 drops to an empty capsule, and swallow.

Personal Care—Prenolone/Prenolone+, Progessence/Progessence Plus (for women only).

Supplements—Power Meal.

Stimulating:

Oils—$^{T}_{F}$Peppermint, TEn-R-Gee, $^{T}_{F}$sage, Teucalyptus[292], Trosemary[292], Tbasil, Tblack pepper, Tfir, Tginger, Tgrapefruit, Torange, Tpatchouli, Trose, TTransformation.

T—Dilute with V-6 Oil to create a massage oil for a stimulating massage. Can also add a few drops of an oil (or of a couple oils) to bath gel, and then add the gel to the bathwater as the tub is filling.

***Comments—Adding a little black pepper to an oil like rosemary can give it a little more power.

Stings: *See Bites/Stings.*

Stomach: *See also Digestive System.*

Oils—$^{T}_{F}$Basil, ^{T}ginger, ^{T}peppermint, ^{T}calamus (supports).

T—Apply to stomach Vita Flex points on feet, or apply as a hot compress over the stomach area.

—Ache

Oils—^{T}Di-Gize (behind ears and down jaw bone), ^{TI}peppermint, ^{T}eucalyptus, ^{T}geranium, ^{T}lavender, ^{T}rosemary.

T—Dilute as necessary, and apply as indicated; or apply over stomach area and on Vita Flex points on the feet.

I—Add 1–2 drops to an empty capsule, and swallow.

—Acid

Oils—^{I}Peppermint

I—Put drop on finger, and place on tongue.

Recipe #1—Put several drops of fresh lemon juice in warm water, and sip slowly.

Supplements—AlkaLime (acid-neutralizing mineral formula).

—Bacteria or Germs

Oils—^{I}Peppermint

I—Add 1–2 drops to an empty capsule, and swallow.

—Bloating

Oils—^{I}Fennel

I—Add 1–2 drops to almond or rice milk, water, or other liquid; drink.

—Cramps

Oils—$^{T}_{F}$Helichrysum, $^{T}_{F}$thyme (general tonic for), ^{T}blue cypress, ^{T}ginger, ^{T}lavender, ^{T}onycha (benzoin), ^{T}rosemary cineol.

T—Apply as a warm compress over stomach area. Dilute as necessary, and apply over stomach area or on Vita Flex points on the feet.

Recipe #2—Flavor water with 5 drops of Di-Gize, and drink for stomach pains **or** add 3 drops basil in a capsule with Di-Gize.

—Tonic

Oils—^{I}Tangerine.

I—Add 1–2 drops to 12–16 oz. of water; drink.

—Upset

Oils—^{TIA}Di-Gize, ^{I}ginger[293].

T—Apply over stomach and colon, behind the ears, on Vita Flex points on the feet

I—Add 1 drop to 8 oz. rice or almond milk, and drink. Place 1–2 drops in an empty capsule, and swallow.

A—Place a couple of drops on the palms of the hands, rub the hands together clockwise, cup hands over nose and mouth, and breathe deeply.

Strength:

Oils—**TA**$_F$Peppermint, **A**cypress, **TA**Hope, **TA**oregano, **TA**patchouli, **TA**Raven, **TA**Roman chamomile (strengthens positive imprinting in DNA), **TA**Sacred Mountain, **TA**White Angelica.

T—Add 1–2 drops to warm bathwater, and bathe. Dilute with V-6 Oil to create a massage oil, and massage onto the skin.

A—Diffuse into the air.

Supplements— NingXia Red, Power Meal, Pure Protein Complete, Wolfberry Crisp Bars.

Strep Throat: *See Throat: Strep.*

Stress: *See also Calming.*

Oils—**AT**Lavender[294], **AT**ylang ylang[295], **T**Stress Away, **T**Tranquil (roll-on), **AT**Peace & Calming, **AT**$_F$bergamot, **AT**lemon[296], **AT**Common Sense, **AT**Aroma Life, **AT**basil, **AT**Believe, **AT**Clarity, **AT**clary sage, **AT**cypress, **AT**elemi, **AT**Evergreen Essence, **AT**frankincense, **AT**geranium, **AT**grapefruit, **AT**Harmony, **AT**Inspiration, **AT**Joy, **AT**marjoram, **AT**neroli, **AT**onycha (benzoin), **AT**pine, **AT**Roman chamomile (relieves stress), **AT**rosewood, **AT**Sacred Mountain, **AT**spruce, **AT**Surrender, **AT**tangerine, **AT**3 Wise Men, **AT**Valor, **AT**White Angelica.

Personal Care—Evening Peace or Sensation Shower Gel, Relaxation or Sensation Massage Oil, Sensation Hand & Body Lotion.

Supplements—ImmuPro, Inner Defense, Master Formula His/Hers, Thyromin, Super B, and Super Cal.

***Comments—You can't change the stressful situations that come, but you can change your response to those situations. Focus on resolution not on recrimination! *(See Forgive)*

—Chemical

Oils—**AT**Lavender, **AT**rosemary, **AT**clary sage, **AT**geranium, **AT**grapefruit, **AT**lemon, **AT**patchouli.

—Emotional Stress

Oils—**AT**Joy, **AT**clary sage, **AT**bergamot, **T**Tranquil (roll-on), **AT**Evergreen Essence, **AT**Forgiveness, **AT**Gathering, **AT**geranium, **AT**ravensara, **AT**sandalwood (layer on navel and chest), **AT**Surrender, **AT**Transformation, **AT**Trauma Life.

—Environmental Stress

Oils—**AT**Bergamot, **AT**geranium, **AT**Roman chamomile, **AT**cypress, **AT**basil, **AT**cedarwood.

—Mental Stress

Oils—**AT**Lavender[294], **AT**bergamot, **AT**grapefruit, **T**Tranquil (roll-on), **AT**basil, **AT**Evergreen Essence, **AT**geranium, **AT**patchouli, **AT**pine, **AT**sandalwood, **AT**Surrender.

—Performance Stress

Oils—**AT**Grapefruit, **AT**bergamot, **T**Tranquil (roll-on), **AT**ginger, **AT**rosemary.

—Physical Stress

Oils—ATPeace & Calming, ATlavender, ATmarjoram, ATbergamot, ATgeranium, ATBelieve, ATfennel, ATGentle Baby, ATHarmony, ATRoman chamomile, ATrosemary, ATthyme, TTranquil (roll-on), ATTrauma Life (calming).

Supplements—ImmuPro.

—Relationship Stress *See also Sex Stimulant.*

Personal Care—Sensation (Hand & Body Lotion, Massage Oil, Bath & Shower Gel) creates an exotic arousal, increasing sexual desire. The fragrance creates a peaceful and harmonious feeling that helps ease relationship stress. Relaxation Massage Oil also creates a peaceful and harmonious feeling. You may want to add jasmine and ylang ylang. .

—Stress That Starts With Tiredness, Irritability, or Insomnia

Blend #1—15 drops clary sage, 10 drops lemon, 5 drops lavender, and 1 oz. V-6 Oil.

Supplements—ImmuPro, Inner Defense, Super B.

Stretch Marks: *See also Pregnancy/Motherhood: Stretch Marks.*

Oils—TGentle Baby, TFlavender, TFmyrrh, Tmandarin, Tneroli.

T—Dilute as necessary, and apply on location.

Blend #1—3 drops rosemary, 15 drops rosewood, and 1¾ oz. hazelnut oil.

Blend #2—6 drops lavender, 4 drops rosewood, 3 drops patchouli, and vitamin E Oil.

***Comments—Patricia Davis recommends adding mandarin and neroli to either rosehip seed oil or almond oil to massage over tummy and hips.

Stroke: *See also Blood: Clots, Blood: Broken Blood Vessels, Brain.*

A stroke occurs when the blood supply to the brain is interrupted. Within a few minutes, brain cells begin to die. The affected area of the brain is unable to function, and one or more limbs on one side of the body become weak and unable to move. Strokes can cause serious disabilities, including paralysis and speech problems.

Oils—ATAroma Life, ATcypress, AThelichrysum, Ifennel[297], ATblack pepper[298], ATcalamus.

A—Inhale oil deeply either directly from bottle or applied to hands, tissue, or a cotton wick. *See Comments under Asthma for a discussion on using* ***plastic nasal inhalers****.*

T—Apply to neck and forehead.

I—Add 1–3 drops to an empty capsule, and swallow.

Supplements—Master Formula His/Hers, NingXia Red, Power Meal, Sulfurzyme, Ultra Young+, Wolfberry Crisp Bars.

—Heat

Oils—TPeppermint, Tlavender

T—Rub on neck and on forehead.

—Muscular Paralysis

Oils—TLavender.

T—Apply on affected muscles, spine, and back of neck.

Blend #1—Mix together equal parts of basil, lavender, and rosemary. Rub spinal column and paralyzed area (*Alternative Medicine—The Definitive Guide*, p. 978).

Personal Guide

Structural Alignment:

> *Valor is considered a "chiropractor in a bottle." It may help to realign the spine and keep the body in balance.*

Oils—TValor, Twintergreen (apply on feet to reduce time and effort necessary for alignments and to increase the amount of time the alignment remains effective), TAroma Siez, Tbasil, Tcypress, Tpeppermint.

T—Dilute as necessary, and apply to spine and to bottoms of feet.

***Comments—**Do the Raindrop Technique**.

Personal Care—Ortho Ease Massage Oil.

Subconscious:

Oils—ATBelieve, ATbalsam fir, ATGratitude, AThelichrysum (uplifts when diffused), ATTransformation, ATwestern red cedar.

A—Inhale directly or applied to hands, tissue, or a cotton wick. Diffuse into the air.

T—Dilute with V-6 Oil to create a massage oil, and massage into the skin. Add 1–2 drops to warm bathwater before bathing.

Sudorific:

S

Oils—TThyme, Thyssop, Tjuniper, Tlavender, TRoman chamomile, Trosemary.

T—Dilute with V-6 Oil to create a massage oil, and apply to the skin.

> *A sudorific is an agent that causes sweating. It may be helpful in times of fever or when toxins need to be released through the skin.*

Sugar:

***Comments—White sugar creates acid in the body.

Supplements—Allerzyme (aids the digestion of sugars, starches, fats, and proteins). NingXia Red (contains 4 of the 8 essential sugars that heal the body and are necessary for cell-to-cell communication).

> *Honey goes into the blood stream faster than sugar and can be harder on the system than sugar. Maple syrup is one of the most perfect sugars because it has equal proportions of positive and negative ions. It also has the same pH as the blood, and it doesn't go into the blood as fast as honey or sugar. Diabetics and pre-diabetics should use blackstrap molasses instead of maple syrup.*

Substitute—Stevia (liquid), Yacon Syrup.

—Remove Addictions to Sugar

Oils—TDill

T—Apply on wrists.

—Stop Eating

Oils—APeace & Calming, APurification.

A—Inhale directly or applied to tissue or a cotton wick.

Supplements—JuvaTone.

Suicide: *See Depression and Emotions.*

Sunburn: *See also Burns.*

Oils—T$_F$Melaleuca, Tlavender TAustralian Blue, Tpeppermint, Ttamanu (mix with helichrysum).

> *My niece came to me in a panic. She had been at the beach all day and had acquired a nasty sunburn on her face, chest, and arms. She was planning to go to a fancy party the next day and decided that she absolutely could not go to the party unless the sunburn was gone. I immediately applied a layer of lavender oil, followed a few minutes later by a layer of peppermint oil. The next day to her amazement the sunburn had vanished and she was able to enjoy her party.*
> ***–Submitted by J. S., Florida (July 2004)***

T—Dilute as necessary, and apply on location.

Recipe #1—Spray or rub with Roman chamomile and lavender. Add 5–6 drops of Roman chamomile to lukewarm bathwater to help reduce the burning sensation.

Recipe #2—Add a little lavender or tamanu oil to some Lavender Hand & Body Lotion.

Blend #1—Put 10 drops of lavender in a 4 oz. glass or plastic spray bottle full of distilled water. Shake well; then spray on location. This is effective for pain and healing.

Supplements—Mineral Essence (can apply directly on affected area).

Personal Care—LavaDerm Cooling Mist (use as often as needed to keep skin cool and moist), A·R·T Skin Care System, Lavender Hand & Body Lotion (later to help maintain moisture).

–Prevent Blistering

Recipe #3—Apply 2–3 drops of lavender with Lavender Hand & Body Lotion.

Sun Screen:

Oils—$^{T}{}_{F}$Helichrysum, ^{T}tamanu[299] (used by Polynesians as a natural sunscreen for centuries).

T—Dilute with V-6 Oil, and apply to the skin.

Personal Care—A·R·T Skin Care System.

Supportive:

Oils—^{TA}Myrrh.

T—Dilute with V-6 Oil to create a massage oil, and massage into the skin. Apply to Vita Flex points on the feet.

A—Diffuse into the air. Inhale directly or applied to hands.

Swelling: *See also Edema (for swelling from water retention), Inflammation.*

Swelling is the enlargement of organs, skin, or other body parts. It is caused by an excess of fluids in the tissues. Swelling can be throughout the body (generalized) or only in a specific part of the body (localized). Swelling can occur due to an injury, infection, or disease.

Oils—^{TI}Tangerine, ^{T}helichrysum, ^{T}lemongrass, ^{T}ocotea.

T—Dilute as necessary, and apply on location.

I—Add 1 drop to 8 oz. of water, and drink.

Blend #1—Layer myrrh, frankincense, balsam fir, and helichrysum directly on location.

Sympathetic Nervous System: *See Nervous System: Sympathetic.*

Sympathy:

Oils—^{AT}Acceptance, ^{AT}Awaken, ^{AT}Present Time.

A—Inhale directly or applied to hands. Diffuse into the air.

T—Apply to auricular emotion points. Add 1–2 drops to warm bathwater, and bathe.

Tachycardia (Rapid Heartbeat): *See Cardiovascular System: Tachycardia.*

Talkative:

Oils—[A]Cypress (for over-talkative).

A—Inhale directly or applied to hands.

Taste:

Oils—[T]Helichrysum, [T]peppermint (for impaired taste).

T—Apply 1 drop on tongue, or on Vita Flex points on the feet.

Supplements—Mineral Essence, Super B, Super C / Super C Chewable (enhances flavor).

Teeth: *See also Oral Conditions.*

—Cavities

Recipe #1—Brush teeth with Thieves. Put a drop on your toothpaste if you can't handle it straight.

Personal Care—Thieves Dentarome/Dentarome Plus Toothpaste, Thieves Fresh Essence Plus Mouthwash, KidScents Toothpaste (for children).

***Comments—*People have had regeneration of their teeth in as little as four months by brushing their teeth with Thieves.*

—Fillings

Recipe #2—To help eliminate toxins from mercury in the system, place 22 drops of balsam fir in a capsule, and take once in the morning and once at night. Can also combine balsam fir with helichrysum and/or frankincense.

Supplements—Super C / Super C Chewable, Cleansing Trio (ComforTone, Essentialzyme, and ICP), Detoxzyme (5 in morning and 5 at night until body says stop! Then back off to 1 or 2 per day).

My husband has very cavity prone teeth that have needed much dental work in the past 5 years. He has been going in for cleanings every 3 months. His dentist had once prescribed a special mouth wash that was supposed to help his decaying teeth. He didn't use the mouthwash regularly enough to see any improvement. About a year ago, he started using Dentarome Plus toothpaste instead of the brand he had been using from the local grocer. That was the only change he made to his dental hygiene routine. At his cleaning in March, his dentist wanted to know what he was doing differently, because his x-rays showed no dental work needed to be done and they didn't have to work as hard to polish his teeth. He told them that all he changed was the toothpaste he was using. They wanted to know if it had fluoride in it, because to be any good (in their eyes) it must have fluoride in it; he brushed them off not wanting to get into the dangers of fluoride with them that day. Then at his cleaning just last week, the dentist had to look at his x-rays twice as well as call on two other colleagues to look at his x-rays to be sure that nothing was being missed because they could not find anything that needed to be fixed. They also told him to come back in six months (instead of 3) for his next cleaning. Now, if I could only get him to use the Fresh Essence Plus mouthwash...

-Submitted by A. Corn
Machesney Park, Illinois (July 2004)

—Gum Surgery

Recipe #3—Helichrysum every 15 minutes for the pain.

—Teething Pain

Oils—[T]German chamomile, [T]Thieves.

—Toothache

Oils—[T,F]Clove, [T]cajeput, [T]melaleuca, [T]Purification (antibacterial), [T]Roman chamomile.

Personal Care—Thieves Dentarome / Dentarome Plus Toothpaste, Thieves Fresh Essence Plus Mouthwash.

—Toothpaste

Oils—[T]Thieves.

*****Comments**—*You may want to put 10-12 drops of Thieves in a 2 oz. spray bottle filled with distilled water. Shake well, then mist in mouth or on toothbrush and brush.*

Personal Care—Thieves Dentarome / Dentarome Plus Toothpaste, Thieves Fresh Essence Plus Mouthwash, KidScents Toothpaste (for children).

Recipe #4—Combine 4 tsp. green or white clay with 1 tsp. salt, 1–2 drops peppermint, and 1–2 drops lemon; mix clockwise.

—Nerve Pain

Recipe #5—Put 1 drop melaleuca in a small amount of water, and hold in mouth for 1–2 minutes to help calm nerves.

T—Dilute as necessary, and apply on location (on gums) and along jawbone. Mix 1–2 drops with 4 oz. water, and use as mouth rinse.

Temperature: *See also Cooling Oils, Fever, Thyroid, Warming Oils.*

Supplements—Thyromin (balances the temperature in the body).

—Lower

Oils—TPeppermint, Tbergamot, Teucalyptus, Tlavender, Tmelissa. TCypress and Trosemary induce sweating to lower temperature indirectly.

T—Use oils in baths; or mix oils with cool water, and sponge over body or area.

—Raise

Oils—TMarjoram, Tthyme, Tonycha (benzoin).

T—Add to V-6 Oil for brisk massage.

*****Comments**—Locally warming (rubefacient) oils like black pepper, juniper, and rosemary help raise temperature in cold extremities.

Tendinitis:

Oils—TWintergreen, Tmarjoram, TPanAway, TRelieve It, Tbasil, Tcypress, Tbalsam fir, Tginger, Tlavender, Tpeppermint, Trosemary.

Supplements—BLM

—Pain Relief

Oils—TWintergreen, TPanAway, Tbalsam fir, Tfrankincense, Tpeppermint.

*****Comments**—If pain and inflammation are results of torn or infected ligaments or tendons, then lemongrass and helichrysum can be helpful when added to any of the above oils.

T—Apply oils in Raindrop fashion on location and apply an ice pack. Can also try alternating cold and hot packs.

> ***Tendinitis Blend***
>
> *This has worked for my tendinitis and for several other people I have given it to. In a 15 ml amber glass bottle, I mix the following essential oils: 3 drops each of helichrysum, pepper, bergamot, and geranium, 5 drops each of Idaho balsam fir and lemongrass, then 3 drops each of hyssop, blue tansy, pine, and myrtle. Then I fill the rest of the bottle with V-6 Mixing Oil. This is applied to the area where the pain is and followed with a layer of peppermint oil. This can be done several times per day. If a sensitivity develops, stop using it for a few weeks.*
>
> ***-Submitted by J. S.***
> ***West Saint Paul, Minnesota (July 2004)***

Tennis Elbow:

▸▸ *Tennis Elbow is the painful inflammation of the tendon on the outer side of the elbow that usually results from excessive strain on and twisting of the forearm.*

Oils—TPanAway, Teucalyptus, Tpeppermint, Thelichrysum, Trosemary, Twintergreen.

T—Dilute as necessary, and apply on location. Apply as cold compress.

Blend #1—10 drops eucalyptus, 10 drops peppermint, 10 drops rosemary, and 1 Tbs. V-6 Oil. Mix and apply; then apply ice pack. Can also try alternating cold and hot packs.

Blend #2—Equal parts lemongrass, helichrysum, marjoram, and peppermint. Mix and apply; then apply ice pack.

Tension:

Oils—**AT**Peace & Calming, **AT**$_F$cedarwood, **T**Stress Away, **AT**lavender, **AT**ylang ylang, **T**Tranquil (roll-on), **AT**basil (nervous), **AT**bergamot (nervous), **AT**frankincense, **AT**Harmony, **AT***Melaleuca ericifolia* (nervous), **AT**Trauma Life (balances and calms), **AT**valerian.

Supplements—SleepEssence (short-term only).

—Relieve

Oils—**T**Tranquil (roll on), **AT**Grapefruit, **AT**Roman chamomile, **AT**Transformation.

Personal Care—Ortho Ease Massage Oil, Relaxation Massage Oil, Prenolone/Prenolone+, Progessence/Progessence Plus.

A—Apply on hands, cup hands over nose and mouth, and breathe deeply; or diffuse. *See COMMENTS under Asthma for a discussion on using* ***plastic nasal inhalers****.*

T—Mix a few drops of oil, or oils of choice, in ½ cup Epsom salts, and dissolve in warm bathwater before bathing. Dilute with V-6 Oil to create a massage oil, and massage into skin.

Testicle/Testes:

›› *The testes are the male reproductive organs. The testes are responsible for producing and storing sperm and male hormones such as testosterone. Hormones produced in the testes are responsible for the development of male characteristics: facial hair, wide shoulders, low voice, and reproductive organs.*

Oils—**TA**$_F$Rosemary.

—Regulation

Oils—**TA**Aroma Siez (combine with Mister), **TA**clary sage, **TA**sandalwood, **TA**geranium, **TA**yarrow.

Personal Care—Prenolone+.

Supplements—Mineral Essence, Prostate Health, Ultra Young+.

T—Dilute as necessary, and apply on location or on Vita Flex points on the feet.

A—Diffuse into the air. Inhale directly or applied to hands, tissue, or a cotton wick.

Thoughts:

Oils—**A**Inspiration (relieves negative), **A**ravensara (lifts emotions).

A—Diffuse into the air. Inhale directly or applied to hands, tissue, or a cotton wick. Wear as perfume or cologne.

Throat: *See also Antibacterial, Antiviral, Colds.*

Oils—**TA**$_F$Cypress, **TA**calamus (helps remove phlegm), **TA**oregano.

***Comments—Myrrh and peppermint are also very effective for removing phlegm and mucus from the throat area.

—Dry

Oils—ITGrapefruit, ITlemon.

—Infection In

Oils—AI F Lemon, TAI F peppermint, TAclary sage, TAoregano.

—Laryngitis *See Laryngitis.*

—Sore

Oils—TAIThieves, T F melaleuca, Toregano, Aeucalyptus, Tbergamot, Tcajeput, Aclary sage, Tgeranium, Tginger, TImmuPower, Alavender, Tmyrrh, TRC, TAsandalwood, Athyme.

Recipe #1—Put 1 drop of Thieves in 32 oz. water, and drink.

Personal Care—Gargle with Fresh Essence Plus Mouthwash.

Supplements—Inner Defense, Thieves Lozenges.

—Strep *See also Antibacterial*

Strep throat is a throat infection caused by streptococci bacteria. This infection causes the throat and tonsils to become inflamed and swollen, resulting in a severe sore throat. Symptoms of strep throat include a sudden severe sore throat, pain when swallowing, high fever, swollen tonsils and lymph nodes, white spots on the back of the throat, skin rash, and sometimes vomiting.

Oils—TAIThieves (rub on throat every time it feels sore; dilute well!), TAgeranium, TAginger, TAhyssop, TAlaurel, TAmelaleuca (combine with Thieves, and dilute), TAoregano, TAravensara (combine with Melrose).

Personal Care—Gargle with Fresh Essence Plus Mouthwash (every hour).

Supplements—Inner Defense, Thieves Lozenges, ImmuPro, Super C / Super C Chewable.

—Tonsillitis

Tonsillitis is inflammation of the tonsils, typically due to infection. Tonsillitis causes the tonsils to become swollen and painful. Symptoms of Tonsillitis include sore throat, red and swollen tonsils, painful swallowing, loss of voice, fever, chills, headache, and white patches on the tonsils.

Oils—TA F Melaleuca, TAThieves, TA F ginger, TAbergamot, TAclove, TAgeranium, TAgoldenrod, TAlavender, Tlemon (gargle), TAonycha (benzoin), TARoman chamomile, TAthyme.

Personal Care—Fresh Essence Plus Mouthwash.

Supplements—Thieves Lozenges.

***Comments—Use caution when considering surgery (tonsillectomy) for recurring tonsillitis, as doctors have discovered that the only area of the body that can synthesize the antibody to poliomyelitis (polio) is the tonsils.

T—Dilute as necessary, and apply 1–2 drops on throat, Vita Flex points on the feet, or lungs. Add 1–2 drops to 4 oz. water, and gargle.

A—Diffuse into the air, and inhale vapors deeply. Inhale directly or applied to hands.

I—Add 1 drop to 8 oz. water (32 oz. for Thieves), and drink.

Thrush: *See Antifungal: Candida.*

Thymus:

The thymus is an organ responsible for the development of T cells needed for immune system functioning. The thymus is located just behind the sternum in the upper part of the chest.

Oils—TThieves, TImmuPower (throat and chest), Telemi, Travensara.

—Stimulates

Oils—T FSpruce, TImmuPower.

Supplements—Ultra Young+ (reverses aging of the thymus gland).

T—Dilute as necessary, and apply as indicated or over thymus and on bottoms of feet.

Thyroid:

›› *The thyroid is a gland located in the front of the neck that plays a key role in regulating metabolism. The thyroid produces and secretes the hormones needed to regulate blood pressure, heart rate, body temperature, and energy production.*

—Dysfunction

Oils—TAClove.

—Normalizes Hormonal Imbalance Of

Oils—TAMyrtle.

—Hyperthyroidism

›› *Hyperthyroidism is when the thyroid gland produces too much of its hormones, typically due to the thyroid becoming enlarged. This can result in a noticeably enlarged thyroid gland (goiter), sudden weight loss, sweating, a rapid or irregular heartbeat, shortness of breath, muscle weakness, nervousness, and irritability.*

Oils—TA FMyrrh, TA Fspruce, TAEndoFlex, TAmyrtle.

Supplements—Sulfurzyme.

Blend #1—Equal parts lemongrass and myrrh. Apply undiluted on thyroid and parathyroid Vita Flex points under big toes; or dilute with a small amount of V-6 Oil, and apply on throat just under the Adam's apple.

Blend #2—Equal parts myrrh and spruce. Apply as directed in **Blend #1** above.

—Hypothyroidism

Oils—TA FMyrtle, TAEndoFlex (on top of big toes), TAclove, TApeppermint, TAspearmint.

***Comments—Combine lemongrass with any or all of these oils, and apply as directed in Blend #1 above.

Supplements—Thyromin (regulates metabolism, balances body temperature, prevents fatigue; *follow directions for use as specified in the Supplements section of the Reference Guide for Essential Oils under Thyromin*).

> *The **thyroid gland** is situated in the neck and regulates the body's metabolic rate.*
>
> *To determine whether or not the thyroid needs help, you must monitor your basal cell temperature. Place a thermometer under your armpit before getting out of bed in the morning, and rest quietly for 10 minutes. A temperature below 97.6° F (36.5° C) may indicate hypothyroidism (low thyroid function), and a temperature above 98° F (36.7° C) may indicate hyperthyroidism.*

***Comments—*One of the signs of thyroid deficiency is rough, dry skin on the bottoms of the feet.*

—Regulation

Oils—TALedum.

—Supports

Oils—TAEndoFlex, TAmyrrh (rub on hands and feet), TAmyrtle.

Supplements—Thyromin (regulates metabolism, balances body temperature, prevents fatigue; *follow directions for use as specified in the Supplements section of the Reference Guide for Essential Oils under*

Thyromin), Cleansing Trio (ComforTone, Essentialzyme, and ICP), EndoGize, MultiGreens (enhances effect of Thyromin), Power Meal.

T—Dilute as necessary, and apply 1–2 drops on base of throat, hands, or Vita Flex points on the feet.

A—Diffuse into the air. Inhale oils applied to hands.

Tinnitus: *See Ears: Tinnitus.*

Tired: *See Energy, Exhaustion, and Fatigue.*

Tissue:

›› *Tissue refers to any group of similar cells that work together to perform a specific function in an organ or in the body. Some types of tissue include muscle tissue, connective tissue, nervous tissue, or epithelial tissue (tissue that lines or covers a surface, such as the skin, or the lining of the blood vessels).*

Oils—ᵀLemongrass, ᵀhelichrysum, ᵀbasil, ᵀelemi (rejuvenates), ᵀlavender, ᵀlime (tightens connective tissue), ᵀmarjoram, ᵀMelrose, ᵀRoman chamomile, ᵀsandalwood.

Personal Care—Essential Beauty Serums (Dry, & Acne-Prone Skin Blends)

Supplements— Power Meal (predigested protein), Pure Protein Complete, True Source (whole food multi-nutrient).

—Anti-inflammatory *See Inflammation*

—Bone and Joint Regeneration

Blend #1—5 drops wintergreen, 2 drops German chamomile, 1 drop blue tansy, 7 drops fir, 5 drops hyssop, 5 drops helichrysum, 4 drops lemongrass, 8 drops sandalwood, 8 drops spruce, and 1 oz. V-6 Oil.

—Cleanses Toxins From

Oils—ᵀFennel.

—Connective Tissue, Weak

Oils—ᵀLemongrass, ᵀAroma Siez, ᵀhelichrysum, ᵀlavender, ᵀpatchouli.

Personal Care—Ortho Ease Massage Oil.

—Deep Tissue Pain

Oils—ᵀDeep Relief (roll-on), ᵀPanAway, ᵀRelieve It, ᵀhelichrysum, ᵀpalo santo.

Personal Care—Ortho Ease and Ortho Sport Massage Oils.

—Repair

Oils—ᵀLemongrass (repairs connective tissue), ᵀelemi (builds), ᵀhelichrysum (scar tissue; reduces tissue pain), ᵀhyssop (scars), ᵀorange, ᵀrosewood, ᵀsage (firms tissue), ᵀRelieve It (deep tissue damage).

Personal Care—A·R·T Skin Care System (unique enzymes that work to repair DNA damage), Rose Ointment (to help maintain, protect, and keep the scab soft), Lavender Hand & Body Lotion (to moisturize and promote healing).

—Regenerate

Oils—ᵀ$_F$Patchouli, ᵀhelichrysum, ᵀlemongrass, ᵀgeranium, ᵀMelrose, ᵀrosehip.

*****Comments**—*Use helichrysum and Melrose together for traumatized tissue (cuts, wounds, and abrasions).*

—Scarring: *See Scarring*

T—Dilute as necessary, and apply on location or on Vita Flex points on the feet. Apply as warm compress. Dilute with V-6 Oil to create a massage oil, and massage on location.

TMJ (Temporomandibular Joint Disorder or TMD):

▸▸ *TMD is a disorder of the temporomandibular joint—the joint connecting the lower jaw to the skull. TMD signs and symptoms include jaw pain or tenderness, difficulty chewing, ear pain, facial pain, difficulty opening and closing the mouth, jaw lock, headache, swelling of the side of the face, and popping or grating sounds when opening or closing the mouth. Some possible causes of TMD are teeth clenching or grinding, osteoarthritis or rheumatoid arthritis, stress, and injury.*

Recipe #1—3 Wise Men. Apply on temple and on side of face, in front of ear and down to the jaw. Cover with ice packs for 10 minutes at a time, 3–4 times a day. May be best to seek advice from a health care professional, especially a dentist.

Tonic:

—Digestive

Oils—**TA**$_F$German chamomile, **TA***Melaleuca quinquenervia*.

Supplements—Digest + Cleanse (very soothing to the digestive system)

—General

Oils—**TA**Lemongrass, **TA**cinnamon bark, **TA**sandalwood, **TA**angelica, **TA**basil, **TA**cajeput, **TA**cardamom, **TA**cistus, **TA**clary sage, **TA**cumin, **TA**galbanum, **TA**geranium, **TA**ginger, **TA**grapefruit, **TA**juniper, **TA**lemon, **TA**lime, **TA**mandarin, **TA**marjoram, **TA**melissa, **TA**Roman chamomile, **TA**mountain savory, **TA**myrrh, **TA**neroli, **TA**nutmeg, **TA**orange, **TA**palmarosa, **TA**patchouli, **TA**spruce, **TA**ylang ylang.

—Heart

Oils—**TA**Thyme, **TA**lavender.

—Nerve

Oils—**TA**$_F$Ravensara, **TA**melaleuca, **TA**clary sage, **TA**carrot, **TA**thyme.

—Skin

Oils—**T**Spearmint, **T**lemon, **T**lime, **T**spikenard.

Personal Care—Essential Beauty Serums (Dry, & Acne-Prone Skin Blends)

—Stomach

Oils—**TA**Tangerine.

—Uterine

Oils—**TA**Jasmine, **TA**thyme.

T—Dilute with V-6 Oil to create a massage oil, and massage into skin and over area of concern. Add 1–2 drops to warm bathwater before bathing. Dilute as necessary, and apply 1–2 drops to area of concern or to Vita Flex points on the feet or hands.

***Comments—The best way to restore tone in a body that is run-down is to apply oils by massage. Baths are next in effectiveness to massage if massage is not possible or in between massages.

Tonsillitis: *See Throat: Tonsillitis.*

Toothache: *See Teeth.*

Toxemia: *See also Antibacterial, Pregnancy/Motherhood: Toxemia/Preeclampsia.*

›› *Toxemia is the general term for toxic substances in the bloodstream. This is typically caused by a bacterial infection in which bacteria release toxins into the blood.*

Oils—TAAroma Life, TAcypress.

Supplements—Rehemogen tincture.

T—Dilute as necessary, and apply 1–2 drops over neck, over heart, or over bottoms of feet. Dilute with V-6 Oil to create a massage oil, and massage on location.

A—Diffuse into the air. Inhale directly or applied to hands.

Toxins: *See Detoxification: Toxins.*

Transition in Life:

Oils—TATransformation, TAAcceptance, TAAwaken (into achieving success), TA basil, TAcypress. May also want to concentrate on the emotional blends of TAValor, TAMotivation, TAGrounding, TARelease, TAHope, and TAJoy (*refer to the pages on "Auricular Emotional Therapy" and "Emotional Release" in the Science and Application section of the Reference Guide for Essential Oils*).

T—Apply to auricular emotion points. Dilute with V-6 Oil to create a massage oil, and massage into skin.

A—Inhale directly or applied to hands. Diffuse into the air.

Trauma: *See also Shock.*

Recipe #1—Release (feet and liver), Joy (heart), 3 Wise Men (crown); use all three blends in succession. May also diffuse. Australian Blue, Envision, Forgiveness, Hope, and Release can also aid in releasing emotional trauma (*Refer to each blend separately in the Blends section of the Reference Guide for Essential Oils for possible applications*). Trauma Life is an excellent blend for helping to cope with shock or emotional trauma. Apply on forehead and on palms; then rub palms together, cup over nose and mouth, and inhale deeply. Others that may help are Valor (on the feet), SARA (on temples), Peace & Calming (on palms; place hands together over heart in prayer position), or Tranquil (roll-on), .

***Comments—Concentrate on relaxing to help release the trauma. Also, if after an emotional or physical trauma you find you don't like the smell of a particular oil, it may be the one you need most to help unlock the trauma. Try exposing yourself to it a little at a time until the healing is finished.

Supplements—ImmuPro, Mineral Essence, Super C / Super C Chewable.

Travel Sickness: *See Motion Sickness, Nausea.*

Tuberculosis (T. B.): *See also Antibacterial, Respiratory System: Blend #5.*

›› *Tuberculosis is a bacterial disease spread through the air (via coughing, spitting, sneezing, etc.). Tuberculosis most commonly infects the lungs, but it can infect other bodily systems as well. Symptoms of Tuberculosis include a chronic cough (often with blood), fever, chills, weakness and fatigue, weight loss, and night sweats. Tuberculosis is contagious and sometimes deadly.*

Oils—AT F *Eucalyptus radiata*, AT F cedarwood, ATmelissa, AT F cypress, AT F thyme linalol, AT F myrtle, ATcajeput, ATlemon, ATpeppermint, ATrosemary verbenon, ATsandalwood.

Recipe #1—Exodus II (on spine and Raven on back with a hot compress), ImmuPower (on spine daily), Raven (1–2 drops in V-6 Oil as a rectal implant), RC (on chest and back—reverse each night with

Raven), rose, rosemary, Thieves (on feet). A hot compress can be used when applying oils to the chest or back. **Do the Raindrop Technique**.

Supplements—ImmuPro, Inner Defense, MultiGreens, Rehemogen Tincture, Super C / Super C Chewable. Do a colon and liver cleanse with Balance Complete or the Cleansing Trio (ComforTone, Essentialzyme, and ICP), and JuvaTone.

Blend #1—1–2 drops each of *Eucalyptus radiata*, myrtle, mountain savory, and ravensara in 1 Tbs. V-6 Oil. Apply as a rectal implant.

***Comments—*Refer to the chapter entitled "How to Use—The Personal Usage Reference" in the Essential Oils Desk Reference under "Tuberculosis" for a specific regimen using the blends and supplements.*

—Airborne Bacteria

Oils—ᴬThieves, ᴬPurification, ᴬRC, ᴬlemongrass[300], ᴬgeranium[300], ᴬRaven, ᴬSacred Mountain.

***Comments—Alternate diffusing different oils to help control the spread of bacteria like *Mycobacterium tuberculosis*.

Blend #2—Equal amounts of cypress and Sacred Mountain. Diffuse.

—Pulmonary

Oils—ᴬᵀ F Oregano, ᴬᵀcypress, ᴬᵀeucalyptus, ᴬᵀInspiration, ᴬᵀravensara.

Blend #3—Equal amounts of frankincense and ImmuPower. Diffuse; or dilute with V-6 Oil, and massage on chest or back. Can also apply to Vita Flex lung points on hands and feet.

A—Diffuse into the air. Add 2–3 drops to a bowl of hot water, and inhale vapors. Inhale directly or applied to hands.

T—Dilute as necessary, and apply on chest, back, or Vita Flex points on the feet. Add 1–2 drops to 1 tsp. V-6 Oil or olive oil, and apply as a rectal implant. Dilute with V-6 Oil to create a massage oil, and massage on chest, back, and feet.

Tumors: *See also Cancer.*

—Antitumoral

▸▸ *An antitumor is a substance used to prevent the development of malignant tumors. A tumor is an abnormal growth of cells in a lump or mass. Some tumors are malignant (cancerous) and some are benign (noncancerous). Benign tumors in most parts of the body do not create health problems. However, both malignant and benign tumors in the brain can cause serious health issues because they press on sensitive areas of the brain.*

Oils—ᵀ F Frankincense (can combine with balsam fir), ᵀledum (may be more powerful than frankincense), ᵀclove (inhibits tumor growth).

T—Apply directly on tumor location.

Supplements—Longevity Capsules (contains clove, orange-high limonene, and frankincense essential oils)

—Lipoma

▸▸ *A lipoma is a fatty tumor that normally grows between the skin and the muscle. Lipomas are not cancerous and are generally harmless.*

Oils—ᵀFrankincense and ᵀclove, ᵀledum, ᵀgrapefruit, ᵀginger.

T—Dilute as necessary, and apply on location and on Vita Flex points on the feet.

Personal Care—Prenolone/Prenolone+, Progessence/Progessence Plus.

Typhoid: *See Antibacterial.*

›› *Typhoid fever is a bacterial infection caused by the bacteria Salmonella typhi. Typhoid is spread through food and water infected with the feces of typhoid carriers. Possible symptoms of typhoid include abdominal pain, severe diarrhea, bloody stools, chills, severe fatigue, weakness, chills, delirium, hallucinations, confusion, agitation, and fluctuating mood.*

Oils—[AT]$_F$Cinnamon bark, [AT]peppermint, [AT]lemon, [AT]Melrose, [AT]mountain savory, [AT]Purification, [AT]Raven, [AT]ravensara, [AT]RC.

A—Diffuse into the air.

T—Dilute with V-6 Oil, and apply over intestines and on Vita Flex points on the feet.

Ulcers:

›› *An ulcer is an open sore either on the skin or on an internal mucous membrane (such as that lining the stomach).*

> *While some sources claim that sixty percent of all **ulcers** are caused by bacteria, F. Batmanghelidj, MD, maintains that the majority of ulcers are only dehydration of the stomach lining. In his book, Your Body's Many Cries for Water, Dr. Batmanghelidj shows that rehydration is the simplest cure for this and many other adverse health conditions.*

Oils—[IT]$_F$Frankincense, [IT]$_F$German chamomile, [IT]$_F$myrrh, [IT]bergamot, [IT]cinnamon bark, [IT]clove, [IT]elemi, [IT]geranium, [IT]lemon, [IT]oregano, [IT]rose, [IT]thyme, [IT]vetiver.

I—Add one drop of oil to rice or almond milk, and take as a dietary supplement.

T—Apply over stomach with a hot compress.

Supplements—Use ComforTone to help destroy the bacteria; then use Essentialzyme, Essentialzymes-4, Master Formula His/Hers.

—Duodenal

›› *A duodenal ulcer is an ulcer in the upper part of the small intestine.*

Oils—[IT]$_F$Frankincense, [IT]$_F$German chamomile, [IT]$_F$myrrh, [IT]bergamot, [IT]cinnamon bark, [IT]clove, [IT]elemi, [IT]geranium, [IT]lemon, [IT]oregano, [IT]rose, [IT]thyme, [IT]vetiver.

I—Add one drop of oil to rice or almond milk, and take as a dietary supplement.

T—Apply over stomach with a hot compress.

Supplements—AlkaLime.

—Gastric *See also Gastritis.*

›› *A gastric ulcer is an ulcer in the stomach.*

Oils—[IT]$_F$Geranium, [IT]bergamot, [IT]frankincense, [IT]geranium, [IT]manuka, [IT]orange, [IT]peppermint.

I—Add one drop of oil to rice or almond milk, and take as a dietary supplement. Add 1 drop as flavoring in food.

T—Applied over stomach with a hot compress. Dilute as necessary, and apply to stomach and Vita Flex points.

Supplements—AlkaLime, Cleansing Trio (ComforTone, Essentialzyme, and ICP), Master Formula His/Hers.

***Comments—*Manuka Honey is said to naturally kill Helicobacter pylori.*

—Leg

›› *An ulcer on the leg may be due to a lack of circulation in the lower extremities or possibly due to a bacterial, fungal, or viral infection.*

Oils—TPurification, TGentle Baby, TMelrose, Tlavender, Tgeranium, TGerman chamomile, Tpatchouli, TRoman chamomile, Trosewood, TSensation.

T—Dilute as necessary, and apply on location.

***Comments—*Dilute oils with V-6 Oil, and massage lower extremities to stimulate circulation. Thyromin may be needed to help with overall circulation.*

Personal Care—Rose Ointment, Sensation Massage Oil.

Blend #1—Equal drops of lavender and either Melrose or Purification applied on location. Can cover with Rose Ointment.

—MOUTH *See also Cankers.*

▸▸ *Mouth ulcers are open, often painful sores that occur in the mouth. Common mouth ulcers include cancer sores and cold sores. Stress, anxiety, fatigue, injury, illness, hormonal changes, and food allergies can often trigger mouth ulcers.*

Oils—TBasil (mouthwash), Tmyrrh, Torange.

T—Dilute as necessary, and apply on location. Add 1–3 drops to 4 oz. water, and use as mouthwash.

Blend #1—1 drop each of sage and clove and 1–3 drops lavender. Apply directly on location.

—PEPTIC

▸▸ *A peptic ulcer is an ulcer that forms in an area of the digestive system where acid is present, such as in the stomach (gastric), esophagus, or upper part of the small intestine (duodenal).*

Recipe #1—Flavor a quart of water with 1 drop of cinnamon bark oil, and sip all day.

Supplements—AlkaLime.

—STOMACH *See GASTRIC above*

—ULCERATIONS

▸▸ *Ulceration is the process of an ulcer being formed or eroding away at the skin or mucous membrane.*

Oils—TLavender, TMelrose, Trose.

T—Dilute as necessary, and apply on location.

***Comments—Cleanse liver and colon (*See Cleansing*).

Personal Care—Rose Ointment.

—VARICOSE ULCERS.

Oils—TMelaleuca, Tgeranium, Tlavender, Teucalyptus, Tthyme, Tyarrow.

T—Dilute as necessary, and apply on location.

Unwind: *See also Calming, Massage.*

Oils—ATLavender, ATPeace & Calming, TTranquil (roll-on).

A—Diffuse into the air. Rub between hands, and inhale deeply,

T—Combine with V-6 Oil or massage oil for a massage. Add 3–5 drops to 1/4 cup Epsom or bath salts, and dissolve in warm bathwater before bathing.

Personal Care—Relaxation Massage Oil, Evening Peace Bath & Shower Gel.

Uplifting:

Oils—ALemon[301], AJoy, ALive with Passion, Aorange, ABelieve, Abergamot, ABrain Power, Afir (emotionally uplifting), Abalsam fir, Agrapefruit, Ahelichrysum, AIdaho tansy, Ajasmine, Alavender, Amyrrh, Aravensara, ASacred Mountain, ASensation, Aspruce, 3 Wise Men, ATransformation, Atsuga, Awintergreen.

A—Diffuse or wear as perfume or cologne. *See Comments under Asthma for a discussion on using **plastic nasal inhalers**.*

Blend #1—3 drops wintergreen, 3 drops lavender, 3 drops orange, 3 drops spruce, and 1 oz. V-6 Oil. Wear a few drops of this blend as a perfume or cologne, or apply it over the heart, on the chest, neck, and/or shoulders, and behind the ears. Can also apply a few drops on both hands, rub hands together, cup hands over nose and mouth, and breathe deeply.

Personal Care—Morning Start Bath & Shower Gel, Sensation Bath & Shower Gel.

Ureter: *See Urinary Tract: Ureter.*

Urinary Tract: *See also Bladder, Kidneys.*

›› *The urinary tract is the collection of organs and tubes responsible for producing and excreting urine. The urinary tract is comprised of the kidneys, ureters, bladder, and urethra.*

Oils—TA FSandalwood, TA Fthyme (infection), TA Fsage, TAbergamot, TAcopaiba, TAImmuPower, TAlavender, TAledum, TAmelaleuca, TApine (antiseptic), TArosemary, TAtarragon.

T—Dilute as necessary, and apply over lower abdomen, lower back, or pubic area. Dilute with V-6 Oil to create a massage oil, and massage on abdomen, lower back, or pubic area. Apply as a warm compress.

A—Diffuse into the air.

—General Stimulant

Oils—TA FEucalyptus, TAbergamot.

T—Dilute as necessary, and apply over lower abdomen, lower back, or pubic area. Dilute with V-6 Oil to create a massage oil, and massage on location. Apply as a warm compress.

A—Diffuse into the air.

—Infection *See also Bladder: Infection.*

Oils—T FCedarwood, TPurification (effective by itself), TImmuPower, TInspiration (effective by itself), Tbergamot, Tcajeput, TDi-Gize, TEndoFlex, Tgeranium, Thyssop, Tjuniper, Tlemongrass, TMelrose, Tonycha, Ttarragon.

T—Apply 2–3 drops of oil directly over bladder. May also apply as a hot compress.

Blend #1—Equal parts sage and Purification.

Blend #2—Equal parts thyme and Melrose.

Blend #3—Equal parts oregano and Thieves.

Blend #4—Equal parts juniper and EndoFlex.

With any of these blends, dilute with V-6 Oil, and massage over lower back and pubic area, or apply with a hot compress.

Supplements—AlkaLime, Inner Defense, K&B Tincture.

Recipe #1—Add 1 drop of mountain savory to 3 droppers of K&B tincture in distilled water, and drink every few hours.

***Comments—*Refer to the chapter entitled "How to Use—The Personal Usage Reference" in the Essential Oils Desk Reference under "Urinary Tract/Bladder Infection" for a unique blend of 14 different oils to specifically help with infection.*

—Stones In

▸▸ *Stones are solid masses that form as minerals and other chemicals crystallize and adhere together. They can form in the bladder or kidneys. While small stones generally cause no problems, larger stones may block the ureters or urethra, causing intense pain and possibly injury.*

Oils—TF Fennel, TF geranium.

T—Apply oils over pubic area and lower back with a hot compress. *See MASTER CLEANSER under Cleansing.*

—Support

Oils—TA Cypress, TA geranium, TA juniper, TA goldenrod, TA juniper, TA laurel, TA melaleuca.

T—Dilute as necessary, and apply over lower abdomen, lower back, or pubic area. Dilute with V-6 Oil to create a massage oil, and massage on location. Apply as a warm compress.

A—Diffuse into the air.

Supplements—K&B Tincture.

—Ureter (Infections In)

▸▸ *Ureters are the two paired tubes by which urine passes from the kidneys to the bladder.*

Oils—TF Lemon, TF myrtle.

T—Apply 2–3 drops of oil directly over bladder. May also apply a hot compress.

Uterus:

▸▸ *The uterus is the female reproductive organ in which a fetus is formed and develops until birth.*

Oils—T Frankincense, T lemon, T cedarwood, T geranium, T jasmine, T myrrh.

—Inflammation

Oils—T Elemi.

—Regeneration of Tissue

Recipe #1—Frankincense, sage, tarragon. Add 1–3 drops of each to 1 tsp. V-6 Oil; insert into vagina, and retain overnight.

Personal Care—PD 80/20, Prenolone/Prenolone +, Progessence/Progessence Plus.

Supplements—FemiGen.

—Uterotonic

Oils—T Thyme.

—Uterine Cancer *See also Cancer.*

Oils—T Frankincense, T geranium, T cedarwood, T Gratitude, T ImmuPower, T lemon, T myrrh.

T—Oils can be applied to the reproductive Vita Flex points on the feet—mostly around the front of the ankle, on either side of the ankle under the ankle bone, and up the Achilles tendon. The most effective application of oils is by vaginal retention implant. Add 2–5 drops of any of these single oils or a combination of any of them to 1 tsp. V-6 Oil; insert into vagina, and retain overnight. A tampon may be used if necessary to help retain the oil.

—Uterine Cysts *See Ovaries: Ovarian Cysts.*

T—Dilute as necessary, and apply on lower abdomen or on Vita Flex points on the feet and ankles. Add 2–5 drops oil to 1 tsp. V-6 Oil, and insert into vagina for overnight retention (a tampon may be used if necessary to help retain the oil).

Vaginal:

—Candida (thrush) *See Antifungal: Candida*

—Infection

▸▸ *Vaginal infections occur when there is a disruption in the normal balance of vaginal organisms, such as the sudden presence of yeast, bacteria, or viruses. Common signs of vaginal infection include redness, swelling, itching, pain, odor, change in discharge color or amount, burning sensation when urinating, and pain or bleeding during intercourse. The most common vaginal infections are yeast infection, trichomoniasis, and bacterial vaginosis.*

Oils—T F Rosemary, T melaleuca, T F rosewood, T F cinnamon bark (be extremely careful; dilute well), T clary sage, T cypress, T eucalyptus, T hyssop, T Inspiration, T juniper, T lavender, T laurel, T Melrose, T myrrh, T mountain savory, T oregano, T sage, T 3 Wise Men, T thyme.

Recipe #1—Apply oregano and thyme along the spine using the Raindrop Technique.

Blend #1—Equal parts oregano, thyme, and Melrose. Dilute with V-6 Oil, and apply as described under **T** (Topical application instructions) below.

Blend #2—3 drops rosemary, 2 drops *Melaleuca quinquenervia*, 2 drops oregano, and 1 drop thyme. Dilute with V-6 Oil, and apply as described under **T** (Topical application instructions) below. Can also apply as a hot compress over lower abdominal area.

Blend #3—5 drops Melrose, 2 drops oregano, and 1 drop thyme in 1 Tbs. V-6 Oil. Use as douche or vaginal retention implant as described under **T** (Topical application instructions) below.

—Inflammation of Vagina *See also Anti-inflammatory*

Oils—T Eucalyptus, T lavender, T melaleuca, T yarrow.

—Retention Implant

***Comments—Used to cleanse and nourish the female reproductive system or as a support when taking products like the FemiGen supplement. Best when done after a colon and liver cleanse using the Cleansing Trio (ComforTone, Essentialzyme, ICP). The following blends can be inserted directly into the vagina with a vaginal syringe (available from Abundant Health). A tampon may be necessary to help retain.

Blend #4—Dilute 2 drops *Melaleuca quinquenervia*, 1 drop lavender, and 1 drop bergamot in 1 Tbs. V-6 Oil. Insert, and retain overnight.

Blend #5—Dilute 2 drops frankincense and 7 drops Purification in 1 Tbs. V-6 Oil. Insert, and retain overnight.

—Vaginitis

▸▸ *Vaginitis is vaginal inflammation, typically due to infection, characterized by redness, swelling, itching, irritation, discharge, and pain of the vaginal area.*

Oils—T F Rosemary, T melaleuca, T F rosewood, T F cinnamon bark (be extremely careful; dilute well), T *Eucalyptus radiata*.

Valerie Worwood suggests the following douche recipe that should be used daily for three days a week only.

Recipe #1—1 drop lavender, 1 drop melaleuca (tea tree), 1 tsp. of vinegar, ½ tsp. lemon juice, and 2½ cups of warm water. Mix thoroughly.

T—Mix desired oil(s) with water, and either use in a douche or in a sitz bath. Desired oil(s) may also be mixed with V-6 Oil and either applied directly, inserted with a vaginal syringe (available from Abundant Health) and retained with a tampon, or by soaking a tampon in mixture, inserting and leaving in all day or night.

Varicose Ulcers: *See Ulcers: Varicose.*

Varicose Veins:

▸▸ *Varicose veins are abnormal swelling of the veins in the legs. They are most often a symptom of poor circulation and of a loss of elasticity of the vascular walls and particularly their valves. If the valves do not work properly, blood accumulates in the veins instead of flowing back to the heart. This accumulation of blood causes the veins to become swollen and twisted. Hemorrhoids are varicose veins of the anus or rectum usually resulting from constipation.*

> *Cleanse the colon.*
>
> *Helichrysum dissolves the coagulated blood inside and outside of the veins. Cypress strengthens the veins. Massage **above** the affected vein toward the heart with helichrysum and cypress every morning and night; wear support hose until healed. It may take from three months to a year to heal completely. It is important to vary the essential oils being used. Try using lavender, juniper or rosemary instead of cypress and helichrysum.* See Diet, Circulatory System.
>
> ***Caution:** Do not rub below the affected area, as rubbing may increase the pressure on the vein*

Oils—$^{T}_{F}$Cypress (as bath oil), $^{T}_{F}$lemongrass, $^{T}_{F}$lemon (tonic for circulatory system), $^{T}_{F}$peppermint, ᵀAroma Life, ᵀAroma Siez, ᵀbasil, ᵀbergamot, ᵀCitrus Fresh, ᵀgeranium, ᵀhelichrysum (especially during pregnancy), ᵀIdaho tansy (helps weak veins), ᵀjuniper, ᵀlavender, ᵀorange, ᵀrosemary, ᵀspikenard, ᵀtangerine, ᵀyarrow.

Personal Care—Cel-Lite Magic (strengthens vascular walls).

Supplements—MultiGreens, Rehemogen Tincture, Super B, Thyromin.

Blend #1—1–3 drops each of lemongrass and Aroma Life with Cel-Lite Magic.

Blend #2—1–3 drops each of basil and Aroma Siez. Massage above the affected vein toward the heart.

***Comments**—Refer to the chapter entitled "How to Use—The Personal Usage Reference" in the Essential Oils Desk Reference under "Varicose Veins" for more specific blend recipes and instructions regarding treatment.

T—Dilute as recommended, and apply oils gently from ankles up the legs. Consistent application of oils for an extended period of time is the key. Wearing support hose and elevating the feet can also help keep blood from pooling in the legs.

Vascular System: *See also Cardiovascular System, Lymphatic System, Arteries, Capillaries, Veins.*

▸▸ *The vascular system refers to the vessels or veins that carry and circulate fluids (blood and lymph) throughout the body.*

Oils—$^{T}_{F}$Lemongrass (strengthens vascular walls), ᵀAroma Life, ᵀcypress, ᵀfrankincense, ᵀhelichrysum.

Personal Care—Cel-Lite Magic (strengthens vascular walls).

—Cleansing *See also Chelation, Metals.*

Oils—ᵀJuva Cleanse.

Supplements—JuvaTone, and MultiGreens work very well together. Essentialzyme, Essentialzymes-4, K&B Tincture, Rehemogen Tincture, Super C, True Source (whole food multi-nutrient).

Blend #1—1–3 drops each of helichrysum and Aroma Life with Cel-Lite Magic Massage Oil. Massage on the body to help dilate the blood vessels and to enhance the chelation of metallics.

T—Dilute with V-6 Oil to create a massage oil, and apply as a full body massage, over heart, and on bottoms of the feet.

Vasodilator: *See Blood: Vasodilator.*

Veins: *See also Cardiovascular System, Vascular System.*

A vein is a blood vessel that carries blood from the capillaries back to the heart. Veins may also have one-way valves on the inside that help keep blood from flowing backwards and pooling in the lower extremities due to gravity.

—Circulation In Vascular Walls of Veins

Oils—T Aroma Life, T cypress, T lemon.

T—Dilute as necessary, and apply on location. Dilute with V-6 Oil to create a massage oil, and massage on location.

—Blood Clot In Veins

Blend #1—Cypress and helichrysum (rub neat on location to dissolve).

Vertigo: *See also Ears, Equilibrium, and Dizziness.*

Vertigo refers to the sensation that the environment and objects around an individual are moving or spinning, usually causing a loss of balance or a feelings of nausea. Vertigo may be caused by ear infections, ear disorders, or motion sickness.

Oils—TA Ginger.

T—Dilute as necessary, and apply around ears and on Vita Flex points on the feet.

A—Inhale directly or applied to hands.

Viral Disease: *See Antiviral: Viral Disease.*

Viruses: *See Antiviral: Viruses.*

Visualization:

Oils—A Awaken, A Dream Catcher, A helichrysum, A palo santo, A PanAway.

A—Diffuse or wear as perfume or cologne.

Vital Centers:

Recipe #1—Oregano and sage may strengthen the vital centers of the body.

Vitamins: *See the Supplements section of the Reference Guide for Essential Oils.*

Supplements—Power Meal, Sulfurzyme (sulfur necessary for proper assimilation of vitamin C), Super B, Super C / Super C Chewable, Super Cal.

Children's Supplements—KidScents MightyVites (chewable vitamin tablets).

Vitiligo: *See Skin: Vitiligo.*

Voice (Hoarse): *See also Laryngitis.*

Oils—T Bergamot, T jasmine.

T—Add 1 drop to 1 oz. (2 Tbs.) water, and gargle.

Blend #1—Add one drop each of Melrose and lemon to 1 tsp. honey. Swish around in mouth for a couple of minutes to liquefy; then swallow.

Void:

Oils—T3 Wise Men (replaces the void).

T—Apply on crown of head.

Vomiting: *See Nausea.*

Oils—IAGinger[302], AT F peppermint, TI F fennel, Tnutmeg, Tblack pepper, Tlavender, TRoman chamomile, Trose.

T—Apply as warm compress over stomach. Dilute with V-6 Oil to create a massage oil, and massage on stomach.

I—Place 1–2 drops in an empty capsule, and swallow.

A—Inhale directly or applied to hands. Diffuse into the air.

Warming Oils: *See also Cooling Oils, Temperature.*

Oils—TCinnamon bark, Toregano, Tthyme, Tonycha (benzoin), Tyuzu.

T—Dilute with V-6 Oil to create a massage oil, and massage briskly into skin.

Warts: *See also Antiviral.*

>> *A wart is a small, firm, hard growth on the skin, usually located on the hands and feet, that is typically caused by a virus.*

Oils—TFrankincense (excellent for more stubborn warts), TMelrose, TThieves, Toregano, Tcinnamon bark, Tclove, Tcypress, Tjasmine, Tlavender, Tlemon (may dilute in 2 tsp. apple cider vinegar).

*My son had a really big **wart** on his hand. I started using lavender and Melrose, and they seemed to help. Then I decided to try something new. I used Melrose, Purification, Thieves, and clove—one drop of each—and rubbed them in one by one, and within a few days the wart was gone. I was so impressed and happy!*

-Submitted by Caroline Rood
Toledo, Ohio (July 2004)

Other—Colloidal silver.

Recipe #1—5 drops cypress, 10 drops lemon, and 2 Tbs. apple cider vinegar. Apply twice daily, and bandage. Keep a bandage on it until the wart is gone.

—Genital

>> *A genital wart is a small, painful wart or cluster of warts located in the genital area or in the mouth or throat. This type of wart is typically spread by contact with the skin through sexual conduct.*

Oils—TFrankincense (excellent for more stubborn warts), Tmelaleuca, Toregano, TThieves, Thyssop, Tthyme.

—Plantar

>> *Plantar warts are painful warts that grow on the bottoms of the feet. They are usually flattened and embedded into the skin due to the pressure caused by walking on them.*

Oils—TOregano.

T—Dilute 1–2 drops of oil in a few drops of V-6 Oil, and apply on location.

*In late October of last year, Cathy brought her 15-year-old daughter to see me for massage therapy. Amanda was dealing with a huge **plantar's wart** grown deep into the ball of her foot. She suffered a great deal of pain with every step, and Cathy was planning to make an appointment for her to see a medical doctor. Cathy also suffered from these warts and had undergone months of treatment at her doctor's office having them repeatedly cut and burned with liquid nitrogen. She was also told you could never get rid of them. I suggested that Amanda rub essential oil of oregano on the infected area, which Amanda did diligently each day, covering it with a bandage. They were amazed that the wart had completely disappeared in 6 weeks and has had no recurrence of the virus. Amanda's only complaint was that she got tired of going to school every day smelling like a pizza.*

-Submitted by Ellie Ayers (July 2004)

Waste: *Refer to the chapter entitled, "Cleansing and Diets" in the Essential Oils Desk Reference for lots of information on cleansing.*

—Eliminating

Oils—T F Lavender (through lymphatic system).

T—Dilute with V-6 Oil to create a massage oil, and massage into the skin.

Supplements—Balance Complete, Cleansing Trio (ComforTone, Essentialzyme, and ICP), Digest + Cleanse. These cleansing products help eliminate toxic waste from the body.

Water Distillation:

Recipe #1—Add 3–5 drops of your favorite oil to the post-filter on your distiller. The oils will help increase the oxygen and frequency of the water. Try lemon or peppermint.

Water Purification:

Oils—IT F Lemon, IT orange.

—Remove Nitrates

›› *Nitrate is a molecule composed of nitrogen and oxygen that shows up in water as a harmful contaminate.*

Oils—IT Peppermint.

I—Add 1 drop to 12–16 oz. of drinking water.

T—Add 1–2 drops to dishwater. Add 1–2 drops to warm bathwater, and bathe. Add 1–2 drops to bowl of water, and use to clean the outside of fruits and vegetables.

Water Retention: *See Edema, Diuretic, and Hormonal Imbalance.*

Weakness: *See also Energy.*

—After Illness

Oils—TA Thyme (physical).

T—Dilute with V-6 Oil to create a massage oil, and massage into the skin.

A—Inhale directly or applied to hands. Diffuse into the air.

Wealth:

Oils—A Abundance, A bergamot.

—Attracts

Oils—A Cinnamon bark.

—Money

Oils—A Ginger, A patchouli.

A—Wear as perfume or cologne. Diffuse into the air.

Weight: *See also Hormonal Imbalance, Obesity, pH Balance.*

›› *Proper exercise and nutrition are the most critical factors for maintaining a healthy weight. Other factors that may influence weight include an individual's metabolism, level of stress, hormonal imbalances, low or high thyroid function, or the level of insulin being produced by the body.*

***Comments—**Proper exercise** is absolutely important!

Oils—**IA**Slique Essence.

Supplements—Enzyme products: Allerzyme (aids the digestion of sugars, starches, fats, and proteins), Detoxzyme (helps maintain and support a healthy intestinal environment), Digest + Cleanse. Balance Complete (an excellent meal replacer, nutritive cleanser providing 11 grams of fiber per serving), Master Formula His/Hers, MultiGreens, Cleansing Trio (ComforTone, Essentialzyme, and ICP), JuvaPower/JuvaSpice, NingXia Red, Pure Protein Complete, Slique Tea, Slique Bar, Slique Gum, Slique Slim Caps.

—CONTROL

Recipe #1—EndoFlex (while taking Thyromin, a drop of EndoFlex under the tongue two or three times a day can help).

Supplements—Balance Complete, Digest + Cleanse, EndoGize, Pure Protein Complete, Thyromin, Wolfberry Crisp Bars.

—EMOTIONS

Oils—Excessive weight may be due to unresolved childhood emotions. Any or all of the following may help: Acceptance, Forgiveness, Inner Child, SARA (*Refer to the "Emotional Release" part of the Science and Application section or to the Blend section of the Reference Guide for Essential Oils for more information on each of these blends*).

—WEIGHT LOSS

Oils—**IA**Slique Essence, **TA**EndoFlex (on throat, under big toes), **TA**Joy, **TA**Motivation.

T—Apply as indicated or to auricular emotion points.

A—Inhale directly. Diffuse into the air.

Blend #1—Put 5 drops lemon[303] and 5 drops grapefruit[303] in 1 gallon of water, and drink during the day. Add more grapefruit to dissolve fat faster.

Blend #2—4 drops lavender, 4 drops basil, 3 drops juniper, 8 drops grapefruit, 5 drops cypress. Mix, and apply to feet, on location, as a body massage, or use in bath. This blend is used to emulsify fat.

Personal Care—Massage whole body with Cel-Lite Magic after showering. If the weight problem is related to a hormonal imbalance, Prenolone/Prenolone+ / Progessence/Progessence Plus combined with Thyromin and EndoFlex may help.

Supplements—Use Balance Complete (to replace 2 meals and to promote proper elimination) to replace breakfast and dinner, ComforTone, Digest + Cleanse, ICP, and Essentialzyme/ Essentialzymes-4 to promote proper elimination of waste material from the bowels, and Thyromin to ensure proper thyroid function. Eat a normal meal at lunch, but watch fat intake. Other products that may help are AlkaLime (improves digestion), JuvaPower/ JuvaSpice, Power Meal, Slique Tea (helps control cravings), Slique Bar, Slique Gum, Slique Slim Caps, Sulfurzyme, Ultra Young+ (may help improve fat-to-lean ratios), Wolfberry Crisp Bars. Master Formula His/Hers is also important to use.

—UNDERWEIGHT

Supplements—Pure Protein Complete. Feed cells with Mineral Essence.

Well Being:

Oils—**A**Citrus Fresh, **A**Idaho tansy, **A**Release (emotional), **A**rose, **A**Transformation.

—FEELING OF

Oils—**A**Harmony, **A**spearmint.

—Promotes

Oils—[A]Eucalyptus, [A]geranium, [A]lavender, [A]lemon, [A]lime.

Supplements—Cleansing Trio (ComforTone, Essentialzyme, and ICP).

A—Diffuse into the air. Inhale directly or applied to tissue or a cotton wick.

Whiplash: *See also Trauma or Shock.*

›› *Whiplash is the over-stretching or tearing of the muscles, ligaments, and/or tendons in the neck and head. This is typically caused by a sudden collision or force pushing the body in one direction, while the head's tendency to remain in the same place causes the head to quickly rock in the opposite direction the body is going.*

Oils—[T]Aroma Siez, [T]Deep Relief (roll-on), [T]PanAway, [T]lemongrass (strained ligaments), [T]marjoram (muscles), [T]wintergreen (bones), [T]Relieve It, [T]basil, [T]helichrysum (bruising), [T]hyssop (inflammation), [T]juniper, [T]Roman chamomile, [T]spruce.

T—Dilute as necessary, and apply on location. Dilute with V-6 Oil to create a massage oil, and gently massage on back of neck, shoulders, and upper back.

Recipe #1—Can also apply valerian, vetiver, helichrysum, clove, and peppermint to the back of the neck (up to the base of the skull) to help calm the sympathetic nervous system and to reduce pain and swelling.

Supplements—Sulfurzyme, Super C / Super C Chewable.

***Comments—Remember to think through every physical aspect of the injury (i.e. muscle damage, nerve damage, inflammation, ligament strain, bone injury, fever, and emotions). Select oils for each area of concern.

Wholeness:

Recipe #1—For one's own spirituality and oneness with the Creator. Apply each of the following blends, one right after the other: Awaken over the heart and on the forehead, Sacred Mountain on the crown of the head and over the thymus, and White Angelica on the shoulders. Then rub hands together, cup hands over nose and mouth, and breathe deeply to inhale the aroma of all three blends together.

Whooping Cough: *See Childhood Diseases: Whooping Cough.*

Withdrawal: *See Addictions.*

Workaholic:

Oils—[A]Basil, [A]geranium, [A]lavender, [A]marjoram.

A—Rub a couple drops between hands, cup hands over nose and mouth, and breathe deeply. Can also be diffused.

Worms: *See also Antifungal: Ringworm, Parasites.*

Oils—[T]Di-Gize (helps expel intestinal worms), [T]lavender, [T]rosemary verbenon, [T]bergamot, [T]melaleuca, [T]peppermint, [T]Roman chamomile, [T]thyme.

T—For intestinal worms, apply a few drops over abdomen with a hot compress, or add to V-6 Oil (½–1 oz.) and use as a retention enema for 15 minutes or more. Can also apply on intestine and colon Vita Flex points on the feet.

Blend #1—Mix 6 drops Roman chamomile, 6 drops eucalyptus, 6 drops lavender, and 6 drops lemon with 2 Tbs. V-6 Oil. Apply 10–15 drops of blend over abdomen with a hot compress, and apply on intestine and colon Vita Flex points on the feet.

Supplements—Cleansing Trio (ComforTone, Essentialzyme, and ICP), Digest + Cleanse, ParaFree.

Worry:

Oils—**A**Bergamot.

A—Diffuse into the air.

Wounds: *See also Cuts, Scarring.*

A wound is a general term for an injury that involves tissue (typically the skin or underlying skeletal muscles) being torn, cut, punctured, scraped, or crushed.

Oils—**T**,**F**Clove (infected wounds), **T**melaleuca, **T**lavender (combine with any of these other oils), **T**Roman chamomile (add to Rose Ointment for an excellent first aid salve), **T**basil[304], **T**The Gift, **T**bergamot, **T**cajeput, **T**cistus (to help reduce scarring), **T**cypress, **T**elemi (infected), **T**eucalyptus, **T**frankincense, **T**galbanum, **T**geranium, **T**juniper, **T**myrrh (infected), **T**onycha (benzoin), **T**peppermint (when wound has closed; will soothe, cool, and reduce inflammation), **T**rose, **T**rosemary, **T**rosewood, **T**sandalwood (for DNA repair), **T**thyme, **T**tsuga.

Blend #1—Lavender with Purification or Melrose.

Recipe #1—First, 1–3 drops of helichrysum on the fresh wound will help stop the bleeding, and a drop of clove will help with pain. Once bleeding is stopped, a drop of lavender (to help start the healing), a drop of Melrose (to help fight infection), and a drop of lemongrass (for possible ligament damage) can be applied. Other oils such as wintergreen, thyme, or sage may also be applied, depending on the extent of the injury. Rose Ointment can then be applied to help seal the wound and to extend the effectiveness of the applied oils; cover it all with a bandage. When changing the bandage, cistus, myrrh, onycha, sandalwood (for DNA repair), or patchouli can be applied to help promote further healing. Thieves, myrrh, or Purification may be necessary to help fight any occurrence of infection.

One Sunday morning I tripped and rammed my foot into a dirty pair of grass clippers, cutting my 4th toe at the base where it joins my foot. I washed it out as best I could with hydrogen peroxide, and then I applied lavender oil and a bandage and went on to church. When I came home, I kept my foot elevated and applied more lavender oil throughout the day. My friend looked at my wound and commented that it wasn't just a gash, it was punctured. That evening I also applied clove oil, along with the lavender oil. I slept with it unbandaged, and then I bandaged it during the day while I was at work. I applied the oils morning and night. I had no infection, and by the following Sunday evening, it was almost totally healed. My friend who looked at it again was amazed, and she's an EMT!

-Submitted by C. Ness
Rapid City, South Dakota (July 2004)

Personal Care—Rose Ointment (seals and protects).

Supplements—Stevia extract (apply on closed wound to help reduce scarring).

—Children (and Infants)

Oils—**T**Lavender and/or **T**Roman chamomile. **T**Helichrysum and **T**peppermint may also be used but are best diluted with lavender or Rose Ointment first to help minimize stinging effect on open wounds.

Blend #2—(for Bruises or Wounds) 1–3 drops each of helichrysum and lavender diluted in 1/8 oz. V-6 Oil.

—Bleeding

Oils—**T**Helichrysum, **T**rose, **T**lemon, **T**lavender.

My husband, Tom, was taking apart a rabbit cage, and the roof with the nails poking through fell on his hand and punctured it. Blood was dripping everywhere, and he was becoming sick with pain and weakness. He applied pressure to the wounds, but it still bled until I applied lavender and PanAway. Before our very eyes it immediately stopped bleeding. It did swell up, but he kept applying lavender and PanAway, and it would take away the pain and bring the swelling down. It was healed in a matter of three days without a trip to the doctor. We feel so blessed to have oils on hand to treat emergencies like this one.

-Submitted by Diana Wolford
Olive Branch, Mississippi (July 2004)

Blend #3—Equal amounts of Roman chamomile, geranium, and lemon. Can alternate with cypress, hyssop, palmarosa, and rose. Apply directly with a compress 2–3 times a day for 3–4 days, and then reduce to once a day until healed.

—Disinfect

Oils—TMelaleuca, Thyssop, TIdaho tansy, Tlavender, Tmountain savory, Tthyme (thymol and linalol).

—Healing *See also Scarring.*

Oils—TBasil[304], Thelichrysum, TThe Gift, Tmyrrh, TIdaho tansy, Tlavender, Tmelaleuca (pus-filled wounds), Tneroli, Tonycha (benzoin), Tpatchouli, Travensara, Tsandalwood, Ttsuga, Tyarrow.

T—Apply directly on wound followed by Rose Ointment.

—Inflammation *See also Anti-Inflammatory*

Oils—TGerman chamomile (helps reduce).

Dr. Marcy Foley maintains that "Each person will have a unique picture which created their healing challenges, and will require that each of these areas be addressed for a complete healing to take place." This is especially true for surface ***wounds*** *where each aspect of the trauma must be considered. For example, there may also be damage to muscles, nerves, ligaments, or bones; there may be infection or inflammation; and there may be an emotion or even fever to deal with. Oils should be considered for each of these different areas as well.*

—Surgical

Oils—TPeppermint (cooling and soothing), TMelrose, TThe Gift, TPurification, TThieves.

Blend #4—3 drops helichrysum, 3 drops frankincense, and 4 drops lavender in 2 tsp. V-6 Oil. Reapply a few drops of blend when changing bandages.

—Weeping

Oils—TMyrrh, TThe Gift, Tjuniper, Tpatchouli, Ttarragon.

Blend #5—5 drops Roman chamomile, 10 drops lavender, 3 drops tarragon, and 2 oz. V-6 Oil. Apply as a hot compress.

T—Dilute as necessary, and apply on location. Apply on location with a warm compress.

Wrinkles: *See Skin: Wrinkles.*

Yeast: *See Antifungal: Candida.*

Yin and Yang:

▸▸ *In Chinese philosophy Yin and Yang are two opposing forces in the universe that, when in harmony, create balance.*

Oils—AYlang ylang (balances)

A—Inhale directly or applied to hands. Diffuse into the air.

Yoga:

Oils—ACedarwood, Asandalwood, Aspruce, Atsuga.

A—Diffuse into the air.

Zest (for life):

Oils—AEn-R-Gee, AMotivation, Anutmeg, ALegacy, ALive with Passion.

A—Diffuse into the air.

Endnotes

Note: *This list contains summaries of research articles referenced in this section. For the full article reference, please see Research References in the appendix of this book. Please note that much of this research is still preliminary, and is meant as an educational reference to guide further research and study. It should not be used to attempt to diagnose or prescribe any medical condition. Consult with a certified medical professional with regard to any medical condition.*

1. Rosemary aroma also was found to enhance quality of memory, compared to control (Moss et al., 2003).
2. In human trials, the aroma of peppermint was found to enhance memory and to increase alertness (Moss et al., 2008).
3. In a small human trial, oral administration of sage lavender oil was found to improve speed of memory as well as alertness and calmness in healthy volunteers, compared to a placebo (Tildesley et al., 2005).
4. A gel with 5% tea tree oil was found to be as effective as a 5% benzoyl peroxide (a common chemical used to treat acne) lotion, with fewer side effects (Bassett et al., 1990).

   A topical gel containing 5% tea tree oil was found to be more effective than a placebo at preventing acne vulgaris lesions and at decreasing severity in patients suffering from acne vulgaris (Enshaieh et al., 2007).

   Tea tree oil and several of its main components were found to be active against *Propionibacterium acnes*, a bacteria involved in the formation of acne. This oil was also found to be active against 2 types of *Staphylococcus* bacteria (Raman et al., 1995).
5. Mice who inhaled lavender were found to have a decreased motility (natural movement) dependent on exposure time. Additionally, mice injected with caffeine (causing a hyperactivity) were found to reduce their movement to near normal levels after inhaling lavender (Buchbauer et al., 1991).
6. Rats with morphine-induced conditioned place preference that received injections of cumin essential oil demonstrated a decreased morphine-induced conditioning, while rats that received a control substance (Tween-80) did not (Khatibi et al., 2008).
7. Inhaled vapor of black pepper oil was found to reduce craving for cigarettes and symptoms of anxiety in smokers deprived from smoking, compared to a control (Rose et al., 1994).
8. Aging rats fed thyme oil or the constituent thymol were found to have higher levels of the antioxidant enzymes superoxide dismutase and glutathione peroxidase in the brain than aging rats not fed the oil or constituent (Youdim et al., 2000).

   Older rats whose diets were supplemented with thyme oil were found to have a higher level of the antioxidant enzymes superoxide dismutase and glutathione peroxidase in the heart, liver, and kidneys than older rats without this supplementation (Youdim et al., 1999).
9. Arzanol, extracted from helichrysum, inhibited HIV-1 replication in T cells and also inhibited the release of proinflammatory cytokines (chemical messengers) in monocytes (Appendino et al., 2007).
10. A formulation of lemongrass and geranium oil was found to reduce airborne bacteria by 89% in an office environment after diffusion for 15 hours (Doran et al., 2009).
11. In human trials, the aroma of peppermint was found to enhance memory and to increase alertness, while ylang ylang aroma was found to increase calmness (Moss et al., 2008).
12. In a small human trial, oral administration of sage lavender oil was found to improve speed of memory as well as alertness and calmness in healthy volunteers, compared to a placebo (Tildesley et al., 2005).
13. Tea tree oil applied to histamine-induced weal and flare in human volunteers was found to decrease the mean weal volume when compared to a control (Koh et al., 2002).

   Tea tree oil was found to reduce swelling during a contact hypersensitivity response in the skin of mice sensitized to the chemical hapten (Brand et al., May 2002).

   Tea tree oil applied to histamine-induced edema (swelling) in mice ears was found to significantly reduce swelling (Brand et al., Jun. 2002).

   Tea tree oil was found to reduce inflammation in the skin of nickel-sensitive human skin exposed to nickel (Pearce et al., 2005).
14. Lavender oil was found to inhibit immediate-type allergic reactions in mice and rats by inhibiting mast cell degranulation (Kim et al., 1999).
15. L-menthol was found to inhibit production of inflammation mediators in human monocytes (a type of white blood cell involved in the immune response) (Juergens et al., 1998).
16. Oils of *Salvia fruticosa* and *Salvia officinalis* were found to inhibit butyrylcholinesterase, an enzyme that has been studied for its potential role in increasing the chances of developing Alzheimer's disease (Savelev et al., 2004).
17. Lavender oil was found to be effective at alleviating agitated behaviors in Chinese patients suffering from dementia (Lin et al., 2007).

   Lavandula angustifolia essential oil demonstrated an ability to inhibit GABA-A receptor channels of rat brain cells (Huang et al., 2008).
18. Subjects who had ylang ylang oil applied to their skin had decreased blood pressure, increased skin temperature, and reported feeling more calm and relaxed, compared to subjects in a control group (Hongratanaworakit et al., 2006).

   In human trials, the aroma of ylang ylang was found to increase calmness (Moss et al., 2008).
19. In human volunteers wearing breathing masks to prevent aroma inhalation, rose oil applied to the skin was found to significantly decrease breathing rate, blood oxygen saturation, and systolic blood pressure, compared to a placebo. And volunteers receiving rose oil rated themselves more calm and relaxed than did subjects receiving the placebo (Hongratanaworakit et al., 2009).
20. Melissa (lemon balm) oil applied topically in a lotion was found to reduce agitation and to improve quality of life factors in patients suffering from severe dementia, compared to those receiving a placebo lotion (Ballard et al., 2002).

21. Oils with aldehyde or phenol as a major component demonstrated a high level of antibacterial activity (Inouye et al., 2001).

    Tea tree, peppermint, and sage oils were found to inhibit oral bacteria, with thymol and eugenol being the most active components of these oils (Shapiro et al., 1994).

    Subjects using a mouthwash containing thymol, menthol, methyl salicylate, and eucalyptol for 6 months were found to not have developed oral bacteria that were resistant to the oils (Charles et al., 2000).

    Thyme oil demonstrated a strong antibacterial effect against staph and *E. coli* bacteria (Mohsenzadeh et al., 2007).

    Cinnamon, thyme, and clove essential oils demonstrated an antibacterial effect on several respiratory tract pathogens (Fabio et al., 2007).

    Cinnamon bark, lemongrass, and thyme oils were found to have the highest level of activity against common respiratory pathogens among 14 essential oils tested (Inouye et al., 2001).

22. MRSA (methicillin-resistant staph) and MSSA (methicillin-sensitive staph) in biofilms (plaque/microcolonies) and 5 of 9 CoNS (coagulase-negative staph) were eradicated by a 5% solution of tea tree oil (Brady et al., 2006).

    66 isolates of *Staphylococcus aureus* (staph), including 64 methicillin-resistant (MRSA) and 33 mupirocin-resistant strains, were inhibited by tea tree essential oil (Carson et al., 1995).

    In a human trial, most patients receiving treatment with *Melaleuca alternifolia* oil placed topically on boils experienced healing or reduction of symptoms; while of those receiving no treatment (control), half required surgical intervention, and all still demonstrated signs of the infection (Feinblatt, 1960).

    Terpinen-4-ol, found in tea tree oil, was found to effectively inhibit MRSA and CoNS, while not exhibiting toxicity to human fibroblast cells (Loughlin et al., 2008).

    Tea tree oil was found to disrupt the cellular membrane and to inhibit respiration in *Candida albicans*, gram-negative *E. coli*, and gram-positive *Staphylococcus aureus* (staph) (Cox et al., 2000).

    Geranium and tea tree demonstrated strong antibacterial effects on *Staphylococcus aureus* (Edwards-Jones et al., 2004).

    Among several oils tested, tea tree (melaleuca), manuka, and eucalyptus demonstrated strong antibacterial activity against detrimental oral bacteria (Hammer et al., 2008).

    Tea tree oil demonstrated an ability to kill *Staphylococcus aureus* (staph) bacteria, both within biofilms and in the stationary growth phase at concentrations below 1% (Kwieciński et al., 2009).

    Tea tree oil and its component terpinen-4-ol were found to demonstrate effective antibacterial activity against *Staphylococcus aureus* (staph) bacteria, superior to the activities of several antibiotic drugs--even against antibiotic resistant strains (Ferrini et al., 2006).

    Tea tree oil and several of its main components were found to be active against *Propionibacterium acnes*, a bacteria involved in the formation of acne. This oil was also found to be active against 2 types of *Staphylococcus* bacteria (Raman et al., 1995).

23. Cinnamon oil exhibited a strong antimicrobial activity against 2 detrimental oral bacteria. Manuka, tea tree, and the component thymol also exhibited antimicrobial potency (Filoche et al., 2005).

    Cinnamon, thyme, and clove essential oils demonstrated an antibacterial effect on several respiratory tract pathogens (Fabio et al., 2007).

    Cinnamon bark, lemongrass, and thyme oils were found to have the highest level of activity against common respiratory pathogens among 14 essential oils tested (Inouye et al., 2001).

24. A formulation of lemongrass and geranium oil was found to reduce airborne bacteria by 89% in an office environment after diffusion for 15 hours (Doran et al., 2009).

    Lemongrass demonstrated ability to inhibit *Helicobacter pylori*, a pathogen responsible for gastroduodenal disease. This pathogen also did not develop resistance to lemongrass after 10 passes (it did develop resistance to the antibiotic drug clarithromycin within the same amount of passes) (Ohono et al., 2003).

    Two components of lemongrass demonstrated antibacterial properties; while the addition of a third component, myrcene, enhanced the anti-bacterial activities even further (Onawunmi et al., 1984).

    Cinnamon bark, lemongrass, and thyme oils were found to have the highest level of activity against common respiratory pathogens among 14 essential oils tested (Inouye et al., 2001).

25. Peppermint and rosemary oils were each found to be more effective at preventing dental biofilm (plaque) formation than chlorhexidine (an antiseptic) (Rasooli et al., 2008).

    Peppermint oil was found to be an effective antibacterial and antioxidant agent (Mimica-Dukić et al., 2003).

    Peppermint oil blended with toothpaste was found to be more effective at lower concentrations in inhibiting the formation of dental plaque than was chlorhexidine (an antiseptic) in human volunteers (Shayegh et al., 2008).

    Peppermint and spearmint oil inhibited resistant strains of *Staphylococcus*, *E. coli*, *Salmonella*, and *Helicobacter pylori* (Imai et al., 2001).

    Subjects using a mouthwash containing thymol, menthol, methyl salicylate, and eucalyptol for 6 months were found to not have developed oral bacteria that were resistant to the oils (Charles et al., 2000).

26. Oregano oil was found to kill antibiotic resistant strains of staph, *E. coli*, *Klebsiella pneumoniae*, *Helicobacter pylori*, and *Mycobacterium terrae* (Preuss et al., 2005).

    Oregano oil was found to inhibit MRSA (Nostro et al., 2004).

27. Lemon Myrtle demonstrated antimicrobial inhibition against staph, *E. coli*, *Pseudomonas aeruginosa*, *Candida*, MRSA, black mold, and others (Hayes et al., 2002).

    Four essential oil samples of *Backhousia citriodora* (lemon myrtle) were found to have antibacterial and antifungal properties (Wilkinson et al., 2003).

28. Basil oil was found to strongly inhibit several multidrug resistant bacteria (Opalchenova et al., 2003).

29. Cinnamon, thyme, and clove essential oils demonstrated an antibacterial effect on several respiratory tract pathogens (Fabio et al., 2007).

30. Peppermint and spearmint oil inhibited resistant strains of *Staphylococcus*, *E. coli*, *Salmonella*, and *Helicobacter pylori* (Imai et al., 2001).

31. A methanol extract from rosemary with 30% carnosic acid, 16% carnosol, and 5% rosmarinic acid was found to be effective against gram-positive and negative bacteria and yeast (Moreno et al., 2006).

32. Rose essential oil demonstrated strong antibacterial activity against several pathogenic bacteria (Ulusoy et al., 2009).

33. *Schinus molle* essential oils demonstrated antibacterial and antifungal activity against a variety of species (Gundidza, 1993).

34. A combination of citricidal and geranium oil demonstrated strong antibacterial effects on MRSA. Geranium and tea tree demonstrated strong antibacterial effects on *Staphylococcus aureus* (Edwards-Jones et al., 2004).

A formulation of lemongrass and geranium oil was found to reduce airborne bacteria by 89% in an office environment after diffusion for 15 hours (Doran et al., 2009).

35. Eucalyptus oil was found to have an anti-inflammatory and mucin-inhibitory effect in rats with lipopolysaccharide-induced bronchitis (Lu et al., 2004).

36. Melaleuca oil inhibited several *Candida* species in vitro (Vazquez et al., 2000).

Eleven types of *Candida* were found to be highly inhibited by tea tree oil (Banes-Marshall et al., 2001).

Tea tree oil was found to alter the membrane properties and functions of *Candida albicans* cells, leading to cell inhibition or death (Hammer et al., 2004).

Tea tree oil was found to disrupt the cellular membrane and to inhibit respiration in *Candida albicans*, gram-negative *E. coli*, and gram-positive *Staphylococcus aureus* (staph) (Cox et al., 2000).

Terpinen-4-ol, a constituent of tea tree oil, and tea tree oil were found to be effective against several forms of vaginal candida infections in rats, including azole-resistant forms (Mondello et al., 2006).

Melaleuca oil at concentrations of .16% was found to inhibit the transformation of *C. albicans* from single-cell yeast to the pathogenic mycelial (multi-cellular strands) form (D'Auria et al., 2001).

Tea tree oil demonstrated fungicidal activity against 4 plant pathogenic fungi (Terzie et al., 2007).

Tea tree oil was found to inhibit 301 different types of yeasts isolated from the mouths of cancer patients suffering from advanced cancer, including 41 strains that are known to be resistant to antifungal drugs (Bagg et al., 2006).

37. Vapor of cinnamon bark oil and cinnamic aldehyde was found to be effective against fungi involved in respiratory tract mycoses (fungal infections) (Singh et al., 1995).

Cinnamon, thyme, oregano, and cumin oils inhibited the production of aflatoxin by *Aspergillus* fungus (Tantaoui-Elaraki et al., 1994).

In a test of 9 oils, clove, followed by cinnamon, oregano, and mace oils, was found to be inhibitory to 2 toxin-producing fungi. It was also shown that whole and ground cloves stored with grain reduced the amount of aflatoxin contamination (Juglal et al., 2002).

38. Clove oil was found to display an antifungal effect against tested *Candida* strains (Chaieb et al., 2007).

Eugenol from clove and thymol from thyme were found to inhibit the growth of *Aspergillus flavus* and *Aspergillus versicolor* at concentrations of .4 mg/ml or less (Hitokoto et al., 1980).

In a test of 9 oils, clove, followed by cinnamon, oregano, and mace oils, was found to be inhibitory to 2 toxin-producing fungi. It was also shown that whole and ground cloves stored with grain reduced the amount of aflatoxin contamination (Juglal et al., 2002).

39. Mice infected with *Candida albicans* who were fed origanum oil or carvacrol diluted in olive oil had an 80% survival rate after 30 days, while infected mice fed olive oil alone all died after 10 days (Manohar et al., 2001).

The vapor of oregano oil was found to be fungicidal against the *Trichophyton mentagrophytes* fungi (a fungi that causes a skin infection known as Malabar itch) (Inouye et al., 2006).

40. Thyme oil was found to inhibit *Candida* species by causing lesions in the cell membrane and by inhibiting germ tube (an outgrowth that develops when the fungi is preparing to replicate) formation (Pina-Vaz et al., 2004).

Cinnamon, thyme, oregano, and cumin oils inhibited the production of aflatoxin by *Aspergillus* fungus (Tantaoui-elaraki et al., 1994).

Eugenol from clove and thymol from thyme were found to inhibit the growth of *Aspergillus flavus* and *Aspergillus versicolor* at concentrations of .4 mg/ml or less (Hitokoto et al., 1980).

41. *Schinus molle* essential oils demonstrated antibacterial and antifungal activity against a variety of species (Gundidza et al., 1993).

In a screening test of essential oils, *Schinus molle* oil demonstrated antifungal activity against several pathogenic fungi (Dikshit et al., 1986).

42. Lemon Myrtle demonstrated antimicrobial inhibition against staph, *E. coli*, *Pseudomonas aeruginosa*, *Candida*, MRSA, black mold, and others (Hayes et al., 2002).

Lemon myrtle oil was found to effectively inhibit 13 bacteria and 8 fungi (Wilkinson et al., 2003).

43. Lemon oil was found to be an effective antifungal agent against 2 bread mold species (Caccioni et al., 1998).

44. Savory oil demonstrated antimicrobial activity against a range of bacteria and yeast, including *E. coli*, MRSA, and *Candida albicans* (Skocibusić et al., 2004).

45. Carrot essential oil was found to demonstrate antifungal activity against yeasts and *Aspergillus* fungi at concentrations that were not cytotoxic to mouse skin dendritic cells (Tavares et al., 2008).

46. Patients with tinea pedis (athlete's foot) were found to have a higher rate of cure and a higher clinical response when treated topically with 25% or 50% tea tree oil solution, compared to control (Satchell et al., 2002).

47. Lavender oil demonstrated both fungistatic (stopped growth) and fungicidal (killed) activity against *Candida albicans* (D'Auria et al., 2005).

48. Peppermint oil was found to have a higher fungistatic and fungicidal activity against various fungi (including *Candida*) than the commercial fungicide bifonazole. Additionally, peppermint oil was found to be an effective antibacterial and antioxidant agent (Mimica-Dukić et al., 2003).

49. Incensole acetate, isolated from frankincense resin, was found to demonstrate an anti-inflammatory and neuro-protective effect in mice with a closed head injury (Moussaieff et al., 2008).

An acetone extract of frankincense was found to decrease arthritic sores, reduce paw edema (swelling), and suppress proinflammatory cytokines (cellular messengers (Fan et al., 2005).

Boswellic acids from frankincense (delivered with sesame seed oil) were found to inhibit TH1 cytokines while potentiating TH2 cytokines, demonstrating their ability to modulate the immune response (Chevrier et al., 2005).

Boswellic acid reduced induced inflammation and tumors in mice (Huang et al., 2000).

Compounds from *Boswellia serrata* were found to carry out anti-inflammatory activity by switching off the proinflammatory cytokines and mediators that initiate the inflammatory process (Gayathri et al., 2007).

Boswellic acid, from frankincense, was found in vitro to prevent expression and activity of several proteins involved in the inflammatory response. In vivo, boswellic acid was found to protect against experimental arthritis (Roy et al., 2006).

Triterpene acids isolated from frankincense were found to exhibit a marked anti-inflammatory activity in TPA-induced inflammation in mice (Banno et al., 2006).

Boswellic extract was found to effect genes related to the inflammatory response in human microvascular cells. Additionally, Boswellic extract was found to reduce inflammation in carrageenan-induced rat paw inflammation (Roy et al., 2005).

50. Inhaled tea tree oil was found to have anti-inflammatory influences on male rats with induced peritoneal inflammation (Golab et al., 2007).

Tea tree oil applied to histamine-induced edema (swelling) in mice ears was found to significantly reduce swelling (Brand et al., 2002).

Melaleuca alternifolia oil was found to mediate the reactive oxygen species (ROS) production of leukocytes (white blood cells), indicating a possible anti-inflammatory activity (Caldefie-Chézet et al., 2004).

Tea tree oil was found to reduce inflammation in the skin of nickel-sensitive human skin exposed to nickel (Pearce et al., 2005).

Melaleuca alternifolia oil was found to reduce reactive oxygen species (ROS) production in neutrophils (a type of white blood cell), indicating an antioxidant effect. It was also found to decrease interleukin-2 (a chemical messenger that helps trigger an inflammatory response) secretion, while increasing the secretion of interleukin-4 (a chemical messenger involved in turning off the inflammatory response) (Caldefie-Chézet et al., 2006).

The water soluble terpinen-4-ol component of tea tree was found to suppress the production of proinflammatory mediators in human monocytes (a type of white blood cell that is part of the human immune system (Hart et al., 2000).

51. Eucalyptus oil was shown to ameliorate inflammatory processes by interacting with oxygen radicals and by interfering with leukocyte activation (Grassmann et al., 2000).

Oils of 3 eucalyptus species (*citriodora*, *tereticornis*, and *globulus*) were found to have analgesic (pain-relieving) and anti-inflammatory properties in rats (Silva et al., 2003).

Eucalyptus oil was found to have an anti-inflammatory and mucin-inhibitory effect in rats with lipopolysaccharide-induced bronchitis (Lu et al., 2004).

Extracts from eucalyptus and thyme were found to have high nitrous oxide (NO) scavenging abilities and were found to inhibit NO production in macrophage cells. This could possibly explain their role in aiding respiratory inflammatory diseases (Vigo et al., 2004).

1,8 cineole (eucalyptol) was found to display an anti-inflammatory effect on rats in several tests and was found to exhibit antinociceptive (pain-reducing) effects in mice, possibly by depressing the central nervous system (Santos et al., 2000).

52. Linalool and linalyl acetate (from lavender and other essential oils) were found to exhibit anti-inflammatory activity in rats subjected to carrageenin-induced edema (inflammation) (Peana et al., 2002).

Oil from *Lavandula angustifolia* was found to reduce writhing in induced writhing in rats and to reduce edema (swelling) in carrageenan-induced paw edema, indicating an anti-inflammatory effect (Hajhashemi et al., 2003).

53. Subtoxic levels of myrrh oil were found to inhibit interleukin (chemical messenger involved in inflammation) in part by inhibiting PGE(2) (prostaglandin E, a lipid compound that has several messenger functions in the body, including in the inflammatory response) (Tipton et al., 2006).

At subtoxic levels, myrrh oil was found to reduce interleukin (chemical signals believed to play a role in the inflammation response) by fibroblast cells in the gums (Tipton et al., 2003).

54. Chamazulene, a chemical in chamomile oil, was found to block formation of leukotriene (a signaling chemical involved in the inflammatory process) in neutrophilic (immune system) granulocytes (white blood cells containing granules). It also demonstrated an antioxidant effect (Safayhi et al., 1994).

55. Methyl salicylate (found in wintergreen or birch oils) was found to inhibit leukotriene C4 (a chemical messenger involved in inflammatory response), while also demonstrating gastroprotective against ethanol-induced gastric injury in rats (Trautmann et al., 1991).

56. Ocotea oil was found to demonstrate anti-inflammatory effects in rats, without damaging gastric mucosa (Ballabeni et al., 2009).

57. A combination of peppermint and caraway oil was found to reduce visceral hyperalgesia (pain hypersensitivity in the gastrointestinal tract) after induced inflammation in rats (Adam et al., 2006).

L-menthol was found to inhibit production of inflammation mediators in human monocytes (a type of white blood cell involved in the immune response) (Juergens et al., 1998).

58. Arzanol, extracted from helichrysum, inhibited HIV-1 replication in T cells and also inhibited the release of proinflammatory cytokines (chemical messengers) in monocytes (Appendino et al., 2007).
59. Clove oil was found to have very strong radical scavenging activity (antioxidant). It was also found to display an antifungal effect against tested *Candida* strains (Chaieb et al., 2007).

    Various essential oils demonstrated an antioxidant effect toward skin lipid squalene oxidized by UV irradiation, with a blend of thyme and clove oil demonstrating the highest inhibitory effect (Wei et al., 2007).
60. Aging rats fed thyme oil or the constituent thymol were found to have higher levels of the antioxidant enzymes superoxide dismutase and glutathione peroxidase in the brain than aging rats not fed the oil or constituent (Youdim et al., 2000).

    Older rats whose diets were supplemented with thyme oil were found to have higher levels of the antioxidant enzymes superoxide dismutase and glutathione peroxidase in the heart, liver, and kidneys than did older rats without this supplementation (Youdim et al., 1999).

    Extracts from eucalyptus and thyme were found to have high nitrous oxide (NO) scavenging abilities and were also found to inhibit NO production in macrophage cells. This could possibly explain their role in aiding respiratory inflammatory diseases (Vigo et al., 2004).

    Various essential oils demonstrated an antioxidant effect toward skin lipid squalene oxidized by UV irradiation, with a blend of thyme and clove oil demonstrating the highest inhibitory effect (Wei et al., 2007).
61. Extracts from rosemary were found to have high antioxidant properties. Rosmarinic acid and carnosic acid from rosemary were found to have the highest antioxidant activities of studied components of rosemary (Almela et al., 2006).

    An ethanol extract of rosemary was found to have an antiproliferative and an antioxidant effect on human leukemia and breast carcinoma cells (Cheung et al., 2007).

    Extracts from rosemary were found to have high antioxidant levels. Additionally, a methanol extract with 30% carnosic acid, 16% carnosol, and 5% rosmarinic acid was found to be effective against gram-positive and gram-negative bacteria and yeast (Moreno et al., 2006).

    In patients with chronic bronchitis, rosemary, basil, fir, and eucalyptus oils were found to demonstrate an antioxidant effect. Lavender was found to promote normalization of lipid levels (Siurin, 1997).
62. Peppermint oil fed to mice prior to exposure to gamma radiation was found to decrease levels of damage from oxidation, compared to mice that were not pretreated with peppermint oil (Samarth et al., 2006).

    Peppermint oil was found to be an effective antibacterial and antioxidant agent (Mimica-Dukić et al., 2003).

    Peppermint extract fed orally to mice demonstrated an ability to protect the testis from gamma radiation damage (Samarth et al., 2009).
63. *Melaleuca alternifolia* oil was found to reduce reactive oxygen species (ROS) production in neutrophils (a type of white blood cell), indicating an antioxidant effect. It was also found to decrease interleukin-2 (a chemical messenger that helps trigger an inflammatory response) secretion, while increasing the secretion of interleukin-4 (a chemical messenger involved in turning off the inflammatory response) (Caldefie-Chézet et al., 2006).

    Melaleuca alternifolia oil was found to mediate the reactive oxygen species (ROS) production of leukocytes (white blood cells), indicating a possible anti-inflammatory activity (Caldefie-Chézet et al., 2004).
64. Arzanol (extracted from helichrysum), at non-cytotoxic concentrations, showed a strong inhibition of TBH-induced oxidative stress in VERO cells (Rosa et al., 2007).
65. Oil from *Abies alba* was found to demonstrate antiradical activity against 2 known free radicals (Yang et al., 2009).
66. Lemon oil and one of its components, gamma-terpinene, were found to inhibit oxidation of low-density lipoprotein (LDL). Oxidation of LDL has been found to increase the risk of atherosclerosis and cardiac disease (Grassmann et al., 2001).
67. Peppermint oil was found to be as effective as Buscopan (an antispasmodic drug) at preventing spasms during a barium enema (a type of enema used to place barium in the colon for X-ray imaging purposes) (Asao et al., 2003).
68. Lavender was found to have a relaxant effect on smooth muscle from guinea-pig ileum (small intestine) (Lis-Balchin et al., 1999).
69. An extract from *Artemisia vulgaris* (mugwort) was found to have antispasmodic and bronchodilating activities in several different animal and animal tissue tests (Khan et al., 2009).
70. Melissa oil demonstrated inhibition of herpes simplex type 1 and type 2 viruses (Schnitzler et al., 2008).
71. Arzanol, extracted from helichrysum, inhibited HIV-1 replication in T cells and also inhibited the release of proinflammatory cytokines (chemical messengers) in monocytes (Appendino et al., 2007).

    Helichrysum was found to have significant antiviral activity against the herpes virus at non-cytotoxic concentrations (Nostro et al., 2003).
72. Tea tree and eucalyptus oil demonstrated an ability to inhibit herpes simplex virus (Schnitzler et al., 2001).
73. Eugenol was found to be virucidal to herpes simplex and to delay the development of herpes-induced keratitis (inflammation of the cornea) in mice (Benencia et al., 2000).
74. In children with *Molluscum contagiosum* (a viral infection causing skin lesions), application of a 10% solution of lemon myrtle oil was found to reduce lesions by more than 90% in 56% of patients, while in children receiving application of a control (olive oil), none had a reduction of lesions greater than 90% (Burke et al., 2004).
75. Herpes simplex viruses pretreated with manuka oil before cell infection were significantly inhibited and had plaque formation reduced by over 98% in cultured monkey kidney cells (Reichling et al., 2005).
76. Peppermint oil demonstrated a direct virucidal activity against herpes type 1 and type 2 viruses (Schuhmacher et al., 2003).

77. An office environment featuring a soothing DVD video presentation and diffused lavender oil was found to reduce anxiety in patients awaiting a gastroscopy procedure, compared to a regular office environment (Hoya et al., 2008).

    Oral supplementation of lavender oil was found to decrease anxiety in females in conditions of low anxiety (Bradley et al., 2009).

    In patients admitted to an intensive care unit, those receiving lavender aromatherapy reported a greater improvement in mood and perceived levels of anxiety, compared to those receiving massage or a period of rest (Dunn et al., 1995).

    Patients being treated with chronic hemodialysis demonstrated less anxiety when exposed to lavender aroma (Itai et al., 2000).

    Lavender oil was found to demonstrate anticonflict effects in mice similar to the anxiolytic (antianxiety) drug diazepam (Umezu, 2000).

    Exposure to lavender odor was found to decrease anxiety in gerbils in the elevated plus maze, with a further decrease in anxiety in females after prolonged (2 week) exposure (Bradley et al., 2007).

78. Female patients waiting for dental treatment were found to be less anxious, more positive, and more calm when exposed to orange oil odor than patients who were not exposed to the orange oil odor (Lehrner et al., 2000).

    Patients waiting for dental treatment were found to be less anxious and to have a better mood when exposed to the odor of lavender or orange oil, compared to control (Lehrner et al., 2005).

79. Lemon oil was found to have an antistress effect on mice involved in several behavioral tasks (Komiya et al., 2006).

    It was found that exposure to lemon oil in rats induced chemical changes in the neuronal circuits involved in anxiety and pain (Ceccarelli et la., 2004).

80. Massage with a carrier oil including Roman chamomile oil was found to enhance the reduction of anxiety, compared to massage with the carrier oil alone (Wilkinson et al., 1999).

81. Two chemical components found in valerian were found to have sedative, sleep-enhancing, and anxiolytic (anxiety-lowering) properties (Marder et al., 2003).

82. Results of a clinical trial indicate that a combination of melissa and valerian oils may have anxiety-reducing properties at some doses (Kennedy et al., 2006).

83. In the elevated plus-maze, copal oil was found to demonstrate anxiolytic effects in rats comparable to the effects of the antianxiety drug diazepam (Curio et al., 2009).

84. Incensole acetate (found in frankincense) was found to open TRPV receptors (a possible channel for emotional regulation) in mice brain (Moussaieff et al., 2008).

85. Lemon oil and one of its components, gamma-terpinene, were found to inhibit oxidation of low-density lipoprotein (LDL) in vitro. Oxidation of LDL has been found to increase the risk of atherosclerosis and cardiac disease (Grassmann et al., 2001).

86. Oral administration of ocotea oil in mice was found to prevent collagen-epinephrine induced thrombosis (blood clots) (Ballabeni et al., 2007).

87. Both fennel oil and its constituent, anethole, were found to significantly reduce thrombosis (blood clots) in mice. They were also found to be free from the prohemorrhagic (increased bleeding) side effect that aspirin (acetylsalicylic acid) has (Tognolini et al., 2007).

88. Clove oil demonstrated an ability to prevent the aggregation of platelets that can lead to blood clots and thrombosis both in vivo and in vitro (Saeed et al., 1994).

89. Treatment of rats with 1,8-cineole (or eucalyptol, found in eucalyptus and rosemary) demonstrated an ability to lower mean aortic pressure (blood pressure)through vascular wall relaxation, without decreasing heart rate (Lahlou et al., 2002).

90. Boswellic acid, from frankincense, was found in vitro to prevent expression and activity of several proteins involved in the inflammatory response. In vivo, boswellic acid was found to protect against experimental arthritis (Roy et al., 2006).

    An acetone extract of frankincense was found to decrease arthritic sores, reduce paw edema (swelling), and suppress proinflammatory cytokines (cellular messengers) (Fan et al., 2005).

91. In patients suffering from arthritis, it was found that a blend of lavender, marjoram, eucalyptus, rosemary, peppermint, and carrier oils reduced perceived pain and depression, compared to control (Kim et al., 2005).

92. Extracts from eucalyptus and thyme were found to have high nitrous oxide (NO) scavenging abilities and to inhibit NO production in macrophage cells. This could possibly explain their role in aiding respiratory inflammatory diseases (Vigo et al., 2004).

    Therapy with 1,8 cineole (eucalyptol) in both healthy and bronchitis-afflicted humans was shown to reduce production of LTB4 and PGE2 (both metabolites of arachidonic acid, a known chemical messenger involved in inflammation) in white blood cells (Juergens et al., 1998).

93. L-menthol was found to inhibit production of inflammation mediators in human monocytes (a type of white blood cell involved in the immune response) (Juergens et al., 1998).

94. The essential oil of rose at concentrations lower than 1% demonstrated relaxant effects on guinea pig trachea comparable to the asthma drug theophylline (Boskabady et al., 2006).

95. An extract from *Artemisia vulgaris* (mugwort) was found to have antispasmodic and bronchodilating activities in several different animal and animal tissue tests (Khan et al., 2009).

96. Clove oil demonstrated an ability to prevent the aggregation of platelets that can lead to blood clots and thrombosis both in vivo and in vitro (Saeed et al., 1994).

97. Both fennel oil and its constituent, anethole, were found to significantly reduce thrombosis (blood clots) in mice. They were also found to be free from the prohemorrhagic (increased bleeding) side effect that aspirin (acetylsalicylic acid) has (Tognolini et al., 2007).

98. Inhaled ylang ylang oil was found to decrease blood pressure and pulse rate and to enhance attentiveness and alertness in volunteers, compared to an odorless control (Hongratanaworaki et al., 2004).

    Subjects who had ylang ylang oil applied to their skin had decreased blood pressure, increased skin temperature, and reported feeling more calm and relaxed, compared to subjects in a control group (Hongratanaworakit et al., 2006).

99. Treatment of rats with 1,8-cineole (or eucalyptol—found in eucalyptus, rosemary, and marjoram) demonstrated an ability to lower mean aortic pressure (blood pressure) through vascular wall relaxation, without decreasing heart rate.

100. Rats fed dill essential oil were found to have reduced total cholesterol, triglyceride, and low-density lipoprotein (LDL) and to have increased levels of high-density lipoprotein (HDL) (Hajhashemi et al., 2008).

101. Clove oil demonstrated an ability to prevent the aggregation of platelets that can lead to blood clots and thrombosis both in vivo and in vitro (Saeed et al., 1994).

102. In mice exposed to whole-body gamma irradiation, only 17% of mice who had been fed peppermint oil died, while 100% of mice who did not receive peppermint oil died. It was also found that mice pre-fed peppermint oil were able to return blood cell levels to normal after 30 days, while control mice were not able to (and, consequently, died), suggesting a protective or stimulating effect of the oil on blood stem cells (Samarth et al., 2004).

103. In a human trial, most patients receiving treatment with *Melaleuca alternifolia* oil placed topically on boils experienced healing or reduction of symptoms, while of those receiving no treatment (control), half required surgical intervention, and all still demonstrated signs of the infection (Feinblatt, 1960).

104. Subjects exposed to 3 minutes of lavender aroma were more relaxed and able to perform math computations faster and more accurately. Subjects exposed to rosemary aroma were more alert and completed math computations faster (but not more accurately) (Diego et al., 1998).

    Subjects who smelled a cleansing gel with lavender aroma were more relaxed and able to complete math computations faster (DField et al., 2005).

105. Several constituents of lemon oil and their metabolites (chemicals made by these chemicals in the body) were found to increase the release of monoamines (various chemicals responsible for neurotransmission and neuromodulation) in rat brain tissue, indicating a possible effect on brain nerve cell behavior (Fukumoto et al., 2006).

    Pretreatment of human and rat astrocyte cells (cells found in the nerve and brain that support the blood-brain barrier and help repair the brain and spinal cord following injuries) with lemon oil was found to inhibit heat-shock induced apoptosis of these cells (Koo et al., 2002).

106. Incensole acetate, isolated from frankincense resin, was found to demonstrate an anti-inflammatory and neuro-protective effect in mice with a closed head injury (Moussaieff et al., 2008).

107. Peppermint oil was found to inhibit apoptosis of astrocytes (the most abundant glial-type [non-neuronal cells that provide support to neuronal cells and form myelin] cell in the brain) when subjected to heat-shock (Koo et al., 2001).

108. Pretreatment of human and rat astrocyte cells (cells found in the nerve and brain that support the blood-brain barrier and help repair the brain and spinal cord following injuries) with lemon oil was found to inhibit heat-shock induced apoptosis of these cells (Koo et al., 2002).

109. Imaging of the brain demonstrated that inhalation of 1,8-cineol (eucalyptol, a constituent of many essential oils—especially eucalyptus, rosemary, and marjoram) increased global cerebral blood flow after an inhalation time of 20 minutes (Nasel et al., 1994).

110. Inhalation of black pepper oil was found to increase cerebral blood flow and to improve the swallowing reflex in elderly patients who had suffered a stroke (Ebihara et al., 2006).

111. Ethanol extract of *Boswellia serrata* demonstrated antiproliferative effects on 5 leukemia and 2 brain tumor cell lines. It was more potent than one type of boswellic acid (AKBA) on 3 leukemia cell lines (Hostanska et al., 2002).

112. Therapy with 1,8 cineole (eucalyptol) in both healthy and bronchitis-afflicted humans was shown to reduce production of LTB4 and PGE2 (both metabolites of arachidonic acid, a known chemical messenger involved in inflammation) in white blood cells (Juergens et al., 1998).

    Extracts from eucalyptus and thyme were found to have high nitrous oxide (NO) scavenging abilities and to inhibit NO production in macrophage cells. This could possibly explain their role in aiding respiratory inflammatory diseases (Vigo et al., 2004).

    Eucalyptus oil was found to have an anti-inflammatory and mucin-inhibitory effect in rats with lipopolysaccharide-induced bronchitis (Lu et al., 2004).

113. Extracts from eucalyptus and thyme were found to have high nitrous oxide (NO) scavenging abilities and to inhibit NO production in macrophage cells. This could possibly explain their role in aiding respiratory inflammatory diseases (Vigo et al., 2004).

114. Inhaling lavender oil was found to lower agitation in older Chinese adults suffering from dementia (Lin et al., 2007).

    Lavandula angustifolia essential oil demonstrated an ability to inhibit GABA-A receptor channels of rat brain cells (Huang et al., 2008).

115. In human trials, ylang ylang aroma was found to increase calmness (Moss et al., 2008).

    Subjects who had ylang ylang oil applied to their skin had decreased blood pressure, increased skin temperature, and reported feeling more calm and relaxed (compared to subjects in a control group) (Hongratanaworakit et al., 2006).

116. In human volunteers wearing breathing masks to prevent aroma inhalation, rose oil applied to the skin was found to significantly decrease breathing rate, blood oxygen saturation, and systolic blood pressure (compared to a placebo). And volunteers receiving rose oil rated themselves as more calm and relaxed than did subjects receiving the placebo (Hongratanaworakit et al., 2009).

    Geraniol and eugenol, 2 components of rose oil (among others), were found to demonstrate antianxiety effects on mice in several tests (Umezu et al., 2002).

117. Melissa (lemon balm) oil applied topically in a lotion was found to reduce agitation and to improve quality of life in patients suffering from severe dementia, compared to those receiving a placebo lotion (Ballard et al., 2002).

118. Female patients waiting for dental treatment were found to be less anxious, more positive, and more calm when exposed to orange oil odor than patients who were not exposed to the orange oil odor (Lehrner et al., 2000).

119. Exposure to lavender oil and to its constituents, linalool and linalyl acetate, was found to decrease normal movement in mice as well as to return mice to normal movement rates after caffeine induced hyperactivity (Buchbauer et al., 1991).

120. Inhaling lavender oil was found to lower agitation in older adults suffering from dementia (Lin et al., 2007).

Exposure to lavender oil, and to its constituents, linalool and linalyl acetate, was found to decrease normal movement in mice and to return mice to normal movement rates after caffeine induced hyperactivity (Buchbauer et al., 1991).

Lavandula angustifolia essential oil demonstrated an ability to inhibit GABA-A receptor channels of rat brain cells (Huang et al., 2008).

Swiss mice fed lavender oil diluted in olive oil were found to be more sedate in several common tests (Guillemain et al., 1989).

121. Lemon oil was found to have an antistress effect on mice involved in several behavioral tasks (Komiya et al., 2006).

122. Two chemical components found in valerian were found to have sedative, sleep-enhancing, and anxiolytic (anxiety-lowering) properties (Marder et al., 2003).

123. Boswellic acids from frankincense were found to induce apoptosis (cell death) in human leukemia cell lines (Xia et al., 2005).

Boswellic acid was found to inhibit DNA and RNA synthesis in human leukemia cells, leading to inhibited cell growth (Shao et al., 1998).

Boswellic acid was found to prevent and to inhibit invasion and metastasis of melanoma (skin pigment) and fibrosarcoma (connective tissue cancer) cells (Zhao et al., 2003).

Boswellic acid was found to cause differentiation in premyelocytic leukemia cells, while inhibiting growth of these cells in mice (Jing et al., 1992).

Boswellic acid was shown to induce apoptosis in 3 leukemia cell lines and to induce differentiation in one leukemia cell line (Jing et al., 1999).

Boswellic acid was found to inhibit the androgen receptors involved in the development and progression of prostate cancer (Yuan et al., 2008).

Boswellic acid induced apoptosis in prostate cancer cells (Lu et al., 2008).

An extract from *Boswellia carterii* was found to induce apoptosis (cell death) in 2 leukemia cell lines (Hunan et al., 1999).

An extract from frankincense was found to produce apoptosis in human leukemia cells (Bhushan et al., 2007).

Boswellic acids demonstrated an antiproliferative and apoptotic effect on liver cancer cells (Liu et al., Dec 2002).

Boswellic acids demonstrated an antiproliferative and apoptotic effect on liver cancer cells (Liu et al., Oct 2002).

124. Alpha-santalol was found to induce apoptosis in human skin cancer cells (Kaur et al., 2005).

Various concentrations of alpha-santalol (from sandalwood) were tested against skin cancer in mice. All concentrations were found to inhibit skin cancer development (Dwivedi et al., 2005).

Alpha-santalol, derived from sandalwood EO, was found to delay and decrease the incidence and multiplicity of skin tumor (papilloma) development in mice (Swivedi et al., 2003).

Pretreatment with alpha-santalol before UVB (ultraviolet B) radiation significantly reduced skin tumor development and multiplicity and induced proapoptotic and tumor-suppressing proteins (Arasada et al., 2008).

A solution of 5% alpha-santalol (from sandalwood) was found to prevent skin tumor formation caused by ultraviolet B (UVB) radiation in mice (Swivedi et al., 2006).

Sandalwood oil was found to decrease skin papilloma (tumors) in mice (Swivedi et al., 1997).

Oral sandalwood oil use enhanced GST activity (a protein in cell membranes that can help eliminate toxins) and acid-soluble SH levels. This suggests a possible chemopreventive action on carcinogenesis (Banerjee et al., 1993).

125. Rats fed diets containing perillyl alcohol (derived from lavender plants) were found to have less incidence of colon tumors and less multiplicity of tumors in the colon, compared to control. Colon tumors of animals fed perillyl alcohol were found to exhibit increased apoptosis of cells compared to control (Reddy et al., 1997).

In tests for mutagenicity, both tea tree and lavender oils were found to not be mutagenic. Lavender oil was also found to have strong antimutagenic activity, reducing mutations of cells exposed to a known mutagen (Evandri et al., 2005).

Mice treated with perillyl alcohol (found in lavender and mint plants) had a 22% reduction in tumor incidence and a 58% reduction in tumor multiplicity during a mouse lung tumor bioassay (Lantry et al., 1997).

Rats with liver tumors that were treated with perillyl alcohol had smaller tumor sizes than did untreated rats, due to apoptosis of cancer cells in treated rats (Mills et al., 1995).

Perillyl alcohol (found in lavender and caraway) and was found to inhibit hyperproliferation of mammary epithelial cells prior to tumorigenisis. (Katdare et al., 1997).

126. Carnosic acid (derived from rosemary) was found to inhibit the proliferation of human leukemia cells in vitro (Steiner et al., 2001).

Rosemary extracts induced CYP (cytochrome P450) activity in liver cells, suggesting a possibility of increased ability to remove toxins (Debersac et al., 2001).

Rosemary extract injected in rats was found to decrease mammary adenocarcinomas in rats (Singletary et al., 1996).

An ethanol extract of rosemary was found to have an antiproliferative effect on human leukemia and breast carcinoma cells, as well as an antioxidant effect (Cheung et al., 2007).

127. Supplementation with caraway was found to inhibit development of aberrant crypt foci (precursors to polyps) in the colorectal area of rats induced to develop aberrant crypt foci (Deeptha et al., 2006).

Perillyl alcohol (found in caraway) was found to inhibit hyperproliferation of mammary epithelial cells prior to tumorigenisis (Katdare et al., 1997).

Rats with liver tumors that were treated with perillyl alcohol had smaller tumor sizes than did untreated rats, due to apoptosis of cancer cells in treated rats (Mills et al., 1995).

Carvone, found in dill and caraway oil, was found to induce the glutathione S-transferase enzyme (which helps to remove toxins from the body) in several target mouse tissues (Zheng et al., 1992).

128. Geraniol (found in lemongrass oil, among others) was found to inhibit colon cancer cell growth, while inhibiting DNA synthesis in these cells (Carnesecchi et al., 2001).

An extract from lemongrass was found to inhibit hepatocarcinogenesis (liver cancer genesis) in rats (Puatanachokchai et al., 2002).

Citral (found in lemongrass, melissa, and verbena oils) was found to induce apoptosis in several cancer cell lines (hematopoietic cells [stem cells that create blood cells]) (Dudai et al., 2005).

Lemongrass oil and its constituent, isointermedeol, were found to induce apoptosis in human leukemia cells (Kumar et al., 2008).

Lemongrass oil was found to inhibit multiple cancer cell lines, both in vitro and in vivo in mice (Sharma et al., 2009).

129. Beta-caryophyllene was found to increase the anticancer activities of paclitaxel (a chemotherapy drug derived from the yew tree) (Legault et al., 2007).

130. Basil and its component, linalool, were found to reduce spontaneous mutagenesis in bacteria cells (Berić et al., 2008).

131. Geraniol (found in geranium and lemongrass oil, among others) was found to inhibit colon cancer cell growth while inhibiting DNA synthesis in these cells (Carnesecchi et al., 2001).

132. Sclareol, from clary sage oil, was found to have a cytostatic effect on human leukemia cell lines (Dimas et al., 1999).

133. In a study of older individuals, it was found that there was a dose-dependent relationship between citrus peel consumption (citrus peels are high in d-limonene) and a lower degree of squamous cell carcinoma (SCC) of the skin (Hakim et al., 2000).

134. Treatment with elemene (found in myrrh oil) was found to increase survival time and to reduce tumor size in patients with malignant brain tumors, as compared with chemotherapy (Tan et al., 2000).

In both in vitro and in vivo studies, elemene (found in myrrh oil) was found to increase apoptosis in laryngeal cancer cells (Tao et al., 2006).

135. Ethanol extract of *Boswellia serrata* demonstrated antiproliferative effects on 5 leukemia and on 2 brain tumor cell lines. It was more potent than 1 type of boswellic acid (AKBA) on 3 leukemia cell lines (Hostanska et al., 2002).

136. Treatment with elemene (found in myrrh oil) was found to increase survival time and to reduce tumor size in patients with malignant brain tumors, as compared with chemotherapy (Tan et al., 2000).

137. Rosemary extract injected in rats was found to decrease mammary adenocarcinomas in rats (Singletary et al., 1996).

An ethanol extract of rosemary was found to have an antiproliferative and an antioxidant effect on human leukemia and breast carcinoma cells (Cheung et al., 2007).

138. Perillyl alcohol (found in lavender and caraway) was found to inhibit hyperproliferation of mammary epithelial cells prior to tumorigenisis. (Katdare et al., 1997).

139. Rats fed diets containing perillyl alcohol (derived from lavender plants) were found to have less incidence of colon tumors and less multiplicity of tumors in the colon, as compared to control. Colon tumors of animals fed perillyl alcohol were found to exhibit increased apoptosis of cells, compared to control (Reddy et al., 1997).

140. Geraniol (found in geranium and lemongrass oil, among others) was found to inhibit colon cancer cell growth, while inhibiting DNA synthesis in these cells (Carnesecchi et al., 2001).

141. Boswellic acids were found to have an antiproliferative and apoptotic effect on human colon cancer cells (Liu et al., 2002).

142. Boswellic acids demonstrated an antiproliferative and apoptotic effect on liver cancer cells (Liu et al., 2002).

143. An extract from lemongrass was found to inhibit hepatocarcinogenesis (liver cancer genesis) in rats (Puatanachokchai et al., 2002).

144. Rats with liver tumors that were treated with perillyl alcohol had smaller tumor sizes than untreated rats, due to apoptosis of cancer cells in treated rats (Mills et al., 1995).

145. Mice treated with perillyl alcohol (found in lavender and mint plants) had a 22% reduction in tumor incidence and a 58% reduction in tumor multiplicity during a mouse lung tumor bioassay (Lantry et al., 1997).

146. Alpha-santalol was found to induce apoptosis in human skin cancer cells (Kaur et al., 2005).

Various concentrations of alpha-santalol (from sandalwood) were tested against skin cancer in mice. All concentrations were found to inhibit skin cancer development (Dwivedi et al., 2005).

Alpha-santalol, derived from sandalwood EO, was found to delay and decrease the incidence and multiplicity of skin tumor (papilloma) development in mice (Dwivedi et al., 2003).

Pretreatment with alpha-santalol before UVB (ultraviolet B) radiation significantly reduced skin tumor development and multiplicity and induced proapoptotic and tumor-suppressing proteins (Arasada et al., 2008).

A solution of 5% alpha-santalol (from sandalwood) was found to prevent skin tumor formation caused by ultraviolet B (UVB) radiation in mice (Dwivedi et al., 2006).

Sandalwood oil was found to decrease skin papilloma (tumors) in mice (Dwivedi et al., 1997).

See pages 25-27 for more detailed application instructions.

147. Boswellic acid was found to prevent and inhibit invasion and metastasis of melanoma (skin pigment) and fibrosarcoma (connective tissue cancer) cells (Zhao et al. 2003).

148. In a human trial in China involving individuals suffering from angina pectoris (heart pain due to restricted blood flow), a preparation of volatile oil fractionated from valerian root was effective in remitting symptoms, decreasing attack frequency, shortening duration, and lowering plasma lipid levels.

149. Older rats whose diets were supplemented with thyme oil were found to have higher levels of the antioxidant enzymes superoxide dismutase and glutathione peroxidase in the heart, liver, and kidneys than did older rats without this supplementation (Youdim et al., 1999).

150. Imaging of the brain demonstrated that inhalation of 1,8-cineol (eucalyptol—a constituent of many essential oils, especially eucalyptus, rosemary, and marjoram) increased global cerebral blood flow after an inhalation time of 20 minutes (Nasel et al., 1994).

151. Colicky infants treated with a fennel oil emulsion were found to exhibit a cessation of colic more frequently than infants treated with the placebo, and the intensity of the colic was significantly lower in the fennel-treated group (Alexandrovich et al., 2003).

    Colicky infants treated with a blend extracted from melissa, German chamomile, and fennel were found to have less crying time than infants treated with a placebo (Savino et al., 2005).

152. Oral administration of German chamomile and melissa extracts was found to delay upper gastrointestinal transit in mice (Capasso et al., 2007).

    Colicky infants treated with a blend extracted from melissa, German chamomile, and fennel were found to have less crying time than infants treated with a placebo (Savino et al., 2005).

153. The use of rosemary, lemon, and peppermint oils in massage demonstrated an ability to reduce constipation and to increase bowel movements in elderly subjects, compared to massage without the oils (Kim et al., 2005).

154. Tea tree oil was found to inhibit 301 different types of yeasts isolated from the mouths of cancer patients suffering from advanced cancer, including 41 strains that are known to be resistant to antifungal drugs (Bagg et al., 2006).

155. Lavender oil demonstrated both fungistatic (stopped growth) and fungicidal (killed) activity against *Candida albicans* (D'Auria et al., 2005).

156. Thyme oil was found to inhibit *Candida* species by causing lesions in the cell membrane and was also found to inhibit germ tube (an outgrowth that develops when the fungi is preparing to replicate) formation (Pina-Vaz et al., 2004).

157. Internal lemongrass capsules were found to reduce cholesterol in some subjects (Elson et al., 1989).

158. Inhalation of lavender and monarda oils was found to reduce cholesterol content and atherosclerotic plaques in the aorta (Nikolaevskii et al., 1990).

159. Rats fed dill essential oil were found to have reduced levels of cholesterol, triglyceride, and low-density lipoprotein (LDL) and increased levels of high-density lipoprotein (HDL) (Hajhashemi et al., 2008).

160. Subjects exposed to 3 minutes of lavender aroma were more relaxed and were able to perform math computations faster and more accurately. (Diego et al., 1998).

    Subjects who smelled a cleansing gel with lavender aroma were more relaxed and were able to complete math computations faster (Field et al., 2005).

161. Incensole acetate, isolated from frankincense resin, was found to demonstrate an anti-inflammatory and neuro-protective effect in mice with closed head injuries (Moussaieff et al., 2008).

162. Eucalyptus oil was found to have an anti-inflammatory and mucin-inhibitory effect on rats with lipopolysaccharide-induced bronchitis (Lu et al., 2004).

163. Basil (*Ocimum gratissimum*) oil was found to facilitate the healing process of wounds in rabbits to a greater extent than did two antibacterial preparations, Cicatrin and Cetavlex (Orafidiya et al., 2003).

164. Lemon oil vapor was found to have a strong antistress and antidepressant effect on mice subjected to several common stress tests (Komiya et al., 2006).

    Lemon oil and its component, citral, were found to decrease depressed behavior in a similar manner to antidepressant drugs in rats involved in several stress tests (Komori et al., Dec. 1995).

    In 12 patients suffering from depression, it was found that inhaling citrus aromas reduced the needed doses of antidepressants, normalized neuroendocrine hormone levels, and normalized immune functioning (Komori et al., May 1995).

165. Incensole acetate (found in frankincense) was found to open TRPV receptors (a possible channel for emotional regulation) in mice brains (Moussaieff et al., 2008).

166. In patients suffering from arthritis, it was found that a blend of lavender, marjoram, eucalyptus, rosemary, peppermint, and carrier oils reduced perceived pain and depression, compared to control (Kim et al., 2005).

    Female students suffering from insomnia were found to sleep better and to have lower levels of depression during weeks they used a lavender fragrance, as compared to weeks they did not use a lavender fragrance (Lee et al., 2006).

167. In 12 patients suffering from depression, it was found that inhaling citrus aromas reduced the needed doses of antidepressants, normalized neuroendocrine hormone levels, and normalized immune functioning (Komori et al., May 1995).

168. Inhaling lavender oil was found to lower agitation in older adults suffering from dementia (Lin et al., 2007).

    Exposure to lavender oil, and to its constituents, linalool and linalyl acetate, was found to decrease normal movement in mice and to return mice to normal movement rates after caffeine-induced hyperactivity (Buchbauer et al., 1991).

    Swiss mice fed lavender oil diluted in olive oil were found to be more sedate in several common tests (Guillemain et al., 1989).

169. Subjects who had ylang ylang oil applied to their skin had decreased blood pressure, increased skin temperature, and reported feeling more calm and relaxed, compared to subjects in a control group (Hongratanaworakit et al., 2006).

170. Melissa (lemon balm) oil applied topically in a lotion was found to reduce agitation and to improve quality of life in patients suffering from severe dementia, compared to those receiving a placebo lotion (Ballard et al., 2002).
171. In animal testing, the essential oil of tarragon demonstrated anticonvulsant and sedative properties at low concentrations (Sayyah et al., 2004).
172. Rosemary extracts induced CYP (cytochrome P450) activity in liver cells, suggesting a possibility of increased ability to remove toxins (Debersac et al., 2001).
173. Three compounds derived from dill and caraway oil (anethofuran, carvone, and limonene) were found to induce the enzyme glutathione S-transferase (involved in transforming or binding to toxins in tissues) in several mice tissues.
174. Oral rosemary extract was found to decrease blood glucose levels, while increasing insulin levels in alloxan-diabetic rabbits (Bakirel et al., 2008).
175. Sage essential oil was found to increase hepatocyte (liver cell) sensitivity to insulin and to inhibit gluconeogenesis (the creation of glucose) in a manner similar to the type 2 diabetes prevention drug, metformin, in mice (Lima et al., 2006).
176. Cuminaldehyde, a component of cumin seed oil, was found to inhibit the activity of aldose reductase (an enzyme that converts glucose into other sugars) and alpha-glucosidase (an enzyme that helps in the digestion of carbohydrates into simple sugars). Inhibiting both of these enzymes has been theorized to aid in controlling diabetes (Lee, 2005).
177. Peppermint oil was found to be as effective as Buscopan (an antispasmodic drug) at preventing spasms during a barium enema (a type of enema used to place barium in the colon for X-ray imaging purposes) (Asao et al., 2003).

     Peppermint oil in enteric-coated capsules was found to relieve symptoms of irritable bowel syndrome better than a placebo (Rees et al., 1979).

     Patients with IBS symptoms who took a peppermint oil formulation in an enteric-coated capsule were found to have a significantly higher reduction of symptoms when compared with IBS patients who took a placebo (Liu et al., 1997).

     When taken internally, an enteric-coated capsule with peppermint and caraway oil was found to reduce pain and symptoms of patients with non-ulcer dyspepsia (indigestion), compared to a control (May et al., 1996).

     A combination of peppermint and caraway oil was found to reduce visceral hyperalgesia (pain hypersensitivity in the gastrointestinal tract) after induced inflammation in rats (Kim et al., 2005).

     The use of rosemary, lemon, and peppermint oils in massage demonstrated an ability to reduce constipation and to increase bowel movements in elderly subjects, compared to massage without the oils (Kim et al., 2005).
178. When taken internally, an enteric-coated capsule with peppermint and caraway oil was found to reduce pain and symptoms in patients with non-ulcer dyspepsia (indigestion), compared to a control (May et al., 1996).

     A combination of peppermint and caraway oil was found to reduce visceral hyperalgesia (pain hypersensitivity in the gastrointestinal tract) after induced inflammation in rats (Kim et al., 2005).
179. Colicky infants treated with a fennel oil emulsion were found to exhibit a cessation of colic more frequently than did infants treated with a placebo, and the intensity of the colic was significantly lower in the fennel-treated group (Alexandrovich et al., 2003).

     Colicky infants treated with a blend extracted from melissa, German chamomile, and fennel were found to have less crying time than infants treated with a placebo (Savino et al., 2005).
180. Lemongrass demonstrated ability to inhibit *Helicobacter pylori*, a pathogen responsible for gastroduodenal disease. This pathogen did not develop resistance to lemongrass after 10 passes (it developed resistance to clarithromycin) (Ohno et al., 2003).
181. Ginger root given one hour before major gynecological surgery resulted in less nausea and fewer incidences of vomiting, compared to control (Nanthakomon et al., 2006).
182. Oregano oil administered orally was found to improve gastrointestinal symptoms in 7 of 11 patients who had tested positive for the parasite *Blastocystis hominis*, and it was found to cause disappearance of this parasite in 8 cases (Force et al., 2000).
183. The use of rosemary, lemon, and peppermint oils in massage demonstrated an ability to reduce constipation and to increase bowel movements in elderly subjects, compared to massage without the oils (Kim et al., 2005).
184. In irritable bowel syndrome patients (IBS) without bacterial overgrowth, lactose intolerance, or celiac disease, peppermint oil was found over a period of 8 weeks to reduce IBS symptoms significantly more than a placebo (Cappello et al., 2007).
185. Peppermint oil was found to be as effective as Buscopan (an antispasmodic drug) at preventing spasms during a barium enema (a type of enema used to place barium in the colon for X-ray imaging purposes) (Asao et al., 2003).
186. In isolated rat ileum tissue, galbanum oil demonstrated an antispasmodic effect against contractions induced by KCl (potassium chloride) (Sadraei et al., 2001).
187. Lavender was found to have a relaxant effect on smooth muscle from guinea pig ileum (small intestine) (Lis-Balchin et al., 1999).
188. Oregano oil administered orally was found to improve gastrointestinal symptoms in 7 of 11 patients who had tested positive for the parasite *Blastocystis hominis*, and it was found to cause disappearance of this parasite in 8 cases (Force et al., 2000).
189. Palmarosa oil and its constituent, geraniol, demonstrated antiparasitic activity against the parasitic roundworm, *Caenorhabditis elegans*, in vitro (Kumaran et al., 2003).
190. Essential oil from *Lavandula angustifolia* demonstrated ability to eliminate protozoal pathogens *Giardia duodenalis*, *Trichomonas vaginalis*, and *Hexamita inflata* at concentrations of 1% or less (Moon et al., 2006).

191. In patients with dyspepsia (indigestion), treatments with capsules containing peppermint and caraway oil were found to decrease pain and pain frequency (Freise et al., 1999).

Children suffering from irritable bowel syndrome (IBS) who received peppermint oil in enteric-coated capsules (encapsulated so the capsules wouldn't open until they reached the intestines) reported a reduced severity of pain associated with IBS (Kline et al., 2001).

Patients with IBS symptoms who took a peppermint oil formulation in an enteric-coated capsule were found to have a significantly higher reduction of symptoms when compared to IBS patients taking a placebo (Liu et al., 1997).

In irritable bowel syndrome (IBS) patients without bacterial overgrowth, lactose intolerance, or celiac disease, peppermint oil was found over a period of 8 weeks to reduce IBS symptoms significantly more than a placebo (Cappello et al., 2007).

192. In patients with dyspepsia (indigestion), treatments with capsules containing peppermint and caraway oil were found to decrease pain and pain frequency (Freise et al., 1999).

193. The scent of grapefruit oil and its component, limonene, was found to affect the autonomic nerves and to reduce appetite and body weight in rats exposed to the oil for 15 minutes 3 times per week (Shen et al., 2005).

194. Inhalation of black pepper oil was found to increase cerebral blood flow and to improve the swallowing reflex in elderly patients who had suffered a stroke (Nasel et al., 1994).

195. Fennel oil was found to reduce contraction frequency and intensity in rat uterus induced to contract (Ostad et al., 2001).

196. Subjects exposed to 3 minutes of lavender aroma were more relaxed and were able to perform math computations faster and more accurately (Diego et al., 1998).

Subjects who smelled a cleansing gel with lavender aroma were more relaxed and were able to complete math computations faster (Field et al., 1995).

197. Patients with alopecia areata (hair loss) that massaged carrier oils containing a blend of thyme, rosemary, lavender, and cedarwood oils into their scalps were more likely to show improvement when compared to a control group that massaged carrier oils alone into their scalps (Hay et al., 1998).

198. A combination of peppermint oil and ethanol was found to have a significant analgesic effect, reducing sensitivity to headache; while a combination of peppermint, eucalyptus, and ethanol was found to relax muscles and to increase cognitive performance in humans (Göbel et al., 1994).

199. Peppermint oil demonstrated a direct virucidal activity against herpes type 1 and type 2 viruses (Schuhmacher et al., 2003).

200. Tea tree and eucalyptus oil demonstrated an ability to inhibit the herpes simplex virus (Schnitzler et al., 2001).

201. Helichrysum was found to have significant antiviral activity against the herpes virus at non-cytotoxic concentrations (Nostro et al., 2003).

202. Eugenol was found to be virucidal to herpes simplex and was found to delay the development of herpes-induced keratitis (inflammation of the cornea) in mice (Benencia et al., 2000).

203. Melissa oil demonstrated inhibition of herpes simplex type 1 and type 2 viruses (Schnitzler et al., 2008).

204. Herpes simplex viruses pretreated with manuka oil before cell infection were significantly inhibited and had plaque formation reduced by over 98% in cultured monkey kidney cells (Reichling et al., 2005).

205. Tea tree oil applied to histamine-induced weal and flare in human volunteers was found to decrease the mean weal volume when compared to a control (Koh et al., 2002).

Tea tree oil applied to histamine-induced edema (swelling) in mice ears was found to significantly reduce swelling (Brand et al., 2002).

Tea tree oil was found to reduce inflammation in the skin of nickel-sensitive human skin exposed to nickel (Pearce et al., 2005).

206. L-menthol was found to inhibit production of inflammation mediators in human monocytes (a type of white blood cell involved in the immune response) (Juergens et al., 1998).

207. Lavender oil was found to inhibit immediate-type allergic reactions in mice and rats by inhibiting mast cell degranulation (Kim et al., 1999).

208. Inhaling lavender oil was found to lower agitation in older adults suffering from dementia (Lin et al., 2007).

209. Growth-retarded pigs receiving a supplementation of oregano leaves and flowers enriched with cold-pressed oregano oil were found to have increased growth, decreased mortality, and higher numbers of immune-system cells and compounds when compared to control pigs who did not receive supplementation (Walter et al., 2004).

210. Boswellic acids from frankincense (delivered with sesame seed oil) were found to inhibit TH1 cytokines while potentiating TH2 cytokines, demonstrating their ability to modulate the immune response (Chevrier et al., 2005).

211. In 12 patients suffering from depression, it was found that inhaling citrus aromas reduced the needed doses of antidepressants, normalized neuroendocrine hormone levels, and normalized immune function (Komori et al, 1995).

213. Basil (*Ocimum gratissimum*) oil was found to facilitate the healing process of wounds in rabbits to a greater extent than did two antibacterial preparations, Cicatrin and Cetavlex (Orafidiya et al., 2003).

214. In a test of 34 different essential oils, patchouli (*Pogostemon cablin*) oil proved to be the insecticide that was most effective against the common house fly (Pavela, 2008).

Both patchouli oil and its constituent, patchouli alcohol (patchoulol), were found to be repellent and insecticidal when applied topically to Formosan termites (Zhu et al., 2003).

215. Clove oil was found to be highly termiticidal (Zhu et al., 2001).

A blend of eugenol, alpha-terpineol, and cinnamic alcohol was found to be insecticidal against American cockroaches, carpenter ants, and German cockroaches (Enan et al., 2001).

216. *Lavandula angustifolia* oil was found to be a potent topical insecticide for the African cotton leafworm larvae (Pavela, 2005).

217. Two basil oils (*Ocimum basilicum* and *O. gratissimum*) were found to be insecticidal against the cowpea weevil (an agricultural pest) beetle and eggs in both a diffused and aromatized powder form (Kéita et al., 2001).
218. Essential oil of *Melaleuca alternifolia* was found to be lethal to more than 80% of *Ixodes ricinus* tick nymphs (carriers or Lyme disease) when they inhaled a 10 microl dose of the oil for 90 minutes or more (Iori et al., 2005).
219. The leaf and fruit oils of *Schinus molle* (pink pepper) demonstrated a repellent and insecticidal activity against two beetles that commonly damage and consume stored grains (Abdel-Sattar et al., 2009).
220. Prepared microcapsules containing rosemary oil were found to be toxic to the larvae of gypsy moths, pests that causes massive defoliation of forests (Moretti et al., 2002).
221. A slow-release citronella formula was found to significantly reduce infection with head lice in elementary school children, compared to a control (Mumcuoglu et al., 2004).

    Citronella oil applied in high concentration was found to effectively repel nymphs of *Amblyomma cajennense* (a type of tick known to carry Rocky Mountain spotted fever) for up to 35 hours (Soares et al., 2009).

    Clove, citronella, and patchouli oils were found to effectively repel 3 species of mosquitoes (with clove being the most effective—demonstrating 100% repellency for 2–4 hours) (Trongtokit et al., 2005).
222. Clove, citronella, and patchouli oils were found to effectively repel 3 species of mosquitoes (with clove being the most effective—demonstrating 100% repellency for 2–4 hours) (Trongtokit et al., 2005).
223. Both patchouli oil and its constituent, patchouli alcohol (patchoulol), were found to be repellent and insecticidal when applied topically to Formosan termites (Zhu et al., 2003).

    Clove, citronella, and patchouli oils were found to effectively repel 3 species of mosquitoes (with clove being the most effective—demonstrating 100% repellency for 2–4 hours) (Trongtokit et al., 2005).
224. Lavender oil was found to be comparable to DEET in its ability to repel ticks (*Hyalomma marginatum*) (Mkolo et al., 2007).

    The infestation of the red bud borer pest was reduced by more than 95% in the grafted buds of apple trees by application of the essential oil of *Lavandula angustifolia* (van Tol et al., 2007).
225. *Citrus hystrix* essential oil was found to be an effective repellent against three types of cockroaches—exhibiting 100% repellency against two types and 87% repellency against the third (Thavara et al., 2007).
226. The leaf and fruit oils of *Schinus molle* (pink pepper) demonstrated repellent and insecticidal activity against two beetles that commonly damage and consume stored grains (Abdel-Sattar et al., 2009).
227. In a small clinical trial, diffusion of lavender oil was found to improve sleep in patients with insomnia more than diffusion of sweet almond oil, which was used as a control (Lewith et al., 2005).

    Female students suffering from insomnia were found to sleep better and to have lower levels of depression during weeks they used a lavender fragrance, compared to weeks they did not use a lavender fragrance (Lee et al., 2006).
228. Subjects suffering from insomnia who took an extract from valerian demonstrated results similar to those of subjects who took oxazepam (an anti-anxiety and anti-insomnia drug) (Ziegler et al., 2002).
229. Older rats whose diets were supplemented with thyme oil were found to have higher levels of the antioxidant enzymes superoxide dismutase and glutathione peroxidase in the heart, liver, and kidneys than did older rats without this supplementation (Youdim et al., 1999).
230. The use of rosemary, lemon, and peppermint oils in massage demonstrated an ability to reduce constipation and to increase bowel movements in elderly subjects, compared to massage without the oils (Kim et al., 2005).
231. Tea tree oil was found to be effective against both lice and dust mites in a mite chamber assay (Williamson et al., 2007).

    Tea tree oil was found to prevent some blood feeding by lice on treated skin; and while not highly effective at the studied dosages, tea tree oil was found to be more effective than DEET at repelling head lice (Canyon et al., 2007).
232. A slow-release citronella formula was found to significantly reduce infection with head lice in elementary school children, compared to a control (Mumcuoglu et al., 2004).
233. Three compounds derived from dill and caraway oil—anethofuran, carvone, and limonene—were found to induce the enzyme glutathione S-transferase (involved in transforming or binding to toxins in tissues) in several mice tissues (Zheng et al., 1992).
234. Rosemary extracts induced CYP (cytochrome P450) activity in liver cells, suggesting a possible increased ability to remove toxins (Debersac et al., 2001).
235. Older rats whose diets were supplemented with thyme oil were found to have higher levels of the antioxidant enzymes superoxide dismutase and glutathione peroxidase in the heart, liver, and kidneys than did older rats without this supplementation (Youdim et al., 1999).
236. A methanol extract of *Boswellia carterii* was found to have a high inhibition rate of hepatitis C virus protease (Hussein et al., 2000).
237. Volunteers completing a battery of tests were found to be more content when exposed to lavender and rosemary aromas. Rosemary aroma also was found to enhance quality of memory, compared to control (Moss et al., 2003).
238. In a small human trial, oral administration of sage lavender oil was found to improve speed of memory as well as alertness and calmness in healthy volunteers, compared to a placebo (Tildesley et al., 2005).
239. In human trials, the aroma of peppermint was found to enhance memory and to increase alertness, while ylang ylang aroma was found to increase calmness (Moss et al., 2008).
240. Subjects who had learned a list of 24 words while exposed to an odor had an easier time relearning the list when exposed to the same odor, compared to those who were exposed to an alternate odor (Smith et al., 1992).

241. A combination of peppermint oil and ethanol was found to have a significant analgesic effect, reducing sensitivity to headache; while a combination of peppermint, eucalyptus, and ethanol was found to relax muscles and to increase cognitive performance in humans (Göbel et al., 1994).

242. Rosemary oil demonstrated a relaxant effect on smooth muscle from the trachea of rabbit and guinea pig (Aqel, 1991).

243. Topical application of 100% tea tree oil was found to produce results similar to topical application of 1% clotrimazole (an antifungal drug) solution on onychomycosis (also known as tinea or fungal nail infection) (Buck et al., 1994).

244. Ginger root given orally to pregnant women was found to decrease the severity of nausea and the frequency of vomiting, compared to control (Vutyavanich et al., 2001).

In a trial of women receiving gynaecological surgery, women receiving ginger root had less incidences of nausea than those who received a placebo. Ginger root has similar results to the antiemetic drug (a drug effective against vomiting and nausea) metoclopramide (Bone et al., 1990).

Ginger root given one hour before major gynecological surgery resulted in lower nausea and fewer incidences of vomiting as compared to the control (Nanthakomon et al., 2006).

245. Pretreatment of human and rat astrocyte cells (cells found in the nerve and brain that support the blood-brain barrier and that help repair the brain and spinal cord following injuries) with peppermint oil was found to inhibit heat-shock induced apoptosis of these cells (Koo et al., 2001).

246. Lavender oil was found to inhibit sympathetic nerve activity, while exciting parasympathetic nerve activity in rats. Linalool, a component of lavender, was shown to have similar effects (Shen et al., 2005).

Lavender oil scent was found to lower sympathetic nerve activity and blood pressure in rats, while elevating parasympathetic nerve activity. It was further found that applying an anosmia-inducing agent (something that causes a loss of smell) eliminated the effects of the lavender oil scent (Tanida et al., 2006).

247. Inhalation of the aroma of lemon essential oil was found to decrease pain response in rats and was also found to modulate the neuronal response to formalin-induced pain (Aloisi et al., 2002).

Several constituents of lemon oil and their metabolites (chemicals made by these chemicals in the body) were found to increase the release of monoamines (various chemicals responsible for neurotransmission and neuromodulation) in rat brain tissue, indicating a possible effect on brain nerve cell behavior (Fukumoto et al., 2006).

Pretreatment of human and rat astrocyte cells (cells found in the nerves and brain that support the blood-brain barrier and help repair the brain and spinal cord following injuries) with lemon oil was found to inhibit heat-shock induced apoptosis of these cells (Koo et al., 2002).

248. In healthy adults, inhalation of essential oils such as pepper, estragon, fennel, and grapefruit had a stimulating effect on sympathetic activity; while inhalation of essential oils of rose or patchouli caused a decrease in sympathetic activity (Haze et al., 2002).

The scent of grapefruit oil and its component, limonene, was found to affect the autonomic nerves, exciting the sympathetic nervous system, and to reduce appetite and body weight of rats exposed to the oil for 15 minutes 3 times per week (Shen et al., 2005).

249. Incensole acetate, isolated from frankincense resin, demonstrated an anti-inflammatory and neuro-protective effect on mice with closed head injuries (Moussaieff et al., 2008).

250. Oral administration of copaiba oil demonstrated antinociceptive (blocks transmission of pain-causing stimuli) activity in rodents (Gomes et al., 2007).

251. Pretreatment of human and rat astrocyte cells (cells found in the nerves and the brain that support the blood-brain barrier and help repair the brain and spinal cord following injuries) with juniper oil was found to inhibit heat-shock induced apoptosis of these cells (Na et al., 2001).

252. 1,8 cineole (eucalyptol) displayed an anti-inflammatory effect on rats in several tests and exhibited antinociceptive (pain-reducing) effects in mice, possibly by depressing the central nervous system (Santos et al., 2000).

253. Female patients waiting for dental treatment were found to be less anxious, more positive, and more calm when exposed to orange oil odor than were patients who were not exposed to the orange oil odor (Lehrner et al., 2000).

254. The scent of grapefruit oil and its component, limonene, was found to affect the autonomic nerves, exciting the sympathetic nervous system, and to reduce appetite and body weight of rats exposed to the oil for 15 minutes 3 times per week (Shen et al., 2005).

255. Tea tree, peppermint, and sage oils were found to inhibit oral bacteria—with thymol and eugenol being the most active components of these oils (Shapiro et al., 1994).

256. Among several oils tested, tea tree (melaleuca), manuka, and eucalyptus demonstrated strong antibacterial activity against detrimental oral bacteria (Takarada et al., 2004).

Tea tree, peppermint, and sage oils were found to inhibit oral bacteria—with thymol and eugenol being the most active components of these oils (Shapiro et al., 1994).

Cinnamon oil exhibited strong antimicrobial activity against two detrimental oral bacteria. Manuka, tea tree, and the component thymol also exhibited antimicrobial potency (Filoche et al., 2005).

257. Peppermint oil blended with toothpaste was more effective at lower concentrations in inhibiting the formation of dental plaque than was chlorhexidine (an antiseptic) in human volunteers (Shayegh et al., 2008).

Subjects using a mouthwash containing thymol, menthol, methyl salicylate, and eucalyptol for 6 months were found to not have developed oral bacteria that were resistant to the oils (Charles et al., 2000).

258. Lavender oil was found to work as an anaesthetic (reducing pain) in rabbit reflex tests (Ghelardini et al., 1999).

    Oil from *Lavandula angustifolia* was found to reduce writhing in induced writhing in rats and to reduce edema (swelling) in carrageenan-induced paw edema, indicating an anti-inflammatory effect (Hajhashemi et al., 2003).

    In patients suffering from arthritis, it was found that a blend of lavender, marjoram, eucalyptus, rosemary, peppermint, and carrier oils reduced perceived pain and depression, compared to control (Kim et al., 2005).

    The odor of lavender combined with relaxing music was found to lessen the intensity of pain following a vascular wound dressing change (Kane et al., 2004).

259. Oils of three eucalyptus species (citriodora, tereticornis, and globulus) were found to have analgesic (pain-relieving) and anti-inflammatory properties in rats (Silva et al., 2003).

    1,8 cineole (eucalyptol) was found to have antinociceptive (pain-reducing) properties similar to morphine. Beta-pinene was found to reverse the effects of morphine in a degree similar to naloxone (a drug used to counter the effects of morphine overdose) (Liape et al., 2007).

    1,8 cineole (eucalyptol) was found to display an anti-inflammatory effect on rats in several tests and was found to exhibit antinociceptive (pain-reducing) effects in mice, possibly by depressing the central nervous system (Santos et al., 2000).

260. Inhalation of the aroma of lemon essential oil was found to decrease pain response in rats and was also found to modulate the neuronal response to formalin-induced pain (Aloisi et al., 2002).

    Rats exposed long-term to lemon essential oil were found to demonstrate different anxiety and pain threshold levels than did untreated rats. It was also found that exposure to lemon oil induced chemical changes in the neuronal circuits involved in anxiety and pain (Ceccarelli et al., 2004).

261. An ethanol extract of rosemary was found to demonstrate antinociceptive (pain-blocking) and anti-inflammatory activity in mice and rats (González-Trujano et al., 2007).

    Rosemary oil was found to have anti-inflammatory and peripheral antinociceptive (pain sensitivity–blocking) properties in mice (Takaki et al., 2008).

    1,8 cineole (eucalyptol) displayed an anti-inflammatory effect on rats in several tests, and exhibited antinociceptive (pain-reducing) effects on mice, possibly by depressing the central nervous system (Santos et al., 2000).

    In patients suffering from arthritis, it was found that a blend of lavender, marjoram, eucalyptus, rosemary, peppermint, and carrier oils reduced perceived pain and depression compared to control (Kim et al., 2005).

262. Beta-caryophyllene (found in clove and copaiba oils) demonstrated anaesthetic (pain-reducing) activity in rats and rabbits (Ghelardini et al., 2001).

263. Oral administration of copaiba oil demonstrated antinociceptive (blocks transmission of pain-causing stimuli) activity in rodents (Gomes et al., 2007).

    Beta-caryophyllene (found in clove and copaiba oils) demonstrated anaesthetic (pain-reducing) activity in rats and rabbits (Ghelardini et al., 2001).

264. The essential oil of laurel (*Laurus nobilis*) reduced pain and inflammation in rats in a manner similar to morphine and piroxicam (an anti-inflammatory drug) in mice and rats (Sayyah et al., 2003).

265. Oregano oil administered orally improved gastrointestinal symptoms in 7 of 11 patients who had tested positive for the parasite *Blastocystis hominis* and caused the disappearance of this parasite in 8 of the patients (Force et al., 2000).

266. Essential oil from *Lavandula angustifolia* demonstrated ability to eliminate protozoal pathogens *Giardia duodenalis*, *Trichomonas vaginalis*, and *Hexamita inflata* at concentrations of 1% or less (Moon et al., 2006).

267. Copaiba oil was found to inhibit the parasite *Leishmania amazonensis* (a protozoa that causes skin lesions) (Santos et al., 2008).

268. Cinnamon, thyme, and clove essential oils demonstrated an antibacterial effect on several respiratory tract pathogens (Fabio et al., 2007).

    Oils with aldehyde or phenol as a major component demonstrated a high level of antibacterial activity (Inouye et al., 2001).

269. Oregano oil was found to kill antibiotic resistant strains of Staph, *E. coli*, *Klebsiella pneumoniae*, *Helicobacter pylori*, and *Mycobacterium terrae* (Preuss et al., 2005).

270. Inhaled ylang ylang oil was found to decrease blood pressure and pulse rate and to enhance attentiveness and alertness in volunteers, compared to an odorless control (Hongratanaworakit et al., 2004).

    Subjects who had ylang ylang oil applied to their skin had decreased blood pressure, increased skin temperature, and reported feeling more calm and relaxed, compared to subjects in a control group (Hongratanaworakit et al., 2006).

271. Ginger root given orally to pregnant women was found to decrease the severity of nausea and frequency of vomiting, compared to control (Vutyavanich et al., 2001).

    Ginger root given one hour before major gynecological surgery resulted in lower nausea and fewer incidences of vomiting, compared to control (Nanthakomon et al., 2006).

    In a trial of women receiving gynaecological surgery, women receiving ginger root had fewer incidences of nausea than did those who received a placebo. Ginger root showed results similar to those of the antiemetic drug (a drug effective against vomiting and nausea) metoclopramide (Bone et al., 1990).

 See pages 25-27 for more detailed application instructions.

272. Jasmine flowers applied to the breast were found to be as effective as the antilactation drug bromocriptine in reducing breast engorgement, milk production, and analgesic (pain relieving drug) intake in women after giving birth (Shrivastave et al., 1988).

273. Female students suffering from insomnia were found to sleep better and to have lower levels of depression during weeks they used a lavender fragrance, compared to weeks they did not use a lavender fragrance (Lee et al., 2006).

In patients suffering from arthritis, a blend of lavender, marjoram, eucalyptus, rosemary, peppermint, and carrier oils was found to reduce perceived pain and depression, compared to control (Kim et al., 2005).

274. In 12 patients suffering from depression, it was found that inhaling citrus aromas reduced the needed doses of antidepressants, normalized neuroendocrine hormone levels, and normalized immune functioning (Komori et al., May 1995).

Lemon oil and its component, citral, were found to decrease depressed behavior in rats involved in several stress tests in a manner similar to antidepressant drugs (Komori et al., Dec. 1995).

Lemon oil vapor was found to have strong antistress and antidepressant effects on mice subjected to several common stress tests (Komiya et al., 2006).

275. Peppermint extract fed orally to mice demonstrated an ability to protect the testis from gamma radiation damage (Samarth et al., 2009).

In mice exposed to whole-body gamma irradiation, only 17% of mice who had been fed peppermint oil died, while 100% of mice who did not receive peppermint oil died. It was also found that mice pre-fed peppermint oil were able to return blood cell levels to normal after 30 days, while control mice were not able to (and consequently died), suggesting a protective or stimulating effect of the oil on blood stem cells (Samarth et al., 2004).

Mice treated with an oral administration of peppermint extract demonstrated a higher ability to tolerate gamma radiation than did untreated mice (Samarth et al., 2003).

276. Pretreatment with alpha-santalol before UVB (ultraviolet-B) radiation significantly reduced skin tumor development and multiplicity and induced proapoptotic and tumor-suppressing protein (Arasada et al., 2008).

A solution of 5% alpha-santalol (from sandalwood) was found to prevent skin-tumor formation caused by ultraviolet-B (UVB) radiation in mice (Dwivedi et al., 2006).

277. *Calophyllum inophyllum* (tamanu) oil was found to demonstrate UV filtering properties in the SPF 18-22 range at low concentrations and was also found to not be cytotoxic to human eye cells at concentrations up to 1% (Said et al., 2007).

278. Subjects who smelled a cleansing gel with lavender aroma were more relaxed and were able to complete math computations faster (Field et al., 2005).

Nurses working in an ICU setting demonstrated decreased perception of stress when receiving a topical application of *Lavandula angustifolia* and *Salvia sclarea* essential oils (Pemberton et al., 2008).

Subjects exposed to 3 minutes of lavender aroma were more relaxed and able to perform math computations faster and more accurately (Diego et al., 1998).

279. Subjects who had ylang ylang oil applied to their skin had decreased blood pressure, increased skin temperature, and reported feeling more calm and relaxed, compared to subjects in a control group (Hongratanaworakit et al., 2006).

280. Lemon oil was found to have an antistress effect on mice involved in several behavioral tasks (Komiya et al., 2006).

281. In human volunteers wearing breathing masks to prevent aroma inhalation, rose oil applied to the skin was found to significantly decrease breathing rate, blood oxygen saturation, and systolic blood pressure, compared to a placebo. And volunteers receiving rose oil rated themselves as more calm and relaxed than did subjects receiving the placebo (Hongratanaworakit et al., 2009).

282. Extracts from eucalyptus and thyme were found to have high nitrous oxide (NO) scavenging abilities and to inhibit NO production in macrophage cells. This could possibly explain their role in aiding respiratory inflammatory diseases (Vigo et al., 2004).

Eucalyptus oil was found to have an anti-inflammatory and mucin-inhibitory effect on rats with lipopolysaccharide-induced bronchitis (Lu et al., 2004).

283. L-menthol was found to inhibit production of inflammation mediators in human monocytes (a type of white blood cell involved in the immune response) (Juergens et al., 1998).

284. Vapor of cinnamon bark oil and cinnamic aldehyde was found to be effective against fungi involved in respiratory tract mycoses (fungal infections) (Singh et al., 1995).

Cinnamon bark, lemongrass, and thyme oils were found to have the highest level of activity against common respiratory pathogens among 14 essential oils tested (Inouye et al., 2001).

285. Linalool, found in several essential oils, was found to inhibit induced convulsions in rats by directly interacting with the NMDA receptor complex (Brum et al., 2001).

286. In a small clinical trial, diffusion of lavender oil was found to improve sleep in patients with insomnia than diffusion of sweet almond oil as a control (Lewith et al., 2005).

Female students suffering from insomnia were found to sleep better and have a lower level of depression during weeks they used a lavender fragrance when compared to weeks they did not use a lavender fragrance (Lee et al., 2006).

287. Two chemical components found in valerian were found to have sedative, sleep-enhancing, and anxiolytic (anxiety lowering) properties (Marder et al., 2003).

288. The scent of grapefruit oil and its component, limonene, was found to affect the autonomic nerves, exciting the sympathetic nervous system, and to reduce appetite and body weight of rats exposed to the oil for 15 minutes three times per week (Shen et al., 2005).

289. Carnosic acid, a diterpene extracted from sage, taken orally was found to significantly inhibit lipid absorption, reduce triglyceride elevation, and reduced the gain of body weight in mice fed a high-fat (olive oil) diet. (Ninomiya et al., 2004).

290. Inhaled vapor of black pepper oil was found to reduce craving for cigarettes and symptoms of anxiety in smokers deprived from smoking compared to a control (Rose et al., 1994).

291. Basil (Ocimum gratissimum) oil was found to facilitate the healing process of wounds in rabbits to a greater extent than two antibacterial preparations, Cicatrin and Cetavlex (Kane et al., 2004).

292. Imaging of the brain demonstrated that inhalation of 1,8-cineol (eucalyptol, a constituent of many essential oils, especially eucalyptus, rosemary, and marjoram) increased global cerebral blood flow after an inhalation-time of 20 minutes (Nasel et al., 1994).

293. In a trial of women receiving gynaecological surgery, women receiving ginger root had less incidences of nausea compared to a placebo. Ginger root has similar results to the antiemetic drug (a drug effective against vomiting and nausea), metoclopramide (Bone et al., 1990).

Ginger root given one hour before major gynecological surgery resulted in lower nausea and fewer incidences of vomiting compared to control (Nanthakomon et al., 2006).

294. Lavender odor was found to reduce mental stress while increasing arousal (Motomura et al., 2001).

Nurses working in an ICU setting demonstrated decreased perception of stress when receiving a topical application of Lavandula angustifolia and Salvia sclaria essential oils (Pemberton et al, 2008).

An office environment featuring a soothing DVD video presentation and diffused lavender oil was found to reduce anxiety in patients awaiting a gastroscopy procedure compared to a regular office environment (Hoya et al., 2008).

295. Subjects who had ylang ylang oil applied to their skin had decreased blood pressure, increased skin temperature, and reported feeling more calm and relaxed compared to subjects in a control group (Hongratanaworakit et al., 2006).

296. Lemon oil vapor was found to have a strong anti-stress and antidepressant effects on mice subjected to several common stress tests (Komiya et al., 2006).

297. Both fennel oil, and its constituent, anethole, were found to significantly reduce thrombosis (blood clots) in mice. They were also found to be free from the prohemorrhagic (increased bleeding) side effect that aspirin (acetylsalicylic acid) has (Tognolini et al., 2007).

298. Inhalation of black pepper oil was found to increase cerebral blood flow and improve the swallowing reflex in elderly patients who had suffered a stroke (Ebihara et al., 2006).

299. Calophyllum inophyllum (tamanu) oil was found to demonstrate UV filtering properties in the SPF 18-22 range at low concentrations, and was also found to not be cytotoxic to human eye cells at concentrations up to 1% (Said et al., 2007).

300. A formulation of lemongrass and geranium oil was found to reduce airborne bacteria by 89% in an office environment after diffusion for 15 hours (Doran et al., 2009).

301. Lemon odor was found to enhance the positive mood of volunteers exposed to a stressor (Kiecolt-Glaser et al., 2008).

302. Ginger root given orally to pregnant women was found to decrease the severity of nausea and frequency of vomiting compared to control (Vutyavanich et al., 2001).

Ginger root given one hour before major gynecological surgery resulted in lower nausea and fewer incidences of vomiting compared to control (Nanthakomon et al., 2006).

303. The scent of grapefruit oil and its component, limonene, was found to affect the autonomic nerves, exciting the sympathetic nervous system, and to reduce appetite and body weight of rats exposed to the oil for 15 minutes three times per week (Shen et al., 2005).

304. Basil (Ocimum gratissimum) oil was found to facilitate the healing process of wounds in rabbits to a greater extent than two antibacterial preparations, Cicatrin and Cetavlex (Orafindiya et al., 2003).

Peace & Calming Saves the Day

My husband works at an elementary school as a LAN technician. Last spring the secretaries union went on strike for 2 weeks. All the other unions in the school district, in a show of support for the secretaries, forbade any of their members to help out with the secretarial duties. That left 3 people in my husband's school (my husband included) who were not union and able to attempt to keep the school running normally. After his first day of secretarial duties, he took in a travel diffuser soaked in Peace & Calming to help calm the kids who were sent to the office because they were troublemakers in their classes as well as to keep himself calm. He still is not sure who the Peace & Calming helped more (him or the kids), but the rest of the 2 weeks were less stressful thanks to the Peace & Calming.

-Submitted by A. Cornn
Machesney Park, Illinois (July 2004)

Appendix

Body Systems Chart

The following chart lists all of the products discussed within this book and indicates which body systems they primarily affect. While this chart does not include every system that could possibly be affected by each product, it attempts to list the primary systems that are most often affected. It is provided to give the beginning aromatherapy student a starting point for personal use and analysis.

Essential Oil/ Blend/Product	Cardiovascular System	Digestive System	Emotional Balance	Hormonal System	Immune System	Muscles and Bones	Nervous System	Respiratory System	Skin and Hair
3 Wise Men			X						
Abundance			X		X			X	
Acceptance			X				X		
AlkaLime	X	X				X			
Allerzyme		X						X	
Angelica			X				X		
Animal Scents Products									X
Anise	X	X		X				X	
Aroma Life	X								
Aroma Siez						X		X	
AromaGuard Deodorants									X
A•R•T System									X
Australian Blue			X						
Awaken			X						
Balance Complete		X							
Basil	X					X			
Believe			X						
Bergamot		X	X						X
BLM						X			
Blue Agave				X		X			
Boswellia Wrinkle Cream									X
Brain Power			X				X		
Breathe Again					X			X	
Cajeput	X							X	
Cardamom		X							
Carrot	X						X		X
Cedar, Western Red									X
Cedarwood							X	X	
Cel-Lite Magic									X
Celery Seed		X				X	X		
Chamomile, German			X				X		X

Essential Oil/ Blend/Product	Cardiovascular System	Digestive System	Emotional Balance	Hormonal System	Immune System	Muscles and Bones	Nervous System	Respiratory System	Skin and Hair
Chamomile, Roman			X				X		X
Christmas Spirit	X		X				X		
Cinnamint Lip Balm									X
Cinnamon Bark					X				
Cistus					X				X
Citronella						X			X
Citrus Fresh			X		X				
ClaraDerm									X
Clarity			X				X		
Clary Sage				X					
Clove	X	X			X			X	
ComforTone		X			X				
Copaiba	X		X			X	X	X	X
Common Sense			X				X		
Coriander		X		X					
CortiStop				X					
Cumin		X			X				
Cypress	X					X			
Cypress, Blue		X			X				
Davana				X					
Deep Relief						X	X		
Detoxzyme		X			X				
Di-Gize		X							
Digest + Cleanse		X							
Dill		X							
Dorado Azul				X			X	X	
Dragon Time			X	X					
Dream Catcher			X						
Elemi									X
Egyptian Gold			X		X				
En-R-Gee			X				X		
EndoFlex				X					
EndoGize		X		X					
Envision			X						
Essentialzyme		X							
Essentialzymes-4		X							
Estro				X					
Eucalyptus						X		X	
Eucalyptus Blue					X			X	
Eucalyptus citriodora								X	
Eucalyptus radiata								X	X
Eucalyptus staigeriana						X		X	X
Evening Peace									X
Evergreen Essence			X						
Exodus II					X				
FemiGen				X					
Fennel		X		X					
Fir								X	

Essential Oil/ Blend/Product	Cardiovascular System	Digestive System	Emotional Balance	Hormonal System	Immune System	Muscles and Bones	Nervous System	Respiratory System	Skin and Hair
Fir, Balsam						X	X		
Fir, Douglas						X		X	
Fir, White			X			X		X	
Fleabane (Conyza)	X			X					
Forgiveness			X						
Frankincense			X		X		X		X
Frankincense, Sacred			X		X		X		X
Galbanum					X				
Gathering			X						
Genesis Lotion			X						X
Gentle Baby			X						X
Geranium			X						X
Ginger		X					X		
GLF		X							
Goldenrod	X			X					
Grapefruit	X								
Grapefruit Lip Balm									X
Gratitude			X						
Grounding			X						
Harmony			X						
Helichrysum	X					X			
Highest Potential			X						
Hinoki			X		X			X	X
Hong Kuai			X		X			X	
Hope			X						
Humility			X						
Hyssop	X						X	X	
ICP	X	X							
Idaho Blue Spruce			X				X	X	
ImmuPower					X				
ImmuPro					X				
Inner Child			X						
Inspiration			X						
Into the Future			X						
Jasmine			X	X					
Joy			X						
Juniper		X	X				X		X
Juva Cleanse		X							
JuvaFlex		X							
JuvaPower		X							
JuvaSpice		X							
JuvaTone		X			X				
K&B		X							
KidScents MightyVites	X		X		X		X		
Lady Sclareol			X						X
Laurel		X			X			X	
LavaDerm Cooling Mist			X						X
Lavandin	X					X		X	

Appendix

Essential Oil/ Blend/Product	Cardiovascular System	Digestive System	Emotional Balance	Hormonal System	Immune System	Muscles and Bones	Nervous System	Respiratory System	Skin and Hair
Lavender	X		X				X		X
Lavender Lotion			X						X
Ledum		X			X				X
Legacy			X						
Lemon		X			X			X	
Lemongrass					X	X			
Lime		X			X			X	
Live with Passion			X				X		
Longevity	X		X						
Longevity Capsules	X				X		X		X
M-Grain						X	X		
Magnify Your Purpose			X				X		
Majestic Essence	X	X			X		X		
Mandarin		X							X
Manuka						X		X	X
Marjoram	X					X			
Master Formula	X		X		X		X		
MegaCal	X					X	X		
Melaleuca					X	X		X	X
Melaleuca Ericifolia								X	X
Melaleuca Quinquenrvia						X		X	
Melissa			X						X
Melrose								X	X
Micromeria					X				
Mineral Essence	X		X	X	X	X	X		
Mister				X					
Morning Start			X						X
Motivation			X				X		
Mountain Savory					X				
MultiGreens	X	X			X	X	X		
Myrrh				X	X		X		X
Myrtle		X		X		X		X	
Neroli		X							X
NingXia Nitro	X	X							
NingXia Red					X				
NingXia Wolfberries		X			X	X			
Nutmeg				X	X		X		
Ocotea	X		X						X
Omega Blue	X						X		
OmegaGize^3	X						X		
Onycha	X		X						X
Orange		X	X		X				X
Orange Blossom Facial Wash									X
Oregano					X	X		X	
Ortho Ease						X			
Ortho Sport						X			
Palmarosa	X		X						X

Essential Oil/ Blend/Product	Cardiovascular System	Digestive System	Emotional Balance	Hormonal System	Immune System	Muscles and Bones	Nervous System	Respiratory System	Skin and Hair
Palo Santo			X		X		X		
PanAway						X	X		
ParaFree		X			X				
Patchouli									X
PD 80/20	X		X	X	X	X			
Peace & Calming			X				X		
Pepper, Black		X					X		
Pepper, Pink					X			X	X
Peppermint		X				X	X	X	X
Petitgrain			X						
Pine			X					X	
Plectranthus Oregano					X	X			
Power Meal	X	X			X	X			
Prenolone			X	X		X	X		X
Present Time			X						
ProGen				X					
Progessence			X	X		X	X		X
Progessence Plus			X	X		X	X		X
Protec				X					
Pure Protein Complete						X			
Purification		X	X						X
Raven								X	X
Ravensara					X			X	
RC								X	
Regenolone				X		X	X		X
Rehemogen	X	X							
Relaxation			X			X			X
Release			X						
Relieve It						X			
Rose			X						X
Rose Ointment									X
Rosemary camphor	X	X				X			
Rosemary cineol					X		X	X	
Rosemary verbenon		X		X					X
Rosewood									X
RutaVaLa			X				X		
Sacred Mountain			X						
Sage				X	X				
Sage Lavender			X	X		X	X	X	X
Sandalwood			X			X	X		X
Sandalwood Moisture Cream									X
SARA			X						
Satin Facial Scrubs									X
SclarEssence		X		X					
Sensation Lotion									X
Sensation Oil Blend			X	X					
SleepEssence	X	X	X			X			

Essential Oil/ Blend/Product	Cardiovascular System	Digestive System	Emotional Balance	Hormonal System	Immune System	Muscles and Bones	Nervous System	Respiratory System	Skin and Hair
Slique Bar		X							
Slique Essence		X	X						
Slique Gum		X							
Slique Tea		X		X					
Slique Slim Caps		X		X					
Spearmint		X	X						
Spikenard			X						X
Spruce			X				X	X	
Stevia	X	X			X				
Stress Away			X		X				
Sulfurzyme					X	X	X		X
Super B	X					X	X		
Super C					X			X	
Super C Chewable					X	X			
Super Cal	X		X			X	X		
Surrender			X				X		
Tangerine			X		X				X
Tansy, Blue							X		
Tansy, Idaho					X				
Tarragon		X					X		
The Gift					X	X			X
Thieves					X				
Thieves Cleaning Prod					X				
Thieves Lozenges					X				
Thyme					X	X			
Thyme linalol								X	X
Thyromin				X					
Tranquil			X				X		
Transformation			X						
Trauma Life			X						
True Source	X				X	X			X
Tsuga	X							X	
Ultra Young+				X	X				
Valerian							X		
Valor			X			X	X		X
Vetiver			X	X			X		X
White Angelica			X						
White Lotus					X				
Wintergreen						X			
Wolfberry Crisp Bars		X			X	X			
Wolfberry Eye Cream									X
Xiang Mao		X			X	X			
Yarrow				X	X				X
Ylang Ylang	X		X	X					
Yuzu		X			X				X

Single Oil Property Chart

The following chart presents some of the properties of each of the single oils. An attempt has been made to indicate the effectiveness of the oils for each property, where supporting information existed. However, this information should not be considered conclusive. It is provided to give the beginning aromatherapy student a starting point for personal use and analysis. Also, keep in mind the applicable safety data when applying an oil for its property. For example, cinnamon bark is one of the best known antiseptics, but it is also extremely irritating to the skin. It may work well to sanitize the bathroom with, but it should be used with extreme caution on the skin.

Essential Oil	A-Bac	A-Cat	A-Dep	A-Fun	A-Inf	A-Infl	A-Mic	A-Par	A-Rhe	A-Sep	A-Spa	A-Vir	Analg	Imm
Angelica		+										+		
Basil	++	+	+		+	+++				+	+	+		
Bergamot					+	+++		+		+	+		+	
Cajeput	+	+			+					+	+		+	
Cardamom										+	+			
Cedarwood				+	+					+				
Chamomile, German	+		+		+	+++				+	+		++	
Chamomile, Roman	+					++		+++			+++		+	
Cinnamon Bark	+		+	+	+	+	++	+		++++	+	+		
Cistus							+			+				+
Citronella	+			+		+				+++	+			
Clary Sage	+		+		+					+	+			
Clove	+++	+		++	+			++	+	+		+++		
Copaiba	++					++++				++			++	
Coriander	++		++		++			+			+		+	
Cumin	+							+		+	++	+		+
Cypress	+				+			+	+	+	+			
Davana					++									
Dill	+	+									+			
Dorado Azul					+									
Elemi		++	++		+					+				
Eucalyptus	++	++++			+	+		+	++	+	++	+++	++	
Eucalyptus Blue					+							+		
Eucalyptus citriodora	++	++		+	++					+		++		
Eucalyptus radiata	++	++			+	+						+++	++	+
Fennel	+	++				+	+	+		+	+			
Fir		+								++			+	
Frankincense		++	++				+				+			+++
Frankincense, Sacred		++	++				+				+			+++
Galbanum		+			+	+	+			+	+	++	++	
Geranium	+++		++	++	+	+				+				
Ginger		++								++			++	
Grapefruit	++									++				
Helichrysum	++	+++		+		++	++			+	+++			
Hinoki	+	+			+							+		
Hong Kuai	+	+			+									
Hyssop	++	++++			+	++		+	+	+	+	+++		
Idaho Blue Spruce					+	+	+				+			
Jasmine		+	++				++				+	+	+	
Juniper					+			+	++	+	+			

Essential Oil	A-Bac	A-Cat	A-Dep	A-Fun	A-Inf	A-Infl	A-Mic	A-Par	A-Rhe	A-Sep	A-Spa	A-Vir	Analg	Imm
Laurel				+						+				
Lavender			++		+	++	+	+	+	+	++		++	
Lavandin	+			+		++				+++	++		++	
Lemon	++				+		++		+	+++	+			++
Lemongrass	+		+	+		++	+			+			++	
Lime	++									++		+		
Mandarin				+						++	+			
Marjoram	+	+		+	+					++	++	+	++	
Melaleuca	+++			++++	+	+		+		+		+++		++
Melaleuca ericifolia	+			+	+		+++							
Melaleuca Quinquenervia	+++			++++		+				+		+++		
Melissa	+		++				+				++	++		
Micromeria	+			+										
Mountain Savory	+++	+		+	++		+++	++		+	+	++	++	++
Myrrh		+		+	+	+++	++	+		+		+++		
Myrtle	+	+++			+					+				
Neroli	+		++		+			+		++	++	+		
Nutmeg						+		+		+				
Ocotea	+				+									
Orange	++		++	+		+				++				
Oregano	+++	+		+++	+++			+++	++	+	+	++	++	++
Palmarosa	+			+			+			+		+		
Patchouli	+		+	+	+	+	+			+		+		
Pepper, Black	+						+			+	+		++	
Peppermint	+	+		+	+	++	+			+	+	+	++	
Petitgrain	+				++	++				+	++			
Pine	+	+		+	++		+			+		+	+	
Plectranthus Oregano	++						+			++				
Ravensara	+	+++		+	+					++		++++		
Rose			++		++	+								
Rosemary	+	+++		+	+		++	+	++	+	+	+	++	
Rosewood	+++		+	++	+		+	+		+	+	++	+	+
Sage	+	+	+	++	+	+	++			+	+	+++		
Sandalwood	+	+++	++	+						++	+			
Spearmint	+			++		++				+	+			
Spikenard	+			+	++	++		++			++			
Spruce		+			+	+++	+		+	+				+
Tangerine														
Tarragon	++				++	++		+		+	++	++		
Thyme	+	+		+++			++	+	++		+	+		++
Valerian	+										++			
Vetiver					+					+	+			+
Idaho Tansy	++				++	++					+	++		+
Xiang Mao	+		+	+		++	+			+			++	
Yarrow						++				++				
Ylang Ylang			+		+					+	+			
Ylang Ylang, Amazonian			+		+					+	+			
Yuzu	+		+											

Glossary

A-Bac (Antibacterial): an agent that prevents bacteria or that destroys bacteria growth.

A-Cat (Anticatarrhal): an agent that helps remove excess catarrh from the body. Expectorants help promote the removal of mucus from the respiratory system.

A-Dep (Antidepressant): an agent that helps alleviate depression.

A-Fun (Antifungal): an agent that prevents and combats fungal infection.

A-Inf (Anti-infectious): an agent that prevents and combats the spread of germs.

A-Infl (Anti-inflammatory): an agent that alleviates inflammation.

A-Mic (Antimicrobial): an agent that resists or destroys pathogenic microorganisms.

A-Par (Antiparasitic): an agent that prevents and destroys parasites.

A-Rhe (Antirheumatic): an agent that helps prevent and relieve rheumatism.

A-Sep (Antiseptic): an agent that destroys and prevents the development of microbes.

A-Spa (Antispasmodic): an agent that prevents and eases spasms or convulsions.

A-Vir (Antiviral): an agent that inhibits the growth of a virus.

Analg (Analgesic): an agent that relieves pain.

Imm (Immune-stimulant): an agent that stimulates the natural defense mechanism of the body.

Single Oil Summary Information

The following chart displays summary information for each of the single oils: botanical name, safety data, and the products (blends, personal care products, bath and shower gels, tinctures, massage oils, and supplements) that contain the single oil. The safety data includes possible skin reactions and conditions where use of that particular oil should be limited or completely avoided (refer to the legend following the Blend Summary Information). **Note:** This safety data is provided for **external use only!**

Single Oil Name	Botanical Name	Safety Data	Products Containing Single Oil
Angelica	*Angelica archangelica* (Umbelliferae)	(GRAS), D, P, PH Dilute 1:1	Awaken, Forgiveness, Grounding, Harmony, Live with Passion, Surrender
Anise	*Pimpinella anisum* (Umbelliferae)	(GRAS), CS Dilute 1:1	Awaken, Di-Gize, Dream Catcher, Allerzyme, ComforTone, Detoxzyme, Digest + Cleanse, Essentialzyme, ICP, JuvaPower, JuvaSpice, ParaFree, Power Meal
Basil	*Ocimum basilicum* (Labiatae)	(GRAS), E*, P*, SI, Dilute 1:1	Aroma Siez, Clarity, M-Grain
Bergamot	*Citrus bergamia* (Rutaceae)	(GRAS), CS*, PH* Dilute 1:1	A·R·T Renewal Serum, Awaken, Believe, Clarity, Dream Catcher, Forgiveness, Gentle Baby, Harmony, Joy, White Angelica, Genesis Hand & Body Lotion, Prenolone, Prenolone+, Progessence, Progessence Plus, Rosewood Moisturizing Shampoo, Rosewood Moisturizing Conditioner, Sandalwood Moisture Cream, Dragon Time Bath Gel, Evening Peace Bath Gel
Cajeput	*Melaleuca leucadendra* (Myrtaceae)	(FA/FL), SI Dilute 1:1	
Calamus	*Acorus calamus (Araceae)*	Dilute 1:4	Exodus II
Caraway	*Carum carvi* (Umbelliferae)	(GRAS), CS, SI, P* Dilute 1:1	Digest + Cleanse
Cardamom	*Elettaria cardamomum* (Zingiberaceae)	(GRAS) Dilute 1:1	Clarity, Transformation
Carrot	*Daucus carota* (Umbelliferae)	(GRAS) Dilute 1:1	Animal Scents Pet Ointment, Rose Ointment
Cassia	*Cinnamomum cassia* (Lauraceae)	(GRAS), CS*, SI*, Dilute 1:4	Exodus II, EndoGize
Cedar, Western Red	*Thuja plicata* (Cupressaceae)	Dilute 1:1	Evergreen Essence, KidScents Lotion
Cedar Leaf	*Thuja occidentalis* (Cupressaceae)	Dilute 1:1	
Cedarwood	*Cedrus atlantica* (Pinaceae)	P	A·R·T Beauty Masque, Australian Blue, Brain Power, Egyptian Gold, Grounding, Inspiration, Into the Future, Live with Passion, Sacred Mountain, SARA, Tranquil, Essential Beauty Serums - Dry Skin Blend & Acne-Prone Skin Blend, KidScents Bath Gel, KidScents Lotion, Sacred Mountain Bar Soap, Peppermint Cedarwood Bar Soap, Progessence Plus, Cel-Lite Magic Massage Oil

Single Oil Name	Botanical Name	Safety Data	Products Containing Single Oil
Celery Seed	*Apium graveolens* (Umbelliferae)	(GRAS), CS, SI, P, Dilute 1:1	GLF, Juva Cleanse
Chamomile (German/Blue)	*Matricaria chamomilla/ recutita* (Compositae)	(GRAS), P, SI	EndoFlex, Surrender, K&B Tincture, A·R·T Day Activator, A·R·T Night Reconstructor, ComforTone, JuvaTone, Omega Blue, OmegaGize[3]
Chamomile (Roman)	*Chamaemelum nobile* (Compositae)	(GRAS), SI	Clarity, Forgiveness, Gentle Baby, Harmony, Joy, JuvaFlex, M-Grain, Motivation, Surrender, Tranquil, ClaraDerm, Genesis Hand & Body Lotion, KidScents Tender Tush, Lemon Sage Clarifying Shampoo, Lemon Sage Clarifying Conditioner, Wolfberry Eye Cream, Dragon Time Bath Gel, Evening Peace Bath Gel, K&B Tincture, Rehemogen Tincture
Cinnamon Bark	*Cinnamomum verum* (Lauraceae)	CS*, P*, SI* Dilute 1:4	Christmas Spirit, Egyptian Gold, Exodus II, Gathering, Magnify Your Purpose, Thieves, Cinnamint Lip Balm, Slique Bar, Thieves Dentarome/Dentarome Plus Toothpaste, Thieves Dentarome Ultra Toothpaste, Thieves Fresh Essence Plus Mouthwash, Thieves Bar Soap, Mineral Essence, Thieves Lozenges
Cistus	*Cistus ladanifer* (Cistaceae)	(FA/FL), P	ImmuPower, The Gift, KidScents Tender Tush
Citronella	*Cymbopogon nardus* (Gramineae)	(GRAS), CS*, P, SI, Dilute 1:1	Purification, Animal Scents Pet Shampoo
Clary Sage	*Salvia sclarea* (Labiatae)	(GRAS), A, P Dilute 1:1	Dragon Time, Into the Future, Lady Sclareol, Live with Passion, SclarEssence, Transformation, Lavender Volume Shampoo, Lavender Volume Conditioner, Prenolone, Prenolone+, Rosewood Moisturizing Shampoo, Rosewood Moisturizing Conditioner, Dragon Time Bath Gel, Evening Peace Bath Gel, Estro Tincture, Cel-Lite Magic Massage Oil, Dragon Time Massage Oil, Ortho Ease Massage Oil, CortiStop (Women's), EndoGize, FemiGen, Transformation
Clove	*Syzygium aromaticum* (Myrtaceae)	(GRAS), CS*, P, SI, Dilute 1:4	Abundance, Deep Relief, En-R-Gee, ImmuPower, Longevity, Melrose, PanAway, Thieves, AromaGuard Deodorants, Essential Beauty Serum - Dry Skin Blend, KidScents Toothpaste, Thieves Dentarome/ Dentarome Plus Toothpaste, Thieves Dentarome Ultra Toothpaste, Thieves Fresh Essence Plus Mouthwash, Thieves Bar Soap, K&B Tincture, BLM, Essentialzyme, Longevity Capsules, Omega Blue, OmegaGize[3], ParaFree, Thieves Lozenges
Copaiba	*Copaifera reticulata or Copaifera L. genus* (Leguminosae)	CS	A·R·T Beauty Masque, Deep Relief, Progessence Plus
Coriander	*Coriandrum sativum* L. (Umbelliferae)	(GRAS), ST Dilute 1:1	A·R·T Renewal Serum, Believe
Cumin	*Cuminus cyminum* (Umbelliferae)	(GRAS), P, PH* Dilute 1:1	ImmuPower, Detoxzyme, ParaFree, Protec
Cypress	*Cupressus sempervirens* (Cupressaceae)	P Dilute 1:1	Aroma Life, Aroma Siez, RC, Cel-Lite Magic Massage Oil, Super Cal

Appendix

Single Oil Name	Botanical Name	Safety Data	Products Containing Single Oil
Cypress, Blue	*Callitris intratropica* (Cupressaceae)		Australian Blue, Brain Power, Essential Beauty Serum - Dry Skin Blend
Davana	*Artemisia pallens* (Compositae)	(FA/FL), P Dilute 1:1	A·R·T Creme Masque, Trauma Life, Lavender Hand & Body Lotion, Lavender Bath Gel
Dill	*Anethum graveolens* (Umbelliferae)	(GRAS), E Dilute 1:1	
Dorado Azul	*Guayafolis officinalis* (Labiatae)		Common Sense
Elemi	*Canarium luzonicum* (Burseraceae)	(FA/FL)	Ortho Sport Massage Oil
Eucalyptus	*Eucalyptus globulus* (Myrtaceae)	(FA/FL) Dilute 1:1	RC, Ortho Ease Massage Oil, Ortho Sport Massage Oil
Eucalyptus Blue	*Eucalyptol natriol azul* (Myrtaceae)		Breathe Again Roll-On
Eucalyptus Citriodora	*Eucalyptus citriodora* (Myrtaceae)	CS Dilute 1:1	RC
Eucalyptus Dives	*Eucalyptus dives* (Myrtaceae)	Dilute 1:1	
Eucalyptus Polybractea	*Eucalyptus polybractea* (Myrtaceae)	Dilute 1:1	
Eucalyptus Radiata	*Eucalyptus radiata* (Myrtaceae)	Dilute 1:1	Raven, RC, Thieves, AromaGuard Deodorants, Ortho Ease Massage Oil, Thieves Dentarome/Dentarome Plus Toothpaste, Thieves Dentarome Ultra Toothpaste, Thieves Fresh Essence Plus Mouthwash, Thieves Bar Soap, Thieves Lozenges
Eucalyptus Staigeriana	*Eucalyptus staigeriana* (Myrtaceae)	Dilute 1:1	Essential Beauty Serum - Acne-Prone Skin Blend
Fennel	*Foeniculum vulgare* (Umbelliferae)	(GRAS), CS, E, P Dilute 1:1	Di-Gize, Dragon Time, JuvaFlex, Mister, SclarEssence, Allerzyme, Detoxzyme, Essentialzyme, JuvaPower, JuvaSpice, Prenolone, Prenolone+, Progessence Cream, Dragon Time Bath Gel, Estro Tincture, K&B Tincture, Dragon Time Massage Oil, CortiStop (Women's), Digest + Cleanse, FemiGen, ParaFree, Power Meal, ProGen
Fir	*Abies alba* (Pinaceae)	(FA/FL), SI Dilute 1:1	Sacred Mountain
Fir, Balsam (Idaho Balsam Fir)	*Abies balsamea* (Pinaceae)	(FA/FL), SI Dilute 1:1	Deep Relief, Egyptian Gold, En-R-Gee, The Gift, Transformation, Animal Scents Pet Ointment, Sacred Mountain Bar Soap, BLM, Slique Slim Caps
Fir, Douglas	*Pseudotsuga menziesii* (Pinaceae)	SI Dilute 1:1	Regenolone
Fir, Red	*Abies magnifica* (Pinaceae)	SI Dilute 1:1	Evergreen Essence
Fir, White	*Abies grandis or Abies concolor* (Pinaceae)	SI Dilute 1:1	Australian Blue, Believe, Evergreen Essence, Gratitude, Grounding, Into the Future, AromaGuard Deodorants

Single Oil Name	Botanical Name	Safety Data	Products Containing Single Oil
Fleabane	*Conyza canadensis* (Compositae)	Dilute 1:1	CortiStop (Women's), EndoGize, Ultra Young+
Frankincense	*Boswellia carterii* (Burseraceae)	(FA/FL)	Abundance, Acceptance, Believe, Brain Power, Common Sense, Egyptian Gold, Exodus II, Forgiveness, Gathering, Gratitude, Harmony, Humility, ImmuPower, Inspiration, Into the Future, Longevity, The Gift, 3 Wise Men, Transformation, Trauma Life, Valor, A·R·T Day Activator, A·R·T Gentle Foaming Cleanser, A·R·T Night Reconstructor, A·R·T Purifying Toner, Boswellia Wrinkle Cream, ClaraDerm, KidScents Tender Tush, Progessence Plus, Protec, Wolfberry Eye Cream, Valor Bar Soap, CortiStop (Women's), Longevity Capsules
Frankincense, Sacred	*Boswellia sacra* (Burseraceae)	(FA/FL)	Transformation
Galbanum	*Ferula gummosa* (Umbelliferae)	(FA/FL)	Exodus II, Gathering, Gratitude, The Gift
Geranium	*Pelargonium graveolens* (Geraniaceae)	(GRAS), CS	A·R·T Creme Masque, A·R·T Renewal Serum, Acceptance, Believe, Clarity, EndoFlex, Envision, Forgiveness, Gathering, Gentle Baby, Harmony, Humility, Joy, JuvaFlex, Lady Sclareol, Release, SARA, Trauma Life, White Angelica, Animal Scents Pet Ointment, AromaGuard Deodorants, Boswellia Wrinkle Cream, Genesis Hand & Body Lotion, Lemon Sage Clarifying Shampoo, Lemon Sage Clarifying Conditioner, Prenolone, Prenolone+, Progessence Cream, Rosewood Moisturizing Shampoo, Rosewood Moisturizing Conditioner, Wolfberry Eye Cream, Animal Scents Pet Shampoo, Dragon Time Bath Gel, Evening Peace Bath Gel, KidScents Bath Gel, KidScents Lotion, Melaleuca Geranium Bar Soap, K&B Tincture, JuvaTone
Ginger	*Zingiber officinale* (Zingiberaceae)	(GRAS), CS, PH Dilute 1:1	Abundance, Di-Gize, Live with Passion, Magnify Your Purpose, Allerzyme, ComforTone, Digest + Cleanse, EndoGize, ICP
Goldenrod	*Solidago canadensis* (Asteraceae)	Dilute 1:1	Common Sense
Grapefruit	*Citrus x paradisi* (Rutaceae)	(GRAS) Dilute 1:1	Citrus Fresh, GLF, Cel-Lite Magic Massage Oil, Power Meal, Slique Essence, Super C
Helichrysum	*Helichrysum italicum* (Compositae)	(GRAS)	Aroma Life, Brain Power, Deep Relief, Forgiveness, GLF, Juva Cleanse, JuvaFlex, Live with Passion, M-Grain, PanAway, Trauma Life, ClaraDerm
Hinoki	*Chamaecyparis obtusa* (Cupressaceae)	Dilute 1:1	
Hong Kuai	*Chamaecyparis formosensis* (Cupressaceae)	P*, Dilute 1:1	
Hyssop	*Hyssopus officinalis* (Labiatae)	(GRAS), E*, HBP*, P*, D-1:1	Egyptian Gold, Exodus II, GLF, Harmony, ImmuPower, Relieve It, White Angelica

Single Oil Name	Botanical Name	Safety Data	Products Containing Single Oil
Jasmine	*Jasminum officinale* (Oleaceae)	(GRAS)	A·R·T Creme Masque, A·R·T Renewal Serum, Clarity, Dragon Time, Forgiveness, Gentle Baby, Harmony, Highest Potential, Inner Child, Into the Future, Joy, Lady Sclareol, Live with Passion, Sensation, The Gift, Genesis Hand & Body Lotion, Lavender Volume Shampoo, Lavender Volume Conditioner, Sensation Hand & Body Lotion, Dragon Time Bath Gel, Evening Peace Bath Gel, Sensation Bath Gel, Dragon Time Massage Oil, Sensation Massage Oil
Juniper	*Juniperus osteosperma* and/or *J. scopulorum* (Cupressaceae)	Dilute 1:1	Di-Gize, Dream Catcher, En-R-Gee, Grounding, Hope, Into the Future, 3 Wise Men, Allerzyme, Morning Start Bath Gel, Morning Start Bar Soap, K&B Tincture, Cel-Lite Magic Massage Oil, Ortho Ease Massage Oil
Laurel	*Laurus nobilis* (Lauraceae)	(GRAS), CS, P* Dilute 1:1	ParaFree
Lavandin	*Lavandula x hybrida* (Labiatae)	(GRAS), E, P*	Purification, Release, Animal Scents Pet Shampoo
Lavender	*Lavandula angustifolia* CT linalool (Labiatae)		A·R·T Beauty Masque, Aroma Siez, Brain Power, Dragon Time, Egyptian Gold, Envision, Forgiveness, Gathering, Gentle Baby, Harmony, M-Grain, Mister, Motivation, RC, RutaVaLa, SARA, Surrender, Tranquil, Trauma Life, A·R·T Gentle Foaming Cleanser, A·R·T Purifying Toner, AromaGuard Deodorants, ClaraDerm, Essential Beauty Serum - Dry Skin Blend, LavaDerm Cooling Mist, Lavender Hand & Body Lotion, Lavender Volume Shampoo, Lavender Volume Conditioner, KidScents Tender Tush, Orange Blossom Facial Wash, Sandalwood Moisture Cream, Wolfberry Eye Cream, Dragon Time Bath Gel, Lavender Bath Gel, Lavender Rosewood Bar Soap, Estro Tincture, Dragon Time Massage Oil, Relaxation Massage Oil, ProGen
Ledum	*Ledum groenlandicum* (Ericaceae)		GLF, Juva Cleanse
Lemon	*Citrus limon* (Rutaceae)	(GRAS), PH*, SI* Dilute 1:1	Citrus Fresh, Clarity, Deep Relief, Forgiveness, Gentle Baby, Harmony, Joy, Raven, Surrender, Thieves, Transformation, A·R·T Gentle Foaming Cleanser, A·R·T Purifying Toner, AromaGuard Deodorants, Genesis Hand & Body Lotion, Animal Scents Pet Shampoo, KidScents Shampoo, Lavender Hand & Body Lotion, Lavender Volume Shampoo, Lavender Volume Conditioner, Lemon Sage Clarifying Shampoo, Lemon Sage Clarifying Conditioner, NingXia Red, Orange Blossom Facial Wash, Thieves Dentarome/Dentarome Plus Toothpaste, Thieves Dentarome Ultra Toothpaste, Thieves Fresh Essence Plus Mouthwash, Dragon Time Bath Gel, Evening Peace Bath Gel, Lavender Bath Gel, Thieves Bar Soap, Lemon Sandalwood Bar Soap, AlkaLime, Digest + Cleanse, JuvaTone, MegaCal, Mineral Essence, MultiGreens, NingXia Red, Power Meal, Slique Essence, Super C, Super C Chewable, Thieves Lozenges, Transformation

Single Oil Name	Botanical Name	Safety Data	Products Containing Single Oil
Lemongrass	*Cymbopogon flexuosus* (Gramineae)	(GRAS), SI* Dilute 1:4	Di-Gize, En-R-Gee, Inner Child, Purification, Allerzyme, Evening Peace Bath Gel, Morning Start Bath Gel, Morning Start Bar Soap, Ortho Ease Massage Oil, Ortho Sport Massage Oil, ICP, MultiGreens, Omega Blue, Slique Slim Caps, Super C, Super Cal
Lime	*Citrus aurantifolia* (Rutaceae)	(GRAS), PH* Dilute 1:1	A·R·T Beauty Masque, Common Sense, Lemon Sage Clarifying Shampoo, Lemon Sage Clarifying Conditioner, AlkaLime, KidScents Mighty Vites
Limette (Combava)	Citrus hystrix (Rutaceae)	PH* Dilute 1:1	Trauma Life
Mandarin	*Citrus reticulata* (Rutaceae)	(GRAS), PH Dilute 1:1	Citrus Fresh, Joy, Dragon Time Bath Gel, KidScents Mighty Vites
Manuka	*Leptospermum scoparium* (Myrtaceae)	Dilute 1:1	Essential Beauty Serum - Acne-Prone Skin Blend
Marjoram	*Origanum majorana* (Labiatae)	(GRAS), P Dilute 1:1	Aroma Life, Aroma Siez, Dragon Time, M-Grain, RC, Dragon Time Bath Gel, Ortho Ease Massage Oil, Ortho Sport Massage Oil, Super Cal
Melaleuca (Tea Tree)	*Melaleuca alternifolia* (Myrtaceae)	(FA/FL), CS Dilute 1:1	Melrose, Purification, Animal Scents Pet Ointment, AromaGuard Deodorants, ClaraDerm, Essential Beauty Serum - Acne-Prone Skin Blend, Rose Ointment, Melaleuca Geranium Bar Soap, Rehemogen Tincture, ParaFree
Melaleuca ericifolia (Rosalina)	*Melaleuca ericifolia* (Myrtaceae)	(FA/FL) Dilute 1:1	Melaleuca Geranium Bar Soap
Melaleuca quinquenervia (Niaouli)	*Melaleuca quinquenervia* (Myrtaceae)	(FA/FL), CS Dilute 1:1	Melrose, AromaGuard Deodorants
Melissa	*Melissa officinalis* (Labiatae)	(GRAS)	Brain Power, Forgiveness, Hope, Humility, Live with Passion, White Angelica, A·R·T Gentle Foaming Cleanser, A·R·T Purifying Toner, MultiGreens
Micromeria	*Micromeria fruticosa* (Labiatae)	P*, SI* Dilute 1:2	
Mountain Savory	*Satureja montana* (Labiatae)	(GRAS), P*, SI* Dilute 1:4	ImmuPower, Surrender
Mugwort	*Artemisia vulgaris* (Asteraceae)	P* Dilute 1:1	Inspiration, ComforTone
Myrrh	*Commiphora myrrha* (Burseraceae)	(FA/FL), P	Abundance, Egyptian Gold, Exodus II, Gratitude, Hope, Humility, The Gift, 3 Wise Men, White Angelica, Animal Scents Pet Ointment, Boswellia Wrinkle Cream, ClaraDerm, Essential Beauty Serum - Dry Skin Blend, Lavender Hand & Body Lotion, Protec, Rose Ointment, Sandalwood Moisture Cream, Lavender Bath Gel, EndoGize, Omega Blue, Thyromin
Myrrh , Biblical Sweet	*Commiphora erythraea* (Burseraceae)	(FA/FL), P	
Myrtle	*Myrtus communis* (Myrtaceae)	Dilute 1:1	EndoFlex, Inspiration, Mister, Purification, RC, JuvaTone, ProGen, Super Cal, Thyromin
Myrtle, Lemon	*Backhousia citriodora* (Myrtaceae)	CS, SI Dilute 1:4	Slique Slim Caps

Single Oil Name	Botanical Name	Safety Data	Products Containing Single Oil
Neroli	*Citrus aurantium bigaradia* (Rutaceae)	(GRAS) Dilute 1:1	Acceptance, Humility, Inner Child, Live with Passion, Present Time
Nutmeg	*Myristica fragrans* (Myristicaceae)	(GRAS), E*, P Dilute 1:2	EndoFlex, En-R-Gee, Magnify Your Purpose, NingXia Nitro, ParaFree, Power Meal
Ocotea	*Ocotea quixos* (Lauraceae)	Dilute 1:1	A·R·T Beauty Masque, A·R·T Creme Masque, Common Sense, Slique Essence, Stress Away Roll-On, Transformation
Onycha	*Styrax benzoin* (Styracaceae)	(FA/FL)	
Orange	*Citrus sinensis* (Rutaceae)	(GRAS), PH* Dilute 1:1	Abundance, Christmas Spirit, Citrus Fresh, Envision, Harmony, Inner Child, Into the Future, Lady Sclareol, Longevity, NingXia Red, Peace & Calming, SARA, Cinnamint Lip Balm, Balance Complete, ImmuPro, Longevity Capsules, Pure Protein Complete, KidScents Mighty Vites, NingXia Red, Power Meal, Slique Bar, Super C, Thieves Lozenges
Oregano	*Origanum compactum* (Labiatae)	(GRAS), SI* Dilute 1:4	ImmuPower, Regenolone, Ortho Sport Massage Oil
Palmarosa	*Cymbopogon martinii* (Gramineae)	(GRAS) Dilute 1:1	Clarity, Forgiveness, Gentle Baby, Harmony, Joy, Animal Scents Pet Ointment, Genesis Hand & Body Lotion, Rose Ointment, Dragon Time Bath Gel, Evening Peace Bath Gel
Palo Santo	*Bursera graveolens* (Burseraceae)		Deep Relief, Transformation
Patchouli	*Pogostemon cablin* (Labiatae)	(FA/FL)	Abundance, Di-Gize, Live with Passion, Magnify Your Purpose, Peace & Calming, Allerzyme, Animal Scents Pet Ointment, Orange Blossom Facial Wash, Rose Ointment
Pepper, Black	*Piper nigrum* (Piperaceae)	(GRAS), SI* Dilute 1:1	Dream Catcher, En-R-Gee, Relieve It, Cel-Lite Magic Massage Oil, NingXia Nitro
Pepper, Pink	*Schinus molle* (Anacardiaceae)	(GRAS), P* Dilute 1:1	
Peppermint	*Mentha piperita* (Labiatae)	(GRAS), CS, HBP, P Dilute 1:2	Aroma Siez, Clarity, Deep Relief, Di-Gize, M-Grain, Mister, PanAway, Raven, RC, Relieve It, SclarEssence, Transformation, A·R·T Purifying Toner, AromaGuard Deodorants, Cinnamint Lip Balm, Lemon Sage Clarifying Conditioner, Mint Satin Facial Scrub, Progessence Plus, Regenolone, Thieves Dentarome/Dentarome Plus Toothpaste, Thieves Dentarome Ultra Toothpaste, Thieves Fresh Essence Plus Mouthwash, Morning Start Bath Gel, Peppermint Cedarwood Bar Soap, Ortho Ease Massage Oil, Ortho Sport Massage Oil, Relaxation Massage Oil, Allerzyme, ComforTone, CortiStop (Women's), Digest + Cleanse, Essentialzyme, Mineral Essence, NingXia Nitro, ProGen, Slique Gum, Thieves Lozenges, Thyromin, Transformation
Petitgrain	*Citrus aurantium* (Rutaceae)	(GRAS) Dilute 1:1	
Pine	*Pinus sylvestris* (Pinaceae)	(FA/FL), SI Dilute 1:1	Evergreen Essence, Grounding, RC, Lemon Sage Clarifying Shampoo, Lemon Sage Clarifying Conditioner

Single Oil Name	Botanical Name	Safety Data	Products Containing Single Oil
Pine, Black	*Pinus nigra* (Pinaceae)	SI	Evergreen Essence
Pine, Lodge Pole	*Pinus contorta* (Pinaceae)	SI	Evergreen Essence
Pine, Piñon	*Pinus edulis* (Pinaceae)	SI	Evergreen Essence
Pine, Ponderosa (Yellow Pine)	*Pinus ponderosa* (Pinaceae)	SI	Evergreen Essence
Plectranthus Oregano	*Plectranthus amboinicus* (Lauraceae)	SI*	
Ravensara	*Ravensara aromatica* (Lauraceae)		ImmuPower, Raven
Rose (Bulgarian)	*Rosa damascena* (Rosaceae)	(GRAS), P	Egyptian Gold, Envision, Forgiveness, Gathering, Gentle Baby, Harmony, Humility, Joy, SARA, Trauma Life, White Angelica, Rose Ointment
Rosehip	*Rosa canina or Rosa rubiginosa* (Rosaceae)	(GRAS)	Animal Scents Pet Ointment, Rose Ointment, Sandalwood Moisture Cream, Wolfberry Eye Cream
Rosemary Cineol	*Rosmarinus officinalis* CT 1,8 cineol (Labiatae)	(GRAS), E*, HBP*, P* Dilute 1:1	En-R-Gee, JuvaFlex, Melrose, Purification, Thieves, Transformation, AromaGuard Deodorants, Thieves Dentarome/Dentarome Plus Toothpaste, Thieves Dentarome Ultra Toothpaste, Thieves Fresh Essence Plus Mouthwash, Evening Peace Bath Gel, Morning Start Bath Gel, Morning Start Bar Soap, Rehemogen Tincture, ComforTone, ICP, JuvaTone, MultiGreens, Thieves Lozenges
Rosemary Verbenon	*Rosmarinus officinalis* CT verbenon (Labiatae)	(GRAS), E*, HBP, P Dilute 1:1	Clarity, Orange Blossom Facial Wash, Sandalwood Moisture Cream
Rosewood	*Aniba rosaeodora* (Lauraceae)	(GRAS)	Acceptance, Clarity, Forgiveness, Gentle Baby, Gratitude, Harmony, Humility, Inspiration, Joy, Lady Sclareol, Magnify Your Purpose, Sensation, Valor, White Angelica, Animal Scents Pet Ointment, AromaGuard Deodorants, Genesis Hand & Body Lotion, KidScents Lotion, KidScents Tender Tush, Progessence Plus, Rose Ointment, Rosewood Moisturizing Shampoo, Rosewood Moisturizing Conditioner, Sandalwood Moisture Cream, Sensation Hand & Body Lotion, Wolfberry Eye Cream, Dragon Time Bath Gel, Evening Peace Bath Gel, Sensation Bath Gel, Lavender Rosewood Bar Soap, Valor Bar Soap, Relaxation Massage Oil, Sensation Massage Oil
Ruta (Rue)	*Ruta graveolens* (Rutaceae)	P*, PH*, SI*	Common Sense, RutaVaLa
Sage	*Salvia officinalis* (Labiatae)	(GRAS), E*, HBP*, P* Dilute 1:1	EndoFlex, Envision, Magnify Your Purpose, Mister, Progessence Cream, Protec, Lemon Sage Clarifying Shampoo, Lemon Sage Clarifying Conditioner, Dragon Time Bath Gel, K&B Tincture, Dragon Time Massage Oil, FemiGen, ProGen
Sage, Spanish (Sage Lavender)	*Salvia lavandulifolia* (Labiatae)	(GRAS) Dilute 1:1	Harmony, Lady Sclareol, SclarEssence

Single Oil Name	Botanical Name	Safety Data	Products Containing Single Oil
Sandalwood	*Santalum album* (Santalaceae)	(FA/FL)	Acceptance, Brain Power, Dream Catcher, Forgiveness, Gathering, Harmony, Inner Child, Inspiration, Lady Sclareol, Live with Passion, Magnify Your Purpose, Release, 3 Wise Men, Transformation, Trauma Life, White Angelica, A·R·T Day Activator, A·R·T Gentle Foaming Cleanser, A·R·T Night Reconstructor, A·R·T Purifying Toner, Boswellia Wrinkle Cream, Essential Beauty Serum - Dry Skin Blend, KidScents Tender Tush, Rosewood Moisturizing Shampoo, Rosewood Moisturizing Conditioner, Sandalwood Moisture Cream, Evening Peace Bath Gel, Lemon Sandalwood Bar Soap, Transformation, Ultra Young+
Spearmint	*Mentha spicata* (Labiatae)	(GRAS), P Dilute 1:2	Citrus Fresh, EndoFlex, GLF, Cinnamint Lip Balm, Thieves Fresh Essence Plus Mouthwash, NingXia Nitro, OmegaGize[3], Relaxation Massage Oil, Slique Essence, Slique Gum, Thyromin
Spikenard	*Nardostachys jatamansi* (Valerianaceae)		Egyptian Gold, Exodus II, Humility, The Gift, Animal Scents Pet Shampoo
Spruce	*Picea mariana* (Pinaceae)	(FA/FL) Dilute 1:1	Abundance, Christmas Spirit, Envision, Gathering, Grounding, Harmony, Hope, Inner Child, Inspiration, Motivation, Present Time, Relieve It, Sacred Mountain, Surrender, 3 Wise Men, Trauma Life, Valor, White Angelica, Sacred Mountain Bar Soap, Valor Bar Soap
Spruce, Colorado Blue	*Picea pungens* (Pinaceae)		Evergreen Essence
Spruce, Idaho Blue	*Picea Pungens* (Pinaceae)	(FA/FL), Dilute 1:1	Believe, Transformation
Tangerine	*Citrus nobilis* (Rutaceae)	(GRAS) Dilute 1:1	Citrus Fresh, Dream Catcher, Inner Child, Peace & Calming, KidScents Shampoo, Relaxation Massage Oil, ComforTone, Slique Essence, Super C
Tansy, Blue	*Tanacetum annuum* (Compositae)	Dilute 1:1	Acceptance, Australian Blue, Dream Catcher, JuvaFlex, NingXia Red, Peace & Calming, Release, SARA, Valor, KidScents Shampoo, KidScents Tender Tush, Dragon Time Bath Gel, Evening Peace Bath Gel, Valor Bar Soap, JuvaTone
Tansy, Idaho	*Tanacetum vulgare* (Compositae)	Dilute 1:1	ImmuPower, Into the Future, Lady Sclareol, ParaFree
Tarragon	*Artemisia dracunculus* (Compositae)	(GRAS), E*, P* Dilute 1:1	Di-Gize, Allerzyme, ComforTone, ICP, Essentialzyme
Thyme	*Thymus vulgaris* (Labiatae)	(GRAS), HBP Dilute 1:4	Longevity, Essential Beauty Serum - Acne-Prone Skin Blend, KidScents Toothpaste, Rehemogen, Longevity Capsules, ParaFree
Thyme linalool	*Thymus vulgaris* CT Linalool (Labiatae)	(GRAS) Dilute 1:2	
Thyme, Red	*Thymus serpyllum* (Labiatae)	(GRAS)	Ortho Ease
Tsuga	*Tsuga canadensis* (Pinaceae)	(FA/FL), SI* Dilute 1:1	RC

Single Oil Name	Botanical Name	Safety Data	Products Containing Single Oil
Valerian	*Valeriana officinalis* (Valerianaceae)	(FA/FL), CS	RutaVaLa, Trauma Life
Vetiver	*Vetiveria zizanioides* (Gramineae)	P	A·R·T Creme Masque, Deep Relief, Lady Sclareol, Thieves Fresh Essence Plus Mouthwash, Melaleuca Geranium Bar Soap, Ortho Ease Massage Oil, Ortho Sport Massage Oil, ParaFree
White Lotus	*Nymphaea lotus* (Nymphaeaceae)		SARA
Wintergreen	*Gaultheria procumbens* (Ericaceae)	E*, P* Dilute 1:2	Deep Relief, PanAway, Raven, Regenolone, Rosewood Moisturizing Shampoo, Rosewood Moisturizing Conditioner, Thieves Dentarome/ Dentarome Plus Toothpaste, Thieves Dentarome Ultra Toothpaste, Ortho Ease Massage Oil, Ortho Sport Massage Oil, BLM, Super Cal
Xiang Mao (Red Lemongrass)	*Cymbopogon citratus* (Gramineae)	(GRAS), SI* Dilute 1:4	
Yarrow	*Achillea millefolium* (Compositae)	CS, P Dilute 1:1	Dragon Time, Mister, Prenolone/ Prenolone+, Progessence Cream, Dragon Time Massage Oil, ProGen
Ylang Ylang	*Cananga odorata* (Annonaceae)	(GRAS), CS Dilute 1:1	Aroma Life, A·R·T Creme Masque, A·R·T Renewal Serum, Australian Blue, Clarity, Common Sense, Dream Catcher, Forgiveness, Gathering, Gentle Baby, Gratitude, Grounding, Harmony, Highest Potential, Humility, Inner Child, Into the Future, Joy, Lady Sclareol, Motivation, Peace & Calming, Present Time, Release, Sacred Mountain, SARA, Sensation, White Angelica, Boswellia Wrinkle Cream, Genesis Hand & Body Lotion, Lemon Sage Clarifying Shampoo, Lemon Sage Clarifying Conditioner, Prenolone/Prenolone+, Sensation Hand & Body Lotion, Dragon Time Bath Gel, Evening Peace Bath Gel, Sensation Bath Gel, Sacred Mountain Bar Soap, Dragon Time Massage Oil, Relaxation Massage Oil, Sensation Massage Oil, FemiGen
Ylang Ylang, Amazonian	*Cananga odorata equitoriana* (Annonaceae)	(GRAS), CS Dilute 1:1	Believe
Yuzu	*Citrus junos* (Rutaceae)	PH, Dilute 1:1	NingXia Red

Single Oil Summary Chart Safety Data Legend:

- A — **Avoid** during and after consumption of **alcohol**
- CS — Could possibly result in **contact sensitization** (redness or irritation of the skin due to repeated application of a substance) (rotate or use different oils)
- CS* — Repeated use can result in **extreme contact sensitization** (rotate between different oils)
- D — **Avoid** if **diabetic**
- E — Use with **caution** if susceptible to **epilepsy** (small amounts or in dilution)
- E* — **Avoid** if susceptible to **epilepsy** (can trigger a seizure)
- HBP — Use with **caution** if dealing with **high blood pressure** (small amounts)
- HBP* — **Avoid** if dealing with **high blood pressure**

Single Oil Summary Chart Safety Data Legend Continued on Next Page...

Single Oil Summary Chart Safety Data Legend (continued):

P	Use with **caution** during **pregnancy** (small amounts or in dilution)
P*	**Avoid** during **pregnancy**
PH	**Photosensitivity**—direct exposure to sunlight after use could cause dermatitis (test first)
PH*	**Extreme photosensitivity**—direct exposure to sunlight after use can cause severe dermatitis (avoid exposing affected area of skin to direct sunlight for 12 hours)
SI	Could possibly result in **skin irritation** (dilution may be necessary)
SI*	Can cause **extreme skin irritation** (dilution highly recommended)
ST	Can cause **stupefication** in high doses (use only small amounts or in dilution)
Dilute	Dilution ratios shown equal Essential Oil:Vegetable Oil

Blend Summary Information

The following chart displays summary information for each of the oil blends: single oils contained in the blend, possible uses or areas of application, and safety data. The safety data includes possible skin reactions and conditions where use of that particular blend should be limited or completely avoided (refer to the legend following the chart). **Note:** This safety data is provided for **external use only!**

Blend Name	Single Oil Contents	Uses/Application Areas	Safety Data
Abundance	Myrrh, frankincense, patchouli, orange, clove, ginger, spruce	Diffuse; Wrists, ears, neck, face; Wallet/urse; Painting; Perfume	CS*, SI Dilute 1:1
Acceptance	Geranium, blue tansy, frankincense, sandalwood, neroli, rosewood (Carrier: Almond oil)	Diffuse; *Liver*, heart, *chest*, face, ears, neck, thymus, wrists; Sacral chakra; Perfume	
Aroma Life	Cypress, marjoram, helichrysum, ylang ylang (Carrier: Sesame seed oil)	Heart; Vita Flex heart points—under left ring finger, under left ring toe, above left elbow, arteries; Spine	
Aroma Siez	Basil, marjoram, lavender, peppermint, cypress	Muscles; Neck; Heart; Vita Flex points; Full-body massage; Bath	Dilute 1:1
Australian Blue	Blue cypress, ylang ylang, cedarwood, blue tansy, white fir	Diffuse; Perfume; Forehead	CS, SI
Awaken	Oil Blends of Joy, Forgiveness, Dream Catcher, Present Time, Harmony	Diffuse; Chest, heart, *forehead*, neck, temples, wrists; Perfume; Full-body massage; Bath	
Believe	Idaho Balsam fir, coriander, bergamot, frankincense, Idaho Blue Spruce, Ylang Ylang, Geranium	Diffuse; *Heart, forehead, temples*; Perfume	Dilute 1:1
Brain Power	Cedarwood, sandalwood, frankincense, melissa, blue cypress, lavender, helichrysum	Diffuse; Neck, throat, nose; Inside of cheeks; Perfume	
Breathe Again *(Roll-on)*	*Eucalyptus staigeriana*, *Eucalyptus globulus*, laurel, rose hip, peppermint, copaiba, *Eucalyptus radiata*, myrtle, manuku, eucalyptus blue	Chest; Under nose	SI, P
Christmas Spirit	Orange, cinnamon bark, spruce	Diffuse; Crown; Perfume; Place on pine boughs or fireplace logs; Add to potpourri	CS*, SI* Dilute 1:1
Citrus Fresh	Orange, tangerine, mandarin, grapefruit, lemon, spearmint	Diffuse; Ears, heart, wrists; Perfume; Full-body massage; Bath; Purify drinking water	SI*, PH* Dilute 1:1
Clarity	Basil, cardamom, rosemary verbenon, peppermint, rosewood, geranium, lemon, palmarosa, ylang ylang, bergamot, Roman chamomile, jasmine	Diffuse; Forehead, neck, temples, wrists; Perfume; Bath	SI, P, PH*
Common Sense	Frankincense, ylang ylang, ocotea, goldenrod, rue, dorado azul, lime	Diffuse	SI, P, PH*
Deep Relief *(Roll-on)*	Peppermint, lemon, balsam fir, copaiba, clove, wintergreen, helichrysum, vetiver, palo santo (Carriers: Fractionated coconut oil and virgin coconut oil)	Directly on pain location; Forehead, neck, temples	

Blend Name	Single Oil Contents	Uses/Application Areas	Safety Data
Di-Gize	Tarragon, ginger, peppermint, juniper, anise, fennel, lemongrass, patchouli	Vita Flex points—feet and ankles; Stomach; Abdomen, bottom of throat; Compress	P, E
Dragon Time	Clary sage, fennel, lavender, marjoram, yarrow, jasmine	Vita Flex points; Diffuse; Abdomen, lower back, location	P
Dream Catcher	Sandalwood, bergamot, ylang ylang, juniper, blue tansy, tangerine, black pepper, anise	Diffuse; Forehead, eyebrows, *temples*, ears, throat chakra; Perfume; Pillow; Bath or sauna	PH
Egyptian Gold	Frankincense, lavender, balsam fir, myrrh, spikenard, hyssop, cedarwood, rose, cinnamon bark	Diffuse; Wrists, ears, neck, temples; Perfume	SI, E Dilute 1:4
En-R-Gee	Rosemary cineol, juniper, nutmeg, balsam fir, black pepper, lemongrass, clove	Diffuse; Wrists, ears, neck, temples, feet; Full-body massage; Perfume	SI*, E Dilute 1:1
EndoFlex	Spearmint, sage, geranium, myrtle, nutmeg, German chamomile (Carrier: Sesame seed oil)	Thyroid, kidneys, liver, pancreas, glands; Vita Flex points	SI, E
Envision	Spruce, geranium, orange, lavender, sage, rose	Vita Flex points; Diffuse; Wrists, *temples*; Bath; Massage	HBP, E, P
Evergreen Essence	Colorado blue spruce (*Picea pungens*), ponderosa pine (*Pinus ponderosa*), pine, red fir (*Abies magnifica*), western red cedar, white fir, black pine (*Pinus nigra*), pinyon pine (*Pinus edulis*), lodgepole pine (*Pinus contorta*), and other conifers	*Diffuse*; Hands, bottoms of feet	CS, SI Dilute 1:1
Exodus II	Cassia, myrrh, cinnamon bark, calamus, hyssop, galbanum, frankincense, spikenard (Carrier: Olive oil)	Vita Flex points; Spine (dilute well)	CS*, SI*, P* Dilute 1:1
Forgiveness	Melissa, geranium, frankincense, rosewood, sandalwood, angelica, lavender, lemon, jasmine, Roman chamomile, bergamot, ylang ylang, palmarosa, helichrysum, rose (Carrier: Sesame seed oil)	Diffuse; *Navel*, heart, ears, wrists; Perfume	
Gathering	Lavender, galbanum, frankincense, geranium, ylang ylang, spruce, cinnamon bark, rose, sandalwood	Diffuse; *Forehead, heart, temples*, neck, thymus, face, chest; Perfume	
Gentle Baby	Rosewood, geranium, palmarosa, lavender, Roman chamomile, ylang ylang, lemon, jasmine, bergamot, rose	Diffuse; Ankles, lower back, abdomen, feet, face, neck; Massage; Perfume; Bath	
GLF	Grapefruit, helichrysum, celery seed, ledum, hyssop, spearmint.	Liver; Vita Flex points on feet	
Gratitude	Balsam fir, frankincense, rosewood, myrrh, galbanum, ylang ylang	Diffuse; *Heart, forehead, temples*; Perfume	Dilute 1:1
Grounding	Fir, spruce, ylang ylang, pine, cedarwood, angelica, juniper	Diffuse; *Brain stem, back of neck, sternum*, temples	SI
Harmony	Lavender, sandalwood, ylang ylang, frankincense, orange, angelica, geranium, hyssop, spruce, sage lavender, rosewood, lemon, jasmine, Roman chamomile, bergamot, palmarosa, rose	Diffuse; Each chakra; Ears, feet, heart; *Energy meridians*, crown; Perfume	P, E*, HBP, PH

Blend Name	Single Oil Contents	Uses/Application Areas	Safety Data
Highest Potential	Oil blends of Australian Blue and Gathering, and single oils of jasmine and ylang ylang	Diffuse; *Heart, forehead, temples*; Perfume	Dilute 1:1
Hope	Melissa, myrrh, juniper, spruce (Carrier: Almond oil)	Diffuse; *Ears*; Chest, heart, temples, solar plexus, neck, feet, wrists; Perfume	
Humility	Rosewood, ylang ylang, geranium, melissa, frankincense, spikenard, myrrh, rose, neroli (Carrier: Sesame seed oil)	Diffuse; *Heart, neck, temples*	
ImmuPower	Hyssop, mountain savory, cistus, ravensara, frankincense, oregano, clove, cumin, Idaho tansy	Diffuse; Throat, chest, spine, feet; Thymus; Veins in neck, under arm pits	SI, P, E Dilute 1:1
Inner Child	Orange, tangerine, jasmine, ylang ylang, spruce, sandalwood, lemongrass, neroli	Diffuse; *Navel, chest, temples, nose*	SI
Inspiration	Cedarwood, spruce, rosewood, myrtle, sandalwood, frankincense, mugwort	Diffuse; *Horns*, crown, shoulders, back of neck	
Into the Future	Clary sage, ylang ylang, white fir, Idaho tansy, juniper, jasmine, frankincense, orange, cedarwood (Carrier: Almond oil)	Diffuse; Bath; Heart, wrists, neck; Compress; Full-body massage	
Joy	Bergamot, ylang ylang, geranium, rosewood, lemon, mandarin, jasmine, Roman chamomile, palmarosa, rose	Diffuse; *Heart*, ears, neck, thymus, temples, forehead, wrists; Bath; Compress; Massage; Perfume	PH*
Juva Cleanse	Helichrysum, ledum, celery seed	Liver; Vita Flex points on feet	SI
JuvaFlex	Fennel, geranium, rosemary cineol, Roman chamomile, blue tansy, helichrysum (Carrier: Sesame seed oil)	Vita Flex points; Feet, spine, LIVER; Full-body massage	SI Dilute 1:1
Lady Sclareol	Rosewood, vetiver, geranium, orange, clary sage, ylang ylang, sandalwood, sage lavender, jasmine, Idaho tansy	On location (by male partner); Massage; Bath; Compress over abdomen; Diffuse, *Perfume*	
Legacy	Ninety-one different essential oils	Vita Flex points; Diffuse; Topically on location	E, P, CS, SI
Live with Passion	Clary sage, ginger, sandalwood, jasmine, angelica, cedarwood, helichrysum, patchouli, neroli, melissa	Wrists, *temples, chest, forehead*; Bath; Perfume or cologne	
Longevity	Thyme, orange, clove, frankincense	Internally as Dietary Supplement	CS, SI, PH Dilute 1:4
M-Grain	Basil, marjoram, lavender, peppermint, Roman chamomile, helichrysum	DIFFUSE; Forehead, crown, shoulders, neck, temples; Vita Flex points; Massage	Dilute 1:1

Blend Name	Single Oil Contents	Uses/Application Areas	Safety Data
Magnify Your Purpose	Sandalwood, rosewood, sage, nutmeg, patchouli, cinnamon bark, ginger	Vita Flex points; Feet, wrists, *temples*; Diffuse; Bath; Massage	E, P, CS, SI
Melrose	Melaleuca (*alternifolia* & *quinquenervia*), rosemary cineol, clove	Diffuse; Forehead, liver; Topically on location	CS, SI Dilute 1:1
Mister	Sage, fennel, lavender, myrtle, peppermint, yarrow (Carrier: Sesame seed oil)	Vita Flex points; Ankles, lower pelvis, prostate (dilute); Compress	P*, E
Motivation	Roman chamomile, spruce, ylang ylang, lavender	Diffuse; Chest, neck; *Solar plexus*, sternum, feet, navel, ears; wrists, palms; Perfume	
PanAway	Wintergreen, helichrysum, clove, peppermint	Compress on spine; Vita Flex on feet; Topically on location	Dilute 1:1
Peace & Calming	Tangerine, orange, ylang ylang, patchouli, blue tansy	Diffuse; Navel, nose, neck, feet; Bath; Perfume	PH
Present Time	Neroli, spruce, ylang ylang (Carrier: Almond oil)	*Thymus*; Neck, forehead	
Purification	Citronella, lemongrass, rosemary cineol, melaleuca, lavandin, myrtle	Diffuse; Vita Flex points; Ears, feet, temples; Topically on location	CS, SI
Raven	Ravensara, lemon, wintergreen, peppermint, *Eucalyptus radiata*	Diffuse; Vita Flex points; Lungs, throat; Pillow; Suppository (diluted)	SI Dilute 1:1
RC	Eucalyptus (*E. globulus*), myrtle, pine, marjoram, *Eucalyptus radiata*, *Eucalyptus citriodora*, lavender, cypress, tsuga, peppermint	DIFFUSE; Chest, back, feet; Sinuses, nasal passages; Ears, neck, throat; Compress; Massage	
Release	Ylang ylang, lavandin, geranium, sandalwood, blue tansy (Carrier: Olive oil)	*Compress on liver*; Ears, feet, Vita Flex points; Perfume	Dilute 1:1
Relieve It	Spruce, Black pepper, hyssop, peppermint	Apply on location of pain	SI, P, E, HBP Dilute 1:1
RutaVaLa	Ruta, valerian, lavender	***Aromatic Use Only!*** Diffuse; Direct inhalation	P*, PH*
Sacred Mountain	Spruce, ylang ylang, fir, cedarwood	Diffuse; *Solar plexus, brain stem*, crown, neck, ears, thymus, wrists; Perfume	SI
SARA	Ylang ylang, geranium, lavender, orange, blue tansy, cedarwood, rose, white lotus (Carrier: Almond oil)	*Energy centers*; Vita Flex points; *Temples, nose*; Places of abuse	
SclarEssence	Clary sage, peppermint, sage lavender, fennel	Internally as dietary supplement	
Sensation	Rosewood, ylang ylang, jasmine	Diffuse; Apply on location; Massage; Bath	
Stress Away *(Roll-on)*	Copaiba, lime, cedarwood, ocotea, lavender	Wrists, temples, neck; Other desired areas	P, SI
Surrender	Lavender, Roman chamomile, German chamomile, angelica, mountain savory, lemon, spruce	*Forehead, rim of ears, nape of neck, chest, solar plexus*; Bath	P, SI
The Gift	Frankincense, balsam fir, jasmine, galbanum, myrrh, cistus, spikenard	Diffuse; Skin, wound location, feet, temples, neck; Bath	SI, P

Blend Name	Single Oil Contents	Uses/Application Areas	Safety Data
Thieves	Clove, lemon, cinnamon bark, *Eucalyptus radiata*, rosemary cineol	Diffuse; Feet, throat, stomach, intestines; Thymus, arm pits (Dilute well for topical uses!)	CS*, SI, P Dilute 1:4
3 Wise Men	Sandalwood, juniper, frankincense, spruce, myrrh (Carrier: Almond oil)	Diffuse; *Crown of head*; Neck, forehead, solar plexus, thymus; Perfume	
Tranquil *(Roll-on)*	Lavender, cedarwood, Roman chamomile (Carriers: Fractionated coconut oil and virgin coconut oil)	Forehead, temples, neck, wrists	
Transformation	Lemon, pepperming, clary sage, sandalwood, Idaho blue spruce, sacred frankincense, cardamom, palo santo, ocotea	Diffuse; *Forehead, heart*	
Trauma Life	Frankincense, sandalwood, valerian, lavender, davana, spruce, geranium, helichrysum, *Citrus hystrix* (leech lime), rose	Diffuse; Spine; Feet, chest, ears, neck, forehead	
Valor	Spruce, rosewood, blue tansy, frankincense (Carrier: Almond oil)	*FEET*; Diffuse; Heart, wrists, solar plexus, neck to thymus, spine; Perfume	
Valor *(Roll-on)*	Spruce, rosewood, frankincense, blue tansy (Carriers: Fractionated coconut oil and virgin coconut oil)	Wrists, solar plexus, neck, spine	
White Angelica	Bergamot, geranium, myrrh, sandalwood, rosewood, ylang ylang, spruce, hyssop, melissa, rose (Carrier: Almond oil)	Diffuse; *Shoulders*, crown, chest, ears, neck, forehead, wrists; Bath; Perfume	PH*

Note: Italicized application areas represent the most effective areas for **emotional applications**.

Safety Data Legend:

A	**Avoid** during and after consumption of **alcohol**
CS	Could possibly result in **contact sensitization** (redness or irritation of the skin due to repeated application of a substance) (rotate or use different oils)
CS*	Repeated use may result in **extreme contact sensitization** (rotate between different oils)
D	**Avoid** if **diabetic**
E	Use with **caution** if susceptible to **epilepsy** (small amounts or in dilution)
E*	**Avoid** if susceptible to **epilepsy** (can trigger a seizure)
HBP	Use with **caution** if dealing with **high blood pressure** (small amounts)
HBP*	**Avoid** if dealing with **high blood pressure**
P	Use with **caution** during **pregnancy** (small amounts or in dilution)
P*	**Avoid** during **pregnancy**
PH	**Photosensitivity**—direct exposure to sunlight after use could cause dermatitis (test first)
PH*	**Extreme photosensitivity**—direct exposure to sunlight after use can cause severe dermatitis (avoid exposing affected area of skin to direct sunlight for 12 hours)
SI	Could possibly result in **skin irritation** (dilution may be necessary)
SI*	Can cause **extreme skin irritation** (dilution highly recommended)
ST	Can cause **stupefication** in high doses (use only small amounts or in dilution)
Dilute	Dilution ratios shown equal Essential Oil:Vegetable Oil

TAXONOMICAL INFORMATION

The following chart is the taxonomical breakdown of the plant families for each of the essential oils found in this book. On the pages following this division chart, there is further information for each family, including the plants within that family that essential oils are derived from, the body systems affected by these essential oils, the properties of these oils, and general uses for these oils.

Division: Embryophyte Siphonogama (plants with seeds)
- Subdivision: Gymnosperm (plants with concentric rings, exposed seeds, & resinous wood)
  - Class: Coniferae (cone-bearing plants) & Taxaceae (yew-like plants)
    - Family: **Pinaceae** (Trees or shrubs with cones and numerous "scales")
      - Genus: Abies (firs, balsam trees), Cedrus (cedars), Pinus (pines), Picea (spruces), Pseudotsuga (false hemlock), Tsuga (hemlocks)
    - Family: **Cupressaceae**
      - Genus: Callitris (blue cypress), Cupressus (cypresses), Juniperus (junipers), Thuja (Arbor vitae or cedars)
- Subdivision: Angiosperm (highly evolved plants with seeds enclosed by fruits)
  - Class: Monocotyledons (plants with one-leaf embryos)
    - Family: **Gramineae, Zingiberaceae**
  - Class: Dicotyledons (plants with multiple-leaf embryos)
    - Family: **Anacardiaceae, Annonaceae, Betulaceae, Burseraceae, Cistaceae, Compositae, Ericaceae, Geraniaceae, Guttiferae, Labiatae, Lauraceae, Myristicaceae, Myrtaceae, Oleaceae, Piperaceae, Rosaceae, Rutaceae, Santalaceae, Styracaceae, Umbelliferae, Valerianaceae**

ANACARDIACEAE (consists of about 850 species in 73 genera of mostly subtropical and tropical resinous trees, shrubs, and climbers; drupe type fruit.)
Body Systems: Lymphatic System, Respiratory System, Water balance
Properties: detoxifying, astringent action
General Uses: congestion (lymphatic, respiratory), hypotension, arthritis, psoriasis
Schinus molle: California pepper tree (Pink pepper)

ANNONACEAE (shrubs, trees, climbers; fragrant flowers; 128 genera, 2000 species; mostly tropical, found in Old World & rain forest)
Body Systems: Cardiovascular System, Nervous System (calming), Hormonal System (aphrodisiac)
Properties: extreme fire and water; nervous sedative, balancing
General Uses: depression, frigidity, impotence, palpitations, skin care
Cananga odorata; two forms exist:
- var. odorata (var. genuina, *Unona odorantissimum*): ylang ylang
- var. macrophylla: cananga

BETULACEAE (shrubs, trees; fruit is one-seeded nut, often winged; includes birches, alders, hornbeams and hazels; 6 genera, 150 species; from northern hemisphere to tropical mountains)
Body Systems: Digestive and Respiratory Systems, Muscles and Bones
Properties: analgesic, draining (lymph), purifying
General Uses: auto intoxication, muscle pain
Betula lenta: sweet birch

BURSERACEAE (means "dry fire"; resinous tropical timber trees; drupe or capsule fruit; 21 genera, 540 species)
Body Systems: Respiratory System (secretions), Emotional Balance (psychic centers),
Skin Properties: cooling, drying, fortifying
General Uses: anti-inflammatory, expectorant, scar tissue (reducing), ulcers, wounds (healing)
Boswellia carterii: frankincense
Bursera graveolens: palo santo
Canarium luzonicum: elemi
Commiphora myrrha: myrrh

CISTACEAE (low shrubs, few herbs; capsule fruit; Cistus species have large flowers; 7 genera, 175 species; Mediterranean, Europe, central Asia and America)
Body Systems: Emotional Balance, Skin (care)
Properties: calming, fortifying, healing
General Uses: anxiety, depression, stress-related disorders, wound healing
Cistus ladanifer: labdanum, cistus

COMPOSITAE (ASTERACEAE) (largest family of flowering plants; inflorescence, small flowers; 1317 genera, 21,000 species; found everywhere, especially around Mediterranean)
Body Systems: Digestive System, Skin
Properties: "perfect balance of etheric and astral forces, promoting realization, reorganization, structure" (Lavabre, *Aromatherapy Workbook*); adaptive, calming, regenerating (note: because of the large variety of plants within this family, the therapeutic activity is very diversified; some plants are neurotoxic)
General Uses: infections, inflammation, regeneration
Achillea millefolium: yarrow

Artemisia dracunculus: tarragon
Artemisia pallens: davana
Artemisia vulgaris: mugwort
Chamaemelum nobile: Roman chamomile
Conyza canadensis: Canadian fleabane
Helichrysum angustifolium (var. *Italicum*): helichrysum
Matricaria recutita: German chamomile
Solidago odora (*Solidago canadensis*): goldenrod
Tanacetum annum: blue tansy
Tanacetum vulgare: wild tansy

CUPRESSACEAE (conifer cypress family, needle-like leaves and cones; 17 genera, 113 species; most in northern temperate zones)
Body Systems: Hormonal, Respiratory, and Nervous Systems
Properties: appeasing, reviving, tonic, warming
General Uses: antirheumatic, astringent, cellulite (reduces), insomnia, nervous tension (reduces), respiration (when inhaled), stress-related conditions
Callitris intratropica: blue cypress
Cupressus sempervirens: cypress
Juniperus communis: juniper
Juniperus scopulorum (*J. osteosperma*): Rocky Mountain juniper
Thuja occidentalis: cedar leaf
Thuja plicata: Western red cedar (leaf)

ERICACEAE (shrubs and small trees with leathery evergreen leaves, fruit berry, drupe or capsule; 103 genera, 3350 species; cosmopolitan centered in northern hemisphere)
Body Systems: Cardiovascular and Digestive Systems
Properties: detoxifying
General Uses: hypertension, kidney and liver stimulant
Ledum groenlandicum: Labrador tea
Gaultheria procumbens: wintergreen

GERANIACEAE (herbs or low shrubs, 14 genera, 730 species; temperate and tropical zones)
Body Systems: Hormonal System, Digestive System (kidneys - excretion, liver & pancreas - metabolism), Nervous System, Emotional Balance
Properties: balancing (nervous system)
General Uses: burns, depression, diabetes, hemorrhage, nervous tension, skin, sore throat, ulcers, wounds
Pelargonium graveolens: geranium

GRAMINEAE (or POACEAE) (nutritious grass family; used for ground covering and food (wheat, rice, corn, barley); large root systems; 737 genera, 7950 species; distributed throughout the world)
Body Systems: Cardiovascular System, Digestive System (stimulant), Respiratory System, Skin
Properties: air purifier, calming, refreshing, sedative
General Uses: air deodorizer, calm digestion, cleanse and balance skin (acne)
Cymbopogon flexuosus: lemongrass
Cymbopogon martinii: palmarosa
Cymbopogon nardus: citronella
Vetiveria zizanoides: vetiver

GUTTIFERAE (or HYPERICACEAE) (trees and shrubs; many useful for timber and edible fruits; 47 genera, 1350 species; tropics)
Body Systems: Muscles and Bones, Skin
Properties: anti-inflammatory, analgesic
General Uses: infections, muscle pain, wounds
Calophyllum inophyllum: tamanu

LABIATAE (LAMIACEAE) (herbs or low shrubs with quadrangular stems; largest of all essential oil–producing plant families; oils are mostly nontoxic and nonhazardous; some antiseptic oils; some oils used for flavoring; most oils helpful for headaches, congestion, muscular problems (analgesic, anti-inflammatory), and stimulating one or more body systems; 224 genera, about 5600 species; main distribution in tropical and warmer temperate regions)
Body Systems: Digestive and Respiratory Systems
Properties: appeases overactive astral body [Lavabre, *Aromatherapy Workbook*], curative, stimulates, warms
General Uses: anemia, diabetes, digestion (poor), headaches, respiratory problems; "good for people with intense psychic activity to prevent exhaustion and loss of self" (Lavabre, *Aromatherapy Workbook*)
Hyssopus officinalis: hyssop
Lavandula angustifolia: lavender
Lavandula x hybrida: lavandin
Melissa officinalis: melissa
Mentha piperita: peppermint
Mentha spicata: spearmint
Ocimum basilicum: basil
Origanum majorana: marjoram
Origanum vulgare: oregano
Pogostemon cablin: patchouli

Rosmarinus officinalis: rosemary several varieties
var. *officinalis*: common rosemary; numerous cultivars and forms;
chemotypes: CT I: camphor; CT II: cineole; CT III: verbenone
Salvia lavendulifolia: Spanish sage
Salvia officinalis: sage *Salvia sclarea*: clary sage
Satureja montana: winter savory
Thymus vulgaris: thyme
chemotypes: linalool; thymol (or geraniol)
Vitex negundo: vitex

LAURACEAE (trees and shrubs with evergreen leaves and aromatic oils; some valued for timber, as ornamentals, or for oils or spices; 45 genera, 200–2500 species; found in tropical and subtropical zones in the Amazons and in Southeast Asia)
Body Systems: Cardiovascular System (cardiac-stimulant, pulmonary-stimulant), Nervous System (regulates), Hormonal System (aphrodisiac), Skin (cellular-regenerative)
Properties: antifungal, antiviral, antibacterial, stimulant, tonic (some oils in this family are irritant)
General Uses: depression, headache, hypotension, scars, sexual debility
Aniba roseodora var. amazonica: Brazilian rosewood, bois de rose
Cinnamomum cassia: cassia
Cinnamomum zeylanicum (*C. verum*): cinnamon bark
Laurus nobilis: laurel
Ravensara aromatica: ravensara

LEGUMINOSEAE (FABACEAE) (the third largest family of flowering plants; 657 genera with about 16,400 species)
Body Systems: Cardiovascular and Respiratory Systems, Emotional Balance, Skin
Properties: antiseptic, physical stimulant; emotionally soothing/warming
General Uses: anxiety, circulation, decongestant (venous), depression
Copaifera reticulata: copaiba

MYRISTICACEAE (plants whose bark produces watery, blood-like exudate; fruit is fleshy with one large seed; 19 genera, about 400 species; found throughout tropics, centered in Malaysia lowland rain forest)
Body Systems: Digestive, Hormonal, and Nervous Systems, Emotional Balance
Properties: analgesic, aphrodisiac, circulation, nervous system stimulant
General Uses: digestion, fatigue (mental and physical), impotence, nervousness, rheumatism
Myristica fragrans: nutmeg

MYRTACEAE (mainly tropical and subtropical plants with dotted leaves and oil glands; fruit is woody capsule or berry with one or many seeds; some have ornamental or showy flowers; many produce valuable timber; 121 genera, 3850 species; found in tropical and warm regions, especially Australia)
Body Systems: Respiratory and Immune Systems
Properties: "balances interaction of four elements (earth, air, fire, water)" (Lavabre, *Aromatherapy Workbook*), antiseptic, stimulant, tonic
General Uses: antiseptic, energy (balances), respiratory (infections), stimulant, tonic
Backhousia citriodora: lemon myrtle
Eucalyptus citriodora: lemon-scented eucalyptus
Eucalyptus dives: peppermint eucalyptus
Eucalyptus globulus: eucalyptus
Eucalyptus polybractea: blue-leaved mallee
chemotype: cineole
Eucalyptus staigeriana: lemon-scented ironbark
Eugenia caryophyllata (*Syzygium aromaticum*): clove bud
Leptospermum scoparium: manuka
Melaleuca alternifolia: tea tree
Melaleuca ericifolia: rosalina
Melaleuca leucadendra: cajeput
Melaleuca quinquenervia: niaouli
Myrtus communis: myrtle (two sub-species exist: green and red)

OLEACEAE (trees or shrubs; including olive and ash; used for timber; 24 genera, 900 species; widely distributed, centered on Asia)
Body Systems: Emotional Balance, Hormonal System (aphrodisiac)
Properties: calming, soothing, uplifting
General Uses: anxiety, depression, frigidity, impotence, stress *Jasminum officinale*: jasmine

PINACEAE (ABIETACEAE) (conifers with male and female cones; 9 genera, 194 species; found in northern hemisphere, temperate climates)
Body Systems: Hormonal, Nervous, and Respiratory Systems; signifies air element
Properties: antiseptic, appeasing, reviving, tonic, warming
General Uses: arthritis, congestion (inhaled), oxygen deficiency, respiratory disorders, rheumatism, stress
Abies alba: fir, silver fir
Abies balsamea: balsam fir
Abies grandis: white fir, giant fir
Cedrus atlantica: Atlas cedarwood
Picea mariana: black spruce

Pinus ponderosa: ponderosa pine
Pinus sylvestris: Scotch pine
Pseudotsuga menziesii: Douglas fir
Tsuga canadensis: hemlock spruce (or tsuga)

PIPERACEAE (pepper family; small trees, shrubs and climbers; small fleshy drupe with single seed; some widely cultivated for condiments; 4 genera, over 2000 species; found throughout tropics, mostly in rainforests)
Body Systems: Cardiovascular, Digestive, and Nervous Systems; root chakra
Properties: drying, heating, stimulant, tonic
General Uses: fevers, indigestion, pain (muscle, tooth), grounding
Piper nigrum: black pepper

ROSACEAE (trees, shrubs, and herbs; some edible fruits; many cultivated for fruits (almond) or flowers (rose); 107 genera, 3100 species; found in temperate climates throughout the world)
Body Systems: Hormonal System (female reproductive); heart chakra
Properties: aphrodisiac, harmonizing, tonic, uplifting
General Uses: emotional shock, frigidity, grief, impotence
Rosa canina: rosehip
Rosa damascena: Bulgarian rose

RUTACEAE (aromatic trees and shrubs; sometimes thorny; dotted, compound leaves with aromatic glands; includes citrus fruits; 161 genera, about 1650 species; found in tropical and warm temperate regions, especially Australia and South Africa)
Body Systems: Digestive (kidneys, liver) and Nervous Systems, Skin
Properties: cooling, refreshing, secretion (fruits), sedative (flowers)
General Uses: inflammation, over-sensitivity, water balance
Citrus aurantifolia: lime
Citrus aurantium: neroli (var. *bigaradia*), petitgrain
Citrus bergamia: bergamot
Citrus hystrix: leech lime
Citrus limon: lemon
Citrus nobilis: tangerine
Citrus x paradisi: grapefruit
Citrus reticulate: mandarin
Citrus sinensis: orange

SANTALACEAE (herbs, shrubs and trees which are semiparasitic on roots and stems of other plants; 36 genera, about 500 species; found in tropical and temperate regions)
Body Systems: Digestive System (excretory balance, genitourinary disinfectant), Nervous System (balances), and Respiratory System (balances)
Properties: balancing, calming, constriction, grounding
General Uses: genitourinary tract infections, impotence, lung congestion, stress-related disorders
Santalum album: East Indian sandalwood, Mysore sandalwood, sandalwood

STYRACACEAE (trees and shrubs with resinous bark used medicinally; used for incense, obtained by wounding tree; 12 genera, 165 species; found in tropical and warm temperate climates in Americas, Malaysia, Mediterranean, and Southeast Asia)
Body Systems: Cardiovascular and Nervous Systems; first chakra
Properties: calming, grounding, soothing
General Uses: hyperactivity
Styrax benzoin: benzoin, onycha

UMBELLIFERAE (APIACEAE) (herbs and a few shrubs, flowers borne in umbels [flowers radiating from a central point, like an umbrella]); some important as food (carrot, celery), while others are very poisonous; some have medicinal actions; 420 genera, 3100 species; found throughout the world, mainly in northern temperate regions)
Body Systems: Digestive System (balances), Hormonal System (stimulates uterus), Respiratory System, Skin (regenerates)
Properties: air element; accumulation (elimination, excretion), secretion
General Uses: gas, glandular problems, spasms
Anethum graveolens: dill
Angelica archangelica: angelica
Apium graveolens: celery
Carum carvi: caraway
Coriandrum sativum: coriander
Cuminum cyminum: cumin
Daucus carota: carrot seed oil
Ferula galbaniflua: galbanum
Foeniculum vulgare: fennel
Pimpinella anisum: aniseed

VALERIANACEAE (herb family; fruit is dry; roots often used medicinally [valium]; 17 genera, 14 species; found throughout the world [except Australia])
Body Systems: Nervous System (calming)

Properties: grounding, sedative; balances upper and lower body
General Uses: anxiety, insomnia, nervous headaches, palpitations, stomach; living in one's head
Nardostachys jatamansi: spikenard
Valeriana officinalis: valerian

ZINGIBERACEAE (ginger family comprising rhizomatous herbs; 53 genera, 1200 species; found mostly in rain forests throughout the tropics, but mainly in Indo-Malaysia)
Body Systems: Digestive and Hormonal Systems, Muscles and Bones
Properties: analgesic, fever-reducing, scurvy (prevents), stimulant, tonic, warming
General Uses: digestive (stimulant), rheumatism, sexual tonic
Elettaria cardamomum: cardamom
Zingiber officinale: ginger

Research References

Abdel-Sattar E, Zaitoun AA, Farag MA, El Gayed SH, Harraz FM (2009 Feb 25). "Chemical composition, insecticidal and insect repellent activity of Schinus molle L. leaf and fruit essential oils against Trogoderma granarium and Tribolium castaneum," Nat Prod Res. Epub ahead of print:1-10.

Abrams SA, Griffin IJ, Hawthorne KM, Liang L, Gunn SK, Darlington G, Ellis KJ (2005 Aug). "A combination of prebiotic short- and long-chain inulin-type fructans enhances calcium absorption and bone mineralization in young adolescents," Am J Clin Nutr. 82(2):471-6.

Alexandrovich I, Rakovitskaya O, Kolmo E, Sidorova T, Shushunov S (2003 Jul-Aug). "The effect of fennel (Foeniculum Vulgare) seed oil emulsion in infantile colic: a randomized, placebo-controlled study," Altern Ther Health Med. 9(4):58-61.

Almela L, Sánchez-Muñoz B, Fernández-López JA, Roca MJ, Rabe V (2006 Jul). "Liquid chromatograpic-mass spectrometric analysis of phenolics and free radical scavenging activity of rosemary extract from different raw material," J Chromatogr A. 1120(1-2):221-9.

al-Zuhair H, el-Sayeh B, Ameen HA, al-Shoora H (1996 Jul-Aug). "Pharmacological studies of cardamom oil in animals," Pharmacol Res. 34(1-2):79-82.

Anderson R.C., Krueger N.A., Byrd J.A., Harvey R.B., Callaway T.R., Edrington T.S., Nisbet D.J. (2009) Effects of thymol and diphenyliodonium chloride against Campylobacter spp. during pure and mixed culture in vitro. Journal of Applied Microbiology. 107: 1258-1268.

Andrews R.E., Parks L.W., Spence K.D. (1980) Some Effects of Douglas Fir Terpenes on Certain Microorganisms. Applied and Environmental Microbiology. 40: 301-304.

Andrian E., Grenier D., Rouabhia M. (2006) Porphyromonas gingivalis-Epithelial Cell Interactions in Periodontitis. Journal of Dental Research. 85: 392-403.

Appendino G, Ottino M, Marquez N, Bianchi F, Giana A, Ballero M, Sterner O, Fiebich BL, Munoz E (2007 Apr). "Arzanol, an anti-inflammatory and anti-HIV-1 phloroglucinol alpha-Pyrone from Helichrysum italicum ssp. microphyllum," J Nat Prod. 70(4):608-12.

Arasada BL, Bommareddy A, Zhang X, Bremmon K, Dwivedi C. (2008 Jan-Feb). "Effects of alpha-santalol on proapoptotic caspases and p53 expression in UVB irradiated mouse skin," Anticancer Res. 28(1A):129-32.

Arias P., Cudeiro J. (2008) Effects of rhythmic sensory stimulation (auditory, visual) on gait in Parkinson's disease patients. Experimental Brain Research. 186: 589-601.

Ariyoshi T., Arakaki M., Ideguchi K., Ishizuka Y. (1975) Studies on the Metabolism of d-Limonene (?-Mentha-1,8-diene). III. Effects of d-Limonene on the Lipids and Drug-Metabolizing Enzmes in Rat Livers. Xenobiotica. 5: 33-38.

Atkinson D.C., Hicks R. (1971) Relationship between the anti-inflammatory and irritant properties of inflammatory exudate. British Journal of Pharmacology. 41: 480-487.

Badia P, Wesensten N, Lammers W, Culpepper J, Harsh J (1990 Jul). "Responsiveness to olfactory stimuli presented in sleep," Physiol Behav. 48(1):87-90.

Bakirel T, Bakirel U, Keleş OU, Ulgen SG, Yardibi H (2008 Feb 28). "In vivo assessment of antidiabetic and antioxidant activities of rosemary (Rosmarinus officinalis) in alloxan-diabetic rabbits," J Ethnopharmacol. 116(1):64-73.

Bakkai F., Averbeck S., Averbeck D., Idaomar M. (2008) Biological effects of essential oils - A review. Food and Chemical Toxicology. 46: 446-475.

Balanehru S., Nagarajan B. (1991) Protective Effect of Oleanolic Acid and Ursolic Acid Against Lipid Peroxidation. Biochemistry International. 24: 981-990.

Ballabeni V, Tognolini M, Giorgio C, Bertoni S, Bruni R, Barocelli E (2009 Oct 13). "Ocotea quixos Lam. essential oil: In vitro and in vivo investigation on its anti-inflammatory properties," Fitoterapia. Epub ahead of print.

Balzer J, Rassaf T, Heiss C, Kleinbongard P, Lauer T, Merx M, Heussen N, Gross HB, Keen CL, Schroeter H, Kelm M (2008 Jun 3). "Sustained benefits in vascular function through flavanol-containing cocoa in medicated diabetic patients a double-masked, randomized, controlled trial," J Am Coll Cardiol. 51(22):2141-9).

Banerjee S, Ecavade A, Rao AR (1993 Feb). "Modulatory influence of sandalwood oil on mouse hepatic glutathione S-transferase activity and acid soluble sulphydryl level," Cancer Lett. 68(2-3):105-9.

Banno N, Akihisa T, Yasukawa K, Tokuda H, Tabata K, Nakamura Y, Nishimura R, Kimura Y, Suzuki T (2006 Sep 19). "Anti-inflammatory activities of the triterpene acids from the resin of Boswellia carterii," J Ethnopharmacol. 107(2):249-53.

Barthelman M., Chen W., Gensler H.L., Huang C., Dong Z., Bowden G.T. (1998) Inhibitory Effects of Perillyl Alcohol on UVB-induced Murine Skin Cancer and AP-1 Transactivation. Cancer Research. 58: 711-716.

Basketter D.A., Wright Z.M., Colson N.R., Patewicz G.Y., Pease C.K.S. (2002) Investigation of the skin sensitizing activity of linalool. Contact Dermatitis. 47: 161-164.

Bastos J.F.A., Moreira I.J., Ribeiro T.P., Medeiros I.A., Antoniolli A.R., de Sousa D.P., Santos M.R.V. (2009) Hypotensive and Vasorelaxant Effects of Cirtonellol, a Monoterpene Alcohol, in Rats. Basic & Clinical Pharmacology & Toxicology. 106: 331-337.

Behnam S, Farzaneh M, Ahmadzadeh M, Tehrani AS (2006). "Composition and antifungal activity of essential oils of Mentha piperita and Lavandula angustifolia on post-harvest phytopathogens," Commun Agric Appl Biol Sci. 71(3 Pt B):1321-6.

Berchtold N.C., Cotman C.W. (1997) Evolution in the Conceptulization of Dementia and Alzheimer's Disease: Greco-Roman Period to the 1960s. Neurobiology of Aging. 19: 173-189.

Berić T, Nikolić B, Stanojević J, Vuković-Gacić B, Knezević-Vukcević J (2008 Feb). "Protective effect of basil (Ocimum basilicum L.) against oxidative DNA damage and mutagenesis," Food Chem Toxicol. 46(2):724-32.

Bezanilla F. (2006) The action potential: From voltage-gated conductances to molecular structures. Biological Research. 39: 425-435.

Birari R.B., Bhutani K.K. (2007) Pancreatic lipase inhibitors from natural sources: unexplored potential. Drug Discovery Today. 12: 879-889.

Bone ME, Wilkinson DJ, Young JR, McNeil J, Charlton S (1990 Aug). "Ginger root--a new antiemetic. The effect of ginger root on postoperative nausea and vomiting after major gynaecological surgery," Anaesthesia. 45(8):669-71.

Bouwstra J.A., Gooris G.S., Dubbelaar F.E.R., Weeheim A.M., Ijzerman A.P., Ponec M. (1998) Role of ceramide 1 in the molecular organization of the stratum corneum lipids. Journal of Lipid Research. 39: 186-196.

Bradford H.F. (1995) Glutamate, GABA, and Epilepsy. Progress in Neurobiology. 47: 477-511.

Bradley BF, Brown SL, Chu S, Lea RW (2009 Jun). "Effects of orally administered lavender essential oil on responses to anxiety-provoking film clips," Hum Psychopharmacol. 24(4):319-30.

Brady A, Loughlin R, Gilpin D, Kearney P, Tunney M (2006 Oct). "In vitro activity of tea-tree oil against clinical skin isolates of methicillin-resistant and -sensitive Staphylococcus aureus and coagulase-negative staphylococci growing planktonically and as biofilms," J Med Microbiol. 55(Pt 10):1375-80.

Brand C, Grimbaldeston MA, Gamble JR, Drew J, Finlay-Jones JJ, Hart PH (2002 May). "Tea tree oil reduces the swelling associated with the efferent phase of a contact hypersensitivity response," Inflamm Res. 51(5):236-44.

Brum LF, Elisabetsky E, Souza D (2001 Aug). "Effects of linalool on [(3)H]MK801 and [(3)H] muscimol binding in mouse cortical membranes," Phytother Res. 15(5):422-5.

Buchbauer G, Jirovetz L, Jäger W, Dietrich H, Plank C (1991 Nov-Dec). "Aromatherapy: evidence for sedative effects of the essential oil of lavender after inhalation," Z Naturforsch [C]. 46(11-12):1067-72.

Bulbring E. (1946) Observations on the Isolated Phrenic Nerve Diaphragm Preparation of the Rat. British Journal of Pharmacology. 1: 38-61.

Burke BE, Baillie JE, Olson RD (2004 May). "Essential oil of Australian lemon myrtle (Backhousia citriodora) in the treatment of molluscum contagiosum in children," Biomed Pharmacother. 58(4):245-7.

Burke Y.D., Stark J., Roach S.L., Sen S.E., Crowell P.L. (1997) Inhibition of Pancreatic Cancer Growth by the Dietary Isoprenoids Farnesol and Geraniol. Lipids. 32: 151-156.

Burt S. (2004) Essential oils: their antibacterial properties and potential applications in foods - a reivew. International Journal of Food Microbiology. 94: 223-253.

Caldefie-Chézet F, Fusillier C, Jarde T, Laroye H, Damez M, Vasson MP, Guillot J (2006 May). "Potential anti-inflammatory effects of Melaleuca alternifolia essential oil on human peripheral blood leukocytes," Phytother Res. 20(5):364-70.

Candan F, Unlu M, Tepe B, Daferera D, Polissiou M, Sökmen A, Akpulat HA (2003 Aug). "Antioxidant and antimicrobial activity of the essential oil and methanol extracts of Achillea millefolium subsp. millefolium Afan. (Asteraceae)," J Ethnopharmacol. 87(2-3):215-20.

Capasso R, Savino F, Capasso F (2007 Oct). "Effects of the herbal formulation ColiMil on upper gastrointestinal transit in mice in vivo," Phytother Res. 21(10):999-1101.

Carlsson L., Larsson A., Lindman H. (2009) Elevated levels of thymidine kinase 1 peptide in serum from patients with breast cancer. Upsala Journal of Medical Sciences. 114: 116-120.
Carnesecchi S., Bradaia A., Fischer B., Coelho D., Scholler-Guinard M., Gosse F., Raul F. (2002) Perturbation by Geraniol of Cell Membrane Permeability and Signal Transduction Pathways in Human Colon Cancer Cells. The Journal of Pharmacology and Experimental Therapeutics. 303: 711-715.
Carnesecchi S., Bras-Goncalves R., Bradaia A., Zeisel M., Gosse F., Poupon M-F., Raul F. (2004) Geraniol, a component of plant essential oils, modulates DNA synthesis and potentiates 5-fluorouracil efficacy on human colon tumor xenografts. Cancer Letters. 215: 53-59.
Carnesecchi S., Langley K., Exinger F., Gosse F., Raul F. (2002) Geraniol, a Component of Plant Essential Oils, Sensitizes Human Colonic Cancer Cells to 5-Flurouracil Treatment. The Journal of Pharmacology and Experimental Therapeutics. 301: 625-630.
Carnesecchi S, Schneider Y, Ceraline J, Duranton B, Gosse F, Seiler N, Raul F (2001 Jul). "Geraniol, a component of plant essential oils, inhibits growth and polyamine biosynthesis in human colon cancer cells," J Pharmacol Exp Ther. 298(1):197-200.
Carreras C.W., Santi D.V. (1995) The Catalytic Mechanism and Structure of Thymidylate Synthase. Anuual Review of Biochemistry. 64: 721-762.
Carroll M.C. (2004) The complement system in regulation of adaptive immunity. Nature Immunology. 5: 981-986.
Carvalho-Freitas MI, Costa M (2002 Dec). "Anxiolytic and sedative effects of extracts and essential oil from Citrus aurantium L," Biol Pharm Bull. 25(12):1629-33.
Cavalieri E., Bergamini C., Mariotto S., Leoni S., Perbellini G., Darra E., Suzuki H., Fato R., Lenaz G. (2009) Involvement of mitochondrial permeability transition pore opening in ?-bisabolol induced apoptosis. FEBS Journal. 276: 3990-4000.
Cavalieri E., Mariotto S., Fabrizi C., de Prati A.C., Gottardo R., Leone S., Berra L.V., Lauro G.M., Ciampa A.R., Suzuki H. (2004) ?-Bisabolol, a nontoxic natural compound, strongly induced apoptosis in glioma cells. Biochemical and Biophysical Research Communications. 315: 589-594.
Ceccarelli I, Lariviere WR, Fiorenzani P, Sacerdote P, Aloisi AM (2004 Mar 19). "Effects of long-term exposure of lemon essential oil odor on behavioral, hormonal and neuronal parameters in male and female rats," Brain Res. 1001(1-2):78-86.
Chaieb K, Zmantar T, Ksouri R, Hajlaoui H, Mahdouani K, Abdelly C, Bakhrouf A (2007 Sep). "Antioxidant properties of the essential oil of Eugenia caryophyllata and its antifungal activity against a large number of clinical Candida species," Mycoses. 50(5):403-6.
Chambers H.F. (2001) The Changing Epidemiology of Staphylococcus aureus?. Emerging Infectious Diseases. 7: 178-182.
Chapman A.G. (1998) Glutamate receptors in epilepsy. Progress in Brain Research. 116: 371-383.
Chapman A.G. (2000) Glutamate and Epilepsy. The Journal of Nutrition. 130: 1043S-1045S.
Charles CH, Vincent JW, Borycheski L, Amatnieks Y, Sarina M, Qaqish J, Proskin HM (2000 Sep). "Effect of an essential oil-containing dentifrice on dental plaque microbial composition," Am J Dent. 13:26C-30C.
Cheung S, Tai J (2007 Jun). "Anti-proliferative and antioxidant properties of rosemary Rosmarinus officinalis," Oncol Rep. 17(6):1525-31.
Chinou IB, Roussis V, Perdetzoglou D, Loukis A (1996 Aug). "Chemical and biological studies on two Helichrysum species of Greek origin," Planta Med. 62(4):377-9.
Chow H.H.S., Salazar D., Hakim I.A. (2002) Pharmacokinetics of Perillic Acid in Humans after a Single Dose Administration of a Citrus Preparation Rich in d-Limonene Content. Cancer Epidemiology, Biomarkers & Prevention. 11: 1472-1476.
Ciftci O., Ozdemir I., Tanyildizl S., Yildiz S., Oguzturk H. (2011) Antioxidative effects of curcumin, ?-myrcene and 1,8-cineole against 2,3,7,8-tetracholorodibenzo-p-dioxin - induced oxidative stress in rats liver. Toxicology and Industrial Health. 27: 447-453.
Clericuzio M., Alagona G., Ghio C., Toma L. (2000) Ab Initio and Density Functional Evaluations of the Molecular Conformations of ?-Caryophyllene and 6-Hydroxy-caryophyllene. Journal of Organic Chemistry. 65: 6910-6916.
Coderch L., Lopez O., de la Maza A., Parra J.L. (2003) Ceramides and Skin Function. American Journal of Clinical Dermatology. 4: 107-129.
Contractor A., Swanson G.T., Sailer A., O'Gorman S., Heinemann S.F. (2000) Identification of the Kainate Receptor Subunits Underlying Modulation of Excitatory Synaptic Transmission in the CA3 Region of the Hippocampus. The Journal of Neuroscience. 20: 8260-8278.
Cooke B., Ernst E. (2000) Aromatherapy: a systematic review. British Journal of General Practice. 50: 493-496.
Crestell T., Monsarrat B., Alvinerie P., Treluyer J.M., Vieira I., Wright M. (1994) Taxol Metabolism by Human Liver Microsomes: Identification of Cytochrome P450 Isozymes Involved in Its Biotransformation. Cancer Research. 54: 386-392.
Cross SE, Russell M, Southwell I, Roberts MS (2008 May). "Human skin penetration of the major components of Australian tea tree oil applied in its pure form and as a 20% solution in vitro," Eur J Pharm Biopharm. 69(1):214-22.
Crowell P.L. (1997) Monoterpenes in breast cancer chemoprevention. Breast Cancer Research and Treatment. 46: 191-197.
Crowell P.L. (1999) Prevention and Therapy of Cancer by Dietary Monoterpenes. J. Nutr. 129:775S-778S.
Crowell P.L., Chang R.R., Ren Z., Elson C.E., Gould M.N. (1991) Selective Inhibition of Isoprenylation of 21-26kDa Proteins by the Anticarcinogen d-Limonene and Its Metabolites. J. Biol. Chem. 266: 17679-17685.
D'Auria FD, Laino L, Strippoli V, Tecca M, Salvatore G, Battinelli L, Mazzanti G (2001 Aug). "In vitro activity of tea tree oil against Candida albicans mycelial conversion and other pathogenic fungi," J Chemother. 13(4):377-83.
Damiani C.E.N., Rossoni L.V., Vassallo D.V. (2003) Vasorelaxant effects of eugenol on rat thoracic aorta. Vascular Pharmacology. 40: 59-66. "
Darra E., Abdel-Azeim S., Manara A., Shoji K., Marechal J-D., Mariotto S., Cavalieri E., Perbellini L., Pizza C., Perahia D., Crimi M., Suzuki H. (2008) Insight into the apoptosis-inducing action of ?-bisabolol towards malignant tumor cells: Involvement of lipid rafts and Bid. Archives of Biochemistry and Biophysics. 476: 113-123.
de Almeida R.N., Araujo D.A.M., Goncalvevs J.C.R., Montenegro F.C., de Sousa D.P., Leite J.R., Mattei R., Benedito M.A.C., de Carvalho J.G.B., Cruz J.S., Maia J.G.S. (2009) Rosewood oil induces sedation and inhibits compound action petential in rodents. Journal of Ethanopharmacology. 124: 440-443.
de Almeida R.N., de Sousa D.P., Nobrega F.F.F., Claudino F.S., Araujo D.A.M., Leite J.R., Mattei R. (2008) Anticonvulsant effect of a natural compound ?,?-epoxy-carvone and its actioin on the nerve excitability. Neuroscience Letters. 443: 51-55.
de Araujo D.A.M., Freitas C., Cruz J.S. (2011) Essential oils components as a new path to understand ion channel molecular pharmacology. Life Sciences. doi: 10.1016/j.lfs.2011.04.020
Debersac P, Heydel JM, Amiot MJ, Goudonnet H, Artur Y, Suschetet M, Siess MH (2001 Sep). "Induction of cytochrome P450 and/or detoxication enzymes by various extracts of rosemary: description of specific patterns," Food Chem Toxicol. 39(9):907-18.
De Carvalho C.C.C.R., da Fonseca M.M.R. (2006) Carvone: Why and how should one bother to produce this terpene. Food Chemistry. 95: 413-422.
de Gruijl F.R. (1999) Skin Cancer and Solar UV Radiation. European Journal of Cancer. 35: 2003-2009.
de Sousa D.P. (2011) Analgesic-like Activity of Essential Oils Constituents. Molecules. 16: 2233-2252.
de Sousa D.P., Goncalves J.C.R., Quintanas-Junior L., Cruz J.S., Araujo D.A.M., de Almeida R.N. (2006) Study of anticonvulsant effect of citronellol, a monoterpene alcohol, in rodents. Neuroscience Letters. 401: 231-235.
Decker K. (1990) Biologically active products of stimulated liver macrophages (Kupffer cells). European Journal of Biochemistry. 192: 245-261.
DeLeo F.R., Otto M., Kreiswirth B.N., Chambers H.F. (2010) Community-associated meticillin-resistant Staphylococcus aureus. The Lancet. 375: 1557-1568.
De-Oliveira A.C.A.X., Ribeiro-Pinto L.F., Paumgartten F.J.R. (1997) In vitro inhibition of CYP2B1 monooxygenase by ?-myrcene and other monoterpenoid compounds. Toxicology Letters. 92: 39-46.
Díaz C, Quesada S, Brenes O, Aguilar G, Cicció JF (2008). "Chemical composition of Schinus molle essential oil and its cytotoxic activity on tumour cell lines," Nat Prod Res. 22(17):1521-34.
Dichter M.A. (1997) Basic Mechanisms of Epilepsy: Targets for Therapeutic Intervention. Epilepsia. 38: S2-S6.
Diggins K.C. (2008) Treatment of mild to moderate dehydration in children with oral rehydration therapy. Journal of the American Academy of Nurse Practitioners. 20: 402-406.
Dikshit A, Naqvi AA, Husain A. (1986 May). "Schinus molle: a new source of natural fungitoxicant," Appl Environ Microbiol. 51(5):1085-8.
Dimpfel W, Pischel I, Lehnfeld R (2004 Sep 29). "Effects of lozenge containing lavender oil, extracts from hops, lemon balm and oat on electrical brain activity of volunteers," Eur J Med Res. 9(9):423-31.

Dolder S., Hofstetter W., Wetterwald A., Muhlbauer R., Felix R. (2006) Effect of Monoterpenes on the Formation and Activation of Osteoclasts In Vitro. Journal of Bone and Mineral Research. 21: 647-655.

Dorman H.J.D., Deans S.G. (2000) Antimicrobial agents from plants: antibacterial activity of plant volatile oils. Journal of Applied Microbiology. 88: 308-316.

Duarte MC, Leme EE, Delarmelina C, Soares AA, Figueira GM, Sartoratto A (2007 May 4). "Activity of essential oils from Brazilian medicinal plants on Escherichia coli," J Ethnopharmacol. 111(2):197-201.

Dunn C, Sleep J, Collett D (1995 Jan). "Sensing an improvement: an experimental study to evaluate the use of aromatherapy, massage and periods of rest in an intensive care unit," J Adv Nurs. 21(1):34-40.

Dwivedi C, Guan X, Harmsen WL, Voss AL, Goetz-Parten DE, Koopman EM, Johnson KM, Valluri HB, Matthees DP (2003 Feb). "Chemopreventive effects of alpha-santalol on skin tumor development in CD-1 and SENCAR mice," Cancer Epidemiol Biomarkers Prev. 12(2):151-6.

Dwivedi C, Valluri HB, Guan X, Agarwal R (2006 Sep). "Chemopreventive effects of alpha-santalol on ultraviolet B radiation-induced skin tumor development in SKH-1 hairless mice," Carcinogenesis. 27(9):1917-22.

Edwards-Jones V, Buck R, Shawcross SG, Dawson MM, Dunn K (2004 Dec). "The effect of essential oils on methicillin-resistant Staphylococcus aureus using a dressing model," Burns. 30(8):772-7.

Enan E (2001 Nov). "Insecticidal activity of essential oils: octopaminergic sites of action," Comp Biochem Physiol C Toxicol Pharmacol. 130(3):325-37.

Engel J. (2001) A Proposed Diagnostic Scheme for People with Epileptic Seizures and with Epilepsy: Report of the ILAE Task Force on Classification and Terminology. Epilepsia. 42: 796-803.

Eriksson K., Levin J.O. (1996) Gas chromatographic-mass spectrometric identification of metabolites from ?-pinene in human urine after occupational exposure to sawing fumes. J. Chromatrography B. 677: 85-98.

Evandri MG, Battinelli L, Daniele C, Mastrangelo S, Bolle P, Mazzanti G (2005 Sep). "The antimutagenic activity of Lavandula angustifolia (lavender) essential oil in the bacterial reverse mutation assay," Food Chem Toxicol. 43(9):1381-7.

Evans J.D., Martin S.A. (2000) Effects of Thymol on Ruminal Microorganisms. Current Microbiology. 41: 336-340.

Fan AY, Lao L, Zhang RX, Zhou AN, Wang LB, Moudgil KD, Lee DY, Ma ZZ, Zhang WY, Berman BM (2005 Oct 3). "Effects of an acetone extract of Boswellia carterii Birdw. (Burseraceae) gum resin on adjuvant-induced arthritis in lewis rats," J Ethnopharmacol. 101(1-3):104-9.

Fearon D.T., Locksley R.M. (1996) The Instructive Role of Innate Immunity in the Acquired Immune Response. Science. 272: 50-54.

Ferrante M, Andreeta A, Landoni MF (2009 Oct 6). "Effect of different penetration enhancers on diclofenac permation across horse skin," Vet J. (Epub ahead of print).

Ferreira-da-Silva F.V., Barbosa R., Moreira-Junior L., dos Santos-Nascimento T., de Oliveira-Martins M.D., Coelho-de-Souza A.N., Cavalcante F.S.A., Ceccatto V.M., de Lemos T.L.G., Magalhaes P.J.C., Lahlou S., Leal-Cardoso J.H. (2009) Effects of 1,8-Cineole on Electrophysiological Parameters of Neurons of the Rat Superior Cervical Ganglion. Clinical and Experimental Pharamacology and Physiology. 36: 1068-1073.

Ferrini AM, Mannoni V, Aureli P, Salvatore G, Piccirilli E, Ceddia T, Pontieri E, Sessa R, Oliva B (2006 Jul-Sep). "Melaleuca alternifolia essential oil possesses potent anti-staphylococcal activity extended to strains resistant to antibiotics," Int J Immunopathol Pharmacol. 19(3):539-44.

Filoche SK, Soma K, Sissons CH (2005 Aug). "Antimicrobial effects of essential oils in combination with chlorhexidine digluconate," Oral Microbiol Immunol. 20(4):221-5.

Force M, Sparks WS, Ronzio RA (2000 May). "Inhibition of enteric parasites by emulsified oil of oregano in vivo," Phytother Res. 14(3):213-4.

Freitas F.P., Freitas S.P., Lemos G.C.S., Vieira I.J.C., Gravina G.A., Lemos F.J.A. (2010) Comparative Larvicial Activity of Essential Oils from Three Medicinal Plants against Aedes aeypti L. Chemistry & Biodiversity. 7: 2801-2807.

Freitas J.C.B.R., Presgrave O.A.F., Fingola F.F., Menezes M.A.C., Paumgartten F.J.R. (1993) Effect of ?-myrcene on pentobarbital sleeping time. Brazilian Journal of Medicine and Biological Research. 26: 519-523.

Fujisawa S., Atsumi T., Kadoma Y., Sakagami H. (2002) Antioxidant and prooxidant action of eugenol-related compounds and their cytotoxicity. Toxicology. 177: 39-54.

Fukumoto S, Sawasaki E, Okuyama S, Miyake Y, Yokogoshi H (2006 Feb-Apr). "Flavor components of monoterpenes in citrus essential oils enhance the release of monoamines from rat brain slices," Nutr Neurosci. 9(1-2):73-80.

Gaetani G.F., Ferraris A.M., Rolfo M., Mangerini R., Arena S., Kirkman H.N. (1996) Predominant role of catalase in the disposal of hydrogen peroxide within human erythrocytes. Blood. 87: 1595-1599.

Gaunt L.F., Higgins S.C., Hughes J.F. (2005) Interaction of air ions and bactericidal vapours to control micro-organisms. Journal of Applied Microbiology. 99: 1324-1329.

Gehrmann J., Matsumoto Y., Kreutzberg G.W. (1995) Microglia: intrinsic immuneffector cell of the brain. Brain Research Reviews. 20: 269-287.

Gertsch J. (2008) Anti-inflammatory cannabinoids in diet. Communicative & Integrative Biology. 1: 26-28.

Gertsch J., Leonti M., Raduner S., Racz I., Chen J-Z., Xie X-Q., Altmann K-H., Karsak M., Zimmer A. (2008) Beta-caryophyllene is a dietary cannabinoid. Proceedings of the National Academy of Sciences. 105: 9099-9104.

Ghelardini C, Galeotti N, Di Cesare Mannelli L, Mazzanti G, Bartolini A (2001 May-Jul). "Local anaesthetic activity of beta-caryophyllene," Farmaco. 56(5-7):387-9.

Ghelardini C, Galeotti N, Salvatore G, Mazzanti G (1999 Dec). "Local anaesthetic activity of the essential oil of Lavandula angustifolia," Planta Med. 65(8):700-3.

Golab M, Skwarlo-Sonta K (2007 Mar). "Mechanisms involved in the anti-inflammatory action of inhaled tea tree oil in mice," Exp Biol Med (Maywood). 232(3):420-6.

Gomes-Carneiro M.R., Dias D.M.M., De-Oliveira A.C.A.X., Paumgartten F.J.R. (2005) Evaluation of mutagenic and antimutagenic activities of ?-bisabolol in the Salmonella/microsome assay. Genetic Toxicology and Environmental Mutagenesis. 585: 105-112.

Goncalves J.C.R., Alves A.M.H., de Araujo A.E.V., Cruz J.S., Araujo D.A.M. (2010) Distinct effects of carvone analogues on the isolated nerve of rats. European Journal of Pharmacology. 645: 108-112.

Goncalves J.C.R., Oliveira F.S., Benedito R.B., de Sousa D.P., de Almeida R.N., Araujo D.A.M. (2008) Antinociceptive Activity of (-)-Carvone: Evidence of Association with Decreased Peripheral Nerve Excitability. Biological and Parmaceutical Bulletin. 31: 1017-1020.

González-Trujano ME, Peña EI, Martínez AL, Moreno J, Guevara-Fefer P, Déciga-Campos M, López-Muñoz FJ (2007 May 22). "Evaluation of the antinociceptive effect of Rosmarinus officinalis L. using three different experimental models in rodents," J Ethnopharmacol. 111(3):476-82.

Goodwin J.S., Atluru D., Sierakowski S., Lianos E.A. (1986) Mechanism of Action of Glucocorticosteroids: Inhibition of T Cell Proliferation and Interleukin 2 Production by Hydrocortisones Is Reversed by Leukotriene B4. Journal of Clinical Investigation. 77: 1244-1250.

Gorwitz R.J., Kruszon-Moran D., McAllister S.K., McQuillan G., McDougal L.K., Fosheim G.E., Jensen B.J., Killgore G., Tenover F.C., Kuehnert M.J. (2008) Changes in the Prevalence of Nasal Colonization with Staphylococcus aureusin the United States, 2001-2004. Journal of Infectious Diseases. 197: 1226-1234.

Grassmann J, Hippeli S, Dornisch K, Rohnert U, Beuscher N, Elstner EF (2000 Feb). "Antioxidant properties of essential oils. Possible explanations for their anti-inflammatory effects," Arzneimittelforschung. 50(2):135-9.

Griesmacher A., Kindhauser M., Andert S.E., Schreiner W., Toma C., Knoebl P., Pietschmann P., Prager R., Schnack C., Schernthaner G., Mueller M.M. (1995) Enhanced Serum Levels of Thiobarbituric-Acid-Reactve Substances in Diabetes Mellitus. The American Journal of Medicine. 98: 469-475.

Grigoleit HG, Grigoleit P (2005 Aug). "Peppermint oil in irritable bowel syndrome," Phytomedicine. 12(8):601-6.

Gundidza M (1993 Nov). "Antimicrobial activity of essential oil from Schinus molle Linn," Cent Afr J Med. 39(11):231-4.

Guo X., Longnecker M.P., Michalek J.E. (2001) Relation of serum tetrachlorodibenzo-p-dioxin concentration to diet among veterans in the Air Force health study with background-level exposure. Journal of Toxicology and Environmental Health, Part A. 63: 159-172.

Gupta A., Myrdal P.B. (2004) Development of perillyl alcohol topical cream formulation. Internation Journal of Pharmaceutics. 269: 373-383.

Gurney A.M. (1994) Mechanisms of Drug-induced Vasodilation. Journal of Pharmacy and Pharmacology. 46: 242-251.

Haag J.D., Lindstrom M.J., Gould M.N. (1992) Limonene-induced Regression of Mammary Carcinomas. Cancer Research. 52: 4021-4026.

Hajhashemi V, Abbasi N (2008 Mar). "Hypolipidemic activity of Anethum graveolens in rats," Phytother Res. 22(3):372-5.

Hakim IA, Harris RB, Ritenbaugh C (2000). "Citrus peel use is associated with reduced risk of squamous cell carcinoma of the skin," Nutr Cancer. 37(2):161-8.

Hammer KA, Carson CF, Riley TV (1996 Jun). "Susceptibility of transient and commensal skin flora to the essential oil of Melaleuca alternifolia (tea tree oil)," J Antimicrob Chemother. 24(3):186-9.

Hart PH, Brand C, Carson CF, Riley TV, Prager RH, Finlay-Jones JJ (2000 Nov). "Terpinen-4-ol, the main component of the essential oil of Melaleuca alternifolia (tea tree oil), suppresses inflammatory mediator production by activated human monocytes," Inflamm Res. 49(11):619-26.

Hay IC, Jamieson M, Ormerod AD (1998 Nov). "Randomized trial of aromatherapy. Successful treatment for alopecia areata," Arch Dermatol. 135(5):1349-52.

Hiramatsu N, Xiufen W, Takechi R, Itoh Y, Mamo J, Pal S (2004). "Antimutagenicity of Japanese traditional herbs, gennoshoko, yomogi, senburi and iwa-tobacco," Biofactors. 22(1-4):123-5.

Holt E. (2005) Doctor sues clinic over Yushchenko poisoning claims. The Lancet. 365: 1375.

Hongratanaworakit T (2009 Feb). "Relaxing effect of rose oil on humans," Nat Prod Commun. 4(2):291-6.

Hongratanaworakit T, Buchbauer G (2006 Sep). "Relaxing effect of ylang ylang oil on humans after transdermal absorption," Phytother Res. 20(9):758-63.

Howard J., Hyman A.A. (2003) Dynamics and mechanics of the microtubule plus end. Nature. 422: 753-758.

Hoya Y, Matsumura I, Fujita T, Yanaga K. (2008 Nov-Dec). "The use of nonpharmacological interventions to reduce anxiety in patients undergoing gastroscopy in a setting with an optimal soothing environment," Gastroenterol Nurs. 31(6):395-9.

Hsu H-Y., Yang J-J., Lin C-C. (1997) Effects of oleanolic acid and ursolic acid in inhibiting tumor growth and enhancing the recovery of hematopoietic system postirradiation in mice. Cancer Letters. 111: 7-13.

Huang MT, Badmaev V, Ding Y, Liu Y, Xie JG, Ho CT (2000). "Anti-tumor and anti-carcinogenic activities of triterpenoid, beta-boswellic acid," Biofactors. 13(1-4):225-30.

Hummel T., Fuschik T., Frasnelli J., Huttenbrink K-B. (2003) Effects of olfactory function, age, and gender on trigeminally mediated sensations: a study based on the lateralization of chemosensory stimuli. Toxicology Letters. 140-141: 273-280.

Hussein G, Miyashiro H, Nakamura N, Hattori M, Kakiuchi N, Shimotohno K (2000 Nov). "Inhibitory effects of sudanese medicinal plant extracts on hepatitis C virus (HCV) protease," Phytother Res. 14(7):510-6.

Ichihashi M., Ueda M., Budiyanto A., Bito T., Oka M., Fukuaga M., Tsuru K., Horikawa T. (2003) UV-induced skin damage. Toxicology. 189: 21-39.

Imai H, Osawa K, Yasuda H, Hamashima H, Arai T, Sasatsu M (2001). "Inhibition by the essential oils of peppermint and spearmint of the growth of pathogenic bacteria," Microbios. 106(Suppl 1):31-9.

Inouye S, Takizawa T, Yamaguchi H (2001 May). "Antibacterial activity of essential oils and their major constituents against respiratory tract pathogens by gaseous contact," J Antimicrob Chemother. 47(5):565-73.

Iori A, Grazioli D, Gentile E, Marano G, Salvatore G (2005 Apr 20). "Acaricidal properties of the essential oil of Melaleuca alternifolia Cheel (tea tree oil) against nymphs of Ixodes ricinus," Vet Parasitol. 129(1-2):173-6.

Itai T, Amayasu H, Kuribayashi M, Kawamura N, Okada M, Momose A, Tateyama T, Narumi K, Uematsu W, Kaneko S (2000 Aug). "Psychological effects of aromatherapy on chronic hemodialysis patients," Psychiatry Clin Neurosci. 54(4):393-7.

Janahmadi M, Niazi F, Danyali S, Kamalinejad M (2006 Mar 8). "Effects of the fruit essential oil of Cuminum cyminum Linn. (Apiaceae) on pentylenetetrazol-induced epileptiform activity in F1 neurones of Helix aspersa," J Ethnopharmacol. 104(1-2):278-82.

Jankovic J. (2008) Parkinson's disease: clinical features and diagnosis. Journal of Neurology, Neurosurgery & Psychiatry. 79: 368-376.

Jefferies H., Coster J., Khalil A., Bot J., McCauley R.D., Hall J.C. (2003) Glutathione. ANZ Journal of Surgery. 73: 517-522.

Jeong H.G. (1999) Inhibition of cytochrome P450 2E1 expression by oleanolic acid: hepatoprotective effects against carbon tetrachloride-induced hepatic injury. Toxicology Letters. 105: 215-222.

Jing Y, Xia L, Han R (1992 Mar). "Growth inhibition and differentiation of promyelocytic cells (HL-60) induced by BC-4, an active principle from Boswellia carterii Birdw," Chin Med Sci J. 7(1):12-5.

Juergens U.R., Dethlefsen U., Steinkamp G., Gillissen A., Repges R., Vetter H. (2003) Anti-inflammatory activity of 1.8-cineol (eucalyptol) in bronchial asthma: a double-blind placebo-controlled trial. Respiratory Medicine. 97: 250-256.

Juergens UR, Stöber M, Vetter H (1998 Dec 16). "The anti-inflammatory activity of L-menthol compared to mint oil in human monocytes in vitro: a novel perspective for its therapeutic use in inflammatory diseases," Eur J Med Res. 3(12):539-45.

Jungersted J.M., Hellgren L.I., Hogh J.K., Drachmann T., Jemec G.B.E., Agner T. (2010) Ceramides and Barrier Function in Healthy Skin. Acta Dermato-Venereologica. 90: 350-353.

Kalemba D., Kunicka A. (2003) Antibacterial and Antifungal properties of Essential Oils. Current Medicinal Chemistry. 10: 813-829.

Kamatou G.P.P., Viljoen A.M. (2010) A Review of the Application and Pharmacological Properties of ?-Bisabolol and ?-Bisabolol-Rich Oils. Journal of the American Oil Chemists' Society. 87: 1-7.

Kane FM, Brodie EE, Coull A, Coyne L, Howd A, Milne A, Niven CC, Robbins R (2004 Oct 28-Nov 10). "The analgesic effect of odour and music upon dressing change," Br J Nurs. 13(19):S4-12.

Kapil A., Sharma S. (1994) Anti-complement activity of oleanolic acid: an inhibitor of C3-convertase of the classical complement pathway. Journal of Pharmacy and Pharmacology. 46: 922-923.

Kato K., Cox A.D., Hisaka M.M., Graham S.M., Buss J.E., Der C.J. (1992) Isoprenoid addition to Ras protein is the critical modification for its membrane association and transforming activity. Proc. Natl. Sci. USA. 89: 6403-6407.

Kaur M, Agarwal C, Singh RP, Guan X, Dwivedi C, Agarwal R (2005 Feb). "Skin cancer chemopreventive agent, {alpha}-santalol, induces apoptotic death of human epidermoid carcinoma A431 cells via caspase activation together with dissipation of mitochondrial membrane potential and cytochrome c release," Carcinogenesis. 26(2):369-80.

Kennedy DO, Little W, Haskell CF, Scholey AB (2006 Feb). "Anxiolytic effects of a combination of Melissa officinalis and Valeriana officinalis during laboratory induced stress," Phytother Res. 20(2):96-102.

Khatibi A, Haghparast A, Shams J, Dianati E, Komaki A, Kamalinejad M (2008 Dec 19). "Effects of the fruit essential oil of Cuminum cyminum L. on the acquisition and expression of morphine-induced conditioned place preference in mice," Neurosci Lett. 448(1):94-8.

Kiecolt-Glaser JK, Graham JE, Malarkey WB, Porter K, Lemeshow S, Glaser R (2008 Apr). "Olfactory influences on mood and autonomic, endocrine, and immune function," Psychoneuroendocrinology. 33(3):328-39.

Kim K-A., Lee J-S., Park H-J., Kim J-W., Kim C-J., Shim I-S., Kim N-J., Han S-M., Lim S. (2004) Inhibition of cytochrome P450 activities by oleanolic acid and ursolic acid in human liver microsomes. Life Sciences. 74: 2769-2779.

Kim MA, Sakong JK, Kim EJ, Kim EH, Kim EH (2005 Feb). "Effect of aromatherapy massage for the relief of constipation in the elderly," Taehan Kanho Hakhoe Chi. 35(1):56-64.

Kim S., Lee J., Jung E., Huh S., Park J-O., Lee J-W., Byun S.Y., Park D. (2008) Mechanisms of depigmentation by ?-bisabolol. Journal of Dermatological Science. doi: 10.1016/j.jdermsci.2008.06.005.

Kite SM, Maher EJ, Anderson K, Young T, Young J, Wood J, Howells N, Bradburn J (1998 May). "Development of an aromatherapy service at a Cancer Centre," Palliat Med. 12(3):171-80.

Klein T.W. (2005) Cannabinoid-Based Drugs As Anti-Inflammatory Therapeutics. Nature Reviews. 5: 400-411.

Kobayashi Y, Takahashi R, Ogino F (2005 Oct 3). "Antipruritic effect of the single oral administration of German chamomile flower extract and its combined effect with antiallergic agents in ddY mice," J Ethnopharmacol. 101(1-3):308-12.

Komiya M, Takeuchi T, Harada E (2006 Sep 25). "Lemon oil vapor causes an anti-stress effect via modulating the 5-HT and DA activities in mice," Behav Brain Res. 172(2):240-9.

Komori T, Fujiwara R, Tanida M, Nomura J (1995 Dec). "Potential antidepressant effects of lemon odor in rats," Eur Neuropsychopharmacol. 5(4):477-80.

Koo HN, Hong SH, Kim CY, Ahn JW, Lee YG, Kim JJ, Lyu YS, Kim HM (2002 Jun). "Inhibitory effect of apoptosis in human astrocytes CCF-STTG1 cells by lemon oil," Pharmacol Res. 45(6):469-73.

Koo HN, Jeong HJ, Kim CH, Park ST, Lee SJ, Seong KK, Lee SK, Lyu YS, Kim HM (2001 Dec). "Inhibition of heat shock-induced apoptosis by peppermint oil in astrocytes," J Mol Neurosci. 17(3):391-6.

Kosaka K., Mimura J., Itoh K., Satoh T., Shimojo Y., Kitajima C., Maruyama A., Yamamoto M., Shirasawa T. (2010) Role of Nrf2 and p62/ZIP in the neurite outgrowth by carnosic acid in PC12h cells. Journal of Biochemistry. 147: 73-81.

Kosaka K., Yokoi T. (2003) Carnosic Acid, a Component of Rosemary (Rosmarinus officinalis L.), Promotes Synthesis of Nerve Growth Factor in T98G Human Glioblastoma Cells. Biological & Pharaceutical Bulletin. 26: 1620-1622.

Kozam G., Mantell G.M. (1978) The Effect of Eugenol on Oral Mucous Membranes. Journal of Dental Research. 57: 954-957.

Kumar A, Malik F, Bhushan S, Sethi VK, Shahi AK, Kaur J, Taneja SC, Qazi GN, Singh J (2008 Feb 15). "An essential oil and its major constituent isointermedeol induce apoptosis by increased expression of mitochondrial cytochrome c and apical death receptors in human leukaemia HL-60 cells," Chem Biol Interact. 171(3):332-47.

Kwieciński J, Eick S, Wójcik K (2009 Apr). "Effects of tea tree (Melaleuca alternifolia) oil on Staphylococcus aureus in biofilms and stationary growth phase," Int J Antimicrob Agents. 33(4):343-7.

Lahlou S., Figueiredo A.F., Magalaes P.J.C., Leal-Cardoso J.H. (2002) Cardiovascular effects of 1,8-cineole, a terpenoid oxide present in many plant essential oils, in normotensive rats. Canadian Journal of Physiology and Pharmacology. 80: 1125-1131.

Lahlou S., Interaminense L.F.L., Magalhaes P.J.C., Leal-Cardoso J.H., Duarte G.P. (2004) Cardiovascular Effects of Eugenol, a Phenolic Compound Present in Many Plant Essential Oils, in Normotensive Rats. Journal of Cardiovascular Pharmacology. 43: 250-257.

Lambert R.J.W., Skandamis P.N., Coote P.J., Nychas G-J.E. (2001) A study of the minimun inhibitory concentration and mode of action of oregano essential oil, thymol and carvacrol. Journal of Applied Microbiology. 91: 453-462.

Lampronti I, Saab AM, Gambari R (2006 Oct). "Antiproliferative activity of essential oils derived from plants belonging to the Magnoliophyta division," Int J Oncol. 29(4):989-95.

Lapczynski A., Bhatia S.P., Letizia C.S., Api A.M. (2008) Fragrance material review on dl-citronellol. Food and Chemical Toxicology. 46: S103-S109.

Larder B.A., Kemp S.D., Harrigan P.R. (1995) Potential Mechanism for Sustained Antiretroviral Efficacy of AZT-3TC Combination Therapy. Science. 269: 696-699.

Leal-Cardoso J.H., Lahlou S., de Souza A.N.C., Criddle D.N., Duarte G.I.B.P., Santos M.A.V., Magalhaes P.J.C. (2002) Inhibitory actions of eugenol on rat isolated ileum. Canadian Journal of Physiology and Pharmacology. 80: 901-906.

Lee HS (2005 Apr 6). "Cuminaldehyde: Aldose Reductase and alpha-Glucosidase Inhibitor Derived from Cuminum cyminum L. Seeds," J Agric Food Chem. 53(7):2446-50.

Lee J., Jun H., Jung E., Ha J., Park D. (2010) Whitening effect of ?-bisabolol in Asian women subjects. International Journal of Cosmetic Science.

Lee SU, Shim KS, Ryu SY, Min YK, Kim SH (2009 Feb). "Machilin A isolated from Myristica fragrans stimulates osteoblast differentiation," Planta Med. 75(2):152-7.

Legault J, Dahl W, Debiton E, Pichette A, Madelmont JC (2003 May). "Antitumor activity of balsam fir oil: production of reactive oxygen species induced by alpha-humulene as possible mechanism of action," Planta Med. 69(5):402-7.

Legault J., Pichette A. (2007) Potentiating effect of ?-caryophyllene on anticancer activity of ?-humulene, isocaryophyllene, and paclitaxel. Journal of Pharmacy and Pharmacology. 59: 1643-1647.

Lehrner J, Eckersberger C, Walla P, Pötsch G, Deecke L (2000 Oct 1-15). "Ambient odor of orange in a dental office reduces anxiety and improves mood in female patients," Physiol Behav. 71(1-2):83-6.

Lewith GT, Godfrey AD, Prescott P (2005 Aug). "A single-blinded, randomized pilot study evaluating the aroma of Lavandula angustifolia as a treatment for mild insomnia," J Altern Complement Med. 11(4):631-7.

Lie J. (2005) Oleanolic acid and ursolic acid: Research perspectives. Journal of Ethnopharmacology. 100: 92-94.

Lim PF, Liu XY, Kang L, Ho PC, Chan YW, Chan SY (2006 Mar 27). "Limonene GP1/PG organogel as a vehicle in transdermal delivery of haloperidol," Int J Pharm 311(12):157-64.

Lima-Accioly P.M., Lavor-Porto P.R., Cavalcante F.S., Magalhaes P.J.C., Lahlou S., Morais S.M., Leal-Cardoso J.H. (2006) Essential Oil of Croton Nepetaefolius and Its Main Constituent, 1,8-Cineole, Block Excitability of Rat Sciatic Nerve In Vitro. Clinical and Experimental Pharmacology and Physiology. 33: 1158-1163.

Lima CF, Azevedo MF, Araujo R, Fernandes-Ferreira M, Pereira-Wilson C (2006 Aug). "Metformin-like effect of Salvia officinalis (common sage): is it useful in diabetes prevention?," Br J Nutr. 96(2):326-33.

Linck V.M., da Silva A.L., Figueiro M., Caramao E.B., Moreno P.R.H., Elisabetsky E. (2010) Effects of inhaled Linalool in anxiety, social interaction and aggressive behavior in mice. Phytomedicine. 17: 679-683.

Linck V.M., da Silva A.L., Figueiro M., Piato A.L., Herrmann A.P., Birck F.D., Moreno P.R.H., Elisabetsky E. (2009) Inhaled linalool-induced sedation in mice. Phytomedicine. 16: 303-307.

Lin PW, Chan WC, Ng BF, Lam LC (2007 May). "Efficacy of aromatherapy (Lavandula angustifolia) as an intervention for agitated behaviours in Chinese older persons with dementia: a cross-over randomized trial," Int J Geriatr Psychiatry. 22(5):405-10.

Lis-Balschin M., Hart S. (1999) Studies on the Mode of Action of the Essential Oil of Lavender (Lavandula angustifolia P. Miller). Phytotherapy Research. 13: 540-542.

Lis-Balchin M, Hart S, Wan Hang Lo B (2002 Aug). "Jasmine absolute (Jasminum grandiflora L.) and its mode of action on guinea-pig ileum in vitro," Phytother Res. 16(5):437-9.

Liu J. (1995) Pharmacology of oleanolic acid and ursolic acid. Journal of Ethnopharmacology. 49: 57-68.

Liu JJ, Nilsson A, Oredsson S, Badmaev V, Duan RD (2002 Oct). "Keto- and acetyl-keto-boswellic acids inhibit proliferation and induce apoptosis in Hep G2 cells via a caspase-8 dependent pathway," Int J Mol Med. 10(4):501-5.

Liu Y., Hartley D.P., Liu J. (1998) Protection against carbone tetrachloride hepatotoxicity by oleanolic acid is not mediated through metallothionein. Toxicology Letters. 95: 77-85.

Livermore D.M. (2002) Multiple Mechanisms of Antimicrobial Resistance in Pseudomonas aeruginosa: Our Worst Nightmare?. Clinical Infectious Diseases. 34: 634-640.

Loew O. (1900) A New Enzyme of General Occurrence in Organisms. Science. 11: 701-702.

Loizzo MR, Tundis R, Menichini F, Saab AM, Statti GA, Menichini F (2007 Sep-Oct). "Cytotoxic activity of essential oils from labiatae and lauraceae families against in vitro human tumor models," Anticancer Res. 27(5A):3293-9.

Longley D.B., Harkin D.P., Johnston P.G. (2003) 5-Fluorouracil: Mechanisms of Action and Clinical Strategies. Nature Reviews. 3: 330-338.

Lu M, Battinelli L, Daniele C, Melchioni C, Salvatore G, Mazzanti G (2002 Mar). "Muscle relaxing activity of Hyssopus officinalis essential oil on isolated intestinal preparations," Planta Med. 68(3):213-6.

Lu XQ, Tang FD, Wang Y, Zhao T, Bian RL (2004 Feb). "Effect of Eucalyptus globulus oil on lipopolysaccharide-induced chronic bronchitis and mucin hypersecretion in rats," Zhongguo Zhong Yao Za Zhi. 29(2):168-71.

Macilwain C. (1993) US Congress urged to back further Agent Orange studies. Nature. 364: 373.

Manohar V, Ingram C, Gray J, Talpur NA, Echard BW, Bagchi D, Preuss HG (2001 Dec). "Antifungal activities of origanum oil against Candida albicans," Mol Cell Biochem. 228(1-2):111-7.

Mans D.R.A., Grivicich I., Peters G.J., Schwartsmann G. (1999) Sequence-dependent Growth Inhibition and DNA Damage Formation by t he Irinotecan-5-Fluorouracil Combination in Human Colon Carcinoma Cell Lines. European Journal of Cancer. 35: 1851-1861.

Marks R. (1995) An Overview of Skin Cancers: Incidence and Causation. Cancer. 75: 607-612.

Maruyama N, Sekimoto Y, Ishibashi H, Inouye S, Oshima H, Yamaguchi H, Abe S (2005 Feb 10). "Suppression of neutrophil accumulation in mice by cutaneous application of geranium essential oil," J Inflamm (Lond). 2(1):1.

Masuda T., Inaba Y., Takeda Y. (2001) Antioxidant Mechanism of Carnosic Acid: Structural Identification of Two Oxidation Products. Journal of Agricultural and Food Chemistry. 49: 5560-5565.

Masukawa Y., Narita H., Sato H., Naoe A., Kondo N., Sugai Y., Oba T., Homma R., Ishikawa J., Takagi Y., Kitahara T. (2009) Comprehensive quantification of ceramide species in human stratum corneum. Journal of Lipid Research. 50: 1708-1719.

Mathews G.C. (2007) The Dual Roles of GABA in Seizures and Epilepsy Generate More Excitement. Epilepsy Currents 7: 28-30.

Mayer M.L. (2005) Glutamate receptor ion channels. Current Opinion in Neurobiology. 15: 282-288.

McCord J.M., Fridovich I. (1969) Superoxide Dismutase: an enzymic function for erytrocuprein (hemocuprein). The Journal of Biological Chemistry. 244: 6049-6055.

McGarvey D.J., Croteau R. (1995) Terpenoid Metabolism. The Plant Cell. 7: 1015-1026.

McGeady P., Wansley D.L., Logan D.A. (2002) Carvone and Perillaldehyde Interfere with the Serum-Induced Formation of Filamentous Structures in Candida albicansat Substantially Lower Concentrations than Those Causing Significant Inhibition of Growth. Journal of Natural Products. 65: 953-955.

McKee M. (2009) The poisoning of Victor Yushchenko. The Lancet. 374: 1131-1132.

Medzhitov R., Janeway C.A. (1997) Innate Immunity: Impact on the adaptive Immune response. Current Opinion in Immunology. 9: 4-9.

Meisler M.H., Kearney J.A. (2005) Sodium channel mutations in epilepsy and other neurological disorders. The Journal of Clinical Investigation. 115: 2010-2017.

Meldrum B.S. (1994) The role of glutamate in epilepsy and other CNS disorders. Neurology. 44: S14-S23.

Meldrum B.S., Akbar M.T., Chapman A.G. (1999) Glutamate receptors and transporters in genetic and acquired models of epilepsy. Epilepsy Research. 36: 189-204.

Melov S., Ravenscroft J., Malik S., Gill M.S., Walker D.W., Clayton P.E., Wallace D.C., Malfroy B., Doctrow S.R., Lithgow G.J. (2000) Extension of Life-Span with Superoxide Dismutase/Catalase Mimetics. Science. 289: 1567-1569.

Mercier B., Prost J., Prost M. (2009) The Essential Oil of Turpentine and Its Major Volatile Fraction (?- and ?-Pinenes): A Review. International Journal of Occupational Medicine and Environmental Health. 22: 331-342.

Mills JJ, Chari RS, Boyer IJ, Gould MN, Jirtle RL (1995 Mar 1). "Induction of apoptosis in liver tumors by the monoterpene perillyl alcohol," Cancer Res. 55(5):979-83.

Milross C.G., Mason K.A., Hunter N.R., Chung W-K., Peters L.J., Milas L. (1996) Relationship of Mitotic Arrest and Apoptosis to Antitumor Effect of Paclitaxel. Journal of the National Cancer Institute. 88: 1308-1314.

Mimura J., Kosaka K., Maruyama A., Satoh T., Harada N., Yoshida H., Satoh K., Yamamoto M., Itoh K. (2011) Nrf2 regulates NGF mRNA induction by carnosic acid in T98G gliobastoma cells and normal human astrocytes. The Journal of Biochemistry. 150: 209-217.

Mitic-Culafic D., Zegura B., Nikolic B., Vukovic-Gacic B., Knezevic-Vukcevic J., Filipic M. (2008) Protective effect of linalool, myrcene and eucalyptol against t-butyl hydroperoxide induced genotoxicity in bacteria and cultured human cells. Food and Chemical Toxicology. 47: 260-266.

Mkolo MN, Magano SR (2007 Sep). "Repellent effects of the essential oil of Lavandula angustifolia against adults of Hyalomma marginatum rufipes," J S Afr Vet Assoc. 78(3):149-52.

Mondello F, De Bernardis F, Girolamo A, Cassone A, Salvatore G (2006 Nov 3). "In vivo activity of terpinen-4-ol, the main bioactive component of Melaleuca alternifolia Cheel (tea tree) oil against azole-susceptible and -resistant human pathogenic Candida species," BMC Infect Dis. 6:158.

Monti D, Chetoni P, Burgalassi S, Najarro M, Saettone MF, Boldrini E (2002 Apr 26). "Effect of different terpene-containing essential oils on permeation of estradiol through hairless mouse skin," Int j Pharm. 237(1-2):209-14.

Monzo M., Rosell R., Sanchez J.J., Lee J.S., O'Brate A., Gonzalex-Larriba J.L., Alberola V., Lorenzo J.C., Nunez L., Ro J.Y., Martin C. (1999) Paclitaxel Resistance in Non-Small Cell Lung Cancer Associated With Beta-Tubulin Gene Mutations. Journal of Clincial Oncology. 17: 1786-1793.

Moreira-Lobo D.C.A., Linhares-Siqueira E.D., Cruz G.M.P., Cruz J.S., de Souza J.L.C., Lahlou S., de Souza A.N.C., Barbosa R., Magalhaes P.J.C., Leal-Cardoso J.H. (2010) Eugenol modifies the excitability of rat sciatic nerve and superior cervical ganglion neurons. Neuroscience Letters. 472: 220-224.

Moreno S, Scheyer T, Romano CS, Vojnov AA (2006 Feb). "Antioxidant and antimicrobial activities of rosemary extracts linked to their polyphenol composition," Free Radic Res. 40(2):223-31.

Morse M.A., Stoner G.D. (1993) Cancer chemoprevention: principles and prospects. Carcinogenesis. 14: 1737-1746.

Moss M, Cook J, Wesnes K, Duckett P (2003 Jan). "Aromas of rosemary and lavender essential oils differentially affect cognition and mood in healthy adults," Int J Neurosci. 113(1):15-38.

Motomura N, Sakurai A, Yotsuya Y (2001 Dec). "Reduction of mental stress with lavender odorant," Percept Mot Skills. 93(3):713-8.

Moussaieff A, Rimmerman N, Bregman T, Straiker A, Felder CC, Shoham S, Kashman Y, Huang SM, Lee H, Shohami E, Mackie K, Caterina MJ, Walker JM, Fride E, Mechoulam R (2008 Aug). "Incensole acetate, an incense component, elicits psychoactivity by activating TRPV3 channels in the brain," FASEB J. 22(8):3024-34.

Muhlbauer R.C., Lozano A., Palacio S., Reinli A., Felix R. (2003) Common herbes, essential oils, and monoterpenes potently modulate bone metabolism. Bone. 32: 372-380.

Mukherjee P.K., Chandra J., Kuhn D.M., Ghannoum M.A. (2003) Mechanism of Fluconazole Resistance in Candida albicansBiofilms: Phase-Specific Role of Efflux Pumps and Membrane Sterols. Infection and Immunity. 71: 4333-4340.

Muller M., Pape H-C., Speckmann E-J., Gorji A. (2006) Effect of Eugenol on Spreading Depression and Epileptiform Discharges in Rat Neocortical and Hippocampal Tissues. Neuroscience. 140: 743-751.

Mumcuoglu KY, Magdassi S, Miller J, Ben-Ishai F, Zentner G, Helbin V, Friger M, Kahana F, Ingber A (2004 Dec). "Repellency of citronella for head lice: double-blind randomized trial of efficacy and safety," Isr Med Assoc J. 6(12):756-9.

Munzel T., Feil R., Mulsch A., Lohmann S.M., Hofmann F., Walter U. (2003) Physiology and Pathophysiology of Vascular Signaling Controlled by Cyclic Guanosine 3',5'-Cyclic Monophosphate-Dependent Protein Kinase. Circulation. 108: 2172-2183.

Nair B. (2001). "Final report on the safety assessment of Mentha Piperita (Peppermint) Oil, Mentha Piperita (Peppermint) Leaf Extract, Mentha Piperita (Peppermint) Leaf, and Mentha Piperita (Peppermint) Leaf Water," Int J Toxicol. 20(Suppl 3):61-73..

Narishetty S.T.K., Panchagnula R. (2004) Transdermal delivey of zidovudine: effect of terpenes and their mechanism of action. Journal of Controlled Release. 95: 367-379.

Narishetty S.T.K., Panchagnula R. (2005) Effects of L-menthol and 1,8-cineole on phase behavior and molecular organization of SC lipids and skin permeation of zidovudine. Journal of Controlled Release. 102: 59-70.

Nasel C, Nasel B, Samec P, Schindler E, Buchbauer G (1994 Aug). "Functional imaging of effects of fragrances on the human brain after prolonged inhalation," Chem Senses. 19(4):359-64.

Nikitin E.S., Balaban P.M. (2000) Optical Recording of Odor-Evoked Responses in the Olfactory Brain of the Naïve and Aversively Trained Terrestrial Snails. Learning & Memory 7: 422-432.

Ninomiya K, Matsuda H, Shimoda H, Nishida N, Kasajima N, Yoshino T, Morikawa T, Yoshikawa M (2004 Apr 19). "Carnosic acid, a new class of lipid absorption inhibitor from sage," Bioorg Med Chem Lett. 14(8):1943-6. Nebert D.W., Russell D.W. (2002) Clinical importance of the cytochromes P450. The Lancet. 360: 1155-1162.

Nostro A, Blanco AR, Cannatelli MA, Enea V, Flamini G, Morelli I, Sudano Roccaro A, Alonzo V (2004 Jan 30). "Susceptibility of methicillin-resistant staphylococci to oregano essential oil, carvacrol and thymol," FEMS Microbiol Lett. 230(2):191-5.

Ohkubo T., Shibata M. (1997) The Selective Capsaicin Antagonist Capsazepine Abolishes the Antinociceptive Action of Eugenol and Guaiacol. Journal of Dental Research. 76: 848-851.

Ohno T, Kita M, Yamaoka Y, Imamura S, Yamamoto T, Mitsufuji S, Kodama T, Kashima K, Imanishi J (2003 Jun). "Antimicrobial activity of essential oils against Helicobacter pylori," Helicobacter. 8(3):207-15.

Olajide OA, Ajayi FF, Ekhelar AI, Awe SO, Makinde JM, Alada AR (1999 Jun). "Biological effects of Myristica fragrans (nutmeg) extract," Phytother Res. 13(4):344-5.

Opalchenova G, Obreshkova D (2003 Jul). "Comparative studies on the activity of basil--an essential oil from Ocimum basilicum L.--against multidrug resistant clinical isolates of the genera Staphylococcus, Enterococcus and Pseudomonas by using different test methods," J Microbiol Methods. 54(1):105-10.

Ostad SN, Soodi M, Shariffzadeh M, Khorshidi N, Marzban H (2001 Aug). "The effect of fennel essential oil on uterine contraction as a model for dysmenorrhea, pharmacology and toxicology study," J Ethnopharmacol. 76(3):299-304.
Paduch R., Kanderfer-Szerszen M., Trytek M., Feidurek J. (2007) Terpenes: substances useful in human healthcare. Archivum Immunologiae et Therapia Experimentalis. 55: 315-327.
Paoletti P., Neyton J. (2007) NMDA receptor subunits: functions and pharmacology. Current Opinion in Pharmacology. 7: 39-47.
Pavela R (2005 Dec). "Insecticidal activity of some essential oils against larvae of Spodoptera littoralis," Fitoterapia. 76(7-8):691-6.
Peana A.T., D'Aquila P.S., Chessa M. L., Moretti M.D.L., Serra G., Pippia P. (2003) (-)-Linalool produces antinociception in two experimental models of pain. European Journal of Pharmacology. 460: 37-41.
Peana A.T., D'Aquila P.S., Panin F., Serra G., Pippia P., Moretti M.D.L. (2002) Anti-inflammatory activity of linalool and linalyl acetate constituents of essential oils. Phytomedicine. 9: 721-726.
Pearce AL, Finlay-Jones JJ, Hart PH (2005 Jan). "Reduction of nickel-induced contact hypersensitivity reactions by topical tea tree oil in humans," Inflamm Res. 54(1):22-30.
Peng SM, Koo M, Yu ZR (2009 Jan). "Effects of music and essential oil inhalation on cardiac autonomic balance in healthy individuals," J Altern Complement Med. 15(1):53-7.
Peters G.J., Backus H.H.J., Freemantle S., van Triest B., Codacci-Pisanelli G., van der Wilt C.L., Smid K., Lunec J., Calvert A.H., Marsh S., McLeod H.L., Bloemena E., Meijer S., Jansen G., van Groeningen C.J., Pinedo H.M. (2002) Induction of thymidylate synthase as a 5-fluorouracil resistance mechanism. Biochimica et Biophysica Acta. 1587: 194-205.
Pichette A, Larouche PL, Lebrun M, Legault J (2006 May). "Composition and antibacterial activity of Abies balsamea essential oil," Phytother Res. 20(5):371-3.
Politano V.T., Lewis E.M., Hoberman A.M., Christian M.S., Diener R.M., Api A.M. (2008) Evaluation of the Developmental Toxicity of Linalool in Rats. International Journal of Toxicology. 27: 183-188.
Preuss HG, Echard B, Enig M, Brook I, Elliott TB (2005 Apr). "Minimum inhibitory concentrations of herbal essential oils and monolaurin for gram-positive and gram-negative bacteria," Mol Cell Biochem. 272(1-2):29-34.
Puatanachokchai R, Kishida H, Denda A, Murata N, Konishi Y, Vinitketkumnuen U, Nakae D (2002 Sep 8). "Inhibitory effects of lemongrass (Cymbopogon citratus, Stapf) extract on the early phase of hepatocarcinogenesis after initiation with diethylnitrosamine in male Fischer 344 rats," Cancer Lett. 183(1):9-15.
Querfurth H.W., LaFeria F.M. (2010) Alzheimer's Disease. The New England Journal of Medicine. 362: 329-344.
Qureshi A.A., Mangels W.R., Din A.A., Elson C.E. (1988) Inhibition of Hepatic Mevalonate Biosynthesis by the Monoterpene, d-Limonene. J. Agric. Food Chem. 36: 1220-1224.
Rao S., Krauss N.E., Heerding J.M., Swindell C.S., Ringel I., Orr G.A., Horwitz S.B. (1994) 3'-(p-Azidobenzamido)taxol Photolabels the N-terminal 31 AminoAcids of ?-Tubulin. The Journal of Biological Chemistry. 269: 3132-3134.
Rao S., Orr G.A., Chaudhary A.G., Kingston D.G.I., Horwitz S.B. (1995) Characterization of the Taxol Binding Site on the Microtubule. The Journal of Biological Chemistry. 270: 20235-20238.
Raphael T.J., Kuttan G. (2003) Effect of naturally occurring triterpenoids glycyrrhizic acid, ursolic acid, oleanolic acid and nomilin on the immune system. Phytomedicine. 10: 483-489.
Rasooli I, Fakoor MH, Yadegarinia D, Gachkar L, Allameh A, Rezaei MB (2008 Feb 29). "Antimycotoxigenic characteristics of Rosmarinus officinalis and Trachyspermum copticum L. essential oils," Int J Food Microbiol. 122(1-2):135-9.
Reddy AC, Lokesh BR (1994). "Studies on anti-inflammatory activity of spice principles and dietary n-3 polyunsaturated fatty acids on carrageenan-induced inflammation in rats," Ann Nutr Metab. 38(6):349-58.
Rees WD, Evans BK, Rhodes J (1979 Oct 6). "Treating irritable bowel syndrome with peppermint oil," Br Med J. 2(6194):835-6.
Reichling J, Koch C, Stahl-Biskup E, Sojka C, Schnitzler P (2005 Dec). "Virucidal activity of a beta-triketone-rich essential oil of Leptospermum scoparium (manuka oil) against HSV-1 and HSV-2 in cell culture," Planta Med. 71(12):1123-7.
Re L., Barocci S., Sonnino S., Mencarelli A., Vivani C., Paolucci G., Scarpantonio A., Rinaldi L., Mosca E. (2000) Linalool modifies the nicotinic receptor-ion channel kinetics at the mouse neuromuscular junction. Pharmacological Research. 42: 177-181.
Reddy B.S., Wang C-X., Samaha H., Lubet R., Steele V.E., Kelloff G.J., Rao C.V. (1997) Chemoprevention of Colon Carcinogenesis by Dietary Perillyl Alcohol. Cancer Research. 57: 420-425.
Ripple G.H., Gould M.N., Stewart J.A., Tutsch K.D., Arzoomanian R.Z., Alberti D., Feierabend C., Pomplun M., Wilding G., Bailey H.H. (1998) Phase I Clinical Trial of Perillyl Alcohol Administered Daily. Clinical Cancer Research. 4: 1159-1164.
Romero-Jiménez M, Campos-Sánchez J, Analla M, Muñoz-Serrano A, Alonso-Moraga A (2005 Aug 1). "Genotoxicity and anti-genotoxicity of some traditional medicinal herbs," Mutat Res. 585(1-2):147-55.
Rose JE, Behm FM (1994 Feb). "Inhalation of vapor from black pepper extract reduces smoking withdrawal symptoms," Drug Alcohol Depend. 34(3):225-9.
Rowinsky E.K., Donehower R.C. (1995) Paclitaxel (Taxol). The New England Journal of Medicine. 332: 1004-1014.
Roy S, Khanna S, Shah H, Rink C, Phillips C, Preuss H, Subbaraju GV, Trimurtulu G, Krishnaraju AV, Bagchi M, Bagchi D, Sen CK (2005 Apr). "Human genome screen to identify the genetic basis of the anti-inflammatory effects of Boswellia in microvascular endothelial cells," DNA Cell Biol. 24(4):244-55.
Saeed SA, Gilani AH (1994 May). "Antithrombotic activity of clove oil," J Pak Med Assoc. 44(5):112-5.
Said T, Dutot M, Martin C, Beaudeux JL, Boucher C, Enee E, Baudouin C, Warnet JM, Rat P (2007 Mar). "Cytoprotective effect against UV-induced DNA damage and oxidative stress: role of new biological UV filter," Eur J Pharm Sci. 30(3-4):203-10.
Samaila D., Toy B.J., Wang R.C., Elegbede J.A. (2004) Monoterpenes Enhanced the Sensitivity of Head and Neck Cancer Cells to Radiation Treatment In Vitro. Anticancer Research. 24: 3089-3096.
Samarth RM, Goyal PK, Kumar A (2004 Jul). "Protection of swiss albino mice against whole-body gamma irradiation by Mentha piperita (Linn.)," Phytother Res. 18(7):546-50.
Samarth RM, Panwar M, Kumar M, Kumar A (2006 May). "Radioprotective influence of Mentha piperita (Linn) against gamma irradiation in mice: Antioxidant and radical scavenging activity," Int J Radiat Biol. 82(5):331-7.
Sampaio, L.F.S., Maia J.G.S., de Parijos A.M., de Souza R.Z., Barata L.E.S. (2011) Linalool from Rosewood (Aniba rosaeodora Ducke) Oil Inhibits Adenylate Cyclase in the Retina, Contributing to Understanding its Biological Activity. Phytotherapy Research. doi: 10.1002/ptr.3518.
Santos AO, Ueda-Nakamura T, Dias Filho BP, Veiga Junior VF, Pinto AC, Nakamura CV (2008 Nov 20). "Effect of Brazilian copaiba oils on Leishmania amazonensis," J Ethnopharmacol. 120(2):204-8.
Santos FA, Rao VS (2000 Jun). "Anti-inflammatory and antinociceptive effects of 1,8-cineole a terpenoid oxide present in many plant essential oils," Phytother Res. 14(4):240-4.
Santos F.A., Rao V.S.N. (1997) Mast cell involvement in the rat paw oedema response to 1,8-cineole, the main constituent of eucalyptus and rosemary oils. European Journal of Pharmacology. 331: 253-258.
Santos F.A., Rao V.S.N. (2001) 1,8-Cineol, a Food Flavoring Agent, Prevents Ethanol-Induced Gastric Injury in Rats. Digestive Diseases and Sciences. 46: 331-337.
Satoh T., Kosaka K., Itoh K., Kobayashi A., Yamamoto M., Shimoho Y., Kitajima C., Cui J., Kamins J., Okamoto S-I., Izumi M., Shirasawa T., Lipton S.A. (2008) Carnosic acid, a catechol-type electrophilic compound, protects neurons both in vitro and in vivothrough activation of the Keap1/Nrf2 pathway via S-alkylation of targeted cysteines on Keap1. Journal of Neurochemistry. 104: 1116-1131.
Savelev SU, Okello EJ, Perry EK (2004 Apr). "Butyryl- and acetyl-cholinesterase inhibitory activities in essential oils of Salvia species and their constituents," Phytother Res. 18(4):315-24.
Sayyah M, Nadjafnia L, Kamalinejad M (2004 Oct). "Anticonvulsant activity and chemical composition of Artemisia dracunculus L. essential oil," J Ethnopharmacol. 94(2-3):283-7.

Sayyah M, Saroukhani G, Peirovi A, Kamalinejad M (2003 Aug). "Analgesic and anti-inflammatory activity of the leaf essential oil of Laurus nobilis Linn," Phytother Res. 17(7):733-6.

Schecter A., Birnbaum L., Ryan J.J., Constable J.D. (2006) Dioxins: An overview. Environmental Research. 101: 419-428.

Schmitt S, Schaefer UF, Doebler L, Reichling J (2009 Oct). "Cooperative interaction of monoterpenes and phenylpropanoids on the in vitro human skin permeation of complex composed essential oils," Planda Med. 75(13):1381-5.

Schnitzler P, Schön K, Reichling J (2001 Apr). "Antiviral activity of Australian tea tree oil and eucalyptus oil against herpes simplex virus in cell culture," Pharmazie. 56(4):343-7.

Schroeter H, Heiss C, Balzer J, Kleinbongard P, Keen CL, Hollenberg NK, Sies H, Kwik-Uribe C, Schmitz HH, Kelm M (2006 Jan 24). "(-)-Epicatechin mediates beneficial effects of flavanol-rich cocoa on vascular function in humans," Proc Natl Acad Sci USA. 103(4):1024-9.

Schroter A., Kessner D., Kiselev M.A., Haub T., Dante S., Neubert R.H.H. (2009) Basic Nanostructure of Stratum Corneum Lipid Matrices Based on Ceramides [EOS] and [AP]: A Neutron Diffraction Study. Biophysical Journal. 97: 1104-1114.

Schuhmacher A, Reichling J, Schnitzler P (2003). "Virucidal effect of peppermint oil on the enveloped viruses herpes simplex virus type 1 and type 2 in vitro," Phytomedicine. 10(6-7):504-10.

Sedmak D.D., Davis D.H., Singh U., van de Winkel J.G.J., Anderson C.L. (1991) Expression of IgG Fc Receptor Antigens in Placenta and on Endothelial Cells in Humans: An Immunohistochemical Study. American Journal of Pathology. 138: 175-181.

Semah F., Picot M-C., Adam C., Broglin D., Arzimanoglou A., Bazin B., Cavalcanti D., Baulac M. (1998) Is the underlying cause of epilepsy a major prognostic factor for recurrence? Neurology. 51: 1256-1262.

Shapiro S., Guggenheim B. (1995) The action of thymol on oral bacteria. Oral Microbiology and Immunology. 10: 241-246.

Shapiro S, Meier A, Guggenheim B (1994 Aug). "The antimicrobial activity of essential oils and essential oil components towards oral bacteria," Oral Microbiol Immunol. 9(4):202-8.

Sharma PR, Mondhe DM, Muthiah S, Pal HC, Shahi AK, Saxena AK, Qazi GN (2009 May 15). "Anticancer activity of an essential oil from Cymbopogon flexuosus," Chem Biol Interact. 179(2-3):160-8.

Shen J, Niijima A, Tanida M, Horii Y, Maeda K, Nagai K (2005 Jun 3). "Olfactory stimulation with scent of grapefruit oil affects autonomic nerves, lipolysis and appetite in rats," Neurosci Lett. 380(3):289-94.

Sherry E, Boeck H, Warnke PH (2001). "Percutaneous treatment of chronic MRSA osteomyelitis with a novel plant-derived antiseptic," BMC Surg. 1:1.

Shibata M., Ohkubo T., Takahashi H., Inoki R. (1989) Modified formalin test: characteristic biphasic pain response. Pain. 38: 347-352.

Sikkema J., de Bont J.A.M., Poolman B. (1995) Mechanisms of Membrane Toxicity of Hydrocarbons. Microbiological Reviews. 59: 201-222.

Silva Brum L.F., Elisabetsky E., Souza D. (2001) Effects of Linalool on [3H] MK801 and [3H] Muscimol Binding in Mouse Cortical Membranes. Phytotherapy Research. 15: 422-425.

Silva Brum L.F., Emanuelli T., Souza D.O., Elisabetsky E. (2001) Effects of Linalool on Glutamate Release and Uptake in Mouse Cortical Synaptosomes. Neurochemical Research. 26: 191-194.

Silva J, Abebe W, Sousa SM, Duarte VG, Machado MI, Matos FJ (2003 Dec). "Analgesic and anti-inflammatory effects of essential oils of Eucalyptus," J Ethnopharmacol. 89(2-3):277-83.

Simons K., Toomre D. (2000) Lipid Rafts and Signal Transduction. Nature Reviews. 1: 31-41.

Singletary K, MacDonald C, Wallig M (1996 Jun 24). "Inhibition by rosemary and carnosol of 7,12-dimethylbenz[a]anthracene (DMBA)-induced rat mammary tumorigenesis and in vivo DMBA-DNA adduct formation," Cancer Lett. 104(1):43-8.

Skocibusić M, Bezić N (2004 Dec). "Phytochemical analysis and in vitro antimicrobial activity of two Satureja species essential oils," Phytother Res. 18(12):967-70.

Skold M., Borje A., Harambasic E., Karlberg A-T. (2004) Contact Allergens Formed on Air Exposure of Linalool. Identification and Quantification of Primary and Secondary Oxidation Products and the Effect on Skin Sensitization. Chemical Research in Toxicology. 17: 1697-1705.

Skold M., Borje A., Matura M., Karlberg A-T. (2002) Studies on the autoxidation and sensitizing capacity of the fragrance chemical linalool, identifying a linalool hydroperoxide. Contact Dermatitis. 46: 267-272.

Skold M., Karlberg A-T., Matura M., Borje A. (2006) The fragrace chemical ?-caryophyllene - air oxidation and skin sensitization. Food and Chemical Toxicology. 44: 538-545.

Smith DG, Standing L, de Man A (1992 Apr). "Verbal memory elicited by ambient odor," Percept Mot Skills. 74(2):339-43.

Soares SF, Borges LM, de Sousa Braga R, Ferreira LL, Louly CC, Tresvenzol LM, de Paula JR, Ferri PH (2009 Oct 7). "Repellent activity of plant-derived compounds against Amblyomma cajennense (Acari: Ixodidae) nymphs," Vet Parasitol. Epub ahead of print.

Sorentino S., Landmesser U. (2005) Nonlipid-lowering Effects of Statins. Current Treatment Options to Cardiovascular Medicine. 7: 459-466.

Sorg O., Zennegg M., Schmid P., Dedosyuk R., Valikhnovskyi R., Gaide O., Kniazevych V., Saurat J-H. (2009) 2,3,7,8-tetrachlorodibenzo-p-dioxin (TCDD) poisoning in Victor Yushchenko: identification and measurement of TCDD metabolites. The Lancet. 374: 1179-1185.

Staubach S., Hanisch F-G. (2011) Lipid rafts: signaling and sorting platforms of cells and their roles in cancer. Expert Review of Proteomics. 8: 263-277.

Steiner M, Priel I, Giat J, Levy J, Sharoni Y, Danilenko M (2001). "Carnosic acid inhibits proliferation and augments differentiation of human leukemic cells induced by 1,25-dihydroxyvitamin D3 and retinoic acid," Nutr Cancer. 41(1-2):135-44.

Stellman J.M., Stellman S.D., Christian R., Weber T., Tomasallo C. (2003) The extent and patterns of usage of Agent Orange and other herbicides in Vietnam. Nature. 422: 681-687.

Stratton S.P., Alberts D.S., Einspahr J.G. (2010) A Phase 2a Study of Topical Perillyl Alcohol Cream for Chemoprevention of Skin Cancer. Cancer Prevention Research. 3: 160-169.

Stratton S.P., Saboda K.L., Myrdal P.B., Gupta A., McKenzie N.E., Brooks C., Salasche S.J., Warneke J.A., Ranger-Moore J., Bozzo P.D., Blanchard J., Einspahr J.G. (2008) Phase 1 Study of Topical Perillyl Alcohol Cream for Chemoprevention of Skin Cancer. Nutrition and Cancer. 60: 325-330.

Sun Y., Olson R., Horning M., Armstrong N., Mayer M., Gouaux E. (2002) Mechanism of glutamate receptor desensitization. Nature. 417: 245-253.

Takada K., Nakane T., Masuda K., Ishii H. (2010) Ursolic acid and oleanolic acid, members of pentacyclic triterpenoid acids, suppress TNF-?-induced E-selectin expression by cultured umbilical vein endothelial cells. Phytomedicine. 17: 1114-1119.

Takarada K, Kimizuka R, Takahashi N, Honma K, Okuda K, Kato T (2004 Feb). "A comparison of the antibacterial efficacies of essential oils against oral pathogens," Oral Microbiol Immunol. 19(1):61-4.

Tanida M, Niijima A, Shen J, Nakamura T, Nagai K (2006 May 1). "Olfactory stimulation with scent of lavender oil affects autonomic neurotransmission and blood pressure in rats," Neurosci Lett. 398(1-2):155-60.

Tantaoui-Elaraki A, Beraoud L (1994). "Inhibition of growth and aflatoxin production in Aspergillus parasiticus by essential oils of selected plant materials," J Environ Pathol Toxicol Oncol. 13(1):67-72.

Tare V, Deshpande S, Sharma RN (2004 Oct). "Susceptibility of two different strains of Aedes aegypti (Diptera: Culicidae) to plant oils," J Econ Entomol. 97(5):1734-6.

Terzi V, Morcia C, Faccioli P, Valè G, Tacconi G, Malnati M (2007 Jun). "In vitro antifungal activity of the tea tree (Melaleuca alternifolia) essential oil and its major components against plant pathogens," Lett Appl Microbiol. 44(6):613-8.

Thomas E.D., Ramberg R.E., Sale G.E., Sparkes R.S., Golde D.W. (1976) Direct Evidence for a Bone Marrow Origin of the Alveolar Macrophages in Man. Science. 192: 1016-1018.

Thorsen M.A., Hildebrandt K.S. (2003) Quantitative determination of phenolic diterpenes in rosemary extracts: Aspects of accurate quantification. Journal of Chromatography A. 995: 119-125.

Tildesley NT, Kennedy DO, Perry EK, Ballard CG, Wesnes KA, Scholey AB (2005 Jan 17). "Positive modulation of mood and cognitive performance following administration of acute doses of Salvia lavandulaefolia essential oil to healthy young volunteers," Physiol Behav. 83(5):699-709.

Tipton DA, Lyle B, Babich H, Dabbous MKh (2003 Jun). "In vitro cytotoxic and anti-inflammatory effects of myrrh oil on human gingival fibroblasts and epithelial cells," Toxicol In Vitro. 17(3):301-10.
Trautmann M, Peskar BM, Peskar BA (1991 Aug 16). "Aspirin-like drugs, ethanol-induced rat gastric injury and mucosal eicosanoid release," Eur J Pharmacol. 201(1):53-8.
Trongtokit Y, Rongsriyam Y, Komalamisra N, Apiwathnasorn C (2005 Apr). "Comparative repellency of 38 essential oils against mosquito bites," Phytother Res. 19(4):303-9.
Trouw L.A., Daha M.R. (2011) Role of complement in innate immunity and host defense. Immunology Letters. 138: 35-37.
Turrens J.F. (2003) Mitochondrial formation of reactive oxygen species. Journal of Physiology.552: 335-344.
Tuszynski M.H. (2007) Nerve Growth Factor Gene Therapy in Alzheimer Disease. Alzheimer Disease & Associated Disorders. 21: 179-189.
Tuszynski M.H., Thal L., Pay M., Salmon D.P., Hoi S.U., Bakay R., Patel P., Blesch A., Vahlsing H.L., Ho G., Tong G., Potkin S.G., Fallon J., Hansen L., Mufson E.J., Kordower J.H., Gall C., Conner J. (2005) A phase 1 clinical trial of nerve growth factor gene therapy in Alzheimer disease. Nature Medicine. 11: 551-555.
Udagawa N., Takahashi N., Akatsu T., Tanaki H., Sasaki T., Nishihara T., Koga T., Martin T.J., Suda T. (1990) Origin of osteoclasts: Mature monocytes and macrophages are capable of differentiating into osteoclasts under a suitable microenvironment prepared by bone marrow-derived stromal cells. Proceedings of the National Academy of Science, USA. 87: 7260-7264.
Umezu T (2000 Jun). "Behavioral effects of plant-derived essential oils in the geller type conflict test in mice," Jpn J Pharmacol. 83(2):150-3.
Umezu T (1999 Sep). "Anticonflict effects of plant-derived essential oils," Pharmacol Biochem Behav. 64(1):35-40.
Uribe S., Ramirez J., Pena A. (1985) Effects of ?-Pinene on Yeast Membrane Functions. Journal of Bacteriology. 161: 1195-1200.
Vaka S.R.K., Murthy S.N., Repka M.A., Nagy T. (2011) Upregulation of Endogenous Neurotophin Levels in the Brain by Intranasal Administration of Carnosic Acid. Journal of Pharmaceutical Sciences. 100: 3139-3145.
van Tol RW, Swarts HJ, van der Linden A, Visser JH (2007 May). "Repellence of the red bud borer Resseliella oculiperda from grafted apple trees by impregnation of rubber budding strips with essential oils," Pest Manag Sci. 63(5):483-90.
Vigo E, Cepeda A, Gualillo O, Perez-Fernandez R (2004 Feb). "In-vitro anti-inflammatory effect of Eucalyptus globulus and Thymus vulgaris: nitric oxide inhibition in J774A.1 murine macrophages," J Pharm Pharmacol. 56(2):257-63.
Vigushin DM, Poon GK, Boddy A, English J, Halbert GW, Pagonis C, Jarman M, Coombes RC (1998). "Phase I and pharmacokinetic study of D-limonene in patients with advanced cancer. Cancer Research Campaign Phase I/II Clinical Trials Committee," Cancer Chemother Pharmacol. 42(2):111-7.
Vuković-Gacić B, Nikcević S, Berić-Bjedov T, Knezević-Vukcević J, Simić D (2006 Oct). "Antimutagenic effect of essential oil of sage (Salvia officinalis L.) and its monoterpenes against UV-induced mutations in Escherichia coli and Saccharomyces cerevisiae," Food Chem Toxicol. 44(10):1730-8.
Vutyavanich T, Kraisarin T, Ruangsri R (2001 Apr). "Ginger for nausea and vomiting in pregnancy: randomized, double-masked, placebo-controlled trial," Obstet Gynecol. 97(4):577-82.
Wallace R.J. (2004) Antimicrobial properties of plant secondary metabolites. Proceedings of the Nutrition Soiciety. 63: 621-629.
Wang T., Takikawa Y., Satoh T., Yoshioka Y., Kosaka K., Tatemichi Y., Suzuki K. (2011) Carnosic acid prevents obesity and hepatic steatosis in ob/ob mice. Hepatology Research. 41: 87-92.
Wei A, Shibamoto T (2007). "Antioxidant activities of essential oil mixtures toward skin lipid squalene oxidized by UV irradiation," Cutan Ocul Toxicol. 26(3):227-33.
Wilkinson JM, Hipwell M, Ryan T, Cavanagh HM (2003 Jan 1). "Bioactivity of Backhousia citriodora: antibacterial and antifungal activity," J Agric Food Chem. 51(1):76-81.
Williamson EM, Priestley CM, Burgess IF (2007 Dec). "An investigation and comparison of the bioactivity of selected essential oils on human lice and house dust mites," Fitoterapia. 78(7-8):521-5.
Wintersberger E. (1996) DNA Damage and Mutagenesis. Biochemical Society Transactions. 25: 303-308.
Wong K-K. (2009) Recent Developments in Anti-Cancer Agents Targeting the Ras/Raf/MEK/ERK Pathway. Recent Patents on Anti-Cancer Drug Discovery. 4: 28-35.
Woolf A. (1999) Essential Oil Poisoning. Clinical Toxicology. 37: 721-727.
Xia L, Chen D, Han R, Fang Q, Waxman S, Jing Y (2005 Mar). "Boswellic acid acetate induces apoptosis through caspase-mediated pathways in myeloid leukemia cells," Mol Cancer Ther. 4(3):381-8.
Xu J., Zhou F., Ji B-P., Pei R-S., Xu N. (2008) The antibacterial mechanism of carvacrol and thymol against Escherichia coli. Letters in Applied Microbiology. 47: 174-179.
Yamato K, Takahashi Y, Akiyama H, Tsuji K, Onishi H, Machida Y (2009 Apr). "Effect of penetration enhancers on transdermal delivery of propofol," Biol Pharm Bull. 32(4):677-83.
Yang GY, Wang W (1994 Sep). "[Clinical studies on the treatment of coronary heart disease with Valeriana officinalis var latifolia]," Zhongguo Zhong Xi Yi Jie He Za Zhi. 14(9):540-2.
Yang SA, Jeon SK, Lee EJ, Im NK, Jhee KH, Lee SP, Lee IS (2009 May). "Radical Scavenging Activity of the Essential Oil of Silver Fir (Abies alba)," J Clin Biochem Nutr. 44(3):253-9.
Yeruva L., Pierre K.J., Elegbede A., Wang R.C., Carper S.W. (2007) Perillyl alcohol and perillic acid induced cell cycle arrest and apoptosis in non small cell lung cancer cells. Cancer Letters. 257: 216-226.
Yoshikawa M., Matsuda H. (2000) Antidiabetogenic activity of oleanolic acid glycosides from medicinal foodstuffs. Biofactors. 13: 231-237.
Youdim KA, Deans SG (1999 Sep 8). "Dietary supplementation of thyme (Thymus vulgaris L.) essential oil during the lifetime of the rat: its effects on the antioxidant status in liver, kidney and heart tissues," Mech Ageing Dev. 109(3):163-75.
Youn L.J., Yoon J.W., Hovde C.J. (2010) A Brief Overview of Escherichia coli O157:H7 and Its Plasmid O157. Journal of Microbiology and Biotechnology. 20: 1-10.
Yuan HQ, Kong F, Wang XL, Young CY, Hu XY, Lou HX (2008 Jun 1). "Inhibitory effect of acetyl-11-keto-beta-boswellic acid on androgen receptor by interference of Sp1 binding activity in prostate cancer cells," Biochem Pharmacol. 75(11):2112-21.
Yu B.P. (1994) Cellular Defenses Against Damage From Reactive Oxygen Species. Physiological Reviews. 74: 139-162.
Yu S.G., Hildebrandt L.A., Elson C.E. (1995) Geraniol, and Inhibitor of Mevalonate Biosynthesis, Suppresses the Growth of Hepatomas and Melanomas Transplanted to Rats and Mice. Journal of Nutrition. 125: 2763-2767.
Yu Y-M., Lin H-C., Chang W-C. (2008) Carnosic acid prevents the migration of human aortic smooth muscle cells by inhibiting the activation and expression of matrix metalloproteinase-9. British Journal of Nutrition. 100: 731-738.
Zamith H.P.S., Vidal M.N.P., Speit G., Paumgartten F.J.R (1993) Absence of genotoxic activity of ?-myrcene in the in vivo cytogenetic bone marrow assay. Brazilian Journal of Medical and Biological Research. 26: 93-98.
Zha C., Brown G.B., Brouillette W.J. (2004) Synthesis and Structure-Activity Relationship Studies for Hydantoins and Analogues as Voltage-Gasted Sodium Channel Ligands. Journal of Medicinal Chemistry. 47: 6519-6528.
Zheng GQ, Kenney PM, Lam LK (1992 Aug). "Anethofuran, carvone, and limonene: potential cancer chemopreventive agents from dill weed oil and caraway oil," Planta Med. 58(4):338-41.
Zheng GQ, Kenney PM, Zhang J, Lam LK (1993). "Chemoprevention of benzo[a]pyrene-induced forestomach cancer in mice by natural phthalides from celery seed oil," Nutr Cancer. 19(1):77-86.
Zhou, J., Tang F., Bian R. (2004) Effect of ?-pinene on nuclear translocation of NF-?B in THP-1 cells. Acta Pharmacol Sin. 25: 480-484.
Zhu BC, Henderson G, Yu Y, Laine RA (2003 Jul 30). "Toxicity and repellency of patchouli oil and patchouli alcohol against Formosan subterranean termites Coptotermes formosanus Shiraki (Isoptera: Rhinotermitidae)," J Agric Food Chem. 51(16):4585-8.
Zore G.B., Thakre A.D., Jadhav S., Karuppayil S.M. (2011) Terpenoids inhibit Candida albicans growth by affecting membrane integrity and arrest of cell cycle. Phytomedicine. doi: 10.1016/j.phymed.2011.03.008.

BIBLIOGRAPHY

Balch, M.D., James, and Phyllis Balch, C.N.C. *Prescription for Nutritional Healing.* Garden City Park, NY: Avery Publishing Group, 1990.
Becker, M.D., Robert O. *The Body Electric.* New York, NY: Wm. Morrow, 1985.
Brown T.L., LeMay H.E., Bursten B.E. Chemistry: The Central Science. 10th ed. Upper Saddle River: Pearson Prentice Hall, 2006.
Burroughs, Stanley. *Healing for the Age of Enlightenment.* Auburn, CA: Burroughs Books, 1993.
Burton Goldberg Group, The. *Alternative Medicine: The Definitive Guide.* Fife, WA: Future Medicine Publishing, Inc., 1994.
Cowan M.K., Talaro K.P. *Microbiology: A Systems Approach. 2nd ed.* New York: McGraw Hill, 2009.
DeVita, Sabina M. *Electromagnetic Pollution. A Hidden Stress to Your System.* Marble Hill, MO: Stewart Publishing Company, 2000.
---------------. *Essential Oils Desk Reference.* Essential Science Publishing. Third Edition, First Printing March 2004.
Fischer-Rizzi, Suzanne. *Complete Aromatherapy Handbook.* New York, NY: Sterling Publishing, 1990.
Foley, Marcy. *Embraced by the Essence! Your Journey into Wellness Using Pure Quality Essential Oils.* Boulder, Colorado: Holistic Wellness Foundation I, April 2000.
Freeman S. *Biological Science. 2nd ed.* Upper Saddle River: Pearson Prentice Hall, 2005.
Gattefosse, Ph.D., Rene-Maurice. *Gattefosse's Aromatherapy.* Essex, England: The C.W. Daniel Company Ltd., 1937 English translation.
Green, Mindy. *Natural Perfumes: Simple Aromatherapy Recipes.* Loveland CO: Interweave Press Inc., 1999.
Guyton A.C., Hall J.E. *Textbook of Medical Physiology. 10th ed.* Philadelphia: W.B. Saunders Company, 2000.
---------------. *Integrated Aromatic Medicine.* Proceedings from the First International Symposium, Grasse, France. Essential Science Publishing, March 2000.
Klug W.S., Cummings M.R., Spencer C., Palladino M.A. *Concepts of Genetics.* San Francisco: Pearson Custom Publishing, 2009.
Lawless, Julia. *The Encyclopaedia of Essential Oils.* Rockport, MA: Element, Inc., 1992.
Lee, M.D., John R. *Natural Progesterone: The Multiple Roles of a Remarkable Hormone.* Sebastopol, CA: BLL Publishing, 1995.
Lewin B. *Essential Genes.* Upper Saddle River: Pearson Prentice Hall, 2006.
Maury, Marguerite. *Marguerite Maury's Guide to Aromatherapy.* C.W. Daniel, 1989.
Pènoël, M.D., Daniel and Pierre Franchomme. *L'aromatherapie exactement.* Limoges, France: Jollois, 1990.
Price, Shirley, and Len Price. *Aromatherapy for Health Professionals.* New York, NY: Churchill Livingstone Inc., 1995.
Price, Shirley, and Penny Price Parr. *Aromatherapy for Babies and Children.* San Francisco, CA: Thorsons, 1996.
Rose, Jeanne. *The Aromatherapy Book: Applications and Inhalations.* Berkeley, CA: North Atlantic Books, 1992.
Ryman, Danièle. *Aromatherapy: The Complete Guide to Plant & Flower Essences for Health and Beauty.* New York: Bantam Books, 1993.
Sheppard-Hanger, Sylla. *The Aromatherapy Practitioner Reference Manual.* Tampa, FL: Atlantic Institute of Aromatherapy, Twelfth Printing February 2000.
Stewart, Ph.D., R.A., David. *A Statistical Validation of Raindrop Technique.* Marble Hill, MO: Care Publications, 2003
Tisserand, Maggie. *Aromatherapy for Women: a Practical Guide to Essential Oils for Health and Beauty.* Rochester, VT: Healing Arts Press, 1996.
Tisserand, Robert. *Aromatherapy: to Heal and Tend the Body.* Wilmot, WI: Lotus Press, 1988.
Tisserand, Robert. *The Art of Aromatherapy.* Rochester, VT: Healing Arts Press, 1977.
Tisserand, Robert, and Tony Balacs. *Essential Oil Safety: A Guide for Health Care Professionals.* New York, NY: Churchill
Tortora G.J., Funke B.R., Case C.L. *Microbiology: An Introduction. 9th ed.* San Francisco: Pearson Benjamin Cummings, 2007.
Livingstone, 1995. Valnet, M.D., Jean. *The Practice of Aromatherapy: a Classic Compendium of Plant Medicines and their Healing Properties.*
Rochester, VT: Healing Arts Press, 1980.
Watson, Franzesca. *Aromatherapy Blends & Remedies.* San Francisco, CA: Thorsons, 1995.
Weaver R.F. *Molecular Biology. 4th ed.* New York: McGraw Hill, 2008.
Wilson, Roberta. *Aromatherapy for Vibrant Health and Beauty: a practical A-to-Z reference to aromatherapy treatments for health, skin, and hair problems.* Honesdale, PA: Paragon Press, 1995.
Worwood, Valerie Ann. *The Complete Book of Essential Oils & Aromatherapy.* San Rafael, CA: New World Library, 1991.
Young, N.D., D. Gary. *An Introduction to Young Living Essential Oils.* Payson, UT: Young Living Essential Oils, 2000.
Young, N.D., D. Gary. *Aromatherapy: The Essential Beginning.* Salt Lake City, UT: Essential Press Publishing, 1995.
Young, Ph.D., Robert O. *One Sickness, One Disease, One Treatment.* Alpine, UT: Self-published, 1995.

Video Listing

---------------. Essential Tips for Happy, Healthy Pets. The Vision Firm, LLC, 2000.
Eaton, Cathy. Raindrop Therapy. Health is Your Wealth Enterprises, 1997.
Woloshyn, Tom. Vita Flex Instruction. Vita-Gem Enterprises, 1998.
Young, ND, D. Gary. Raindrop Technique. Young Living Essential Oils, 2000.

INDEX

The following index has been manually verified and adjusted to increase its effectiveness and reduce its length. Due to the extent that the single oils are listed throughout this reference guide, we thought it best to list only the most relevant page numbers for each single oil listing. The single oils are all listed in bold print to make it easy to identify them. All other page numbers that are listed in bold print are the most relevant for their respective listing.

3 Wise Men 42, 171, 180, 186, 198, 202, 246, 299, 309, 312, 323, 327, 329, 356, 357, 364, 368, 372, 375, 384, 385, 389, 390, 391, 392, 408, 409, 412, 434, 441, 442, 463, 464, 466, 482, 496, 499, 509, 510, 514, 516, 519, 543, 555, 556, 557, 560, 567

A

Abandoned 187, **298**, 391. *See also* Emotions
Abrasions 95, 188
Abscess 57, 68, 78, 89, 100, **298**, 455. *See also* Antifungal, Antibacterial, Infection, Oral Conditions
Absent Minded **298**. *See also* memory
Absorption 296
Abundance **149**, 263, 267, 272, 284, 285, 298, 317, 320, 322, 343, 355, 373, 375, 394, 423, 430, 464, 466, 475, 479, 520, 543, 553, 555, 557, 558, 560, 563
Abuse 179, 197, **299**, 391, 485
Acceptance **150**, 166, 173, 178, 180, 186, 298, 299, 302, 308, 309, 324, 326, 329, 332, 333, 334, 335, 344, 347, 356, 357, 373, 374, 376, 384, 386, 388, 389, 390, 391, 392, 398, 400, 408, 409, 412, 413, 416, 417, 418, 421, 434, 437, 438, 441, 444, 445, 446, 454, 457, 461, 463, 464, 466, 472, 475, 477, 480, 482, 483, 485, 488, 495, 496, 502, 510, 521, 543, 555, 558, 559, 560, 563
Accidents **299**. *See also* Emotions
Aches/Pains 33, 49, 60, 62, 63, 66, 69, 71, 73, 78, 80, 91, 95, 105, 118, 121, 130, 152, 218, 246, 299, 447, 497, 498
Acid/Acidic 245, 251, 257, 267, 300, 336, 348, 351, 363, 405, 420, 463, 474, 498
Acidosis **299**, 300, 306, 351, 363, 406, 420, 463, 474. *See also* Alkaline, pH Balance
Acne 50, 51, 52, 55, 57, 62, 69, 70, 71, 78, 79, 86, 89, 94, 95, 96, 103, 111, 114, 119, 120, 121, 122, 132, 134, 277, **300**, 301, 346, 488. *See also* Hormonal Imbalance, Scarring, Skin, Stress
Actinic Keratosis 489
Addictions 112, 183, 258, 259, **302**, 413, 494
Addison's Disease 303, 304. *See also* Adrenal Glands
Adenitis 303. *See also* Lymphatic System
Adrenal Glands 33, 100, 105, 115, 116, 124, 125, 136, 137, 165, 181, 283, 300, 303, 305, 393, 421, 437, 438, 480. *See also* Endocrine System, Lupus, Thyroid
Adversity 205
Aftershave 153, 171, **304**, 440, 489. *See also* Skin
Agent Orange Poisoning **305**
Aging 76, 77, 94, 117, 119, 186, 210, 212, 221, 235, 251, 253, 260, 286, **305**, 415, 474, 488, 489, 492. *See also* Wrinkles
Agitation 50, **346**. *See also* Calming
AIDS 285, 286, 300, **305**. *See also* Antiviral
Air 306, 373, 494
Airborne Bacteria 157, **306**, 511. *See also* Antibacterial
Air purification 9, 157, 192
Air Travel 297
Alcohol 259, 278, 302, 561, 567
Alcoholism 80, **302** . *See also* Addictions
Alertness 158, **306**, 442
AlkaLime **245**, 300, 306, 307, 317, 318, 326, 336, 338, 348, 351, 363, 366, 371, 379, 380, 381, 382, 395, 401, 405, 406, 418, 420, 423, 428, 429, 433, 444, 456, 463, 475, 498, 512, 513, 514, 521, 543, 556, 557
Alkaline/Alkalize 245, 267, 299, 300, **306**, 311, 317, 336, 348, 350, 351, 364, 405, 463. *See also* Acidosis, pH Balance
Alkalosis 48, 307, 463 . *See also* pH Balance
Allergies 53, 57, 69, 76, 77, 89, 90, 98, 111, 123, 153, 193, 194, 246, 251, 255, 279, 296, **307**, 333, 351, 370, 386, 423, 427, 437, 488
Allerzyme **246**, 302, 303, 318, 327, 346, 379, 395, 400, 401, 406, 408, 418, 423, 432, 501, 521, 543, 552, 554, 555, 556, 557, 558, 560
Alone (feeling) **308**. *See also* Emotions
Alopecia Areata **308**, 415. *See also* Hair
Aluminum Toxicity 302, 308
Alzheimer's Disease 9, 10, 120, 121, 207, 277, 308, 436, 461. *See also* Brain, Memory, Pineal Gland, Pituitary Gland
Amazonian Ylang Ylang *See* Ylang Ylang, Amazonian
Amenorrhea 61, 100, 134, 403
Amino Acids 255, 258, 271, 284, 285, 286, 309
Amnesia **309**. *See also* Memory
Amygdala 10, 40, 65
Anaerobic Bacteria 188
Analgesic 11, 14, 50, 51, 56, 61, 62, 63, 68, 71, 72, 75, 78, 88, 91, 94, 96, 111, 113, 118, 121, 126, 133, 135, **309**, 469, 549–551, 568, 569, 570, 572. *See also* Pain
Anchoring 73, 74, 75
Anemia 53, 91, **309**, 569
Anesthesia 106, **310**. *See also* Pain
Aneurysm 127, 310. *See also* Blood, Cardiovascular System
Angelica **47**, 543, 549, 552
Anger 48, 55, 57, 58, 82, 103, 113, 126, 136, 152, 153, 183, 194, 206, 310, 347, 389, 439. *See also* Calming, Liver
Angina 80, 87, 107, **311**, 352. *See also* Cardiovascular System
Animals 9, 88, 161, 188, 197, **311**, 386, 493
Animal Scents Pet Ointment **214**, 311, 343, 362, 552, 554, 555, 557, 558, 559
Animal Scents Pet Shampoo **214**, 311, 553, 555, 556, 560
Anise **48**, 543, 552

Index

Ankles 387
Anorexia 47, 63, 132, 386. *See also* Eating Disorders
Antacid 245
Anthrax 129, **315**. *See also* Antibacterial
Antiallergic 94
Antianxiety 131
Antiarthritic 72
Antiasthmatic 84
Antibacterial 8, 11, 14, 15, 20, 26, 33, 49, 50, 52, 53, 54, 58, 60, 61, 62, 63, 64, 65, 66, 67, 68, 70, 71, 79, 82, 88, 91, 92, 94, 95, 96, 97, 98, 99, 100, 103, 104, 106, 108, 109, 112, 113, 114, 115, 116, 118, 119, 120, 122, 123, 125, 126, 127, 128, 129, 131, 135, 137, 163, 196, 201, 298, 300, 301, 306, 315, 422, 466, 512, 549–551, 570
Antibiotic **316**, 350. *See also* Antibacterial
Anticancerous 8, 76, 77, 90, 91, 107, 118, 120, 128, 133, 255. *See also* Cancer: Anticancerous
Anticarcinogenic 113
Anticatarrhal 51, 68, 71, 72, 76, 77, 82, 84, 85, 111, 118, 121, 122, **316**, 354, 549–551. *See also* Congestion
Anticoagulant 47, 82, 88, 126, **316**, 357. *See also* Blood
Anticonvulsive 60, 88
Antidandruff 131
Antidepressant 58, 68, 76, 77, 79, 81, 85, 88, 90, 98, 104, 107, 121, 123, 136, 137, **317**, 375, 386, 470, 549–551. *See also* Depression
Antidiarrheal 106
Antifungal 8, 11, 18, 48, 53, 55, 58, 60, 61, 63, 64, 66, 70, 71, 87, 88, 90, 94, 96, 97, 98, 99, 100, 103, 104, 106, 108, 109, 111, 112, 116, 118, 119, 122, 123, 127, 128, 129, 149, 163, 298, **317**, 549–551, 570
Antihemorrhaging 116. *See also* Blood: Hemorrhaging
Antihistamine 11, 52, 88, 94, 98, 126, **307**. *See also* Allergies
Anti-infectious 8, 15, 18, 20, 33, 49, 50, 51, 52, 55, 56, 57, 58, 61, 65, 66, 68, 70, 71, 76, 77, 78, 83, 84, 88, 93, 94, 95, 96, 97, 100, 101, 102, 104, 110, 111, 114, 116, 118, 119, 121, 124, 125, 127, 128, 129, 476, 549–551. *See also* Infection, Antibacterial, Antifungal, Antiviral
Anti-inflammatory 14, 18, 47, 49, 50, 51, 52, 56, 57, 58, 60, 61, 62, 63, 65, **67**, 68, **69**, 70, 71, 73, 76, 77, 78, 84, 87, 88, 91, 96, 98, 101, 102, 103, 105, 106, 111, 112, 113, 114, 118, 121, 122, 123, 124, 125, 126, 127, 128, 129, 133, 134, 135, 190, 195, 300, 301, **319**, 330, 406, 469, 549–551, 568, 569. *See also* Antioxidant
Antimicrobial 18, 33, 51, 52, 58, 59, 65, 78, 88, 94, 97, 98, 103, 109, 112, 115, 121, 129, 130, 239, 240, 241, 265, 316, **320**, 373, 549–551. *See also* Antibacterial, Antifungal, Antiviral
Antimutagenic 88, 90, 116, 120
Antineuralgic 51, 115
Antioxidant 20
Antioxidants 8, 49, 56, 58, 61, 63, 64, 82, 84, 90, 96, 100, 106, 118, 128, 186, 216, 217, 219, 229, 230, 234, 235, 238, 242, 253, 255, 263, 267, 271, 272, 278, 279, 280, 281, 285, 305, **320**
Antiparasitic 8, 50, 52, 57, 58, 61, 64, 72, 84, 96, 100, 103, 104, 105, 108, 119, 128, 129, 255, 270, **320**, 549–551. *See also* Parasite
Antirheumatic 11, 55, 56, 63, 70, 75, 125, 133, **320**, 549–551, 569. *See also* Arthritis
Antiseptic 8, 11, 14, 18, 20, 26, 33, 48, 49, 50, 51, 52, 54, 55, 56, 58, 59, 60, 61, 62, 64, 65, 68, 70, 71, 72, 73, 74, 75, 76, 77, 78, 79, 80, 81, 84, 86, 87, 88, 90, 91, 92, 93, 94, 95, 96, 98, 100, 101, 102, 103, 104, 105, 106, 107, 108, 109, 110, 111, 113, 114, 115, 116, 120, 121, 122, 128, 129, 130, 132, 133, 134, 135, 136, 137, 156, 157, 188, 201, 228, 236, 239, 240, 241, 306, **321**, 381, 469, 549–551, 570. *See also* Antibacterial, Antifungal, Antiviral
Antisexual 95, **321**
Antispasmodic 14, 18, 48, 49, 50, 51, 52, 56, 57, 58, 60, 63, 64, 67, 71, 72, 75, 78, 82, 84, 85, 86, 88, 94, 95, 98, 100, 104, 107, 108, 111, 112, 113, 114, 118, 120, 121, 122, 124, 125, 127, 128, 131, 132, 133, 136, 137, **321**, 380, 495, 549–551
Antitoxic 64, 88, 111, 426
Antitumoral 8, 11, 52, 56, 61, 76, 77, 88, 90, 101, 110, 112, 121, **321**, 511. *See also* Tumors, Cancer
Antiviral 8, 11, 15, 26, 49, 53, 58, 61, 64, 65, 68, 69, 70, 71, 78, 82, 84, 90, 92, 94, 96, 98, 100, 103, 104, 108, 109, 112, 113, 115, 116, 119, 127, 128, 129, 149, 156, 163, 201, 306, **321**, 350, 358, 549–551, 570
Anxiety 49, 50, 55, 58, 63, 66, 73, 74, 75, 81, 84, 85, 89, 91, 92, 93, 95, 98, 104, 107, 111, 115, 123, 130, 132, 136, 153, 166, 167, 176, 191, 199, 200, 202, 312, 314, **323**, 328, 467, 568, 570, 572. *See also* Calming
Apathy 85, **323**. *See also* Depression
Aphrodisiac 52, 64, 104, 111, 116, 117, 121, **323**, 570, 571
Apnea **324**
Appetite 47, 50, 52, 64, 80, 84, 87, 105, 107, 111, 112, 122, 128, 134, 324
Application Notes 295
Applications 25–28
Argumentative 310, **324**. *See also* Calming
Arms-Flabby **324**
AromaGuard Deodorants **215**, 374, 455, 488, 543, 553, 554, 555, 556, 557, 558, 559
Aroma Life **151**, 207, 310, 324, 325, 336, 337, 338, 341, 351, 352, 353, 354, 357, 397, 417, 419, 421, 430, 431, 439, 441, 442, 469, 472, 477, 480, 483, 487, 488, 499, 500, 510, 517, 553, 555, 557, 561, 563
Aroma Siez 33, 35, **152**, 187, 195, 325, 330, 331, 332, 341, 346, 357, 371, 374, 388, 402, 417, 431, 446, 447, 448, 449, 458, 467, 482, 484, 495, 501, 505, 508, 517, 522, 552, 553, 556, 557, 558, 563
Aromatic 352, 543
Arousing 184, 198, 486
Arrythmia **352**
A·R·T Beauty Masque 489, 491, 552, 553, 556, 557, 558
A·R·T Creme Masque 491, 492, 554, 555, 556, 558, 561
A•R•T Creme Masque **210**
A·R·T Day Activator 553, 555, 560
A•R•T Day Activator **209, 210**
Arterial Vasodilator **324**. *See also* Arteries
Arteries 95, 136, **324**, 353
Arteriosclerosis 55, 118, 300. *See also* Arteries
A·R·T Gentle Foaming Cleanser 555, 556, 557, 560
A•R•T Gentle Foaming Cleanser **211**
Arthritis 33, 51, 55, 56, 62, 63, 65, 73, 80, 84, 86, 89, 91, 95, 105, 107, 113, 118, 120, 121, 124, 125, 127, 128, 132, 134, 190, 195, 231, 232, 233, 277, 285, 300, 312, **325**, 346, 568, 570. *See also* Acidosis
A·R·T Night Reconstructor 553, 555, 560
A•R•T Night Reconstructor 212
A·R·T Purifying Toner 343, 357, 555, 556, 557, 558, 560
A•R•T Purifying Toner **212**
A·R·T Renewal Serum 490, 552, 553, 555, 556, 561
A•R•T Renewal Serum **213**
A·R·T Skin Care System 300, 305, 357, 438, 472, 474, 482, 488, 490, 492, 502, 508
A•R•T Skin Care System **209–213, 543**
Ashamed **326**. *See also* Emotions
Assault **326**. *See also* Emotions
Assimilating Food **327**
Asthenia 121
Asthma 51, 52, 65, 67, 69, 70, 73, 74, 75, 76, 77, 78, 82, 84, 87, 89, 91, 95, 98, 101, 103, 107, 108, 113, 115, 116, 117, 118, 120, 121, 129, 130, 193, 231, 232, 233, **327**, 454. *See also* Respiratory System
Astringent 55, 58, 59, 60, 65, 73, 74, 75, 79, 84, 86, 90, 101, 103, 106, 111, 112, 121, 130, 134, **328**, 568, 569

Athlete's Foot 70, 95, 96, 101, **328**. *See also* Antifungal
Attention Deficit Disorder (ADD/ADHD) 90, 205, 308, **328**
Attitude 186, 204
Aura 42, 206, **328**, 359, 463
Auricular Emotional Therapy Chart 41
Auricular Internal Body Points - Chart 32
Auricular Therapy 25
Australian Blue **152**, 176, 310, 351, 353, 358, 365, 366, 389, 420, 473, 486, 487, 501, 510, 543, 552, 554, 560, 561, 563
Autism **328**
Auto-Immune System 59, 304, **328**, 416. *See also* AIDS, Grave's Disease, Hashimoto's Disease, Lupus
Autonomic Nervous System 67, 128
Autonomic Nervous System Chart 38
Avoidance **328**. *See also* Emotions
Awake **329**. *See also* Alertness
Awaken 150, 153, 163, 165, 180, 181, 199, 207, 267, 304, 323, 328, 329, 332, 341, 356, 365, 367, 368, 372, 373, 375, 384, 388, 394, 398, 400, 412, 440, 442, 446, 452, 454, 460, 466, 471, 485, 489, 496, 502, 510, 522, 543, 552, 563
Awaken the Mind, Spirit **329**
Awaken the Past **329**
Awareness 134, 198, 206, **329**, 337, 485, 496

B

Babies/Children 171, 172, 227, 296, **329**, 360, 467. *See also* Children/Infants
Back 33, 73, 313, **329–330**
Backaches 131, 231, 232, 233
Bacteria 33, 58, 62, 73, 104, 120, 129, 130, 156, 188, 192, 215, 239, 277, 280, 300, 306, 340, 373, 466, 475, 498, 511, 512. *See also* Antibacterial
Bad Breath (Halitosis) 122, 241
Balance 18, 33, 68, 78, 81, 89, 99, 117, 120, 121, 122, 123, 124, 125, 131, 134, 135, 153, 157, 164, 165, 166, 170, 174, 175, 185, 198, 199, 200, 203, 205, 206, 235, 241, 242, 245, 250, 253, 255, 267, 280, 296, 299, 300, 323, 332, 336, 339, 363, 387, 388, 389, 402, 405, 406, 414, 421, 439, 443, 464, 496, 501, 568, 569, 570, 571, 572
Balance Complete **247**, 252, 260, 261, 269, 270, **273**, 283, 300, 302, 305, 306, 317, 318, 327, 348, 363, 364, 366, 367, 371, 377, 378, 379, 381, 382, 400, 401, 405, **406**, 408, 412, 418, 423, 433, 434, 436, 438, 454, 463, 468, 475, 511, 520, 521, 543, 558
Baldness 118, **333**. *See also* Hair
Balsam Fir *See* Fir, Balsam
Basal Cell Temperature **281**, 437, 507
Basil **49**, 543, 549, 552
Bath 26, 152, 153, 157, 159, 163, 166, 172, 181, 182, 188, 191, 216, 220, 225, 228, 237, 296, 305, **333**, 446, 493, 497, 509
Bath Gel Base **216**, 296, 333
Beard **413**
Bed Wetting 259, 335. *See also* Bladder
Be-Fit 263, 264, 267, 272, 273, 284, 285
Belching 161, **333**
Believe **154**, 173, 204, 329, 341, 347, 376, 390, 391, 392, 407, 443, 466, 480, 496, 499, 500, 501, 543, 552, 553, 554, 555, 560, 561, 563
Bereavement **333**
Bergamot **50**, 543, 549, 552
Betrayed (Feeling) 187, **333**. *See also* Emotions
Bibilical Sweet Myrrh *See* Myrrh, Biblical Sweet
Birthing 171
Bites 49, 50, 62, 76, 77, 111, 128, **333**, 426
Bitterness **334**. *See also* Emotions
Black Pepper *See* Pepper, Black
Bladder 86, 92, 103, 116, 134, 259, **334**, 514
Blame **335**. *See also* Emotions
Bleeding 59, 79, 82, 107, 112, 311, 337, 403, 523
Blending Essential Oils 22–24, 296, 297
Blend Summary Information 563
Blindness 397
Blisters 98, **335**, 427, 502
BLM **248**, 311, 312, 326, 330, 331, 340, 341, 346, 354, 371, 432, 434, 447, 448, 450, 461, 497, 504, 543, 553, 554, 561
Bloating 56, 161, 198, 246, 251, 379, 498
Blocked (Emotionally) **389**. *See also* Emotions
Blood 10, 48, 53, 57, 65, 73, 82, 91, 191, 203, 231, 232, 233, 245, 255, 264, 267, 273, 278, 283, 285, 286, 300, 306, 308, 309, 310, 317, 335, 336, 340, 350, 352, 364, 366, 376, 378, 393, 396, 401, 415, 420, 431, 437, 461, 463, 474, 491, 500, 501, 517
Blood-Brain Barrier 10, 14, 76, 77, 309
Blood Clots 62, 106, 231, 232, 233, 325, **337**, 500, 518
Blood Pressure 69, 89, 91, 92, 95, 115, 118, 136, 137, 277, **336**
Blood Sugar 231, 232, 233, 246, 248, 267, 272, 277, 283, 285, **338**, 375, 378, 418
Blood Type Information **335**
Blood Vessels 337
Blue Agave **248**, 543
Blue Cypress *See* Cypress, Blue
Bodygize 378
Body Systems 104, 323, **339**, 416
Body Systems Chart **543–550**
Boils 50, 52, 57, 59, 78, 89, 95, 96, **339**
Bonding **339**, 359
Bone Density 231, 232, 233
Bones 33, 49, 56, 60, 62, 63, 65, 69, 71, 73, 74, 75, 79, 80, 82, 88, 92, 96, 98, 103, 104, 107, 108, 109, 113, 121, 122, 124, 125, 129, 133, 134, 135, 152, 154, 160, 173, 187, 190, 195, 205, 230, 231, 232, 233, 235, 245, 248, 264, 266, 267, 271, 272, **273**, 278, 279, 280, 283, 284, 285, 311, 312, **339**, 348, 349, 350, 456, 497, 508, 524, 543–550, 568, 569, 572
Boredom **341**
Boswellia Wrinkle Creme **216**, 305, 488, 489, 491, 492, 493, 543, 555, 557, 560, 561
Botanical Names 552–564
Bowel 52, 64, 127, 249, 250, 255, **341**, 351, 366, 379, 491, 521. *See also* Digestive System
Boxed in (Feeling) **341**
Brain 59, 66, 67, 154, 158, 191, 203, 205, 271, 308, 322, 324, **341**, 348, 375, 417, 430, 436, 446, 450, 452, 454, 461, 464, 494
Brain Power **154**, 159, 298, 299, 305, 309, 313, 324, 368, 375, 394, 399, 407, 430, 441, 442, 450, 451, 452, 463, 464, 484, 494, 514, 543, 552, 554, 555, 556, 557, 560, 563
Breast 132, 231, 232, 233, **342**, 343, 348, 375, 432, 467, 471. *See also* Cancer, Pregnancy/Motherhood
Breath 52, 61
Breathe Again 343, 368, 423, 479, 487, 488
Breathing 136, 137, 469. *See also* Respiratory System
Bronchitis 48, 49, 50, 51, 52, 55, 56, 59, 61, 62, 65, 68, 69, 71, 73, 74, 75, 76, 77, 78, 82, 87, 89, 90, 95, 96, 97, 98, 101, 103, 107, 108, 112, 113, 115, 116, 117, 118, 120, 121, 122, 129, 130, 193, 201, **343**, 479. *See also* Respiratory System
Bruises 47, 52, 57, 84, 89, 95, 103, 127, 160, 188, 190, 201, 340, **344**, 488, 523
Bugged (Feeling) **344**. *See also* Emotions
Bugs (Repel) **344**, 427. *See also* Bites, Insect
Building 178, 183
Bulimia **344**, 386. *See also* Eating Disorders
Bumps 160, 190, **344**
Bunions 116, **344**. *See also* Bursitis
Burdens 344, 389. *See also* Emotions
Burns 57, 69, 73, 79, 89, 95, 96, 100, 116, 117, 125, 188, 225, 295, **345**, 476, 501, 569
Bursitis 51, 277, 344, **346**

C

Caffeine 302, **346**
Cajeput **51**, 543, 549, 552
Calamus 552
Calcification 314
Calcium 264, 265, 277, 280, 285, 300, **346**, 374, 460. *See also* Hormonal Imbalance
Callouses 401. *See also* Skin
Calming 14, 18, 47, 54, 55, 56, 57, 63, 68, 71, **77**, 80, 95, 97, 99, 100, 103, 104, 111, 121, 122, 126, 131, 132, 136, 137, 151, 152, 153, 154, 157, 172, 191, 199, 202, 203, 204, 205, 226, 228, 231, 236, 242, 310, 311, **346**, 541, 568, 570, 571
Calories **277**
Cancer 48, 62, 76, 77, 79, 90, 101, 110, 116, 183, 232, 233, 285, 286, 300, **347**, 375, 378, 401, 441, 476, 511, 515. *See also* Chemicals, tumors, Radiation
Candida 50, 69, 96, 101, 109, 113, 118, 119, 122, 123, 124, 125, 129, 130, 188, 201, 251, 300, 378, 407, 423. *See also* Antifungal
Cankers 188, 201, **351**, 513. *See also* Acidosis
Capillaries 65, 91, 92, 279, 310, 338, **351**, 352, 399, 431. *See also* Cardiovascular System
Caraway **51**, 552
Carbohydrates 277, 378, 407
Carbuncles 50, 76, 77, 89, 95, **351.** *See also* Boils
Cardamom **52**, 543, 549
Cardiac Muscle **447**
Cardiotonic 88, 129, **353.** *See also* Cardiovascular System
Cardiovascular System 48, 49, 51, 53, 62, 63, 65, 72, 75, 81, 82, 84, 88, 89, 96, 106, 107, 109, 122, 130, 136, 137, 151, 157, 186, 245, 256, 260, 261, 263, 264, 266, 267, 269, 270, 271, 272, 274, 277, 278, 280, 283, **351**, 543–550, 568, 569, 570, 571. *See also* Arteries, Blood, Capillaries, Veins
Carminative 53
Carpal Tunnel Syndrome **354.** *See also* Inflammation
Carrot **53**, 543
Cartilage 122, 248, **340**
Cassia **53**, 552
Catalysts 245, **395**
Cataracts **397.** *See also* Eyes
Catarrh (Mucus) 51, 59, 67, 73, 74, 75, 76, 77, 78, 80, 85, 95, 101, 103, 112, 120, 122, 134, 551. *See also* Anticatarrhal, Congestion
Cats **311**
Cavities 240, **503.** *See also* Oral Conditions, Teeth
Cedar Leaf **54**, 552
Cedar, Western Red **54**, 543, 552
Cedarwood **55**, 543, 549, 552
Celery Seed 543, 553
Celibacy 95, **354**
Cel-Lite Magic **217**, 310, 325, 338, 352, 355, 358, 368, 397, 398, 406, 439, 440, 448, 492, 517, 521, 543, 552, 553, 555, 556, 558
Cells 19, 61, 104, 109, 112, 122, 149, 194, 205, 210, 212, 231, 232, 233, 236, 237, 245, 248, 265, 272, 273, 277, 278, 279, 281, 283, 284, 285, 296, 301, 308, 309, 320, 325, 337, **355**, 373, 395, 400, 401, 415, 436, 437, 439, 457, 466, 474, 476
Cellulite 55, 64, 65, 81, 91, 92, 111, 118, 126, 134, **355**, 400, 569
Centering 68, 84
Central Nervous System 56, 71, 91
Chakras (Energy Centers) 42, 43, 50, 79, 105, 112, 120, 122, 174, 175, 202, 296, 308, 332, **356**, 471, 571
Chamomile, German (Blue) **56**, 543, 549, 553
Chamomile, Roman **57**, 544, 549, 553
Change (Personal) 203, **357.** *See also* Emotions
Charley Horse **357**, 447. *See also* Muscles
Cheeks **357**
Chelating/Chelation 82, 151, 183, 302, 310, **357**, 517. *See also* Detoxification
Chelex Tincture 250, 553
Chemical Constituents 10, 11–15
Chemicals 82, 296, 306, 347, **358**, 415, 417, 491, 499. *See also* Metals
Chemotherapy **477**
Chicken Pox 70, 358. *See also* Childhood Diseases
Chiggers 427. *See also* Insect
Childbirth 61, 63, 68, 85, 122, 217. *See also* Pregnancy/Motherhood
Childhood Diseases **358**, 446, 522
Childhood Issues/Emotions 389, 390, 521
Children 58, 67, 92, 94, 103, 157, 162, 179, 191, 205, 227, 296, 339, 344, **359**, 360, 380, 414, 417, 428, 456, 518, 523. *See also* Childhood Diseases, Hyperactive
Chills 80, 107, 112, 118, 121, **362**
Chiropractor **205**
Chivalry 409
Chlorophyll 267, **362**
Chocolate **261**
Cholera 51, 62, 112, 116, 118, 131, **362.** *See also* Antibacterial
Cholesterol 61, 92, 107, 118, 251, 286, 337, **363**, 473
Christmas Spirit **155**, 299, 315, 352, 375, 386, 390, 416, 430, 483, 544, 553, 558, 560, 563
Chronic Fatigue 300, **363**, 395. *See also* Acidosis, Hormonal Imbalance
Cigarettes 9, **364**, 466, 475. *See also* Smoking
Cinnamint Lip Balm **217**, 434, 490, 544, 553, 558, 560
Cinnamon Bark **58**, 544, 549, 553
Circulation 15, 58, 62, 63, 64, 65, 78, 86, 92, 104, 105, 107, 109, 112, 117, 118, 121, 122, 126, 129, 130, 151, 182, 190, 206, 308, 310, 330, 336, 338, 415, 437, 449, 469, 517, 518, 570. *See also* Cardiovascular System
Circulatory System 33, 61, 65, 81, 82, 115, 121, 132, 151, 300, 517. *See also* Cardiovascular System
Cirrhosis 85, **364**, 435. *See also* Liver
Cistus **59**, 544, 549, 553
Citronella **60**, 544, 549, 553
Citrus Fresh **157**, 180, 266, 272, 279, 285, 299, 301, 306, 311, 315, 343, 346, 347, 352, 361, 373, 375, 386, 387, 388, 390, 401, 428, 430, 439, 450, 470, 478, 517, 521, 544, 555, 556, 557, 558, 560, 563
ClaraDerm **217**, 342, 393, 467, 468, 472, 488, 491, 544, 553, 555, 556, 557
Clarity 49, 91, 92, 93, 154, 155, **158**, 165, 166, 170, 171, 181, 186, 187, 188, 200, 281, 298, 300, 302, 306, 309, 324, 329, 337, 352, 363, 364, 368, 372, 375, 384, 391, 394, 399, 400, 407, 417, 421, 430, 437, 439, 441, 442, 446, 452, 461, 467, 472, 487, 488, 497, 544, 552, 553, 555, 556, 558, 559, 561, 563
Clarity of Thoughts **364**
Clary Sage **60**, 544, 549, 553
Cleaning 27, 104, 228, **422**, 475
Cleansing 72, 82, 84, 86, 91, 92, 96, 182, 183, 188, 216, 228, 236, 240, 249, 255, 258, 267, 300, 308, 316, 337, 345, 349, **364**, 365, 367, 375, 376, 378, 400, 411, 431, 435, 437, 439, 454, 491, 508, 513, 516, 517. *See also* Housecleaning
Cleansing Trio 302, 303, 305, 306, 308, 309, 310, 325, 327, 348, 349, 352, 358, 363, 364, 366, 367, 368, 371, 377, 378, 381, 382, 393, 406, 412, 418, 423, 431, 433, 435, 436, 437, 439, 444, 446, 460, 461, 462, 468, 470, 475, 484, 486, 503, 508, 511, 512, 516, 520, 521, 522, 523
Clearing 199, 200, 389
Closed Minded **365**
Clothes 27, **365**, 422, 475
Clove **61**, 544, 549, 553
Club Foot **401**
Cockroaches 427. *See also* Insects
Coffee (Stop Drinking) 259, 302, **365.** *See also* Addictions
Coldness (Emotional) **390**
Colds 47, 49, 51, 54, 58, 59, 60, 62, 63, 65, 69, 70, 71, 73, 74, 75, 76, 77, 80, 84, 90, 91, 92, 95, 96, 98, 103, 107, 108, 111, 112, 115, 116, 118, 121, 127, 129, 130, 131, 134, 178, 193, 194,

201, 277, 312, 350, 359, **365**, 417. *See also* Antiviral, Coughs, Congestion
Cold Sores 50, 66, 89, 95, 96, 98, 188, 193, 201, **366**. *See also* Herpes Simplex
Colic 47, 50, 52, 53, 54, 58, 63, 64, 67, 72, 80, 95, 98, 100, 104, 107, 112, 113, 131, 136, 308, 314, 359, **366**. *See also* Children/Infants
Colitis 48, 52, 82, 118, 128, 129, 130, 246, **366**. *See also* Colon
Collagen 209, 216, 305, 437, 492
Colloidal Minerals **265**
Colon 36, 249, 255, 300, 302, 321, 348, 349, 352, **366**, 417, 454, 513, 517. *See also* Diverticulitis
Colonic 250, 403
Coma **367**, 452
Comforting 95, 107, 112, 171, **367**
ComforTone 161, 179, 184, 246, **249**, 251, 253, 254, 256, 257, 258, 259, 260, 271, 272, 278, 285, 300, 302, 303, 305, 306, 307, 308, 309, 310, 318, 324, 325, 327, 346, 348, 349, 352, 358, 363, 364, 366, 367, 368, 371, 377, 378, 379, 380, 381, 382, 393, 395, 397, 406, 412, 414, 418, 419, 423, 431, 433, 435, 436, 437, 438, 439, 444, 446, 460, 461, 462, 463, 466, 467, 468, 470, 475, 484, 486, 503, 508, 511, 512, 516, 520, 521, 522, 523, 544, 552, 553, 555, 557, 558, 559, 560
Common Sense 442, 443, 499, 544, 558, 563
Compassion **367**
Complexion 50, 91, 92, 107. *See also* Skin
Compresses 26, 298, 303, 314, 455
Concentration (Poor) 49, 84, 98, 129, 130, 155, 337, **368**
Concussion **368**. *See also* Brain
Confidence 42, 85, 86, 104, 136, 151, 182, 186, 205, 206, **368**, 390
Confusion 135, **368**
Congestion 55, 56, 64, 71, 73, 80, 85, 95, 111, 118, 121, 193, 194, **368**, 568, 570. *See also* Anticatarrhal
Conjunctivitis 85, **397**. *See also* Eyes
Consciousness 89, **369**
Constipation 48, 53, 67, 72, 95, 107, 112, 122, 126, 136, 246, 249, 251, 277, 300, 360, 366, 379, 380, 468, 517. *See also* Digestive System
Contact Sensitization 561, 567
Contagious Diseases **369**
Contractions 85
Control 339, **369**
Convalescence 63
Convulsions 79, 89, 484, 551. *See also* Seizure
Cooking **27**, 80, 242
Cooling Oils 225, **369**, 405, 571. *See also* Temperature
Copal 62, 544, 549, 553
Copper 484
Coriander **63**, 544, 549, 553
Corns 350, 401. *See also* Feet, Warts
Corrective 103
Cortisol 250, 375
Cortisone 124, 125, **370**, 437
CortiStop (Women) **250**, 252, 301, 375, 396, 402, 403, 421, 544, 553, 554, 555, 558
Coughs 47, 48, 50, 51, 52, 54, 55, 58, 59, 65, 66, 68, 69, 73, 74, 75, 76, 77, 78, 80, 84, 85, 86, 90, 96, 98, 101, 103, 107, 112, 115, 121, 122, 130, 194, 201, 307, 312, **370**
Courage 57, 62, 72, 80, 104, 151, 186, 205, 206, **370**, 391
Cows **312**
Cradle Cap 360. *See also* Children/Infants
Cramps 33, 61, 65, 66, 78, 80, 82, 89, 95, 127, 134, 161, 162, 246, 249, 251, 264, 348, **371**, 381, 447, 497, 498. *See also* Digestive System, Hormonal Imbalance, Menstruation, Muscles, PMS
Creates Sacred Space **371**
Creativity 84, 154, 463
Crohn's Disease 351, **371**
Croup **360**
Crown Chakra 42, 202. *See also* Chakras
Crying 360
Cumin **64**, 544, 549, 553
Cushing's Disease **304**. *See also* Adrenal Glands
Cuts 57, 66, 68, 70, 73, 78, 84, 95, 96, 100, 107, 115, 116, 119, 121, 132, 188, 192, 201, 214, 277, 312, 364, **372**, 488. *See also* Tissue, Wounds
Cypress **64**, 544, 549, 553
Cypress, Blue **65**, 544, 554
Cystic Fibrosis **372**, 454
Cystitis (Bladder Infection) 50, 51, 54, 55, 56, 57, 62, 69, 70, 71, 72, 73, 92, 103, 115, 118, 122, 129, 130, 134
Cysts 65, **456**

D

Dandruff 55, 70, 89, 95, 111, 118, 120, 121, 414
Davana **66**, 544, 549, 554
Day Dreaming **372**
Deafness 64, 133
Death (of Loved One) **372**. *See also* Emotions
Debility 52, 64, 91, 92, 93, 105, 121, **372**
Decongestant 33, 49, 56, 57, 65, 81, 84, 93, 94, 96, 103, 111, 120, 126, 134, 194, 330, **373**, 439, 473. *See also* Congestion
Deep Relief 160, 319, 330, 331, 354, 357, 417, 418, 434, 447, 448, 457, 458, 459, 487, 495, 497, 508, 522, 544, 553, 554, 555, 556, 558, 561
Defeated **390**. *See also* Emotions
Degenerative Disease **373**
Dehydration **373**, 399, 512
Delivery 172, 468
Denial **373**
Dental Abscess **455**
Dental Infection 62, **374**. *See also* Oral Conditions
Dentarome/Dentarome Plus Toothpaste 298, 413, 456, 503, 504
Deodorant 60, 65, 70, 104, 106, 111, 114, 123, 215, **374**, 455
Deodorizing 60, 103, 115, **374**
Depletion **374**
Depression 42, 49, 50, 57, 58, 61, 73, 76, 77, 79, 81, 85, 86, 89, 93, 98, 104, 107, 108, 111, 113, 114, 118, 119, 120, 122, 123, 129, 130, 131, 132, 136, 176, 187, 191, 206, 231, 232, 233, 284, 308, 317, **374**, 390, 404, 421, 551, 568, 569, 570. *See also* Diet
Deprogramming **376**
Dermatitis 57, 71, 82, 84, 86, 97, 107, 111, 121, 129, 277, 346, 488. *See also* Skin
Despair **376**
Despondency **377**
Detoxification 79, 82, 86, 90, 182, 183, 251, 255, 363, **377**, 379, 395, 406, 435, 568, 569. *See also* Chelation, Cleansing, Housecleaning
Detoxzyme **251**, 318, 327, **378**, 379, 395, 408, 503, 521, 544, 552, 553, 554
DHEA 231, 271, 283
Diabetes 66, 69, 79, 115, 118, 136, 248, 277, 300, 364, **378**, 415, 501, 569
Diaper Rash 89, 171, 223, 360. *See also* Children/Infants
Diarrhea 52, 53, 54, 59, 61, 62, 63, 65, 69, 76, 77, 79, 80, 96, 100, 101, 103, 104, 105, 107, 111, 112, 113, 122, 123, 126, 127, 130, 246, 251, 265, 300, 380, 468. *See also* Digestive System
Diet 300, 317, 349, **378**, 379, 400, 415, 454, 463, 517. *See also* Blood, Fasting, Food, Cleansing
Diffuser 26
Diffusing Oils 202, 306, 379, 478
Digest + Cleanse 247, **251**, 269, **273**, 300, 302, 305, 306, 307, 308, 317, 318, 327, 336, 346, 348, 355, 363, 364, 366, 367, 368, 371, 375, 377, 378, 379, 381, 382, 393, 400, 401, 405, 406, 408, 412, 418, 423, 433, 434, 437, 438, 454, 460, 463, 468, 474, 475, 509, 520, 521, 523, 544, 552, 554, 555, 556, 558

Digestive System 39, 48, 49, 50, 52, 56, 57, 58, 60, 61, 62, 63, 64, 66, 67, 72, 79, 80, 81, 84, 86, 87, 90, 91, 92, 94, 96, 98, 100, 101, 103, 104, 105, 106, 107, 108, 109, 111, 112, 113, 117, 119, 120, 123, 126, 128, 129, 130, 134, 135, 138, 161, 172, 183, 198, 245, 246, **247**, 249, 251, 252, 253, 254, 255, 256, 257, 258, 259, 260, **263**, 267, 271, 272, 274, 277, 285, 286, 300, 313, 317, 318, 361, 367, 371, 379, 407, 408, 428, 437, 509, 543–550, 568, 569, 570, 571, 572. *See also* Bowel, Colon, Giardia, Hiccoughs/Hiccups, Stomach, Ulcers
Digestive Tract Chart 39
Di-Gize **161**, 184, 246, 249, 250, 251, 253, 254, 256, 257, 258, 259, 260, 307, 312, 315, 318, 320, 321, 330, 333, 347, 348, 363, 364, 366, 368, 371, 379, 380, 381, 382, 408, 434, 439, 445, 450, 451, 456, 460, 466, 467, 470, 473, 479, 498, 514, 522, 544, 552, 554, 555, 556, 557, 558, 560, 564
Dill 66, 544, 549, 554
Dilution 562, 567
Diphtheria 76, 77, 81, **382**
Direct Application - Guidelines 25
Disappointment **383**
Discouragement **383**
Disease 58, 70, 80, 86, 96, 103, 296, 463, 474, 490
Dishwater **27**
Disinfectant 27, 61, 81, 83, 91, 106, 120, 124, 125, 133, **383**, 422, 524
Diuretic 33, 48, 52, 55, 59, 65, 68, 72, 73, 74, 75, 78, 79, 81, 84, 86, 87, 95, 100, 106, 111, 112, 120, 128, 130, 131, 133, 135, 383, 387. *See also* Antibacterial, Antifungal, Antiviral
Diverticulitis 48, 366. *See also* Colon
Dizziness 52, 126, **383**, 518
DNA 209, 210, 212, 305, 355, 364, **384**, 413, 439, 499
Dogs **312**
Dorado Azul 544
Doubt 347
Down Syndrome **384**
Dragon Time **162**, 189, 232, 233, 235, 253, 255, 263, 271, 352, 374, 396, 398, 402, 403, 404, 405, 417, 421, 425, 433, 441, 442, 444, 467, 468, 472, 473, 488, 544, 553, 554, 556, 557, 561, 564
Dragon Time Bath & Shower Gel **218**, 374, 402, 403, 404, 489, 552, 553, 554, 555, 556, 557, 558, 559, 560, 561
Dragon Time Massage Oil **219**, 255, 374, 403, 404, 421, 467, 553, 554, 556, 559, 561
Dream Catcher 153, **162**, 171, 181, 199, 341, 356, 368, 369, 372, 374, 375, 383, 384, 390, 392, 398, 441, 451, 496, 518, 544, 552, 556, 558, 560, 561, 564
Dreams 123, 154, 162, 163, 166, 170, 190, 191, 203
Dream State 61, **384**
Driving 159, 165, 329
Dropsy 134
Drowning in Own Negativity **384**
Drowsiness 450
Drugs **303**, 415. *See also* Addictions
Dying **384**
Dysentery 51, 59, 62, 63, 79, 85, 98, 101, 103, 112, **385**. *See also* Digestive System
Dysmenorrhea 100, 131, 134, 371, 403
Dyspepsia (Impaired Digestion) 52, 54, 62, 63, 64, 67, 81, 87, 92, 94, 101, 103, 104, 107, 112, 114, 118, 127, 128, 129. *See also* Digestive System
Dysuria 112

E

Earache 49, 58, 72, 89, 188, 189, 313, 361, **385**
Ears 69, 71, 97, 116, 119, 296, 313, 322, **385**, 518
Eating Disorders 81, **386**
Eczema 50, 57, 58, 79, 82, 85, 86, 89, 97, 98, 101, 111, 119, 120, 121, 123, 134, 277, 346, **387**, 488, 490. *See also* Skin
Edema 65, 90, 92, 126, 134, **387**, 502. *See also* Hormonal Imbalance, Inflammation
Egyptian Gold **163**, 315, 317, 322, 411, 437, 464, 544, 552, 553, 554, 555, 556, 557, 559, 560, 564
Electrical Balance 296, 308
Electrical Energies 205, 206, 332, 356, 394
Electrical Problems in the Body **387**. *See also* Balance
Electrolytes 278, **388**
Elemi 67, 544, 549, 554
Elevating 103, 117, 130, 134, 173
Emergency Oils **388**
Emmenagogue 403
Emotional Balance 42, 47, 50, 57, 58, 63, 73, 75, 76, 77, 79, 83, 85, 86, 89, 99, 106, 107, 108, 109, 110, 114, 115, 117, 121, 122, 123, 124, 125, 126, 132, 133, 136, 137, 150, 153, 154, 155, 157, 159, 162, 163, 164, 165, 166, 167, 169, 170, 172, 173, 174, 175, 176, 178, 179, 180, 181, 182, 183, 184, 185, 186, 188, 190, 191, 192, 195, 196, 197, 199, 200, 202, 203, 204, 205, 207, 218, 219, 221, 225, 226, 228, 232, 233, 235, 237, 238, 260, 263, 264, 266, 271, 275, 280, 296, 332, 417, 499, 510, 543–550, 567, 568, 569, 570
Emotional Blocks 166, 182
Emotional Release/Cleansing **42–43**, 206, 339, 376, 388
Emotions 18, 42, 50, 52, 57, 58, 59, 65, 79, 85, 98, 99, 104, 109, 121, 122, 124, 125, 126, 130, 133, 152, 164, 166, 174, 176, 179, 181, 185, 191, 194, 199, 200, 203, 299, 300, 308, 309, 326, 328, 334, 335, 337, 339, 344, 347, 357, 372, 384, **388**, 474, 521, 524
Emphysema 67, **392**. *See also* Respiratory System
Empowering 73, 74, 75, 154, 164, 166, 175, 176, 185, 186, 188, 196, 205, **393**
Endocrine System 50, 56, 66, 112, 118, 119, 165, 303, 393, 403, 411, 437, 438, 464, 494. *See also* Adrenal Glands, Thyroid, Pituitary Gland, Lupus, etc.
EndoFlex 162, **165**, 189, 253, 268, 272, 281, 284, 285, 303, 305, 318, 329, 334, 370, 372, 374, 383, 387, 393, 396, 398, 402, 403, 406, 411, 412, 416, 421, 430, 431, 437, 438, 439, 443, 453, 459, 461, 472, 473, 479, 507, 514, 521, 544, 553, 555, 557, 558, 559, 560, 564
EndoGize 252, 304, 305, 318, 330, 370, 372, 375, 393, 402, 403, 404, 406, 411, 412, 416, 421, 422, 430, 438, 459, 461, 486, 508, 521, 544, 552, 553, 555, 557
Endometriosis 69, 71, **393**, 421. *See also* Hormonal Imbalance
Endurance **393**
Enema, Retention 234, 350
Energizing 154, 155, 185, 203, 229, 399
Energy 63, 65, 69, 73, 80, 85, 86, 91, 92, 93, 105, 110, 111, 112, 130, 150, 164, 165, 175, 189, 197, 203, 251, 263, 267, 268, 272, 277, 284, 285, 308, 332, 336, 354, 394, 439, 468, 570
Energy Centers 33, 43, 174, 332, **356**. *See also* Chakras
Enhancing 58, 91
Enlightening **394**
En-R-Gee 153, 159, **164**, 267, 268, 278, 281, 284, 303, 329, 351, 392, 393, 394, 400, 430, 441, 442, 475, 497, 524, 544, 553, 554, 556, 557, 558, 559, 564
Enteritis 51, **395**
Enuresis 129
Envision 150, 153, 155, 163, **166**, 178, 180, 181, 264, 266, 267, 268, 272, 278, 284, 285, 299, 332, 347, 351, 369, 388, 390, 394, 445, 466, 472, 510, 544, 555, 556, 558, 559, 560, 564
Enzymes 251, 253, 277, 317, 327, 336, 367, 379, 393, **395**, 407, 408, 521
Epidemics 86
Epilepsy 49, 52, 64, 100, 131, 450, 484, 561, 567. *See also* Seizure
Episiotomy 172, 468
Epstein Barr 322, 363, **395**, 423. *See also* Antiviral, Chronic Fatigue, Hypoglycemia, Mononucleosis
Equilibrium 136, 137, 199, **395**, 518

Erysipelas 98
Essential Beauty Serums **219,** 305, 399, 488, 492, 493, 508, 509, 552
  Acne-Prone Skin Blend **220,** 300, 301, 552, 554, 557, 560
  Dry Skin Blend **220,** 474, 552, 553, 554, 556, 557, 560
  Oily Skin Blend 560
Essential Oils **395**
Essentialzyme 161, 179, 184, 245, **247,** 249, 250, **253,** 256, 259, 271, 272, **273,** 277, 278, 280, 281, 285, 300, 303, 305, 306, 307, 308, 309, 310, 313, 317, 318, 320, 324, 325, 327, 336, 346, 348, 349, 352, 358, 363, 364, 366, 367, 368, 371, 372, 377, 378, 379, 380, 381, 382, 393, 395, 397, 406, 408, 410, 412, 414, 418, 419, 423, 426, 431, 432, 433, 435, 436, 437, 438, 439, 444, 446, 449, 459, 460, 461, 462, 463, 466, 467, 468, 470, 474, 475, 484, 486, 493, 503, 508, 511, 512, 516, 517, 520, 521, 522, 523, 544, 552, 553, 554, 558, 560
Essentialzymes-4 253, 300, 303, 305, 307, 313, 317, 318, 320, 324, 327, 346, 367, 372, 379, 380, 381, 395, 397, 406, 407, 408, 410, 414, 419, 426, 432, 449, 459, 463, 466, 468, 470, 474, 490, 493, 512, 517, 521, 544
Estradiol 121, 198
Estrogen 48, 120, 231, 234, 250, 254, 255, 263, **395,** 414, 421
Estro Tincture 189, **254,** 263, 396, 421, 467, 544, 553, 554, 556
Eucalyptus 68, 544, 549, 554
Eucalyptus Blue 69
Eucalyptus Citriodora 544, 549, 554
Eucalyptus Dives 70, 554
Eucalyptus Polybractea 70, 554
Eucalyptus Radiata 71, 544, 549, 554
Eucalyptus Staigeriana 71, 544, 554
Euphoria 61, 85, 86, 103, **396**
Evening Peace Bath & Shower Gel **220,** 323, 333, 374, 389, 426, 448, 478, 489, 493, 499, 513, 544, 552, 553, 555, 556, 557, 558, 559, 560, 561
Evergreen Essence **166,** 315, 321, 323, 327, 392, 499, 544, 552, 554, 558, 559, 560, 564
Excitement 198
Exercise 271, 284, 300, 336, 449, 497, 521
Exfoliating 237
Exhaustion 58, 62, 63, 64, 68, 93, 121, 231, 232, 233, **396.** *See also* Energy
Exodus 167, 168, 179, 252, 256, 273, 279, 421, 555, 556, 560
Exodus II **167,** 179, 201, 256, 279, 305, 320, 343, 365, 368, 371, 373, 392, 404, 408, 410, 413, 423, 425, 465, 466, 467, 470, 480, 510, 544, 552, 553, 555, 557, 560, 564
Expectorant 11, 21, 47, 51, 52, 55, 59, 67, 68, 70, 71, 72, 73, 74, 75, 76, 77, 78, 82, 95, 96, 100, 103, 106, 111, 115, 116, 118, 130, 551, 568
Expression (Self Expression) 390, **396**
Eyes 53, 61, 72, 92, 93, 117, 127, 133, 243, 268, 295, 300, 301, 390, **396–398,** 492

F

Face 229, 236, 237
Facial Oils **399,** 488. *See also* Skin
Fainting 49, 89, 105, **399,** 486. *See also* Shock
Faith 166, **399**
Fasting 284, 349, 378, **400**
Fat 122, 126, 151, 255, 271, 284, 286, 300, 303, 346, 355, **400.** *See also* Cellulite, Diet, Weight
Father (Problems With) 389, 390, 392, **400**
Fatigue 33, 49, 60, 62, 81, 84, 105, 113, 114, 115, 116, 118, 120, 123, 129, 136, 152, 204, 246, 281, 330, 349, **400,** 423, 442, 448, 570. *See also* Energy
Fatty Deposits **401.** *See also* Cellulite, Fat, Weight
Fear 63, 104, 123, 126, 181, 189, 190, 205, 328, 347, 389, 391, **401.** *See also* Anxiety, Calming
Feet 25, 115, 194, 296, 359, **401,** 519
Feet, Vita Flex Chart 31
Females 72, 136, 137, 232, 254, 332, 338, 391, 421, 486, 516, 571
Female Specific Conditions 61, **401.** *See also* Hormonal Imbalance, Infertility, Ovaries, Pregnancy/Motherhood, Uterus
FemiGen 189, 232, 233, 252, 255, 263, 281, 301, 309, 341, 349, 350, 351, 353, 371, 393, 396, 401, 402, 403, 404, 405, 411, 421, 425, 456, 467, 515, 516, 544, 553, 554, 559, 561
Fennel 71, 544, 549, 554
Fertility 48, 98, 402, **405.** *See also* Female Specific Conditions, Male Specific Conditions
Fever 18, 49, 50, 52, 54, 55, 58, 60, 65, 69, 70, 71, 72, 73, 74, 75, 80, 84, 86, 87, 90, 91, 92, 98, 100, 107, 109, 111, 113, 114, 117, 121, 123, 127, 134, 135, 179, 300, 361, **405,** 501, 504, 524, 571, 572
Fiber 255, 285, 379, **406,** 408
Fibroids 231, 232, 233, **406.** *See also* Hormonal Imbalance
Fibromyalgia **406,** 421
Fibrositis 120, **407.** *See also* Fibromyalgia
Fillings **503**
Finger **407**
Fir 72, 544, 549, 554
Fir, Balsam 73, 545, 554
Fir, Douglas 74, 545, 554
Fir, Idaho Balsam *See* Fir, Balsam
Fir, Red 554
Fir, White 75, 545, 554
Flatulence (Gas) 47, 48, 52, 56, 62, 63, 64, 67, 72, 78, 80, 87, 89, 92, 101, 103, 104, 105, 107, 112, 114, 123, 126, 134, 135, 380. *See also* Digestive System
Fleabane 75, 545, 555
Fleas 115, 313
Flexibility 248
Flies 127, 314
Flu 51, 58, 60, 62, 63, 64, 69, 71, 73, 74, 75, 80, 87, 96, 103, 107, 112, 113, 115, 116, 118, 121, 127, 129, 130, 135, 178, 193, 194, 201, 277, 350, 361, 417, 423. *See also* Influenza
Fluids 72. *See also* Edema, Diuretic
Focus 104, 131, 155, 170, 199, 337, 390, **407**
Food 253, 317, 342, 348, 378, 407, 421. *See also* pH Balance
Food Poisoning 91, 113, **408**
Forehead **408**
Forgive (and Forget) 168, 169, 389, **408**
Forgiveness 42, **168,** 171, 173, 177, 178, 180, 198, 200, 246, 259, 298, 299, 302, 303, 304, 309, 310, 326, 333, 334, 335, 344, 346, 347, 352, 356, 357, 376, 388, 389, 390, 391, 392, 394, 408, 410, 412, 417, 429, 436, 437, 442, 451, 454, 455, 456, 463, 464, 466, 468, 478, 480, 485, 499, 510, 521, 545, 552, 553, 555, 556, 557, 558, 559, 560, 561, 564
Formaldehyde **409**
Fortifying **409**
Frankincense 76, 545, 549, 555
Frankincense, Sacred 77, 545, 549, 555
Freckles 127, **409**
Free Radicals 273, 309, 320, 397, **409.** *See also* Antioxidant
Frequency 9, **9–11,** 168, 169, 177, 178, 194, 206, 245, 296, 348, 355, 390, 394, 520
Fresh Essence Plus Mouthwash 413, 456, 503, 504, 506
Frigidity 61, 85, 105, 117, 136, **409,** 433, 486, 568, 570, 571. *See also* Libido, Sex Stimulant
Frustration 136, 137, 194, **409**
Fungus 33, 58, 70, 95, 96, 101, 104, 188, 192, 245, 300, 317, 320, 340, 348, 422, 427, 463, 475, 551. *See also* Antifungal

G

Galbanum 545, 549, 555
Gallbladder 52, 53, 57, 65, 79, 82, 93, 119, 126, 134, 172, 251, **410**
Gallstones 50, 69, 81, 89, 91, 92, 105, 134

Gangrene 68, 345, **410**
Gas 52, 113, 246, 251, 255, 380, 571. *See also* Digestive System
Gastritis 57, 129, 135, 380. *See also* Digestive System
Gathering 163, **169**, 171, 176, 186, 188, 266, 298, 309, 323, 341, 347, 368, 372, 374, 376, 377, 383, 388, 390, 391, 392, 407, 409, 412, 441, 444, 461, 463, 464, 466, 468, 480, 487, 493, 496, 499, 545, 553, 555, 556, 559, 560, 561, 564
General Tonic **410**
Genesis Hand & Body Lotion **221**, 304, 305, 306, 360, 415, 463, 486, 488, 489, 490, 492, 493, 545, 552, 553, 555, 556, 558, 559, 561
Genitals 61, **410**, 440, 519
Gentle Baby **171**, 180, 300, 302, 339, 343, 346, 352, 359, 367, 374, 376, 381, 389, 390, 391, 412, 417, 421, 423, 432, 441, 442, 468, 469, 471, 472, 478, 482, 483, 488, 490, 493, 495, 500, 513, 545, 552, 553, 555, 556, 558, 559, 561, 564
Gentleness **411**
Geranium 78, 545, 549, 555
German Chamomile *See* Chamomile, German.
Germs 73, 91, 104, 239, 240, 280, **411**, 498, 551. *See also* Antibacterial, Antifungal, Antiviral
Ginger 79, 545, 549, 555
Gingivitis 101, 102, 112, 117, 120, 130, 241, 455. *See also* Oral Conditions
Glands (Swollen) 56, 78
Glandular System 120, 122, 124, 125, **411**. *See also* Endocrine System
Glaucoma 397. *See also* Eyes
GLF **172**, 302, 305, 310, 349, 375, 377, 379, 381, 410, 434, 435, 436, 454, 459, 479, 494, 545, 553, 555, 556, 560, 564
Glucose 63, 67, 277
Glycemic index **248**
Goals 154, 166, 170, 175, 177, 185, 190, 191, 203, 390
Goiter **411**. *See also* Endocrine System
Goldenrod 80, 545, 555
Gonorrhea 50, 69, 76, 77, 112
Gout 49, 56, 63, 72, 84, 87, 91, 105, 107, 112, 115, 118, 127, 134, 135, 277, 346, **411**
Grapefruit 81, 545, 549, 555
Grapefruit Lip Balm 545
GRAS 295, 552
Gratitude 173, 347, 376, 388, 392, 423, 456, 473, 496, 501, 515, 545, 554, 555, 557, 559, 561, 564
Grave's Disease **412**. *See also* Thyroid
Grief/Sorrow 84, 126, 181, 391, **412**, 439, 571
Grounding 42, 65, 73, 74, 75, 124, 125, 126, 130, 131, 132, 152, 154, 166, 170, **173**, 176, 177, 196, 200, 202, 203, 204, 246, 280, 299, 310, 376, 383, 389, 390, 391, 392, **412**, 467, 472, 487, 495, 510, 545, 552, 554, 556, 558, 560, 561, 564, 571, 572
Growth (Hair) **414**
Guilt 392, **412**
Gulf War Syndrome **413**
Gum Disease 456. *See also* Oral Conditions
Gum/Grease Removal 91, 92
Gums 65, 101, 102, 121, 123, 130, 188, 201, 277, **413**, 503. *See also* Oral Conditions

H

Habits **413**. *See also* Addictions
Hair 57, 91, 92, 114, 118, 119, 125, 135, 136, 223, 227, 277, 333, 346, **413**, 543–550
Hair Loss 54, 55, 87, 89, 118, 120, 121, 136, 231, 232, 233, 414, 415
Halitosis 52, 62, 105, 111, 113, 456. *See also* Oral Conditions
Hands **415**. *See also* Skin
Hand, Vita Flex Chart 30
Hangovers **416**
Happiness 85, 94, 108, **416**
Harmonizing 78, 121, 122, 123, 571
Harmony 42, 153, **174**, 186, 188, 192, 195, 246, 253, 254, 257, 258, 263, 266, 280, 296, 298, 299, 302, 307, 308, 309, 310, 323, 324, 325, 332, 339, 346, 352, 356, 357, 368, 372, 374, 376, 377, 383, 387, 389, 390, 391, 412, 416, 429, 444, 455, 456, 463, 464, 465, 467, 468, 471, 474, 478, 480, 499, 500, 505, 521, 545, 552, 553, 555, 556, 558, 559, 560, 561, 564
Harmony in Body Systems **416**
Harshness **416**
Hashimoto's Disease **416**. *See also* Thyroid
Hate 183, 194, 389, **417**
Hay Fever 51, 69, 71, 89, 307, 454. *See also* Allergies
Headaches 49, 51, 52, 60, 62, 64, 67, 76, 77, 82, 86, 89, 92, 95, 104, 111, 113, 117, 118, 121, 123, 129, 130, 135, 152, 160, 187, 206, 231, 232, 233, 246, **417**, 423, 426, 443, 569, 570, 572. *See also* Migraine Headaches
Healing 62, 69, 76, 77, 91, 96, 110, 156, 166, 178, 182, 188, 190, 223, 225, 277, 301, 340, 345, **418**, 524, 568
Health 69, 89, 91, 149, **418**
Hearing 82
Heart 58, 71, 73, 89, 98, 104, 107, 108, 112, 114, 118, 122, 127, 136, 137, 151, 163, 170, 207, 264, 284, 296, 299, 310, 313, 324, 325, 338, 349, 352, 356, 375, 391, 466, 480, 509, 517. *See also* Cardiovascular System
Heartburn 52, 91, 107, 112, 113, 161, 251, 381. *See also* Digestive System
Heat 297, 500
Helichrysum 82, 545, 549, 555
Helicobacter pylori 95
Hematoma 82, **419**. *See also* Bruise
Hemoglobin 325, 337, 349
Hemorrhaging 65, 76, 77, 117, 338, 402, **419**, 469, 569. *See also* Blood
Hemorrhoids 49, 56, 61, 65, 73, 79, 98, 101, 102, 103, 111, 113, 122, 135, 151, 206, **419**, 517
Hemostat 151
Hepatic 53, 56, 94
Hepatitis 62, 85, 90, 118, 435. *See also* Liver
Herbicide 305
Hernia 61, 63, 133, **419**
Herniated Discs 330
Herpes 69, 70, 76, 77, 89, 101, 116
Herpes Simplex 66, 71, 98, 117, 366, **420**
Herpes Zoster 66, 486
hGH 283, 284
Hiatal Hernia 419
Hiccoughs 49, 94, 122, 128, 361, **420**
High Blood Pressure 76, 77, 89, 119, 151, 206, 324, **336**, 353, 469, 561, 567. *See also* Blood
Highest Potential **175**, 323, 356, 372, 374, 389, 390, 391, 392, 401, 407, 441, 487, 545, 556, 561, 565
Hinoki 83, 545, 549, 555
HIV **305**
Hives 89, 111, 113, **420**
Hoarseness 85, 90
Home 178, 192
Honey 396, 423, 501
Hong Kuai 83, 549, 555
Hoof Rot 314
Hope 42, 79, 85, **176**, 177, 182, 192, 198, 204, 205, 246, 299, 310, 323, 324, 344, 347, 352, 367, 374, 375, 376, 377, 383, 389, 390, 391, 392, 394, 399, 401, 409, 412, 421, 426, 429, 441, 457, 468, 471, 499, 510, 545, 556, 557, 560, 565
Hormonal Imbalance 48, 61, 66, 79, 300, 301, 346, 371, 393, 401, **421**, 453, 507, 520, 521
Hormonal System 48, 61, 63, 66, **67**, 72, 75, 81, 85, 100, 101, 103, 105, 119, 120, 121, 132, 135, 136, 137, 162, 165, 189, 198, 218, 219, 232, 233, 234, 235, 237, 238, 248, 250, 252, 254, 255, 266, 271, 273, 276, 277, 280, 281, 283, 363, 406, **421**,

440, 543–550, 568, 569, 570, 571, 572. *See also* Endocrine System
Hormone-like 56, 57, 75
Hormones 72, 121, 122, 123, 126, 134, 198, 232, 254, 283, 284, 296, 393, 402, 415, 460
Horses 188, 311, **314**, 315
Hot Flashes 113, 162, 165, 189, 402, 453. *See also* Female Specific Conditions
Housecleaning **422**
HPV **66**
HRT Tincture 349
Human Growth Hormone (hGH) 400, 464
Humility **177**, 180, 204, 299, 310, 324, 388, 389, 390, 409, 418, 429, 454, 478, 496, 545, 555, 557, 558, 559, 560, 561, 565
Hydrating 109, 198, 221, 225, 399
Hyperactivity 58, 191, 205, 301, 328, 346, 361, 571. *See also* Calming
Hyperpnea (Abnormal Rapid Breathing) 136, 480. *See also* Respiratory System
Hypertension (High Blood Pressure) 62, 71, 81, 98, 112, 122, 134, 135, 136, 191, 285, **336**, 353, 415, 569
Hyperthyroidism 101, 124, 125, 412, 416, **507**
Hypnotic 94, 131
Hypoglycemia 69, 231, 232, 233, 248, 277, 317, 322, 378, 407, **423**, 450, 474. *See also* Blood, Protein
Hypotension 126, 568, 570
Hypothalamus 65, 119, 154, 163
Hypothyroidism 103, 317, 415, 450, 507
Hyssop **84**, 545, 549, 555
Hysterectomy 263, 421
Hysteria 89, 95, 96, 100, 104, 113, **423**

I

ICP 249, 250, **255**, 259, 271, 272, 278, 285, 300, 303, 305, 306, 307, 308, 309, 310, 318, 325, 327, 346, 348, 349, 351, 352, 358, 363, 364, 366, 367, 368, 371, 377, 378, 379, 380, 381, 382, 393, 395, 397, 406, 408, 412, 418, 419, 423, 431, 433, 435, 436, 437, 438, 439, 444, 446, 460, 461, 462, 468, 470, 475, 477, 484, 486, 503, 508, 511, 512, 516, 520, 521, 522, 523, 545, 552, 555, 557, 559, 560
Idaho Blue Spruce *See* Spruce, Idaho Blue
Idaho Balsam Fir *See* Fir, Balsam
Idaho Tansy *See* Tansy, Idaho
Idaho Tansy Floral Water 314
Identity 179, **390**
IGF-1 **284**
Illness **22**, 256
Immune-stimulant 58, 61, 76, 77, 96, 108, 110, 132, 306, **549–551**
Immune System 8, 20, 33, 58, 59, 62, 64, 66, **69**, 76, 77, 78, 87, 90, 91, 92, 96, 99, 100, 101, 103, 104, 105, 108, 109, 110, 112, 116, 118, 120, 126, 127, 129, 130, 133, 135, 138, 149, 150, 154, 156, 157, 164, 168, 173, 178, 179, 199, 200, 201, 204, 239, 249, 251, 256, 257, 259, 260, 261, 263, 264, 266, 267, 268, 269, 271, 272, 273, 277, 278, 279, 280, 283, 284, 285, 286, 305, 313, 322, 373, 375, **423**, 437, 439, 444, 543–550, 551, 570
ImmuneTune 168, 179, 256, 279, 305, 378, 446, 553, 556, 558
ImmuPower 178, 179, 200, 201, 256, 279, 300, 304, 305, 307, 309, 315, 317, 318, 320, 322, 325, 327, 328, 332, 343, 347, 348, 349, 350, 363, 371, 385, 386, 392, 395, 402, 405, 406, 410, 423, 425, 427, 430, 435, 437, 438, 444, 449, 465, 467, 473, 506, 507, 510, 511, 514, 515, 545, 553, 555, 557, 558, 559, 560, 565
ImmuPro **256**, 304, 305, 306, 307, 322, 328, 348, 351, 363, 375, 378, 395, 410, 412, 416, 423, 425, 428, 438, 444, 446, 449, 471, 499, 500, 506, 510, 511, 545, 558
Impetigo 491. *See also* Skin
Impotence 61, 62, 80, 81, 105, 117, 122, 136, 137, **424**, 486, 568, 570, 571
Incisional Hernia **419**
Indifference 85, **424**
Indigestion 47, 50, 52, 56, 64, 67, 78, 80, 89, 94, 98, 113, 131, 136, 161, 246, 381, 571. *See also* Digestive System
Infants 58, 107, **296**
Infection 33, 50, 58, 59, 60, 61, 62, 63, 68, 71, 73, 74, 75, 76, 77, 82, 86, 87, 89, 91, 92, 95, 97, 98, 101, 102, 103, 104, 105, 107, 109, 111, 115, 116, 117, 118, 120, 122, 123, 127, 128, 129, 130, 134, 135, 136, 137, 178, 188, 193, 201, 246, 259, 313, 314, 315, 316, 318, 322, 335, 340, 343, 345, 365, 386, 402, 410, 418, **424**, 425, 431, 440, 454, 456, 466, 470, 476, 479, 506, 514, 516, 523, 524, 551, 569, 570, 571. *See also* Antibacterial, Antifungal, Antiviral
Infectious Disease 50, **425**, 444
Inferiority **425**
Infertility 231, 232, 233, 401, 402, 421, **425**, 440. *See also* Female Specific Conditions, Hormonal Imbalance, Male Specific Conditions
Inflammation 33, 50, 53, 61, 68, 69, 71, 75, 76, 77, 78, 79, 96, 101, 102, 112, 113, 120, 134, 231, 232, 233, 234, 298, 303, 319, 330, 340, 343, 350, 354, 366, 386, 398, 415, 431, 440, 454, 458, 474, 486, 487, 488, 504, 515, 516, 524, 551, 568, 571. *See also* Anti-inflammatory
Influenza 65, 81, 89, 90, 97, 112. *See also* Antiviral, Colds, Respiratory System
Inhalation, Methods for 26
Injuries 89, 118, 135, 188, 314, 342, 418, **426**, 497. *See also* Cuts, Pain, Scarring, tissue, Wounds
Inner Child 42, 173, 178, **179**, 198, 246, 299, 376, 377, 389, 390, 391, 412, 426, 454, 462, 488, 496, 521, 545, 556, 557, 558, 560, 561, 565
Inner Defense 256, 304, 306, 322, 348, 351, 363, 375, 378, 395, 410, 412, 416, 423, 424, 425, 431, 438, 439, 444, 446, 464, 465, 479, 499, 500, 506, 511, 514
Inner Knowing **426**
Insanity **426**
Insect Bites 49, 50, 51, 61, 62, 72, 88, 89, 95, 98, 136, 188, 192
Insecticidal 11, 51, 60, 70, 91, 94, 96, 111, 122, 427
Insect Repellent 49, 50, 55, 65, 68, 70, 79, 89, 91, 192, 427
Insects 111, 192, 333, 334, **426**, 445, 463
Insomnia 49, 50, 57, 58, 59, 61, 65, 79, 89, 94, 95, 97, 98, 103, 104, 107, 114, 116, 123, 126, 129, 130, 131, 132, 136, 157, 191, 231, 232, 233, 300, 421, **428**, 493, 500, 569, 572
Inspiration 173, 178, 180, 181, 186, 198, 207, 309, 310, 329, 335, 365, 374, 376, 377, 390, 392, 412, 416, 429, 463, 464, 467, 478, 480, 482, 487, 496, 499, 505, 511, 514, 516, 545, 552, 555, 557, 559, 560, 565
Inspiring 152, 153, 176
Insulin 63, 67, 285, 378
Integration, Brain **342**
Intelligence 129, 130
Intestinal Parasites 50, 54, 65, 91
Intestines, Problems 49, 51, 52, 94, 95, 123, 126, 128, 136, 137, 248, 251, 255, 257, 375, 460. *See also* Digestive System
Into the Future 150, 153, 163, 166, 181, 188, 199, 204, 205, 309, 329, 357, 391, 396, 463, 464, 467, 469, 496, 545, 552, 553, 554, 555, 556, 558, 560, 561, 565
Invigorating 52, 90, 91, 113, 153, 181, 231, **428**
Ions **428**, 501
Iris 69, 71, **398**
Iron 351, 415, **429**
Irritability 58, 63, 94, 95, 126, 200, 246, **429**, 500. *See also* Calming
Irritable Bowel Syndrome (IBS) 48, 113, 127, 246, 382. *See also* Digestive System
Isoprene Unit **11**
Itching 127, 217, 246, 358, 415, 427, **429**, 491

J

Jasmine 85, 545, 549, 556
Jaundice (Liver Disease) 56, 76, 77, 79, 107, 121, 127, 133, 361, 435. *See also* Liver
Jealousy **429**
Jet Lag 81, 329, **430**
Jock Itch 440
Joints 33, 51, 57, 71, 73, 74, 75, 95, 105, 124, 125, 134, 248, **430**, 437, 457, 458, 508. *See also* Rotator Cuff, Shoulder, Tennis Elbow
Joy 42, 104, 150, 151, 153, 169, 181, 198, 199, 205, 207, 246, 263, 284, 299, 302, 303, 304, 310, 312, 323, 324, 328, 339, 346, 347, 352, 357, 374, 375, 376, 377, 383, 385, 389, 390, 391, 392, 394, 396, 412, 416, 417, 429, 430, 433, 436, 437, 438, 439, 441, 444, 454, 465, 466, 468, 471, 474, 477, 480, 482, 483, 484, 485, 487, 496, 499, 510, 521, 545, 552, 553, 555, 556, 557, 558, 559, 561, 565
Joyous **430**
Juniper 86, 545, 549, 556
Juva Cleanse 172, **182**, 257, 258, 285, 307, 308, 309, 337, 347, 349, 350, 352, 375, 377, 382, 410, 411, 434, 435, 436, 454, 461, 473, 517, 545, 553, 555, 556, 565
JuvaFlex 172, 183, 195, 246, 249, 250, 251, 253, 254, 256, 257, 258, 259, 267, 268, 277, 281, 284, 302, 305, 310, 314, 320, 349, 375, 377, 379, 381, 410, 411, 430, 431, 434, 435, 436, 439, 452, 479, 545, 553, 554, 555, 559, 560, 565
JuvaPower 172, **257**, 258, 285, 300, 302, 306, 375, 433, 484, 545, 552, 554
JuvaPower/JuvaSpice 302, 366, 367, 375, 381, 382, 385, 395, 437, 446, 454, 461, 475, 484, 490, 495, 521
JuvaSpice **258**, 285, 545, 552, 554
JuvaTone 161, 172, 184, 246, 249, 250, 251, 253, 254, 256, 257, 258, 267, 281, 284, 300, 302, 303, 308, 309, 311, 325, 327, 337, 348, 349, 352, 364, 365, 377, 381, 382, 395, 406, 412, 418, 431, 434, 435, 436, 437, 446, 461, 462, 463, 468, 470, 475, 489, 495, 501, 511, 517, 545, 553, 555, 556, 557, 559, 560

K

K&B Tincture **259**, 430, 431, 514, 515, 517, 545, 553, 554, 555, 556, 559
Kidneys 49, 54, 56, 61, 72, 81, 86, 90, 92, 127, 128, 133, 134, 165, 255, 259, 300, 303, 305, 308, 314, **430**, 464, 569, 571. *See also* Diuretic
Kidney Stones 72, 79, 86, 123, 134, 135, 314, 431
KidScents Bath Gel **222**, 359, 552, 555
KidScents Lotion **222**, 305, 359, 440, 489, 552, 555, 559
KidScents Mighty Mist 266, 285, 309, 442, 484
KidScents Mighty Vites **259**, 266, 285, 309, 359, 429, 442, 484, 518, 545, 557, 558
KidScents Shampoo **223**, 359, 414, 415, 556, 560
KidScents Tender Tush **223**, 359, 361, 491, 553, 555, 556, 559, 560
KidScents Toothpaste **224**, 359, 413, 456, 503, 504, 553, 560
Knee Cartilage Injury **432**

L

Labor 85, **432**, 468, 469. *See also* Pregnancy/Motherhood
Lactation (Secretion of Breast Milk) 56, 72, **432**, 470. *See also* Pregnancy/Motherhood
Lactose Intolerance **432**
Lady Sclareol 184, 253, 323, 394, 409, 416, 421, 422, 433, 437, 478, 481, 486, 545, 553, 555, 556, 558, 559, 560, 561, 565
Laryngitis 51, 52, 65, 70, 76, 77, 85, 89, 90, 107, 121, 129, **432**, 506
Laundry 422. *See also* Housecleaning
Laurel 87, 545, 550, 556
LavaDerm Cooling Mist **225**, 345, 502, 545, 556
Lavandin 88, 545, 550, 556
Lavender 88, 546, 550, 556
Lavender Bath & Shower Gel 225, 554, 556, 557
Lavender Hand & Body Lotion 226, 546, 554, 556, 557
Lavender Lip Balm 226, 434, 490
Lavender Rosewood Moisturizing Soap **226**, 333, 389, 488, 556, 559
Lavender Volume Conditioner 227, 413, 414, 415, 474, 553, 556
Lavender Volume Shampoo **227**, 413, 414, 415, 474, 553, 556
Laxative 80, 105, 111, 126, 128, 255, **433**
Layering Oils **296**
Learning **77**
Ledum 89, 546, 556
Legacy 421, 524
Legs 33, 57, 135, 314, 371, 387, 512, 517
  Restless **433**
Lemon 90, 546, 550, 556
Lemon Balm *See* Melissa
Lemongrass 91, 546, 550, 557
Lemon Myrtle *See* Myrtle, Lemon
Lemon Sage Clarifying Conditioner 553, 555, 556, 557, 558, 559, 561
Lemon Sage Clarifying Shampoo 553, 555, 556, 557, 558, 559, 561
Lemon Sandalwood Cleansing Soap **228**, 333, 375, 394, 488
Lemon Sandalwood CleansingSoap 556, 560
Leprosy 101
Lethargy 85, **433**
Leucorrhea 71, 130
Leukocyte 91, 92
Libido (Low) 231, 232, 233, 277, 409, 421, **433.** *See also* Frigidity, Sex Stimulant
Lice 115, **434**
Life 5 245, 246, 251, 253, 254, 257, 258, 260, 271, 283, 298, **300**, **306**, **307**, **317**, **318**, **322**, **349**, 359, **363**, **366**, **371**, **379**, **380**, **381**, **382**, **406**, **432**, **435**
Ligaments 73, 92, 104, 314, 341, **434**, 458, 524. *See also* Muscles
Limbs (Aching) 126
Lime 92, 546, 550, 557
Limette 93, 557
Limping (Animals) **313**
Lipid Metabolism **443**
Lipoma **511.** *See also* Tumors
Lips 89, 217, 222, 226, **434**
Listlessness 93, **434.** *See also* Calming
Liver 14, 42, 52, 53, 56, 57, 65, 67, 75, 79, 81, 82, 85, 86, 87, 90, 91, 92, 93, 94, 95, 113, 116, 117, 118, 119, 120, 121, 126, 127, 133, 135, 151, 165, 172, 182, 183, 194, 251, 253, 257, 258, 268, 272, 283, 284, 285, 299, 300, 302, 305, 308, 349, 355, 375, 406, **434**, 435, 454, 461, 486, 513, 569, 571
Live with Passion 150, 153, 163, 176, 181, 182, 185, 188, 199, 267, 272, 273, 284, 285, 347, 368, 370, 374, 388, 390, 392, 433, 445, 466, 468, 514, 524, 546, 552, 553, 555, 556, 557, 558, 560, 565
Longevity 72, 95, 186, 252, 260, 261, 268, 305, 436, 439, 546, 553, 555, 558, 560, 565
Longevity Capsules 186, 247, 252, 257, **260**, 269, 270, 273, 283, 305, 320, 338, 341, 352, 363, 377, 409, 418, 423, 430, 434, **435**, 436, 511, 546, 553, 558, 560
Loss 65, **391**
Loss of Loved One **436**
Loss of Smell **436**
Lou Gehrig's Disease 9, 10, 277, **436.** *See also* Alzheimer's Disease, Brain, Multiple Sclerosis, Parkinson's Disease, Pineal Gland, Pituitary Gland
Love 42, 50, 80, 85, 86, 89, 181, 182, 323, **437**, 471, 485
Low Blood Pressure 84, 120, 127, 300, **337**
Lumbago 122, **437.** *See also* Back
Lungs 50, 65, 69, 72, 84, 103, 115, 116, 194, 349, 479, 571. *See also* Respiratory system

Lupus 62, 285, 303, 393, **437.** *See also* Adrenal Glands, Digestive System, Endocrine System, Immune System, Thyroid
Lyme Disease **439.** *See also* Antibacterial, Insect
Lymphatic System 33, 52, 56, 81, 82, 89, 90, 91, 92, 120, 122, 126, 134, 151, 157, 183, 201, 300, 303, 411, **439,** 568. *See also* Immune System
Lymphoma 349. *See also* Cancer

M

Magnesium 277, 280
Magnify Your Purpose 150, 166, 176, 181, 182, 186, **187,** 198, 263, 264, 267, 268, 272, 273, 278, 281, 284, 285, 328, 357, 376, 391, 392, 393, 445, 472, 546, 553, 555, 558, 559, 560, 566
Majestic Essence Chocolates **261,** 320, 351, 378, 382, 546
Malaria 49, 50, 69, 91, 112, **440**
Males Specific Conditions 136, 137, 189, 332, 391, 422, **440,** 486. *See also* Aftershave, Impotence, Skin, Sterility
Mandarin 93, 546, 550, 557
Manna Bars 248, 250, 261, 264, 268, 272, 284, 285
Manuka 94, 546, 557
Maple Syrup **364,** 501
Marjoram 95, 546, 550, 557
Massage 26, 152, 153, 157, 166, 172, 181, 182, 184, 187, 188, 194, 199, 278, 348, **440,** 509, 513
Master Cleanser 302, 327, 339, **364,** 367, 400, 405, 411, 430, 433, 468
Master Formula Hers **263,** 401, 402, 404, 456, 471
Master Formula Hers/His 266, 272, 278, 285, 304, 309, 320, 332, 336, 348, 355, 363, 372, 379, 384, 394, 401, 423, 426, 429, 435, 440, 446, 460, 465, 466, 486, 499, 500, 512, 521, 546
Master Formula His **263,** 273, 440, 473
Mastitis (Breast Infection) **343,** 470
Measles 63, 69, **358.** *See also* Childhood Diseases
Measurements **23**
Medication 278, **441**
Meditation 10, 54, 55, 59, 68, 76, 77, 78, 84, 110, 122, 123, 130, 131, 135, 163, 180, 203, 207, **441,** 496
MegaCal 264, 280, 348, 546, 556
Melaleuca Ericifolia (Rosalina) 97, 546, 550, 557
Melaleuca Geranium Moisturizing Soap **228,** 555, 557, 561
Melaleuca Leucadendron *See* Cajeput
Melaleuca Quinquenervia (Niaouli) 97, 546, 550, 557
Melaleuca (Tea Tree) 96, 546, 550, 557
Melanoma 350, **441.** *See also* Cancer
Melissa 98, 546, 550, 557
Melrose 188, 193, 195, 235, 298, 312, 313, 314, 315, 316, 317, 318, 319, 321, 324, 325, 339, 344, 345, 347, 351, 364, 366, 372, 378, 385, 386, 393, 401, 402, 410, 413, 422, 424, 426, 427, 432, 444, 455, 456, 465, 475, 476, 477, 479, 482, 488, 489, 490, 491, 492, 497, 506, 508, 512, 513, 514, 516, 518, 519, 523, 524, 546, 553, 557, 559, 566
Memory 42, 49, 62, 80, 91, 92, 93, 113, 114, 118, 119, 121, 158, 179, 194, 197, 202, 298, 308, 309, 337, 355, **441,** 485
Meningitis 76, 77
Menopause 47, 48, 57, 65, 72, 89, 107, 120, 135, 255, 353, 403, 405, 421. *See also* Female Specific Conditions
Menorrhagia 403, **404**
Menstruation 49, 52, 56, 59, 60, 63, 65, 79, 84, 85, 95, 98, 100, 105, 112, 113, 117, 118, 120, 121, 122, 123, 127, 128, 131, 133, 162, 301, 371, 403, 417. *See also* Female Specific Conditions
Mental Alertness/Activity 155, 159, 164, **442.** *See also* Alertness, Energy, Memory, Brain, Stress
Mental Difficulties/Fatigue 49, 52, 108, 167, 204, 277, 400, **442,** 499
Mercury 377, 503
Metabolism 33, **69,** 84, 120, 122, 165, 263, 264, 267, 271, 281, 283, 375, 393, **443,** 460, 569
Metals 82, 296, 306, 357, 363, 377, 417, **442,** 461, 477, 517. *See also* Detoxification, Chelation
M-Grain 187, 298, 346, 352, 374, 396, 398, 402, 417, 418, 421, 441, 442, 445, 450, 470, 472, 483, 488, 546, 552, 553, 555, 556, 557, 558, 565
Mice (Repel) 192, **443**
Micromeria 99, 546, 550, 557
Migraine Headaches 49, 57, 60, 63, 64, 69, 81, 87, 89, 95, 98, 113, 123, 131, 187, 300, 417, 421. *See also* Headaches
Mildew 192, **443**
Mind 49, 54, 57, 58, 73, 74, 75, 102, 104, 108, 109, 114, 117, 119, 151, 154, 162, 163, 166, 167, 170, 173, 176, 190, 199, 200, 203, 204, 307, 323, 391, 416, **443.** *See also* Alertness, Brain, Energy, Memory, Mental
Mineral Essence 245, 253, 254, 257, 258, 264, **265,** 277, 281, 284, 298, 300, 302, 304, 305, 306, 307, 309, 313, 318, 320, 326, 338, 340, 345, 346, 351, 352, 363, 367, 371, 373, 374, 375, 378, 379, 381, 384, 386, 388, 394, 395, 402, 405, 406, 412, 416, 418, 421, 423, 442, 444, 446, 447, 448, 449, 450, 451, 452, 460, 463, 466, 484, 486, 491, 502, 503, 505, 510, 521, 546, 553, 556, 558
Minerals (deficiency) 258, 263, 264, 265, 266, 271, 278, 285, 317, 345, 346, 354, 377, 379, 442, **444**
Miscarriage 127, 421, **470.** *See also* Pregnancy/Motherhood
Mister 162, 189, 235, 253, 255, 263, 264, 273, 332, 350, 352, 374, 396, 398, 401, 402, 403, 405, 417, 421, 422, 424, 425, 433, 439, 440, 441, 442, 444, 467, 472, 473, 488, 505, 546, 554, 556, 557, 558, 559, 561, 566
Mites 96
Moisturizing 212, 216, 217, 219, 229, 230, 231, 232, 234, 235, 238, 242, 488. *See also* Antifungal
Mold 9, 192, 422, **444,** 475
Moles **444**
Moment **444**
Money 80, 111
Mono (Mononucleosis) 116, 395, **444.** *See also* Antiviral, Chronic Fatigue, Epstein-Barr
Monoterpenes 11
Mood Elevation Protocol **391**
Mood Swings 255, **444.** *See also* Hormonal Imbalance
Morning Sickness 113, 161, **470.** *See also* Pregnancy/Motherhood
Morning Start Bath & Shower Gel **228,** 333, 374, 375, 394, 489, 514, 546, 556, 557, 558, 559
Morning Start Moisturizing Soap **229,** 556, 557, 559
Mosquitoes 66, 334, **445.** *See also* Insect
Mother (Problems with) 299, 389, 391, 392, **445,** 467, 469
Mothers (Expectant) 79, 171
Motion Sickness 80, 113, **445.** *See also* Nausea
Motivation 150, 153, 163, 166, 182, 186, **189,** 190, 267, 279, 302, 328, 341, 369, 375, 390, 391, 394, 396, 401, 445, 454, 466, 468, 472, 510, 521, 524, 546, 553, 556, 560, 561, 566
Mountain Savory 99, 546, 550, 557
Mouth 89, 101, 102, 107, 120, 130, 351, 513
Mouthwash 277
MRSA **445,** 497. *See also* Antibacterial
MSM 227, 232, 243, 271, 277, 278, 457
Mucolytic 65, 70, 82, 84, 118
Mucus 66, 80, 81, 84, 85, 89, 100, 107, 120, 193, 296, 343, 454, 551. *See also* Congestion
Mugwort 100, 557
MultiGreens 245, 252, 263, 264, 267, 271, 272, 273, 277, 279, 281, 284, 285, 363, 546, 556, 557, 559
Multiple Sclerosis (M.S.) 9, 10, 277, 436, **445,** 450. *See also* Myelin Sheath
Mumps 359. *See also* Childhood Diseases
Muscles 33, 49, 51, 56, 57, 60, 63, 65, 69, 71, 73, 74, 75, 80, 82, 85, 86, 88, 91, 92, 93, 95, 96, 98, 103, 104, 105, 107, 108, 109, 110, 112, 113, 118, 121, 122, 129, 130, 132, 134, 135, 152, 154, 160, 173, 187, 190, 195, 198, 205, 230, 231, 232, 233, 235, 245, 248, 264, 266, 267, 271, 272, **273,** 277, 278, 279,

280, 283, 285, 286, 312, 314, 321, 330, 346, 353, 357, 371, 375, 431, 434, **447**, 458, 495, 497, 500, 524, 543–550, 568, 569, 571, 572
Muscles and Bones 200
Muscular Dystrophy 286, **449**
Music **44–46**
Mutation (of Cells) **296**, 320, 474
Myelin Sheath 342, 445, **449**
Myrrh 101, 546, 550, 557
Myrrh, Biblical Sweet 102, 557
Myrtle 102, 546, 550, 557
Myrtle, Lemon 103, 557

N

Nails 57, 91, 92, 95, 277, 346, **450**
Narcolepsy **450**
Nasal 69, 71, **454.** *See also* Nose
Nasopharynx 69
Nausea 52, 54, 62, 63, 72, 80, 89, 98, 105, 111, 112, 113, 119, 123, 128, 187, 249, 348, **450**, 519. *See also* Motion Sickness, Pregnancy/Motherhood, Vomiting
Neat (Applying Oils) 295
Neck 71, 236, 296, 322, 417, 448, **450**
Negative Dreams 162
Negative Emotions 42, 174, 187, 188, 194, 197, 202, **392**
Negative Energies 34, 202, 206
Negative Ions 9, 306, 379, 428, 429, 452, 478, 493
Negativity 10, 180, **451**
Nephritis **431**
Neroli 104, 546, 550, 558
Nerves 33, 57, 59, 73, 79, 86, 90, 91, 93, 100, 113, 114, 116, 118, 122, 127, 129, 130, 134, 160, 179, 191, 203, 234, 264, 271, 308, 330, 354, 395, 446, **451**, 453, 479, 486, 504, 509, 524
Nervine 66, 98, 114, 126, 127, 130
Nervous Fatigue/Tension 55, 84, 85, 89, 94, 97, 98, 107, 109, 115, 117, 118, 122, 130, 569
Nervousness 58, 63, 66, 67, 81, 85, 91, 92, 93, 110, 132, 200, 314, 451, 570
Nervous System 18, 20, 28, 36, 47, 53, 55, 56, 57, 58, 63, **67**, 73, 76, 77, 80, 84, 86, 89, 93, 94, 98, 100, 101, 102, 105, 109, 110, 112, 113, 118, 120, 121, 122, 124, 125, 126, 127, 131, 132, 150, 154, 155, 157, 159, 160, 165, 173, 186, 187, 188, 190, 191, 196, 200, 203, 205, 232, 233, 235, 260, 261, 263, 264, 266, 267, 269, 270, 277, 278, 280, 346, 396, **451**, 466, 543–550, 568, 569, 570, 571. *See also* Lou Gehrig's Disease, Carpal Tunnel Syndrome, Multiple Sclerosis, Paralysis, Parkinson's Disease
Nettles 62
Neuralgia (Severe pain along nerve) 56, 57, 60, 63, 79, 95, 105, 112, 121, 135, 451, 486. *See also* Nervous System
Neuritis 57, 62, 135, 452. *See also* Nervous System
NeuroGen 556, 558
Neurological Problems 342, 452. *See also* Nervous System
Neuromuscular 128, **453**
Neurotonic 129. *See also* Nervous System
Neutralizing 245
Newborn 171
Niacin flush 278, 420
Niaouli *See* Melaleuca Quinquenervia
Night Sweats 120, **453.** *See also* Hot Flashes, Hormonal Imbalance
NingXia Nitro **267**, 394, 558, 560
NingXia Red 247, 250, 252, 261, 264, 267, **268**, 269, 270, 272, 273, 283, 284, 285, 302, 305, 306, 309, 311, 320, 322, 326, 328, 335, 348, 352, 355, 359, 363, 373, 375, 379, 382, 394, 396, 400, 404, 406, 409, 418, 423, 431, 434, 435, 436, 438, 447, 454, 499, 500, **501**, 521, 546, 556, 558, 560, 561
Ningxia Wolfberries 305, 320, 348, 423
Nose 65, 365, **453**
Nose and Olfactory System Chart **40**
Notes (Oil Blending) 24, 297
Nourishing 198, 242
Nursing 52, 67, 432, 470. *See also* Pregnancy/Motherhood
Nutmeg 105, 546, 550, 558
Nutrients 271, 278, 283, 300, 373, 395, 402, 466, 491

O

Obesity 72, 81, 86, 94, 107, 118, 126, 134, 324, **454**. *See also* Diet, Weight
Obsessiveness **454**
Ocotea 319, 325, 383
Odors 9, 95, 188, 192, 339, 401, **455.** *See also* Deodorant
Office, Reducing errors in **158**
Oil (Grease Removal) 91, 92
Olfactory System Chart **40**
Omega Blue **247**, 252, 257, 261, **268**, **269**, **273**, **283**, 298, 302, 306, 308, 309, **320**, 341, 351, 352, 368, 375, 390, 401, 404, 405, 407, 418, **434**, **435**, **436**, 437, 441, 442, 446, **449**, 451, 461, 471, 484, 546, 553, 557
OmegaGize3 **270**, 298, 302, 307, 308, 309, 320, 341, 351, 352, 368, 375, 390, 401, 404, 405, 407, 418, 434, 435, 436, 437, 441, 442, 446, 449, 451, 461, 471, 484, **546**, 553, 560
Onycha 106, 546, 558
Opening (to receive) 130, 134, 166, 173, 356, 369, **455**, 463
Opposition 205, **455**
Optimism 85, 86
ORAC 260, 320
Oral Hygiene 280
Oral Infections 119, **455**
Orange 107, 546, 550, 558
Orange Blossom Facial Wash **229**, 237, 301, 480, 488, 490, 491, 493, 546, 556, 558, 559
Oregano 108, 546, 550, 558
Organs 271, 281, 296
Ortho Ease 33, 35, 152, 161, 190, **229**, 278, 280, 311, 312, 319, 326, 330, 332, 340, 346, 352, 354, 371, 406, 412, 426, 432, 447, 448, 449, 457, 458, 483, 497, 501, 505, 508, 546, 553, 554, 556, 557, 558, 560, 561
Ortho Sport 152, 161, 190, **230**, 278, 280, 311, 319, 331, 332, 340, 346, 352, 354, 371, 406, 412, 426, 432, 434, 440, 447, 448, 449, 457, 458, 486, 497, 508, 546, 554, 557, 558, 561
Osteoarthritis **326**
Osteomyelitis 340, **456.** *See also* Bones
Osteoporosis 134, 264, 300, 308, 421, **456.** *See also* Bones
Otitis 118
Ovaries 49, 65, 103, 118, 350, 393, 404, 421, **456**, 464. *See also* Female Specific Conditions, Hormonal Imbalance
Overbearing 199
Overcome and Release Unpleasant, Difficult Issues in Life 190, 205, 310, 400, **457**
Overeating 387, **457.** *See also* Eating disorders
Overexertion **480**
Overweight 246, **457.** *See also* Obesity, Weight
Overwhelmed 391, **457**
Oxidation **320**
Oxygen 8, 10, 73, 92, 122, 154, 169, 186, 190, 231, 232, 233, 245, 265, 296, 300, 306, 308, 320, 335, 342, 355, 373, 401, **457**, 463, 464, 480, 492, 497, 520, 570

P

Pain 33, 60, 62, 63, 65, 66, 72, 73, 74, 75, 76, 77, 78, 80, 82, 85, 91, 95, 105, 110, 111, 112, 124, 125, 127, 128, 130, 134, 152, 190, 195, 205, 218, 246, 251, 265, 298, 311, 312, 313, 314, 316, 322, 326, 330, 331, 340, 341, 345, 352, 392, 403, 413, 447,

452, **457**, 460, 469, 481, 487, 504, 508, 523, 551, 568, 569, 571
Painting 27, **459**
Palmarosa **109**, 546, 550, 558
Palo Santo 110, 547, 558
Palpitations 87, 98, 104, 107, 118, 127, 133, 136, **353**, 568, 572. *See also* Cardiovascular System
PanAway 187, 190, 195, 235, 255, 278, 280, 311, 319, 320, 325, 326, 329, 330, 331, 339, 340, 341, 344, 346, 351, 352, 353, 374, 388, 392, 406, 407, 411, 417, 418, 426, 434, 447, 448, 450, 452, 457, 458, 459, 460, 469, 483, 487, 497, 504, 508, 518, 522, 523, 547, 553, 555, 558, 561, 566
Pancreas 57, 63, 65, 72, 75, 79, 82, 284, 296, 375, 378, 393, 396, **459**, 569
Pancreatitis 459. *See also* Pancreas
Panic 323. *See also* Anxiety, Calming
Pap Smears (Abnormal) **402**
ParaFree 250, 256, 259, **270**, 315, 318, 322, 379, 381, 382, 426, 460, 467, 523, 547, 552, 553, 554, 557, 558, 560, 561
Paralysis 52, 250, 382, 446, **460**, 500. *See also* Nervous System
Parasites 48, 50, 55, 57, 60, 61, 62, 72, 84, 100, 104, 115, 126, 128, 130, 161, 249, 251, 270, 296, 315, 381, **460**, 551. *See also* Digestive System
Parasympathetic Nervous System 38, 92, 95, 428. *See also* Nervous System
Parathyroid 132, 165, 393, **460**
Parkinson's Disease 9, 10, 133, 277, 436, **461**. *See also* Brain, Pineal Gland, Pituitary Gland, Alzheimer's Disease
Passion 185
Past **461**
Patchouli **110**, 547, 550, 558
PD 80/20 250, **271**, 308, 341, 375, 403, 404, 406, 432, 433, 440, 446, 452, 456, 467, 473, 474, 486, 489, 490, 493, 515, 547
Peace 57, 58, 79, 86, 89, 96, 104, 108, 119, 136, 166, 170, 176, 191, 205, 346, **462**. *See also* Calming
Peace & Calming 173, 178, **191**, 196, 200, 205, 207, 255, 299, 302, 303, 309, 310, 311, 312, 313, 314, 319, 324, 325, 326, 341, 344, 346, 347, 352, 361, 362, 364, 365, 370, 374, 375, 376, 377, 388, 389, 390, 400, 404, 412, 417, 428, 429, 434, 437, 444, 446, 448, 451, 461, 462, 468, 471, 478, 480, 484, 493, 494, 495, 497, 499, 500, 501, 505, 510, 513, 541, 547, 558, 560, 561, 566
Pediculosis 87
Pelvic Pain Syndrome **462**
Pepper, Black **111**, 547, 550, 558
Peppermint **113**, 547, 550, 558
Peppermint Cedarwood Moisturizing Soap **231**, 333, 389, 488, 552, 558
Pepper, Pink **112**, 547, 558
Perfume/Cologne **25**, 70, 376
Perineum **172**
Periodontal (Gum) Disease 96, 130, 201, 241, 277. *See also* Oral Conditions
Personal Growth **462**
Personality (Multiple) 462
Perspiration 60, 65, 84, 114, **462**
Pest Troubles **463**. *See also* Insect, Mice
Petitgrain **114**, 547, 550, 558
Petrochemicals 154, 405
Pets 214
Pharyngitis 81, 130, **463**
pH Balance 198, 217, 219, 222, 223, 229, 230, 234, 235, 238, 242, 245, 251, 267, 299, 306, 307, 317, 318, 336, 348, 373, 379, 407, 420, **463**, 474, 520. *See also* Acidosis, Alkalosis
Pheromones 11
Phlebitis 82, 89, 353. *See also* Cardiovascular System
Phosphorus 277, 460
Photosensitivity 295, 360, 562, 567
Physical Body 205, 296
Piles 62, 63
Pimples 277, 346, 386. *See also* Acne
Pine **115**, 547, 550, 558
Pineal Gland 10, 14, 42, 55, 65, 76, 77, 78, 89, 122, 124, 125, 154, 165, 169, 308, 375, 393, 436, 461, **463**, 480, 492
Pine, Black 559
Pine, Lodge Pole 559
Pine, Piñon 559
Pine, Ponderosa (Yellow Pine) 559
Pink Eye **397**. *See also* Eyes
Pituitary Gland 10, 14, 65, 76, 77, 118, 119, 122, 154, 163, 165, 169, 284, 308, 393, 400, 436, 461, **464**, 492. *See also* Endocrine System
Plague 62, 86, 117, 118, 201, **464**. *See also* Antibacterial
Plantar Wart **519**
Plaque 240, 241, 271, 310
Plectranthus Oregano **109**, **547**, 559
Pleurisy 65, 129, **464**. *See also* Antibacterial, Antiviral, Respiratory System
PMS 48, 61, 72, 104, 255, 263, 371, 404, 421, 423. *See also* Female Specific Conditions
Pneumonia 51, 76, 77, 97, 108, 115, 116, 193, 194, 201, **465**. *See also* Antibacterial, Respiratory System
Poison Oak/Ivy 62, **465**
Poisons 95, 296
Pollution **465**. *See also* Purification
Polyps 367, 454, 466. *See also* Colon, Nose
Positive Feelings 10, 175, 185, **466**
Positive Ions 394, 428, 429. *See also* Ions
Postpartum Depression 471
Potassium Deficiency 258, 265, 277, 280, 300, **466**
Potential 154, 175, 181, 206, 329, **466**
Power **467**
Power Meal 246, 248, 250, 251, 253, 254, 256, 257, 258, 259, 261, 264, 266, 267, 268, **271**, 273, 278, 280, 284, 298, 299, 300, 302, 306, 307, 308, 309, 311, 318, 326, 327, 336, 340, 348, 352, 353, 363, 371, 373, 375, 378, 393, 394, 396, 400, 401, 406, 407, 408, 423, 430, 431, 432, **434**, **435**, 438, 440, 443, 444, 446, 447, 448, 449, 452, 454, 461, 470, 474, 477, 497, 499, 500, 508, 518, 521, 547, 552, 554, 555, 556, 558
Power Surges 162. *See also* Hot Flashes
Prayer 10, 180, **467**, 496
Pregnancy 68, 85, 94, 171, 296, 401, 403, 432, **467**, 500, 562, 567
Pregnenolone **231**, 234, 271, 445, 471
Premature (Babies) **361**
Pre-menopause 61, 72
Pre-menstrual 81, 89, 128, 301
Prenolone/Prenolone+ **231**, 235, 250, 252, 254, 300, 301, 305, 326, 327, 341, 342, 353, 354, 357, 363, 371, 375, 389, 393, 396, 401, 402, 403, 404, 405, 409, 421, 424, 425, 432, 433, 436, 440, 446, 452, 456, 467, 471, 473, 474, 486, 488, 489, 490, 493, 497, 505, 511, 515, 521, 547, 552, 553, 554, 555, 561
Present Time 42, **191**, 246, 299, 310, 368, 372, 376, 377, 383, 389, 390, 401, 409, 412, 429, 430, 437, 438, 441, 444, 452, 454, 455, 456, 461, 467, 469, 494, 495, 502, 547, 558, 560, 561, 566
Pressure 246, 251, 338
Pride **472**
Procrastination 150, 187, 189, **472**
ProGen 252, 264, 547, 554, 556, 557, 558, 559, 561
Progessence Cream **232**, 252, 300, 301, 305, 326, 341, 342, 349, 350, 351, 353, 354, 357, 363, 371, 375, 389, 393, 401, 402, 403, 404, 405, 409, 418, 421, 425, 432, 433, 436, 446, 452, 456, 467, 471, 473, 486, 488, 489, 490, 493, 497, 505, 511, 515, 521, 547, 552, 554, 555, 559, 561
Progessence Plus Serum **233**, 300, 301, 305, 326, 341, 342, 349, 350, 351, 353, 354, 357, 363, 371, 375, 389, 393, 401, 402, 403,

404, 405, 409, 418, 421, 425, 432, 433, 436, 446, 452, 456, 467, 471, 473, 486, 488, 489, 493, 497, 505, 511, 515, 521, 547
Progesterone 120, 231, 232, 234, 250, 341, 353, 363, 396, 421, 445, 471, **472**
Prosperity 149, **473**
Prostate 49, 65, 76, 77, 101, 103, 134, 162, 189, 234, 350, 433, **473**
Prostate Cancer 48, **474.** *See also* Cancer
Prostate Health 272, 370, 393, 405, 411, 421, 422, 424, 425, 440, 473, 474, 505
Prostatitis 124, 125, 135
Protec **234,** 273, 350, 405, 406, 456, 467, 473, 474, 547, 553, 555, 557, 559
Protection 62, 162, 166, 178, 196, 197, 205, 206, 210, 299, **474,** 496
Protein 253, 267, 271, 277, 285, 303, 306, 307, 336, 337, 346, 348, 350, 374, 378, 397, 400, 407, 423, 463, **474**
Provera **353**
Psoriasis 50, 51, 54, 55, 82, 89, 103, 129, **474,** 488, 568. *See also* Skin
Psychic 68, 92, **475**
Puberty **475**
Pulmonary 86, 103, 108, **480.** *See also* Respiratory System
Pure Protein Complete **273,** 309, 336, 378, 394, 407, 423, 447, 448, 449, 474, 499, 508, 521, 547, 558
Purification 55, 69, 72, 86, 91, 92, 93, 135, 192, 246, 250, 256, 298, 300, 302, 303, 306, 307, 313, 315, 316, 318, 320, 321, 325, 333, 334, 339, 345, 365, 370, 373, 374, 385, 386, 388, 402, 409, 422, 424, 427, 443, 454, 455, 460, 462, 465, 466, 475, 482, 492, 494, 501, 503, 511, 512, 513, 514, 516, 519, 523, 524, 547, 553, 556, 557, 559, 566
Purifying 55, 58, 71, 84, 96, 114, 120, 165, 231, 236, 306, 369, 373, 496, 568
Pus **476.** *See also* Antibacterial, Infection, Anti-infectious

Q

Quinsy 112

R

Radiation 98, 113, 347, 415, **476.** *See also* Cancer
Raindrop Technique 25, **33–39,** 179, 205, 313, 314, 315, 322, 330, 331, 371, 378, 406, 446
Rashes 57, 58, 68, 89, 95, 96, 109, 123, 188, 223, 307, 361, 491. *See also* Skin
Raven 155, **193,** 194, 300, 307, 316, 317, 324, 327, 339, 343, 365, 368, 370, 372, 392, 396, 423, 424, 425, 459, 465, 479, 480, 499, 510, 511, 512, 547, 554, 556, 558, 559, 561, 566
Ravensara 116, 547, 550, 559
Raynaud's Disease **477**
RC 155, 193, 194, 300, 307, 315, 316, 317, 320, 322, 324, 327, 339, 340, 343, 350, 352, 365, 366, 368, 370, 372, 374, 392, 396, 411, 425, 439, 444, 454, 459, 465, 479, 480, 487, 488, 495, 497, 506, 510, 511, 512, 547, 553, 554, 556, 557, 558, 560, 566
Refreshing 50, 52, 65, 79, 90, 93, 94, 114, 153, 198, 237, 571
Regenerating 79, 82, 86, 88, 92, 96, 98, 111, 117, 119, 122, 171, 188, 225, 234, 301, 340, 349, 373, 436, **477,** 488, 503, 508, 515, 568, 571
Regenolone **234,** 326, 432, 438, 451, 452, 487, 488, 547, 554, 558, 561
Regulating 90, 121, 131, 136, 355
Rehemogen Tincture **273,** 279, 309, 325, 337, 349, 358, 364, 431, 436, 510, 511, 517, 547, 553, 557, 559, 560
Rehydrating 305, 489, 512
Rejection 187, 392, **477**
Rejuvenating 68, 98
Relationships 85, 136, 137, **478,** 500
Relaxation 173, 191, 205, 333, 371, 374, 389, 428, 440, 447, **478,** 547
Relaxation Massage Oil **235,** 416, 478, 499, 500, 505, 513, 556, 558, 559, 560, 561
Relaxation/Relaxing 18
Relaxing 33, 56, 57, 65, 73, 74, 75, 79, 80, 95, 104, 111, 119, 123, 131, 136, 137, 152, 153, 157, 171, 172, 173, 174, 196, 197, 199, 202, 220, 226, 485, 510
Release 42, 150, **194,** 195, 197, 246, 250, 256, 259, 267, 284, 299, 310, 323, 339, 344, 346, 364, 366, 374, 376, 388, 389, 390, 391, 392, 410, 412, 416, 417, 426, 430, 431, 434, 435, 457, 462, 463, 478, 491, 495, 510, 521, 547, 555, 556, 560, 561, 566
Release Negative Trauma **478**
Relieve It 134, 190, 195, 255, 320, 329, 330, 331, 339, 340, 341, 352, 353, 370, 372, 417, 421, 426, 441, 442, 447, 448, 449, 452, 457, 458, 459, 467, 472, 483, 488, 504, 508, 547, 555, 558, 560, 566
Relieving 152, 185
Repair 209, 210
Repellent 93, 132
Reproductive System 72, 85, 119, 232, 255, 263, 393, **405,** 464, 516
Resentment 347, **478**
Respiration 136, 324, 569
Respiratory Infections 69
Respiratory System 19, 33, 47, 48, 50, 51, 55, 62, 63, 65, 67, 69, 70, 71, 73, 74, 75, 76, 77, 81, 82, 83, 84, 85, 87, 88, 89, 90, 91, 92, 95, 96, 97, 98, 103, 104, 106, 108, 112, 113, 115, 116, 118, 120, 121, 122, 124, 125, 127, 129, 130, 135, 150, 152, 156, 178, 188, 193, 194, 196, 246, 279, 322, 327, 343, 392, 457, **479,** 488, 510, 543–550, 551, 568, 569, 570, 571. *See also* Bronchitis, Pleurisy, Pneumonia
Restlessness 94, 131, **480,** 493. *See also* Calming
Restorative 78, 92
Retardation (Mental) **442**
Retina 398
Revitalizing 91, 94, 167, 176, 228, 329, 399
Reviving 98, 570
Rheumatic Fever 47, 80, 128, 320, **481**
Rheumatism 50, 51, 52, 53, 54, 55, 56, 58, 62, 63, 65, 69, 73, 74, 75, 78, 80, 84, 86, 89, 91, 95, 105, 107, 108, 110, 112, 113, 118, 120, 121, 124, 125, 127, 129, 130, 131, 132, 133, 134, 135, 190, 277, 346, 448, 551, 570, 572. *See also* Muscles, Arthritis
Rheumatoid Arthritis 112, 115, 300, **326**
Rhinitis 49, 59, 121, **481**
Rhinopharyngitis 116, 463, **481**
Rickets 308
Right Brain **342**
Ringworm 79, 95, 101, **481.** *See also* Antifungal
Ritalin 191
Ritual Abuse 197, **299,** 485
Rituals 55
RNA 355, 364, 413
Romance 184, 198, 237
Roman Chamomile *See* Chamomile, Roman
Romantic Touches **481**
Root Canal 298
Rosacea (Acne Rosacea) **301, 481.** *See also* Acne
Rosalina *See* Melaleuca Ericifolia
Rose 116, 547, 550, 559
Rosehip 117, 559
Rosemary Camphor 547
Rosemary Cineol 117, 547, 550, 559
Rosemary Verbenon 118, 547, 559
Rose Ointment 189, **235,** 300, 305, 319, 321, 339, 361, 415, 429, 465, 474, 488, 489, 491, 492, 508, 513, 523, 524, 547, 552, 557, 558, 559
Rosewood 119, 547, 550, 559
Rosewood Moisturizing Conditioner 552, 553, 555, 559, 560, 561
Rosewood Moisturizing Shampoo 552, 553, 555, 559, 560, 561
Rotator Cuff 341

Rubefacient 111, 132
Rubella **359**
RutaVaLa 196, 301, 321, 346, 347, 376, 428, 451, 480, 493, 547, 556, 559, 561, 566

S

Sacred Frankincense *See* Frankincense, Sacred
Sacred Mountain 171, 196, 200, 207, 264, 299, 310, 315, 328, 357, 364, 372, 375, 377, 383, 388, 389, 393, 401, 412, 429, 439, 454, 467, 474, 479, 480, 481, 483, 484, 495, 496, 499, 511, 514, 522, 547, 552, 554, 560, 561, 566
Sacred Mountain Moisturizing Soap **236**, 333, 488, 552, 554, 560, 561
Sacredness 196, **481**
Saddle Sores 314
Sadness 107, 126, **482**
Safety Data 552–564, 563–567
Sage 120, 547, 550, 559
Sage Lavender (Sage, Spanish) 121, 547, 559
Saint Vitus Dance (Chorea) **482**
Sandalwood 121, 547, 550, 560
Sandalwood Moisture Creme 229, 236, 301, 304, 305, 374, 488, 489, 490, 492, 493, 547, 552, 556, 557, 559, 560
Sanitation **482.** *See also* Antibacterial, Antifungal, Antiviral
SARA 42, **197**, 246, 299, 376, 389, 390, 391, 426, 457, 462, 485, 510, 521, 547, 552, 555, 556, 558, 559, 560, 561, 566
Satin Facial Scrub **237**, 305, 457, 480, 488, 489, 491, 492, 493, 547, 558
Sauna 115
Scabies 50, 52, 87, 115, 127. *See also* Skin
Scabs 70
Scalp 52
Scarlet Fever 415
Scar/Scarring 65, 76, 77, 78, 82, 84, 89, 94, 100, 104, 117, 135, 217, 219, 229, 230, 234, 235, 238, 242, 277, 300, 345, **482**, 524, 568, 570
Schmidt's Syndrome **304.** *See also* Adrenal Glands
Sciatica 52, 56, 76, 77, 82, 122, 124, 125, 127, 128, 129, 133, 190, 195, **483**
SclarEssence 198, 253, 342, 396, 402, 403, 405, 421, 424, 433, 440, 485, 486, 497, 547, 553, 554, 558, 559, 566
Scoliosis 205, **483**, 488. *See also* Back
Scours 312
Scrapes 116, 188, 214, **483.** *See also* Cuts, Wounds
Scratches 95, 214
Scurvy 80, 90, 91, 107, 115, 130, **483**, 572
Seborrhea 277, 300
Security 65, 108, 109, 150, 157, 166, 174, 176, 196, **483**
Sedative/Sedating 14, 47, 50, 55, 60, 63, 68, 71, 73, 74, 75, 76, 77, 79, 84, 88, 91, 94, 95, 97, 98, 103, 104, 106, 107, 110, 111, 116, 121, 126, 131, 132, 135, 136, 137, 196, 346, 375, 571, 572. *See also* Calming
Seductive 184
Seizure 312, 369, **484**
Self Adjustment **485**
Self Esteem 42, 136, 182, 205, 206, 337, 349, 474, **485**
Self Hypnosis **485**
Self Pity 187, **485**
Sensation 188, **198**, 300, 323, 374, 391, 405, 433, 437, 462, 481, 485, 488, 513, 514, 547, 556, 559, 561, 566
Sensation Bath & Shower Gel **237**, 333, 375, 389, 436, 437, 478, 481, 486, 489, 499, 514, 556, 559, 561
Sensation Hand & Body Lotion **237**, 304, 305, 323, 389, 416, 436, 437, 440, 478, 481, 486, 488, 489, 499, 500, 547, 556, 559, 561
Sensation Massage Oil **238**, 300, 323, 375, 389, 416, 436, 437, 478, 481, 486, 490, 499, 556, 559, 561
Sensitivity 307, **399**
Sensory System (Senses) 104, 113, 134, 237, 328, 329, **485.** *See also* Awareness
Sexual Abuse 120, 197, 299, 391, **485**
Sexual Energies 132, 136, 137
Sexual Problems 56, 117, 136, 137, 570
Sexual Stimulant 58, 80, 85, 111, 394, 409, 416, 422, 433, 478, **485**, 572
Shingles 79, 95, 116, **486.** *See also* Antiviral, Childhood Diseases
Shock 57, 63, 95, 96, 98, 104, 113, 126, 132, 136, 137, 158, 399, **486**, 510, 522, 571. *See also* Fainting
Shoulder (Frozen) **487**
Single Oil Property Chart **549–551**
Single Oil Summary Information Chart **552–564**
Sinus 82, 103, **487**
Sinusitis 51, 55, 62, 68, 69, 71, 73, 80, 95, 97, 103, 115, 116, 118, 121, 193, 201, **488.** *See also* Respiratory System
Skeletal System 205. *See also* Bones
Skin 14, 50, 51, 52, 53, 54, 55, 56, 57, 58, 60, 61, 62, 63, 65, 66, 68, 69, 70, 71, 76, 77, 78, 79, 82, 85, 86, 89, 90, 91, 92, 94, 95, 96, 97, 99, 101, 102, 103, 104, 106, 107, 108, 109, 111, 113, 115, 117, 118, 119, 120, 121, 122, 123, 126, 130, 131, 132, 134, 135, 136, 137, 171, 172, 184, 188, 193, 198, 200, 205, 209, 210, 211, 212, 213, 214, 215, 216, 217, 218, 219, 221, 222, 223, 224, 225, 226, 228, 229, 230, 231, 232, 233, 234, 235, 236, 237, 238, 242, 258, 277, 278, 283, 284, 300, 304, 305, 306, 307, 345, 350, 361, 378, 379, 395, 401, 437, 440, 472, **488**, 491, 492, 501, 509, 543–550, 549, 561, 567, 568, 569, 570, 571. *See also* Acne, Allergies, Boils, Bruises, Burns, cancer, Cuts, Dermatitis, Eczema, Facial Oils, Feet, Moles, Psoriasis, Wounds, Wrinkles
Sleep 56, 62, 96, 123, 131, 132, 153, 162, 163, 165, 170, 196, 199, 284, 302, 313, 324, 358, 428, 450, 480, **493**
SleepEssence 346, 478, 493, 505
Slimming and Toning Oils **494.** *See also* Weight
Slique Bar **274**, 324, 454, 521, **548**, 553, 558
Slique Essence **275**, 324, 454, 521, **548**, 555, 556, 558, 560
Slique Gum **276**, 324, 454, 521, **548**, 558, 560
Slique Slim Caps **276**, 324, 454, 521, **548**, 554, 557
Slique Tea 276, 320, 324, 326, 351, 352, 421, 454, 521, 548
Slivers (Splinters) 201, **494**
Smell-Loss of 49, **494**
Smoke 192
Smoking 62, 278, 303, 370, **494.** *See also* Addictions, Air Pollution, Purification
Snake Bites 49, 72, 111, 315, **334**
Snoring **495**
Solar plexus 71, 119, 124, 125
Soothing 57, 60, 71, 107, 119, 123, 126, 156, 166, 171, 173, 196, 223, 237, 242, 305, 382, 489, **495**, 570, 571
S-ORAC 320
Sores 57, 62, 66, 69, 70, 73, 76, 77, 79, 95, 112, 115, 120, 130, 131, 135, 312, 351, 378, **495.** *See also* Antibacterial, Antifungal, Antiviral, Cuts, Wounds
Sore Throat 50, 51, 61, 70, 73, 79, 80, 84, 91, 92, 96, 101, 107, 135, 193, 194, 201, 280, 569. *See also* Throat
Soul 176
Spacing Out **495**
Spasms 49, 52, 63, 64, 65, 72, 85, 95, 104, 107, 126, 128, 152, 160, 190, 249, 321, 352, 353, 357, 367, 382, 448, **495**, 551, 571. *See also* Digestive System, Muscles, Antispasmodic
Spearmint 122, 548, 550, 560
Speech 308
Spiders 192, 334, 427
Spikenard **123**, 548, 550, 560
Spina Bifida **495**
Spine 34, 119, 129, 130, 205, 322, 330, 331, 332, 486, **496**, 501. *See also* Back

Spiritual 54, 55, 76, **77**, 78, 79, 86, 101, 102, 104, 110, 136, 153, 154, 168, 170, 174, 180, 181, 202, 203, 204, 205, 207, 296, 329, 398, **496**, 522
Spleen 87, 95, 348, **496**
Splinters 201
Split Ends **415**
Sports 152, 160, 190, 426, **497.** *See also* Aches/Pains, Bones, Injuries, Muscles, Tissue
Spousal Abuse **299**
Sprains 80, 85, 89, 95, 112, 117, 119, 120, 127, 132, 133, 135, 160, 190, 448. *See also* Muscles
Spruce **124,** 548, 550, 560
Spruce, Colorado Blue 560
Spruce, Idaho Blue **124, 545, 549, 560**
Spurs, Bone 193, 340, **497.** *See also* Bones
Stabilizing 132, 154, 164, 173, 176, 181, 185, 186
Stains 91, 92, **497.** *See also* Housecleaning
Stamina 112
Staph Infection 76, 77, 95, 118, 123, **497**
Sterility 79, 98, 121, 405, **497**
Sterilizing 88
Stevia/Stevia Select **274, 277,** 378, 408, 423, 459, 501, 548
Stiffness 62, 63, 332, **448**
Stimulant 56, 93
Stimulating 11, 21, 33, 48, 49, 52, 55, 59, 60, 62, 63, 64, 65, 67, 68, 69, 72, 73, 74, 75, 80, 81, 82, 86, 90, 93, 94, 95, 96, 99, 100, 105, 109, 111, 112, 114, 115, 117, 121, 122, 127, 128, 132, 133, 153, 157, 158, 203, 204, 304, 328, 353, 354, 355, 369, 423, 436, 442, 459, **497,** 507, 569, 570, 571, 572
Stings 49, 62, 88, 89, **334,** 427 *See also* Bites/Stings, Insects
Stomach 66, 82, 107, 118, 123, 126, 127, 129, 130, 135, 161, 246, 277, 278, 371, **498,** 509, 513, 572. *See also* Digestive System
Stomachaches 58, 136, 313
Stomachic 47, 52, 53, 58
Stomatitis 130
Strain 120
Strength 72, 166, 176, 177, 196, 199, 206, **499**
Strengthening 65, 68, 104, 178, 185, 204, 304, 328, 339, 353, 443, 474
Strep 76, 77, 95, 118, 201, 240
Strep Throat **506.** *See also* Throat
Stress 50, 57, 58, 63, 68, 71, 73, 76, 77, 78, 79, 81, 84, 89, 91, 94, 95, 104, 107, 109, 115, 118, 121, 123, 126, 129, 130, 131, 132, 151, 152, 153, 162, 171, 174, 187, 191, 199, 204, 278, 300, 313, 317, 351, 379, 380, 392, 415, 418, 429, 442, **499,** 541, 568, 569, 570, 571. *See also* Calming
Stress Away 346, 376, 389, 478, 493, 499, 505, 558
Stretch Marks 89, 94, 101, 104, 126, 171, 217, 219, 229, 230, 234, 235, 238, 242, 343, 472, **500.** *See also* Pregnancy/Motherhood
Stroke 313, **500.** *See also* Blood, Brain
Structural Alignment **501**
Studying 158
Stupification 562, 567
Styptic 134
Subconscious **501**
Sudorific 300, 301, **501**
Sugar 240, 248, 259, 271, 302, 303, 317, 346, 348, 364, 378, 396, 407, 408, 418, 423, **501**
Suicide/Suicidal 176, 299, 376, **392.** *See also* Depression, Emotions
Sulfur **271,** 277, 346, 415, 449, 490
Sulfurzyme 246, 251, 264, 266, 267, 271, 273, **277,** 280, 284, 298, 300, 304, 307, 308, 310, 311, 312, 326, 328, 340, 348, 352, 353, 354, 371, 378, 379, 380, 396, 397, 401, 406, 407, 410, 412, 413, 415, 416, 421, 423, 430, 435, 437, 445, 446, 447, 449, 450, 451, 452, 457, 458, 461, 474, 475, 487, 489, 490, 500, 507, 518, 521, 522, 548
Sunburn 53, 89, 95, 96, 125, 127, 133, 135, 225, 265, 345, **501.** *See also* Burns
Sunlight 295
Sun Screen 82, 125, 210, 345
Sunstroke 89
Super B 252, **278,** 298, 299, 301, 304, 306, 311, 320, 324, 327, 348, 351, 352, 353, 355, 394, 397, 414, 415, 421, 423, 444, 445, 446, 451, 452, 460, 499, 500, 503, 517, 518, 548
Super C 151, 179, 250, 256, **278,** 299, 302, 303, 306, 307, 310, 317, 318, 320, 321, 322, 326, 327, 330, 340, 348, 349, 350, 388, 393, 395, 397, 398, 405, 406, 410, 412, 416, 423, 424, 425, 426, 430, 431, 435, 438, 441, 444, 446, 479, 483, 491, 495, 503, 506, 510, 511, 517, 518, 522, 548, 555, 556, 557, 558, 560
Super Cal 252, **280,** 307, 326, 340, 341, 346, 348, 349, 351, 354, 363, 371, 407, 412, 420, 421, 446, 447, 448, 450, 452, 458, 466, 499, 518, 548, 553, 557, 561
Super C Chewable 179, **279,** 299, 302, 303, 306, 307, 310, 317, 318, 320, 321, 322, 326, 327, 330, 340, 348, 349, 350, 388, 393, 395, 397, 398, 405, 407, 410, 412, 416, 423, 424, 425, 426, 430, 431, 435, 438, 441, 444, 446, 447, 479, 483, 491, 495, 503, 506, 510, 511, 518, 522, 548, 556
Supporting 78, 149, 165, 166, 176, 181, 203, 248, 339, 354, 459, **502,** 507, 515
Surgery 190, 413, 415, 418, 458, 503, **524**
Surrender 180, 199, 259, 299, 302, 310, 323, 346, 367, 389, 390, 392, 395, 407, 410, 428, 429, 443, 451, 467, 499, 548, 552, 553, 556, 557, 560, 566
Sweating 121, **405,** 501
Swelling 112, 126, 298, 398, 440, **502.** *See also* Edema, Inflammation
Sympathetic Nervous System 38, 429. *See also* Nervous System
Sympathy 392, **502**
Syphilis 76, 77, 101, 415

T

Tachycardia (Rapid Heartbeat) 89, 104, 118, 123, 136, 353. *See also* Cardiovascular System
Talkative **503**
Tamanu 125
Tangerine **126,** 548, 550, 560
Tansy, Blue **126,** 548, 560
Tansy, Idaho 548, 550, 560
Tarragon **128,** 548, 550, 560
Taste **503**
Taxonomical Information **568–573, 573–578, 582**
Teeth 224, 240, 264, 362, 364, 377, **503.** *See also* Oral Conditions
Teething 57, 58, 201, **362,** 503
Temperature **504.** *See also* Cooling Oils, Fever, Thyroid, Warming Oils
Tendonitis 134, 277, **504**
Tendons 73, 104, 504
Tennis Elbow **504**
Tension 47, 50, 56, 57, 62, 65, 73, 74, 75, 76, 77, 78, 79, 81, 89, 95, 104, 109, 123, 131, 152, 153, 154, 160, 191, 199, 202, 448, 467, **505**
Terpenes 11
Testicles 118, 119, 393, 464, **505**
Testosterone 120, 121, 198, 231, 234, 414, 415
Tests, Increasing Scores 158
The Gift **200,** 418, 423, 523, 524, 548, 566
Thieves 178, 179, 193, 194, 200, 201, 239, 246, 250, 256, 259, 277, 279, 280, 298, 299, 300, 303, 304, 305, 306, 313, 314, 315, 316, 318, 320, 322, 327, 335, 338, 343, 344, 348, 351, 363, 365, 366, 369, 370, 372, 375, 377, 378, 388, 392, 393, 395, 396, 398, 408, 410, 417, 418, 422, 423, 424, 425, 426, 431, 437, 438, 439, 444, 455, 456, 459, 464, 465, 467, 477, 479, 480, 487, 492, 494, 495, 503, 506, 507, 511, 514, 519, 523, 524, 548, 553, 554, 556, 559, 567
Thieves AromaBright Toothpaste **238**
Thieves Cleaning Products **239,** 548

Thieves Cleansing Soap **239,** 333, 375, 426, 488, 553, 554, 556
Thieves Dental Floss 239
Thieves Dentarome/Dentarome Plus Toothpaste **240,** 553, 554, 556, 558, 559, 561
Thieves Dentarome Ultra Toothpaste **240,** 553, 554, 556, 558, 559, 561
Thieves Foaming Hand Soap 241
Thieves Fresh Essence Plus Mouthwash **241,** 553, 554, 556, 558, 559, 560, 561
Thieves Household Cleaner **239**
Thieves Lozenges **280,** 322, 366, 370, 506, 548, 553, 554, 556, 558, 559
Thieves Spray 239
Thieves Waterless Hand Purifier 242
Thieves Wipes 239
Thoughts **505**
Thread Veins 104
Throat 51, 61, 65, 69, 89, 91, 98, 107, 113, 120, 130, 194, 350, **505.** *See also* Antibacterial, Antiviral, Colds
Thrombosis 135
Thrush 50, 89, 96, 101, 117, 362. *See also* Antifungal
Thyme 33, **128,** 548, 550, 560
Thyme Linalol **129,** 548, 560
Thyme, Red 560
Thymus 42, 68, 124, 125, 165, 284, 296, 305, 307, 308, 393, **506**
Thyroid 62, 90, 109, 165, 231, 232, 233, 264, 267, 281, 284, 296, 303, 317, 322, 336, 393, 407, 412, 416, 425, 437, 438, 460, 464, 504, **507**
Thyromin 232, 233, 235, 252, 267, 272, 277, **281,** 284, 285, 302, 304, 305, 306, 309, 311, 317, 318, 324, 326, 327, 328, 352, 355, 370, 374, 375, 376, 393, 394, 395, 401, 406, 407, 412, 414, 415, 416, 421, 423, 438, 443, 449, 450, 459, 466, 467, 493, 499, 504, 507, 517, 521, 548, 557, 558, 560
Ticks 96, 313, **334**
Tinnitus 386
Tissue 11, 14, 19, 65, 68, 72, 78, 79, 82, 92, 96, 98, 107, 111, 117, 119, 120, 134, 167, 188, 190, 195, 225, 234, 241, 245, 271, 279, 281, 306, 314, 319, 345, 353, 357, 372, 375, 437, 446, 448, 457, 459, 463, 469, 488, 492, 497, 508, 515, 568
TMJ (Temporomandibular Joint Disorder) **509**
Tobacco 259, 302
Tongue 120
Tonic 18, 47, 48, 51, 52, 53, 56, 58, 59, 60, 64, 73, 74, 75, 78, 79, 80, 81, 86, 90, 91, 92, 93, 94, 95, 96, 98, 100, 101, 104, 105, 107, 109, 111, 112, 121, 123, 124, 125, 126, 129, 130, 135, 136, 498, **509,** 569, 570, 571, 572
Tonsillitis 50, 76, 77, 80, 81, 84, 96, 129, 362. *See also* Throat
Toothache 51, 57, 58, 61, 62, 63, 112, 113, 127, 128, 133, **509.** *See also* Teeth
Tooth decay 277
Toxemia 472, **510.** *See also* Antibacterial, Pregnancy/Motherhood
Toxins 9, 11, 36, 52, 67, 72, 82, 84, 86, 111, 122, 161, 245, 249, 253, 296, 298, 300, 301, 303, 308, 364, 367, 373, 377, 437, 457, 477, 491, 501, 503, 508, 520. *See also* Detoxification
Tranquil 202, 299, 301, 310, 311, 312, 324, 341, 347, 376, 442, 452, 461, 462, 465, 467, 478, 480, 493, 497, 499, 500, 505, 510, 513, 548, 552, 553, 556, 567
Tranquilizing 58, 104, 131, 132
Transformation 203, 302, 309, 310, 323, 324, 333, 341, 344, 346, 356, 357, 364, 368, 369, 373, 376, 377, 384, 389, 390, 391, 392, 393, 396, 399, 408, 412, 413, 425, 433, 436, 451, 455, 457, 461, 462, 463, 466, 478, 482, 485, 496, 497, 499, 501, 505, 510, 514, 521, 548, 552, 553, 554, 555, 556, 558, 559, 560, 567
Transition in Life **510**
Trauma 48, 93, 132, 194, 197, 204, 205, 299, 313, 384, 390, 454, 485, **510,** 522. *See also* Shock
Trauma Life 198, **204,** 299, 309, 310, 311, 313, 324, 326, 346, 347, 361, 367, 372, 374, 376, 377, 389, 390, 392, 399, 444, 457, 462, 463, 464, 478, 480, 493, 499, 500, 505, 510, 548, 554, 555, 556, 557, 559, 560, 561, 567
Travel Sickness 313, **510.** *See also* Motion Sickness, Nausea
True Source 257, **282,** 298, 304, 305, 306, 308, 310, 320, 322, 325, 328, 340, 341, 348, 351, 352, 353, 363, 373, 375, 378, 395, 396, 397, 405, 407, 412, 416, 423, 426, 430, 438, 441, 442, 444, 446, 458, 517, 548
Tsuga **130,** 548, 560
Tuberculosis (T.B.) 55, 62, 65, 69, 76, 77, 89, 103, 108, 112, 113, 117, 122, 127, 129, 133, 193, **510.** *See also* Antibacterial, Respiratory system
Tumors 62, 73, 79, 112, 127, 234, 285, 342, 347, 349, 350, **511.** *See also* Cancer
Typhoid 58, 76, 77, 89, 91, **512**

U

Ulcers 50, 57, 61, 62, 68, 69, 76, 77, 79, 86, 95, 101, 102, 107, 112, 117, 134, 135, 246, **512,** 568, 569
Ultraviolet Rays/Radiation 111, 210, 295
Ultra Young+ 252, 268, 278, 281, **283,** 298, 306, 340, 352, 367, 375, 394, 400, 405, 406, 421, 422, 423, 449, 450, 452, 464, 465, 484, 489, 492, 493, 500, 505, 507, 521, 548, 555, 560
Unwind **513.** *See also* Calming, Massage, Relaxing
Uplifting 15, 49, 50, 52, 81, 82, 93, 94, 99, 101, 102, 107, 114, 127, 129, 130, 152, 154, 155, 166, 175, 181, 185, 186, 188, 198, 202, 229, 392, 496, **514,** 570, 571
Ureter 91, 103, **514.** *See also* Urinary Tract
Urethritis 112
Urinary Tract 50, 51, 55, 65, 69, 73, 79, 81, 86, 90, 107, 115, 123, 128, 129, 130, 134, 135, 246, **514.** *See also* Bladder, Kidneys, Ureter
Urine 52, 56
Uterus 85, 98, 107, 129, 130, 350, 401, 468, 469, 509, **515,** 571

V

V-6 Oil 33, 34, **242,** 296, 303, 307, 311, 395
Vaginal 50, 96, 101, 129, 318, 393, 402, 405, **516**
Vaginitis 58, 69, 71, 118, 119, 123, 135, **516**
Valerian **131,** 548, 550, 561
Valor 29, 33, 34, 36, 42, 151, 153, 166, 169, 171, 182, 195, 198, 205, 207, 246, 256, 266, 267, 268, 273, 278, 279, 280, 284, 298, 299, 302, 304, 305, 308, 310, 312, 313, 323, 324, 325, 326, 329, 330, 331, 332, 333, 334, 335, 339, 340, 341, 342, 344, 346, 352, 354, 367, 368, 370, 372, 374, 375, 376, 377, 378, 383, 384, 385, 386, 387, 388, 389, 390, 391, 392, 394, 396, 400, 401, 406, 408, 409, 412, 429, 430, 436, 437, 438, 441, 443, 444, 445, 447, 452, 454, 455, 457, 460, 461, 467, 468, 471, 474, 480, 482, 483, 484, 485, 487, 488, 494, 497, 499, 501, 510, 548, 555, 559, 560, 567
Valor Moisturizing Soap **242,** 555, 559, 560
Varicose Ulcers 513. *See also* Ulcers
Varicose Veins 50, 65, 82, 91, 92, 113, 135, **517**
Vascular System 81, 92, 338, 500, **517.** *See also* Cardiovascular System, Lymphatic System, Arteries, Capillaries, Veins
Vasoconstrictor 65
Vasodilator 18, 91, 95, 325, 338. *See also* Blood
Veins 517, 518. *See also* Cardiovascular System, Vascular System
Venereal Disease 54, 55, 112
Venom 426
Vertigo 52, 98, 112, **518.** *See also* Ears, Equilibrium, Dizziness
Vetiver **132,** 548, 550, 561
Viral Disease 51, 84, 87, 95, 96, 101, 104, 116, 193, 373, 435, 486, **518.** *See also* Antiviral
Viruses 33, 58, 69, 104, 112, 119, 129, 130, 156, 179, 201, 300, 322, 331, 332, 363, 423, 453, 518, 519, 551. *See also* Antiviral

Vision 162, 181, 390, 392, 397, **398**
Visions 162
Visualization 162, **518**
Vita Flex Therapy 25, **28–31**
VitaGreen (see MultiGreens) 267, 298, 300, 304, 306, 307, 317, 318, 320, 324, 326, 328, 336, 337, 338, 348, 349, 350, 351, 355, 358, 362, 363, 371, 372, 378, 379, 394, 395, 397, 400, 401, 402, 404, 405, 406, 412, 414, 416, 420, 421, 423, 425, 430, 431, 435, 438, 440, 441, 446, 447, 449, 450, 459, 460, 461, 463, 470, 471, 474, 486, 497, 508, 511, 517, 521
Vital Centers 33, 120, **518**
Vitamins 217, 219, 227, 229, 230, 234, 235, 238, 242, 259, 263, 271, 277, 278, 279, 285, 312, 372, 378, 415, **518**
Vitex 132
Voice (Hoarse) **518.** *See also* Laryngitis
Void **519**
Vomiting 49, 52, 62, 72, 98, 105, 111, 112, 113, 127, 133, **519.** *See also* Nausea

W

Warming 58, 60, 80, 91, 95, 107, 132, 133, **519**, 569, 570, 572. *See also* Cooling Oils, Temperature
Warts 54, 55, 58, 62, 76, 77, 96, 112, 350, 401, **519.** *See also* Antiviral
Waste 253, **520**, 521
Water 317, 358, 378, 419, 512
Water Distillation **520**
Water Purification 91, 475, **520**
Water Retention 55, 65, 81, 86, 89, 92, 94, 95, 107, 111, 118, 126, 135, 300, 387, 421, 438, 464, **520.** *See also* Edema, Diuretic, Hormonal Imbalance
Weakness 33, 129, 130, **520**, 523. *See also* Energy
Wealth **520**
Weight 111, 123, 165, 232, 233, 271, 277, 336, 400, 415, 454, **520**. *See also* Hormonal Imbalance, Obesity, pH Balanc
Weight Control 231
Well Being 69, 79, 89, 91, 92, 93, 123, 127, 157, 174, **521**
Western Red Cedar *See* Cedar, Western Red
Whiplash **522.** *See also* Trauma, Shock
White Angelica 29, 34, 42, 153, 196, 198, 205, 206, 207, 246, 299, 323, 328, 329, 352, 374, 389, 390, 391, 392, 394, 401, 408, 412, 429, 439, 441, 466, 471, 474, 478, 496, 499, 522, 548, 552, 555, 557, 559, 560, 561, 567
White Fir *See* Fir, White
White Lotus 133, 548, 561
Wholeness **522**
Whooping Cough (Pertussis) 48, 49, 61, 65, 82, 89, 108, 129, 359, **522.** *See also* Childhood Disease
Wintergreen 133, 548, 561
Wisdom 85
Withdrawal 64, 81, **303.** *See also* Addictions
Wolfberry 209, 232, 271, 277, 283, 284, 285, 305, 306, 320, 397
Wolfberry, Benefits **285**
Wolfberry Crisp Bars 250, 261, 264, 266, 267, 272, 283, 284, **285**, 305, 320, 322, 348, 352, 353, 396, 401, 404, 423, 447, 454, 499, 500, 521, 548
Wolfberry Eye Creme **243**, 305, 492, 493, 548, 553, 555, 556, 559
Workaholic **522**
Worms 50, 72, 100, 127, **522.** *See also* Antifungal, Parasites
Worry **523**
Wounds 50, 52, 57, 59, 61, 62, 65, 68, 69, 70, 73, 74, 75, 76, 77, 78, 79, 84, 86, 89, 96, 101, 102, 107, 111, 112, 116, 117, 119, 123, 125, 128, 129, 130, 134, 135, 192, 277, 315, 425, 476, 477, **523**, 568, 569
Wrinkles 53, 59, 68, 78, 101, 102, 104, 107, 111, 117, 171, 209, 216, 221, 231, 232, 233, 277, 305, 488. *See also* Skin

X

Xiang Mao 135, 548, 561
X-ray 297

Y

Yacon Syrup 378, 408, 423, 459, 501
Yarrow 134, 548, 550, 561
Yeast 245, 251, 300, **317**, 318, 348, 463. *See also* Antifungal
Yin and Yang 134, **524**
Ylang Ylang 136, 548, 550, 561
Ylang Ylang, Amazonian 137, 550, 561
Yoga 122, 130, **524**
Yuzu 137

Z

Zest (for life) **524**
Zinc 484